General and Systematic
Pathology

For Churchill Livingstone:

Publisher: Laurence Hunter
Project Editor: Barbara Simmons
Copy Editor: Ruth Swan
Production Controllers: Debra Barrie, Nancy Arnott
Designer: Erik Bigland
Indexer: Monica Trigg

General and Systematic Pathology

Edited by

J. C. E. Underwood MD FRCPath

Joseph Hunter Professor of Pathology,
University of Sheffield Medical School;
Honorary Consultant Histopathologist,
Central Sheffield University Hospitals,
Sheffield
UK

Illustrated by Robert Britton and Peter Lamb

SECOND EDITION

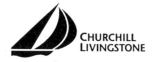
CHURCHILL
LIVINGSTONE

EDINBURGH LONDON NEW YORK PHILADELPHIA SYDNEY TORONTO 1996

CHURCHILL LIVINGSTONE
A Medical Division of Harcourt Brace and Company Limited

© Pearson Professional Limited 1996
© Harcourt Brace and Company Limited 1998

D is a registered trademark of Harcourt Brace and
Company Limited

First Edition 1992
Second Edition 1996
Reprinted 1998

ISBN 0443 05282 4

International Edition second edition 1996
    Reprinted 1997
    Reprinted 1998

ISBN 0 443 05632 3

British Library of Cataloguing in Publication Data
A catalogue record for this book is available from the British Library.

Library of Congress Cataloging in Publication Data
A catalog record for this book is available from the Library of
Congress.

Medical knowledge is constantly changing. As new information
becomes available, changes in treatment, procedures, equipment and
the use of drugs become necessary. The editor, contributors and the
publishers have, as far as it is possible, taken care to ensure that the
information given in this text is accurate and up to date. However,
readers are strongly advised to confirm that the information,
especially with regard to drug usage, complies with current
legislation and standards of practice.

The
publisher's
policy is to use
**paper manufactured
from sustainable forests**

Produced by Addison Wesley Longman China Limited, Hong Kong
GCC/03

Preface

This textbook, intended primarily for medical students, presents pathology in the context of modern medicine and of advances in cellular and molecular biology.

Part 1 (Basic Pathology) deals with the nature and causes of disease and the role of pathology in clinical practice. Disease mechanisms are covered in Part 2. A clear understanding of the cellular and molecular defects involved in disease is important before learning in detail about the specific conditions affecting individual organs or body systems covered in Part 3.

After each major heading within a chapter, where it is considered appropriate, there is a summary panel of key facts serving two purposes: first, to provide the reader with a framework of basic knowledge on which the subsequent details can be placed; second, to assist revision by scanning the text. Where relevant, there are comments on treatment and its relationship to the pathological features of a disease. Each chapter ends with references to review articles and specialist texts for further reading.

Medical schools in many countries are using increasingly the principles of problem-oriented learning in their curricula. This encourages learning through enquiry and exploration. With this in mind, each of the chapters in Part 3 includes a table relating clinical problems (i.e. signs and symptoms) to the pathological abnormalities responsible for them. This approach may be useful as a diagnostic aid, but more importantly it provides a basis for the learning of pathology through clinical experience. Students are also encouraged to augment their learning of pathology by using the two companion textbooks—*MCQ Companion to General and Systematic Pathology* and *Case Studies in General and Systematic Pathology;* the latter is particularly relevant to problem-oriented learning.

Increasingly, the structural abnormalities in disease are being revealed by modern medical imaging techniques such as computerised tomography, ultrasound and magnetic resonance. This aspect of "morbid anatomy", often neglected in pathology textbooks and in medical teaching, is included here to emphasise the utility of images of structural pathology in clinical diagnosis.

The book ends with a glossary of words used frequently in pathology, but which, by usage, have a meaning different from that to be found in most dictionaries or in the public domain.

This new edition of *General and Systematic Pathology* builds on the success of the first edition which was adopted widely as the recommended textbook on pathology for medical undergraduates in many countries. All chapters have been revised and updated with advances in biomedical knowledge. Three new chapters have been introduced — 'Genetic and environmental causes of disease' (Chapter 3), 'Diagnostic pathology in clinical practice' (Chapter 4) and 'Ageing and death' (Chapter 12). A team of International Advisers has been established to ensure that, as far as possible, this and future editions accord with the developments in medical curricula internationally.

I continue to welcome comments from medical students and their teachers that will lead to further improvements in future editions.

Sheffield
1996

J.C.E.U.

Acknowledgements

First, I am grateful to many students and pathologists from various countries who provided comments on the first edition. Their advice has been very useful in planning this second edition. I thank especially all of the International Advisers who devoted so much time to critically appraising the first edition from the perspective of medical education in their own countries; their suggestions have been immensely helpful.

As editor I am very grateful to all contributors for extensively revising and updating their chapters, particularly when the competing demands on their time have increased so dramatically since the first edition was prepared. As editor, and on behalf of all contributors, I thank the staff at Churchill Livingstone for their constant guidance and help, with only a brief respite between publication of the first edition and the planning of this new edition. I thank Peter Lamb for producing the new artwork. I am grateful to Dr Roy Jennings for dealing with my numerous queries about microbiological matters.

As with the first edition, I acknowledge the unfailing support I have enjoyed from my colleagues in the University of Sheffield Department of Pathology, many of whom are contributors, during the preparation of this new edition. I acknowledge also that they have contributed over many years to a departmental slide collection from which many of the illustrations are taken. My secretary, Brenda Barrass, has cheerfully accepted the extra work related to the preparation of this edition and shielded me from other matters during times when I was fully preoccupied with it.

My work on this edition would not have been possible without the constant encouragement, support and understanding of my wife, Alice, and of my family.

Sheffield
1996

J.C.E.U.

International Advisers

The following individuals have made a valuable contribution to the development of the second edition of this textbook. In utilising their extensive knowledge of their countries' medical curricula and the teaching of pathology, it is hoped that this textbook will prove a valuable learning resource internationally. Their contribution is gratefully recognised.

Professor J W Arends
Department of Pathology
University of Limburg
Maastricht
The Netherlands

Professor Y Collan
Department of Pathology
University of Turku
Turku
Finland

Professor J P Cruse
Department of Anatomical Pathology
University of Cape Town
Cape Town
South Africa

Dr H Goldman
Professor of Pathology
Harvard Medical School
Boston
United States of America

Professor Lai-Meng Looi
Department of Pathology
University of Malaya
Kuala Lumpur
Malaysia

Professor R Machinami
Department of Pathology
University of Tokyo
Tokyo
Japan

Professor T L Miko
Department of Histopathology
Szent-Györgyi University Medical School
Szeged
Hungary

Professor H K Muller
Department of Pathology
University of Tasmania
Hobart
Australia

Dr K Ramnarayan
Professor of Pathology
Kasturba Medical College
Manipal
India

Professor R H Riddell
Department of Anatomical Pathology
McMaster University Medical Centre
Hamilton
Canada

Contributors

D W K Cotton BSc PhD BM MD MRCPath
Reader in Pathology, University of Sheffield;
Honorary Consultant, Central Sheffield University
Hospitals, Sheffield

A J Coup MB ChB FRCPath
Consultant Histopathologist, Barnsley District General
Hospital, Barnsley, South Yorkshire; Honorary Clinical
Lecturer in Pathology, University of Sheffield, Sheffield

S S Cross BSc MB BS MD MRCPath
Senior Lecturer, Department of Pathology, University of
Sheffield Medical School; Honorary Consultant, Central
Sheffield University Hospitals Trust, Sheffield

M F Dixon MD FRCPath
Reader in Gastrointestinal Pathology, University of
Leeds, Leeds

P J Gallagher MD PhD FRCPath
Reader in Pathology, University of Southampton;
Honorary Consultant Pathologist, Southampton
University Hospital, Southampton

J R Goepel MB ChB FRCPath
Senior Lecturer in Pathology, University of Sheffield;
Honorary Consultant Pathologist, Weston Park Hospital
and Central Sheffield University Hospitals, Sheffield

M Greaves MD FRCP FRCPath
Professor of Haematology and Honorary Consultant
Haematologist, University of Aberdeen, Aberdeen

A J Howat MB BS MRCPath
Consultant Histopathologist, Royal Preston Hospital,
Preston; formerly Senior Lecturer in Pathology,
University of Sheffield, Sheffield

J W Ironside BMSc MBChB MRCPath
Senior Lecturer in Pathology, University of Edinburgh;
Honorary Consultant Neuropathologist, Western General
Hospital, Edinburgh

K A MacLennan DM FRCPath
Reader in Tumour Pathology, Consultant Histopathologist,
St James's University Hospital, Leeds

M A Parsons MB ChB FRCPath
Senior Lecturer and Honorary Consultant in Ophthalmic
Pathology; Director, Ophthalmic Sciences Unit, University
of Sheffield

J R Shortland BSc MB ChB PhD FRCPath
Honorary Clinical Lecturer, University of Sheffield;
Consultant Histopathologist, Northern General Hospital,
Sheffield

T J Stephenson MD MHSM MRCPath
Consultant Histopathologist, Central Sheffield Hospitals
Trust, Sheffield; Honorary Clinical Lecturer, University
of Sheffield

R A Walker MD FRCPath
Reader in Pathology, University of Leicester, Leicester

M Wells BSc MD FRCPath
Professor of Gynaecological Pathology, University of
Leeds; Honorary Consultant Pathologist, St James's
University Hospital, Leeds

Contributors

Contents

Part 1

BASIC PATHOLOGY

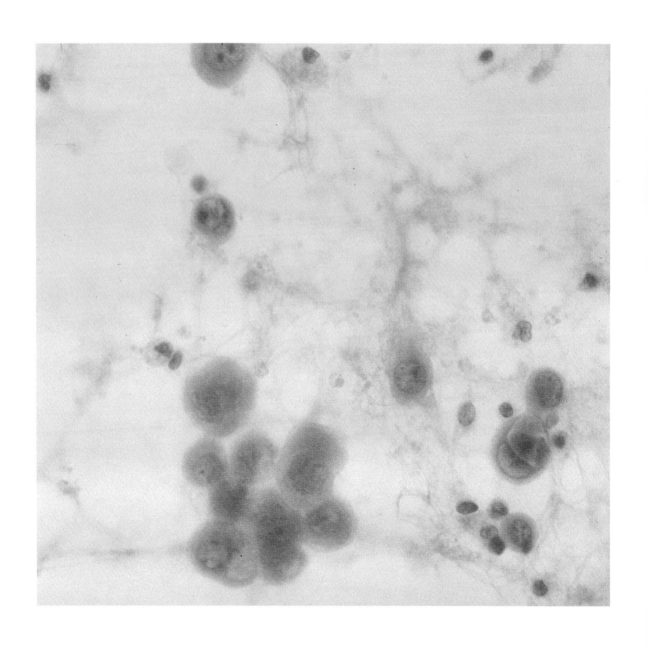

1

Introduction to pathology

Pathology is the *scientific study of disease*. In clinical practice and medical education, pathology also has a wider meaning: pathology constitutes a large body of scientific knowledge, ideas and investigative methods essential for the understanding and practice of modern medicine.

Pathology is not synonymous with the morphology of diseased tissues; this is an outmoded perception. Pathology includes knowledge and understanding of the *functional* and *structural* changes in disease, from the molecular level to the effects on the individual.

Pathology is continually subject to change, revision and expansion as the application of new scientific methods illuminates our knowledge of disease.

The ultimate goal of pathology is the identification of the *causes* of disease, a fundamental objective that leads the way to disease prevention.

HISTORY OF PATHOLOGY

The evolution of concepts about the causes and nature of human disease reflects the prevailing ideas about the explanation for all worldly events and the techniques available for their investigation (Table 1.1). Thus, the early dominance of *animism*, in the philosophies of Plato and Pythagoras, resulted in the attribution of disease to the adverse influences of immaterial or supernatural forces; it was therefore assumed that nothing could be learnt from the objec-

tive examination of the corpses of those who succumbed. Even when the clinical significance of many abnormal physical signs and postmortem findings was established early in the long history of medicine, the nature of the underlying disease was thought to be due to an excess or deficiency of the various *humors*— phlegm, black bile, and so on. These concepts are now firmly and irrevocably consigned to medical antiquity.

Morbid anatomy

The first opportunity for the scientific study of disease came from the thorough internal examination of the body after death. *Autopsies* (necropsies or postmortem examinations) have been performed scientifically from about 300 BC and have revealed much information that has helped to clarify the nature of many diseases. As these examinations were confined initially to the gross (rather than microscopic) examination of the organs, this period is regarded as the era of *morbid anatomy*. During the 19th century in Germany, major contributions were made by Rokitansky and Aschoff, who meticulously performed and documented many thousands of autopsies and correlated their findings with the clinical signs and symptoms of the patients and with the natural history of a wide variety of diseases.

Microscopy and cellular pathology

Pathology, and indeed medicine as a whole, was revolutionised by the application of *microscopy* to the

Table 1.1 Historical relationship between the hypothetical causes of disease and the dependence on techniques for their elucidation

Hypothetical cause of disease	Techniques supporting causal hypothesis	Period
Animism	None	Primitive, though the ideas persist in some cultures
Magic	None	Primitive, though the ideas persist in some cultures
Humors (excess or deficiency)	Early autopsies and clinical observations	c. 300 BC to c.1500 AD
Spontaneous generation (abiogenesis)	Analogies with decomposing matter	Prior to 1800 AD
Environmental	Modern autopsy Cellular pathology (e.g. microscopy) Toxicology Microbiology Epidemiology	1850 to present
Genetic	Molecular pathology (e.g. DNA analysis) and clinical observations on inherited defects	20th century

study of diseased tissues from about 1800. Prior to this, it was postulated that diseases arose by a process of *spontaneous generation*; that is, by a process of metamorphosis independent of any external cause or other influence. This notion seems ridiculous to us today, but 200 years ago nothing was known of bacteria, viruses, ionising radiation, carcinogenic chemicals, and so on. So Pasteur's demonstration that micro-organisms in the environment could contaminate and impair the quality of wine was a major landmark in our perception of the environment and our understanding of its possible adverse effects, and it has had an enormous impact on medicine.

Rudolf Virchow (1821–1902), a German pathologist and ardent advocate of the microscope, recognised that the cell was the smallest viable constituent unit of the body and contrived a new and lasting set of ideas about disease — *cellular pathology*. The light microscope enabled him to see changes in diseased tissues at a cellular level and his observations, extended further by electron microscopy, have had a profound influence. That does not mean to say that Virchow's cell pathology theory is immutable. Indeed, current advances in biochemistry are revolutionising our understanding of many diseases at a molecular level; we now have biochemical explanations for many of the cellular and clinical manifestations of disease.

Molecular pathology

The impact of *molecular pathology* is exemplified by the advances being made in our knowledge of the biochemical basis of congenital disorders and cancer. Techniques with relatively simple principles (less easy in practice) can reveal the change of a single nucleotide in genomic DNA resulting in the synthesis of the defective gene product that may be the fundamental lesion in a particular disease (Ch. 3).

Cellular and molecular alterations in disease

As a result of the application of modern scientific methods, we now have a clearer understanding of the ways in which diseases can be attributed to disturbances of normal cellular and a molecular mechanisms (Table 1.2). It is by continuing to study disease in this way that knowledge can be advanced and treatment improved.

THE SCOPE OF PATHOLOGY

Pathology is the foundation of medical science and

practice. Without pathology, the practice of medicine would be reduced to myths and folklore.

Clinical and experimental pathology

Scientific knowledge about human diseases is derived from observations on patients or, by analogy, from experimental studies on animals and cell cultures. The greatest contribution comes from the study in depth of tissue and body fluids from patients.

Clinical pathology

Clinical medicine is based on a longitudinal approach to a patient's illness — the patient's history, the examination and investigation, the diagnosis, and the treatment. Clinical pathology is more concerned with a cross-sectional analysis at the level of the disease itself, studied in depth — the cause and mechanisms of the disease, and the effects of the disease upon the various organs and systems of the body. These two perspectives are complementary and inseparable: clinical medicine cannot be practised without an understanding of pathology; pathology is meaningless if it is bereft of clinical implications.

Experimental pathology

Experimental pathology is the observation of the effects of manipulations on experimental systems such as animal models of disease or cell cultures. Fortunately, advances in cell culture technology have reduced the usage of laboratory animals in medical research and experimental pathology. However, it is extremely difficult to reproduce in cell cultures the physiological milieu that prevails in the intact human body.

Subdivisions of pathology

Pathology is a vast subject with many ramifications. In practice, however, it can be split into major subdivisions:

- *histopathology:* the investigation and diagnosis of disease from the examination of tissues
- *cytopathology:* the investigation and diagnosis of disease from the examination of isolated cells
- *haematology:* the study of disorders of the cellular and coagulable components of blood
- *microbiology:* the study of infectious diseases and the organisms responsible for them

Table 1.2	Examples of the involvement of cellular and extra-cellular components in disease	
Component	Normal function	Examples of alterations in disease
Cellular		
Nucleus	Genes encoded in DNA	Inherited or spontaneous mutations (e.g. inherited metabolic disorders, cancer)
		Site of viral replication
Mitochondria	Oxidative metabolism	Mutations of mitochondrial DNA
		Enzyme defects
Lysosomes	Enzymic degradation	Metabolic storage disorders
		Defects in microbial killing
Cell membrane	Functional envelope of cell	Defects in ion transfer (e.g. cystic fibrosis, hereditary spherocytosis)
Adhesion molecules	Cellular adhesion	Altered expression in inflammation
		Decreased expression in neoplasia
HLA substances	Immune recognition	Aberrant expression associated with autoimmune disease
		Haplotypes correlate with risk of some diseases
Receptors	Specific recognition	Hormone receptors cause cells to respond to physiological or pathological hormone levels
		Lymphocyte receptors enable immune responses to antigens
Secreted products		
Collagen	Mechanical strength of tissues	Integrity of wounds Inherited defects (e.g. osteogenesis imperfecta)
Immunoglobulins	Antibody activity in immune reactions	Deficiency leads to increased infection risk
		Secreted by myeloma cells
		Specific antibody activity may be in response to infection or a marker of autoimmune disease
Nitric oxide	Endothelium-derived relaxing factor causing vasodilatation, inhibition of platelet aggregation and of proliferation	Increased levels in endotoxic shock and in asthma
Hormones	Control of specific target cells	Excess or deficiency due to disease of endocrine organs
Cytokines	Regulation of inflammatory and immune responses and of cell proliferation	Increased levels in inflammatory, immunological and reparative tissue reactions
Free radicals	Microbial killing	Inappropriate or excessive production causes tissue damage

- *immunology:* the study of the specific defence mechanisms of the body
- *chemical pathology:* the study and diagnosis of disease from the chemical changes in tissues and fluids
- *genetics:* the study of abnormal chromosomes and genes
- *toxicology:* the study of the effects of known or suspected poisons
- *forensic pathology:* the application of pathology to legal purposes (e.g. investigation of death in suspicious circumstances).

These subdivisions are more important professionally (because each requires its own team of specialists) than educationally. The subject must be taught and learnt in an integrated manner, for the body and its diseases make no distinction between these conventional subdivisions.

This book, therefore, adopts a multidisciplinary

approach to pathology. In the systematic section, the normal structure and function of each organ is summarised, the pathological basis for clinical signs and symptoms is described, and the clinical implications of each disease are emphasised.

TECHNIQUES OF PATHOLOGY

Our knowledge of the nature and causation of disease has been disclosed by the continuing application of technology to its study.

Gross pathology

Before microscopy was applied to medical problems (c. 1800), observations were confined to those made with the unaided eye, and thus was accumulated much of our knowledge of the *morbid anatomy* of disease. Gross or macroscopic pathology is the modern nomenclature for this approach to the study of disease and, especially in the autopsy, it is still an important investigative method. The gross pathology of many diseases is so characteristic that, when interpreted by the experienced pathologist, a fairly confident diagnosis can often be given prior to further investigation by, for example, light microscopy.

Light microscopy

Advances in the optical quality of lenses have resulted in a wealth of new information about the structure of tissues and cells in health and disease that can be gleaned from their examination by light microscopy.

If solid tissues are to be examined by light microscopy, the sample must first be thinly sectioned to permit the transmission of light and to minimise the superimposition of tissue components. These sections are routinely cut from tissue hardened by permeation with and embedding in wax or, less often, transparent plastic. For some purposes (e.g. histochemistry, very urgent diagnosis) sections have to be cut from tissue that has been hardened rapidly by freezing. The sections are stained to help distinguish between different components of the tissue (e.g. nuclei, cytoplasm, collagen).

Histochemistry

Histochemistry is the study of the chemistry of tissues, usually by microscopy of tissue sections after they have been treated with specific reagents so that the features of individual cells can be visualised.

Immunohistochemistry and immunofluorescence

Immunohistochemistry and immunofluorescence employ antibodies (immunoglobulins with antigen specificity) to visualise substances in tissue sections or cell preparations; these techniques use antibodies linked chemically to enzymes or fluorescent dyes respectively. Immunofluorescence requires a microscope specially modified for ultraviolet illumination and the preparations are often not permanent (they fade). For these reasons, immunohistochemistry has become more popular; in this technique, the end product is a deposit of opaque or coloured material that can be seen with a conventional light microscope and does not deteriorate. The repertoire of substances detectable by these techniques has been greatly enlarged by the development of *monoclonal antibodies*.

Electron microscopy

Electron microscopy has extended the range of pathology to the study of disorders at an organelle level, and to the demonstration of viruses in tissue samples from some diseases.

Biochemical techniques

Biochemical techniques applied to the body's tissues and fluids in health and disease are now one of the dominant influences on our growing knowledge of pathological processes. The clinical role of biochemistry is exemplified by the importance of monitoring fluid and electrolyte homeostasis in many disorders. Serum enzyme assays are used to assess the integrity and vitality of various tissues; for example, raised levels of cardiac enzymes in the blood indicate damage to cardiac myocytes.

Haematological techniques

Haematological techniques are used in the diagnosis and study of blood disorders. These techniques range from relatively simple cell counting, which can be performed electronically, to assays of blood coagulation factors.

Cell cultures

Cell cultures are widely used in research and diagnosis. They are an attractive medium for research because of the ease with which the cellular environment can be modified and the responses to it monitored. Diagnostically, cell cultures are used to prepare chromosome spreads for *cytogenetic analysis*.

Medical microbiology

Medical microbiology is the study of diseases caused by organisms such as bacteria, fungi, viruses and parasites. Techniques used include direct microscopy of appropriately stained material (e.g. pus), cultures to isolate and grow the organism, and methods to identify correctly the cause of the infection. In the case of bacterial infections, the most appropriate antibiotic can be selected by determining the sensitivity of the organism to a variety of agents.

Molecular pathology

Many important advances are now coming from the science of molecular pathology revealing defects in the chemical structure of molecules arising from errors in the genome, the sequence of bases that directs amino acid synthesis. Using *in situ hybridisation* it is possible to render the presence of specific genes or their messenger RNA visible in tissue sections or cell preparations. Minute quantities of nucleic acids can be amplified by using the *polymerase chain reaction* using oligonucleotide primers specific for the genes being studied.

Molecular pathology is manifested in various conditions, for example: abnormal haemoglobin molecules, such as in sickle cell disease (Ch. 23); abnormal collagen molecules in osteogenesis imperfecta (Ch. 3); and alterations in the genome governing the control of cell and tissue growth, now believed to play an important part in the development of tumours (Ch. 11).

GENERAL AND SYSTEMATIC PATHOLOGY

Pathology is best taught and learnt in two stages:

- *general pathology:* the mechanisms and characteristics of the principal types of disease process (e.g. congenital versus acquired diseases, inflammation, tumours, degenerations)
- *systematic pathology:* the descriptions of specific diseases as they affect individual organs or organ systems (e.g. appendicitis, lung cancer, atheroma).

General pathology

General pathology is our current understanding of the causation, mechanisms and characteristics of the major categories of disease.

These processes are covered in Part 2 of this textbook and many specific diseases mentioned by way of illustration. It is essential that the principles of general pathology are understood before an attempt is made to study systematic pathology. General pathology is the foundation of knowledge that has to be laid down before one can begin to study the systematic pathology of specific diseases.

Systematic pathology

Systematic pathology is our current knowledge of specific diseases as they affect individual organs or systems. ('Systematic' should not be confused with 'systemic' in this context. Systemic pathology would be characteristic of a disease that pervaded *all* body systems!) Each specific disease can usually be attributed to the operation of one or more categories of causation and mechanism featuring in general pathology. Thus, acute appendicitis is acute inflammation affecting the appendix; carcinoma of the lung is the result of carcinogenesis acting upon cells in the lung, and the behaviour of the cancerous cells thus formed follows the pattern established for malignant tumours; and so on.

Systematic pathology is covered in Part 3 of this textbook.

LEARNING PATHOLOGY

There are two apparent difficulties that face the new student of pathology: *language* and *process*. Pathology, like most branches of science and medicine, has its own vocabulary of special terms: these need to be learnt and understood not just because they are the language of pathology; they are also a major part of the language of clinical medicine. The student must not confuse the learning of the language with the learning of the mechanisms of disease and their effects on individual organs and patients. For example, the term 'hyperplasia' means an increase in the size of an organ due to the proliferation of its constituent cells; this definition must be learnt before the student attempts to learn about the process of hyperplasia. In this book, each important term will be clearly defined in the main text or the glossary or both.

Disease mechanisms constitute general pathology, knowledge that can be applied to related diseases occurring in different organs or systems. It is absolutely vital to understand general pathology before attempting to study systematic pathology in depth. Systematic pathology deals more with specific diseases; the rules of general pathology apply, but there are many variations peculiar to the same disease process affecting different organs.

A logical and orderly way of thinking about diseases and their characteristics must be cultivated; for each entity the student should be able to run through the list of chief characteristics that apply to any disease:

- incidence
- aetiology
- pathogenesis
- pathological and clinical features
- complications and sequelae
- prognosis
- treatment.

Our knowledge about many diseases is still incomplete, but at least such a list will serve to prompt the memory and enable students to organise their knowledge.

Pathology is learnt through a variety of media; in addition to this textbook the student will no doubt have a fairly comprehensive course of relatively didactic lectures perhaps supplemented by tutorials, problem-solving-oriented practical classes involving the gross and microscopic examination of diseased tissues, demonstrations, and postmortem teaching. If a student's curriculum lacks one or more of these features it should not be considered in any way deficient; there is no prescribed way of teaching the subject and each medical school will have evolved its own scheme based on local factors. Nevertheless, students of pathology should be encouraged to avail themselves of every opportunity to learn about diseases. Even the bedside, operating theatre and outpatient clinic provide ample opportunities for further experience of pathology; hearing a diastolic cardiac murmur through a stethoscope should prompt the listening student to consider the pathological features of the narrowed mitral valve orifice (mitral stenosis) responsible for the murmur, and the effects of this stenosis on the lungs and the rest of the cardiovascular system.

Pathology in the problem-oriented integrated medical curriculum

Although medicine, surgery, pathology and other disciplines are frequently taught as separate subjects in the curriculum, students must develop an integrated understanding of disease. Diseases are compartmentalised in this way only so that all aspects can be taught in sufficient depth to provide a full and working understanding. In practice, no such boundaries exist.

To encourage this integrated attitude, in this textbook the pathological basis of common clinical signs is frequently emphasised so that students can develop an interface between their everyday clinical experiences and their knowledge of pathology.

In general, the development of a clinicopathological understanding of disease can be pursued by two equally legitimate and complementary approaches:

- problem-oriented
- disease-oriented.

In learning pathology, the disease-oriented approach is more relevant because medical practitioners require knowledge of diseases (e.g. pneumonia, cancer, ischaemic heart disease) so that correct diagnoses can be made and the most appropriate treatment given.

The problem-oriented approach

Historically, before diseases had been properly characterised, the problems caused by diseases constituted all that was known about them. The classification of disease was based almost entirely upon symptomatology supported by a limited range of clinical signs.

The problem-oriented approach is still the first step in the clinical diagnosis of disease. In many illnesses, symptoms alone suffice for diagnosis. In other illnesses, the diagnosis has to be supported by clinical signs (e.g. abnormal heart sounds). In some instances, the diagnosis can be made conclusively only by special investigations (e.g. laboratory analysis of blood or tissue samples, imaging techniques).

The links between *diseases* and the *problems* they produce are emphasised in the systematic chapters (Part 3) and are exemplified here (Table 1.3).

Justifications for the problem-oriented approach are that:

- Patients present with 'problems' rather than 'diagnoses'.
- Some clinical problems lack a known pathological basis (this is true particularly of psychiatric conditions such as depressive illness).
- Clinical treatment is often directed towards relieving the patient's problems rather than curing their disease (which may either remit spontaneously or be incurable).

The disease-oriented approach

Modern pathological understanding of illnesses is based on a disease-oriented approach; knowledge of diseases and their clinical manifestations is fundamental to good medical practice.

Table 1.3   The problem-oriented approach: examples of combinations of clinical problems and their pathological basis

Problems	Pathological basis (diagnosis)	Comment
Weight loss and haemoptysis	Lung cancer or tuberculosis	Can be distinguished by finding either cancer cells or mycobacteria in sputum
Dyspnoea and ankle swelling	Heart failure	Due to, for example, valvular disease
Chest pain and hypotension	Myocardial infarction	Should be confirmed by ECG and serum assay of cardiac enzymes
Vomiting and diarrhoea	Gastroenteritis	Specific microbial cause can be determined
Headache, impaired vision and microscopic haematuria	Hypertension	May be due to various causes or, more commonly, without evident cause
Headache, vomiting and photophobia	Subarachnoid haemorrhage or meningitis	Can be distinguished by other clinical features and examination of cerebrospinal fluid

The disease-oriented approach has also proved to be the most successful manner in which to impart pathological knowledge. It would be possible to compose a textbook of pathology in whch the chapters were entitled, for example, 'Cough', 'Weight loss', 'Headaches' and 'Pain' (these being problems), but the reader would be unlikely to come away with a clear understanding of the diseases. This is because one disease may cause a variety of problems — for example, cough, weight loss, headaches and pain — and may therefore crop up in several chapters. Consequently, this textbook, like most textbooks of pathology (and, indeed, of medicine) adopts a disease-oriented approach.

MAKING DIAGNOSES

Diagnosis is the act of naming a disease in an individ-

ual patient. The diagnosis is important because it enables the patient to benefit from treatment that is known, or is at least likely, to be effective from observing its effects on other patients with the same disease.

The process of making diagnoses involves:

- taking a clinical history to document *symptoms*
- examining the patient for *clinical signs*
- if necessary, performing *investigations* guided by the provisional diagnosis based on signs and symptoms.

When this process is carried out in an individual patient, proof or strong suspicion of a particular disease eventually emerges as the diagnosis. If the diagnosis is still uncertain, a pragmatic approach to the problem can be adopted by observing the effects of a specific treatment or some other intervention.

Although experienced clinicians can diagnose many patients' diseases quite rapidly (and possibly reliably), the student will find that it is helpful to adopt a formal strategy based on a series of logical steps leading to the gradual exclusion of various possibilities and the emergence of a single diagnosis. For example:

- First decide which organ or body system is likely to be affected by the disease.
- From the signs and symptoms, decide which general category of disease (inflammation, tumours, etc.) is likely to be present.
- Then, using other factors (age, gender, previous medical history, etc.), compute a diagnosis or a small number of possibilities for investigation. ·
- Investigations should be performed only if the outcome of each one can be expected to resolve the diagnosis, or influence management if the diagnosis is already known.

This strategy can be refined and presented in the form of decision trees or diagnostic algorithms, but these details are outside the scope of this book.

Diagnostic pathology

In living patients we investigate and diagnose their illness by applying pathological methods to the examination of *tissue biopsies* and *body fluids*. Subject to ethical constraints, and if there are clinical indications to do so, it may be possible to obtain a series of samples from which the course of the disease can be monitored.

The applications of pathology in clinical diagnosis and patient management are described in Chapter 4.

Autopsies

Autopsy (necropsy and postmortem examination are synonymous) means to 'see for oneself'. In other words, rather than relying on clinical signs and symptoms and the results of diagnostic investigations during life, here is an opportunity for direct inspection and analysis of the organs.

Autopsies are useful for:

- determining the *cause of death*
- *audit* of the accuracy of clinical diagnosis
- *education* of undergraduates and postgraduates
- *research* into the causes and mechanisms of disease
- gathering accurate *statistics* about disease incidence.

The clinical use of information from autopsies is described in Chapter 4.

For the medical undergraduate and postgraduate, the autopsy is an important medium for the learning of pathology. It is an unrivalled opportunity to correlate clinical signs with their underlying pathological explanation.

PATHOLOGY AND THE SOCIAL CONTEXT

Although pathology, as practised professionally, is a laboratory-based clinical discipline focused on the care of individual patients and the advancement of medical knowledge, our ideas about the causes of disease, disability and death have wide implications for society.

Causes and agents of disease

There is socially (and politically) relevant controversy about what actually constitutes the *cause* of a disease. Critics argue that the science of pathology leads to the identification of merely the *agents* of some diseases rather than their underlying causes. For example, the bacterium *Mycobacterium tuberculosis* is the infective agent resulting in tuberculosis but, because many people exposed to the bacterium alone do not develop the disease, social deprivation and malnutrition (both of which are epidemiologically associated with the risk of tuberculosis) might be regarded by some as the actual causes. Without doubt, the marked fall in the incidence of many serious infectious diseases during the 20th century has been achieved at least as much through improvements in housing, hygiene, nutrition and sewage treatment as by specific immunisation and antibiotic treatment directed at the causative organisms. This distinction between agents and causes is developed further in Chapter 3.

The health of a nation

Because the methods used in pathology enable reliable diagnoses to be made, either during life by, for example, biopsy or after death by autopsy, the discipline has an important role in documenting the incidence of disease in a population. Cancer registration data is most reliable when it is based on histologically proven diagnoses; this happens in most cases. Epidemiological data derived from death certificates is notoriously unreliable unless verified by autopsy. The pathologically-based information thus obtained can be used to determine the true incidence of a disease in a population and the resources for its prevention and treatment can be deployed accordingly where they will achieve the greatest benefit.

Preventing disability and premature death

Laboratory methods are used increasingly for the detection of early disease by population screening. The prospects of cure are invariably better the earlier a disease is detected.

The incidence of death from cancer of the cervix is lowered by screening programmes; in many countries, women have their cervix scraped at regular intervals and the exfoliated cells are examined microscopically to detect the earliest changes associated with development of cancer. Although screening for breast cancer is primarily by mammography (X-ray imaging of the breast), any abnormalities are further investigated either by examining cells aspirated from the suspicious area or by histological examination of the tissue itself.

2

Characteristics, classification and incidence of disease

WHAT IS DISEASE?

A disease is a condition in which the presence of an abnormality of the body causes a loss of normal health (dis-ease). The mere presence of an abnormality is insufficient to imply the presence of disease unless it is accompanied by ill health, although it may denote an early stage in the development of a disease. The word *disease* is, therefore, synonymous with ill health and illness.

Each separately named disease is characterised by a distinct set of features (cause, signs and symptoms, morphological and functional changes, etc.). Many diseases share common features and are thereby grouped together in disease classification systems.

Disease is the clinical manifestation, through signs and symptoms, of an underlying abnormality. The abnormality may be structural or functional or both. In many instances the abnormality is obvious and well characterised (e.g. a tumour); in other instances the patient may be profoundly unwell but the nature of the abnormality is relatively poorly defined (e.g. depressive illness).

Limits of normality

Normal is virtually impossible to define as a single discrete state for any biological characteristic. Apart from differences between individuals, the human body changes naturally during fetal development, childhood, puberty, pregnancy (gender permitting), ageing, etc.

Most quantifiable biological characteristics are normally distributed, in statistical terms, about an average value. There are no constant numbers that can be used to define a normal height, weight, serum sodium concentration, etc. Normality, when quantifiable, is expressed as a numerical range, usually encompassed by two standard deviations (for a 'normally' distributed feature) either side of the mean (Ch. 4). The probability that a measurable characteristic is abnormal increases the nearer it is to the limits of the normal range, but just because it lies outside the normal range does not necessarily denote abnormality — merely that it is very probably abnormal.

A distinction must be drawn also between what is usual and what is normal. It is usual to find atheroma (Ch. 13) in an elderly individual—but is it normal? In contrast, atheroma in a young person is so unusual that it would be regarded as abnormal and worthy of further investigation.

Responses to the environment

The natural environment of any species contains potentially injurious agents to which the individual or species must either adapt or succumb.

Adaptation

Adaptation of the individual to an adverse environment is well illustrated by the following examples. Healthy mountaineers ascending rapidly to the rarified atmosphere at high altitudes develop 'mountain sickness'; they recover by a process of adaptation (increased haemoglobin, etc.), but failure to do so can result in death from heart failure. Fair-skinned people get sunburnt from excessive exposure to ultraviolet light from the sun; some adapt by developing a protective tan, but untanned individuals run a higher risk of skin cancer if they persist in unprotected exposure to the sun for long periods. Environmental micro-organisms are a common cause of disease; those individuals who develop specific defences against them (e.g. antibodies) can resist the infection, but those who fail to adapt may succumb.

Disease: failure of adaptation

Susceptibility of a species to injurious environmental factors results either in its extinction or, over a long period, the favoured selection of a new strain of the species better adapted to withstand such factors. However, this holds true only if the injury manifests itself in the early years of life, thus thwarting propagation of the abnormal susceptibility by reproduction. If the injury manifests only in later life or if a lifetime of exposure to the injurious agent is necessary to produce the pathological changes, then the agent produces no evolutionary pressure for change.

An arguable interpretation of disease is that it represents a set of abnormal bodily responses to agents for which, as yet, the human species has little or no tolerance. The study of human pathology is not ordinarily concerned with the evolutionary impact of disease, but the geographic and racial distribution of some diseases provides evidence for the importance of this continuing process.

Ageing and adaptation

One of the main features of ageing is progressive inability of the individual to adapt to new or worsening environmental threats (Ch. 12). This is exemplified by the gradual impairment of immune responses, resulting in:

- re-emergence of dormant infections such as tuberculosis and herpes zoster

- failure to mount an effective immune response to newly encountered pathogens.

Tumours occur more commonly in the elderly. This could be due to the intrinsic delay, often decades, between exposure to the causative agent(s) and the clinical presentation of the resulting tumour. However, another possibility is that, with ageing, the body either deals less effectively with environmental carcinogens, or fails to eradicate deviant cells, or the carcinogenic process is augmented by cumulative spontaneous mutations.

Disease as an adaptive advantage

It is paradoxical for a disease to have beneficial effects on the individual. However, a few diseases, in addition to their deleterious effects, confer adaptive protection against specific environmental pathogens. This advantage may explain the high prevalence of a disease in areas where the specific pathogen for another disease is endemic.

The best examples are the sickle cell gene (HbS) and the glucose-6-phosphate dehydrogenase (G6PD) deficiency gene which confer protection against malaria by creating a hostile environment for the plasmodium parasite within red cells.

CHARACTERISTICS OF DISEASE

> ► *Aetiology*: the cause of a disease
> ► *Pathogenesis*: the mechanism causing the disease
> ► *Pathological and clinical manifestations*: the structural and functional features of the disease
> ► *Complications and sequelae*: the secondary, systemic or remote consequences of a disease
> ► *Prognosis*: the anticipated course of the disease in terms of cure, remission, or fate of the patient
> ► *Epidemiology*: the incidence and population distribution of a disease

All diseases have a set of characteristic features enabling them to be better understood, categorised and diagnosed. For many diseases, however, our knowledge is still incomplete or subject to controversy. The characteristics of any disease are (Fig. 2.1):

- aetiology (or cause)
- pathogenesis (or mechanism)
- morphological, functional and clinical changes (or manifestations)
- complications and sequelae (or secondary effects)
- prognosis (or outcome)
- epidemiology (or incidence).

The aetiology and pathogenesis of a disease may be combined as *aetiopathogenesis*.

Aetiology

The aetiology of a disease is its *cause*: the initiator of the subsequent events resulting in the patient's illness. Diseases are caused by a variable interaction between *host* (e.g. genetic) and *environmental* factors. Environmental causes of diseases are called *pathogens*, though this term is used commonly only when referring to bacteria; bacteria capable of causing disease are pathogenic bacteria and those that are harmless are non-pathogenic.

General categories of aetiological agents include:

- genetic abnormalities
- infective agents, e.g. bacteria, viruses, fungi, parasites
- chemicals
- radiation
- mechanical trauma.

Some diseases are due to a combination of causes, such as genetic factors and infective agents; such diseases are said to have a *multifactorial aetiology*.

Sometimes the aetiology of a disease is unknown, but the disease is observed to occur more commonly in people with certain constitutional traits, occupations, habits or habitats; these are regarded as *risk factors*. These factors may provide a clue to an as yet unidentified aetiological agent. Other risk factors may simply have a permissive effect, facilitating the development of a disease in that individual: examples include malnutrition, which favours infections.

In the absence of any known cause, a disease is usually classified aetiologically as *primary, idiopathic, essential, spontaneous* or *cryptogenic*; all these terms have the same meaning although they are often used in special contexts (e.g. essential hypertension, spontaneous pneumothorax, cryptogenic cirrhosis). In each instance the precise initial cause awaits discovery.

Some agents can cause more than one disease depending on the circumstances; for example, ionising radiation can cause either rapid deterioration leading to death, scarring of tissues, or tumours.

Identification of the causes of disease

In terms of causation, diseases may be:

- entirely genetic
- multifactorial (genetic and environmental interplay)
- entirely environmental.

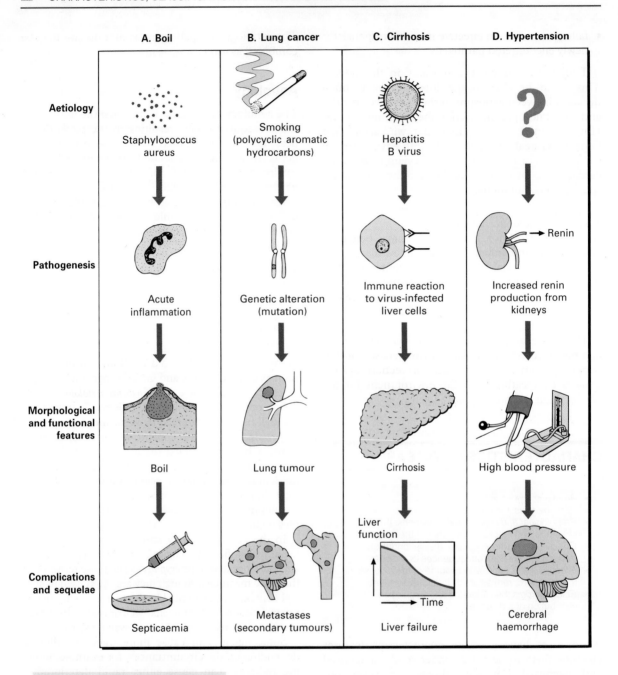

Fig. 2.1 Characteristics of disease

The relationship between aetiology, pathogenesis, morphological and functional manifestations, and complications and sequelae is exemplified by four diseases. **A.** Boil. **B.** Lung cancer. **C.** Cirrhosis. **D.** Hypertension.

Most common diseases have an entirely environmental cause, but genetic influences in disease susceptibility are being increasingly discovered, and many diseases with no previously known cause are being shown to be due to genetic abnormalities (see Ch. 3); this is the reward of applying the principles of clinical genetics and the new techniques of molecular biology to the study of human disease. The extent to which a disease is due to genetic or environmental causes can often be deduced from some of its main features or its association with host factors.

Features pointing to a significant genetic contribution to the occurrence of a disease include a high incidence in particular families or races, or an association with an inherited characteristic (e.g. gender, blood group, histocompatibility haplotypes). Diseases associated with particular occupations or geographic regions tend to have an environmental basis; the most abundant environmental causes of disease are microbes (bacteria, viruses, fungi, etc.).

Host predisposition to disease

Many diseases are the *predictable* consequence of exposure to the initiating cause; host factors make relatively little contribution. This is particularly true of physical injury: the immediate results of mechanical trauma or radiation injury are dose-related; the outcome can be predicted from the strength of the injurious agent.

Other diseases are the *probable* consequence of exposure to causative factors, but they are not inevitable. This is exemplified by infections with potentially harmful bacteria: the outcome can be influenced by various host factors such as nutritional status, genetic influences and pre-existing immunity.

Some diseases occur more commonly in individuals with a congenital predisposition. For example, ankylosing spondylitis (Ch. 25), a disabling inflammatory disease of the spinal joints of unknown aetiology, occurs more commonly in individuals with the HLA-B27 haplotype.

Some diseases predispose patients to the risk of developing other diseases. Diseases associated with an increased risk of cancer are designated *premalignant conditions;* for example, hepatic cirrhosis predisposes to hepatocellular carcinoma and ulcerative colitis predisposes to carcinoma of the large intestine. The histologically identifiable antecedent lesion from which the cancers directly develop is designated the *premalignant lesion.*

Some diseases predispose to others because they have a permissive effect allowing environmental agents, that are not normally pathogenic, to cause disease. This is best exemplified by *opportunistic infections* in patients with impaired defence mechanisms resulting in infection by organisms not normally harmful (i.e. non-pathogenic) to man (Ch. 9). Patients with leukaemia or the acquired immune deficiency syndrome (AIDS), organ transplant recipients, or other patients treated with cytotoxic drugs or steroids, are susceptible to infections such as pneumonia due to *Aspergillus* fungi, cytomegalovirus, or *Pneumocystis carinii.*

Causes and agents of disease

It is argued that a distinction should be made between the *cause* and the *agent* of a disease; for example, tuberculosis is caused, arguably, not by the tubercle bacillus (*Mycobacterium tuberculosis*) but by poverty, social deprivation and malnutrition — the tubercle bacillus is 'merely' the agent of the disease, the underlying cause is adverse socio-economic factors. There is, in fact, incontrovertible evidence that the decline in incidence in many serious infectious diseases is attributable substantially to improvements in hygiene, sanitation and general nutrition rather than to immunisation programmes or specific antimicrobial therapy. Such arguments are of relevance here only to emphasise that the socio-economic status of a country or individual may influence the prevalence of the environmental factor or the host susceptibility to it. In practice, causes and agents are conveniently embraced by the term *aetiology.*

Causal associations

A causal association is a marker for the risk of developing a disease, but it is not necessarily the actual cause of the disease. The stronger the causal association, the more likely it is to be the aetiology of the disease. Causal associations become more powerful if:

- they are *plausible*, supported by experimental evidence
- the presence of the disease is associated with *prior exposure* to the putative cause
- the risk of the disease is *proportional* to the level of exposure to the putative cause
- *removal* of the putative cause lessens the risk of the disease.

The utility of these statements is exemplified by reference to the association between lung cancer and cigarette smoking. Lung cancer is more common in smokers than in non-smokers; the risk of lung cancer is proportional to cigarette consumption; population groups that have reduced their cigarette consumption (e.g. doctors) show a commensurate reduction in their rate of lung cancer.

Causal associations may be neither exclusive nor absolute. For example, because some heavy cigarette smokers never develop lung cancer, smoking cannot alone be regarded as a *sufficient* cause; other factors are required. Conversely, because some non-smokers develop lung cancer, smoking cannot be regarded as a *necessary* cause; other causative factors must exist.

Causal associations tend to be strongest with infections. For example syphilis, a venereal disease, is always due to infection by the spirochaete

Treponema pallidum; there is no other possible cause for syphilis; syphilis is the only disease caused by *Treponema pallidum*.

Koch's postulates

An infective (e.g. bacterial, viral) cause for a disease is not usually regarded as proven until it fulfils the requirements of the postulates enunciated by Robert Koch (1843–1910), a German bacteriologist and Nobel prizewinner in 1905. The postulates requiring satisfaction are:

- The organism must be sufficiently abundant in every case to account for the disease.
- The organism associated with the disease can be cultivated artificially in pure culture.
- The cultivated organism produces the disease upon inoculation into another member of the same species.
- Antibodies to the organism appear during the course of the disease.

The last postulate was added subsequently to Koch's list. Although Koch's postulates have lost their novelty, their relevance is undiminished. However, each postulate merits further comments because there are notable exceptions:

- In some diseases the causative organism is very sparse. A good example is tuberculosis, where the destructive lung lesions contain very few mycobacteria; in this instance, the destruction is caused by an immune reaction prompted by the presence of the organism.
- Cultivation of some organisms is remarkably difficult, yet their role in the aetiology of disease is undisputed. *Treponema pallidum* is the cause of syphilis, but it has defied all attempts at cultivation outside the body.
- Ethics prohibit attempts to transmit a disease from one person to another, but animals have been used successfully as surrogates for human transmission.
- Immunosuppression may lessen the antibody response and also render the host extremely susceptible to the disease. In addition, if an antibody is detected it should be further classified to confirm that it is an *IgM* class antibody, denoting recent infection, rather than an *IgG* antibody, denoting long-lasting immunity due to previous exposure to the organism.

Pathogenesis

The pathogenesis of a disease is the *mechanism* through which the aetiology (cause) operates to pro-

duce the pathological and clinical manifestations. Groups of aetiological agents often cause disease by acting through the same common pathway of events. Examples of pathogeneses of disease include:

- inflammation: a response to many micro-organisms and other harmful agents causing tissue injury
- degeneration: a deterioration of cells or tissues in response to, or failure of adaptation to, a variety of agents
- carcinogenesis: the mechanism by which cancer-causing agents result in the development of tumours
- immune reactions: undesirable effects of the body's immune system.

These pathways of disease development constitute our knowledge of general pathology, and their description forms the first part of this textbook.

Latent intervals and incubation periods

Few aetiological agents cause signs and symptoms immediately after exposure. Usually, some time elapses. In the context of carcinogenesis, this time period is referred to as the *latent interval*; it is often two or three decades. In infectious disorders (due to bacteria, viruses, etc.), the period between exposure and the development of disease is called the *incubation period*; it is often measured in days or weeks, and each infectious agent is usually associated with a characteristic incubation period.

The reason for discussing these time intervals here is that it is during these periods that the pathogenesis of the disease is being enacted, culminating in the development of pathological and clinical manifestations that cause the patient to seek medical help.

Structural and functional manifestations

The aetiological agent (cause) acts through a pathogenetic pathway (mechanism) to produce the *manifestations* of disease, giving rise to clinical signs and symptoms (e.g. weight loss, shortness of breath) and the abnormal features or *lesions* (e.g. carcinoma of the lung) to which the clinical signs and symptoms can be attributed. The pathological manifestations may require biochemical methods for their detection and, therefore, should not be thought of as only those structural abnormalities evident to the unaided eye or by microscopy. The biochemical changes in the tissues and the blood are, in some instances, more important than the structural changes, many of which may appear relatively late in the course of the disease.

Although each separately named disease has its own distinctive and diagnostic features, it is possible to generalise about the range of structural and functional abnormalities, alone or combined, resulting in ill health.

Structural abnormalities

Common general structural abnormalities causing ill health are:

- space-occupying lesions (e.g. tumours) destroying, displacing or compressing adjacent healthy tissues
- deposition of an excessive or abnormal material in an organ (e.g. amyloid)
- abnormally sited tissue (e.g. tumours, heterotopias) as a result of invasion, metastasis or developmental abnormality
- loss of healthy tissue from a surface (e.g. ulceration) or from within a solid organ (e.g. infarction)
- obstruction to normal flow within a tube (e.g. asthma, vascular occlusion)
- rupture of a hollow viscus (e.g. aneurysm, intestinal perforation).

Other structural abnormalities, visible only by light or electron microscopy, are very common and, even though they do not directly cause clinical signs or symptoms, they are nevertheless diagnostically useful and often specific manifestations of disease. For this reason, the morphological study of diseased tissues is very rewarding for patient management and for clinical research. At an ultrastructural level (electron microscopy), one might see alien particles such as viruses in the affected tissue; there could be abnormalities in the number, shape, internal structure or size of tissue components such as intracellular organelles or extracellular material. By light microscopy, abnormalities in cellular morphology or tissue architecture can be discerned. With the unaided eye, changes in the size, shape or texture of whole organs can be discerned either by direct inspection or by indirect means such as radiology.

Functional abnormalities

Examples of functional abnormalities causing ill health include:

- excessive secretion of a cell product (e.g. nasal mucus in the common cold, hormones having remote effects)

- insufficient secretion of a cell product (e.g. insulin lack in diabetes mellitus)
- impaired nerve conduction
- impaired contractility of a muscular structure.

What makes patients feel ill?
The 'feeling' of illness is usually due to one or a combination of common symptoms:

- pain
- fever
- nausea
- malaise.

Each of these common symptoms has a pathological basis and, in those conditions that remit spontaneously, all that is required for treatment is symptomatic relief.

In addition to the general symptoms of disease, there are other specific expressions of illness which help to focus attention, diagnostically and therapeutically, on a particular organ or body system. Examples include:

- altered bowel habit (diarrhoea or constipation)
- abnormal swellings
- shortness of breath
- skin rash (which may or may not itch).

The symptoms of disease (the patient's presenting complaints) invariably have an identifiable scientific basis. This is important to know because often nothing more than symptomatic treatment is required, because either the disease will remit spontaneously (e.g. the common cold) or there is no prospect of recovery (e.g. disseminated cancer). Examples of known mediators of symptoms are listed in Table 2.1.

Lesions

A lesion is the structural or functional abnormality responsible for ill health. Thus, in a patient with myocardial infarction, the infarct or patch of dead heart muscle is the lesion; this lesion is in turn a consequence of another lesion — occlusion of the supplying coronary artery by a thrombus (coronary artery thrombosis). A lesion may be purely biochemical, such as a defect in haemoglobin synthesis in a patient with a haemoglobinopathy.

Of course, not all diseases have overtly visible lesions associated with them, despite profound consequences for the patient; for example, schizophrenia and depressive illness yield nothing visibly abnormal in the brain using conventional methods.

Table 2.1   Examples of the known mediators of the symptoms of disease

Symptom	Mediators	Comment
Pain	Free nerve endings stimulated by mechanical, thermal or chemical agents (e.g. bradykinin, 5-HT, histamine; prostaglandins enhance sensitivity)	May signify irritation of a surface (e.g. peritoneum), distension of a viscus (e.g. bladder), ischaemia (e.g. angina), erosion of a tissue (e.g. by tumour) or inflammation
Swelling	Increased cell number or size, or abnormal accumulation of fluid or gas	Common manifestation of inflammation and of tumours
Shortness of breath (dyspnoea)	Increased blood CO_2 or, to a lesser extent, decreased blood O_2 concentration	Usually due to lung disease, heart failure or severe anaemia
Fever (pyrexia)	Interleukin-1 (IL-1) released by leukocytes acts on thermoregulatory centre in hypothalamus, mediated by prostaglandins (PG)	IL-1 release frequently induced by bacterial endotoxins Aspirin reduces fever by blocking PG synthesis
Weight loss	Inadequate food intake or catabolic state mediated by humoral factors from tumours	Common manifestation of cancer, not necessarily of the alimentary tract or disseminated
Bleeding	Weakness or rupture of blood vessel wall or coagulation defect	Coagulation defects lead to spontaneous bruising or prolonged bleeding after injury
Diarrhoea	Malabsorption of food results in osmotic retention of water in stools Decreased transit time, possibly due to humoral effects Damage to mucosa impairing absorption and exuding fluid	Most commonly due to infective causes not requiring specific treatment other than fluid replacement
Itching	Mast cell degranulation and release of histamine	Manifestation of, for example, allergy
Cough	Neuropeptide release in response, usually, to irritation of respiratory mucosa	Common manifestation of respiratory tract disease
Vomiting	Stimulation of vomiting centre in medulla, usually by afferent vagal impulses	Usuallly denotes upper gastrointestinal disease (e.g. gastroenteritis), but may be due to CNS lesions
Cyanosis	Reduced oxygen content of arterial haemoglobin	Due to either respiratory disease, cardiac failure or congenital shunting

Pathognomonic abnormalities

Pathognomonic features are restricted to a single disease, or disease category, and without them the diagnosis is impossible or uncertain. For example, Reed–Sternberg cells are said to be pathognomonic of Hodgkin's disease; they are exceptionally rare in any other condition. Similarly, the presence of *Mycobacterium tuberculosis*, in the appropriate context, is pathognomonic of tuberculosis.

Pathognomonic abnormalities are extremely useful clinically, because they are absolutely diagnostic. Their presence leaves no doubt about the diagnosis. Unfortunately, some diseases are characterised only by a combination of abnormalities, none of which on its own is absolutely diagnostic; it is the particular combination that is diagnostic. Diseases characterised by multiple abnormalities are called *syndromes* (see p. 23).

Complications and sequelae

Diseases may have *prolonged*, *secondary* or *distant* effects. Examples include the spread of an infective organism from the original site of infection, where it had provoked an inflammatory reaction, to another part of the body, where a similar reaction to it will occur. Similarly, malignant tumours arise initially in one organ as primary tumours, but tumour cells eventually permeate lymphatics and blood vessels and thereby spread to other organs to produce secondary tumours or metastases. The course of a disease may be prolonged and complicated if the body's capacity for defence, repair or regeneration is deficient.

Sometimes, a succession of complications of a disease may lead to anatomically remote consequences. Diseases have no respect for anatomical or systematic boundaries.

Prognosis

The prognosis forecasts the known or likely *course of the disease* and, therefore, the fate of the patient. When we say that the 5-year survival prospects for carcinoma of the lung are about 5%, this is the prognosis of that condition. Sometimes we can be very specific because the information available about an individual patient and his disease may enable an accurate forecast; for example, a patient who presents with a carcinoma of the lung that has already spread to the liver, bones and the brain very probably (and unfortunately) has a 6-month survival prospect of nil.

The prognosis of any disease is of course subject to influence by medical or surgical intervention. So one must distinguish between the prognosis of a disease that is allowed to follow its natural course and the prognosis of the same disease in a group of patients receiving appropriate therapy.

In assessing the long-term prognosis of a chronic disease, it is important to compare the survival of a group of patients with actuarial data for comparable populations without the disease. The survival data for the group with the disease should be corrected to allow for deaths that are likely to occur from other diseases.

Remission and relapse

Not all chronic diseases pursue a relentless course. Some are punctuated by periods of quiescence when the patient enjoys relatively good health. *Remission* is the process of conversion from active disease to quiescence. Later, the signs and symptoms may reappear; this is the process of *relapse*. Some diseases may oscillate through several cycles of remission and relapse before the patient is cured of or succumbs to the disease. Diseases characterised by a tendency to remit and relapse include chronic inflammatory bowel disease (Crohn's disease and ulcerative colitis) and treated acute lymphoblastic leukaemia (particularly in childhood).

The tendency of some diseases to go through cycles of remission and relapse makes it difficult to be certain about prognosis in an individual case.

Morbidity and mortality

The *morbidity* of a disease is the sum of the effects upon the patient. The morbidity of a disease may or may not result in *disability* of the patient. For example, a non-fatal myocardial infarct (heart attack) leaves an area of scarring of the myocardium, impairing its contractility and predisposing to heart failure: this is the morbidity of the disease in that particular patient. The heart failure manifests itself with breathlessness, restricting the patient's activities: this is the patient's disability.

The *mortality* of a disease is the probability that death will be the end result. Mortality is expressed usually as a percentage of all those patients presenting with the disease. For example, the mortality rate of myocardial infarction could be stated as 50% under defined circumstances.

Disability and disease

Many diseases result in only transient disability; for example, influenza or a bad cold may necessitate time off work for an employed person. Some diseases, however, are associated with a significant risk of permanent disability; in such cases, treatment is intended to minimise the risk of disability. Some investigations and treatments carry a small risk of harm, often permanent, and the risk of disability must be outweighed by the potential benefit to the patient.

As a general rule, the earlier a disease is diagnosed, the smaller the risk of disability either from the disease itself or from necessary treatment. This is one of the main objectives of screening programmes for various conditions (e.g. for cancers of the cervix and breast). The objective assessment, preferably measurement, of disability is important in the evaluation of the impact of a disease or the adverse effects of its treatment. There is, for example, a balance between the longevity of survival from a disease and the quality of life during the period of survival after diagnosis: a treatment that prolongs life may be unacceptable because it prolongs suffering; treatment that makes a patient more comfortable, but does not prolong life and may actually shorten it, may be more acceptable. The measure that takes account of the duration and quality of survival is QALYs (*quality-adjusted life years*), and enables scientifically based judgements about the impact of diseases, treatments and preventive measures.

NOMENCLATURE OF DISEASE

▶ Uniform nomenclature facilitates communication and enables accurate epidemiological studies
▶ Many standard conventions are used to derive names of diseases
▶ Eponymous names commemorate, for example, discoverer or signify ignorance of cause or mechanism
▶ Syndromes are defined by the aggregate of signs and symptoms

Before proceeding to a detailed discussion of disease it is important to clarify the meaning of some of the common terms, prefixes and suffixes used in the nomenclature of diseases and their pathological features.

Primary and secondary

The words *primary* and *secondary* are used in two different ways in the nomenclature of disease:

1. They may be used to describe the *causation* of a disease. Primary in this context means that the disease is without evident antecedent cause. Other words which have the same meaning in this context are essential, idiopathic and cryptogenic. Thus, primary hypertension is defined as abnormally high blood pressure without apparent cause.

Secondary means that the disease represents a complication or manifestation of some underlying lesion. Thus, secondary hypertension is defined as abnormally high blood pressure as a consequence of some other lesion (e.g. renal artery stenosis).

2. The words primary and secondary may be used to distinguish between the initial and subsequent *stages* of a disease, most commonly in cancer. The primary tumour is the initial tumour from which cancer cells disseminate to cause secondary tumours elsewhere in the body.

Acute and chronic

Acute and chronic are terms used to describe the *dynamics* of a disease. Acute conditions have a rapid onset, often but not always followed by a rapid resolution. Chronic conditions may follow an acute initial episode, but often are of insidious onset, and have a prolonged course lasting months or years. Subacute, a term not often used now, is intermediate between acute and chronic. These terms are most often used to qualify the nature of an inflammatory process. However, they can be used to describe the dynamics of any disease. The words may be used by patients to describe some symptoms, e.g. an 'acute' pain being sharp or severe.

Benign and malignant

Benign and malignant are emotive terms used to classify certain diseases according to their likely *outcome*. Thus, benign tumours remain localised to the tissue of origin and are very rarely lethal unless they compress some vital structure (e.g. brain), whereas malignant tumours invade and spread from their origin and are commonly lethal. Benign hypertension is relatively mild elevation of blood pressure that develops gradually and causes insidious injury to the organs of the body. This situation contrasts with malignant hypertension, in which the blood pressure rises rapidly and causes severe symptoms and tissue injury (e.g. headaches, blindness, renal failure, cerebral haemorrhage).

Prefixes

Commonly used prefixes and their meanings are:

- *ana-*, meaning absence (e.g. anaphylaxis)
- *dys-*, meaning disordered (e.g. dysplasia)
- *hyper-*, meaning an excess over normal (e.g. hyperthyroidism)
- *hypo-*, meaning a deficiency below normal (e.g. hypothyroidism)
- *meta-*, meaning a change from one state to another (e.g. metaplasia).

Suffixes

Commonly used suffixes and their meanings are:

- *-itis*, meaning an inflammatory process (e.g. appendicitis)
- *-oma*, meaning a tumour (e.g. carcinoma)
- *-osis*, meaning state or condition, not necessarily pathological (e.g. osteoarthrosis)
- *-oid*, meaning bearing a resemblance to (e.g. rheumatoid disease)
- *-penia*, meaning lack of (e.g. thrombocytopenia)
- *-cytosis*, meaning increased number of cells, usually in blood (e.g. leukocytosis)
- *-ectasis*, meaning dilatation (e.g. bronchiectasis)
- *-plasia*, meaning a disorder of growth (e.g. hyperplasia)
- *-opathy*, meaning an abnormal state lacking specific characteristics (e.g. lymphadenopathy).

Eponymous names

An eponymous disease or lesion is named after a person or place associated with it. Eponymous names are used commonly either when the nature or cause of the disease or lesion is unknown, or when long-term usage has resulted in the name becoming part of the language of medicine, or to commemorate the person who first described the condition. Examples include:

- Graves' disease: primary thyrotoxicosis
- Paget's disease of the nipple: infiltration of the skin of the nipple by cells from a cancer in the underlying breast tissue

- Crohn's disease: a chronic inflammatory disease of the gut affecting most commonly the terminal ileum and causing narrowing of the lumen
- Hodgkin's disease: a neoplasm of lymph nodes characterised by the presence of Reed–Sternberg cells
- Reed–Sternberg cells: large cells with bilobed nuclei and prominent nucleoli which are virtually diagnostic of Hodgkin's disease.

Syndromes

A syndrome is an aggregate of signs and symptoms or a combination of lesions without which the disease cannot be recognised or diagnosed. Syndromes often have eponymous titles. Examples include:

- Cushing's syndrome: hyperactivity of the adrenal cortex resulting in obesity, hirsutism, hypertension, etc. (Cushing's *disease* is this syndrome resulting specifically from a pituitary tumour secreting ACTH)
- nephrotic syndrome: albuminuria, hypoalbuminaemia and oedema; this syndrome can result from a variety of glomerular and other renal disorders.

Numerical coding systems

Standard numerical codes, rather than names, are often used in epidemiological studies. Each disease or disease group is designated a specific number. The most widely used systems are ICD (International Classification of Disease, a World Health Organization System), SNOP and SNOMED (Systematized Nomenclature of Pathology, Systematized Nomenclature of Medicine, systems devised by the American College of Pathologists).

PRINCIPLES OF DISEASE CLASSIFICATION

> ► Classifications aid diagnosis and learning
> ► Subject to change with advances in medical knowledge
> ► Diseases may be classified by a variety of complementary methods

Diseases do not occur to conform to any classification. Disease classifications are creations of medical science and are justified only by their utility. Classifications are useful in diagnosis to enable a

name (disease or disease category) to be assigned to a particular illness.

Disease classification at a relatively coarse level of categorisation is unlikely to change quickly. However, the more detailed the level of classification, the more likely it is to change as medical science progresses. For example, the general classification of disease into categories such as inflammatory and neoplastic (see below) is long established, yet in the 1970s four separate new classifications for lymphomas (tumours of lymph nodes) were introduced!

General classification of disease

The most widely used general classification of disease is that based on pathogenesis or disease mechanisms. Most diseases can be assigned a place in the following classification:

- congenital
  - genetic
  - non-genetic
- acquired
  - inflammatory
  - vascular
  - growth disorders
  - injury and disordered repair
  - metabolic and degenerative disorders.

Two important points must be made here. First, the above classification is not the only possible classification of disease. Second, many diseases share characteristics of more than one of the above categories.

Patients might prefer the following disease classification:

- recovery likely
  - with residual disability
  - without residual disability
- recovery unlikely
  - with pain
  - without pain.

This classification is perfectly legitimate, but it is not particularly useful either as a diagnostic aid or for categorisation according to the underlying pathology.

Congenital diseases

Congenital abnormalities (genetic/chromosome disorders and malformations) occur in approximately 5% of births in the UK. They comprise:

- malformations in 3.5%

- single gene defects in 1%
- chromosome aberrations in 0.5%.

Common malformations include congenital heart defects, spina bifida and limb deformities. Single gene defects include conditions such as phenylketonuria and cystic fibrosis. Chromosomal aberrations are exemplified by Turner's syndrome (XO sex chromosomes) and Down's syndrome (trisomy 21 — three copies of chromosome 21). The risk of chromosomal abnormalities increases with maternal age: for example, the risk of a child being born with Down's syndrome, the commonest chromosome abnormality, is estimated at 1 in 1500 for a 25-year-old mother, rising to 1 in 30 at the age of 45 years.

Congenital diseases are initiated before birth, but some may not cause clinical signs and symptoms until adult life. Congenital diseases may be due to genetic defects, either inherited from the parents, or genetic mutations before birth, or to external interference with normal embryonic and fetal development. An example of a genetic defect is cystic fibrosis, which is a disorder of cell membrane transport inherited as an autosomal recessive abnormality. Examples of non-genetic defects include congenital diseases such as deafness and cardiac abnormalities resulting from fetal infection by maternal rubella (German measles) during pregnancy.

The natural consequence of an abnormal pregnancy is a miscarriage or spontaneous abortion. However, some abnormal pregnancies escape natural elimination and may survive to full-term gestation unless there is medical intervention.

Acquired diseases

Acquired diseases are due to environmental causes. Most diseases in adults are acquired.

Acquired diseases are further classified according to their pathogenesis.

Inflammatory diseases
Inflammation (Ch. 10) is a physiological response of living tissues to injury. Diseases in which an inflammatory reaction is a major component are classified accordingly. They are usually named from the organ affected followed by the suffix '-itis'. Thus the following are all examples of inflammatory diseases:

- tonsillitis (tonsils)
- appendicitis (appendix)
- dermatitis (skin)
- arthritis (joints).

There are, however, potentially confusing exceptions to the nomenclature. For example, tuberculosis, leprosy and syphilis are infections characterised by an inflammatory reaction. Pneumonia and pleurisy refer to inflammation of the lung and pleura respectively.

Each separate inflammatory disease has special features determined by:

- the cause
- precise character of the body's response
- organ affected.

Vascular disorders
Vascular disorders (Chs 8 and 13) are those resulting from abnormal blood flow to, from, or within an organ. Blood vessels are vital conduits. Any reduction in flow through a vessel leads to *ischaemia* of the tissue it supplies. If the ischaemia is sustained, then death of the tissue or *infarction* results. Vascular disorders have become major health problems in developed countries. Examples include:

- myocardial infarction ('heart attack')
- cerebral infarction or haemorrhage ('stroke')
- limb gangrene
- shock and circulatory failure.

Growth disorders
Diseases characterised by abnormal growth include adaptation to changing circumstances. For example, the heart enlarges (by hypertrophy) in patients with high blood pressure, and the adrenal glands shrink (by atrophy) if a disease of the pituitary gland causes loss of ACTH production. The most serious group of diseases characterised by disordered growth is neoplasia or new growth formation, leading to the formation of solid tumours (Ch. 11) and leukaemias (Ch. 23).

The suffix '-oma' usually signifies that the abnormality is a solid tumour. Exceptions include 'granuloma' and 'atheroma'; these are not tumours.

Injury and repair
Mechanical injury or trauma leads directly to disease, the precise characteristics of which depend upon the nature and extent of the injury. The progress of disease is influenced by the body's reaction to it. In particular, repair mechanisms may be defective due to senility, malnutrition, excessive mobility, presence of foreign bodies, and infection. This subject is discussed in detail in Chapter 6.

Metabolic and degenerative disorders
Metabolic and degenerative disorders are numerous

and heterogeneous. Some metabolic disorders are congenital (inborn errors of metabolism) and are inherited via defective parental genes. Other metabolic disorders are acquired (e.g. diabetes mellitus, gout), although there may be a degree of genetic predisposition, and some are abnormalities secondary to disease (e.g. hypercalcaemia due to hyperparathyroidism). Degenerative disorders are characterised by a loss of the specialised structure and function of a tissue; as such this category could include almost every disease, but the designation is reserved for those conditions in which degeneration appears to be the primary or dominant feature and the cause poorly understood. These disorders are discussed in detail in Chapter 7.

Iatrogenic diseases

The broad meaning of iatrogenic disease is any ill health induced by a medical practitioner's words or actions. Currently, iatrogenic diseases are restricted to those attributable to practitioners' *actions*. However, the suggestion that *words* could induce harm is not as fanciful as it seems. For example, a patient with a relatively trivial respiratory complaint is likely to be alarmed when asked by a doctor, who mistakenly suspects lung cancer, 'How much weight have you lost?' and 'Have you coughed up any blood?' The disturbing suggestions implicit in the line of questioning cause iatrogenic 'dis-ease' in the patient. (While it is perfectly reasonable to consider the possibility of lung cancer, such questions are better asked in the less prejudicial form of 'What's been happening to your weight recently?' and 'Have you noticed anything about your sputum?')

All medical intervention is associated with some risk to the patient. The probability that harm might result must be outweighed by the probability that the patient will benefit. If harm results, litigation may follow. However, there is a considerable difference between harm resulting from culpable negligence and that resulting from appropriate intervention justified by the clinical circumstances.

The scope of iatrogenic diseases is very wide (Table 2.2). It includes harm resulting from investigations and treatment, from drugs and surgery. It is said, with justification, that in the 20th century surgery has become safer but medicine has become more dangerous. Adverse drug reactions constitute a major category of iatrogenic disease and surveillance arrangements are in force in many countries, for example the 'yellow card' system of reporting to the Committee on the Safety of Medicines in the UK.

Table 2.2 Examples of iatrogenic diseases	
Causative agent	Resulting disease or abnormality
Radiation (therapeutic)	Skin erythema Fibrous scarring Neoplasia
Radiation (diagnostic)	Neoplasia Fetal malformations
Blood transfusion and blood products (e.g. clotting factor concentrates)	Hepatitis (due to viruses) Haemolysis (if mismatched blood) AIDS (due to HIV)
Penicillin	Allergy
Aspirin and other non-steroidal anti-inflammatory drugs	Gastric ulceration
Chloramphenicol	Aplastic anaemia
Chlorpromazine	Cholestatic jaundice
Steroid therapy	Cushing's syndrome

Adverse drug reactions

Adverse drug reactions can be categorised as follows:

- dose-dependent or predictable (type A)
- unpredictable (type B).

Dose-dependent drug reactions occur predictably in any person taking a sufficient dose of the drug. For example, paracetamol always produces hepatic necrosis if, unwisely, a sufficiently large dose is taken. Similarly, steroids can cause Cushing's syndrome (obesity, hirsutism, osteoporosis, etc.) in any patient receiving doses in excess of the usual bodily requirements. Often, the adverse effects disappear when the dosage is reduced, and mortality tends to be low.

Unpredictable adverse drug reactions are due to:

- idiosyncrasy or allergy
- permissive effects.

One of the commonest idiosyncratic drug reactions is due to allergy to penicillin. Another common example is cholestatic jaundice induced by chlorpromazine. Idiosyncratic reactions are due to unexpected metabolic or immunological responses to the drug. This type of drug reaction merits withdrawal of the drug and substitution of alternative therapy. The mortality is higher than that associated with predictable reactions.

In unpredictable adverse drug reactions where the effect is *permissive*, the drug itself produces no harm, but it predisposes the patient to other diseases. For example, some antibiotic therapy may be complicated by pseudomembranous colitis (Ch. 15) because it permits overgrowth of *Clostridium difficile* in the colon. Steroids and other immunosuppressive agents predispose to infections by organisms that would not normally be harmful (e.g. *Pneumocystis carinii* pneumonia, cytomegalovirus pneumonia).

EPIDEMIOLOGY

> ▶ Epidemiology is the 'pathology of populations'
> ▶ Measured by incidence, prevalence, remission and mortality rates of a disease
> ▶ Variations may provide clues to aetiology and guide optimal deployment of resources

Epidemiology is the study of disease in populations. Epidemiology concerns also the identification of the causes and modes of acquisition of disease. Epidemiology involves the recording and analysis of data about disease in groups of people rather than in the individual person only.

Knowledge about the occurrence of a disease is important for:

- providing aetiological clues
- planning preventive measures
- provision of adequate medical facilities
- setting up population screening (if relevant).

Epidemiological clues to the causes of disease

Epidemiology, sometimes referred to as the 'pathology of populations', often provides important clues to the causes of a disease. If, for example, in a particular geographical region or group of individuals the actual incidence of a disease exceeds the expected incidence, this suggests that the disease may be due to:

- a genetic predisposition more prevalent in that population, or
- an environmental cause more prevalent in that geographical region or group of individuals, or
- a combination of genetic and environmental factors.

The analysis of epidemiological data can be very arduous. Humans live in a complex environment, often modified by their own action. Populations subject to epidemiological study vary in their ethnic origins, their age distribution, their occupational histories and their lifestyles. These variations and the concomitant variations in disease incidence provide fertile opportunities for epidemiological study.

Epidemiologically derived clues about the causes of a disease invariably require direct confirmation by laboratory testing.

Disease incidence, prevalence, remission and mortality rates

Incidence, prevalence, remission and mortality rates are numerical data about the impact of a disease on a population:

- the *incidence rate* is the number of new cases of the disease occurring in a population of defined size during a defined period
- the *prevalence rate* is the number of cases of the disease to be found in a defined population at a stated time
- the *remission rate* is the proportion of cases of the disease that recover
- the *mortality rate* is the number or percentage of deaths from a disease in a defined population.

From these four measures one can deduce much about the behaviour of a disease (Fig. 2.2). Chronic (long-lasting) diseases have a high prevalence: although the incidence of new cases might be low, the total number of cases in the population accumulates. Diseases with relatively acute manifestations may have a high incidence but a low prevalence, because cases have either high remission rates (e.g. chickenpox) or high mortality rates (e.g. lung cancer).

In comparing the occurrence of a disease in different populations, epidemiologists have to standardise the data to eliminate any bias due to the average age of the population and its life expectancy. Diseases that are more common in the elderly may be relatively rare in some populations, simply because most of the people do not live long enough to develop them.

Migrant populations are especially useful to epidemiologists, enabling them to separate the effects of genetic (racial) factors and the environment (e.g. diet). If a migrant population, formerly suffering a high incidence of a disease, moves to a low incidence area and their disease reduces to the same incidence as that enjoyed by their new neighbours, this finding suggests that an environmental factor is responsible. If, alternatively, the high incidence of the disease persists in a population that has migrated to a low incidence area, this finding suggests that genetic factors are more likely to be responsible.

Population
sample

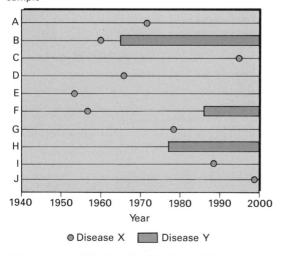

Fig. 2.2   Disease incidence and prevalence

A population sample of 10 individuals (A to J), all born in
1940, is followed for 60 years to determine the relative
incidence and prevalence of two diseases. Disease X is an
acute illness with no long-term effects; it has a very high
incidence (affecting 90% in this sample), but a low
prevalence because at any one time the number of cases to
be found is very low. Disease Y is a chronic illness; it has a
lower incidence (affecting only 30% in this sample), but a
relatively high prevalence (from 1980 onwards in this
sample) because of the accumulation of cases.

Data capture

Data on the frequency of diseases are more likely to be
in the form of mortality statistics rather than actual
disease incidence. The reason is that, unless legislation requires cases of the disease under study to be
formally notified to some register, the most reliable
data are likely to be derived from official death
certificates. This means that, if a disease does not
often have a fatal outcome, mortality data will severely
underestimate its incidence. The only common
exceptions to this are certain infectious diseases, designated as *notifiable* in the UK, and cancers, for which
many developed countries have registries.

In countries with well-developed health care systems, the epidemiology of many serious diseases
should be relatively easy to determine from statistical
data already held on databases (e.g. cancer registries);
retrospective studies are usually possible. In countries with relatively poor systems, however, it may be
necessary to search actively for the disease in order
to determine its true incidence and the distribution
in the general population; most studies have to be
done prospectively.

Geographic variations

Although many diseases occur worldwide, there are
many geographic variations (Fig. 2.3), even within
one country. There are considerable differences
between so-called developed and developing countries. For example, cardiovascular disorders, psychiatric illness and some cancers predominate in
countries such as the USA and the UK, but these
conditions are much less common in most of Africa
and Asia. In developing countries, the major health
problems are due to infections and malnutrition.

Historical changes in disease incidence and mortality

Changes in disease incidence with time (Fig. 2.4)
reflect variation in the degree of exposure to the
cause, or preventive measures such as immunisation.
Changes in mortality additionally reflect the success
of treatment.

The reduced incidence of serious infections (e.g.
typhoid, cholera, tuberculosis, smallpox) is the result
of improved sanitation and, in some instances, the
introduction of immunisation programmes. Indeed,
it is arguable that sanitation, particularly sewerage
and the provision of fresh water supplies, has had a
much greater impact on the incidence of these diseases than have advances in medical science.
Mortality from bacterial infections is also much
reduced due to the advent of antibiotic therapy.
Many viral infections elude specific treatment, but

Country

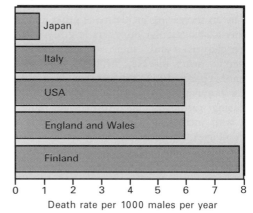

**Fig. 2.3   Geographic variations in disease
incidence: fatalities from ischaemic heart disease**

World Health Organization (WHO) data.

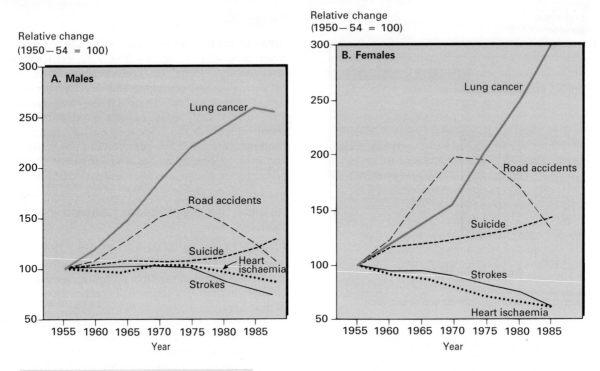

Fig. 2.4 Variations in death rates with time

A. Males. **B.** Females. Changing patterns of death rates from disease are exemplified by reference to five common conditions. Note the dramatic rise in deaths from lung cancer (attributable to smoking); the arrested increase in deaths due to road accidents (probably due to seat belt and other traffic legislation); the steady rise in suicides (probably due to social factors); and the sustained fall in deaths from ischaemic heart disease and strokes (probably due to dietary changes and other interventions). Data from WHO survey of developed countries: Europe, USSR, Australasia, Canada, USA, Israel and Japan.

mass immunisation has led to a considerable reduction in their incidence.

During the 19th and 20th centuries, the declining incidence in serious infections has been accompanied by an increasing incidence of other conditions, notably cardiovascular disorders (e.g. hypertension, atherosclerosis) and their complications (e.g. ischaemic heart disease, strokes). The apparent increase is partly due to the fact that the average age of the population in most developed countries is increasing; cardiovascular disorders are more common with increasing age, unlike infections which afflict all ages. Nevertheless, irrespective of this age-related trend, there is a genuine increased incidence of these disorders. This increase is almost certainly due to changes in diet (e.g. fat content) and lifestyle (e.g. smoking, lack of exercise). Intervention by reducing dietary and behavioural risk factors has begun to yield a beneficial reduction in the risk of developing the complications of cardiovascular disorders.

Historical changes in the incidence of neoplastic diseases (i.e. tumours) can provide vital clues to their aetiology. For example, a dramatic increase in the incidence of a formerly uncommon tumour may be the result of exposure to a new environmental hazard. Historical changes led to the discovery of the association between ionising radiation and many types of cancer, and between smoking and lung cancer.

Socio-economic factors

Socio-economic factors undoubtedly influence the incidence of certain diseases and the host response to them. Overcrowding encourages the spread of infections, leading to the rapid development of epidemics. Economic hardship is commonly accompanied by malnutrition (Ch. 7), a condition causing ill health directly and also predisposing to infections.

A particularly sensitive and widely used indicator of the socio-economically related health of a population is the *infant mortality rate*. This rate varies

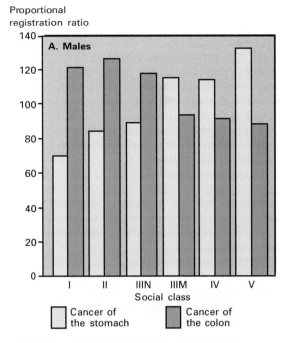

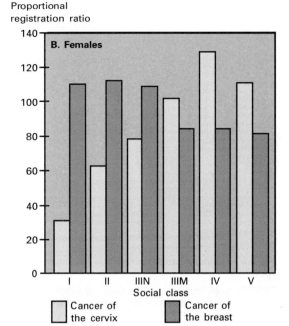

Fig. 2.5   Social class and cancer incidence

A. Males. **B.** Females. With some types of cancer there are correlations between social class and cancer incidence. In females, an increased risk of cancer of the cervix occurs in lower social classes; the converse applies in colonic cancer. These differences are almost certainly attributable to behavioural and environmental factors. Data from Office of Population Censuses and Surveys, UK, 1975. (IIIN = class III, non-manual; IIIM = class III, manual)

considerably between countries, but in general the rate is lower in countries regarded as being developed.

Some correlations between social class and cancer incidence are summarised in Figure 2.5. In some instances the cause of the correlation is obvious; in others, it awaits elucidation.

Occupational factors

The association of a disease with a particular occupation can reveal the specific cause. Well-documented associations include:

- coal-worker's pneumoconiosis due to coal dust inhalation
- asbestosis due to asbestos dust inhalation
- skin cancer due to lubricating oils
- nasal sinus cancer due to hardwood dust
- bladder cancer due to aniline dye manufacture.

It is important to identify occupational hazards so that they can be minimised. Furthermore, in many countries, patients disabled by occupational diseases may be entitled to compensation.

Hospital and community contrasts

Medical students often develop a biased impression of the true incidence of diseases because most of their training takes place in a hospital environment. The patients and diseases they see are selected rather than representative; only those cases requiring hospital investigation or treatment are sent there. In the case of most diseases, even in countries with well-developed health services, patients remain in the community. For example, patients seen by a community medical practitioner are most likely to have psychiatric illness, upper respiratory tract infections, and musculoskeletal problems. The general hospital cases are more likely to be patients with cardiovascular diseases, proven or suspected cancer, drug overdoses, severe trauma, etc.

Common causes of death

Death is inevitable. In many people surviving into their seventies and eighties, death may be preceded by a variable period of senility during which there is

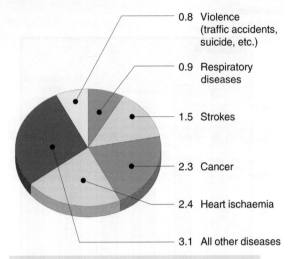

0.8 Violence (traffic accidents, suicide, etc.)

0.9 Respiratory diseases

1.5 Strokes

2.3 Cancer

2.4 Heart ischaemia

3.1 All other diseases

Fig. 2.6 Common causes of death in developed countries

Deaths in millions from each cause. Data (for 1986) from WHO survey of developed countries: Europe, USSR, Australasia, Canada, USA, Israel and Japan.

cumulative deterioration of the structure and function of many organs and body systems (Ch. 12). Unless an acute episode of serious illness supervenes, the accumulated deterioration of the body reduces its viability until it reaches the point where death supervenes. In almost every case, however, there is a final event that tips the balance and is registered as the immediate cause of death. In younger individuals dying prematurely, death is usually more clearly attributable to a single cause in an otherwise reasonably healthy individual.

In developed countries, such as the USA and in Europe, diseases of the cardiovascular system account for the vast majority of deaths (Fig. 2.6). Cancer, in general, is the second commonest cause of death. It is estimated that a newborn infant in these countries has a 1 in 3 chance of ultimately dying in adult life of ischaemic heart disease, and a 1 in 5 chance of ultimately dying of cancer. In some famine-ridden countries, newborn infants have similar probabilities of dying from diarrhoeal diseases and malnutrition in childhood.

FURTHER READING

Alderson M 1983 An introduction to epidemiology, 2nd edn. Macmillan, London

Barker D J P, Hall A J 1991 Practical epidemiology. Churchill Livingstone, Edinburgh

D'Arcy P F, Griffin J P (eds) 1986 Iatrogenic diseases, 3rd edn. Oxford University Press, Oxford

3

Genetic and environmental causes of disease

CAUSES OF DISEASE

> ► Diseases are due to genetic, environmental or
>   multifactorial causes
> ► Role of genetic and environmental factors can be
>   determined by epidemiological observations, family
>   studies or laboratory investigations
> ► Some diseases with a genetic basis may not appear
>   until adult life
> ► Some diseases with environmental causes may
>   cause their effects during embryogenesis

In terms of causation, diseases may be:

- entirely *genetic* — either inherited or acquired
  defects
- *multifactorial* — interaction of genetic and
  environmental factors
- entirely *environmental* — no genetic component to
  risk of disease.

Features pointing to a significant genetic contribution to the cause of a disease include a high incidence in particular families or races, or an association with a known inherited feature (e.g. gender, blood group, histocompatibility antigens). Environmental factors are suggested by disease associations with occupations or geography. Ultimately, however, only laboratory investigation can provide irrefutable identification of the cause of a disease. The extent to which a disease is due to genetic or environmental causes can often be deduced from some of its main features (Table 3.1).

Predisposing factors and precursors of disease

Many diseases are the *predictable* consequence of exposure to the initiating cause; host (i.e. genetic) factors make relatively little contribution to the out-come. This is particularly true of physical injury: the results of mechanical trauma and radiation injury are largely dose-related; the effect is directly proportional to the physical force.

Other diseases are the *probable* consequence of exposure to causative factors, but they are not absolutely inevitable. For example, infectious diseases result from exposure to potentially harmful environmental agents (e.g. bacteria, viruses), but the outcome is often influenced by various host factors.

Some diseases *predispose* to others: for example, ulcerative colitis predisposes to carcinoma of the colon and hepatic cirrhosis predisposes to hepatocellular carcinoma. Diseases predisposing to cancer are called *premalignant conditions*; lesions from which cancers can develop are called *premalignant lesions*. Some diseases occur most commonly in those individuals with a congenital predisposition. For example, ankylosing spondylitis, a disabling inflammatory disease of the spinal joints of unknown aetiology, is much more common in people with the HLA-B27 tissue antigen (see Ch. 25).

Some diseases predispose to others because they have a *permissive effect* allowing environmental agents, that are not normally pathogenic, to cause disease. For example, *opportunistic infections* occur in those patients with impaired defence mechanisms, allowing infection by normally non-pathogenic organisms (see Ch. 9).

Aetiology and age of disease onset

Do not assume that all diseases manifest at birth have an inherited or genetic basis; as noted previously (see Ch. 2), diseases present at birth are classified into those with a genetic basis (further subdivided into those in which the genetic abnormality is inherited and those in which the genetic abnormality is acquired during gestation) and those without a genetic basis. Conversely, although most

Table 3.1	Clues to a disease being caused by either genetic or environmental factors	
Disease characteristic	Genetic cause	Environmental cause
Age of onset	Usually early (often in childhood)	Any age
Familial incidence	Common	Unusual (unless family exposed to same environmental agent)
Remission	No (except by gene therapy)	Often (when environmental cause can be eliminated)
Incidence	Relatively rare	Common
Clustering	In families	Temporal or spatial or both
Linkage to inherited factors	Common	Relatively rare

adult diseases have an entirely environmental cause, genetic influences to disease susceptibility and vulnerability to environmental agents are being increasingly discovered.

The incidence of many diseases rises with age because:

- Probability of contact with an environmental cause increases with duration of exposure risk.
- The disease may depend on the cumulative effects of one or more environmental agents.
- Impaired immunity with ageing increases susceptibility to some infections.

Multifactorial aetiology of disease

Many diseases with no previously known cause are being shown to be due to an interplay of environmental factors and genetic susceptibility (Fig. 3.1). These discoveries are the rewards of detailed family studies and, in particular, application of the new techniques of molecular genetics. Diseases of adults in which there appears to be a significant genetic component include:

- breast cancer
- Alzheimer's disease
- type 1 (insulin-dependent) diabetes mellitus
- osteoporosis
- coronary atherosclerosis.

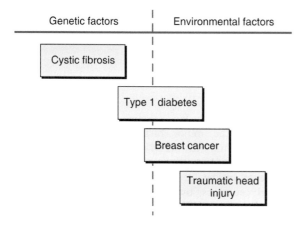

Fig. 3.1 Proportionate risk of disease due to genetic or environmental factors

Some conditions are due solely to genetic (e.g. cystic fibrosis) or environmental (e.g. traumatic head injury) factors. An increasing number of other diseases (e.g. type 1 diabetes, breast cancer) are being shown to have a genetic component to their risk, particularly in cases diagnosed at a relatively young age.

One of the reasons why there may be only slow progress in characterising the genetic component of the diseases listed above and others is that two or more genes may be involved. Pursuing the genetic basis of these *polygenic disorders* requires complex analyses.

Evidence for genetic and environmental factors

Genetic contributions to disease incidence are more obvious when any putative environmental factors are either widely prevalent (most individuals are exposed) or non-existent (no known or plausible agents). The epidemiologist Geoffrey Rose has exemplified this by suggesting that if every individual smoked 40 cigarettes a day, we would never discover that smoking was responsible for the high incidence of lung cancer; however, any individual (especially familial) variation in susceptibility to lung cancer would have to be attributed to genetic differences. An environmental cause, such as smoking, is easier to identify when there are significant variations in exposure which can be correlated with disease incidence; indeed, it was the individual variations in cigarette-smoking habit that enabled Doll and Hill to demonstrate a strong aetiological link to lung cancer risk.

Family studies

Potent evidence for the genetic cause of a disease, with little or no environmental contribution, comes from observations of its higher than expected incidence in families, particularly if they are affected by a disease that is otherwise very rare in the general population. Such diseases are said to 'run in families'.

Having identified the abnormality in a family, it is then important to provide *genetic counselling* so that parents can make informed decisions about future pregnancies. The precise mode of inheritance (see p. 40) will determine the proportion of family members (i.e. children) likely to be affected. Because inherited genetic disorders are either sex-linked or autosomally dominant or recessive, not all individuals in one family will be affected even if the disease has no environmental component.

Studies on twins
Observations on the incidence of disease in monozygotic (identical) twins are particularly useful in disentangling the relative influences of 'nature and nurture'; of greatest value in this respect are identical twins who, through unfortunate family circum-

stances, are reared in separate environments. Uncommon diseases occurring in both twins are more likely to have a genetic component to their aetiology, especially if the twins have been brought up and lived in different environments.

Studies on migrants

The unusually high incidence of a particular disease in a country or region could be due either to the higher prevalence of a genetic predisposition in the racial or ethnic group(s) in that country or to some environmental factor such as diet or climatic conditions. Compelling evidence of the relative contributions of genetic and environmental factors in the aetiology and pathogenesis of a disease can be yielded by observations on disease incidence in migrant populations (Fig. 3.2). For example, if a racial group with a low incidence of a particular disease migrates to another country in which the disease is significantly more common, there are two possible outcomes leading to different conclusions:

1. If the incidence of the disease in the migrant racial group rises, it is likely that environmental factors (e.g. diet) are responsible for the high incidence in the indigenous population.

2. If the incidence of the disease in the migrant racial group remains low, it is more likely that the higher incidence in the indigenous population is due to genetic factors.

Most observations on disease incidence in migrant populations have been made on neoplastic disorders (cancer). This is because cancer is a major illness, likely to be reliably diagnosed by biopsy, and, in many countries, documented in cancer registries. As disease registration systems improve, it may be possible to investigate the aetiology of a wider range of diseases in this way.

Association with gene polymorphisms

Within the human population there are many normal genetic variations or *polymorphisms*. The effect of some of these genetic polymorphisms is obvious: examples are skin, hair, and eye colour, body habitus, etc. When possessed by large groups of people of common ancestry, a cluster of polymorphic variants constitutes racial characteristics. In other instances the polymorphism has no visible effects: examples are blood groups and HLA antigens (see below); these are evident only by laboratory testing.

The polymorphisms of greatest relevance to disease susceptibility are:

- HLA antigens
- blood groups
- cytokine genes.

HLA antigens
Clinical and experimental observations on the fate of organ transplants led to the discovery of genes known as the major histocompatibility complex (MHC). In humans, the MHC genes reside on chromosome 6 and are designated *HLA genes* (human leukocyte antigen genes). HLA genes are expressed on cell surfaces by the presence of substances referred to as 'antigens', not because they normally operate as antigens in the host that bears them, but because of their involvement in graft rejection (Ch. 9). The body does not normally react to these substances, because it is immunologically tolerant of them and they are recognised as 'self' antigens.

HLA antigens are grouped into classes, principally:

- Class I antigens expressed on the surface of all nucleated cells. In all diploid cells there are pairs

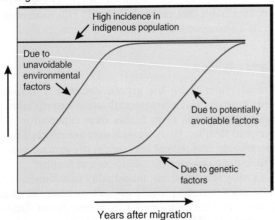

Incidence of disease
in migrants

Fig. 3.2 Clues to genetic and environmental causes from disease incidence in migrants

When people with a low incidence of a disease migrate to a country in which the indigenous population has a high incidence, any change in the incidence of the disease in the migrants provides important clues to the role of genetic and environmental factors in causing the disease. A rapid rise in incidence would attribute the disease to unavoidable environmental factors such as climate or widely prevalent micro-organisms. A more gradual rise would be due to factors such as diet, over which there may be some initial cultural resistance to change. No change in disease incidence attributes the high incidence to genetic factors in the indigenous population. The distinctions are rarely as clear-cut as in this graphic example.

of allelic genes at each of three loci: these genes are known as A, B and C. The normal role of class I antigens is to enable cytotoxic T-lymphocytes to recognise and eliminate virus-infected cells.

- Class II antigens expressed on the surface of those cells that interact with T-lymphocytes by physical contact, such as antigen-presenting cells (e.g. Langerhans' cells). The pairs of allelic genes at each of three loci are known as DP, DQ, and DR. The normal role of class II antigens is the initiation of immune responses.

Diseases may be associated with HLA antigens because:

- some infective micro-organisms bear antigens similar to those of the patient's HLA antigens and thereby escape immune recognition and elimination
- the immune response to an antigen on an infective micro-organism cross-reacts with one of the patient's HLA antigens, thus causing tissue damage
- the gene predisposing to a disease is closely linked (genetic linkage — Ch. 7) to a particular HLA gene.

Diseases associated with HLA antigens are listed in Table 3.2. They are all chronic inflammatory or immunological disorders. In some instances the association is so strong that HLA testing is important diagnostically: the best example is the association of HLA-B27 with ankylosing spondylitis (Ch. 25).

Autoimmune diseases (diseases in which the body's immunity destroys its own cells) are most frequently associated with specific HLA antigens. The combination of HLA-DR3 and HLA-B8 is particularly strong in this regard, but it must be emphasised that it is present in only a minority of patients with autoimmune disease. Autoimmune diseases also illustrate a separate feature of the association between HLA antigens and disease. Normally, HLA class II antigens are not expressed on epithelial cells. However, in organs affected by autoimmune disease, the target cells for immune destruction are often found to express class II antigens. This expression enables their immune recognition and facilitates their destruction.

Blood groups
Blood group expression is directly involved in the pathogenesis of a disease only rarely; the best example is haemolytic disease of the newborn due to rhesus antibodies (Ch. 23). A few diseases show a weaker and indirect association with blood groups. This association may be due to genetic linkage; the blood group determinant gene may lie close to the gene directly involved in the pathogenesis of the disease.

Examples of blood-group-associated diseases include:

- duodenal ulceration and group O
- gastric carcinoma and group A.

Cytokine genes
There is quite strong evidence linking the incidence or severity of chronic inflammatory diseases to polymorphisms within or adjacent to cytokine genes. Cytokines are important mediators and regulators of inflammatory and immunological reactions; it is logical, therefore, to explore the possibility that enhanced or abnormal expression of cytokine genes may be relevant.

Table 3.2 Examples of diseases associated with HLA antigens

Disease	HLA antigen(s)	Comments
Allergic disorders (e.g. eczema, asthma)	A23	Requires environmental allergen
Ankylosing spondylitis	B27	Associated in c. 90% of cases
Coeliac disease	DR3, B8	Gluten sensitivity
Graves' disease (primary thyrotoxicosis)	DR3, B8	Due to thyroid-stimulating immunoglobulin
Hashimoto's thyroiditis	DR5	Aberrant HLA class II expression on thyroid epithelium
Insulin-dependent (juvenile onset) **diabetes mellitus**	DR3, DR4, B8	Probable viral injury to β-cells in pancreatic islets
Rheumatoid disease	DR4	Autoimmune disease

Although associations have been found between a tumour necrosis factor (TNF) gene polymorphism and Graves' disease of the thyroid (see Ch. 17) and systemic lupus erythematosus (see Ch. 25), the TNF gene resides on chromosome 6 between the HLA classes I and II loci, linkage with which may explain an indirect association between TNF gene polymorphism and disease. However, independent of HLA polymorphisms, there are associations between interleukin-1 gene cluster (chromosome 2) polymorphisms and chronic inflammatory diseases. The associations seem to be more with disease severity than with susceptibility.

Gender and disease

Gender, like any other genetic attribute of an individual, may be directly or indirectly associated with disease. An example of a direct association, other than the absurdly simple (e.g. carcinoma of the uterus and being female), is haemophilia. Haemophilia is an inherited X-linked recessive disorder of blood coagulation. It is transmitted by females to their male children. Haemophilia is rare in females because they have two X chromosomes, only one of which is likely to be defective. Males always inherit their single X chromosome from their mothers; if the mother is a haemophilia carrier, half her male children will have the disease.

Some diseases show a predilection for one of the sexes. For example, autoimmune diseases (e.g. rheumatoid disease, systemic lupus erythematosus) are generally more common in females than in males; the reason for this is unclear. Atheroma and its consequences (e.g. ischaemic heart disease) tends to affect males earlier than females, but after the menopause the female incidence catches up with that in males. Females are more prone to osteoporosis, a common cause of bone weakening, particularly after the menopause.

In some instances the sex differences in disease incidence are due to social or behavioural factors. The higher incidence of carcinoma of the lung in males is due to the fact that they smoke more cigarettes than do women. Differences in alcohol consumption explain the higher incidence of cirrhosis of the liver in males.

Racial differences

Like gender, racial differences in disease incidence may be genetically determined or attributable to behavioural or environmental factors (Table 3.3). Racial differences may also reflect adaptational responses to the threat of disease. A good example is provided by malignant melanoma (Ch. 24). Very strong evidence implicates ultraviolet light in the causation of malignant melanoma of the skin; the highest incidence is in Caucasians living in parts of the world with high ambient levels of sunlight, such as Australia. The tumour is, however, relatively uncommon in Africa, despite its high sunlight levels, because the indigenous population has evolved with an abundance of melanin in the skin; they are classified racially as blacks and benefit from the protective effect of the melanin in the skin.

Some abnormal genes are more prevalent in certain races. For example, the cystic fibrosis gene is carried by 1:20 Caucasians, whereas this gene is rare in blacks and Asians. Conversely, the gene causing sickle cell anaemia is more common in blacks than in any other race.

Other diseases in different races may be due to socio-economic factors. Perinatal mortality rates are thought to be an accurate monitor of the socio-economic welfare of a population. Regrettably, the perinatal mortality rate is much higher in certain racial groups, but this outcome is due almost entirely to their social circumstances and is, therefore, theoretically capable of improvement.

Parasitic infestations are more common in tropical climates, not because the races predominantly dwelling there are more susceptible, but often because the parasites cannot complete their lifecycles without other hosts that survive only in the prevailing environmental conditions.

Table 3.3	Associations between disease and race	
Disease	Racial association	Explanation
Cystic fibrosis	Caucasians	Defective gene more prevalent in Caucasians
Sickle cell anaemia (HbS gene)	Blacks	Sickle cells resist malarial parasitisation HbS gene more common in blacks in areas of endemic malaria
Skin cancers	Caucasians	Fair skin contains less melanin to protect against harmful effects of UV light

GENETIC ABNORMALITIES IN DISEASE

▶ Genetic abnormalities may be inherited, acquired during conception or embryogenesis, or acquired during post-natal life
▶ Genetic abnormalities inherited or prenatally acquired are often associated with congenital metabolic abnormalities or structural defects
▶ Polygenic disorders result from interaction of two or more abnormal genes
▶ Neoplasms (tumours) are the most important consequences of post-natally acquired genetic abnormalities

Table 3.4   Landmarks in genetics and molecular biology

Date	Discovery
1940s	Genes encoded by combinations of only 4 nucleotides in nuclear DNA
1950s	Complementary double-stranded helical structure of DNA
	46 chromosomes in humans
	DNA polymerase enzyme
1960s	Plasmids — providing a mechanism for transfer of genes to bacteria
	Lyon hypothesis
	Restriction endonucleases
1970s	Recombinant DNA technology
	Chromosome banding
	Hybridisation techniques
	Southern blotting
1980s	Gene polymorphisms
	Polymerase chain reaction
	Transgenic mice
	Gene therapy

Advances in genetics and molecular biology have revolutionised our understanding of the aetiology and pathogenesis of many diseases and, with the advent of gene therapy, may lead to their amelioration in affected individuals (Table 3.4).

Defective genes in the germ-line (affecting all cells) and present at birth, because of either inherited or acquired abnormalities, cause a wide variety of conditions, such as:

• *metabolic defects* (e.g. cystic fibrosis, phenylketonuria)
• *structural abnormalities* (e.g. Down's syndrome)
• *predisposition to tumours* (e.g. familial adenomatous polyposis, retinoblastoma, multiple endocrine neoplasia syndromes).

Genetic damage after birth, for example due to ionising radiation, is not present in the germ-line and causes neither obvious metabolic defects affecting the entire individual, because the defect is concealed by the invariably larger number of cells with normal metabolism, nor structural abnormalities, because morphogenesis has ceased. The main consequence of genetic damage after birth is, therefore, tumour formation (see Ch. 11). There is, however, increasing evidence to suggest that cumulative damage to mitochondrial genes contributes to ageing (see Ch. 12).

Gene structure and function

Nuclear DNA

Each of the 23 paired human chromosomes contains, on average, approximately 10^7 base (nucleotide) pairs arranged on the double helix of DNA; genes are encoded in a relatively small proportion of this DNA. To accommodate this length of DNA within the relatively small nucleus, the DNA is tightly folded. The first level of compaction involves wrapping the double helix around a series of *histone* proteins; the bead-like structures thus formed are *nucleosomes*. At the second level of compaction, the DNA strands are coiled to form a *chromatin* fibre and then tightly looped. During metaphase, when the duplicated chromosomes separate to form the nuclei of two daughter cells, the DNA is even more tightly compacted.

During DNA synthesis (S phase) the bases are copied by complementary nucleotide pairing. Any copying errors are at risk of being inherited by the daughter cells and may result in disease. Copying during DNA synthesis starts in a co-ordinated way at approximately 1000 places along an average chromosome.

Nuclear genes
Genes are encoded by combinations of four nucleotides (adenine, cytosine, guanine, thymine) within DNA. Nuclear DNA is double-stranded with complementary specific bonding between nucleotides on the *sense* and *anti-sense* strands — adenine to thymine, guanine to cytosine — the anti-sense strand thereby serving as a template for synthesis of the sense strand. Most of the DNA in eukaryotic (nucleated, e.g. mammalian) cells is within nuclei; a relatively smaller amount resides in mitochondria.

The nuclear DNA in human cells is distributed between 23 pairs of chromosomes: 22 are called *autosomes*; 1 pair are *sex chromosomes* (XX in females, XY in males). Only approximately 10% of nuclear DNA encodes functional genes; the remainder comprises a large quantity of anonymous variable and repetitive sequences distributed between genes and between segments of genes. These non-coding sequences include *satellite DNA* which is highly repetitive and located at specific sites along the chromosomes (e.g. telomeres); the function of these sequences is unknown, but they may be important for maintaining chromosome structure.

The segments of genes encoding for the final product are known as *exons*; the segments of anonymous DNA between exons are called *introns* (Fig. 3.3). The exons comprise a sequence of *codons*, triplets of nucleotides each encoding for an amino acid via messenger RNA (mRNA). In addition, there are start and stop codons defining the limits of each gene. During mRNA synthesis from the DNA template, the introns are spliced out and the exons may be rearranged.

Gene linkage and recombination

Linkage and recombination are important processes enabling tracing of genes associated with disease. During meiosis there is exchange of chromosomal material between maternally and paternally derived chromosomes. Adjacent genes on the same chromosome are unlikely to be separated by this process and are said to show a high degree of *linkage*. When exchange of chromosomal material does occur, the result is called *recombination*. The distance between genes can be expressed in *centimorgans* (after a

geneticist called T H Morgan); one centimorgan is the distance between two gene loci showing recombination in 1 in 100 gametes.

These processes of linkage and recombination are not only responsible for the balance between familial characteristics and individual diversity, but are also important phenomena enabling defective genes to be identified, even when their precise function or sequence is unknown, by tracking neighbouring DNA in affected individuals and families.

Gene transcription and translation

The normal flow of biochemical information is that a messenger RNA transcript is made corresponding to the nucleotide sequence of the gene encoded in the DNA (in RNA, uracil replaces thymine). The RNA transcript comprises nucleotide sequences encoding only the exons of the gene. The RNA is then translated into a sequence of amino acids specified by the code and the protein is assembled.

Under some circumstances, however, the flow of genetic information is reversed. In the presence of *reverse transcriptase*, an enzyme present in some RNA viruses, a DNA copy can be made from the RNA (Fig. 3.4).

Homeotic genes

Research on the fruitfly (*Drosophila*) has revealed that their genome contains four homeotic gene complexes characterised by the presence of sequences designated *homeobox genes*. The corresponding genes in mammals are designated *hox* genes; in the human genome, these genes are designated *pax* (*p*aired bo*x*)

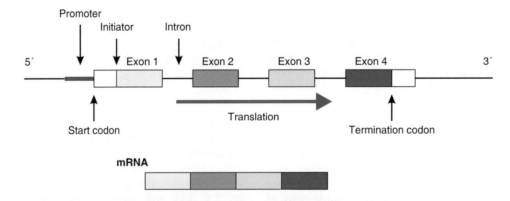

Fig. 3.3 Simplified structure of a gene and its mRNA product

Upstream of the gene is a promoter DNA sequence through which, by specific binding with regulating proteins, the translation of the gene is controlled. Start and termination codons mark the limits of the gene, bounded by untranslated sequences. The encoding portion of the gene is divided into exons, four in this example, interspersed with introns which do not appear in the mRNA product.

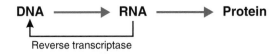

Fig. 3.4 Reverse transcription of DNA from RNA

Normally, the genetic information encoded in DNA is transcribed to RNA and translated into amino acids from which the protein is synthesised. However, some RNA viruses contain reverse transcriptase, an enzyme which produces a DNA transcript of the RNA; this may then be incorporated into the genome of the cell, possibly altering permanently its behaviour and potentially leading to tumour formation (see Ch. 11).

genes. Experiments on the fruitfly show that these homeotic genes play a major role in *embryogenesis*. Defects in homeotic genes could, therefore, result in major *congenital malformations*. For example, defects in *hox* genes in mice are associated with a congenital malformation resembling spina bifida.

Mitochondrial genes

Most inherited disorders are carried on abnormal genes within nuclear DNA. There are, however, a small but significant number of genetic abnormalities inherited through mitochondrial DNA. Mitochondrial DNA differs from nuclear DNA in several important respects; it is characterised by:

- circular double-stranded conformation
- high rate of spontaneous mutation
- few introns
- maternal inheritance.

The structure of mitochondrial DNA resembles that of bacterial DNA and it is postulated that eukaryotic cells acquired mitochondria as a result of an evolutionary advantageous symbiotic relationship with bacteria.

Because the head of the fertilising spermatozoon consists almost entirely of its nucleus, the mitochondria of an individual are derived from the cytoplasm of the mother's ovum. Thus, mitochondrial disorders are transmitted by females, but may be expressed in males and females.

The genes in mitochondrial DNA encode mainly for enzymes involved in oxidative phosphorylation. Therefore, defects of these enzymes resulting from abnormal mitochondrial genes tend to be associated with clinicopathological effects in tissues with high energy requirements, notably neurones and muscle cells. Examples of disorders due to inheritance of defective mitochondrial genes include *familial mitochondrial encephalopathy* and *Kearns–Sayre syndrome*.

Mitochondria and ageing

Because mitochondria play a key role in intracellular oxygen metabolism, it is hypothesised that defects of mitochondrial genes and the enzymes encoded by them could lead to the accumulation of free oxygen-radical mediated injury. Such injury could include damage to nuclear DNA, thus explaining not only the phenomenon of ageing (Ch. 12) but also the higher incidence of neoplasia in the elderly (Ch. 11).

Gene therapy

During the next decade, significant advances are anticipated in the specific treatment of genetic disorders (such as inherited metabolic disorders and cancer). This is the relatively new clinical science of gene therapy.

There are two approaches. First, it may be possible to replace a defective gene with a normal copy. This would be an ideal solution to the problem of inherited disorders such as cystic fibrosis. Indeed, attempts are being made to correct the respiratory tract problems in cystic fibrosis by local gene therapy applied by inhalation to the airways. Second, the function of an abnormal gene may be abrogated by administering anti-sense RNA; this is being attempted experimentally for tumours.

Techniques applied to the study of genetic disorders

Genetic disorders can be studied at various complementary levels:

- population
- family
- individual
- cell
- chromosomes
- genes.

At the population level, one is seeking variations in disease that cannot be ascribed to environmental factors; the study of migrant populations is particularly useful in disentangling the relative contributions made by genetic and environmental factors to the incidence of a disease (see p. 34). In families and individuals, one is seeking evidence of the mode of inheritance — whether it is sex-linked or autosomal, whether it is dominant or recessive (see p. 40); in diseases in which the abnormality is poorly characterised, studies of linkage with neighbouring genes (positional genetics) can lead to elucidation of the structure and function of defective and normal proteins. In cells, expression of the protein can be studied. It is, however, in the study of chromosomes and genes that the greatest advances have been made in recent years.

Modes of inheritance in families

> ▶ May be inherited as autosomal or sex-linked genes
> ▶ Genes coding for abnormalities may be dominant or recessive
> ▶ Abnormal genes may be detected either directly from the presence of the gene itself or the defective product, or indirectly by virtue of its linkage with a detectable polymorphism

Although some inborn errors are attributable to genetic mutations, most are inherited through parental genes. Genes located on autosomes (chromosomes other than the sex chromosomes) are *autosomal*; genes on the sex chromosomes are *sex-linked*. By studying the pattern of inheritance in an affected family (Fig. 3.5), it is possible to classify the mode of transmission as either:

● *dominant*—only one abnormal copy of the paired gene (allele) is necessary for expression of the disease
● *recessive*—both copies of the paired gene are required to be abnormal for expression of the disease.

Single gene defects inherited as an autosomal dominant are almost twice as common as autosomal recessive disorders. A minority of single gene defects are sex-linked. Most inborn errors of *metabolism* are autosomal recessive disorders, whereas inherited disorders resulting in *structural* defects are autosomal dominant disorders; there are, however, exceptions to these general tendencies. A few inherited disorders are sex-linked; haemophilia (Ch. 23) is a notable example.

Fig. 3.5 Patterns of inheritance of abnormal genes

A. Autosomal dominant. Only one abnormal copy of the gene needs to be inherited for the disease to be expressed; thus, both homozygous and heterozygous individuals are affected. **B. Autosomal recessive**. Both copies of the gene must be abnormal for the disease to be expressed; thus, homozygous individuals are affected and heterozygous individuals are asymptomatic carriers. **C. Sex chromosome-linked**. In this example, a defective gene (e.g. for haemophilia) is located on the X chromosome. In females, the other normal X chromosome corrects the abnormality, but females can be asymptomatic carriers. In males, the disease is expressed because there is no normal X chromosome to correct the abnormality.

A. Autosomal dominant

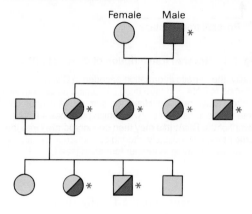

B. Autosomal recessive

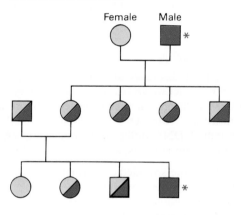

C. Sex chromosome (X)-linked

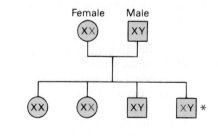

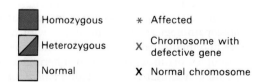

◼ Homozygous	∗ Affected
◪ Heterozygous	X Chromosome with defective gene
◻ Normal	X Normal chromosome

Homozygous and heterozygous states

The two genes at an identical place (locus) on a pair of chromosomes are known as *alleles*. Individuals with identical alleles at a particular locus are said to be *homozygous*. If the alleles are not identical, the term used is *heterozygous*. Dominant genes are expressed in heterozygous individuals because only one abnormal copy of the gene is required. However, by definition, recessive genes are expressed only in homozygous individuals because both copies of the gene must be abnormal. The importance of this situation is that a parent carrying only one copy of a recessive abnormal gene (who is, therefore, heterozygous for this gene) appears to be normal. If the other parent is also heterozygous for this abnormal gene, then the disease will be inherited and expressed, on average, by 25% of their children. There is a higher incidence of homologous autosomal recessive heterozygosity in related individuals and, for that reason, there is a greater risk of inherited abnormalities in the children of closely related parents (e.g. cousins). Marriage between close relatives is, therefore, prohibited by law or discouraged by tradition in many communities.

One problem in tracing genetic disorders through families is that the gene may show variable expression or *penetrance*. Although an abnormal gene is present, it may not necessarily always manifest itself and, when it does, the abnormality may be only slight.

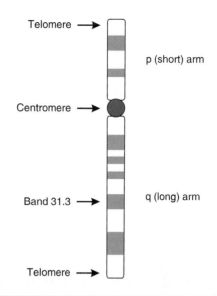

Fig. 3.6   Structure of a chromatid after banding

The centromere is a constriction at which the chromatids are joined. The short arm is designated 'p' (petit) and the long arm is 'q'. The arms terminate in telomeres rich in repetitive sequences. The dark bands are numbered in order from the centromere to the tip of each arm; sub-bands are preceded by a decimal point (for example, the cystic fibrosis gene locus is on chromosome 7 and designated 7q31.3).

Chromosomal analysis

The chromosomal constitution of a cell or individual is known as the *karyotype*. The 46 chromosomes in human nuclei can be seen more clearly during mitosis, especially in metaphase, when they separate. To obtain a sufficient number of cells in metaphase, a drug called colchicine can be added to the culture medium in which they are growing; this inhibits polymerisation of tubulin, preventing formation of the mitotic spindle along which the chromosomes migrate and thus blocking cell division in metaphase. The chromosomes can be:

- counted
- banded by staining
- grouped according to size, banding, etc.
- probed for specific DNA sequences.

Counting reveals disorders associated with abnormal numbers of chromosomes (e.g. trisomy in, for example, Down's syndrome). Banding is a technique revealing, at a fairly gross level, the structure of a chromosome (Fig. 3.6). The most widely used technique is *G-banding*; the chromosomes are first partially digested with trypsin and then treated with Giemsa stain. This reveals alternating light and dark bands characteristic to each chromosome; the light bands comprise *euchromatin* (gene-rich DNA); the dark bands comprise *heterochromatin* (rich in repetitive sequences).

The size, characteristic banding, and position of the centromere enable each pair of chromosomes to be identified according to a scheme in which they are numbered from 1 to 22 (the sex chromosomes, X or Y, are not identified by number).

Probing for specific DNA sequences (either genes or repetitive sequences) can be done by incubating either chromosome spreads or interphase nuclei with complementary DNA sequences labelled with a reporter molecule such as a radioactive isotope (located by autoradiography) or a non-isotopic label such as an enzyme (revealed by incubation with its substrate), an antigen (revealed by a specific antibody), or a fluorescent dye (revealed by ultraviolet microscopy). These powerful techniques enable individual genes to be mapped to chromosomes.

Molecular analysis of genetic disorders

With the techniques of molecular biology it is now possible to identify precisely the genetic abnormality in many disorders. Formerly, this identification could be done only at the level of the gene product (e.g. the defective protein or enzyme); now it is possible to locate which part of which chromosome is defective, and even to determine the gene sequence.

The motivation to study these conditions at the genetic level of detail is twofold:

- to identify accurately the abnormality so that it can be detected for use in prenatal diagnosis and in parental counselling
- to improve our understanding of the expression of defective and normal genes.

This approach is yielding important advances, but many inherited disorders are not yet completely characterised at the genetic level.

Prenatal detection can be achieved by the molecular analysis of *chorionic villus biopsies* in cases known to be at risk.

Functional and positional genetics

There are two possible strategies for the elucidation of the genetic abnormality in genetic diseases — functional and positional (Fig. 3.7). Which strategy is used depends on the nature of the genetic disorder and, in particular, whether the key biochemical abnormality is known.

If the biochemical abnormality resulting from the genetic defect is known, then the chromosomes or DNA from them can be probed with a complementary DNA sequence corresponding to the gene being investigated. The sequence can be deduced from the amino acid sequence of the known gene product. This is the strategy of functional genetics.

If the biochemical abnormality is not known, it can be determined by an alternative strategy of positional genetics (also called *reverse genetics*). 'Positional' in this context refers to the position of the abnormal gene in relation to well characterised neighbouring genes with which it is linked on the same chromosome. The neighbouring genes will probably be inherited along with the defective gene, so that by

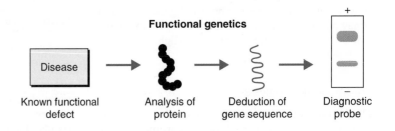

Functional genetics

Disease → Known functional defect → Analysis of protein → Deduction of gene sequence → Diagnostic probe

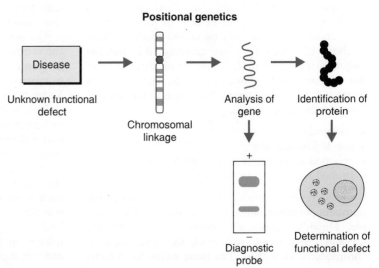

Positional genetics

Disease → Unknown functional defect → Chromosomal linkage → Analysis of gene → Identification of protein → Diagnostic probe → Determination of functional defect

Fig. 3.7 Functional and positional genetics

Functional genetics is the strategy employed to investigate a genetic disorder in which the biochemical defect is known. This enables determination of the amino acid sequence of the abnormal protein and deduction of the DNA sequence. A complementary DNA probe can then be synthesised and used, for example, in diagnostic testing for the abnormality. **Positional genetics** is employed when the biochemical defect associated with the genetic disorder is unknown. However, the abnormal gene can be located by studying its linkage with neighbouring genes in affected individuals. The gene can then be analysed and the protein encoded by it deduced from the DNA sequence. Complementary DNA can be used as a diagnostic probe and the function of the defective protein can be determined.

studying the affected and unaffected individuals it may be possible to determine the DNA sequence of the defective gene and deduce the amino acid sequence of the gene product.

Genetic linkages

Immediately prior to meiosis leading to the production of haploid germ cells (ova and spermatozoa) from their diploid precursors, there is a random interchange of DNA segments between the homologous paternally or maternally derived chromosomes to form new, recombinant chromosomes. The process of interchange occurs over such short lengths of DNA that only those genes lying adjacent on chromosomes are likely to remain together and be inherited through successive generations. This phenomenon is useful in positional genetics only if the genes and their products are polymorphic; *polymorphic genes* show natural (and normal) variations in their base sequences and protein products — HLA substances (Ch. 2) are good examples. This polymorphism enables the gene and its immediate neighbours to be mapped through a family and to the chromosomal level (Fig. 3.8).

DNA polymorphisms

Although polymorphic genes are useful for the mapping of abnormalities, it must be remembered that most of the DNA in chromosomes is redundant or anonymous; it does not encode any genes and has no phenotypic manifestations. However, because it lacks any function, this anonymous DNA tolerates a higher frequency of polymorphic variation than the DNA in which genes are encoded. In human nuclear DNA, these random polymorphic variations occur in approximately 1 in 200 base pairs. These variations are inherited and can be used to map the inheritance of neighbouring linked genes, even though the neighbouring genes may not have been fully characterised.

These polymorphisms comprise:

- RFLP (restriction fragment length polymorphisms)
- VNTR (variable number of tandem repeats)
- satellites — mini- and micro-.

Polymorphic variations arise as a result of:

- substitution of a single base on the DNA strand, thus abolishing a recognition site for a restriction enzyme
- presence of variable numbers of tandem repeats of base sequences, thus giving restriction fragments of corresponding variable size.

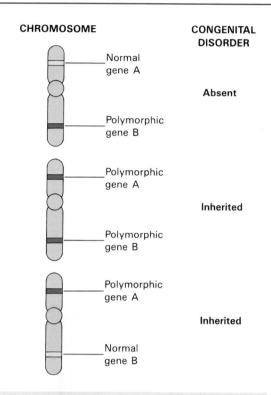

Fig. 3.8   Identification of the chromosome locus for an inherited disease by genetic linkage

Prior to meiosis there is interchange of segments of DNA between homologous chromosomes, but adjacent genes are unlikely to be separated by this process. Polymorphic (variant) DNA sequences for normal genes (e.g. for blood groups) or restriction fragment length polymorphism in 'anonymous' DNA may be used as markers for the inheritance of a congenital disease, if the abnormal gene for the disease is on the same part of the same chromosome as the polymorphic marker. In this simplified example showing homologous chromosomes from three different individuals, two of whom are affected by the disease, the evidence favours the abnormal gene being very close to the polymorphic gene A.

Variations in anonymous DNA are detected, not by using its polymorphic products (it has none), but by determining the variations in size of the smaller DNA fragments produced by incubation with *restriction enzymes*. These enzymes, derived from bacteria, break DNA strands at specific points by virtue of the ability of the enzymes to recognise specific sequences of bases. By electrophoretic separation of the broken DNA strands according to their size, it is possible to detect polymorphic differences between individuals (Fig. 3.9).

RFLP analysis is proving useful not only in mapping the chromosomal location of the abnormal

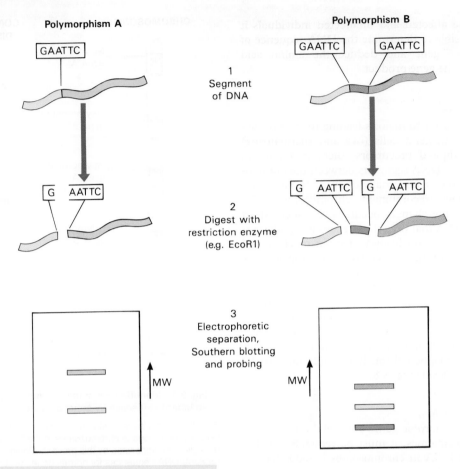

Fig. 3.9   Restriction fragment length polymorphism

Homologous regions of anonymous DNA from two individuals are shown. The polymorphic variations can be detected as follows: *Step 1*. The DNA is isolated. *Step 2*. The DNA is incubated with a restriction enzyme (EcoR1 in this example) that specifically recognises and splits DNA at sites only where there is a GAATTC base sequence. One such site exists in polymorphism A; an additional site is present in polymorphism B. *Step 3*. The enzymatically-digested DNA fragments are loaded on to a gel and separated in an electric field according to their molecular sizes. After absorption on to a sheet of nitrocellulose filter paper (Southern blot), the location of the fragments of the polymorphous region can be visualised by probing with a radioactive complementary DNA strand. (MW = molecular weight)

genes of inborn metabolic errors, but also in forensic science, in cases of alleged rape or disputed paternity, because of its claimed individual uniqueness.

Polymerase chain reaction

The polymerase chain reaction (PCR) technique is being used increasingly for the prenatal identification of genetic polymorphisms associated with congenital diseases when the precise base sequence of the polymorphic gene is known (e.g. in cystic fibrosis). The technique is specially applicable to prenatal diagnosis because it enables the abnor-

mal gene to be amplified biochemically from only minute starting samples, even a single cell.

The PCR technique has wide applications in molecular medicine. It is a method of specifically amplifying predetermined segments of DNA from a small sample. The specificity is determined by *primers*, short DNA sequences complementary to the known flanking regions of the DNA segment being sought. The amplification is achieved by using a type of *DNA polymerase* enzyme that can withstand the cyclical heating of the reaction mixture necessary to separate the DNA strands and then cooling to permit DNA synthesis. The reaction mixture must also contain free *nucleotides* for incorporation into the newly synthesised DNA segments. Within a few hours the DNA segment, if present in the starting sample, will have been amplified about 1 million-fold. Its identity can be confirmed by gel electrophoresis to determine its size, and by absorption on to a special film (Southern blotting), where it can be probed with labelled (e.g. radioactive) complementary DNA to verify that it has the appropriate nucleotide sequence for the polymorphic gene.

Diseases due to genetic defects

The important role of genetic abnormalities in carcinogenesis and tumour pathology is covered in Chapter 11. Here we deal with non-neoplastic disorders associated with:

- abnormalities of chromosome numbers
- single gene defects
- fragile chromosomes.

Abnormal chromosome numbers

Abnormal chromosome numbers are usually obvious in karyotypic analyses and are frequently associated with grossly evident morphological abnormalities (Table 3.5). If three, rather than the normal pair, of a particular chromosome are present, the abnormality is referred to as *trisomy*. If only one of the normally paired chromosomes is present, this is *monosomy*. A complete triploid karyotype resulting from fertilisation of the ovum by two haploid sets of paternal chromosomes is often associated with formation of a partial hydatidiform mole (see Ch. 19).

Autosomes
The commonest numerical autosomal abnormality is Down's syndrome ('mongolism'); the features are listed in Table 3.5. The risk of a child being affected by Down's syndrome increases dramatically with maternal age (Fig. 3.10). In most cases, the abnormality is trisomy 21. Some of the consequences may be attributable to an increased level of gene products encoded on chromosome 21; for example, patients with Down's syndrome develop changes in their brains similar to those seen in Alzheimer's disease, characterised by deposition of an amyloid glycoprotein, the gene for which resides on chromosome 21 (see Ch. 26).

Sex chromosomes
Numerical aberrations of sex chromosomes may be characterised by absence of one of the usual pair, as

in Turner's syndrome (X), or extra sex chromosomes, as in Klinefelter's syndrome (XXY). These relatively uncommon conditions are usually associated with abnormalities of sexual development and, therefore, may not be obvious until puberty.

Single gene defects

Single gene defects usually cause discrete biochemical or structural abnormalities. For example, most of the inherited metabolic disorders (inborn errors of metabolism) are due to single gene defects (see Ch. 7).

As a rule (there are exceptions) single gene abnormalities resulting in structural manifestations (e.g. tumours) in adult life are inherited in a dominant manner; those resulting in biochemical abnormalities (e.g. enzyme deficiencies) in childhood are inherited in a recessive manner (Table 3.5).

Single gene defects may result from:

- deletion of the gene
- point mutation (substitution of a nucleotide)
- insertion or deletion (addition or removal of one or more nucleotides resulting in a shift of the reading sequence)

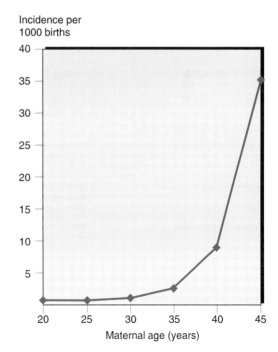

Fig. 3.10   Down's syndrome and maternal age
The risk of a child being born with Down's syndrome increases dramatically with maternal age.

Table 3.5 Examples of genetic diseases

Disease	Genetic defect	Frequency per 1000 births	Features
AUTOSOMAL SINGLE GENE ABNORMALITIES			
Autosomal dominant			
Neurofibromatosis	Defective neurofibromin gene on chromosome 17	0.25	Multiple nerve sheath tumours Skin pigmentation (*café au lait*)
Familial adenomatous polyposis	Mutated APC gene on chromosome 5	0.1	Numerous benign colorectal polyps with increased risk of colorectal carcinoma
Huntington's disease	Excess tandem CAG repeats at locus on chromosome 4	0.2	Adult onset Unco-ordinated movement (chorea) Dementia
Autosomal recessive			
Phenylketonuria	Phenylalanine hydroxylase deficiency	0.2–0.5	Neurological abnormalities
Cystic fibrosis	Cell membrane transport defect	0.5–0.6	Chest infections Pancreatitis
Albinism	Tyrosinase deficiency	0.025	Absence of melanin pigmentation Increased risk of skin cancer from UV light exposure
ABNORMAL CHROMOSOME NUMBERS			
Sex chromosomes			
Turner's syndrome	45, X	0.1	Female gender Webbed neck Broad chest Increased elbow angle Undeveloped ovaries
Klinefelter's syndrome	47, XXY	1.3	Male gender with female habitus
Autosomes			
Down's syndrome (mongolism)	47, trisomy 21 (in c. 95% cases)	1.4	Upward slanting eyes Flat nasal bridge Single palmar crease Mental subnormality Congenital heart defects
Patau's syndrome	47, trisomy 13	0.1	Microcephaly Small eyes Cleft palate Low-set ears
FRAGILE CHROMOSOMES			
Ataxia telangiectasia	High frequency of non-random translocations	*	Vascular dilatations on skin Ataxia (unco-ordinated movement) Predisposition to tumours
Bloom syndrome	High frequency of non-random trranslocations	*	Vascular dilatations on skin Immune deficiency Predisposition to tumours
Fragile X syndrome	Fragile site on Xq27.3	0.5	High forehead Prominent jaw Mental retardation More severe in males
X-LINKED DISORDERS			
Duchenne muscular dystrophy	Dystrophin deficiency	0.3[a]	Progressive muscular weakness
Haemophilia	Factor 8 deficiency	0.1[a]	Tendency to bleed
Glucose-6-phosphate dehydrogenase (G6PD) deficiency	G6PD deficiency	[b]	Haemolysis Resistance to malaria

*reliable frequency data not available
[a]frequency in males
[b]considerable inter-racial variation

- fusion of a gene with another (by chromosomal translocation).

These possibilities are illustrated in Figure 3.11.

X-linked single gene disorders
In addition to conditions due to abnormal numbers of sex chromosomes (see p. 46), there are disorders due to defective genes carried on the sex chromosomes. However, because females carry two X chromosomes they only rarely develop disorders due to abnormal X chromosome genes; both X chromosomes would have to carry the same defective gene for the abnormality to appear, and that is relatively improbable. In most instances, the normal X chromosome compensates for the genetic defect on its unhealthy partner.

One of the paired X chromosomes is randomly inactivated in early embryogenesis; this is the *Lyon hypothesis* (after the geneticist Mary Lyon). Thus, approximately half of the cells of a female express genes on the maternally-derived X chromosome, and the other cells express genes on the paternally-derived partner. Females inheriting a defective gene on one X chromosome are therefore cellular mosaics: some cells are normal, others are defective.

Fragile sites and chromosomal translocations

Some individuals have an inherited predisposition to chromosomal translocations (Table 3.5); that is, there is a tendency for chromosomal material to be exchanged between one chromosome and another. These translocations depend on the presence of 'fragile sites' at specific locations on the affected chromosomes. Translocations are often involved in the molecular pathogenesis of cancer (see Ch. 11); it is, therefore, not surprising that individuals with these rare conditions associated with an increased risk of translocations have a significantly increased risk of developing tumours.

Although they are rare, study of these conditions enables a better understanding of the functional role of the genes involved in translocations and in the tumours and other abnormalities resulting from them.

ENVIRONMENTAL FACTORS

Most diseases are due to environmental causes, such as infective agents, rather than to genetic abnormalities.

Gene deletion

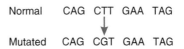

Normal

Deleted

?

Consequence: • absent gene product

Point mutation

Normal   CAG CTT GAA TAG
                    ↓
Mutated   CAG CGT GAA TAG

Consequences: • absent gene product
                       • false stop codon—truncated protein
                       • altered stop codon—elongated protein
                       • altered splicing signal

Insertion or deletion

Normal   CAG CTT GAA TAG

Insertion CAG CGT TGA ATA G...
                    ↑
Consequence: • frame shift

Fusion

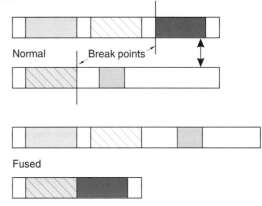

Normal   Break points

Fused

Consequences: • new protein encoded by fused genes
                       • no product

Fig. 3.11 Genetic abnormalities associated with disease

The molecular consequence of a genetic abnormality depends on whether the resulting nucleotide sequence corresponds either to a codon for an alternative amino acid (*mis-sense* mutations) or to a premature stop codon (*nonsense* mutations).

Infective agents

The main classes of infective agent are:

- bacteria
- viruses
- yeasts and fungi
- parasites.

In addition there is some evidence for the existence of infectious proteins (called *prions*) as a possible cause of neurodegenerative disease, in particular the rare Creutzfeldt–Jakob disease.

Infective agents often demonstrate tissue specificity. Some organisms selectively infect particular organs or body systems. For example, the hepatitis viruses (A, B and C) apparently infect and harm only the liver and no other organ; they are said to be hepatotropic viruses. In contrast, *Staphylococcus aureus* is capable of producing injury in almost any tissue.

The mode of transmission often reflects the environmental preferences of the micro-organisms. For example, *venereal infections* are acquired through intimate foreplay or sexual intercourse and are caused by a relatively small group of organisms that have a preference for the warm moist micro-environment prevailing in the genital regions. *Anaerobic bacteria*, such as clostridia and bacteroides, have a preference for the hypoxic environment of tissue with an impaired blood supply.

Bacteria

Not all bacterial infections are of immediate environmental origin; they all come from the environment but may have colonised the body harmlessly long before they cause disease in that particular individual. Soon after birth the surface of the skin, gut and vagina become colonised by a range of bacteria that are beneficial to the host; these normally-present bacteria are *commensals*. However, if the body's resistance is impaired, these commensal bacteria can enter the tissues, causing disease. Other bacteria causing disease are not normally present in the body.

Not all bacteria are capable of causing disease. Those that are capable are called *pathogenic bacteria* and their ability to do so is related to their *virulence*.

Bacteria usually cause disease through the production of enzymes and toxins that injure host tissues. They may also cause tissue damage indirectly by prompting a defensive reaction in excess of that justified by their innate capacity to injure. For example, most of the tissue destruction seen in pulmonary tuberculosis is due to the body's reaction to the causative bacterium rather than to any bacterial enzymes or toxins.

Bacterial lesions are often localised within a particular tissue. However, if bacteria are found within the blood, the patient is said to have *bacteraemia*. If the bacteria within the blood are proliferating and producing a systemic illness, then the patient is said to have *septicaemia*; this is a very serious condition with a high mortality.

Bacteria constitute a very large group of organisms subdivided according to their characteristics (Table 3.6) and causing a wide variety of diseases. The correct classification of a bacterium causing a clinical infection is important so that the most appropriate antibiotic can be administered without delay and so that the epidemiology of the infection can be monitored. The major classification of bacteria is according to shape — e.g. *bacilli* (rods) and *cocci* (spheres) — and staining characteristics — e.g. *Gram-negative* and *Gram-positive*; thus there are Gram-negative bacilli and cocci and there are Gram-positive bacilli and cocci. In addition, there are other major categories, such as spirochaetes and mycobacteria. Some bacteria are capable of surviving hostile conditions by forming *spores*.

Although bacteria are widely prevalent, the prevention and therapy of bacterial infections have been great triumphs of modern medicine. Successful preventive measures have included general improvements in sanitation (drinking water, drainage, etc.) as well as the development of specific vaccines and a range of antibiotics. Coincident with the major advances in medical microbiology, immunisation and antimicrobial chemotherapy, there has been an increased incidence of troublesome endemic hospital-acquired (*nosocomial*) infections. The organisms causing these infections are often resistant to a wide range of antibiotics and are particularly difficult to eradicate.

The harmful effects (pathogenicity) of bacteria are mediated by (Fig. 3.12):

- pili and adhesins
- toxins
- aggressins
- undesirable consequences of immune responses.

Bacterial pili and adhesins
Pili, or *fimbriae*, are slender processes on the surface of some bacteria. They are coated with recognition molecules called *adhesins*. Pili and their adhesin coats serve two functions:

- sexual interaction between bacteria: sex pili
- adhesion to body surfaces: adhesion pili.

Table 3.6 Examples of diseases caused by bacteria

Bacterium	Classification	Diseases
Staphylococci S. aureus	Gram-positive cocci	1 Boils, carbuncles, impetigo of skin; abscesses in other organs following septicaemia 2 Staphylococcal toxin causes scalded skin syndrome, food poisoning and toxic shock syndrome
S. epidermidis		Skin commensal causing disease only in immunosuppressed hosts
Streptococci S. pyogenes	Gram-positive cocci β-haemolytic	1 Cellulitis, otitis media, pharyngitis 2 Streptococcal toxin causes scarlet fever 3 Immune complex glomerulonephritis
S. pneumoniae (pneumococcus)	α-haemolytic	Pneumonia, otitis media
S. viridans	α-haemolytic	Mouth commensal causing bacterial endocarditis on previously damaged valves
Neisseria N. gonorrhoeae	Gram-negative cocci	Venereally transmitted genital tract infection
N. meningitidis		Meningitis
Corynebacteria C. diphtheriae	Gram-positive bacilli	Pharyngitis with toxin production causing myocarditis and paralysis
Clostridia C.tetani	Anaerobic Gram-positive bacilli	Wound infection producing an exotoxin causing muscular spasm (tetanus)
C. perfringens (welchii)		Gas and toxin-producing infection of ischaemic wounds (gas gangrene)
C. difficile		Toxin causes pseudomembranous colitis
Bacteroides	Anaerobic Gram-negative bacilli	Wound infections
Enterobacteria Shigellae (e.g. S. sonnei)	Gram-negative bacilli	Colitis with diarrhoea
Salmonellae (e.g. S. typhi)		Enteritis with diarrhoea sometimes complicated by septicaemia
Parvobacteria Haemophilus influenzae	Gram-negative bacilli	Pneumonia, bronchitis, meningitis, otitis media
Bordetella pertussis		Bronchitis (whooping cough)
Pseudomonas P. aeruginosa	Gram-negative bacillus	Pneumonia, wound infections, and septicaemia in immunosuppressed hosts
Vibrios V. cholerae	Gram-negative bacillus	Severe diarrhoea due to exotoxin activating cAMP (cholera)
Mycobacteria M. leprae	Acid/alcohol-fast bacilli	Chronic inflammation, the precise character and outcome determined by the host immune response (leprosy)
M. tuberculosis		Chronic inflammation, the precise character and outcome determined by the host immune response (tuberculosis)

Table 3.6 *cont'd*

Bacterium	Classification	Diseases
Spirochaetes *Treponema pallidum*	Spiral bacteria	Venereally transmitted genital tract infection, leading to secondary and tertiary lesions in other organs (syphilis)
Borrelia burgdorferi		Lyme disease
Leptospira interrogans (serotype *icterohaemorrhagiae*)		Weil's disease
Actinomyces *A. israelii*	Gram-positive filamentous bacterium	Mouth commensal causing chronic inflammatory lesions of face, neck or lungs
Chlamydiae *C. psittaci*	Obligate intracellular bacteria	Causes psittacosis, from infected birds; pneumonia
C. trachomatis		Various subtypes causing trachoma (keratoconjunctivitis), urethritis, salpingitis, Reiter's syndrome, and lymphogranuloma venereum
Rickettsiae *Coxiella burnetii*	Obligate intracellular bacteria	Causes Q ('query') fever, from infected animals; pneumonia, endocarditis
Mycoplasma *M. pneumoniae*	Bacteria without cell wall	Pneumonia, often described as atypical
cAMP=cyclic adenosine monophosphate		

Adhesion pili are the means by which bacteria stick to body surfaces. These processes enable them to become fixed and thereby infect that site. Pili are a feature predominantly of Gram-negative bacteria (e.g. enterobacteria causing gastrointestinal infections, neisseriae causing meningitis and genital infections). A few Gram-positive bacteria also possess pili, notably β-haemolytic streptococci, enabling them to adhere to the pharyngeal mucosa.

Host factors rendering some individuals more susceptible to certain types of infection include polymorphisms of the glycoproteins on cell surfaces to which the adhesin-coated pili stick. These include blood group substances.

Bacterial toxins
There are two categories of bacterial toxins:

• exotoxins
• endotoxins.

These toxins are responsible for many of the local and remote effects of bacteria. The toxins can be neutralised by specific antibodies.

Exotoxins. These are enzymes secreted by bacteria and have local or remote effects. Their effects tend to be more specific than those of endotoxins. Examples of exotoxin-mediated effects of bacterial include:

• pseudomembranous colitis due to *Clostridium difficile*
• neuropathy and cardiomyopathy due to *Corynebacterium diphtheriae*
• tetanus due to tetanospasmin produced by *Clostridium tetani*
• scalded skin syndrome due to *Staphylococcus aureus*
• diarrhoea due to activation of cyclic-AMP by *Vibrio cholerae*.

The genes directing the synthesis of exotoxins are usually an intrinsic part of the bacterial genome. In a few instances, however, bacteria acquire the gene in the form of a *plasmid*, a loop of DNA that can convey genetic information from one bacterium to another; this is also a mechanism by which bacteria can acquire resistance to an antibiotic. Genes encoding for exotoxins can also be transmitted by *phages*: these are viruses that affect bacteria. The toxin produced

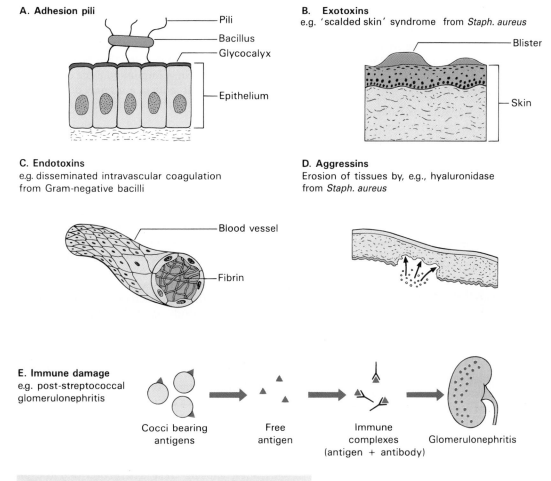

A. Adhesion pili

- Pili
- Bacillus
- Glycocalyx
- Epithelium

B. Exotoxins
e.g. 'scalded skin' syndrome from *Staph. aureus*

- Blister
- Skin

C. Endotoxins
e.g. disseminated intravascular coagulation from Gram-negative bacilli

- Blood vessel
- Fibrin

D. Aggressins
Erosion of tissues by, e.g., hyaluronidase from *Staph. aureus*

E. Immune damage
e.g. post-streptococcal glomerulonephritis

Cocci bearing antigens → Free antigen → Immune complexes (antigen + antibody) → Glomerulonephritis

---

Fig. 3.12   Pathogenesis of diseases caused by bacteria

Various factors may be responsible for the local and remote effects of a bacterial infection. Not all factors are relevant to every bacterial infection. **A.** Adhesion pili. **B.** Exotoxins. **C.** Endotoxins. **D.** Aggressins. **E.** Immune damage.

---

are viruses that affect bacteria. The toxin produced by *Corynebacterium diphtheriae* is encoded on a gene conveyed to the bacterium by a phage; strains of this and other organisms synthesising exotoxins are known as *toxigenic*.

Occasionally, disease results from the ingestion of preformed exotoxin; this is the mechanism in some cases of food poisoning. A typical, but fortunately rare, example is botulism due to contamination of food with a neurotoxin from *Clostridium botulinum*. Toxins acting upon the gut are often referred to as *enterotoxins*.

Endotoxins. These are lipopolysaccharides from the cell walls of Gram-negative bacteria (e.g. *Escherichia coli*). They are released on death of the bacterium. The most potent is lipid A, a powerful activator of:

- the complement cascade — causing inflammatory damage
- the coagulation cascade — causing disseminated intravascular coagulation
- interleukin-l (IL-l) release from leukocytes — causing fever.

When these effects are severe, in an overwhelming infection, the patient is said to suffer from *endotoxic shock*. The patient is feverish and hypotensive; cardiac and renal failure may ensue. Disseminated intravascular coagulation may be evinced by bruising and prolonged bleeding from venepuncture sites, as well as more serious internal manifestations. Bilateral adrenal haemorrhage, particularly associated with overwhelming meningococcal infection (Waterhouse – Friderichsen syndrome), is a dramatic consequence of endotoxic shock.

Aggressins

These are bacterial enzymes with predominantly local effects, altering the tissue environment in a way that favours the growth and spread of the organism. In this way, aggressins inhibit or counteract host resistance. Examples include:

- *coagulase* from *Staphylococcus aureus* — inducing coagulation of fibrinogen to create a barrier between the focus of infection and the inflammatory reaction
- *streptokinase* from *Streptococcus pyogenes* — digesting fibrin to enable the organism to spread within the tissue
- *collagenase* and *hyaluronidase* — digesting connective tissue substances, thus facilitating the invasion of the organism into the host tissues.

Some bacterial enzymes have brought great benefit to medicine, notably the restriction enzymes (endonucleases) that are used to break DNA at specific points into smaller fragments prior to electrophoretic separation (see p. 44), and streptokinase used to dissolve thrombi in patients with blood vessel thrombosis.

Undesirable consequences of immune responses

Bacteria can indirectly cause tissue injury by inducing an immune response that harms the host. Fortunately, this mechanism is rare and most immune responses to bacteria are helpful to the host.

Immune responses can harm host tissues by three possible mechanisms:

- *Immune complex formation.* Soluble antigens from the bacteria combine with host antibody to form insoluble immune complexes in the patient's blood. These complexes can usually be removed by phagocytic cells lining the vascular sinusoids of the liver and spleen, causing no further harm. However, under certain conditions the complexes can become entrapped in the walls of blood vessels, notably the glomeruli of the kidney (causing glomerulonephritis), and capillaries in the skin (causing cutaneous vasculitis). Post-streptococcal glomerulonephritis (Ch. 21) is a good example of this phenomenon.
- *Immune cross-reactions.* The host tissues of some individuals have antigenic similarities to some bacteria. The defensive antibody response to some bacteria can, therefore, cross-react with normal tissue antigens; rheumatic fever (Ch. 13) is a good example.
- *Cell-mediated immunity.* The degree of tissue destruction seen in tuberculosis is not attributable to the organism itself but to the host's immune

reaction to the organisms. Without much host immunity, *Mycobacterium tuberculosis* induces the formation of small granulomas that can become widely disseminated and thus be fatal. In the presence of host immunity, if the organism gains a foothold, it induces a severely destructive tissue reaction in which the organisms are extremely sparse.

Viruses

Viruses are submicroscopic infectious particles consisting of a nucleic acid core and a protein coat. They can be broadly divided into RNA and DNA viruses according to the type of nucleic acid core, but there are many further subdivisions (Table 3.7).

Viruses can survive outside cells, but they always require the biochemical machinery of cells for their multiplication. Viruses show more evidence of tissue specificity than do bacteria. The ability to infect a cell type depends upon the virus binding to a substance on the cell surface; for example, human immunodeficiency virus (HIV) — the AIDS virus — selectively infects a subpopulation of T-lymphocytes expressing the CD4 (CD=cluster differentiation antigen) substance on their surface.

Some viruses circulate in the blood to reach other organs from their portal of entry; this process is called *viraemia*. For example, the polio virus enters the body through the gastrointestinal tract, eventually causing a viraemia to reach spinal motor neurones, causing their destruction and the patient's paralysis.

The possible general pathological effects of viruses are:

- acute tissue damage exciting an immediate inflammatory response
- slow virus infections causing chronic tissue damage
- transformation of cells to form tumours.

The clinical manifestations of viral infections are, therefore, protean. Slow virus infections are a known or postulated cause of several neurodegenerative disorders (Ch. 26). The ability of some viruses to transform normal cells into cells capable of forming tumours is covered in Chapter 11. For many diseases where the cause is still unknown, a viral aetiology is inevitably being considered.

DNA and RNA viruses

The properties and behaviour of viruses differ according to their nucleic acid content. Unlike cells

Table 3.7 Examples of diseases caused by viruses

Disease	Virus classification	Features
AIDS (acquired immune deficiency syndrome)	HIV (human immunodeficiency virus) (RNA retrovirus)	Infects CD4 T-helper lymphocytes causing lymph node enlargement, immune suppression, and opportunistic infections
Coryza (common cold)	Rhinovirus (RNA)	Inflammation of nasal mucosa
Genital herpes	Herpes simplex virus II DNA	Sexually transmitted infection causing inflammation of genitalia
Herpetic stomatitis	Herpes simplex virus I DNA	Latent infection in nerve ganglia re-activated to cause vesicles in skin around mouth
Infectious mononucleosis (glandular fever)	Epstein–Barr (EB) virus (herpes group; DNA)	Fever, pharyngitis, generalised lymph node enlargement EB virus also associated with Burkitt's lymphoma (with malaria as co-factor) and nasopharyngeal carcinoma
Measles	Paramyxovirus (RNA)	Fever, skin rash, respiratory tract inflammation Can be fatal in association with malnutrition
Mumps	Paramyxovirus (RNA)	Fever, salivary gland inflammation and, occasionally, pancreatitis and orchitis
Poliomyelitis	Enterovirus (RNA)	Enteric infection initially, then viraemia, from which anterior horn cells become infected, causing paralysis
Rabies	Rhabdovirus (RNA)	Acute encephalomyelitis
Rotavirus diarrhoea	Reovirus (RNA)	Fever, vomiting and diarrhoea
Rubella (German measles)	Togavirus (RNA)	Fever, lymph node enlargement, skin rash, rhinitis; usually mild Maternal rubella associated with high risk of fetal malformations
Squamous epithelial tumours (e.g. warts, probably carcinoma of cervix)	Human papillomavirus (DNA)	Transformation of cells causing their uncontrolled growth
Varicella (chickenpox)	Herpes group (DNA)	Fever, vesicular skin rash Latent infection of dorsal nerve root ganglia; can be re-activated later causing herpes zoster (shingles)

(e.g. bacteria, plant and animal cells), viruses contain either DNA or RNA, never both; the viral nucleic acid can be either single- or double-stranded.

Viruses with a DNA core are capable of surviving in the nucleus of the cell they infect, taking advantage of the biochemical machinery there to maintain the DNA of the host cell. The DNA of some viruses can become integrated into the DNA of the host cell. These properties enable DNA virus infections to become latent, reactivated under certain circumstances, and possibly result in neoplastic transformation of the cell (see Ch. 11).

RNA viruses have high mutation rates because their RNA polymerase, which copies the viral genome, is incapable of detecting and repairing transcription errors. These mutations lead to changes in antigenicity, enabling RNA viruses often to evade host immunity. Some RNA viruses contain reverse transcriptase (see p. 38); this enzyme produces a DNA copy of the virus which can then become integrated in the genome of the host cell.

Tissue specificity
Unlike bacteria, viruses are incapable of replication outside cells. Therefore, a key factor in determining whether an individual becomes infected is the ability of the virus to enter the cells of the body. There are two alternative mechanisms:

- entry by interaction with a specific cellular receptor
- fusion directly with the cell membrane.

Many viruses show a high degree of tissue specificity, infecting a limited range of organs or cell types. This is known as *tropism*, and invariably results from the fact that the virus must bind first to a specific receptor present on a limited range of cells. Some receptors are, however, widely distributed and enable a virus to infect a wide variety of cell types.

Examples of receptor-mediated virus infection include:

- CD4 receptors on T-helper lymphocytes which bind HIV
- complement receptors which bind Epstein–Barr virus
- cell adhesion molecule ICAM-1 which binds rhinovirus
- sialic acid receptors which bind influenza virus.

Pathogenesis of cell injury

Viruses can produce tissue injury by a variety of mechanisms (Fig. 3.13):

- *Direct cytopathic effect.* Cells harbouring viruses may be damaged by their presence. This effect can often be demonstrated in cell cultures where, after incubation with the virus, a cytopathic effect is observed: the cells swell and die. This effect is mediated by injury to the cell membranes, causing fatal ionic equilibration with respect to the extracellular electrolyte concentrations, or by depriving the cell of its nucleotides and amino acids. An example of a directly cytopathic virus is hepatitis A virus (Ch. 16).
- *Induction of immune response.* Some viruses do not harm cells directly but cause new antigens to appear on the cell surface. These new virus-associated antigens are recognised as foreign by the host's immune system and the virus-infected cells are destroyed. A consequence of this phenomenon is that, if the immune response is weak or non-existent, the virus-infected cells are not harmed. This situation may benefit the patient because their infected cells are not destroyed, but on the other hand the patient becomes an asymptomatic and apparently healthy carrier of the virus, capable of infecting other people. A good example is hepatitis B virus (Ch. 16).
- *Incorporation of viral genes into the host genome.* This phenomenon underlies the ability of some viruses to induce tumours (Ch. 11). Genes of DNA viruses can become directly incorporated into the host genome, but the genes of RNA viruses require the action of reverse transcriptase enzymes to produce a DNA transcript that can be

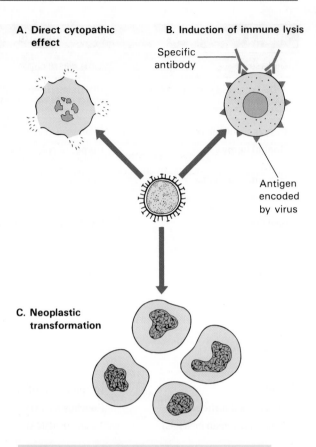

Fig. 3.13 Pathogenesis of diseases caused by viruses

A. Directly cytopathic viruses, injuring or killing cells infected by them. **B.** Immune destruction of virus-infected cells. However, in the absence of an effective immune response, the cell may tolerate the virus infection. **C.** Incorporation of viral genes into host cell genome. This incorporation may transform the cell into a neoplastic state.

inserted. RNA viruses with reverse transcriptase activity are called *retroviruses*.

There are few effective therapeutic remedies against viral infections. There are vaccines for immunisation against particularly serious or common viral infections, but once the infection has developed there are few instances where specific treatment is either available or justified. One of the body's own antiviral mechanisms — *interferon production* — can be used in some instances. Interferons are produced by virus-infected cells and, in vitro, can be shown to interfere with or inhibit viral replication. Interferons can now be produced in large amounts by genetic engineering and are being evaluated in the treatment of potentially serious viral infections.

Yeasts and fungi

Yeasts and fungi constitute a relatively heterogeneous collection of micro-organisms causing disease (Table 3.8). The diseases caused by yeasts and fungi are known as *mycoses*.

Fungal infections are less common than bacterial or viral infections. However, they assume a special importance in patients with impaired immunity; in these patients, otherwise harmless fungi take advantage of the opportunity to infect a defenceless host. This situation is known as *opportunistic infection* and is shared by a few viruses and bacteria.

The usual tissue reaction to yeasts and fungi is inflammation, often characterised by the presence of granulomas and sometimes also eosinophils.

Mycotoxins

Mycotoxins are toxins produced by fungi. The mycotoxins of greatest medical relevance are the *aflatoxins* produced by *Aspergillus flavus*. Food stored in warm humid conditions can become infected with this fungus, thus contaminating the food with aflatoxins. Animals ingesting sufficiently high doses will develop acute hepatic damage. In man the greatest problem is the increased risk of hepatocellular carcinoma due to ingestion of relatively small doses.

Parasites

Parasites differ from other infectious agents in that they are nucleated unicellular or multicellular living organisms deriving sustenance from their hosts. It is not unusual for a parasite to be harboured within the body without causing any disease.

Parasites are the most heterogeneous group of infectious agents (Tables 3.9–3.12). Due to their requirement for particular environmental conditions and, in some instances, other hosts for their life-cycle, parasitic infections are generally more common in the tropics.

Parasites are subdivided into:

- *protozoa*: unicellular organisms
- *helminths*: worms (roundworms, tapeworms and flukes).

Parasites, particularly helminths, have complex and exotic life-cycles requiring more than one host (Fig. 3.14). Furthermore, within one host there may be successive involvement of more than one organ. Humans may either be *definitive hosts* or *inadvertent intermediate hosts*.

The tissue reactions to parasites are extremely variable. If an inflammatory reaction is prompted, it is often characterised by the presence of eosinophils and granulomas. Two parasites are associated with an increased risk of tumours: *Schistosoma haematobium* is associated with bladder cancer, and *Clonorchis sinensis* is associated with bile duct cancer.

Chemical agents as a cause of disease

The study of environmental chemicals causing disease is *toxicology*. The range of possible harmful

---

Table 3.8   Examples of diseases caused by yeasts and fungi

Organism	Classification	Disease
Aspergillus species	Fungus	Common environmental fungus Allergic asthma; fungal infection of lung cavity (mycetoma); pneumonia (invasive aspergillosis) in immunosuppressed hosts
Candida albicans	Yeast	Oral and vaginal commensal causing local disease (thrush) or systemic disease (septicaemia) in immunosuppressed hosts, diabetics, and if local bacterial flora are altered by antibiotics
Cryptococcus neoformans	Fungus (yeast-like)	From bird droppings Causes systemic infection (cryptococcosis) in immunosuppressed hosts
Histoplasma capsulatum	Fungus (yeast-like)	From bird and bat droppings Causes acute or chronic lung infections; systemic infection in immunosuppressed hosts
Pneumocystis carinii	Fungus (yeast-like)	Often present in normal lungs Causes pneumonia in immunosuppressed hosts, notably in AIDS cases

Table 3.9   Protozoal causes of disease

Disease	Parasite	Vector/route	Comment
Amoebiasis	*Entamoeba histolytica*	Faecal–oral spread of amoebic cysts	Causes amoebic dysentery and 'amoebomas'
Cryptosporidiosis	*Cryptosporidium*	Faecal–oral	Intestinal infection causing diarrhoea and weight loss; common in AIDS
Giardiasis	*Giardia lamblia (intestinalis)*	Faecal–oral	Intestinal infection causing diarrhoea and weight loss
Leishmaniasis	*Leishmania* sp.	Sandfly	Cutaneous and visceral leishmaniasis (kala-azar) caused by different species
Malaria	*Plasmodium* sp.	Female anopheline mosquito	Acute fever; *P. falciparum* often fatal
Toxoplasmosis	*Toxoplasma gondii*	Cats are definitive hosts	Man is inadvertent host; infection from animal faeces or contaminated meat; lesions in various organs
Trichomoniasis	*Trichomonas vaginalis*	Venereal transmission between humans	Venereal disease
Trypanosomiasis			
African	*Trypanosoma gambiense* and *rhodesiense*	Tsetse fly	'Sleeping sickness'
American	*Trypanosoma cruzi*	Reduviid bug	Chagas' disease

Table 3.10   Diseases due to trematodes (flukes)

Disease	Trematode	Vector/source	Life-cycle
Clonorchiasis	*Clonorchis sinensis*	Water snails then fish	Eggs from faeces ingested by snail and hatch, releasing miracidia which then develop into cercariae; cercariae penetrate fish skin and then encyst to be ingested by human; metacercariae enter bile ducts where they mature
Fascioliasis	*Fasciola hepatica*	Water snails then fish	As for clonorchiasis
Schistosomiasis (bilharzia)	*Schistosoma haematobium* *S. japonicum* *S. mansoni*	Water snails	Eggs from faeces or urine hatch in water releasing miracidia which penetrate skin of snail; snail releases cercariae which penetrate human skin; schistosomules travel in blood to mature in portal vein (*S. mansoni/ aponicum*) or bladder veins (*S. haematobium*) where they lay eggs; these cause granulomas and fibrosis

chemical agents in the environment is enormous and considerable effort is expended in their identification and safe handling. All new drugs, food additives, pesticides, etc. must be exhaustively tested for safety before they can be introduced for general use. There is insufficient space to give a comprehensive list of all chemicals that are known to be harmful. The cellular mechanisms of chemical injury are described in Chapter 6.

Corrosive effects

Strong acids (e.g. sulphuric acid) and alkalis (e.g. sodium hydroxide) have a direct corrosive effect on tissues. They cause digestion or denaturation of proteins, and thus damage the structural integrity of the tissue. Powerful oxidising agents, such as hydrogen peroxide, have a similar effect.

If accidentally applied to the skin, corrosive agents

Table 3.11   Diseases due to nematodes (roundworms)

Disease	Nematode	Vector/source	Life-cycle
Ascariasis	*Ascaris lumbricoides*	Faecal–oral	Intestinal parasite; larvae penetrate mucosa, travel to lungs in blood, penetrate alveoli, ascend airways to be swallowed into gut
Dracunculiasis (Guinea worm)	*Dracunculus medinensis*	Water containing infected cyclops	Larvae ingested and enter blood, then migrate through tissues, eventually reaching skin to form a blister containing mature worm so long that it can be withdrawn by winding round a stick
Hookworm	*Ancylostoma duodenale*	Faecal–soil–cutaneous (or faecal–soil–oral)	Eggs hatch in warm soil, larvae penetrate skin and travel in blood to lungs, then swallowed; larvae may also be ingested
	Necator americanus	Faecal–soil–cutaneous	Cycle as for *A. duodenale,* but without option of being ingested
Cutaneous larva migrans	*Ancylostoma braziliense*	Faecal–soil–cutaneous	Localised skin lesion
Threadworm	*Enterobius vermicularis*	Faecal–oral	Intestinal infestation
Trichinosis	*Trichinella spiralis*	Meat containing larvae	Larvae enter blood from gut and form encysted larvae in muscles
Toxocariasis	*Toxocara canis* or *cati*	Canine/feline faecal–oral	Eggs ingested and release larvae in gut, which then enter blood, causing granulomatous inflammation in various organs
Filariasis **Loa-loa**	*Loa loa*	*Chrysops* flies	Similar life-cycle to onchocerciasis but adult worms migrate freely
Lymphatic filariasis (elephantiasis)	*Wuchereria bancrofti*	Mosquito	Microfilariae ingested by bloodsucking mosquitoes; mature larvae injected into human skin; adults develop in and block lymphatic channels, causing lymphatic oedema
Onchocerciasis	*Onchocerca volvulus*	Blackfly	Microfilariae ingested by bloodsucking blackflies, mature larvae injected into human skin; adults develop locally, releasing microfilariae into blood

Table 3.12   Diseases due to cestodes (tapeworms)

Disease	Cestode	Vector/source	Life-cycle
Cysticercosis	*Taenia solium*	Infected pork	Usually asymptomatic intestinal parasites but *T. solium* may form cysticerci (encysted larvae) in humans in muscle and brain
	Taenia saginata	Infected beef	
Vitamin B$_{12}$ deficiency	*Diphyllobothrium latum*	Fish	Humans infected by ingesting fish infected by feeding upon water fleas carrying cestode eggs
Hydatid disease	*Echinococcus granulosus*	Dog	Cattle, pigs and sheep are usual intermediate hosts; humans infected by ingesting parasite eggs which release onchosphere, eventually forming hydatid cyst in liver, lung, etc.

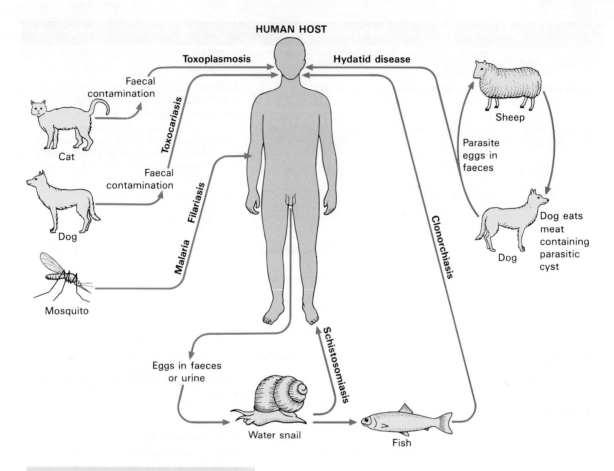

Fig. 3.14   Examples of parasite life-cycles

Simplified diagrammatic summary of the roles of hosts and vectors in the life-cycle of some parasitic diseases.

cause the epidermis and underlying tissues to become necrotic and slough off, leaving an ulcer with a raw base that eventually heals by cellular regeneration.

Metabolic effects

The metabolic effects of chemicals causing disease are usually attributable to interaction with a specific metabolic pathway. However, the harmful metabolic effects of some chemicals affect many organs. Alcohol (ethanol) is a good example: it causes drowsiness and impaired mentation, liver damage, pancreatitis, etc.

The widespread effects of some chemicals are due either to the ubiquity of a particular metabolic pathway or to the multiple effects of a single agent on different pathways.

Some chemicals are directly toxic. Others are relatively harmless until they have been converted into an active metabolite within the body.

Membrane effects

If cells had an Achilles heel, it would be the membrane that invests them. The cell membrane is not merely a bag to prevent spillage of the cytoplasm; it has numerous specific functions. In particular, it bears many receptors and channels for the selective binding and transport of natural substances. These structures are vulnerable to injurious chemicals and their damage can severely disrupt the function of the cell.

Mutagenic effects

Chemical agents or their metabolites that bind to or alter DNA can result in genetic alterations (e.g. base substitutions) called *mutations*. Chemicals acting in this way are classified as *mutagens*. Mutagens have two serious consequences:

* They can affect embryogenesis, leading to

congenital malformations (Ch. 5). Agents acting in this way are said to be *teratogenic*.
- They may be *carcinogenic*, leading to the development of tumours (Ch. 11).

Allergic reactions

Large molecules (e.g. peptides and proteins) may induce immune responses if the body's immune system recognises them as foreign substances. Very small molecules are unlikely to be antigenic, but they may act as *haptens*; that is, they are too small to constitute antigens on their own, but do so by binding to a larger molecule such as a protein. The allergic reaction to chemicals may be mediated by antibodies or by cells, such as lymphocytes (Ch. 9), causing tissue damage.

Smoking

Tobacco smoking is, without doubt, a major cause of illness and premature death. Almost 400 years ago it was condemned by King James I of England as *'loathsome to the eye, harmful to the brain, dangerous to the lungs, and in the black stinking fume thereof, nearest resembling the horrible Stygian smoke of the pit that is bottomless'*! Epidemiological studies during the latter half of the 20th century provide irrefutable evidence of the causal relationship between smoking and a range of neoplastic and non-neoplastic disorders including:

- carcinoma of the lung
- carcinoma of the larynx
- carcinoma of the bladder
- carcinoma of the cervix
- ischaemic heart disease
- gastric ulcers
- chronic bronchitis and emphysema.

Paradoxically, the addictive component of tobacco smoke (nicotine) is probably the least harmful constituent. Carcinogens within the polycyclic aromatic hydrocarbon fraction of the smoke are responsible for the increased incidence of tumours of the respiratory tract and other sites in smokers. The carbon monoxide in the inhaled smoke is probably responsible for endothelial hypoxia accelerating the development of atheroma.

Alcohol

It is still controversial whether alcohol (ethyl alcohol) in moderation can have beneficial effects on health. Some epidemiological studies suggest that regular consumption of one or two units per day can slightly reduce the risk of premature death from ischaemic heart disease. This apparent relationship between mortality and alcohol consumption is referred to as the J-shaped curve; the line plotted to show the relationship graphically is J-shaped. However, on balance, alcohol consumption exceeding this modest allowance is probably responsible for more harm than good.

Alcohol is incriminated in the aetiology of diseases including:

- hepatic cirrhosis
- gastritis
- cardiomyopathy
- chronic pancreatitis
- fetal alcohol syndrome (due to maternal consumption)
- encephalopathy.

Alcohol is also a factor in many road traffic accidents and in physical injury by assault.

Drugs

Many of the drugs used in therapy have a risk of adverse effects. Some of these drugs and others are also used (abused) for 'recreational' purposes.

Adverse effects of drugs

Iatrogenic disease is a major problem in modern medicine. Many of the drugs and other treatments (e.g. surgery, radiotherapy) commonly employed have adverse as well as beneficial effects. The mechanism of the adverse effect varies according to the chemistry of the drug, its metabolism, and the condition of the patient (see Ch. 2).

Drug abuse

Drug abuse is a major social and medical problem in developed countries. The medical harm that results may be due directly to the abused drug or to coincidental problems. For example, intravenous drug abusers are harmed not only by the effects of the self-administered drugs, but also by viruses transmitted by sharing equipment with infected addicts. Human immunodeficiency virus (HIV, causing AIDS) and hepatitis C virus (HCV, causing chronic liver disease) are particularly common.

Physical agents as a cause of disease

Tissue damage by mechanical injury is obvious and direct. The mediation of thermal or radiation injury is more complex.

Mechanical injury

Mechanical injury to tissues is called *trauma* (although by common usage this word has acquired a wider meaning, e.g. 'psychological trauma'). Cells and tissues are disrupted by trauma, causing cell and tissue loss. Depending on the tissue, regeneration may be possible. The reaction of different tissues to trauma is described in Chapter 6.

Thermal injury

The body is more tolerant of reductions in body temperature than of increases. Indeed, cooling of tissues and organs is commonly used for their short-term preservation prior to transplantation. For major cardiac surgery the body is often cooled to reduce the metabolic requirements of vital organs, such as the brain, when the circulation is temporarily arrested. Accidental *hypothermia* is a common medical emergency in the elderly during winter in countries such as the UK; however, recovery is usually possible unless the body temperature has fallen below 28°C.

Increased body temperature is known as *pyrexia*. In infections, it is usually mediated by the action of interleukins on the hypothalamus. Body temperatures above 40°C are associated with increasing mortality. Enzyme systems are severely disturbed, with severe metabolic consequences.

Local heating of the skin causes increasing local damage. Heat coagulates proteins and thereby disrupts the structure and function of cells. As the temperature rises, burns occur in the following ascending order of severity:

- first degree: skin erythema (redness) only
- second degree: epidermal necrosis and blistering of the skin
- third degree: epidermal and dermal necrosis.

Thermal injury is commonly used in surgery to coagulate tissues and arrest bleeding; this is the technique of *diathermy*.

Radiation injury

Potentially harmful radiation is a source of considerable alarm because it is invisible and there is no immediate sensation of its presence.

The effects depend upon the type of radiation, the dose and the type of tissue. Cell and tissue injury from radiation is described in detail in Chapter 6.

Ionising radiation

The harmful effects of ionising radiation are:

- at high doses, immediate clinical effects due to tissue damage from the production of free radicals
- injury to rapidly dividing cell populations (e.g. haemopoietic cells)
- inflammatory reactions leading to scarring of tissues due to the induction of fibrosis (e.g. radiation stricture of the bowel)
- neoplasia (solid tumours and leukaemias).

The injury to rapidly dividing cells is immediate and becomes evident clinically within a few days or weeks (anaemia, bleeding, etc.). Fibrosis takes longer to appear: usually months or even years. Neoplasia occurs only decades after radiation; leukaemias tend to occur earlier than solid tumours.

Despite these serious adverse effects of radiation, it is widely used in medicine for diagnostic imaging of tissues (e.g. chest X-ray, radionuclide scanning) and for therapy (e.g. irradiation of tumours).

Non-ionising radiation

Ultraviolet (UV) light, particularly UVB, is harmful to the skin. It would almost certainly harm deeper tissues if it was not for the skin acting as a screen. UV light causes:

- skin tumours (e.g. melanoma; Ch. 11)
- dermal elastosis (Ch. 12).

FURTHER READING

Alderson M 1983 An introduction to epidemiology, 2nd edn. Macmillan, London

D'Arcy P F, Griffin J P (eds) 1986 Iatrogenic diseases, 3rd edn. Oxford University Press, Oxford

Khaw K T 1994 Genetics and environment: Geoffrey Rose revisited. Lancet 343: 838–839

Mims C A, Playfair J H L, Roi H I M, Wakelin D, Williams R 1993 Medical microbiology. Mosby, St Louis

Peter W, Gilles H M 1989 A colour atlas of tropical medicine and parasitology, 3rd edn. Wolfe Medical, London

Raffle P A B, Lee W R, McCallum R I (eds) 1987 Hunter's Diseases of the occupations. Hodder & Stoughton, London

Streiner D L, Norman G R, Blum H M 1989 Epidemiology. Decker, Toronto

Thompson M W, McInnes R R, Willard H F 1991 Genetics in medicine, 5th edn. W B Saunders, Philadelphia

Trent R J 1993 Molecular medicine. Churchill Livingstone, Edinburgh

Weatherall D J 1991 The new genetics and clinical practice, 3rd edn. Oxford University Press, Oxford

4

Diagnostic pathology in clinical practice

Laboratory techniques play an important part in the diagnosis and treatment of disease in patients. Many of the tests performed in pathology laboratories are diagnostic, quantitative measurements or prognostic, but these are complemented by expert advice on the interpretation of the results. Microbiologists are also involved in formulating policies designed to prevent spread of infection in hospitals; haematologists have clinical responsibilities for treating patients with haematological malignancies and other disorders.

In this chapter the general principles of diagnostic tests, quantitative measurements and prognostic tests are given and these are then related to the specific roles of clinical chemistry, cytogenetics, cytopathology, haematology, histopathology, immunology, microbiology and autopsies.

TYPES OF LABORATORY TESTS

> ▶ Diagnostic tests assign patients to diagnostic categories
> ▶ Quantitative tests may assist in diagnosis, prognosis or management
> ▶ Effectiveness of diagnostic tests can be expressed as accuracy (the proportion of cases correctly diagnosed) and sensitivity (the proportion of cases of the disease detected by the test)
> ▶ 'Normal ranges' for quantitative tests assume normal (Gaussian) distribution of values; 5% of normal individuals have results lying outside this range

Diagnostic tests

Diagnostic tests are those which are made on a sample from a patient, the result allocating the case to a diagnostic grouping; an example would be a fine-needle aspirate of a lesion of the breast which is sent for cytopathological examination and classified into a benign or malignant (i.e. cancer) category. Quantitative measurements, such as haemoglobin concentration or arterial blood oxygen tension, may be used in the clinician's diagnostic process but they do not by themselves assign a patient to a particular diagnostic category. A diagnostic test may be based on:

- *quantitative measurement,* such as the level of β human chorionic gonadotrophin in the diagnosis of trophoblastic disease
- *subjective assessment,* based on past experience such as a cytopathologist's assessment of a fine-needle aspirate of the breast.

The ideal diagnostic test would produce complete separation between two diagnostic categories; usually, however, there is some overlap. This problem can be illustrated by taking as an example a screening test for colorectal carcinoma which makes measurements on a sample of faeces (many attempts have been made to devise such a test using measurements of blood contained in the faeces and other parameters). An ideal diagnostic test would produce complete separation of patients with and without colorectal carcinoma (Fig. 4.1). The majority of real diagnostic tests do not provide complete separation between diagnostic categories and there is overlap (Fig. 4.2).

The effectiveness of a diagnostic test can be expressed using a number of different parameters:

- A *true positive* (TP) result is a positive result from the test under consideration which is confirmed by the real outcome of the situation (e.g. a fine-needle aspirate of the breast (FNAB) which is reported as malignant and the subsequently excised breast tissue contains invasive carcinoma; Table 4.1).

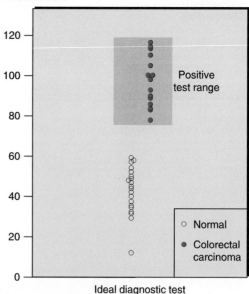

Units of measurement

Fig. 4.1 Distribution graph for an ideal diagnostic test

There is complete separation of the population into those with colorectal carcinoma (shaded area) and those without. In this example a measurement of above 70 units would indicate that the subject had colorectal carcinoma and a measurement below 60 units would indicate that the subject did not have colorectal carcinoma.

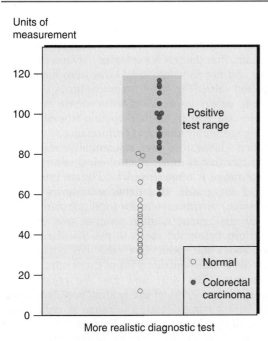

Units of measurement

Fig. 4.2 Distribution graph of a more realistic diagnostic test

In this example there is a range of values between 60 and 80 units where there are subjects with and without colorectal carcinoma.

Table 4.1   True and false test results in fine-needle aspiration of the breast (FNAB)

Actual outcome	Test result from FNAB Benign	Malignant
Benign	True negative	False positive
Malignant	False negative	True positive

- A *true negative* result (TN) is a negative test result confirmed by a negative real outcome.
- A *false positive* result (FP) is a positive test result which has a negative real outcome (e.g. a FNAB which is reported as malignant but the subsequently excised breast tissue shows no evidence of malignancy).
- A *false negative* result (FN) is the reverse of this.

These can be combined into the following measures:

$$\text{Accuracy} = \frac{(TN + TP)}{(TN + TP + FN + FP)} \cdot 100$$

$$\text{Sensitivity} = \frac{(TP)}{(TP + FN)} \cdot 100$$

$$\text{Specificity} = \frac{(TN)}{(TN + FP)} \cdot 100$$

$$\begin{array}{l}\text{Predictive value} \\ \text{of positive result}\end{array} = \frac{(TP)}{(TP + FP)} \cdot 100$$

$$\begin{array}{l}\text{Predictive value} \\ \text{of negative result}\end{array} = \frac{(TN)}{(TN + FN)} \cdot 100$$

The desired values of these for a particular test will vary according to the action taken on the result. A malignant FNAB result can result in a surgeon excising the breast (mastectomy) so the specificity and predictive value of a positive result must be as close to 100% as possible. In contrast if a disease has a relatively safe, non-toxic treatment (such as a course of antibiotics) but the consequences of not detecting the disease can be fatal (e.g. bacterial meningitis) then the sensitivity and predictive value of a negative result should be as high as possible. In most situations there is a direct 'trade-off' between sensitivity and specificity and a suitable threshold has to be set that will give the best overall performance (Fig. 4.3).

In many medical situations a continuous biological spectrum is arbitrarily divided into a number of discrete categories which will always lead to some apparent misclassification but is necessary to give information on which clinicians can base their management decisions (e.g division of intraepithelial neoplasia of the uterine cervix into three categories, see Ch. 19).

A laboratory's performance in diagnostic tests should be monitored by a formal *audit process* and by use of appropriate positive and negative controls in tests.

Quantitative measurements

Many tests in pathology do not categorise results into discrete groups but give a quantitative result which is interpreted in relation to a 'normal' range of values. Examples of such tests include measurement of haemoglobin concentration, electrolyte concentrations and blood oxygen and carbon dioxide levels.

The measures of performance for such tests differ from diagnostic grouping tests. In quantitative tests the *accuracy* of the measurement (how close the measured value is to the 'true' value determined by a more accurate or absolute method) and the *reproducibility* of the measurement (what variation there is

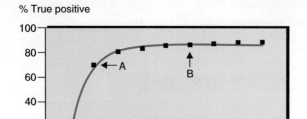

Fig. 4.3 Receiver operator curve for a diagnostic test showing the trade-off between the true and false positive results

If the threshold for the test is set at A then there would be 70% true positives and 20% false positives. At a threshold set at B there would be 60% false positives but the true positives would only increase to 85%.

when measuring the same sample many times) are important parameters. These can be assessed by using reference samples with 'known' values and putting these through the measurement system at regular intervals; most laboratories will have their own reference samples which are used frequently

(internal quality assurance), and graphs of single measurement and running mean values will be used to ensure that the test is performing within expected limits and not showing 'drift' away from the central expected value (Fig. 4.4). Many countries also have *external quality assurance schemes* where reference samples are sent to all participating laboratories to ensure acceptable analytical performance.

When a laboratory gives a quantitative result for a parameter that is under physiological control a reference range is often given to facilitate interpretation of the result. If a parameter shows normal (Gaussian) distribution in the local population then the 'normal' range is often given as two standard deviations below the mean to two standard deviations above the mean. If a value lies outside this range then it lies outside 95% of the results for that population (Fig. 4.5) and may be regarded as abnormal, but 2.5% of the healthy population will have values lying outside the range at either end. Thus, all the details of the individual case must be considered, including other measurements, since a number of results at the top end of the 'normal' range could be more significant than a single result just above the 'normal' range. If the distribution is not Gaussian then it may require normalisation by transformation, or non-parametric methods must be used.

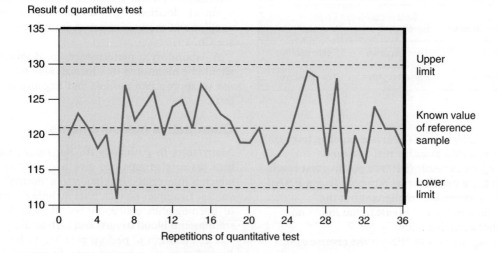

Fig. 4.4 Internal quality assurance graph for a quantitative pathological test

A reference sample is used for each test; tests A and B lie outside the acceptable range and the process of the test would have to be investigated for sources of errors (e.g. out of date reagents, contamination, etc.).

Relative
probability

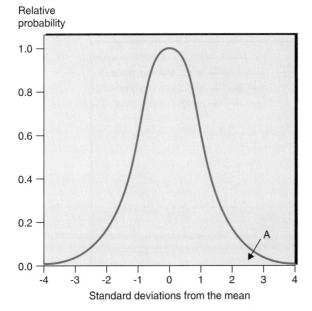

Standard deviations from the mean

Fig. 4.5   Quantitative measurement with a normal (Gaussian) distribution in the population

The result at A lies more than 2 standard deviations away from the mean and so may be regarded as abnormal, but 2.5% of the normal population will have values in this area.

Prognostic tests

In many tumours assignment to a diagnostic category (e.g. adenoma or carcinoma) gives an indication of the prognosis for the individual patient but within such groupings (e.g. colorectal carcinoma) there may be wide variation in the biological behaviour of the tumour. In order to plan appropriate treatment and to be able to give useful information and counselling to individual patients many prognostic pathological tests have been developed.

In tumour pathology one of the most predictive prognostic tests is *staging* of the tumour (extent of spread) which is always assessed in the histopathological examination of specimens. One of the best examples of this is Dukes' staging of colorectal carcinoma (Ch. 11 and Ch. 15). The *histological type* of tumour has important prognostic implications, particularly in some organs; subjects with papillary thyroid carcinoma have a life expectancy which is the same as the rest of the general population without the tumour whereas subjects with anaplastic thyroid carcinoma have a median survival of a few months. The *grade* of the tumour, an assessment of its degree of differentiation and proliferative activity, also has predictive value.

In tumours which produce substances which enter the blood or urine (e.g. alpha-fetoprotein produced by testicular teratomas, see Ch. 20) then measurement of the levels of these at the time of diagnosis may be predictive of prognosis (and can be used in follow-up). Tests which have yet to establish themselves in routine prognostic pathology include the detection of oncogene and anti-oncogene products (Fig. 4.6). When evaluating any new prognostic test the significance for the individual patient has to be considered; a test which shows a statistically significant difference between two large groups of patients may not assign individual cases to a prognostic category with a sufficient degree of certainty to be useful in management decisions or patient information.

SPECIALISED TESTS

▶ Clinical chemistry: measurement and interpretation of substances in blood, other body fluids and tissues
▶ Cytogenetics: analysis of chromosomal and genetic abnormalities
▶ Cytopathology: diagnostic interpretation of the morphology and other characteristics of cells; commonly used in cancer screening and diagnosis
▶ Haematology: diagnosis of diseases of the bone marrow and blood; blood transfusion
▶ Histopathology: diagnostic interpretation of tissue samples
▶ Immunology: investigation of immunological responses
▶ Microbiology: detection and identification of viruses, bacteria, fungi and parasites

Clinical chemistry

Methods in clinical chemistry detect and measure subcellular substances—usually in the blood but also in other bodily fluids and tissue:

- blood
  — serum
  — plasma
  — red blood cells
- urine
- faeces
- gastric contents/aspirate
- effusions (e.g. pleural, pericardial).

The range of molecules measured is constantly expanding, ranging through electrolytes (such as sodium and potassium), larger inorganic molecules

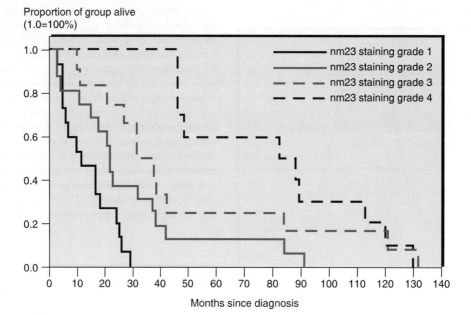

Fig. 4.6   Prognostic indices

nm23 is a putative anti-oncogene which is thought to suppress metastasis. This Kaplan–Meier graph shows the length of survival for patients with deep malignant melanomas according to grade of staining with an antibody directed against the product of nm23 gene. Those cases with strong staining (grade 4) survive for longer than those with least staining (grade 1). Such a test could give useful information about prognosis if studies with large numbers of patients confirmed these results. (Data courtesy Dr Janice Royds, Sheffield)

(urea), proteins (including many enzymes) and exogenous molecules (such as carbon monoxide and drugs):

- *blood gases*: e.g. oxygen, carbon dioxide
- *electrolytes*: e.g. sodium, potassium
- *smaller organic molecules*: e.g. urea, creatinine
- *hormones*: e.g. thyroid stimulating hormone, prolactin
- *non-enzymatic proteins*: e.g. albumin, lipoproteins
- *enzymes*: e.g. aspartate transaminase, amylase
- *drugs*: e.g. lithium, digoxin.

Since many of the tests in clinical chemistry are quantitative, the laboratories have extensive programmes of internal and external quality control, and laboratory reports quote reference ranges. For many tests ranges appropriate for the age and sex of the patient may be quoted.

As with all pathological tests the clinician with direct responsibility for the patient must decide whether a particular test is an appropriate investigation and what sample is most appropriate for that test. These considerations are especially important in clinical chemistry where large automated machines can measure a wide range of substances on a single sample and, if not used selectively, may generate non-essential data which may be difficult to interpret and require unnecessary further investigations.

The type of sample and the circumstances in which it is taken are also important. It is outside the scope of this chapter to give specific recommendations for individual tests but examples of inappropriate samples would be blood taken for glucose analysis shortly after a large carbohydrate-rich meal, blood taken for electrolyte analysis from a vein in an arm receiving an intravenous infusion, and blood taken for a digoxin level immediately after a dose of the drug.

The interpretation of results also requires knowledge about the substances being assayed and the advice of a specialist clinical chemist is often useful. An example of this is the use of cardiac enzymes measured to determine whether a myocardial infarct has occurred. The enzymes lactate dehydrogenase, aspartate transaminase and creatine phosphokinase normally reside intracellularly in muscle cells; if muscle is damaged then the enzymes gain entry to the blood and elevated levels may be detected. The interpretation of these assays requires knowledge about the time course of the enzyme release and the possible sites of enzyme release. The enzymes are not released immediately when the myocytes become hypoxic because the cell membranes take some time to break down; Figure 4.7 shows typical curves of the enzymes in blood after a myocardial infarct; it can also be seen from this graph that total creatine kinase and aspartate transaminase reach their peaks earlier than lactate dehydrogenase. The interpretation of the enzyme results will thus require knowledge of these properties and an estimate of when the ischaemic myocardial event is likely to have occurred in the patient. Cardiac muscle is not the only tissue to contain these enzymes, they are also present in skeletal muscle, but different forms of the enzymes (iso-enzymes) are present in the different sites. If an assay is used which measures the total amount of these enzymes then damage to skeletal muscle would produce elevations. Thus, if a patient had been found collapsed at home and had been lying on the floor, measurement of the iso-enzymes,

such as creatine kinase MB, or muscle proteins would be required to ascertain whether an ischaemic myocardial event had precipitated the collapse. Similar interpretative considerations apply to all tests in clinical chemistry.

Cytogenetics

Cytogenetics is playing a more important role in clinical pathology (Ch. 3) and discrete genetic abnormalities are being identified in specific tumours (Ch. 11). The number and form of chromosomes is called the *karyotype*; this can be examined using a sample of peripheral blood. Phytohaemagglutinin is added to the blood which stimulates the T-lymphocytes to divide, colchicine is then added to arrest the dividing cells in metaphase when the chromosomes will be most easily visible. The chromosomes may be stained by several methods but the most common is the Giemsa method which produces alternate light and dark bands when the preparation is viewed by light microscopy (G-banding); the patterns of banding allow identification of each chromosome and visualisation of missing or additional material of about 4000 kilobases or more. Abnormalities may be divided into:

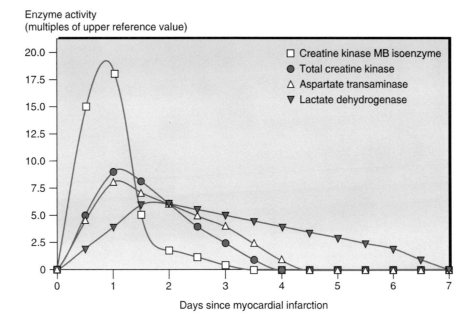

Fig. 4.7 Enzyme assays

Levels of the enzymes creatine kinase (total and MB iso-enzyme), aspartate transaminase and lactate dehydrogenase at time intervals after a myocardial infarct.

- numerical abnormalities
  - — aneuploidy
  - — polyploidy
- structural abnormalities
  - — translocation
  - — deletion and ring chromosome
  - — duplication
  - — inversion
  - — isochromosome
  - — centric fragment.

The number of chromosomal abnormalities associated with specific tumours is growing rapidly; currently there are over 30 human tumour types associated with non-random chromosomal abnormalities. One of the chromosomal abnormalities with the strongest association with a malignancy is the Philadelphia chromosome in chronic myeloid leukaemia. This abnormality is a reciprocal translocation between chromosome 9 and 22 resulting in the translocation of the *abl* oncogene to a breakpoint cluster region which results in a hybrid gene producing a novel protein which may be responsible for the neoplastic transformation (see Ch. 23). Another chromosomal abnormality strongly associated with a specific tumour is the 13q14 microdeletion seen in retinoblastoma.

As more of these abnormalities are found it becomes increasingly important to send tumour samples for cytogenetic analysis as a diagnostic/prognostic procedure. Cytogenetic analysis requires fresh tissue which has been placed in an appropriate transport medium and which must be transported rapidly to the cytogenetics laboratory. It is important to send appropriate samples which might include 'normal' background tissue as well as tumour; the most appropriate staff to do this might be the histopathologists if they receive the specimen fresh before immersion in a fixative solution. The investigation of individual genetic abnormalities is described in Chapter 3.

Cytopathology

Cytopathology specimens consist of single cells or clumps of cells which are dissociated from their surrounding tissues (Fig. 4.8). The technique is used mainly for the investigation and diagnosis of malignancy. The cells are distributed on glass slides, either by the person who takes the sample smearing them directly onto the slide at the time the sample is taken or by centrifugation methods in the laboratory. The slides are stained by an appropriate method, which is most often the Papanicolaou technique, and examined by light microscopy. Since the cells are dissociated from their surrounding tissue some features that are used in histopathological diagnosis, such as invasion and other architectural abnormali-

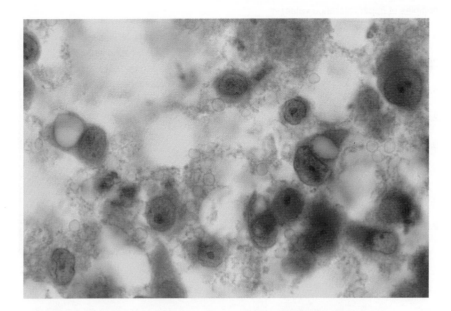

Fig. 4.8 Cytological preparation of a fine-needle aspirate of a breast carcinoma

The specimen consists of dissociated cells with no surrounding tissue.

ties, are not available for assessment. The main features used in cytopathological diagnosis are:

- variation in size of nuclei (nuclear pleomorphism)
- increased staining of DNA in the nucleus (nuclear hyperchromatism)
- ratio of nuclear area to cytoplasmic area (by subjective assessment).

Cells may be collected for cytological examination from epithelium shed or scraped from a body surface (*exfoliative cytology*) or by aspirating cells through a fine bore needle into a syringe (*aspiration cytology*). Many cytopathological specimens are taken to assess dysplasia or malignancy in tissues but infective pathologies may also be diagnosed by this method (for example *Pneumocystis carinii* pneumonia in immunosuppressed patients may be detected by cytological examination of alveolar washings).

Cancer screening

Cervix
One of the most frequent uses of cytopathological techniques is in the detection and assessment of dysplasia and neoplasia in the uterine cervix (see Ch. 19). The surface of the cervix is relatively accessible by speculum examination and cells are scraped from the surface at the junction between the squamous and glandular epithelium (the transformation zone) using a spatula. The cells are spread directly onto a glass slide, fixed and sent to the cytopathology laboratory where they are stained using the Papanicolaou technique. Cells from areas of dysplasia or neoplasia are recognised by their abnormal nuclear (*dyskaryotic*) features and the degree of abnormality is graded in a range from mild to severe. Mild abnormalities represent early dysplastic or reactive changes in the cervical epithelium which may regress, so the usual management for those women is surveillance by further smears. More severe changes (Fig. 4.9) represent marked dysplasia or carcinoma; women whose smears show such changes are referred to gynaecologists for further assessment and probable surgical treatment. In many countries cervical cytology is performed as a screening programme; the aim is to take samples at regular intervals from all women who are at risk of developing cervical cancer (which is most women with a uterus who have had sexual intercourse) and to detect early abnormalities which can be treated before invasive carcinoma has developed. The method of cytopathological examination of cells from the uterine cervix is effective in detecting the abnormalities but most cervical screening programmes have not been totally effective because a

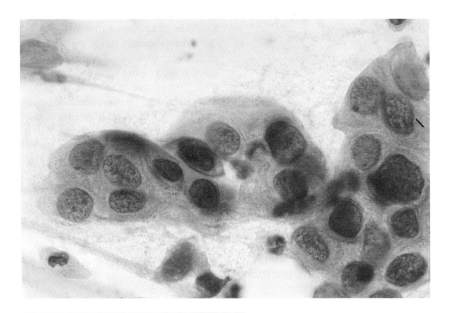

Fig. 4.9 Smear of cervical epithelial cells

There is nuclear hyperchromatism and pleomorphism consistent with a severe degree of dysplasia or actual carcinoma.

significant proportion of women have failed to attend for screening.

Breast

Another common use of cytopathology is the diagnosis of lesions in the breast. Palpable lesions in the breast are easily aspirated with a fine gauge needle and syringe and mammographically-detected impalpable lesions may be sampled using stereotactic radiographic sampling methods. The results of auditing cytopathological diagnosis of breast lesions have shown that a high degree of specificity and sensitivity can be obtained which is important if the service is to be clinically useful. In most centres the positive predictive value of a malignant cytopathological diagnosis is 100% (i.e. there are no false positives, so if this corresponds with the surgeon's clinical diagnosis and any mammographic findings then definitive surgery, such as wide local excision or mastectomy, may be undertaken without further diagnostic tests). Fine-needle aspiration of breast lesions has thus replaced needle core biopsy (which caused more pain and trauma to the patient), surgical biopsy of lesions (which required a longer hospital stay, possibly with a general anaesthetic) and intra-operative frozen section diagnosis (which did not allow full counselling of the patient before definitive treatment). It also has considerable cost savings to a breast disease service since it is performed as an outpatient procedure and the cost of specimen preparation is less than paraffin-embedded histology.

Haematology

Haematology covers diseases of the blood; the pathology of these is described in Chapter 23. The work of haematologists is usually divided into three areas:

- diagnosis of haematological disorders
- management of haematological disorders
- blood transfusion.

The diagnosis of haematological disorders is based on clinical history and examination, measurement of parameters in the blood, microscopic examination of blood films and often microscopic examination of bone marrow aspirates and trephine samples.

Automated machines measure many parameters in a sample of blood; the most common are:

- heamoglobin concentration
- red cell count
- packed cell volume (haematocrit)
- mean cell volume

- mean cell haemoglobin
- mean cell haemoglobin concentration
- white cell count and differential count
- platelet count
- coagulation times
  — prothrombin time
  — activated partial thromboplastin time
  — thrombin time
- fibrinogen concentration.

Such machines can produce a plethora of data and the same problems of interpretation may occur as described in the section on clinical chemistry above, but in haematology many of the parameters (e.g. haemoglobin, red cell count and mean cell volume) are linked and need to be examined together when making a diagnosis. Other measurements, such as of serum ferritin or cyanocobalamin (vitamin B_{12}), may need to be made to confirm the diagnosis.

Examination of the blood film can reveal abnormalities of red blood cell shape and size (e.g. anisocytosis, poikilocytosis, macrocytosis — see Ch. 23) and abnormal white blood cells such as blast cells in leukaemia. Some features, such as rouleaux formation by red blood cells, may suggest abnormalities in the non-cellular components of blood (in this case possible overproduction of antibodies or immunoglobulin).

Bone marrow examination

Samples of the bone marrow may be taken by insertion of a relatively large bore needle into a site, such as the iliac bone, and aspiration by a syringe. At the same time a tissue sample of marrow can be sampled with a trephine needle. A smear of aspirated cells, stained by the Giemsa method, allows identification of cells, and their relative proportions may be quantified. This is an integral part of the diagnosis of leukaemia and assessment of its response to treatment (see Ch. 23). Trephine samples of bone marrow retain the architecture of the tissue and allow assessment of the overall cellularity, amount of reticulin and site of different cell types; such samples are essential in diseases which produce fibrosis of the bone marrow, such as myelofibrosis or metastatic prostatic carcinoma, since aspirates will usually produce a very low cellular yield.

Blood transfusion

The primary purpose of blood transfusion is the supply of a product for the treatment of patients. The blood products which can be supplied include:

- red cell concentrates, for rapid correction of anaemia
- fresh frozen plasma, to replace coagulation factors
- platelets, for treatment of thrombocytopenia
- plasma fractions
  — albumin, to correct hypoalbuminaemia
  — immunoglobulin, for passive immunisation
  — factors VIII and IX, to treat or prevent bleeding in haemophilia A or B.

Primary concerns in the operation of a blood transfusion laboratory will include an error-free system of cross-matching (since a mismatched transfusion may prove fatal), safeguards against transmission of microbiological agents (such as HIV, hepatitis B and C) by transfusion, and balancing supply and demand of the products.

Histopathology

Histopathology involves the macroscopic examination of tissue with selection of tissue samples for light microscopic examination. Histopathology is usually the primary mode of diagnosis for tumours and also gives prognostic information by grading and staging of surgical resection specimens. Diagnosis of infective and inflammatory conditions can also be made as, for instance, the detection of *Helicobacter pylori* in gastric biopsies or the diagnosis of inflammatory conditions of the skin.

Most diagnostic histopathology is performed on haematoxylin and eosin-stained sections of paraffin-wax-embedded tissue. The tissue removed by surgical excision or biopsy is placed in a solution of fixative (most commonly formaldehyde) and transported to the histopathology laboratory. On receipt it is examined by the laboratory staff; a macroscopic description is given and tissue is selected for light microscopic examination. Larger specimens, where most of the tissue will not be examined by light microscopy, are assessed and sampled by medically-trained staff who are familiar with a wide range of macroscopic appearances and have a detailed knowledge of anatomy. The samples taken will vary but in a resection specimen would include samples of:

- tumour (for histogenetic pattern of differentiation and grading)
- resection margins
- lymph nodes
- background tissue.

The samples of tissue are processed by machine into paraffin wax, a process involving progressive dehydration through increasingly pure solutions of alcohol which is usually carried out overnight. The wax-embedded tissue samples are then mounted on a microtome and sections of 5–7 μm thickness are cut, mounted on glass slides and stained. These slides are interpreted by expert pathologists and reports are issued to the clinicians who sent the specimens. The reports are tailored to the type of specimen and the clinical details given on the request form. If a tumour is being examined the report will include the type of tumour, its grade (well, moderate or poorly differentiated), its stage (how far it has spread locally, whether any vascular invasion is detected and whether any sampled lymph nodes contain tumour) and comments on the surrounding tissue (e.g. whether there is dysplasia in background epithelium).

Although haematoxylin and eosin is the most commonly used stain there are other stains which may be used to investigate specific features of the tissue. Many of these are standard tinctorial procedures (Table 4.2).

Immunohistochemistry

An increasingly commonly used technique is *immunohistochemistry*. In this method antibodies are used which have been raised artificially to specific substances of interest (e.g. low molecular weight cytokeratins in a suspected epithelial tumour) and these bind to the specific substances if they are present in the tissue section. The bound antibody is then visualised using one of a variety of methods, such as antibodies against the initial anti-

Table 4.2 Commonly used stains in histopathology

Stain	Use
Haematoxylin and eosin	Routine stain for histological sections
Masson's trichrome	Fibrous tissue
Perls'	Haemosiderin
Masson–Fontana	Melanin
Modified Giemsa	Helicobacter
Ziehl–Neelsen	Acid-fast bacilli
Gram	Bacteria
Periodic acid Schiff	Glycogen, fungi
Grocott's silver stain	Fungi
Alcian blue	Acidic mucin
Periodic acid Schiff with diastase	Neutral mucin

body and a dye complex such as diaminobenzidine. Immunohistochemistry is useful in:

- typing tumours which are poorly differentiated and so are difficult to categorise from appearances on haematoxylin and eosin staining
- typing of lymphomas
- classification of glomerulonephritis.

In situ hybridisation (ISH)

DNA probes can be constructed which will bind to specific DNA or messenger RNA (mRNA) in tissue sections. The DNA probes are single-stranded sequences of DNA from tens to thousands of kilobases long and are labelled with radioisotopes, or now more commonly biotin or digoxigenin, to visualise the site of hybridisation using a colorimetric or fluorescent agent. The DNA in the tissue section is made into a single-stranded form, by conditions such as strong alkalis, and the probe will bind to complementary sequences in the target DNA or mRNA. This technique is useful for detecting infectious agents in tissue sections, such as cytomegalovirus or Epstein–Barr virus. It can also be used to detect production (rather than simply storage) of proteins in cells by detection of the mRNA for the specific protein.

Electron microscopy

Electron microscopy may be used to visualise subcellular detail in tissue samples. In the past this technique was used for detecting features of differentiation in tumours (such as melanosomes in malignant melanomas) but immunohistochemistry has largely replaced this function. Electron microscopy is still used in the classification of glomerulonephritis, where the site and nature of immune complexes in the glomerular basement membrane may be visualised (see Ch. 21).

Immunology

Immunology is concerned with the immune response, both antibody and cell mediated, in health and disease. The range of antibodies and cellular features that can be detected and measured has increased so much in recent years that many centres have a separate immunology department to deal with these. The various tests may be divided into those measuring antibodies and those measuring cells.

Immunoglobulins and antibodies

The overall levels of antibodies of certain classes can be measured but this is of little diagnostic use except in generalised immunodeficiencies such as hypogammaglobulinaemia. Detection or measurement of antibodies directed against specific antigens is important in the diagnosis and assessment of *autoimmune diseases*. Samples of a patient's serum are placed on tissue sections and any bound antibody can be visualised by applying further antibodies against human immunoglobulin (or a specific subclass) to which is attached an immunofluorescent dye. Auto-antibodies detected in this way include antinuclear antibodies found in systemic lupus erythematosus. To detect auto-antibodies bound to the patient's own tissues a sample of tissue is taken from the patient (this might be skin or a renal biopsy), antibodies against human immunoglobulins are applied to the biopsy and any bound antibody visualised by immunofluorescent or other techniques. This technique is used in the assessment of glomerulonephritis (see Ch. 21) and bullous skin disorders (pemphigus, pemphigoid, dermatitis herpetiformis, etc., see Ch. 24).

Lymphocytes

There are now antibodies to the specific antigens of most subsets of lymphocytes, such as T-cells or B-cells, T-suppressor cells, T-helper cells, etc., and in conjunction with other techniques (such as fluorescence activated cell sorting—FACS) the number of lymphocytes in each subclass can be measured. These measurements can give important information about a patient's immune status. In acquired immune deficiency syndrome (AIDS) there is selective destruction of T-helper cells by the human immunodeficiency virus (HIV) so that a reduction in the T-helper cell/T-suppressor cell ratio in HIV-positive subjects can indicate the onset of AIDS (see Ch. 9). In organ transplantation the detection of acute cellular rejection is important if appropriate immunosuppressive therapy is to be given in time to prevent loss of the graft. Rejection is primarily detected by histological examination of a biopsy of the graft (e.g. kidney) but measurement of the T-cell helper/suppressor ratio provides useful additional information and, with more specific subtyping of lymphocytes, such tests may eventually replace graft biopsy.

Microbiology

Microbiology involves the detection and identification

of micro-organisms including viruses, bacteria, fungi, protozoa and helminths. These may be detected by direct examination of a sample from a patient or by culture of such a sample to increase the number of organisms before using a detection method. Evidence of infection can also be inferred from serological tests for an antibody response to the organism. The susceptibility of cultured organisms to therapeutic agents, such as antibiotics, will also be assessed and microbiologists have wider responsibilities for general control of infection in hospitals and the community.

Direct detection methods in microbiology include:

- direct microscopy (by light or electron microscopy)
- specific antibody detection methods (visualised by enzyme-linked immunosorbent assay [ELISA], radio-immunoassay or immunofluorescence)
- nucleic acid hybridisation technology with labelled probes or the polymerase chain reaction (PCR).

These methods give rapid results, which can be very useful to clinicians. Examples of direct detection include the identification of *Pneumocystis carinii* in bronchoalveolar washings from immunosuppressed patients (such as those with AIDS), immunofluorescent detection of *Cryptosporidia* in faeces, and immunofluorescent detection of respiratory syncytial virus in nasopharyngeal aspirates.

Viruses

Viruses are obligate intracellular parasites and so can be grown only in a cellular culture, such as 'immortal' cells derived from tumours or cultures with a finite life-span derived from embryonic tissues. The presence of a virus may be detected by the presence of a cytopathic effect, by haemadsorption/haemagglutination or by the direct methods described above. The identity of the virus is confirmed by neutralisation of the cytopathic effect or haemadsorption/haemagglutination by antibodies raised against specific viruses. Serological tests are often used to diagnose viral infection: such tests involve the measurement of antibodies against specific viruses using a detection system such as ELISA, radio-immunoassay, immunofluorescence or complement fixation tests. A detectable level of virus-specific IgM or a four-fold rise in the titre of other classes of virus-specific antibody is an indication of recent infection with that virus.

Bacteria

Bacteria may be cultivated in cell-free media. For most purposes the medium used is solid rather than liquid ('broth'). Most solid culture media are based on agar, to which blood or other nutrients are added. Where it is wished to identify a specific pathogen existing in the presence of other bacteria, substances may be incorporated which will inhibit the growth of these other bacteria while not affecting the specific pathogen being sought ('selective media'). For any given type of specimen a range of media is chosen which will support the growth of all pathogens relevant to the clinical condition. Cultures are then incubated at appropriate temperatures and atmospheric conditions (i.e. aerobic and anaerobic). Most bacteria will grow within a few days and can then be identified by:

- the specific conditions in which they have grown
- morphology of their colonies on the culture plate
- by *Gram staining* of samples from the cultured colonies
- biochemical tests (such as the breakdown of carbohydrates)
- enzyme production (e.g. coagulase production by *Staphylococcus aureus*)
- serological tests of antigenic structure.

Some bacteria require specialised media and prolonged incubation in order to produce detectable colonies (for example *Mycobacterium tuberculosis* may need up to 8 weeks' incubation on Löwenstein–Jensen medium). The *susceptibility* of bacteria to antibiotics may be determined by various methods, most commonly by observing inhibition of bacterial growth around antibiotic-impregnated filter-paper discs placed on culture plates prior to incubation (Fig. 4.10). Microbiologists should provide advice on the empirical choice of antibiotics in cases where treatment may need to begin before the results of susceptibility tests are available.

Fungi

Fungi are grown on simple media (such as glucose peptone agar or blood agar with antibiotics to inhibit bacterial overgrowth) in aerobic conditions. Cultured fungi are identified by the method of spore production (asexual and sexual), morphology of the colony, morphology of vegetative and aerial hyphae, biochemical reactions and antigenic structure.

Parasites

Diseases caused by parasites are major problems in

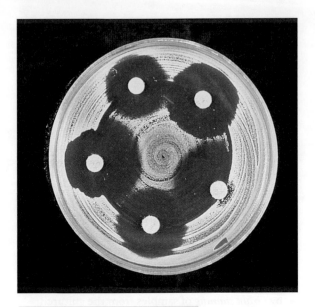

Fig. 4.10   Antibiotic sensitivities

A culture plate with antibiotic-impregnated discs on it showing inhibition of growth of bacteria around the discs and thus sensitivity to those antibiotics.

many countries, particularly those with tropical climates in which the vectors (e.g. insects) thrive. Parasites may be identified in, for example, tissue samples or faeces by their often distinctive morphology.

Precautions

When requesting microbiological tests it is especially important to send suitable specimens. Such samples should come from the likely site of infection, should not contain contaminants, should not contain substances likely to inhibit growth (such as antibiotics), should be put into a suitable container (which may contain a transport medium) and should be transported rapidly to the microbiology laboratory. If septicaemia is suspected but no focus of infection has been identified then multiple samples including blood and urine should be sent before systemic antibiotic therapy is started. The risk to staff looking after patients with microbiological infections, or handling specimens from them, is roughly classified according to the degree of hazard (Table 4.3). Most infective agents are included in category 2 (according to the scheme used in the UK). If a patient potentially has a category 3 pathogen then all samples should be marked as such since laboratories receiving these samples will have to take special precautions in handling them (this includes samples sent for non-microbiological investigations).

Hospital-acquired infections

Hospitals contain many patients with microbiological infections and there is considerable potential for spread to other patients. All hospitals should have agreed procedures for preventing the spread of infec-

Table 4.3   Categories of risk (in the UK) for infectious organisms*

Category	Risk	Examples
1	An organism that is most unlikely to cause human disease	Algae
2	An organism that may cause human disease and may be a hazard to those handling it, but is unlikely to spread to the community and effective prophylaxis or treatment is usually available	*Staphylococcus aureus, Escherichia coli*
3	An organism that may cause severe human disease and present a serious hazard to those handling it. It may present a risk of spread to the community but there is usually effective prophylaxis available	Hepatitis B virus, *Mycobacterium tuberculosis, Salmonella typhi*
4	An organism that causes severe human disease and is a serious hazard to those handling it. It may present a high risk of spread to the community and there is usually no effective prophylaxis or treatment	Lassa fever virus, Marburg virus

*Adapted from: Categorisation of pathogens according to hazard and categories of containment 1990, 2nd edn. ACDP, HMSO

tion including adequate sterilisation and disinfection, and isolation or barrier nursing when required. Such policies will have been formulated in consultation with the microbiologists of the hospital. The microbiological laboratory will be in a position to detect outbreaks of particular infections if there is suitable monitoring of laboratory results. An increasing problem in hospitals is the emergence of bacteria which are resistant to antibiotics, and this can be limited by the development of protocols for antibiotic usage.

AUTOPSIES

▶ May be performed for legal or medical purposes
▶ Information from autopsies is useful for clinical audit, education, medical research and allocation of resources
▶ Diagnostic discrepancies are revealed by autopsies in approximately 30% of cases

In most countries autopsies fall into two main categories:

1. those performed under the instruction of a legal authority
2. those performed with permission from the deceased's relatives for gathering further information about the nature and extent of the deceased's disease.

Medicolegal autopsies

Medicolegal autopsies are performed to determine the cause of death and to collect evidence that may be used in the prosecution of those alleged to be responsible for the death. In many cases of murder the cause of death (e.g. bullet wounds or stab wounds) is obvious and most of the work of the pathologist is the collection of evidence such as trace evidence confirming contact between the deceased and the person accused of the murder (e.g. blood stains, tissue beneath the deceased's fingernails, semen in body orifices) or evidence to link a specific weapon with the deceased's wounds (e.g. retrieval of bullets from wounds).

Clinical autopsies

Non-medicolegal (clinical) autopsies performed on patients who die in hospital may appear to be diagnostic tests that have been performed too late, but much useful information can be gathered from these procedures. Many studies have shown that the certified cause of death given by the clinicians with primary responsibility for the patient shows a discrepancy with the cause identified at autopsy, to the extent of being in a different organ system in about 30% of cases. The hospital autopsy is therefore very useful in providing more accurate data about the cause of death; this is important for *clinical audit*, for *education* of clinicians, and for national *allocation of health resources* if the cause of death is used as an index of the prevalence of disease (which it is in many countries including the UK). The hospital autopsy is also useful in defining the extent of disease and response to treatment. If a patient has had a malignant tumour, such as malignant melanoma, which has spread to other sites in the body and that patient has then received systemic treatment it is then important to have the most accurate data available about the organs to which the tumour had spread and whether the therapy had had any apparent effect on the tumour. Modern methods of in vivo imaging, such as computerised axial tomography and nuclear magnetic resonance, may provide some of this data but if the patient dies an autopsy is a simple and cost effective method of gathering accurate data.

The rate of autopsies on patients dying in hospital has shown a decline in most countries over the past decade; this will inevitably lead to loss of much useful information about human disease.

Autopsy techniques

Performing an autopsy is a relatively cheap, low technology procedure which has not changed much since the pioneering work of Virchow in the 19th century. A midline incision from the neck to symphysis pubis is made and the thoracic and abdominal organs are removed. The scalp is reflected from the skull and the cranium is opened to remove the brain. All the organs are dissected in detail by a medically-trained pathologist and the macroscopic appearances and weights are recorded; samples may be taken for microscopic examination, clinical chemistry analysis or microbiological culture. Return of the organs to the body cavities and reconstruction of the body produces an acceptable cosmetic result so that relatives can view the body after autopsy. More limited examination of the body can still generate useful information and so the examination may be limited (by the deceased's relatives' wishes) to certain areas of the body. This may allow an autopsy examination to be performed where permission would otherwise be refused (e.g. exclusion of examination of the cranial cavity in a patient who had received chemotherapy and had no hair, making any scalp incision clearly visible). The ultimate limited autopsy is the *needle autopsy* where percutaneous samples of organs are taken for histological examination using a needle core biopsy needle or fine-needle aspiration techniques; such a technique is useful to assess liver disease in cases of hepatitis B or C where risk of infection may preclude a full autopsy.

FURTHER READING

Connor J M, Ferguson-Smith M A 1993 Essential medical genetics, 4th edn. Blackwell Scientific Publications, Oxford

Cross S S, Cotton D W K 1993 The hospital autopsy. Butterworth-Heinemann, Oxford

Hoffbrand A V, Pettit J E 1993 Essential haematology, 3rd edn. Blackwell Scientific Publications, Oxford

Mayne P D 1994 Clinical chemistry in diagnosis and treatment, 6th edn. Edward Arnold, London

Roitt I 1994 Essential immunology, 8th edn. Blackwell Scientific Publications, Oxford

Sleigh J D, Timbury M C 1994 Notes on medical bacteriology, 4th edn. Churchill Livingstone, Edinburgh

Timbury M C 1994 Notes on medical virology, 10th edn. Churchill Livingstone, Edinburgh

Underwood J C E 1987 Introduction to biopsy interpretation and surgical pathology, 2nd edn. Springer-Verlag, Berlin

Part 2

DISEASE MECHANISMS

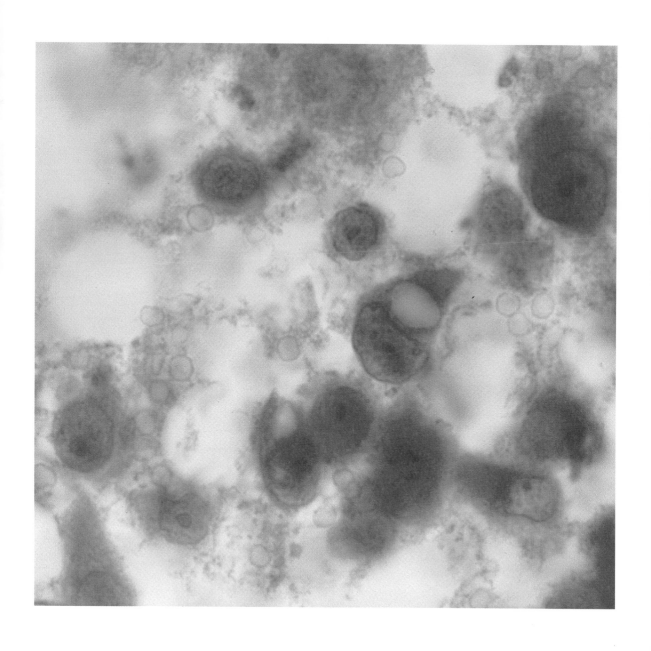

5

Disorders of growth, differentiation and morphogenesis

Growth, differentiation and *morphogenesis* are the processes by which a single cell, the fertilised ovum, develops into a large complex multicellular organism, with co-ordinated organ systems containing a variety of cell types, each with individual specialised functions. Growth and differentiation continue throughout adult life, as many cells of the body undergo a constant cycle of death, replacement and growth in response to normal (physiological) or abnormal (pathological) stimuli.

There are many stages in human embryological development at which anomalies of growth and/or differentiation may occur, leading to major or minor abnormalities of form or function, or even death of the fetus. In post-natal and adult life, some alterations in growth or differentiation may be beneficial, as in the development of increased muscle mass in the limbs of workers engaged in heavy manual tasks. Other changes may be detrimental to health, as in cancer, where the outcome may be fatal.

This chapter explores the wide range of abnormalities of growth, differentiation and morphogenesis which may be encountered in clinical practice, relating them where possible to specific deviations from normal cellular functions or control mechanisms.

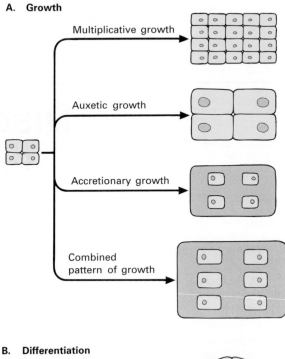

A. Growth

Multiplicative growth

Auxetic growth

Accretionary growth

Combined pattern of growth

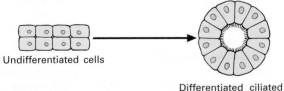

B. Differentiation

Undifferentiated cells

Differentiated ciliated cells in bronchus

DEFINITIONS

Growth

Growth is the process of increase in size resulting from the synthesis of specific tissue components. The term may be applied to populations, individuals, organs, cells, or even subcellular organelles such as mitochondria.

Types of growth in a tissue (Fig. 5.1A) are:

- *Multiplicative*, involving an increase in numbers of cells (or nuclei and associated cytoplasm in syncytia) by mitotic cell divisions. This type of growth is present in all tissues during embryogenesis.
- *Auxetic*, resulting from increased size of individual cells, as seen in growing skeletal muscle.
- *Accretionary*, an increase in intercellular tissue components, as in bone and cartilage.
- *Combined patterns* of multiplicative, auxetic and accretionary growth as seen in embryological development, where there are differing directions and rates of growth at different sites of the

---

Fig. 5.1   Growth and differentiation

A. Types of growth in a tissue. **B.** Differentiation of undifferentiated cells into ciliated cells in bronchus.

---

developing embryo, in association with changing patterns of cellular differentiation.

Differentiation

Differentiation is the process whereby a cell develops an overt specialised function or morphology which distinguishes it from its parent cell. Thus, differentiation is the process by which genes are expressed selectively and gene products act to produce a cell with a specialised function (Fig. 5.1B). After fertilisation of the human ovum, and up to the eight-cell stage of development, all of the embryonic cells are apparently identical. Thereafter, cells undergo several stages of differentiation in their passage to fully differentiated cells, such as, for example, the ciliated epithelial cells lining the respiratory passages of the nose and trachea. Although the changes at each stage of differentiation may be minor, differentiation can be said to have occurred only if there has been *overt* change in cell morphology (e.g. development of a skin epithelial cell from an ectodermal cell), or an alteration in the specialised function of a cell (e.g. the synthesis of a hormone).

Morphogenesis

> ▶ Complex process of embryological development
> ▶ Responsible for formation of shape and organisation of body organs
> ▶ Involves cell growth and differentiation, and relative movement of cell groups
> ▶ Programmed cell death (apoptosis) removes unwanted features

Morphogenesis is the highly complex process of development of structural shape and form of organs, limbs, facial features, etc. from primitive cell masses during embryogenesis. For morphogenesis to occur, primitive cell masses must undergo co-ordinated growth and differentiation, with movement of some cell groups relative to others, and focal programmed cell death (apoptosis) to remove unwanted features.

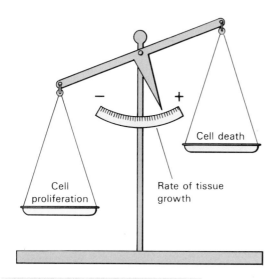

Fig. 5.2   Cell proliferation and death

Growth rate is determined by the balance between cell proliferation and cell death.

CELL TURNOVER

In both fetal and adult life, tissue growth depends upon the balance between the increase in cell numbers, due to cell proliferation, and the decrease in cell numbers due to cell death (Fig. 5.2).

In fetal life, growth is rapid and all cell types proliferate, but even in the fetus there is constant cell death, some of which is an essential (and genetically programmed) component of morphogenesis. In postnatal and adult life, however, the cells of many tissues lose their capacity for proliferation at the high rate of the fetus, and cellular replication rates are variably reduced. Some cells continue to divide rapidly and continuously, some divide only when stimulated by the need to replace cells lost by injury or disease, and others are unable to divide whatever the stimulus.

Regeneration

> ▶ Process of replacing injured or dead cells
> ▶ Cell types vary in regenerative ability
> ▶ *Labile cells*: very high regenerative ability and rate of turnover (e.g. intestinal epithelium)
> ▶ *Stable cells*: good regenerative ability but low rate of turnover (e.g. hepatocytes)
> ▶ *Permanent cells*: no regenerative ability (e.g. neurones)

Regeneration enables cells or tissues destroyed by injury or disease to be replaced by functionally identical cells. The ability of cells to proliferate governs their regenerative potential. Mammalian cells fall into three classes according to their regenerative ability:

- labile
- stable
- permanent.

Labile cells proliferate continuously in post-natal life; they have a short life-span and a rapid 'turnover' time. Their high regenerative potential means that lost cells are rapidly replaced. However, the high cell turnover renders these cells highly susceptible to the toxic effects of radiation or drugs (such as anti-cancer drugs) which interfere with cell division. Examples of labile cells include:

- haemopoietic cells of the bone marrow, and lymphoid cells
- epithelial cells of the skin, mouth, pharynx, oesophagus, the gut, exocrine gland ducts, the cervix and vagina (squamous epithelium),

endometrium, urinary tract (transitional epithelium), etc.

The high regenerative potential of the skin is exploited in the treatment of patients with skin loss due to severe burns. The surgeon removes a layer of the split skin which includes the dividing basal cells from the unburned donor site, and fixes it firmly to the burned graft site where the epithelium has been lost (see Ch. 6). Dividing basal cells in the graft and the donor site ensure regeneration of squamous epithelium at both sites, enabling rapid healing in a large burned area where regeneration of new epithelium from the edge of the burn would otherwise be prolonged.

Stable cells (sometimes called 'conditional renewal cells') divide very infrequently under normal conditions, but are stimulated to divide rapidly when such cells are lost. This group includes cells of the liver, endocrine glands, bone, fibrous tissue and the renal tubules.

Permanent cells normally divide only during fetal life and they cannot be replaced when lost. Cells in this category include neurones, cardiac muscle cells and skeletal muscle (although skeletal muscle cells do have a very limited capacity for regeneration).

The cell cycle

Successive phases of progression of a cell through its cycle of replication are defined with reference to DNA synthesis and cellular division. Unlike the synthesis of most cellular constituents, which occurs throughout the interphase period between cell divisions, DNA synthesis occurs only during a limited period of the interphase; this is the *S phase* of the cell cycle. A further distinct phase of the cycle is the cell-division stage or *M phase* (Fig. 5.3) comprising nuclear division (mitosis) and cytoplasmic division (cytokinesis). Following the M phase, the cell enters the *first gap (G_1) phase* and, via the S phase, the *second gap (G_2) phase* before entering the M phase again.

Some cells (e.g. some of the stable cells) may 'escape' from the G_1 phase of the cell cycle by temporarily entering a G_0 'resting' phase; others 'escape' permanently to G_0 by a process of *terminal differentiation*, with loss of potential for further division and death at the end of the lifetime of the cell; this occurs in permanent cells, such as neurones.

Molecular events in the cell cycle

At the molecular level, growth is stimulated initially by the receptor-mediated actions of *growth factors* — e.g. epidermal growth factor (EGF), platelet-derived growth factor (PDGF) and insulin-like growth factors (IGF-1 and IGF-2) — on cells in the quiescent G_0 phase of the cell cycle (Fig. 5.3) via intracellular second messengers. Stimuli are transmitted to the nucleus of the cell, where transcription factors are activated, leading to the initiation of DNA synthesis followed by cell division.

The process of cell cycling is modified by the actions of the *cyclin* family of proteins, which activate

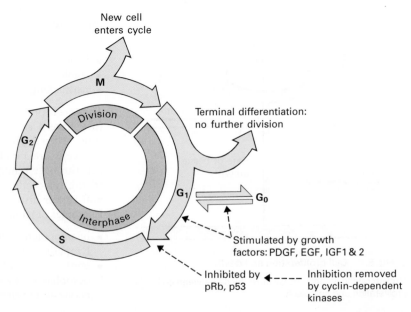

Fig. 5.3 The cell cycle

The four main stages of the cell cycle are the M phase (mitosis and cytokinesis, i.e. cell division), and the interphase stages G_1 (gap 1), S phase (DNA synthesis) and G_2 (gap 2). Cells may enter a resting phase (G_0), which may be of variable duration, followed by re-entry into the G_1 phase. Some cells may terminally differentiate from the G_1 phase, with no further cell division and death at the end of the normal lifetime of the cell. The sites at which growth factors and inhibitors act are shown.

(by phosphorylation) a number of proteins involved in DNA replication, mitotic spindle formation and other events in the cell cycle. Thus, for example, the inhibitory (antimitotic) action of the retinoblastoma gene product pRb is itself inhibited by the phosphorylating action of a cyclin-dependent kinase (Fig. 5.3); removal of this growth-inhibiting action of the retinoblastoma gene allows growth to proceed (see Ch. 11).

Duration of cell cycle

In mammals, different cell types divide at very different rates, with observed cell cycle times (also called generation times) ranging from as little as eight hours, in the case of gut epithelial cells, to 100 days or more, exemplified by hepatocytes in the normal adult liver. The principal difference between rapidly dividing cells and those which divide slowly is the time spent in the G_1 phase of the cell cycle; some cells remain in the G_1 phase for days or even years. In contrast, the duration of S, G_2 and M phases of the cell cycle is remarkably constant, and independent of the rate of cell division.

Therapeutic interruption of cell cycle

Many of the drugs used in the treatment of cancer affect particular stages within the cell cycle (Fig. 5.4). These drugs inhibit the rapid division of cancer cells,

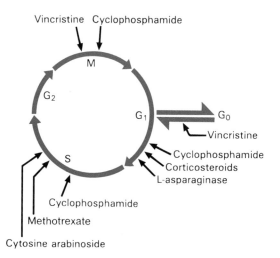

Fig. 5.4 Pharmacological interruption of the cell cycle

The sites of action in the cell cycle of drugs that may be used in the treatment of cancer.

although there is often inhibition of other rapidly dividing cells, such as the cells of the bone marrow and lymphoid tissues. Thus, anaemia, a bleeding tendency and suppression of immunity may be clinically important side-effects of cancer chemotherapy.

Cell death in growth and morphogenesis

It seems illogical to think of cell death as a component of normal growth and morphogenesis, although we recognise that the loss of a tadpole's tail, which is mediated by genetically-programmed cell death, is part of the metamorphosis of a frog. Cell death is a paradox of growth, and it is now clear that cell death has an important role in the development of an embryo, and in the regulation of tissue size throughout life. Alterations in the rate at which cell death occurs are important in situations such as hormonal growth regulation, immunity and neoplasia.

Apoptosis

The term *apoptosis* is used to define the type of individual cell death which is related to growth and morphogenesis, but which appears to have an opposite function in regulating the size of a cell population. Apoptosis is a biochemically specific mode of cell death characterised by activation of non-lysosomal endogenous endonuclease which digests nuclear DNA into smaller DNA fragments. Morphologically, apoptosis is recognised as death of scattered single cells which form rounded, membrane-bound bodies; these are eventually phagocytosed (ingested) and broken down by adjacent unaffected cells.

The coincidence of both mitosis and apoptosis within a cell population ensures a continuous renewal of cells, rendering a tissue more adaptable to environmental demands than one in which the cell population is static.

Apoptosis can be triggered by factors outside the cell or it can be an autonomous event ('programmed cell death'). In embryological development, there are three categories of autonomous apoptosis:

- morphogenetic
- histogenic
- phylogenetic.

Morphogenetic apoptosis is involved in alteration of tissue form. Examples include:

- interdigital cell death responsible for separating the fingers (Fig. 5.5)
- cell death leading to the removal of redundant epithelium following fusion of the palatine

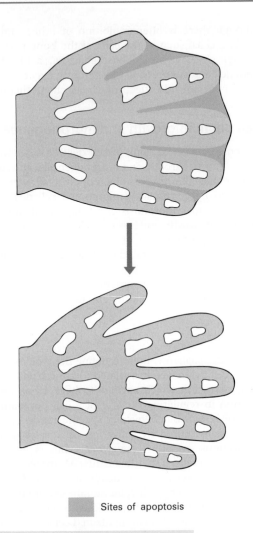

Sites of apoptosis

Fig. 5.5   Morphogenesis by apoptosis

Genetically programmed apoptosis (individual cell death) causing separation of the fingers during embryogenesis.

processes during development of the roof of the mouth
- cell death in the dorsal part of the neural tube during closure, required to achieve continuity of the epithelium, the two sides of the neural tube and the associated mesoderm.

Failure of morphogenetic apoptosis in these three sites is a factor in the development of *syndactyly* (webbed fingers), *cleft palate* (see p. 106) and *spina bifida* (see p. 105), respectively.

Histogenic apoptosis occurs in the differentiation of tissues and organs, as seen, for example, in the hormonally-controlled differentiation of the accessory reproductive structures from the Müllerian and

Wolffian ducts. In the male, for instance, anti-Müllerian hormone produced by the Sertoli cells of the fetal testis causes regression of the Müllerian ducts (which in females form the fallopian tubes, uterus and upper vagina) by the process of apoptosis.

Phylogenetic apoptosis is involved in removing vestigial structures from the embryo; structures such as the pronephros, a remnant from a much lower evolutionary level, are removed by the process of apoptosis.

Regulation of apoptosis

When cells within tissues are stimulated to divide by mitogens the tissues enter a high turnover state, in which mitotic activity is accompanied by some degree of coincident apoptosis (Fig. 5.6). The ultimate fate of individual cells within the tissue—whether the cell will survive or undergo apoptosis—depends upon the balance between apoptosis inducers (survival inhibitors) and apoptosis inhibitors (survival factors). Although apoptosis can be induced by diverse signals in a variety of cell types, a few genes appear to regulate a final common pathway. The most important of these are the members of the *bcl-2* family (*bcl-2* was originally identified at the t (14;18) chromosomal breakpoint in follicular B-cell lymphoma, and it can inhibit many factors which induce apoptosis). The *bax* protein (also in the *bcl-2* family) forms *bax–bax* dimers which enhance apoptotic stimuli. The ratio of *bcl-2* to *bax* determines the cell's susceptibility to apoptotic stimuli, and constitutes a 'molecular switch' which determines whether a cell will survive, leading to tissue expansion, or undergo apoptosis.

The study of factors regulating apoptosis is of considerable importance in finding therapeutic agents to enhance cell death in malignant neoplasms.

SYSTEMIC GROWTH DISORDERS

The most obvious indication of growth of an individual is an increase in height, which is largely a function of longitudinal skeletal growth. The most rapid normal growth occurs during fetal life, when the embryo undergoes the equivalent of some 42 cell divisions in progressing from a fertilised ovum to term (at 40 weeks), with only five more cell divisions needed to achieve adult size. In the first 2 months of embryological life, differing rates of growth, death and migration of cells are responsible for morphogenesis (development of form) within the developing fetus. Maximal growth velocity, however, does not occur until about 20 weeks' gestation (for body

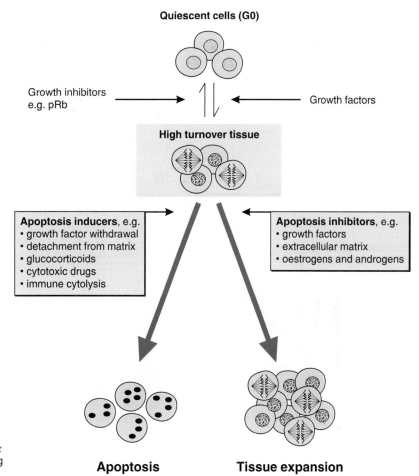

Fig. 5.6   Control of tissue growth by induction or inhibition of apoptosis

Quiescent (mitotically inactive) cells in G_0 are recruited into a high turnover (mitotically active) state by growth factors (see Fig. 5.3). Their subsequent fate depends on the presence or absence of apoptosis inducers or inhibitors. The inducers and inhibitors are mediated by the *bax* and *bcl-2* proteins respectively, among others.

length) and 34 weeks (for body weight); growth velocity then slows until term.

Despite apparently precise genetic programming of growth, marked variations in birth size can occur due to either normal physiological processes or disease. In infancy and childhood there may be variations in height between individuals of the same sex, but the most important normal variations are those between the heights of the two sexes. In childhood, girls are typically shorter than boys, but they become temporarily taller than boys as a result of their pre-pubertal growth spurt (9 cm/year), which starts at around 10.5 years of age. The boys' growth spurt starts at about 12.5 years, but the higher growth velocity (10.3 cm/year) results in their overtaking the girls in height at about 14 years, and accounts for the final height advantage in boys.

Within an individual, different parts of the body do not follow the same pattern as longitudinal growth. Children have relatively larger heads compared with the trunk and legs than do adults. The reproductive organs grow little before puberty, but then increase rapidly in size. Lymphoid organs grow maximally before puberty, and their growth velocity decreases before skeletal growth velocity.

Growth is controlled by and susceptible to variations in:

- hormones and growth factors
- genetic factors
- nutrition
- environmental factors
- disease.

Endocrinological growth control and its disorders

Cells may be stimulated into growth by the action of hormones and growth factors (Fig. 5.7). *Hormones*

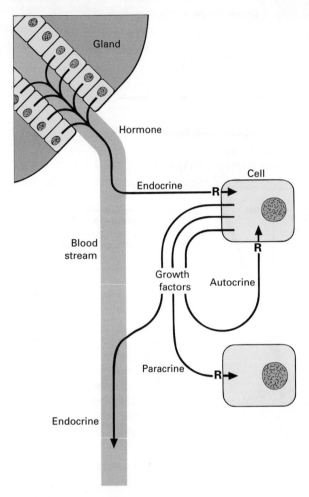

Fig. 5.7 Endocrine, paracrine and autocrine mechanisms of hormones and growth factors

In each case, the hormone and growth factors have their effects through specific receptors (**R**).

are synthesised and stored in specific tissues (glands) and released into the blood to exert their effect on distant target cells; this is the *endocrine* mechanism. *Growth factors* are synthesised in many different cell types throughout the body. They often act on the cell in which they are synthesised (an *autocrine* mechanism), or on nearby cells in the same tissue (a *paracrine* mechanism), but they may have additional endocrine actions on distant cells via the blood stream.

Individual hormones and growth factors require highly specific cellular receptors to mediate their actions on target cells. Steroid hormone receptors are intracellular, but receptors for peptide hormones and growth factors are located on the cell membrane. A high concentration of a receptor renders a cell highly susceptible to the actions of a hormone or growth factor; conversely, the absence of a receptor leads to hormone or growth factor insensitivity.

Post-natal growth

In post-natal life, growth is controlled by an endocrine pathway which regulates total body size (Fig. 5.8). Growth hormone (GH) is central to the endocrine control of post-natal growth.

The release of GH from the pituitary is regulated by the opposing actions of hypothalamic growth hormone releasing factor (GRF) and the inhibitory hormone somatostatin. Growth hormone acts via intermediary hormones — the somatomedins, insulin-like growth factor 1 (IGF-1) and insulin-like growth factor 2 (IGF-2); these are predominantly (but not exclusively) synthesised in the liver. Somatomedins may also be released from the liver under the influence of insulin, sex-steroid hormones, thyroid hormone and nutritional factors. Growth hormone may have a minor direct anabolic effect on non-skeletal tissues, but here too IGF-1 and IGF-2 are quantitatively more important.

Again, it is important to appreciate that each of the above hormone actions is mediated via individual specific cellular receptor proteins, the concentration of which principally determines the sensitivity of the target cell to the hormone.

Reduced growth

Reduced GH production due to hypopituitarism (of whatever pathological cause) in childhood leads to dwarfism which can be corrected by regular GH injections given before puberty arrests skeletal growth by epiphyseal fusion. Dwarfism due to GH deficiency is characterised by normal body proportions, in contrast to the effects of reduced thyroid hormones (see below).

Reduced GH receptors are a feature of the rare Laron dwarfism. Although circulating GH concentrations are high, the liver is insensitive to GH, and circulating somatomedins are greatly reduced. Treatment with GH will not increase growth rate.

Reduced thyroid hormone secretion causes a reduction in hepatic IGF-1 secretion. In the resultant dwarfism, the head is of normal size but the limbs are stunted because bone ossification is reduced. Treatment with GH has no effect, but thyroxine is corrective if given before puberty.

Block between GH and IGF-1 release may occur in malnutrition or emotionally-based growth retardation, although the metabolite-mobilising actions of GH are maintained. IGF-1 levels correlate positively

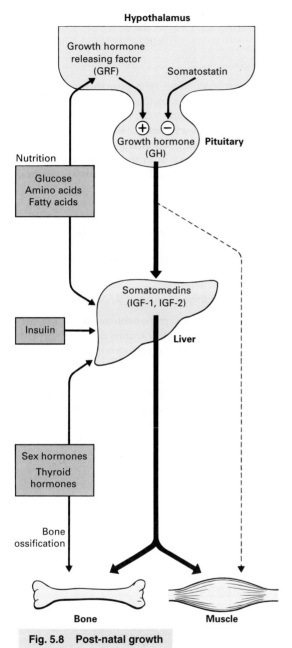

Hypothalamus

Growth hormone releasing factor (GRF)

Somatostatin

$\oplus$ $\ominus$
Growth hormone (GH) **Pituitary**

Nutrition

Glucose
Amino acids
Fatty acids

Somatomedins
(IGF-1, IGF-2)

Liver

Insulin

Sex hormones
Thyroid
hormones

Bone
ossification

Bone

Muscle

Fig. 5.8   Post-natal growth

The hormonal control of post-natal growth is mediated by
hypothalamic and pituitary hormones, and liver
somatomedins — the insulin-like growth factors 1 and 2 (IGF-1
and IGF-2).

with the protein content of the diet and nitrogen balance.

Inhibition of growth by corticosteroids may occur with
endogenous corticosteroids, e.g. Cushing's disease,
or with exogenous corticosteroids used, for example,
in the treatment of asthma or leukaemia.

Increased growth
Increased GH secretion from a normal pituitary or a
pituitary tumour results in increased IGF-1 and
increased growth. Before puberty this causes *gigantism*; after puberty, longitudinal skeletal growth cannot occur (due to maturation and ossification with
resulting epiphyseal fusion), but the hands, feet and
head increase in size to produce *acromegaly*.

Increased sex-steroid hormone secretion in childhood
may lead to precocious puberty, with an initial
increase in height resulting from a premature rise in
pubertal IGF-1 levels. However, epiphyseal fusion in
long bones is accelerated, and the final height may
be *below* normal.

Embryo and fetal growth

The mechanisms of endocrinological growth control
in the first few weeks of embryological life are as yet
unknown, although it is likely that autocrine and
paracrine actions of growth factors are involved.

The control of growth later in fetal life is very different from that in the post-natal child. The fetus is a
self-contained unit with respect to growth, as maternal peptide and thyroid hormones do not cross the
placenta in physiologically significant concentrations
and, although sex-steroid hormones and other
steroids do cross the placenta, they are generally
metabolised into inactive forms.

The fetus produces its own GH, but this is not
used to promote growth as the GH receptor is greatly reduced in the fetus (particularly in the liver).
Fetal growth does not require a pituitary, a hypothalamus or even a head, and anencephalic human fetuses often attain normal weights for gestational age.

Although fetal growth is not GH-mediated,
somatomedins (particularly IGF-2 in the fetus) are
important, although they are not yet under GH control. Other growth factors, such as epidermal growth
factor (EGF), platelet-derived growth factor (PDGF),
transforming growth factor beta (TGF-β) and nerve
growth factor (NGF), are probably also involved.

The most important growth-regulating hormone
in the fetus is, without doubt, *insulin* (Fig. 5.9). As
in the adult, blood insulin concentrations in the
fetus are controlled by glucose concentrations, and
both insulin and glucose are required for normal
metabolic functions of the fetus and the placenta.
In addition, however, insulin directly stimulates
the production of growth factors (in particular the
somatomedin, IGF-II) in cells, and these act on the

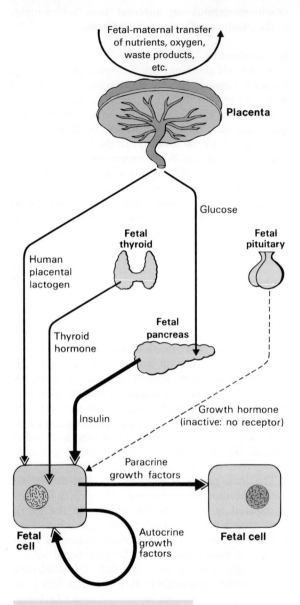

Fig. 5.9   Fetal growth regulation

Insulin is the major hormone stimulating growth in the fetus; its action is mediated by growth factors. Growth hormone receptors are not present during most of fetal life. Placental and thyroid hormones are also important.

IGF-2-synthesising cells and adjacent cells, by autocrine and paracrine mechanisms respectively, to stimulate growth. Additional, but relatively less important, effects on growth factor synthesis are stimulated by human placental lactogen (HPL) — a hormone which has marked structural similarity to

GH, and is synthesised by the placenta — and fetal thyroid hormones.

Birthweight

Many factors may affect fetal growth rate and ultimate size (Table 5.1). Although insulin levels are crucial, the most common causes of low birthweight are premature delivery (before 40 weeks' gestation) and genetically controlled small size (a small baby born to small parents). It is therefore important to relate the birthweight first to gestational age and then to allow for parental size.

Reduced growth
Reduced fetal insulin production may lead to a low birthweight e.g. 1.2–2 kg (normal mean 3 kg). The causes are uncommon, and include:

- fetal diabetes mellitus.
- pancreatic agenesis (failure of development)

Reduced fetal insulin receptors, with resultant insensitivity to circulating insulin, causes a similar growth reduction (the rare Leprechaun syndrome).

Increased growth
Increased growth occurs due to increased circulating insulin levels in the fetus (hyperinsulinaemia).

Diabetic mothers may have heavy infants, although birth lengths are not usually increased. Increased glucose diffuses passively into the fetus from the

Table 5.1 Factors affecting fetal growth rate and size		
Factors	Examples
Decreased growth	
Genetic	Small parents
	Racial origin (e.g. pygmies)
Endocrine	Reduced fetal insulin or insulin receptor levels (rare)
Nutrition	Maternal intake <1500 kcal/day
Intra-uterine environment	Placental disease
	Decreased oxygen (high altitude)
	Maternal smoking
	Maternal alcohol consumption
	Maternal drug abuse
	Infection
Increased growth	
Endocrine	Fetal hyperinsulinaemia (e.g. in maternal diabetes mellitus)

mother, stimulating fetal insulin secretion. The increased weight is due mainly to excess fat.

Infants with hyperinsulinaemia associated with the rare condition *nesidioblastosis* (an uncontrolled proliferation of pancreatic endocrine cells) or Beckwith–Weidemann syndrome (see below) are more obviously overgrown, e.g. birthweight 4.5–5.5 kg (normal mean 3 kg).

Genetic factors in growth control

The most important genetic factors which regulate the height of an individual are:

- *parental height*, probably mediated by multifactorial genetically controlled endocrinological factors
- the *sex* of the individual, mediated by sex-steroid hormones (as discussed above).

As such a large number of hormones, growth factors, receptors, enzymes and other proteins play a coordinated role in normal growth, it is not surprising that a wide range of chromosomal abnormalities can interfere with normal growth. Some of these conditions are inherited; others are the results of sporadic gene mutation or chromosomal aberration. Some conditions are incompatible with life; others are compatible with a normal life modified only by reduced stature.

Primary genetically-mediated growth abnormalities are classified into two broad groups, according to whether growth of the limbs and/or trunk with respect to the head is *proportionate* or *disproportionate*.

Proportionate alterations of skeletal growth

Autosomal chromosomes
Proportionate alterations of skeletal growth may result from abnormalities of autosomal chromosomes including:

- *pygmies*: genetically-mediated inability to make the somatomedin IGF-1 (chromosome 12)
- *Down's syndrome* (mongolism): short stature associated with trisomy 21 (extra 21 chromosome)
- *Beckwith–Weidemann syndrome*: increased growth due to a rare duplication of the short arm of chromosome 11 (carrying the genes for insulin and the somatomedin IGF-2).

Sex chromosomes (X and Y)
Sex chromosome abnormalities leading to proportional abnormalities of skeletal growth include:

- *Turner's syndrome*: females have an XO rather than XX genotype. In its most extreme form, girls have no ovaries, and lack of oestrogens prevents a normal pubertal growth spurt.
- *Pseudohypoparathyroidism*: a very rare X-linked dominant condition characterised by tissue insensitivity to parathyroid hormone (PTH), probably due to reduced or absent PTH receptors.

Disproportionate alterations of skeletal growth

Disproportionate shortness of stature at birth is often the result of the genetically-mediated *osteochondrodysplasias* (specific disorders of growth of bone and/or cartilage). These can be classified into two groups, depending upon whether the disproportionate shortness of limbs is, or is not, accompanied by a significantly shortened spine. Examples of these conditions include:

Achondroplasia
Achondroplasia, the most common of the osteochondrodysplasias, is an autosomal dominant condition (although there are many sporadic cases). The genetically-mediated defect is considered to be a primary disturbance of endochondral ossification which occurs in early life and is well established by birth (although severely affected fetuses may die towards the end of pregnancy). Achondroplastics, if they survive the neonatal period, usually reach adult life but with reduced stature. Mildly affected cases are usually of normal intelligence, but this may be reduced in more severe cases.

Achondroplastics have variably severe shortening of the limbs (hypomelia or micromelia), with long bones as little as half the normal length. Epiphyses are greatly enlarged, and the shafts of long bones widen to surround the enlarged epiphyses at the ends of long bones. Accompanying changes in the base of the skull may cause narrowing of the foramen magnum, with spinal cord compression. The spine itself is not shortened.

Rare osteochondrodysplasias
Many (but not all) of these rare conditions have an autosomal recessive mode of inheritance. They include severe conditions such as achondrogenesis, which is incompatible with life, and conditions such as pseudoachondroplasia, where the spine is shortened in addition to the limbs.

Nutritional factors in growth control

Maternal nutrition, surprisingly, has a very small

influence on human *fetal size*, and even severe food deprivation results in little more than a 200–300 g reduction in birthweight. In the Dutch winter famine of 1944, birthweight declined only when maternal nutritional input was less than 1500 kcal per day, and then by no more than 500 g.

The fetus is, however, highly susceptible to placental disorders such as infection or to partial detachment, both of which reduce the fetal intake of nutrients and impair gas exchange; the result, if not fatal, may be a severe reduction in birthweight. Small local defects, such as small haemangiomas, do not affect placental function, and hence do not affect growth.

In *post-natal life*, growth may be severely affected by low or poorly-balanced nutritional intake. Starvation, in the form of kwashiorkor (protein deprivation) or marasmus (protein and total calorie deprivation) (Ch. 7), severely disturbs growth endocrinology, producing a negative nitrogen balance as part of a catabolic state.

Environmental factors in growth control

Fetal growth can be affected by several physiological and pathological environmental factors:

- *Uterine size.* The size of the uterus is an important constraining influence on fetal size, as shown in classical experiments by Walton and Hammond in 1938 in which reciprocal hybrids of the huge Shire horse and the tiny Shetland pony grew much larger in the uterus of the Shire horse than the Shetland pony. Clinical observations of humans suggest that the uterine effect on fetal growth occurs late in gestation, and does not affect the fetus during early pregnancy.
- *Altitude.* Infants born at an altitude of 15 000 feet (4570 m) have a birthweight 16% less than infants born at 500 feet (150 m); this is due to decreased intra-uterine oxygen availability.
- *Maternal smoking.* The effect of smoking 20 cigarettes per day is to reduce birthweight by about 200 g (about 7%), probably by reducing uterine blood flow.
- *Maternal alcohol abuse.* This retards fetal growth, and catch-up growth does not occur. Fetuses may be microcephalic, with hypotonia and mental retardation. Cardiac atrial septal defects are common, and there may be altered facies (facial features). This is the 'fetal-alcohol syndrome'.
- *Maternal drug abuse.* About half of the fetuses exposed to heroin have a low birthweight. The mechanism is uncertain, but it may involve co-existent socio-economic factors rather than a direct effect of heroin. The newborn infants often develop withdrawal symptoms.

Post-natal environmental growth effects can be seen in children from unstable home backgrounds (e.g. emotional deprivation, physical abuse), who may have a reduced rate of growth. Catch-up growth occurs following hospitalisation, without medication.

Effect of intercurrent disease on growth

The commonest growth alterations in childhood are those which are caused indirectly by a wide range of diseases, which decrease growth for the duration of the illness and are followed by a period of 'catch-up' growth. These diseases include common bacterial and viral illnesses experienced by many children. Some are relatively short-lived and the decreased growth may not be noticed. However, with increasing severity and chronicity of the illness it is more likely that the growth disturbance will be noticeable and clinically significant. Thus, severe growth disturbance may be present in chronic cardiovascular or respiratory disease, renal disease, hepatic cirrhosis, chronic gastrointestinal disease (e.g. coeliac disease, Crohn's disease), and chronic infections such as AIDS, malaria or tuberculosis.

The effect of intercurrent diseases may compound growth disturbances due to the nutritional or environmental factors discussed above, and/or primary endocrinological or genetic growth disorders.

NORMAL AND ABNORMAL GROWTH IN SINGLE TISSUES

Within an individual organ or tissue, increased or decreased growth takes place in a range of physiological and pathological circumstances as part of the adaptive response of cells to changing requirements for growth.

Increased growth: hypertrophy and hyperplasia

> - Hyperplasia and hypertrophy are common tissue responses
> - May be physiological (e.g. breast enlargement in pregnancy) or pathological (e.g. prostatic enlargement in elderly men)
> - Hypertrophy: increase in cell size without cell division
> - Hyperplasia: increase in cell number by mitosis

The response of an individual cell to increased functional demand is to increase tissue or organ size (Fig. 5.10) by:

- increasing its size without cell replication (hypertrophy)
- increasing its numbers by cell division (hyperplasia)
- a combination of these.

The stimuli for hypertrophy and hyperplasia are very similar, and in many cases identical; indeed, hypertrophy and hyperplasia commonly co-exist. In permanent cells (p. 82) hypertrophy is the only adaptive option available under stimulatory conditions. In some circumstances, however, permanent cells may increase their DNA content (ploidy) in hypertrophy, although the cells arrest in the G_2 phase of the cell cycle without undergoing mitosis; such a circumstance is present in severely hypertrophied hearts, where a large proportion of cells may be polyploid.

An important component of hyperplasia, which is often overlooked, is a *decrease* in cell loss by apoptosis; the mechanisms of control of this decreased apoptosis are unclear, although they are related to the factors causing increased cell production (Fig. 5.6).

Physiological hypertrophy and hyperplasia

Examples of physiologically increased growth of tissues include:

- *Muscle hypertrophy* in athletes, both in the skeletal muscle of the limbs (as a response to increased

muscle activity) and in the left ventricle of the heart (as a response to sustained outflow resistance).
- *Hyperplasia of bone marrow cells* producing red blood cells in individuals living at high altitude. This is stimulated by increased production of the growth factor, erythropoietin.
- *Hyperplasia of breast tissue* at puberty, and in pregnancy and lactation, under the influence of several hormones, including oestrogens, progesterone, prolactin, growth hormone and human placental lactogen.
- *Hypertrophy and hyperplasia of uterine smooth muscle* at puberty and in pregnancy, stimulated by oestrogens.
- *Thyroid hyperplasia* as a consequence of the increased metabolic demands of puberty and pregnancy.

In addition to such physiologically increased tissue growth, hypertrophy and hyperplasia are also seen in tissues in a wide range of *pathological* conditions.

Repair and regeneration

The proliferation of myofibroblasts in scar tissue and the regeneration of specialised cells within a tissue are the important components of the response to tissue damage at various sites.

Skin
The healing of a skin wound is a complex process involving the removal of necrotic debris from the wound and repair of the defect by hyperplasia of capillaries, myofibroblasts and epithelial cells. Figure 5.11 illustrates some of these events, most of which are mediated by growth factors.

When tissue injury occurs there is haemorrhage into the defect from damaged blood vessels; this is controlled by normal haemostatic mechanisms, during which platelets aggregate and thrombus forms to plug the defect in the vessel wall. Because of interactions between the coagulation and complement systems, inflammatory cells are attracted to the site of injury by chemotactic complement fractions. In addition, platelets release two potent growth factors, platelet-derived growth factor (PDGF) and transforming growth factor beta (TGF-β), which are powerfully chemotactic for inflammatory cells, including macrophages; these migrate into the wound to remove necrotic tissue and fibrin.

In the *epidermis*, PDGF acts synergistically with epidermal growth factor (EGF) and the

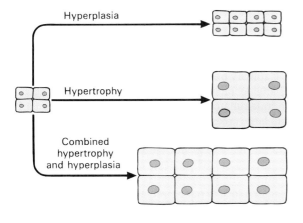

Fig. 5.10 Hyperplasia and hypertrophy

In hypertrophy, cell size is increased. In hyperplasia, cell number is increased. Hypertrophy and hyperplasia may co-exist.

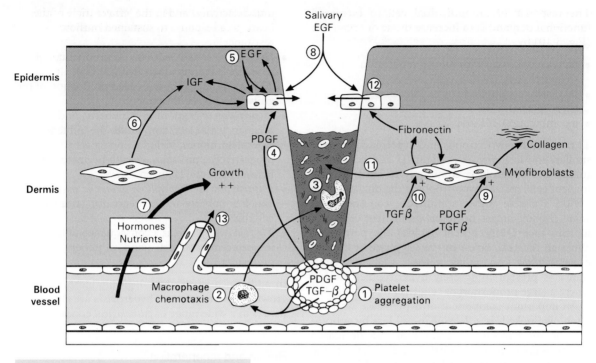

Fig. 5.11 Factors mediating wound healing

A wound is shown penetrating the skin, and entering a blood vessel. (**1**) Blood coagulation and platelet degranulation, releasing platelet-derived growth factor (PDGF) and transforming growth factor beta (TGF-β). (**2**) PDGF and TGF-β are chemotactic for macrophages, which migrate into the wound to phagocytose bacteria and necrotic debris (**3**). *In the epidermis*: (**4**) the released PDGF activates epidermal basal epithelial cells, which are also under autocrine and paracrine stimulation by epidermal growth factor (EGF) and insulin-like growth factors (IGF), (**5**), some derived from dermal myofibroblasts (**6**). Nutrients and oxygen (**7**) and circulating hormones and growth factors diffusing from blood vessels (including insulin, thyroxine, IGF-1 and IGF-2), and EGF (**8**) from saliva (if the wound is licked) all contribute to epidermal growth. *In the dermis*: (**9**) PDGF and TGF-β stimulate cell division in myofibroblasts, and (**10**) TGF-β stimulates these cells to produce collagen and fibronectin. Fibronectin stimulates migration of dermal myofibroblasts (**11**) and epidermal epithelial cells (**12**). Angiogenic growth factors (not shown) stimulate the proliferation and migration of new blood vessels into the area of the wound (**13**).

somatomedins (IGF-1 and IGF-2) to promote the progression of basal epithelial cells through the cycle of cell proliferation (p. 82). PDGF acts as a 'competence factor' to move cells from their 'resting' phase in G_0 to G_1. EGF and IGFs then act sequentially in cell progression from the G_1 phase to that of DNA synthesis. Thereafter, the cell is independent of growth factors. In the epidermis, EGF is derived from epidermal cells (autocrine and paracrine mechanisms), and is also present in high concentrations in saliva when the wound is licked. IGF-1 and IGF-2 originate from the circulation (endocrine mechanisms) and from the proliferating cell and adjacent epidermal and dermal cells (autocrine and paracrine mechanisms).

In the *dermis*, myofibroblasts proliferate in response to PDGF (and TGF-β); collagen and fibronectin secretion is stimulated by TGF-β, and

fibronectin then aids migration of epithelial and dermal cells.

Capillary budding and proliferation are stimulated by angiogenic factors. The capillaries ease the access of inflammatory cells and fibroblasts, particularly into large areas of necrotic tissue.

Hormones (e.g. insulin and thyroid hormones) and nutrients (e.g. glucose and amino acids) are also required. Lack of nutrients or vitamins, the presence of inhibitory factors such as corticosteroids or infection, or a locally poor circulation with low tissue oxygen concentrations, may all materially delay wound healing; these factors are very important in clinical practice.

Liver

In severe chronic hepatitis (see Ch. 16) extensive

hepatocyte loss is followed by scarring, as is the case in the skin or other damaged tissues. Hepatocytes, like the skin epidermal cells, have massive regenerative potential, and surviving hepatocytes may proliferate to form nodules. Hyperplasia of hepatocytes and fibroblasts is presumably mediated by a combination of hormones and growth factors, although the mechanisms are far from clear. Regenerative nodules of hepatocytes and scar tissue are the components of cirrhosis of the liver.

Heart
Myocardial cells are permanent cells (p. 82), and so cannot divide in a regenerative response to tissue injury. In myocardial infarction, a segment of muscle dies and, if the patient survives, it is replaced by hyperplastic myofibroblast scar tissue. As the remainder of the myocardium must work harder for a given cardiac output, it undergoes compensatory hypertrophy (without cell division) (see Fig. 5.12). Occasionally, there may be right ventricular hypertrophy as a result of left ventricular failure and consequent pulmonary hypertension.

Non-regenerative hypertrophy and hyperplasia

Many conditions are characterised by hypertrophy or hyperplasia of cells. In some instances, this is the principal feature of the condition from which the disease is named. The more common examples are summarised in Table 5.2. For more detail, consult the relevant chapters.

Apparently autonomous hyperplasias

In some apparently hyperplastic conditions, cells appear autonomous, and continue to proliferate rapidly despite the lack of a demonstrable stimulus or control mechanism. The question then arises as to whether these should be considered to be hyperplasias at all, or whether they are autonomous and hence neoplastic. If the cells can be demonstrated to be monoclonal (derived as a single clone from one cell), then this suggests that the lesion may indeed be neoplastic, but clonality is often difficult to establish.

Three examples are:

- *psoriasis*, characterised by marked epidermal hyperplasia (Ch. 24)
- *Paget's disease of bone*, in which there is hyperplasia of osteoblasts and osteoclasts resulting in thick but weak bone (Ch. 25)
- *fibromatoses*, which are apparently autonomous proliferations of myofibroblasts, occasionally forming tumour-like masses, exemplified by

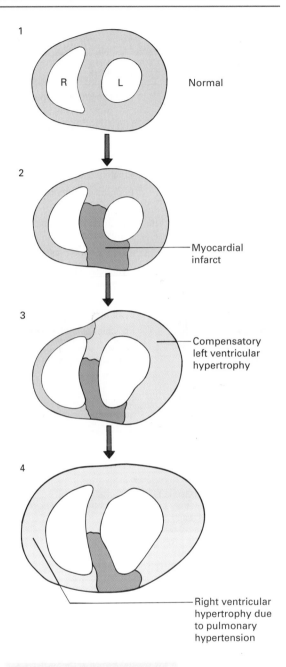

Fig. 5.12 Cardiac hypertrophy

A horizontal slice through the myocardium of the left (L) and right (R) ventricles. (1) Normal. (2) Area of anteroseptal left ventricular infarct. (3) Compensatory hypertrophy of the surviving left ventricle. (4) Right ventricular hypertrophy secondary to left ventricular failure and pulmonary hypertension.

palmar fibromatosis (Dupuytren's contracture), desmoid tumour, retroperitoneal fibromatosis and Peyronie's disease of the penis.

Table 5.2 Examples of non-regenerative hypertrophy and hyperplasia

Organ/tissue	Condition	Comment
Myocardium	Right ventricular hypertrophy	Response to pulmonary valve stenosis, pulmonary hypertension or ventricular septal defect (Ch. 13)
	Left ventricular hypertrophy	Response to aortic valve stenosis or systemic hypertension (Ch. 13)
Arterial smooth muscle	Hypertrophy of arterial walls	Occurs in hypertension (Ch. 13)
Capillary vessels	Proliferative retinopathy	Complication of diabetes mellitus (Ch. 26)
Bone marrow	Erythrocyte precursor hyperplasia	Response to increased erythropoietin production (due to e.g. hypoxia) (Ch. 23)
Cytotoxic T-lymphocytes	Hyperplastic expansion of T-cell populations	Involved in cell-mediated immune responses (Fig. 5.13)
Breast	Juvenile hyperplasia (females)	Exaggerated pubertal enlargement (Ch. 18)
	Gynaecomastia (males)	Due to high oestrogen levels (e.g. in cirrhosis, iatrogenic, endocrine tumours) (Ch. 18)
Prostate	Epithelial and connective tissue hyperplasia	Relative excess of oestrogens stimulates oestrogen-sensitive central zone (Ch. 20)
Thyroid	Follicular epithelial hyperplasia	Most commonly due to a thyroid-stimulating antibody (Graves' disease) (Ch. 17)
Adrenal cortex	Cortical hyperplasia	Response to increased ACTH production (e.g. from a pituitary tumour or, inappropriately, from a lung carcinoma) (Ch. 17)
Myointimal cells	Myointimal cell hyperplasia in atheromatous plaques	Myointimal cells in plaques proliferate in response to platelet-derived growth factor (Ch. 13)

Decreased growth: atrophy

> ► Atrophy: decrease in size of an organ or cell
> ► Organ atrophy may be due to reduction in cell size or number or both
> ► May be mediated by apoptosis
> ► Atrophy may be physiological (e.g. post-menopausal atrophy of uterus)
> ► Pathological atrophy may be due to decreased function (e.g. an immobilised limb), loss of innervation, reduced blood or oxygen supply, nutritional impairment or hormonal insufficiency

Atrophy is the decrease in size of an organ or cell by reduction in cell size and/or reduction in cell numbers, often by a mechanism involving apoptosis (pp. 83–84). Tissues or cells affected by atrophy are said to be atrophic or atrophied. Atrophy is an important adaptive response to a decreased requirement of the body for the function of a particular cell or organ. It is important to appreciate that for atrophy to occur there must be not only a cessation of growth but also an active reduction in cell size and/or a decrease in cell numbers, mediated by apoptosis.

Atrophy occurs in both physiological and pathological conditions.

Physiological atrophy

Physiological atrophy occurs at times from very early embryological life, as part of the process of morphogenesis, into late old age, where its results are regarded as the bane of existence (Table 5.3).

Pathological atrophy

There are several categories of pathological condition in which atrophy may occur.

Decreased function

As a result of decreased function as, for example, in a limb immobilised as a consequence of a fracture, there may be marked muscle atrophy (due to decrease in muscle fibre size). Extensive physiotherapy may be required to restore the muscle to its former bulk, or to prevent the atrophy.

In extreme cases of 'disuse' atrophy of a limb,

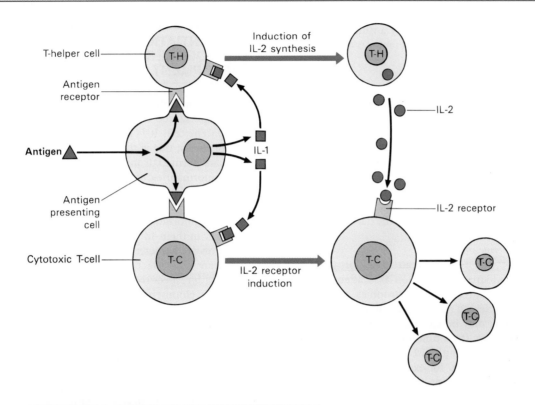

Fig. 5.13   Interleukins and cytotoxic T-cell hyperplasia

Cytotoxic T-cell hyperplasia is mediated by presentation of an antigen by an antigen-presenting cell (a macrophage) to T-helper and T-cytotoxic cells. Interleukin-1 (IL-1) acts on these cells via membrane receptors, stimulating the production of interleukin-2 (IL-2) by the T-helper cell, and of IL-2-receptors by T-cytotoxic cells. IL-2 from the T-helper cells stimulates the now receptive T-cytotoxic cell to multiply.

Table 5.3 Tissues involved in physiological atrophy	
Embryo and fetus	**Early adult**
Branchial clefts	Thymus
Notochord	
Thyroglossal duct	**Late adult and old age**
Müllerian duct (males)	Uterus, endometrium
Wolffian duct (females)	(females)
	Testes (males)
Neonate	Bone (particularly females)
Umbilical vessels	Gums
Ductus arteriosus	Mandible (particularly
Fetal layer adrenal cortex	edentulous)
	Cerebrum
	Lymphoid tissue

bone atrophy may lead to osteoporosis and bone weakening; this is also a feature of conditions of prolonged weightlessness, such as occurs in astronauts.

Loss of innervation
Loss of innervation of muscle causes muscle atrophy, as is seen in nerve transection or in poliomyelitis, where there is loss of anterior horn cells of the spinal cord. In paraplegics, loss of innervation to whole limbs may also precipitate 'disuse' atrophy of bone, which becomes osteoporotic.

Loss of blood supply
This may cause atrophy as a result of tissue hypoxia, which may also be a result of a sluggish circulation. Epidermal atrophy is seen, for example, in the skin of the lower legs in patients with circulatory stagnation related to varicose veins or with atheromatous narrowing of arteries.

'Pressure' atrophy
This occurs when tissues are compressed, either by exogenous agents (atrophy of skin and soft tissues overlying the sacrum in bedridden patients producing 'bed sores') or endogenous factors (atrophy of a

blood vessel wall compressed by a tumour). In both of these circumstances a major factor is actually local tissue hypoxia.

Lack of nutrition
Lack of nutrition may cause atrophy of adipose tissue, the gut and pancreas and, in extreme circumstances, muscle. An extreme form of systemic atrophy similar to that seen in severe starvation is termed 'cachexia'; this may be seen in patients in the late stages of severe illnesses such as cancer. In some wasting conditions, such as cancer, cytokines such as tumour necrosis factor (TNF) are postulated to influence the development of cachexia.

Loss of endocrine stimulation
Atrophy of the 'target' organ of a hormone may occur if endocrine stimulation is inadequate. For example, the adrenal gland atrophies as a consequence of decreased ACTH secretion by the anterior pituitary; this may be caused by destruction of the anterior pituitary (by a tumour or infarction), or as a result of the therapeutic use of high concentrations of corticosteroids (in, for example, the treatment of cancer), with consequent 'feedback' reduction of circulating ACTH levels.

Hormone-induced atrophy
This form of atrophy may be seen in the skin, as a result of the growth-inhibiting actions of corticosteroids. When corticosteroids are applied topically in high concentrations to the skin, they may cause dermal and epidermal atrophy which may be disfiguring. All steroids, when applied topically, may also be absorbed through the skin to produce systemic side-effects, e.g. adrenal atrophy when corticosteroids are used.

Decreased growth: hypoplasia

> ► Hypoplasia: failure of development of an organ
> ► Process is related to atrophy
> ► Failure of morphogenesis

Although the terms 'hypoplasia' and 'atrophy' are often used interchangeably, the former is better reserved to denote the failure in attainment of the normal size or shape of an organ as a consequence of a developmental failure. Hypoplasia is, therefore, a failure in morphogenesis, although it is closely related to atrophy in terms of its pathogenesis. An example of hypoplasia is the failure in development of the legs in adult patients with severe spina bifida and neurological deficit in the lower limbs.

DIFFERENTIATION AND MORPHOGENESIS IN HUMAN DEVELOPMENT

Differentiation is the process whereby a cell develops an overt specialised function which was not present in the parent cell. It is an important component of morphogenesis; this is the means by which limbs or organs are formed from primitive groups of cells. Thus, abnormalities of differentiation often lead to abnormal morphogenesis and fetal abnormality. It must be remembered, however, that growth also plays an important role in morphogenesis; cells which vary in their differentiation may have very different growth characteristics. Variations in differentiation may also affect the ability of some cells to migrate with respect to others. Thus, normal embryological development requires highly co-ordinated processes of differentiation, growth and cell migration which together comprise morphogenesis.

Control of normal differentiation

> ► Embryonic differentiation of cells is controlled by genes, systemic hormones, position within the fetus, local growth factors and matrix proteins
> ► Maintenance of differentiated state is dependent upon persistence of some of these factors
> ► Differentiation and morphogenesis may be disturbed by environmental factors (e.g. teratogens)

A fertilised ovum may develop into a male or female, a human or a blue whale; the outcome depends on the structure of the genome. There are many similarities between the corresponding cell types in different species. Individual cell types are distinct only because, in addition to the many functional proteins required by all cell types for 'household' functions of respiration, repair, etc., each cell also produces a specific set of specialised proteins which are appropriate for only one cell type and one species.

Most differentiated cells contain the same genome as in the fertilised ovum. This has been demonstrated elegantly by injecting the nucleus of a differentiated tadpole gut epithelial cell into an unfertilised frog ovum, the nucleus of which was destroyed using ultraviolet light; the result was a normal frog with the normal variety of differentiated cell types (Fig. 5.14).

There are very few exceptions to the rule that differentiated cells contain an identical genome to that of the fertilised ovum. In man, for example, they include B- and T-lymphocytes which have antigen-

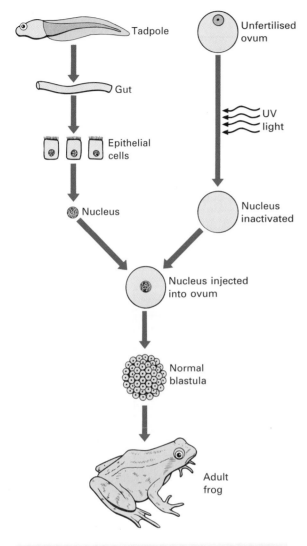

Fig. 5.14   Potential of the genome of somatic cells

Differentiated cells from the gut of a tadpole have the complete genome and potential for control of production of the whole frog. (After J B Gurdon)

receptor genes rearranged to endow them with a large repertoire of possible receptors (see Ch. 9).

Transcriptional control

As most differentiated cells have an identical genome, differences between them cannot be due to amplification or deletion of genes. The cells of the body differ because they *express* different genes; genes are selectively switched on or off to control the synthesis of gene products.

The synthesis of a gene product can in theory be controlled at several levels:

- *transcription*: controlling the formation of mRNA
- *transport*: controlling the export of mRNA from the nucleus to the ribosomes in the cytoplasm
- *translation*: controlling the formation of gene product within the ribosomes.

In fact, many of the important 'decision' stages of differentiation in embryogenesis are under transcriptional control, and the manufacture of gene product is proportional to the activity of the gene.

For a cell to differentiate in a particular way, given that it contains the potential of activation of the whole of the genome, some groups of genes must be switched on and other groups off. There is now ample evidence that the regulation of transcription of several (or many) individuals within a group of genes is mediated by the gene products of a small number of 'control' genes, which may themselves be regulated by the product of a single 'master' gene (Fig. 5.15).

Positional control in early embryogenesis

Some insight into possible control mechanisms in human differentiation and morphogenesis has been gained from observations of the fruitfly, *Drosophila*. Disturbances of single 'master' genes in *Drosophila* have been shown to result in major malformations, such as the development of legs on the head in place of antennae, mediated by the response of many controlled genes to the alteration in 'master' gene product. Such a *homeotic* mutation (the transformation of one body part into another part which is usually found on a different body segment) highlights the importance of another factor in the control of differentiation and morphogenesis, namely the three-dimensional spatial co-ordinates (position) of a cell within an embryo at a given time.

In *Drosophila*, a group of genes, which individually cause a range of homeotic mutations, have been found to share a 60-amino-acid sequence domain which is common to genes controlling normal larval segmentation. This sequence, named the *homeobox*, has also been demonstrated in vertebrates, including humans (see Ch. 3). Homeobox-containing genes are transcriptional regulators influencing morphogenesis. Parts of human anatomy appear to be constructed on a segmental basis, for example rows of somites, teeth and limb segments, and here it is probable that homeobox-containing genes have an important morphogenetic role.

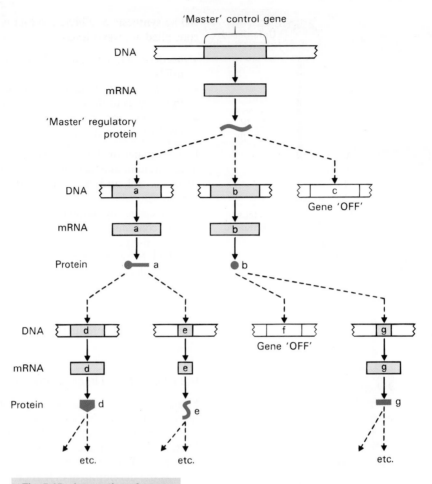

Fig. 5.15   Interaction of genes

A single master gene produces a regulatory protein which switches genes **a** and **b** on and gene **c** off; these in turn switch on or off a cascade of other genes.

Cell determination

The homeobox-containing genes, and other genes which regulate embryogenesis, act on the embryo at a very early stage, before structures such as limbs have begun to form. Nonetheless, by observing the effects of selective marking or obliteration of cells, a 'fate map' of the future development of cells in even primitive embryos can be constructed. Thus, some of the cells of somites become specialised at a very early stage as precursors of muscle cells, and migrate to their positions in primitive limbs. These muscle-cell precursors resemble many other cells of the limb rudiment, and it is only after several days that they differentiate and manufacture specialised muscle proteins. Thus, long before they differentiate, the developmental path of these cells is planned; such a

cell which has made a developmental choice before differentiating is said to be *determined*. A determined cell must:

- have differences which are heritable from one cell generation to another
- be committed and commit its progeny to specialised development
- change its internal character, not merely its environment.

Determination therefore differs from differentiation, in which there must be *demonstrable* tissue specialisation.

Some cells which are determined, but not differentiated, may remain so for adult life; good examples are the *stem cells*, such as bone marrow haemopoietic cells or basal cells of the skin, which proliferate continuously and produce cells committed to a particular form of differentiation.

Cell position and inductive phenomena

Even before fertilisation, ova have cytoplasmic determinants of polarity; the manner in which major morphogenetic positional changes may occur under the influence of a small number of controlling genes has been discussed above. As the fields of cells over which spatial chemical signals act are generally small, large-scale changes to the whole individual occur early, and more specific minor features of differentiation within small areas of an organ or limb are specified later and depend on the position of the cell within the structure. Simple changes may occur in response to a diffusible substance (such as vitamin A in the developing limb bud), and serve to control local cell growth and/or differentiation according to the distance from the source. Additional differentiation changes may, however, occur as a result of more complex cellular interactions.

Many organs eventually contain multiple distinct populations of cells which originate separately but later interact. The pattern of differentiation in one cell type may be controlled by another, a phenomenon known as *induction*. Examples of induction include:

- the action of mesoderm on ectoderm at different sites to form the various parts of the neural tube
- the action of mesoderm on the skin at different sites to form epithelium of differing thickness and accessory gland content
- the action of mesoderm on developing epithelial cells to form branching tubular glands
- the action of the ureteric bud (from the mesonephric duct) to induce the metanephric blastema in kidney formation.

Inductive phenomena also occur in cell migrations, sometimes along pathways which are very long, controlled by generally uncertain mechanisms (although it is known, for example, that migrating cells from the neural crest migrate along pathways which are defined by the host connective tissue). Inductive phenomena control the differentiation of the migrating cell when it arrives at its destination—neural crest cells differentiate into a range of cell types, including sympathetic and parasympathetic ganglion cells, and some cells of the neuro-endocrine (APUD) system.

Maintenance and modulation of an attained differentiated state

Once a differentiated state has been attained by a cell, it must be maintained. This is achieved by a combination of factors:

- 'cell memory' inherent in the genome, with inherited transcriptional changes
- interactions with adjacent cells, through secreted paracrine factors
- secreted factors (autocrine factors) including growth factors and extracellular matrix.

Even in the adult, minor changes to the differentiated state may occur if the local environment changes. These alterations to the differentiated state are rarely great, and most can be termed *modulations*, i.e. reversible interconversions between closely related cell phenotypes. An example of a modulation is the alteration in synthesis of certain liver enzymes in response to circulating corticosteroids.

In the neonatal stage of development, cell *maturation* may involve modulations of the differentiated state. Examples are:

- the production of surfactant by type II pneumonocytes under the influence of corticosteroids.
- the synthesis of vitamin K-dependent blood-clotting factors by the hepatocyte
- gut maturation affected by epidermal growth factor (EGF) in milk.

Normal differentiation and morphogenesis: summary

Differentiation

During development of an embryo, determination and differentiation occur in a cell by transcriptional modifications to the expression of the genome, without an increase or decrease in numbers of genes present. The factors involved are summarised in Figure 5.16. Expression of individual genes within the genome is *modified* during development by:

- positional information carried by a small number of 'control' gene products, causing local alterations in growth and differentiation
- migrations of cells and modifications mediated by adjacent cells (paracrine factors) or endocrine factors.

Once attained, the differentiated state is *maintained* or *modulated* by:

- paracrine factors (interactions with adjacent cells)

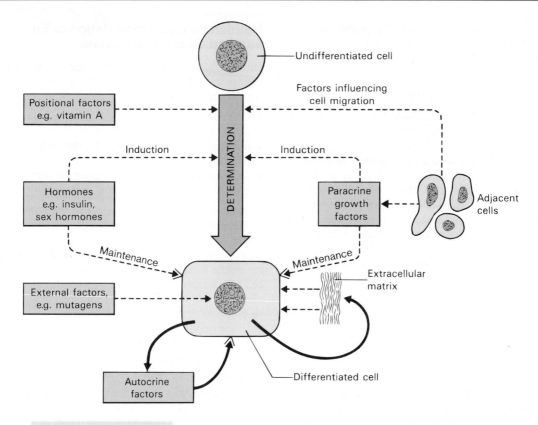

Fig. 5.16 Differentiation

Factors affecting determination, differentiation, maintenance and modulation of the differentiated state of a cell during embryogenesis include positional factors, hormones, paracrine growth factors and external factors such as teratogens. With the exception of positional factors, all of these are important in influencing the differentiated state of cells in post-natal and adult life.

● autocrine factors, such as growth factors and the extracellular matrix secreted by the cell.

External factors may cause alterations to the differentiated state of the cell, either during development or at any stage of adult life.

Morphogenesis

The main features of morphogenesis are summarised in Figure 5.17.

Congenital disorders of differentiation and morphogenesis

The processes involved in human conception and development are so complex that it is perhaps remarkable that any normal fetuses are produced; the fact that they are produced is a result of the tight controls of growth and morphogenesis which are involved at all stages of development.

The usual outcome of human conception is abortion; 70–80% of all human conceptions are lost, largely as a consequence of chromosomal abnormalities (Fig. 5.18). The majority of these abortions occur spontaneously in the first 6–8 weeks of pregnancy, and in most cases the menstrual cycle might appear normal, or the slight delay in menstruation causes little concern. Chromosomal abnormalities are present in 3–5% of live-born infants, and a further 2% have serious malformations which are not associated with chromosomal aberrations. The most common conditions in these two categories are illustrated in Table 5.4.

Chromosomal abnormalities affecting whole chromosomes

Autosomal chromosomes

The three most common autosomal chromosome defects involve the presence of additional whole

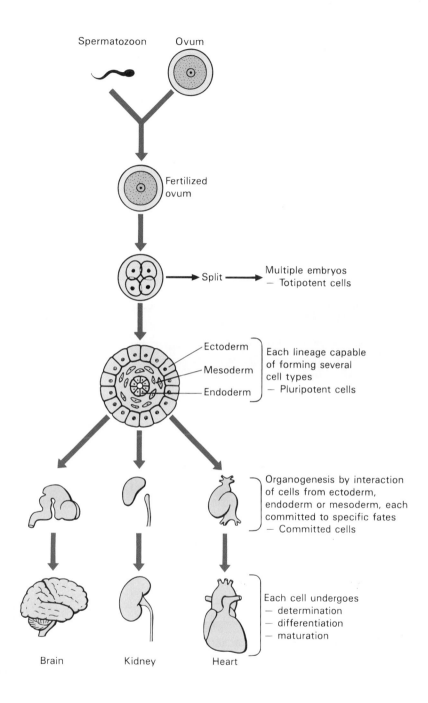

Fig. 5.17 Major steps in morphogenesis

chromosomes (trisomy). As the genome of every cell in the body has an increased number of genes, gene product expression is greatly altered and multiple abnormalities result during morphogenesis.

Trisomy 21 (Down's syndrome) affects approximately 1 in 1000 births; it is associated with mental retarda-

tion, a flattened facial profile, slanting eyes (producing a 'mongoloid' appearance) and prominent epicanthic folds. The hands are short, with a transverse 'simian' (i.e. monkey-like) palmar crease. There are also abnormalities of the ears, trunk, pelvis and phalanges. The incidence increases with maternal age.

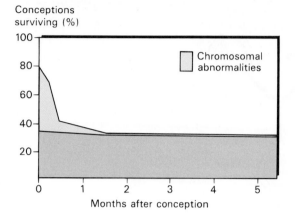

Fig. 5.18   Fate of human conceptions

Between 70 and 80% of human conceptions are lost by spontaneous abortion in the first 6–8 weeks of pregnancy, most as a consequence of chromosomal abnormality. Chromosomal abnormalities are present in 3–5% of live-born infants. (After Witschi 1969)

Table 5.4 Incidence of some congenital abnormalities	
Chromosomal abnormality	Incidence per 1000 live births
Down's syndrome (47,+21)	1.4
Klinefelter's syndrome (47,XXY)	1.3
Double Y male (47,XYY)	<1
Multiple X female (47,XXX)	<1
Major malformations	Incidence per 1000 stillbirths + live births
Congenital heart defects	6
Pyloric stenosis	3
Spina bifida	2.5
Anencephaly	2
Cleft lip (± cleft palate)	1
Congenital dislocation of the hip	1

Trisomy 18 (Edwards' syndrome) affects 1 in 5000 births. It is associated with ear and jaw, cardiac, renal, intestinal and skeletal abnormalities.

Trisomy 13 (Patau's syndrome) affects 1 in 6000 births, with microcephaly and microphthalmia, hare lip and cleft palate, polydactyly, abnormal ears, 'rocker-bottom' feet, and cardiac and visceral defects.

Sex chromosomes

Chromosomal disorders affecting the sex chromosomes (X and Y) are relatively common, and usually induce abnormalities of sexual development and fer-

tility. In general, variations in X chromosome numbers cause greater mental retardation.

Klinefelter's syndrome (47,XXY) affects 1 in 850 male births. There is testicular atrophy and absent spermatogenesis, eunuchoid bodily habitus, gynaecomastia, female distribution of body hair and mental retardation. Variants of Klinefelter's syndrome (48,XXXY, 49,XXXXY, 48,XXYY) are rare, and have cryptorchidism and hypospadias, in addition to more severe mental retardation and radio-ulnar synostosis.

Double Y males (47,XYY) form 1 in 1000 male births; they are phenotypically normal, although most are over six feet tall. Some are said to have increased aggressive or criminal behaviour.

Turner's syndrome (gonadal dysgenesis; 45,X) occurs in 1 in 3000 female births. About one-half are mosaics (45,X/46,XX) and some have 46 chromosomes and two X chromosomes, one of which is defective. Turner's syndrome females may have short stature, primary amenorrhoea and infertility, webbing of the neck, broad chest and widely spaced nipples, cubitus valgus, low posterior hairline and coarctation of the aorta.

Multiple X females (47,XXX, 48,XXXX) comprise 1 in 1200 female births. They may be mentally retarded, and have menstrual disturbances, although many are normal and fertile.

True hermaphrodites (most 46,XX, some 46,XX/ 47,XXY mosaics) have both testicular and ovarian tissue, with varying genital tract abnormalities.

Parts of chromosomes

The loss (or addition) of even a small part of a chromosome may have severe effects, especially if 'controlling' or 'master' genes are involved, as these affect many other genes. An example of a congenital disease in this group is *cri-du-chat syndrome* (46,XX, 5p- or 46,XY, 5p-). This rare condition (1 in 50 000 births) is associated with deletion of the short arm of chromosome 5 (5p-), and was so named because infants have a characteristic cry like the miaow of a cat. There is microcephaly and severe mental retardation; the face is round, there is gross hyperteleorism (increased distance between the eyes) and epicanthic folds.

Single gene alterations

All of the inherited disorders of single genes are transmitted by autosomal dominant, autosomal recessive or X-linked modes of inheritance (see Ch. 3). There are more than 2700 known Mendelian disorders; 80–85% of these are familial, and the remainder are the result of new mutations. The alteration of expression of gene product constitutes at least a modulation of cell differentiation, and some have important effects on growth and morphogenesis.

Single gene disorders fall into four categories, discussed below.

Enzyme defects

An altered gene may result in decreased enzyme synthesis, or the synthesis of a defective enzyme (Ch. 7). This may lead to accumulation of the enzyme substrate, for example:

- accumulation of galactose and consequent tissue damage in galactose-1-phosphate uridyl transferase deficiency
- accumulation of phenylalanine, causing mental abnormality, in phenylalanine hydroxylase deficiency
- accumulation of glycogen, mucopolysaccharides, etc. in lysosomes in the enzyme deficiency states of the lysosomal storage disorders.

A failure to synthesise the end products of a reaction catalysed by an enzyme may block normal cellular function. This occurs, for example, in albinism, caused by absent melanin production due to tyrosinase deficiency.

Defects in receptors or cellular transport

The lack of a specific cellular receptor causes insensitivity of a cell to substances such as hormones. In one form of male pseudohermaphroditism, for example, insensitivity of tissues to androgens, caused by lack of androgen receptor, prevents the development of male characteristics during fetal development.

Cellular transport deficiencies may lead to conditions such as cystic fibrosis (Ch. 7), a condition in which there is a defective cell membrane transport system across exocrine secretory cells.

Non-enzyme protein defects

Failure of production of important proteins, or production of abnormalities in proteins, has widespread effects. Thus, sickle cell anaemia is caused by the production of abnormal haemoglobin, and Marfan's syndrome and Ehlers–Danlos syndrome are the result of defective collagen production.

Adverse reactions to drugs

The apparently innocuous condition of glucose-6-phosphate dehydrogenase (G6PD) deficiency does not result in disease until the antimalarial drug, primaquine, is administered; severe haemolytic anaemia then results. The prevalence of G6PD deficiency in the tropics may reflect evolutionary selective pressure, as the deficiency may confer a degree of protection against malarial parasitisation of red blood cells.

Functional aspects of developmental disorders

Abnormalities can occur at almost any stage of fetal development; the mechanisms by which the anomaly occurs are sometimes unknown. In most cases the genetic defect is unknown, although the majority are almost certainly the result of transcriptional alterations to an intact genome.

Embryo division abnormalities

Monozygotic twins (or multiple births) result from the separation of groups of cells in the early embryo, well before the formation of the primitive streak. On occasion, there is a defect of embryo division, resulting in:

- *Siamese twins*: the result of incomplete separation of the embryo, with fusion of considerable portions of the body (or minor fusions which are easily separated).
- *Fetus in feto*: one of the fused twins develops imperfectly and grows on the other, either externally or within the abdominal cavity. It is possible that some extragonadal 'teratomas' in neonates belong to this group.

Teratogen exposure

Physical, chemical or infective agents can interfere with growth and differentiation, resulting in fetal abnormalities; such agents are known as *teratogens*. The extent and severity of fetal abnormality depend on the nature of the teratogen and the developmental stage of the embryo when exposed to the teratogen. Thus, if exposure occurs at the stage of early organogenesis (4–5 weeks' gestation) then the effects on developing organs or limbs are severe.

Clinical examples of teratogenesis include the severe and extensive malformations associated with use of the drug thalidomide (absent/rudimentary limbs, defects of the heart, kidney, gastrointestinal tract, etc.), and the effects of rubella (German measles) on the fetus (cataracts, microcephaly, heart defects, etc.). Some other teratogens are listed in Table 5.5.

Failure of cell and organ migration

Failure of migration of cells may occur during embryogenesis.

Kartagener's syndrome. In this rare condition there is a defect in ciliary motility, due to absent or abnormal dynein arms, the structures on the outer doublets of cilia which are responsible for ciliary movement. This affects cell motility during embryogenesis, which often results in situs inversus

Table 5.5 Teratogens and their effects	
Teratogen	Teratogenic effect
Irradiation	Microcephaly
Drugs	
Thalidomide	Amelia/phocomelia (absent/rudimentary limbs), heart, kidney, gastrointestinal and facial abnormalities
Folic acid antagonists, e.g. 4 amino PGA	Anencephaly, hydrocephalus, cleft lip/palate, skull defects
Anticonvulsants	Cleft lip/palate, heart defects, minor skeletal defects
Warfarin	Nasal/facial abnormalities
Testosterone and synthetic progestagens	Virilisation of female fetus, atypical genitalia
Alcohol	Microcephaly, abnormal facies, oblique palpebral fissures, growth disturbance
Infections	
Rubella	Cataracts, microphthalmia, microcephaly, heart defects
Cytomegalovirus	Microcephaly
Herpes simplex	Microcephaly, microphthalmia
Toxoplasmosis	Microcephaly

(congenital lateral inversion of the position of body organs resulting in, for example, left-sided liver and right-sided spleen). Complications in later life include bronchiectasis and infertility due to sperm immobility.

Hirschsprung's disease is a condition leading to marked dilatation of the colon and failure of colonic motility in the neonatal period, due to absence of Meissner's and Auerbach's nerve plexuses. It results from a selective failure of craniocaudal migration of neuroblasts in weeks 5–12 of gestation. It is, interestingly, ten times more frequent in children with trisomy 21 (Down's syndrome), and is often associated with other congenital anomalies.

Undescended testis (cryptorchidism) is the result of failure of the testis to migrate to its normal position in the scrotum. Although this may be associated with severe forms of Klinefelter's syndrome (e.g. 48,XXXY) it is often an isolated anomaly in an otherwise normal male. There is an increased risk of neoplasia in undescended testes.

Anomalies of organogenesis

▶ *Agenesis (aplasia):* failure of development of an organ or structure within it
▶ *Atresia*: failure of the development of a lumen in a normally tubular structure
▶ *Hypoplasia*: failure of an organ to attain its normal size
▶ *Maldifferentiation (dysgenesis):* failure of normal organ differentiation or persistence of primitive embryological structures
▶ *Ectopia (heterotopia):* development of mature tissue in an inappropriate site

Agenesis (aplasia)
The failure of development of an organ or structure is known as agenesis (aplasia). Obviously, agenesis of some structures (such as the heart) is incompatible with life, but agenesis of many individual organs is recorded. These include:

● *Renal agenesis*. This may be unilateral or bilateral (in which case the affected infant may survive only a few days after birth). It results from a failure of the mesonephric duct to give rise to the ureteric bud, and consequent failure of metanephric blastema induction.
● *Thymic agenesis* is seen in Di George syndrome, where there is failure of development of T-lymphocytes, and consequent severe deficiency of cell-mediated immunity. Recent evidence suggests that there is failure of processing of stem cells to T-cells as a result of a defect in the thymus anlage.
● *Anencephaly* is a severe neural tube defect in which the cerebrum, and often the cerebellum, are absent (see Ch. 26). The condition is lethal.

Atresia
Atresia is the failure of development of a lumen in a normally tubular epithelial structure. Examples include:

● *oesophageal atresia*, which may be seen in association with tracheo-oesophageal fistulae, as a result of anomalies of development of the two structures from the primitive foregut
● *biliary atresia*, which is an uncommon cause of obstructive jaundice in early childhood
● *urethral atresia*, a very rare anomaly, which may be associated with recto-urethral or urachal

fistula, or congenital absence of the anterior abdominal wall muscles ('prune belly' syndrome).

Hypoplasia

A failure in development of the normal size of an organ is termed hypoplasia. It may affect only part of an organ, e.g. segmental hypoplasia of the kidney. A relatively common example of hypoplasia affects the osseous nuclei of the acetabulum causing congenital dislocation of the hip, due to a flattened roof to the acetabulum.

Maldifferentiation (dysgenesis, dysplasia)

Maldifferentiation, as its name implies, is the failure of normal differentiation of an organ, which often retains primitive embryological structures. This disorder is often termed 'dysplasia', although this is a potential cause of confusion, as the more common usage of the term dysplasia implies the presence of a pre-neoplastic state (p. 108).

The best examples of maldifferentiation are seen in the kidney ('renal dysplasia') as a result of anomalous metanephric differentiation. Here, primitive tubular structures may be admixed with cellular mesenchyme and, occasionally, smooth muscle.

Ectopia and heterotopia

Ectopic and heterotopic tissues are usually small areas of mature tissue from one organ (e.g. the gastric mucosa) which are present within another tissue (e.g. Meckel's diverticulum) as a result of a developmental anomaly. Another clinically important example is endometriosis, in which endometrial tissue is found around the peritoneum in some women, causing abdominal pain at the time of menstruation.

Complex disorders of growth and morphogenesis

Three examples of complex, multifactorial defects of growth and morphogenesis will be discussed: neural tube defects, disorders of sexual differentiation, and cleft palate and related disorders.

Neural tube defects

The development of the brain, spinal cord and spine from the primitive neural tube is highly complex and, not surprisingly, so too are the developmental disorders of the system (Fig. 5.19).

Neural tube malformations are relatively common in the United Kingdom and are found in about 1.3% of aborted fetuses, and 0.1% of live births. There are

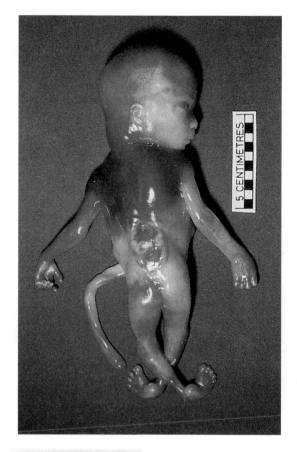

Fig. 5.19   Spina bifida

Dorsal view of a fetus from a pregnancy terminated after prenatal diagnosis of spina bifida. Extending from the lower thoracic to the sacral region there is an oval defect due to failure of spinal canal formation. Deformity and hypoplasia of the legs results from neurological deficit.

regional differences in incidence, and social differences, the condition being more common in social class V than in classes I or II. The pathogenesis of these conditions — anencephaly, hydrocephalus and spina bifida — is uncertain and probably multifactorial (see Ch. 26).

Disorders of sexual differentiation

Disorders of sexual differentiation are undoubtedly complex, and involve a range of individual chromosomal, enzyme and hormone receptor defects. The defects may be obvious and severe at birth, or they may be subtle, presenting with infertility in adult life.

Chromosomal abnormalities causing ambiguous or abnormal sexual differentiation have already been discussed (p. 102).

Female pseudohermaphroditism, in which the genetic sex is always female (XX), may be due to exposure of the developing fetus to the masculinising effects of excess testosterone or progestagens, causing abnormal differentiation of the external genitalia. The causes include:

- an enzyme defect in the fetal adrenal gland, leading to excessive androgen production at the expense of cortisol synthesis (with consequent adrenal hyperplasia due to feedback mechanisms which increases ACTH secretion)
- exogenous androgenic steroids from a maternal androgen-secreting tumour, or administration of androgens (or progestagens) during pregnancy.

Male pseudohermaphroditism, in which the genetic sex is male (XY), may be the result of several rare defects:

- testicular unresponsiveness to human chorionic gonadotrophin (hCG) or luteinising hormone (LH), by virtue of reduction in receptors to these hormones; this causes failure of testosterone secretion
- errors of testosterone biosynthesis in the fetus, due to enzyme defects (may be associated with cortisol deficiency and congenital adrenal hyperplasia)
- tissue insensitivity to androgens (androgen receptor deficiency)

- abnormality in testosterone metabolism by peripheral tissues, in 5 α-reductase deficiency
- defects in synthesis, secretion and response to Müllerian duct inhibitory factor
- maternal ingestion of oestrogens and progestins.

These defects result in the presence of a testis which is small and atrophic, and a female phenotype.

Cleft palate and related disorders
Cleft palate, and the related cleft (or hare) lip, are relatively common (about 1 per 1000 births). Approximately 20% of children with these disorders have associated major malformations. The important stages of development of the lips, palate, nose and jaws occur in the first nine weeks of embryonic life. From about five weeks' gestational age the maxillary processes grow anteriorly and medially, and fuse with the developing fronto-nasal process at two points just below the nostrils, forming the upper lip. Meanwhile, the palate develops from the palatal processes of the maxillary processes, which grow medially to fuse with the nasal septum in the midline at about nine weeks.

Failure of these complicated processes may occur at any stage, producing small clefts or severe facial

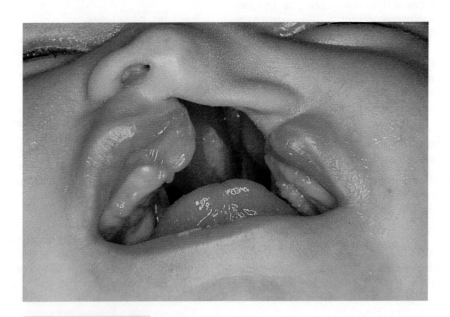

Fig. 5.20 Cleft palate
There is a large defect involving the upper lip, the upper jaw and the palate. (Courtesy of Mr D Willmott, Sheffield)

deficits (Fig. 5.20). A cleft lip is commonly unilateral but may be bilateral; it may involve the lip alone, or extend into the nostril or involve the bone of the maxilla and the teeth. The mildest palatal clefting may involve the uvula or soft palate alone, but can lead to absence of the roof of the mouth. Cleft lip and palate occur singly or in combination, and severe combined malformations of the lips, maxilla and palate can be very difficult to manage surgically.

Recently, lip and palate malformations have been extensively studied as a model of normal and abnormal states of morphogenesis in a complicated developmental system. It appears from the relatively high incidence of these malformations that the control of palatal morphogenesis is particularly sensitive to both genetic and environmental disturbances:

- genetic: e.g. Patau's syndrome (trisomy 13) is associated with severe clefting of the lip and palate
- environmental: e.g. the effects of specific teratogens such as folic acid antagonists or anticonvulsants, causing cleft lip and/or palate.

Recent experimental evidence has suggested that several cellular factors are involved in the fusion of the fronto-nasal and maxillary processes. The differentiation of epithelial cells of the palatal processes is of paramount importance in fusion of the processes. It is thought that the most important mechanism is mediated by mesenchymal cells of the palatal processes; these induce differentiation of the epithelial cells (p. 99), to form either ciliated nasal epithelial cells or squamous buccal epithelial cells, or to undergo programmed cell death by apoptosis (p. 83) to allow fusion of underlying mesothelial cells. Positional information of genetic and chemical (paracrine) nature is important in this differentiation, and is mediated via mesenchymal cells (and possibly epithelial cells). In addition, the events may be modified by the actions of epidermal growth factor (EGF) and other growth factors through autocrine or paracrine mechanisms (p. 99), and the endocrine actions of glucocorticoids and their intercellular receptors.

As yet, the precise way in which all of these factors interact in normal palatal development or cleft palate is unclear. In the mouse, it is known that physiological concentrations of glucocorticoids, their receptors and EGF are required for normal development, but that altered concentrations may precipitate cleft palate.

ACQUIRED DISORDERS OF DIFFERENTIATION AND GROWTH

Metaplasia

> ▶ Metaplasia is an acquired form of altered differentiation
> ▶ Transformation of one mature differentiated cell type into another
> ▶ Reversible response to altered cellular environment
> ▶ Affects epithelial or mesenchymal cells
> ▶ May undergo further indirect transformation to neoplasia via dysplasia (e.g. squamous cell carcinoma associated with squamous metaplasia in bronchi)

Metaplasia (transdifferentiation) is the reversible transformation of one type of terminally differentiated (epithelial or mesenchymal) cell into another fully differentiated cell type. Metaplasia often represents an adaptive response of a tissue to environmental stress, and is presumed to be due to the activation and/or repression of groups of genes involved in the maintenance of cellular differentiation. The metaplastic tissue is better able to withstand the adverse environmental changes.

Examples of metaplasia in *epithelial* tissues include a change to squamous epithelium (squamous metaplasia) in:

- ciliated respiratory epithelium of the trachea and bronchi in smokers
- ducts of the salivary glands and pancreas, and bile ducts in the presence of stones
- transitional bladder epithelium in the presence of stones, and in the presence of ova of the trematode *Schistosoma haematobium*
- transitional and columnar nasal epithelium in vitamin A deficiency.

Another example is the replacement of normal squamous epithelium of the oesophagus by columnar glandular epithelium (glandular metaplasia) in patients with reflux of gastric acid into the oesophagus. This is the condition of Barrett's oesophagus.

Examples of metaplasia in *mesenchymal* tissues are bone formation (osseous metaplasia):

- following calcium deposition in atheromatous arterial walls
- in bronchial cartilage
- following longstanding disease of the uveal tract of the eye.

Metaplasia does not itself necessarily progress to

malignancy, although the environmental changes which initially caused the metaplasia may also induce dysplasia and, if persistent, progression to tumour formation.

Metaplasia is sometimes said to occur in tumours as, for example, in squamous or glandular 'metaplasia' which may occur in transitional carcinomas of the bladder. These examples of transdifferentiation certainly do occur in tumours, but the term 'metaplasia' is best reserved for changes in non-neoplastic tissues.

Dysplasia

> ▶ Dysplasia is characterised by increased cell growth (e.g. more mitoses visible than normal), presence of atypical morphology (e.g. abnormally large nuclei), and altered differentiation (e.g. cellular immaturity)
> ▶ May be caused by chronic physical or chemical injury
> ▶ May be reversible only in early stages
> ▶ Dysplastic lesions are often pre-neoplastic

Dysplasia is a *premalignant* condition characterised by increased cell growth, the presence of cellular atypia, and altered differentiation. Early mild forms of dysplasia may be reversible if the initial stimulus is removed, but severe dysplasia will progress to a malignant neoplasm unless it is adequately treated.

Dysplasia may be caused by longstanding irritation of a tissue, with chronic inflammation, or by exposure to carcinogenic substances.

In affected tissues, dysplasia may be recognised by:

- evidence of increased growth, such as increased tissue bulk (e.g. increased epithelial thickness), and increased numbers of mitoses
- presence of cellular atypia, with pleomorphism (variation in the size and shape of cells and their nuclei), a high nuclear/cytoplasmic ratio and increased nuclear DNA (recognised by hyperchromatism, i.e. more darkly stained nuclei)
- altered differentiation, as the cells often appear more primitive than normal. For example, dysplastic squamous epithelium may not show the normal differentiation from basal cells to flattened surface cells of the skin; this appearance is described as showing 'loss of epithelial polarity'.

Dysplasia may occur in tissue which has coincident metaplasia (e.g. dysplasia developing in metaplastic squamous epithelium from the bronchus of smokers). Dysplasia may also develop without co-existing metaplasia, for example in squamous epithelium of

the uterine cervix, glandular epithelium of the stomach, or the liver.

Dysplasia may be present for many years before a malignant neoplasm develops, and this observation can be used to screen populations at high risk of developing tumours.

The term 'dysplasia' is sometimes used misleadingly to denote the failure of differentiation of an organ which may retain primitive embryological structures. To avoid confusion, it is better to substitute the terms 'maldifferentiation' or 'dysgenesis' for this condition (see p. 105).

Neoplasia

> ▶ Neoplasia is characterised by abnormal, unco-ordinated and excessive cell growth
> ▶ Persists after initiating stimulus has been withdrawn
> ▶ Associated with genetic alterations
> ▶ Neoplastic cells influence behaviour of normal cells by the production of hormones and growth factors

The word 'neoplasia' literally means 'new growth', and the lesion so produced is termed a *neoplasm* (Ch. 11). A neoplasm is an abnormal tissue mass, the excessive growth of which is unco-ordinated with that of normal tissues, and which persists after the removal of the neoplasm-inducing stimulus. The term *tumour* is often used to denote a neoplasm.

This chapter has so far only considered examples of alterations in growth and differentiation as a response to genetically programmed stimuli required in organ or embryonic development, or as a response to alterations in the environment or work load of a cell or tissue. Growth and differentiation, when appropriately controlled, are beneficial, allowing the body to respond flexibly to various environmental stimuli. In contrast, however, neoplasms result from uncontrolled growth and often disordered differentiation, which is excessive and purposeless. The growth of neoplasms continues in an autonomous manner, in the absence of normal physiological stimuli and without normal negative feedback mechanisms to arrest the cellular proliferation.

Numerous factors have been implicated in the development of human tumours, and these are discussed in detail in Chapter 11. It should be noted, however, that there are multiple steps in the development of neoplasms, and that many of these involve subversion of the normally controlled mechanisms of growth and cellular differentiation, e.g. hormones, growth factors and growth-factor-simulating proteins such as some of the oncoproteins.

FURTHER READING

Alberts B, Bray D, Lewis J, Raff M, Roberts K, Watson J D 1989 Molecular biology of the cell, 2nd edn. Garland Publishing, New York

Berry C L 1989 Paediatric Pathology, 2nd edn. Springer Verlag, London

Keeling J W 1987 Fetal and neonatal pathology. Springer Verlag, London

Lodish H, Darnell J, Baltimore D 1990 Molecular cell biology, 3rd edn. Scientific American Books, New York

Oltvai Z N, Korsmeyer S J 1994 Checkpoints of dueling dimers foil death wishes. Cell 79: 189–192

Thompson C B 1995 Apoptosis in the pathogenesis and treatment of disease. Science 267: 1456–1462

Waterfield M D (ed) 1989 Growth factors. British Medical Bulletin

6

Responses to cellular injury

CELLULAR INJURY

> ► Numerous causes: physical and chemical agents including products of micro-organisms
> ► Various mechanisms: disruption, membrane failure, metabolic interference (respiration, protein synthesis, DNA), free radicals
> ► May be reversible, or end in cell death

Many agents can injure cells, but they can be classified into a small number of groups. Their mechanisms of action are also often very similar; widely differing agents may act through an identical final common pathway at the cellular level.

Causative agents

A wide range and variety of physical, chemical and biological agents may be associated with cellular injury; some examples are given in Table 6.1. Major causes of cellular injury include:

• trauma
• thermal injury, hot or cold
• poisons
• drugs
• infectious organisms
• ionising radiation.

Physical agents

Trauma and thermal injury result in cell death by disrupting cells and denaturing proteins, and also by causing local vascular thrombosis with consequent tissue ischaemia or infarction (Ch. 8). Missile injury combines these effects, as much energy is dissipated into tissues around the track. Blast injuries are the result of shearing forces, where structures of differing density and mobility are moved with respect to one another; traumatic amputation is a gross example.

Chemical and biological agents

Cells may be injured by contact with drugs and other chemicals; the latter may include enzymes and toxins secreted by micro-organisms.

Drugs and poisons
Numerous naturally occurring and synthetic chemicals can cause cellular injury; the effect is usually dose related, but in a few instances the effect is exacerbated by constitutional factors.

Some are highly toxic systemic metabolic poisons, while others exert their damage locally; the latter group includes caustic liquids applied to skin or mucous membranes, or gases that injure the lung. Furthermore, some substances produce one effect locally and another systemically. For example, some drugs are potentially caustic, and care needs to be taken to avoid extravasation into soft tissues when giving them by intravenous injection; diazepam is an example.

Caustic agents cause rapid local cell death due to their extreme alkalinity or acidity, in addition to having a corrosive effect on the tissue by digesting proteins.

Infectious organisms
The mechanisms of tissue damage produced by infectious organisms are varied, but with many bacteria it is their metabolic products or secretions that are harmful (see Ch. 3). Thus, the host cells receive a chemical insult which may be toxic to their metabolism or membrane integrity. In addition there will often be a host inflammatory response that may itself prove chemically damaging. Intracellular agents like viruses often result in the physical rupture of infected cells, but further local tissue damage may be the result of host immune reactions rather than infection. It follows that the cellular response to injury caused by infections will depend upon a combination of the damage inflicted by the agent both directly and indirectly, as a result of the host response to the agent.

Mechanisms of cellular injury

Cells may be damaged either reversibly or irre-

Table 6.1 Examples of causes of cellular injury and their mode of action	
Example agent	Mode of action
Trauma (e.g. road traffic accident)	Mechanical disruption of tissue
Carbon monoxide inhalation	Prevents oxygen transport
Contact with strong acid	Coagulates tissue proteins
Paracetamol overdose	Metabolites bind to liver cell proteins and lipoproteins
Bacterial infections	Toxins and enzymes
Ionising radiation (e.g. X-rays)	Damage to DNA

versibly in a variety of ways (Fig. 6.1). The effect on a tissue will depend on:

- the duration of the injury
- the nature of the injurious agent
- the proportion and type of cells affected
- the ability of the tissues to regenerate.

If the injury is fatal to the cells, then they may undergo necrosis. This often has the appearance of coagulative necrosis and at this stage it may not be possible to deduce the nature of the initiating cause. Alternatively, intracellular damage may trigger apoptosis (see pp. 83–84).

It is postulated that the influx of calcium ions may be a final common pathway resulting from several initial mechanisms of cellular injury. However, this may be only one aspect of the ionic equilibration (loss of normal ionic gradient across cell membranes) that characterises irreversible cell injury.

Mechanical disruption

Cells can be damaged, sometimes fatally, by direct mechanical force. This happens when tissues are incised surgically or accidentally; the cell membranes are ruptured, the cytoplasm spills out, and recovery is impossible. Freezing also damages cells mechanically because intracellular and cell membranes are perforat-ed by the ice crystals. Cells can also rupture as a result of osmotic imbalance across the cell membrane. This could be produced by a rapid change in the osmotic pressure of the extracellular or intracellular fluid.

Failure of membrane integrity

Cell membrane damage is an important mode of cellular injury for which there are several possible mechanisms:

- complement-mediated cytolysis
- perforin-mediated cytolysis
- specific blockage of ion channels
- failure of membrane ion pumps
- alteration of membrane lipids
- cross-linking of membrane proteins.

Cell membrane damage is one of the consequences of *complement activation* (Ch. 9); some of the end products of the complement cascade (C5b, 8 and 9) have cytolytic activity. Another recently discovered effector of cytolysis is *perforin*, a mediator of lymphocyte cytotoxicity, that causes damage to the cell membrane of the target cells, such as those infected by viruses.

Intramembrane channels permit the controlled entry and exit of specific ions. Blockage of these channels is sometimes used therapeutically. For

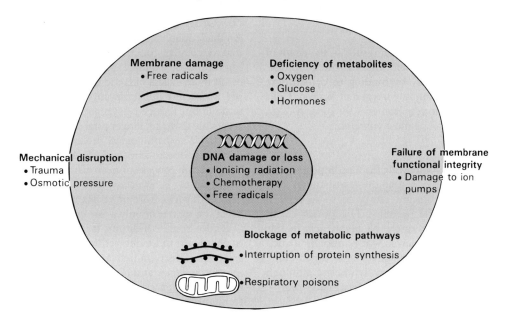

Fig. 6.1 Mechanisms of cellular injury

Different agents can injure the various structural and functional components of the cell. Some cells with specific function are selectively prone to certain types of injury.

example, verapamil is a calcium channel blocker used in the treatment of hypertension and ischaemic heart disease. Used in inappropriate circumstances or at high dosage, however, the calcium channel blockage may have toxic effects.

Membrane pumps that are responsible for maintaining, for example, the relatively high potassium and low sodium concentrations within cells are dependent on an adequate supply of ATP. Any chemical agents that deplete ATP, either by interfering with mitochondrial oxidative phosphorylation or by consuming ATP in their metabolism, will compromise the integrity of the membrane pumps and expose the cell to the risk of lysis. The Na/K ATPase in cell membranes can be directly inhibited by ouabain.

Just as disastrous for the cell is biochemical alteration of the lipoprotein bilayer forming the cell membrane. This can result from reactions with either the phospholipid or protein moieties. Membrane phospholipids may be altered through peroxidation by activated oxygen species, such as free radicals (see below), and by phospholipases. Membrane proteins may be altered by cross-linking induced by free radicals.

Blockage of metabolic pathways

Cell injury may be a consequence of specific interference with intracellular metabolism, effected usually by relative or total blockage of one or more pathways.

Cellular respiration
Prevention of oxygen utilisation results in the death of many cells due to loss of their principal energy source. Cyanide acts in this way by binding to cytochrome oxidase and thus interrupting oxygen utilisation. Cells with higher metabolic requirements for oxygen (e.g., cardiac myocytes) will be most vulnerable.

Protein synthesis
Cell function and viability will also be compromised if protein synthesis is blocked at the translational level because there is a constant requirement to replace enzymes and structural proteins. The potent toxin, ricin, derived from the castor oil plant, acts in this manner at the ribosomal level. Many antibiotics, such as streptomycin, chloramphenicol and tetracycline, act by interfering with protein synthesis, although toxic effects by this mechanism are fortunately rare.

DNA damage or loss

Damage to DNA may not be immediately evident unless it involves a region of the genome that is being actively transcribed. Cell populations that are constantly dividing (i.e. labile cells such as intestinal epithelium and haemopoietic cells) are immediately affected by a dose of radiation sufficient to alter their DNA. Other cell populations may require a growth or metabolic stimulus before the DNA damage is revealed. Since non-lethal DNA damage may be inherited by daughter cells, a clone of transformed cells with abnormal growth characteristics may be formed; this is the process of neoplastic transformation that results in tumours (Ch. 11).

Normal erythrocytes are particularly sensitive to injury because they lack a nucleus and, therefore, the DNA template essential for repair. This will also be the fate of any cell in which the nucleus is severely damaged, or when mitosis is attempted but its completion is blocked. The latter is the result of DNA strand breaks or cross-linkages; ionising radiation and some cytotoxic drugs used in cancer therapy have this effect. Damaged cells are deleted by apoptosis.

Deficiency of essential metabolites

By definition, a deficiency of any essential metabolite, such as a vitamin, oxygen, glucose or a hormone (Ch.7), leads inevitably to cell injury. As vitamin E has an anti-oxidant effect, this may be protective in any situation characterised by the release of free oxygen radicals.

Oxygen deprivation
An inadequate supply of oxygen is potentially damaging to cellular function. Even though there is the option of, for example, anaerobic glycolysis this may result in an excess of lactic acid and an intolerably low pH. Complete but temporary lack of oxygen, or continuous but reduced oxygenation, will often result in reversible damage; longer total oxygen deprivation will be fatal. The pathological process resulting from lack of oxygen due to impaired blood supply is *ischaemia*. The specific process of necrosis resulting from lack of blood supply is *infarction*. The duration necessary for cell death varies from one tissue to another, but for the brain is a matter of only a few minutes.

Under some conditions it is possible for the onset of cell death to be delayed until blood flow has been restored. This paradoxical phenomenon is known as *reperfusion injury* and may be due to the generation of reactive oxygen species free radicals and to damage to membrane calcium pumps. Cells damaged in this way probably undergo apoptosis rather than necrosis.

Glucose deprivation
Glucose is another important metabolite and source

of energy. Some cells, cerebral neurones for example, are dependent upon it and have high requirements. In diabetes mellitus, there is inadequate utilisation of glucose due to an absolute or relative lack of insulin.

Hormone deficiency
Reduced concentrations of a trophic hormone result in involution of its target cells (Ch. 5). The organ containing the target cells shrinks (*atrophy*) through the process of apoptosis which causes cell loss (Ch. 5). Apoptosis is a normal physiological process, but it may be present to an abnormal degree in a target organ in pathological circumstances such as destruction of the organ synthesising its trophic hormone.

Free radicals
Free radicals are atoms or groups of atoms with an unpaired electron (denoted as a superscript dot); as such, they may enter into chemical bond formation. They are highly reactive, chemically unstable, generally present only at low concentrations, and tend to participate in, or initiate, chain reactions.

Free radicals can be generated by two principal mechanisms:

- Deposition of energy, e.g. ionisation of water by radiation. An electron is displaced, resulting in free radicals. This is discussed further under the mode of action of ionising radiation later in this chapter.
- Interaction between oxygen, or other substances, and a free electron in relation to oxidation–reduction reactions. In this instance the superoxide radical ($O_2^{\cdot-}$) could be generated.

The consequences of free radical formation include the following:

- A chain reaction may be initiated in which other free radicals are also formed. A common final event is damage to polyunsaturated fatty acids, which are an essential component of cell membranes.
- The free radical may be scavenged by endogenous or exogenous anti-oxidants, e.g. sulphydryl compounds such as cysteine.
- Superoxide radicals may be inactivated by the copper-containing enzyme, superoxide dismutase, which generates hydrogen peroxide; catalase then mops this up to form water.

The clinicopathological events involving free radicals include:

- toxicity of some poisons (e.g. carbon tetrachloride)
- oxygen toxicity
- tissue damage in inflammation
- intracellular killing of bacteria.

Cells irreversibly damaged by free radicals are deleted by apoptosis.

Cellular appearances following injury

The agents and mechanisms mentioned above cause a variety of histological abnormalities, although very few are specific for each agent. Two patterns of sublethal cellular alteration seen fairly commonly are hydropic change and fatty change.

Hydropic change

The descriptive term hydropic change is applied to cells when the cytoplasm becomes pale and swollen due to the accumulation of fluid. Minor degrees of intracellular oedema are called cloudy swelling; a further increase in fluid and swelling of organelles results in the cytoplasm appearing vacuolated. Hydropic change is generally the result of disturbances of metabolism such as hypoxia or chemical poisoning. These changes are reversible, although they may herald irreversible damage if the causal injury is persistent.

Fatty change

Vacuolation of cells is often due to the accumulation of lipid droplets as a result of a disturbance to ribosomal function and uncoupling of lipid from protein metabolism. The liver is commonly affected in this way by several causes, such as hypoxia, alcohol or diabetes. There may be many small vacuoles, or they may coalesce to form one large vacuole filling the cell and displacing the nucleus. Moderate degrees of fatty change (steatosis) are reversible, but severe fatty change may not be.

Necrosis

> ► Death of tissues: causes include ischaemia, metabolic, trauma
> ► Coagulative necrosis in most tissues; colliquative in brain
> ► Tuberculosis shows caseous necrosis
> ► Gangrene is necrosis with putrefaction: it follows vascular occlusion or certain infections
> ► Fibrinoid necrosis: arterioles in malignant hypertension
> ► Fat necrosis: in pancreatitis, or after trauma

Death of cells or tissues in a living organism is referred to as necrosis, irrespective of the cause. It is a pathological process following cellular injury, and often involves a solid mass of tissue (Fig. 6.2). Several distinct types of necrosis are recognised:

- coagulative
- colliquative
- caseous
- gangrene
- fibrinoid
- fat necrosis.

The type of tissue and nature of the causative agent determine the type of necrosis.

Coagulative necrosis

Coagulative necrosis is the most common form of necrosis and occurs in almost all organs. Following devitalisation, the cells retain their outline as their proteins coagulate and metabolic activity ceases. The gross appearance will depend in part on the cause of cell death, and in particular on any vascular alteration such as dilatation, or cessation of flow. To begin with, the texture of the tissue will be normal or firm, but later it may become soft as a result of digestion by macrophages. This can have disastrous con-

sequences in necrosis of the myocardium following infarction, as there is a risk of rupture of the ventricle (Ch. 13).

Microscopic examination of an area of necrosis shows a variable appearance depending on the time interval since tissue death. In the first few hours, there will be no abnormality of staining. Subsequently, there will be progressive loss of nuclear staining until it ceases to be haematoxyphilic; this is accompanied by loss of cytoplasmic detail. The collagenous stroma is much more resistant to dissolution. The result is that, histologically, the tissue retains a faint outline of its structure until such time as the damaged area is removed by phagocytosis (or sloughed off a surface), and is then repaired or regenerated, according to the organ involved. The presence of necrotic tissue usually evokes an inflammatory response; this is independent of the reaction to the initiating cause of the necrosis.

Colliquative necrosis

Colliquative necrosis is seen in the brain because of its lack of any substantial supporting stroma; thus, necrotic neural tissue is liable to total liquefaction. There will be a glial reaction around the periphery,

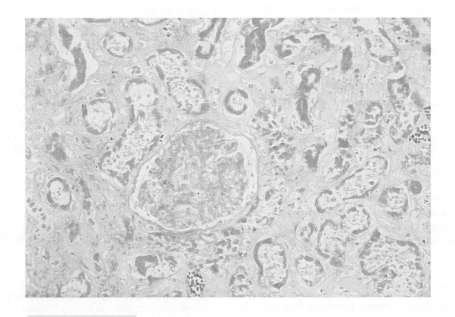

Fig. 6.2 Necrosis

Histology of part of a kidney deprived of its blood supply by an arterial embolus (see Ch. 8). Cellular and nuclear detail has been lost. This is an example of coagulative necrosis.

and the site of necrosis will be marked eventually by a cyst.

Caseous necrosis

Tuberculosis is characterised by caseous necrosis, a pattern of necrosis in which the dead tissue lacks any structure. Routine histological staining shows an amorphous eosinophilic area stippled by haematoxyphilic nuclear debris. Though not confined to tuberculosis, nor invariably present, caseation in a biopsy should always raise the possibility of this important disease.

Gangrene

Gangrene is necrosis with putrefaction of the tissues, sometimes as a result of the action of certain bacteria, notably clostridia. The affected tissues appear black, because of the deposition of iron sulphide from degraded haemoglobin. Thus, ischaemic necrosis of the distal part of a limb may proceed to gangrene if complicated by an appropriate infection. As clostridia are very common in the bowel, intestinal necrosis is particularly liable to proceed to gangrene; it can be seen as a complication of appendicitis, or incarceration of a hernia if the blood supply is impeded. These are examples of 'wet' gangrene. In contrast, 'dry' gangrene is usually seen in the toes, as a result of gradual arterial or small vessel obstruction in atherosclerosis or diabetes mellitus, respectively. In time, a line of demarcation develops between the gangrenous and adjacent viable tissues.

In contrast to the above, primary infection with certain bacteria or combinations of bacteria may result in similar putrefactive necrosis. Gas gangrene is the result of infection by *Clostridium perfringens*, while synergistic gangrene follows infection by combinations of organisms, such as *Bacteroides* and *Borrelia vincenti*.

Fibrinoid necrosis

In the context of malignant hypertension, arterioles are under such pressure that there is necrosis of the smooth muscle wall. This allows seepage of plasma into the media with consequent deposition of fibrin. The appearance is termed fibrinoid necrosis. With haematoxylin and eosin staining, the vessel wall is a homogeneous bright red. Fibrinoid necrosis is sometimes a misnomer because the element of necrosis is inconspicuous or absent. Nevertheless, the histological appearance is distinctive and its close resemblance to necrotic tissue perpetuates the name of this lesion.

Fat necrosis

Fat necrosis may be due to:

- direct trauma to adipose tissue and extracellular liberation of fat
- enzymatic lysis of fat due to release of lipases.

Following trauma to adipose tissue, the release of intracellular fat elicits a brisk inflammatory response, with polymorphs and macrophages phagocytosing the fat, proceeding eventually to fibrosis. The result may be a palpable mass, particularly at a superficial site such as the breast.

In acute pancreatitis, there is release of pancreatic lipase (Ch. 16). As a result, fat cells have their stored fat split into fatty acids, which then combine with calcium to precipitate out as white soaps. In severe cases, hypocalcaemia can ensue.

Apoptosis

▶ Individual cell deletion in physiological growth control and in disease
▶ Activated or prevented by a variety of stimuli
▶ Reduced apoptosis contributes to cell accumulation, e.g. neoplasia
▶ Increased apoptosis results in excessive cell loss, e.g. atrophy

Apoptosis is a mechanism of cell death quite different from necrosis (Table 6.2). Also called *programmed cell death*, it is an energy-dependent process for deletion of unwanted individual cells. It has a role in morphogenesis (Ch. 5), and is the mechanism for continuing control of organ size, maintaining normal size in the face of cell turnover, or a reduction during atrophy. Unwanted or defective cells also undergo apoptosis: thus lymphocyte proliferation in germinal centres and the thymus is followed by apoptosis of unwanted cells. Factors controlling apoptosis include substances outside the cell and internal metabolic pathways:

- *Inhibitors* include growth factors, cell matrix, sex steroids, some viral proteins.
- *Inducers* include growth factor withdrawal, loss of matrix attachment, glucocorticoids, some viruses, free radicals, ionising radiation.

Exposure to inducers or withdrawal of inhibitors initiates activation of *endogenous proteases* and *endonucleases*. These result in degradation of the cytoskeletal

Table 6.2 Comparison of cell death by apoptosis and necrosis		
Feature	Apoptosis	Necrosis
Induction	May be induced by physiological or pathological stimuli	Invariably due to pathological injury
Extent	Single cells	Cell groups
Biochemical events	Energy-dependent fragmentation of DNA by endogenous endonucleases	Impairment or cessation of ion homeostasis
	Lysosomes intact	Lysosomes leak lytic enzymes
Cell membrane integrity	Maintained	Lost
Morphology	Cell shrinkage and fragmentation to form apoptotic bodies with dense chromatin	Cell swelling and lysis
Inflammatory response	None	Usual
Fate of dead cells	Ingested (phagocytosed) by neighbouring cells	Ingested (phagocytosed) by neutrophil polymorphs and macrophages

framework, fragmentation of DNA and loss of mitochondrial function. The cell shrinks, retaining an intact plasma membrane (Fig. 6.3), but alteration of this membrane rapidly induces phagocytosis. Dead cells not phagocytosed break into smaller membrane-bound fragments called *apoptotic bodies*. There is no inflammatory reaction to apoptotic cells. Various diseases may be associated with reduced or increased apoptosis.

Reduced apoptosis

The product of p53 gene checks the integrity of the genome before mitosis: defective cells are switched to apoptosis instead. In contrast, *bcl*-2 protein inhibits apoptosis. It follows that loss of p53 function or excess *bcl*-2 expression may result in failure of initiation of apoptosis with resulting cell accumulation: both these defects are recorded in neoplasia

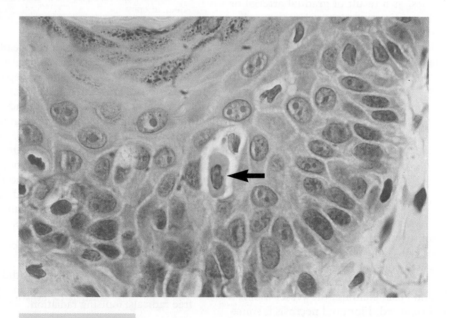

Fig. 6.3 Apoptosis

Histology of skin from a case of graft-versus-host disease (see Ch. 9) in which there is individual cell death (arrowed) in the epidermis as a result of immune injury.

(Ch. 11). Autoimmune disease (Ch. 9) might reflect failure of induction of apoptosis in lymphoid cells directed against host antigens; in systemic lupus erythematosus alterations are reported in the *Fas* lymphocyte surface receptor, which is critical in apoptosis induction in lymphocytes. Certain viruses enhance their survival by inhibition of apoptosis of cells they infect, and latent infection by Epstein–Barr virus upregulates *bcl-2*.

Increased apoptosis

Diseases in which increased apoptosis is probably important include acquired immune deficiency syndrome (AIDS), neurodegenerative disorders and some blood disorders characterised by low numbers of peripheral cells. In AIDS, human immunodeficiency virus proteins may activate CD4 on uninfected T-helper lymphocytes, inducing apoptosis with resulting immunodepletion. Apoptosis is probably the mode of cell death in reperfusion injury (Ch. 8) and exposure to ionising radiation (p. 127).

HEALING, REPAIR AND REGENERATION

> ▶ Cells can be divided into labile, stable or permanent populations; only labile and stable cells can be replaced if lost
> ▶ Complex tissue architecture may not be reconstructed
> ▶ Healing is restitution with no, or minimal, residual defect, e.g. superficial skin abrasion, incised wound healing by first intention
> ▶ Repair is necessary when there is tissue loss: healing by second intention

The ultimate consequences of an injury will depend upon many factors. The most important of these is the capability of cells to replicate in order to replace those that are lost, coupled with the ability to replace complex architectural structures.

Structures such as intestinal villi that depend largely on the epithelium for their shape can be rebuilt. However, complex arrangements such as the renal glomeruli cannot be reconstructed if destroyed.

Cell renewal

Once adult life is reached, cells can be classified into three populations according to their potential for renewal:

• *Labile cells* have a good capacity to regenerate.

Surface epithelial cells are typical of this group; they are constantly being lost from the surface and replaced from deeper layers.
• *Stable cell populations* divide at a very slow rate under physiological conditions, but still retain the capacity to divide when necessary. Hepatocytes and renal tubular cells are good examples.
• Nerve cells and striated muscle cells are regarded as *permanent* because they have no capacity to divide.

Stem cells

Cells lost through injury or normal senescence are replaced from the *stem cell pool* present in many labile and stable populations. When stem cells undergo mitotic division, one of the daughter cells progresses along a differentiation pathway according to the needs and functional state of the tissue; the other daughter cell retains the stem cell characteristics. Stem cells are a minority population in many tissues and are often located in discrete compartments: in the epidermis, stem cells are in the basal layer immediately adjacent to the basement membrane; in intestinal mucosa, the stem cells are near the bottom of the crypts.

The ability of a tissue to regenerate may be dependent on the integrity of the stem cell population. Stem cells are particularly vulnerable to radiation injury; this can result either in their loss, thus impairing the regenerative ability of the tissue, or in mutations propagated to daughter cells with the risk of neoplastic transformation.

Complete restitution

Loss of part of a labile population of cells can be completely restored. For example, consider the result of a minor skin abrasion (Fig. 6.4). The epidermis is lost over a limited area, but at the margins of the lesion there remain cells that can multiply to cover the defect. In addition the base of the lesion probably transects the neck of sweat glands and hair follicles; cells from here can also proliferate and contribute to healing. At first, cells proliferate and spread out as a thin sheet until the defect is covered. When they form a confluent layer, the stimulus to proliferate is switched off; this is referred to as *contact inhibition*, and controls both growth and movement. Once in place, the epidermis is rebuilt from the base upwards until it is indistinguishable from normal. This whole process is called *healing*.

Contact inhibition of growth and of movement are important control mechanisms in normal cells; in neoplasia (Ch. 11) these control mechanisms are

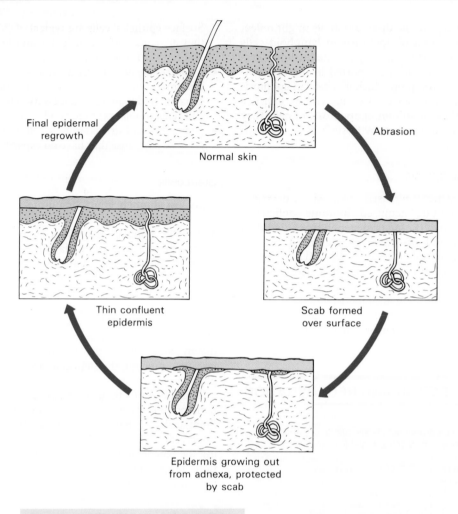

Final epidermal
regrowth

Normal skin

Abrasion

Thin confluent
epidermis

Scab formed
over surface

Epidermis growing out
from adnexa, protected
by scab

Fig. 6.4   Healing of a minor skin abrasion

The scab, a layer of fibrin, protects the epidermis as it grows to cover the defect. The scab
is then shed and the skin is restored to normal.

lost, allowing the continued proliferation of tumour
cells.

The contribution of adnexal gland cells to regeneration is made use of in plastic surgery when using split skin grafts. The whole of the epidermis is removed and positioned as the donor graft, but the necks of adnexa are left in place to generate a replacement at the donor site.

Organisation

▶ The repair of specialised tissues by the formation of
  a fibrous scar
▶ Occurs by the production of granulation tissue and
  removal of dead tissue by phagocytosis

Organisation is the name given to the process whereby specialised tissues are repaired by the formation of mature fibrovascular connective tissue. Granulation tissue is formed in the early stages, often on the basis of fibrin, and any dead tissue is removed by phagocytic cells such as neutrophil polymorphs and macrophages. The granulation tissue contracts and gradually accumulates collagen to form the scar.

Organisation is a common consequence of pneumonia, inflammation of the alveoli of the lung in which inflammatory exudate fills the alveoli. The exudate subsequently becomes organised. Organisation also occurs when a volume of tissue dies as a result of cessation of its blood supply (an infarct). In all instances, the organised area is firmer than normal, and shrunken or puckered.

Granulation tissue

> ▶ A repair phenomenon
> ▶ Loops of capillaries, supported by myofibroblasts
> ▶ Inflammatory cells may be present
> ▶ Actively contracts to reduce wound size; this may result in a stricture later

When specialised tissue is destroyed, it cannot be reconstructed; a stereotyped response then follows, a process known as *repair*. Capillary endothelial cells proliferate and grow into the area to be repaired; initially they are solid buds but soon they open into vascular channels. The vessels are arranged as a series of loops arching into the damaged area. At the same time, fibroblasts are stimulated to divide and to secrete collagen; they also acquire bundles of muscle filaments and attachments to adjacent cells and stroma. These modified cells are called myofibroblasts, and display features and functions of both fibroblasts and smooth muscle cells. As well as secreting a collagen framework, they play a fundamental role in wound contraction. This combination of capillary loops and myofibroblasts is known as granulation tissue. The name derives from the appearance of the base of a skin ulcer; when the repair process is observed, the capillary loops are just visible and impart a granular texture. Such a name is less appropriate for an internal repair, but is used despite this. Granulation tissue must not be confused with a granuloma (an aggregate of epithelioid histiocytes).

Wound contraction and scarring

Wound contraction plays a considerable role in reducing the volume of tissue for repair; the tissue defect may be reduced by 80%. It is the result of the contraction of *myofibroblasts* in the granulation tissue. These are attached to each other and to the adjacent ground substance, so that granulation tissue as a whole contracts and draws together the surrounding tissues. Collagen is secreted at the same time and forms a local scar in place of the specialised tissues lost.

Although wound contraction serves a very useful function, it can also lead to problems. If the tissue damage is circumferentially around the lumen of a tube such as the gut, subsequent contraction may progress until it causes obstruction due to a *stricture*. Similarly, burns to the skin can be followed by considerable contraction, with resulting cosmetic damage and, often, impaired mobility.

Outcome of injuries in different tissues

Having considered the general principles of healing and repair, the particular outcome of injuries to a variety of tissues will be considered.

Skin

The process of healing of a skin wound depends on the size of the defect.

Incised wound: healing by first intention
An incision such as that made by a surgical scalpel causes very little damage to tissues on either side of the cut. If the two sides of the wound can be brought together accurately, then healing can proceed with the minimum of delay or difficulty (Fig. 6.5). It is obvious that at least some small blood vessels will have been cut, but these will be occluded by thrombosis, and close apposition of wound edges will help. Fibrin precipitated locally will then link across the

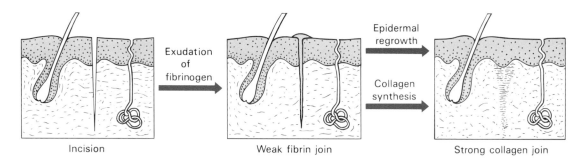

Fig. 6.5 Skin incision healed by first intention
As little or no tissue has been lost, the apposed edges of the incision are joined by a thin layer of fibrin, which is ultimately replaced by collagen covered by surface epidermis.

two sides. Coagulated blood on the surface forms the scab, and helps to keep the wound clean. This join is very weak, but is formed rapidly and is a framework for the next stage. It is important that it is not disrupted, and sutures, sticking plaster or other means of mechanical support are invaluable aids. Over the next few days, capillaries proliferate sufficiently to bridge the tiny gap, and fibroblasts secrete collagen as they migrate into the fibrin network. If the sides of the wound are very close, then such migration is minimal, as would be the amount of collagen and vascular proliferation required. By about ten days, the strength of the repair is sufficient to enable removal of sutures. The only residual defect will be the failure to reconstruct the elastic network in the dermis.

While these changes are proceeding in the dermis, the basal epidermal cells proliferate to spread over any gap. If the edges of the wound are gaping, then the epidermal cells will creep down the sides. Eventually, when the wound is healed, these cells will usually stop growing and be resorbed, but occasionally they will remain and grow to form a keratin-filled cyst (implantation dermoid).

Tissue loss: healing by second intention
When there is tissue loss or some other reason why the wound margins are not apposed, then another mechanism is necessary for repair. For example, if there is haemorrhage locally, then this will keep the sides apart and prevent healing by first intention; infection will have a similar effect in addition to its own particular consequences. A local loss of an epithelial covering is referred to as an *ulcer*. This is a purely descriptive term and does not imply any particular cause, such as trauma, inflammation or neoplasia. The response will be characterised by:

- phagocytosis to remove any debris
- granulation tissue to fill in defects and repair specialised tissues lost
- epithelial regeneration to cover the surface (Fig. 6.6).

The timescale will depend upon the volume of the defect, since this determines the amount of granulation tissue to be generated and the area to cover with epithelium. Quite large expanses of tissue can be removed if necessary, and the defect left to heal by second intention. The final cosmetic result will depend upon how much tissue loss there has been, as this will affect the amount of scarring.

Keloid nodules
Dermal injury is sometimes followed by excessive

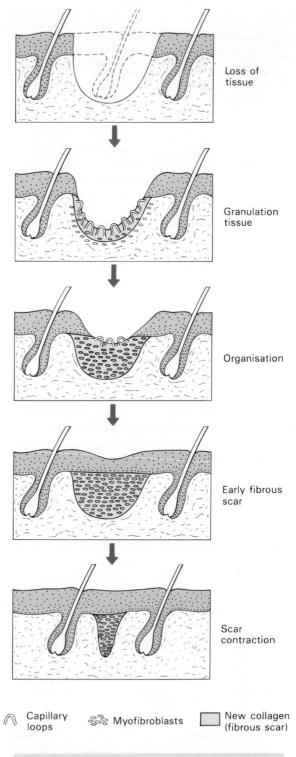

Loss of tissue

Granulation tissue

Organisation

Early fibrous scar

Scar contraction

⋀ Capillary loops   ⟋⟍⟋ Myofibroblasts   ▢ New collagen (fibrous scar)

Fig. 6.6 Skin wound repaired by second intention

The tissue defect becomes filled with granulation tissue, which eventually contracts, leaving a small scar.

fibroblast proliferation and collagen production. This phenomenon is genetically determined, and is particularly prevalent among blacks. A mass several centimetres across may follow surgery or injury, particularly burns.

Gastrointestinal tract

The fate of an intestinal injury depends upon its depth.

Mucosal erosions

An erosion is defined as loss of part of the thickness of the mucosa. Viable epithelial cells are immediately adjacent to the defect, and rapidly proliferate to regenerate the mucosa. Such an erosion can be covered in a matter of hours, provided that the cause has been removed. Notwithstanding this remarkable speed of recovery, it is possible for a patient to lose much blood from multiple gastric erosions before they heal. In such a patient, if endoscopy to identify the cause of haematemesis is delayed, the erosions may no longer be present, and thus escape detection.

Mucosal ulceration

Ulceration is loss of the full thickness of the mucosa, and often the defect goes much deeper to penetrate the muscularis propria; further complications are discussed in Chapter 15. The principles of repair have been outlined above. Destroyed muscle cannot be regenerated, and the mucosa must be replaced from the margins. The outcome of mucosal ulceration is discussed below with reference to a gastric ulcer, but colonic ulcers show similar features. Damaged blood vessels will have bled and, in time, the surface will be covered by a layer of fibrin. Macrophages then migrate in to remove any dead tissue by phagocytosis. Meanwhile, granulation tissue is produced in the ulcer base, as capillaries and myofibroblasts proliferate. Also, the mucosa will begin to regenerate at the margins and spread out on to the floor of the ulcer.

If the cause persists, the ulcer becomes chronic and there is a continuing oscillation between further ulceration and repair. This may result in considerable destruction of the gastric wall. If healing ever proceeds far enough, the fibrous scar tissue that has replaced muscle will contract, with distortion of the stomach and possible obstruction. Any larger arteries that lie in the path of the advancing ulceration are at risk of rupture, with resulting haemorrhage. However, there may be a zone of inflammation around the ulceration, and if this abuts the vessel it results in a reactive proliferation of the vascular inti-

ma. This feature is referred to as *endarteritis obliterans* on account of the obliteration of the lumen; it has nothing specifically to do with end arteries.

Bone

> ▶ Haematoma organised and dead bone removed
> ▶ Callus formed, then replaced by trabecular bone
> ▶ Finally remodelled
> ▶ Fracture healing delayed if bone ends are mobile, infected, very badly misaligned or avascular

Fracture healing

The cellular mechanisms involved in the healing of a fracture are closely related to the repair process in other tissues, although they are modified for the special environment of bone. Immediately after the fracture, there will be haemorrhage within the bone from ruptured vessels in the marrow cavity, and also around the bone in relation to the periosteum. A *haematoma* at the fracture site facilitates repair by providing a foundation for the growth of cells (Fig. 6.7). There will also be devitalised fragments of bone, and probable soft tissue damage nearby. The opening phases of repair will thus be removal of necrotic tissue and organisation of the haematoma. The latter takes a special form, as the capillaries will be accompanied by fibroblasts and osteoblasts. These lay down bone in an irregularly woven pattern. The mass of new bone, sometimes with islands of cartilage, is called *callus*; that which lies within the medullary cavity is internal callus, while that in relation to the periosteum is external callus. The latter is helpful as a splint, although it will need to be resorbed eventually. Woven bone is subsequently replaced by more orderly, lamellar bone; this in turn is gradually remodelled according to the direction of mechanical stress.

Problems with fracture healing

Several factors can delay, or even arrest, the repair of a fracture:

* movement
* interposed soft tissues
* gross misalignment
* infection
* pre-existing bone disease.

Movement between the two ends, apart from causing pain, also results in excessive callus and prevents or slows down tissue union. If continued, movement will prevent bone formation, and collagen is laid down instead to give fibrous union; the result is the

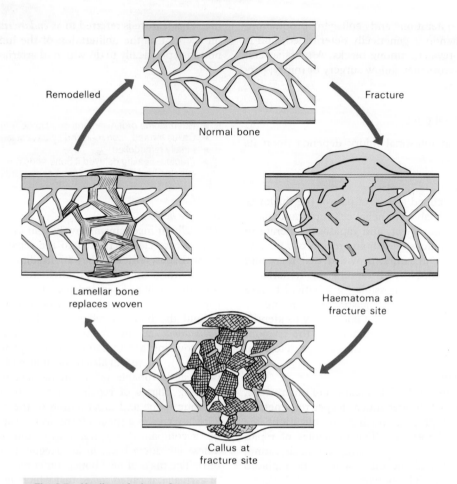

Remodelled

Fracture

Normal bone

Lamellar bone
replaces woven

Haematoma at
fracture site

Callus at
fracture site

Fig. 6.7   Healing of a bone fracture

The haematoma at the fracture site gives a framework for healing. It is replaced by a
fracture callus, which is subsequently replaced by lamellar bone, which is then remodelled
to restore the normal trabecular pattern of the bone.

formation of a false joint at the fracture site. Movement of a lesser degree gives rise to excessive callus which takes a long time to be resorbed and may impinge on adjacent structures.

Interposed soft tissues between the broken ends delay healing at least until they have been removed, and there is an increased risk of non-union.

Gross misalignment also slows the rate of healing and will prevent a good functional result, leading to increased risk of accelerated degenerative disease (osteoarthrosis) in adjacent joints.

Infection at the fracture site will delay healing and there is the additional risk of chronic osteomyelitis. Infection is more likely if the skin over the fracture is broken; this is referred to as a *compound fracture.*

If the bone broken was not normal, the break is called a *pathological fracture*. Abnormal bone is at risk of fracture after an impact force that is trivial compared to that necessary to break a normal bone, or it may break spontaneously. Pathological fracture may be the result of a primary disorder of bone, or the secondary involvement of bone by some other condition, such as metastatic carcinoma. In most instances, a pathological fracture will heal satisfactorily, but sometimes treatment of the underlying cause will be required first.

Liver

Hepatocytes have excellent regenerative capacity, although they are a stable population and replicate only slowly. The hepatic architecture, however, cannot be satisfactorily reconstructed if severely damaged. Consequently, conditions that simply result in hepatocyte loss may be followed by complete restitution, whereas damage destroying both the hepatocytes and architecture may not. In the latter situation, the imbalance between hepatocyte regeneration and failure to reconstruct the architecture may proceed to cirrhosis (Fig. 6.8).

Kidney

The kidney is similar to the liver with respect to tissue injury, in that it has an epithelium that can be regenerated but an architecture that cannot. Loss of tubular epithelium following an ischaemic episode or exposure to toxins may result in clinical renal failure, but in general there is sufficient surviving epithelium to repopulate the tubules and enable normal renal function to return. Inflammatory or other damage resulting in destruction of the glomerulus is likely to be permanent or result in glomerular scarring, with loss of filtration capacity. Similarly, interstitial inflammation is liable to proceed to fibrosis and, thus, impaired reabsorption from tubules into the circulation.

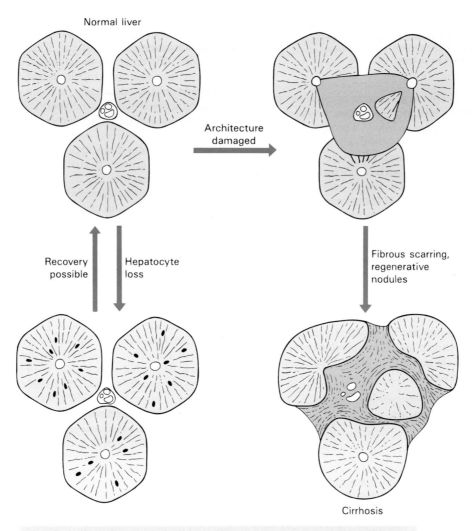

Fig. 6.8 Consequences of liver injury depending on extent of tissue damage

Loss of only scattered liver cells, or even small groups, can be restored without architectural disturbance. However, if there is confluent loss of liver cells and architectural damage, the liver heals by scarring and nodular regeneration of liver cells, resulting in cirrhosis.

Muscle

Cardiac muscle fibres and smooth muscle cells are a permanent population; vascular smooth muscle may be different, in that new vessels can be formed. This means that damaged muscle is replaced by scar tissue. However, if the contractile proteins only are lost, then it is possible to synthesise new ones within the old endomysium. Voluntary muscle has a limited capacity for regeneration from satellite cells.

Neural tissue

> ▶ Central nervous system does not repair effectively
> ▶ Peripheral nerves show Wallerian degeneration (Ch. 26) distal to trauma; variable recovery depending on alignment and continuity
> ▶ May produce amputation neuroma

There is no effective regeneration of neurones in the central nervous system. Glial cells, however, may proliferate in response to injury, a process referred to as *gliosis*.

Peripheral nerve damage affects axons and their supporting structures, such as Schwann cells. If there is transection of the nerve, axons degenerate proximally for a distance of about one or two nodes; distally, there is Wallerian degeneration followed by proliferation of Schwann cells in anticipation of axonal regrowth. If there is good realignment of the cut ends, the axons may regrow down their previous channels (now occupied by proliferated Schwann cells); however, full functional recovery is unusual. When there is poor alignment or amputation of the nerve, the cut ends of the axons still proliferate, but in a disordered manner, to produce a tangled mass of axons and stroma called an *amputation neuroma*. Sometimes, these give rise to painful sensations and have to be removed.

Modifying influences

> ▶ Damage to fetus or infant may affect subsequent development
> ▶ In general, children heal rapidly
> ▶ In old age, reserve capacity is reduced and there may be co-existent disease, such as ischaemia
> ▶ Vitamin C deficiency impairs collagen synthesis
> ▶ Malnutrition impairs healing and resistance to disease
> ▶ Excess steroids, advanced malignancy, and local ischaemia impair healing
> ▶ Denervation increases tissue vulnerability

The description of tissue injury and repair given above applies to an otherwise healthy adult. This will not always be the case. Various factors can impair healing and repair:

- age, both very young and elderly
- disorders of nutrition
- neoplastic disorders
- Cushing's syndrome and steroid therapy
- diabetes mellitus and immunosuppression
- vascular disturbance
- denervation.

Age

Early in life, cellular injury is likely to impair or prevent the normal growth and development of an organ. Organogenesis is at risk if there is impaired function, differentiation or migration of the precursor cells. For example, rubella infection or thalidomide administration in early pregnancy can result in congenital abnormalities; therapeutic doses of irradiation are associated with microcephaly and mental retardation.

Similar considerations apply to childhood, in that there may be growth disturbance following tissue damage. For example, the distal pulmonary airways may be permanently damaged by severe infection or mechanical stress, as in whooping cough. High doses of irradiation will result in loss of replicating cells and in local failure to grow; the affected area will then be smaller in proportion to the rest of the body. On the other hand, wound healing proceeds rapidly in healthy children, and fractures unite more quickly than in adults.

The physiology of ageing is poorly understood, but at least one characteristic is a reduced ability to repair damaged tissues. Connective tissues gradually lose their elasticity, renal function loses its reserve capacity, bones fail to maintain their strength, and cerebral nerve cells are lost. A possible consequence of this is a more substantial effect from the same insult when compared with that in a younger adult. Wound healing is often delayed in old age because of ischaemia or other significant disease. As a result of this, the patient may suffer further complications while recovering from the first incident.

Disorders of nutrition

Wound healing is profoundly influenced by the ability to synthesise protein and collagen. The latter is dependent on vitamin C for the hydroxylation of proline as a step in collagen synthesis. Scurvy (vitamin C deficiency) leads to wound healing of greatly reduced strength; capillaries are also fragile and thus haemorrhages occur.

Protein malnutrition, whether due to dietary deficiency or the consequence of protein loss, also impairs wound healing. In addition, severe malnutrition reduces the ability to respond to infection; tissue damage may then proceed unimpeded with a fatal outcome. For example, measles is generally a transient problem in well-nourished children, but is frequently fatal in the malnourished.

Neoplastic disorders

In advanced malignant neoplastic disease with widely disseminated tumours, or gastrointestinal symptoms such as dysphagia, the patient is malnourished. However, a catabolic state with profound weight loss may be an early feature of some cancers. Such patients show evidence of impaired healing, and this may compromise the recovery from attempted surgical removal of the lesion.

There may also be evidence of impaired healing localised to the vicinity of the tumour. Skin stretched over a superficial tumour will often break down and ulcerate, and it is necessary to treat the tumour to promote healing of the ulcer. A pathological fracture of bone through a metastatic deposit of tumour may not heal unless the tumour is dealt with first; in practice, the management often includes irradiation to the tumour and internal fixation of long bones.

Cushing's syndrome and steroid therapy

Excessive circulating corticosteroids, whether they result from tumour or from therapeutic administration, have two effects on tissue injury.

- Due to their immunosuppressive actions, the consequences of injury or infection may be more severe.
- Steroids impair healing by interfering with the formation of granulation tissue and, thus, wound contraction.

Diabetes mellitus and immunosuppression

Both diabetes mellitus and immunosuppression increase susceptibility to infection by low-virulence organisms, and put the patient at risk of tissue damage. The normal healing responses are possible, although they may be impaired by continuing infection. Diabetes may affect polymorph function, and may also result in occlusion of small blood vessels and cause neuropathy.

Vascular disturbance

An adequate vascular supply is essential for normal cellular function. An impaired supply can result in ischaemia or infarction and is discussed in Chapter 8. In the context of tissue injury and repair, it is worth stating that what is an adequate supply for resting tissue may prove inadequate if the demand increases. For example, in coronary artery disease, the blood flow may be sufficient for the resting state, but not for exertion when the cardiac output increases. This induced deficit of oxygen may then result in tissue damage.

Another effect of a reduced vascular supply is impaired healing. This occurs because hypoxia and reduced local nutrition result in poorer tissue regrowth or repair.

Denervation

An intact nerve supply supports the structural and functional integrity of many tissues. In addition, nerves have a role in mediating the inflammatory response which is part of the host mechanism for limiting the effects of injury. Denervated tissues may become severely damaged, probably through a combination of unresponsiveness to repeated minor trauma, and lack of awareness of intercurrent infection or inflammation. Thus, patients with conditions such as peripheral neuropathy or leprosy may develop ulceration of the foot (neuropathic ulcers); with intervention and care to prevent further injury, healing is possible. A neuropathic joint (Charcot's joint) may be damaged unwittingly and progressively beyond repair.

INJURY DUE TO IONISING RADIATION

- ▶ Electromagnetic and particulate: background, accidental, occupational and medical exposure
- ▶ Indirect effect of oxygen radicals and hydroxyl ions on DNA
- ▶ Rapidly dividing cell populations show early susceptibility
- ▶ Chronic effects: fibrosis and increased tumour risk
- ▶ Tumour induction roughly proportional to dose received

Radiation is now generally perceived by the public as harmful. In the European Community it is now mandatory that medical practitioners using radiation for investigating or treating patients have a core of knowledge relevant to radiation protection. This section seeks to give certain aspects of this core, particularly in relation to:

- nature of ionising radiation and its interaction with tissue
- genetic and somatic effects of ionising radiation.

Definition and sources

Radiation of medical importance is largely restricted to that which causes the formation of ions on interaction with matter (ionising radiation). The exception to this is some ultraviolet light. Ionising radiation includes:

- electromagnetic radiation: X-rays and gamma-rays
- particulate radiation: alpha particles, beta particles (electrons), neutrons.

Electromagnetic radiation

Only part of the electromagnetic spectrum produces ionising events. The production of ions requires a photon of high energy and thus of short wavelength, in practice shorter than that of ultraviolet light. If the photon is produced artificially, the radiation is called an X-ray. If it is emitted as a result of the disintegration of an unstable atom, it is referred to as a gamma-ray.

Particulate radiation

As well as photons, certain subatomic particles may also produce ionisation. These include alpha particles (helium nuclei), beta particles (electrons) and neutrons. The distinction between beta particles and electrons is the same as that between gamma-rays and X-rays; beta particles are produced through the process of radioactive decay, whereas electrons are a structural component of atoms that may be artificially projected as a beam.

Units of dose

Various units have been used for measuring radiation; the current unit of *absorbed dose* is the gray (Gy). It is equivalent to 100 rads, the previous unit, and is the usual measure of therapeutic irradiation when a uniform type of irradiation is administered to a specified tissue.

However, different forms of irradiation vary in the biological effect produced (alpha particles are about 20 times more damaging than beta particles or X-rays), and tissues differ in their sensitivity (Table 6.3). Therefore, when subjects are exposed to

Table 6.3 Relative sensitivities of different tissues to harmful effects of ionising radiation

Tissue	Factor
Gonads	0.25
Breasts	0.15
Haemopoietic tissue	0.12
Lungs	0.12
Liver	0.06
Thyroid	0.03
Bone	0.03
Other organs (total)	0.24
	Total for body = 1.00

a mixture of different forms of radiation to several tissues, it is useful to make mathematical corrections for comparative purposes, and express the result as the *effective dose equivalent*, measured in sieverts (Sv): this is equivalent to 100 rem, the previous unit (Fig. 6.9).

Another relevant unit is a measure of the rate of disintegration of unstable atoms. One becquerel (Bq) is one emission per second; it replaces the curie (Ci); one Ci equals 3.7×10^{10} Bq. The becquerel is not itself a measure of dose, because it expresses only a rate of disintegration irrespective of the nature or energy of the products of disintegration. However, for any particular atom the latter is known, so the dose can be calculated.

Background radiation

Everyone is exposed to background radiation from their environment. In the United Kingdom the average annual dose is 2.5 mSv, which comes from:

- natural sources (87%)
- artificial sources (13%).

Over 90% of the artificial component is from medical usage, such as diagnostic X-rays, with only a small contribution from nuclear-weapons-testing fallout and the nuclear power industry (including its accidents). The natural component is made up from cosmic, terrestrial, airborne and food sources. The most locally variable among these is the airborne radiation, which derives mainly from radon and radon daughters; these diffuse out of the ground and are commoner in certain types of rock, such as granite. In the United Kingdom, there are 100-fold differences from one place to another. Some draught-proofed homes in areas of high natural airborne radiation accumulate radon to concentrations exceeding acceptable industrial limits, thereby placing occupants at risk of lung disease from radiation.

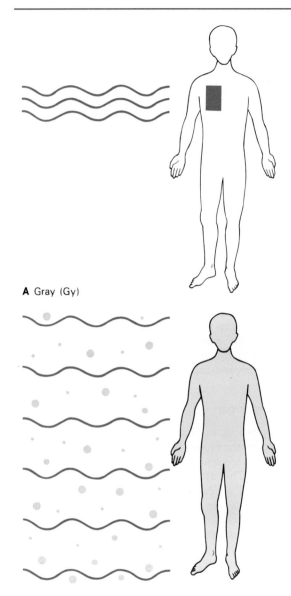

A Gray (Gy)

B Effective dose equivalent in sievert (Sv)

Fig. 6.9 Units of dose of irradiation

A. The gray (Gy) is a measure of absorbed dose.
B. The sievert (Sv) measures the radiation dose corrected for different types of radiation and the differing sensitivities of tissues to them.

Mode of action

When radiation passes through tissue, any collisions within it will be randomly distributed amongst its components. However, it seems that direct damage as a result of ionisation of proteins or membranes does not make a major contribution to the biological end result. Water is the most prevalent molecule, and following ionisation several types of short-lived but highly reactive radicals are formed such as H˙ and hydroxyl radical OH˙. In a well-oxygenated cell, oxygen radicals will also be formed, e.g. hydroperoxyl radical, HO_2˙ and superoxide radical O_2˙$^-$.

These radicals then interact with macromolecules, of which the most significant are membrane lipids and DNA.

DNA damage

The types of radiation-induced DNA damage include:

- strand breaks
- base alterations
- cross-linking.

Breakage of the DNA strand (Fig. 6.10) is a common result of irradiation. When only one strand is broken, repair can generally be accomplished accurately; however, double-strand breaks may prove impossible to repair because there is no template.

Base alterations are also frequent, such that the DNA strand no longer transcribes correctly. The result may be non-readable, or may read incorrectly.

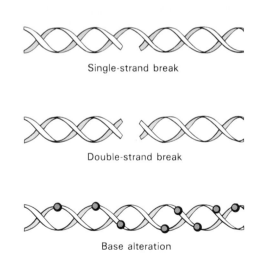

Single-strand break

Double-strand break

Base alteration

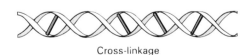

Cross-linkage

Fig. 6.10 DNA damage by irradiation

Single-strand breaks can be reconstituted by DNA repair enzymes, because the complementary strand forms a template. The other injuries are less easily remedied. Cross-linkage is lethal.

DNA strand cross-linking occurs when irradiation fuses the complementary strands, resulting in an inability to separate and thus to make a new copy. DNA replication is therefore blocked. This effect is also the mechanism of action of alkylating agents, hence their description as 'radiomimetic drugs'.

The consequences of DNA damage depend on its nature and extent, and on the results of any attempts at repair. Irreversibly damaged cells are deleted by apoptosis. Mammalian cells given about 1.5 Gy of X-rays will show extensive base damage and about 1000 strand breaks, some 50 of which will be double-strand; two-thirds of the cells will die. However, there are repair enzyme systems to cope with ionising radiation and similar damage from ultraviolet light. If these are deficient, as in the condition xeroderma pigmentosum, the patient will show increased radiosensitivity. This results in the induction of excessive radiation damage and tumours of the skin from normal light exposure.

Effects on tissues

Despite knowledge of the molecular events following irradiation, there is continuing debate about how these are translated into the observed tissue responses. The immediate physico-chemical events and consequent biomolecular damage are over in a few milliseconds; the varied outcomes are manifest in hours to years.

DNA damage may have three possible consequences:

- cell death, either immediately or at the next attempted mitosis
- repair and no further consequence
- a permanent change in genotype.

The dose given will influence this outcome, as will the radiosensitivity of the cell. Tissue and organ changes will reflect the overall reactions in the component parts.

Acute effects

Acute effects of irradiation are generally the result of cell killing and the interruption of successful mitotic activity. Hierarchical cell organisations, such as the bone marrow or gut epithelium, which have a dividing stem cell population and daughter cells of finite life expectancy, will show the most pronounced effects. In essence, the supply of functioning differentiated cells is cut off or suspended. In addition, there is vascular endothelial damage, resulting in fluid and protein leakage rather like that of the inflammatory response (Ch. 10).

Chronic effects

Chronic effects of irradiation are the result of a number of possible factors, and the contribution of each is contentious. Vascular endothelial cell loss will result in exposure of the underlying collagen. This will prompt platelet adherence and thrombosis, which is subsequently incorporated into the vessel wall and is associated with the intimal proliferation of endarteritis obliterans. A possible result of this is long-term vascular insufficiency with consequent atrophy and fibrosis.

However, the observed atrophy may simply be a function of continuing cell loss over a long period of time, reflecting an inherently slow rate of proliferation of cells in the tissue concerned. If this is the case, the vascular alterations are part of the chronic radiation process, but not the cause of the atrophy.

The cellular alterations induced by irradiation are permanent. The limits of tissue tolerance cannot be exceeded even if many years have elapsed. In addition to the effects mentioned above, radiation-induced mutation of the genome causes an increased risk of neoplastic transformation (see below).

Bone marrow

Haemopoietic marrow is a hierarchical tissue which maintains the blood concentration of functional cells of limited life span by a constant high rate of mitotic activity. The effect of irradiation is to suspend renewal of all cell lines. Subsequent blood counts will fall at a rate corresponding to the physiological survival of cells; granulocytes will be reduced after a few days but erythrocytes survive much longer.

The ultimate outcome will depend on the dose received, and will vary from complete recovery to death from marrow failure (unless a marrow transplant is successful). In the long-term survivor, there is a risk of leukaemia. Localised heavy irradiation will not alter the blood count, but it will result in local loss of haemopoiesis and fibrosis of the marrow cavity.

Intestine

The surface epithelial lining of the small intestine is renewed every 24–48 hours. A significant dose of irradiation will therefore result in loss of protective and absorptive functions over a similar timescale; diarrhoea and the risk of infection then follow. If a high dose is given to a localised region, the mucosa will regrow, although often with a less specialised cell type, and with the probability of mutations in the remaining cells. The muscle coat will also have been damaged, and there is the risk of granulation tissue causing the formation of a stricture later.

Skin

The changes in the skin reflect its composition from epithelium, connective tissue and blood vessels. Epidermis will suffer the consequences of cessation of mitosis, with desquamation and hair loss. Provided enough stem cells survive, hair will regrow, and any defects in epidermal coverage can be re-epithelialised. The regenerated epidermis will lack rete ridges and adnexa. Damage to keratinocytes and melanocytes results in melanin deposition in the dermis where it is picked up by phagocytic cells; these tend to remain in the skin and result in local hyperpigmentation (post-inflammatory pigmentation). Some fibroblasts in the dermis will be killed, while others are at risk of an inability to divide, or to function correctly. As a consequence, the dermis is thinned, and histology shows bizarre, enlarged fibroblast nuclei.

The vessels show various changes depending on their size. Endothelial cell loss or damage is the probable underlying factor; these cells develop vacuoles. Small and thin-walled vessels will leak fluid and proteins, and mimic the inflammatory response; in the long term, they can be permanently dilated and tortuous (telangiectatic). Larger vessels develop intimal proliferation and may permanently impair blood flow.

In summary, the skin is at first reddened with desquamation, and subsequently shows pigmentation. Later, it is thinned with telangiectasia; if damage is too severe, it will break down and ulcerate (radionecrosis).

Gonads

Germ cells are very radiosensitive, and permanent sterility can follow relatively low doses. Also of great significance is the possibility of mutation in germ cells, which could result in passing on defects to the next generation; this is a teratogenic effect.

Lung

Ionising radiation is one of several agents that can damage alveoli, culminating in fibrosis (Ch. 14). Inhaled radioactive materials induce pulmonary tumours.

Kidney

Renal irradiation results in gradual loss of parenchyma and impaired renal function. Systemic effects include the development of hypertension.

Whole body irradiation

Whole body irradiation can be the result of accidental or therapeutic exposure to high or low doses. The consequences can mostly be predicted (Fig. 6.11). At very high doses, death occurs rapidly with convulsions, suggesting a cerebral effect. At doses below this, the clinical picture is dominated in the first few days by gastrointestinal problems, and later by bone marrow suppression; either of these may prove fatal. In the long term, there is the risk of neoplasia.

Therapeutic usage of total body irradiation is mainly for the deliberate ablation of the bone marrow prior to transplantation of marrow, using either stored marrow from the patient or from another donor.

Ionising radiation and tumours

There is no doubt that ionising radiation causes tumours (Ch. 11). This is now firmly established for relatively high doses, but with low-dose irradiation some uncertainty remains.

There is a roughly linear relationship between the dose received and the incidence of tumours. The mechanism is incompletely understood, but the fundamental event is mutation of the host cell DNA; it is unlikely that a single point mutation is sufficient and more probably many will be present. As the radiation dose increases, so a greater number of cells will be lethally irradiated, thus reducing the number surviving and thus at risk of undergoing neoplastic transformation.

The dose–response information comes from several different sources, including animal experiments and observations on patients or populations exposed to irradiation. Thus, children who received irradiation to the thyroid gland show an incidence of tumours corresponding to the dose received. Occupational exposure to radon gas in mines also shows a correlation with the risk of lung tumours. For a given dose, the risk of neoplasia varies between tissues (Table 6.4).

Common to all these observations is a time delay between exposure to radiation and development of the tumour. Studies of Japanese survivors of the atomic bombs show significant numbers of cases of leukaemia by about six years, with a mean delay of 12.5 years and thereafter a decreasing incidence. For solid cancers, however, the mean delay has been 25 years and there is a continuing increased incidence in these people four decades later; in absolute numbers, there have now been many more solid cancers than leukaemias (Fig. 6.12).

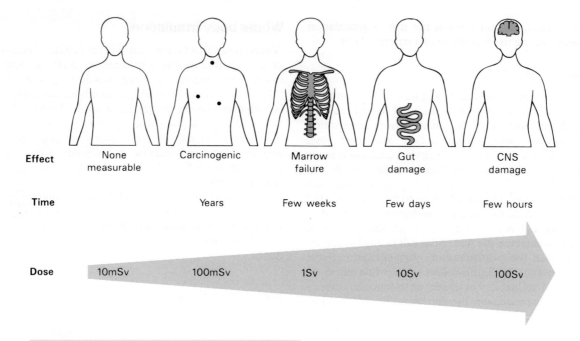

Effect	None measurable	Carcinogenic	Marrow failure	Gut damage	CNS damage
Time		Years	Few weeks	Few days	Few hours
Dose	10mSv	100mSv	1Sv	10Sv	100Sv

Fig. 6.11   Consequences of whole body irradiation

As the dose increases, so do the severity and immediacy of the effects.

Table 6.4   Relative lifetime risk of fatal cancer from a standard dose of ionising radiation

Tissue	Risk factor (Sv^{-1})
Lung	1 in 80
Female breasts	1 in 90
Haemopoietic tissue	1 in 360
Bone	1 in 2000
Thyroid	1 in 4000
Other organs (total)	1 in 43
Total for body = 1 in 20	

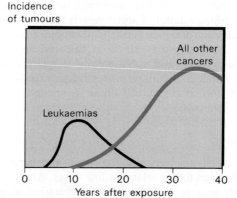

Fig. 6.12   Tumours in atom bomb survivors

There is a latent interval between exposure to radiation and the detection of the tumours. This is relatively short for leukaemias, but up to several decades for solid tumours.

While it is tempting simply to extrapolate the higher-dose data back down to low-dose ranges, it is very much more difficult to prove that this is justified. The problem is that the number of tumours expected is very small, so it is unlikely that any study will generate enough data such that the number of tumours exceeds the confidence limits of the analysis. This does not prove that there is a threshold below which tumours do not occur. On the contrary, there is every reason to believe that any increase in radiation gives a corresponding increase in risk; however, for low doses this risk cannot be measured with precision. It is possible that children are at a greater risk than are adults for any given dose.

Ultraviolet light

Ultraviolet light has a range of wavelengths:

- UVA 320–400 nm
- UVB 290–320 nm.

UVB is associated with sunburn and can also cause skin tumours; although not ionising, it damages

DNA by inducing pyrimidine dimers and thus strand linkage. UVA probably induces non-dimer damage, and also inhibits DNA repair processes. The tumours produced are basal cell and squamous cell carcinomas, and malignant melanomas. Melanin pigmentation, itself induced by ultraviolet light, is protective against these effects.

Far-UV (210–290 nm) is very toxic and is used in germicide lamps. However, the solar radiation in this range is filtered out by the ozone layer.

Principles of radiation protection

In view of the risk of harm from ionising radiation, it is important that it is used safely and only when there are no suitable alternatives. The International Commission on Radiological Protection (ICRP) has published recommendations with three central requirements:

- No practice shall be adopted unless its introduction produces a net benefit.
- All exposures shall be kept as low as reasonably achievable, economic and social factors being taken into account.
- The dose equivalent to individuals shall not exceed the limits recommended for the appropriate circumstances by the Commission.

In view of the risk of harm from ionising radiation, it is important that it is used in a discriminating manner that takes into account other alternatives. In the European Community, the Protection of Persons Undergoing Medical Examination or Treatment (POPUMET) regulations require the doctor to consider whether a procedure, or an investigation, involving irradiation is justifiable in each and every circumstance.

The second requirement is sometimes referred to as the ALARA principle. This emphasises that doses should be 'as low as reasonably achievable, not simply kept below dose limits'.

Therapeutic irradiation: radiotherapy

> ► Fractionation enables higher dose to be given
> ► Typical tumours treated: basal cell carcinoma of skin, squamous carcinoma of larynx, malignant lymphoma, seminoma of testis
> ► Effects and complications are delineated by the fields given

Like most effective treatments in medicine, radiotherapy carries certain risks of undesirable or unpredictable side-effects. This means that it tends to be reserved for serious or life-threatening conditions, or palliation of incurable diseases. The most common effect required from irradiation is the ability to kill cells; this is used in the treatment of tumours. Sometimes, the object is to induce fibrosis or vascular occlusion, as in the treatment of vascular malformations.

Radiation may be given with the intention of producing a cure, generally of a tumour. Usually, the idea is to give as high a dose as possible to the tumour, while producing the least possible damage to adjacent normal tissues. Some tumours are relatively radiosensitive, so that the therapeutic margin between tumour cell kill and tissue damage is wide; but in others the normal tissue tolerance is the limiting factor. The actual tumours given radical treatment will vary from one institution to another but a few examples are discussed below.

Basal cell carcinoma of the skin is very common and often managed by radiotherapy, although local excision is also effective. Squamous carcinoma of the larynx is usually irradiated in the first instance, because this preserves voice production. Squamous carcinoma of the uterine cervix is a tumour that may be managed by primary surgery or radiotherapy (Fig. 6.13). Localised malignant lymphoma is often irradiated, whereas generalised lymphoma is treated by chemotherapy. Metastatic seminoma of testis in para-aortic lymph nodes is usually irradiated, illustrating that radical treatment is possible even when metastases are present. Seminoma is an example of a very radiosensitive tumour. Carcinoma of the breast is usually treated by surgery, but as local recurrence is a risk, patients often proceed to post-operative radical radiotherapy.

Even when there is no hope of cure, there is much that can be done to relieve symptoms. Palliative radiotherapy is often given to treat metastatic tumour deposits, such as painful bone secondaries.

Fractionation

A higher dose of radiation may be given without increasing side-effects if it is divided into a number of fractions and given on different days. In practice, it is common to treat on only five days a week, so that a dose divided into 25 fractions would be given over five weeks. Each treatment fraction induces tissue damage, but is followed by attempts at repair. Normal cells included in the treated tissue volume are better able to repair effectively than are neoplastic cells. This means that there is a differential cell killing of more tumour cells than normal cells.

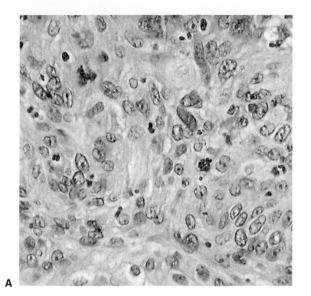

A

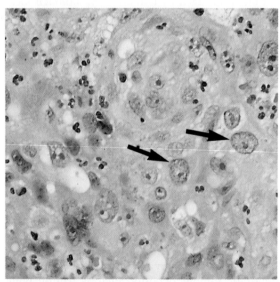

B

Fig. 6.13 Effect of radiation on carcinoma of the cervix

A. Before irradiation.
B. One week after high-dose irradiation, showing injury to the tumour cells (note bloating of arrowed nuclei) and the induced inflammatory reaction.

Palliative treatment is often a lower dose given as fewer larger fractions, in order to get a more rapid response.

Response modifiers

In addition to the benefits of fractionating treatment,

there has been considerable interest in modifying the tissue response to radiation. There are often conflicting interests, in that an increased sensitivity is required in the tumour and increased resistance in the normal tissue.

The most common reason for reduced sensitivity in a tumour is a low oxygen tension. The probable explanation is the central role of oxygen radicals in mediating the biological impact of ionising radiation; a lower oxygen concentration means, quite simply, that fewer oxygen radicals are generated. Many tumours have a poorly developed vascular network, resulting in hypoxic areas; patients are also often anaemic, which increases the problem. Nothing can be done about the tumour vascularity, but blood transfusion can correct anaemia.

Radiosensitisers are drugs that diffuse into tissues, including avascular areas, and, by mimicking the effect of oxygen, enhance the response. Though they are under investigation, none is in current use. The nearest equivalent is the use of psoralens to enhance the efficacy of ultraviolet light in the management of psoriasis, a skin disease. Hyperbaric oxygen and hyperthermia have both been used, but neither has passed into routine practice.

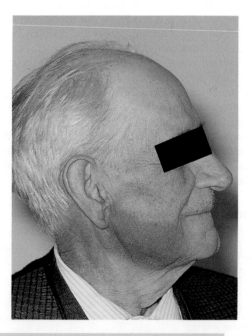

Fig. 6.14 Skin erythema due to therapeutic radiation

Skin erythema is an immediate reaction to radiation.

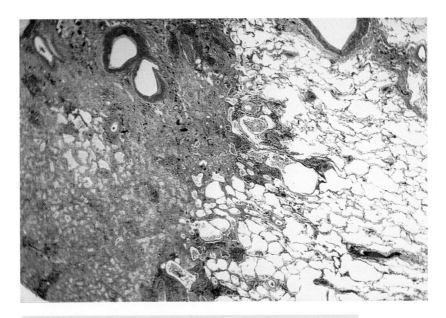

Fig. 6.15 Histology of lung fibrosis due to therapeutic radiation

Note the abrupt demarcation between the solid scarred lung (left) and the adjacent normally aerated lung (right); this is due to the sharp cut-off at the edge of the irradiated field, to minimise the extent of damage to adjacent structures.

Complications of radiotherapy

The complications of radiotherapy can be deduced from the effects of irradiation on tissues as described above, but a few may be mentioned in the context of therapy.

Irrespective of the part of the body treated, nausea and vomiting are very common side-effects of radiotherapy. The mechanism is not understood, but it is more likely to occur when large volumes of tissue are treated.

Major and minor salivary glands are liable to undergo permanent atrophy after irradiation. If treatment has been given from both sides of the body then this can result in a troublesome dry mouth.

Depending on the type of irradiation, the skin will receive a proportion of any dose given to any internal target. Certain techniques result in skin-sparing, and radionecrosis is unlikely unless the skin itself is the target of irradiation. However, skin reactions are very common and range from the expected acute inflammatory phases to residual pigmentation. All these phenomena will be strictly delineated by the margins of the treatment field with its straight edges (Fig. 6.14). They can thus be distinguished from other diseases.

Fibrosis is a late manifestation in irradiated tissue and will also be restricted to the treated field (Fig. 6.15). Most treatment techniques take care to avoid clinical consequences from such fibrosis, but occasionally an individual patient will show an excessive reaction, such as a stricture of the bowel. Sometimes, fibrosis is the desired objective of therapy, as in the treatment of intracerebral vascular malformations by inducing scarring.

FURTHER READING

Cheeseman K H, Slater T F 1993 Free radicals in medicine. British Medical Bulletin 49: 479–724

Cotton D W K 1995 Death: the cell. Progress in Pathology 2: in press

Hall P A 1992 Differentiation, stem cells and tumour histogenesis. Recent Advances in Histopathology 15: 1–15

Hancock B W, Bradshaw J D 1986 Lecture notes on clinical oncology, 2nd edn. Blackwell Scientific Publications, Oxford, p 33

National Radiological Protection Board 1989 Living with radiation. HMSO, London

7

Disorders of metabolism and homeostasis

Metabolic disorders, congenital or acquired, are well-defined abnormalities of metabolic pathways, often having considerable clinical effects. Congenital metabolic disorders are usually the result of inherited enzyme deficiencies.

Closely related are conditions characterised by perturbations of the body's *homeostatic mechanisms* maintaining the integrity of fluids and tissues. Such conditions are almost always acquired and their effects can be diverse.

INBORN ERRORS OF METABOLISM

> ► Single-gene defects due to inherited or spontaneous mutations
> ► Usually manifested in infancy or childhood
> ► May result in: defective amino acid metabolism; pathological effects of an intermediate metabolite; impaired membrane transport; synthesis of a defective protein

The concept of inborn errors of metabolism was formulated by Sir Archibald Garrod in 1908 as a result of his studies on a condition called alkaptonuria, a rare inherited deficiency of homogentisic acid oxidase.

Inborn errors (inherited congenital defects) of metabolism are important causes of illness presenting in infancy. Some require prompt treatment to avoid serious complications. Others defy treatment. All deserve accurate diagnosis so that parents can be counselled about the inherited risk to further pregnancies. Inborn metabolic errors are potentially chronic problems, because the primary abnormality is innate rather than due to any external cause that could be eliminated by treatment.

Inborn errors of metabolism are *single-gene defects* resulting in the absence or deficiency of an enzyme or the synthesis of a defective protein. Single-gene defects occur in about 1% of all births, but the diseases caused by them show geographic variations in incidence; this is exemplified by the high incidence of thalassaemias — due to defects in haemoglobin synthesis (Ch. 23) — in Mediterranean regions. These variations reflect the prevalence of specific abnormal genes in different populations.

Inborn errors of metabolism have four possible consequences:

- accumulation of an intermediate metabolite (e.g. homogentisic acid in alkaptonuria)
- deficiency of the ultimate product of metabolism (e.g. melanin in albinos)

- synthesis of an abnormal and less effective end product (e.g. haemoglobin S in sickle cell anaemia)
- failure of transport of the abnormal synthesised product (e.g. α_1-antitrypsin deficiency).

Accumulation of an intermediate metabolite may have toxic or hormonal effects. However, in some conditions the intermediate metabolite accumulates within the cells in which it has been synthesised, causing them to enlarge and compromising their function or that of neighbouring cells; these conditions are referred to as *storage disorders* (e.g. Gaucher's disease). Other inborn metabolic errors lead to the production of a protein with defective function; for example, the substitution of just a single amino acid in a large protein can have considerable adverse effects (e.g. haemoglobinopathies).

The genetic basis of the inheritance of these disorders is discussed in Chapter 3.

Inherited metabolic disorders may be classified according to the principal biochemical defect (e.g. amino acid disorder) or the consequence (e.g. storage).

Amino acid metabolism

Several inherited disorders of amino acid metabolism involve defects of enzymes in the phenylalanine/tyrosine pathway (Fig. 7.1).

Phenylketonuria

This autosomal recessive disorder affects approximately 1 in 10 000 infants. It is due to a deficiency of *phenylalanine hydroxylase*, an enzyme responsible for the conversion of phenylalanine to tyrosine (Fig. 7.1).

In the UK and many other countries the clinical effects of phenylketonuria are now seen only very rarely, because it is detected by screening all newborn infants and treated promptly. Testing is done by analysing a drop of blood, dried on to filter paper, for phenylalanine (Guthrie test). If phenylketonuria is not tested for in this way and the affected infant's diet contains usual amounts of phenylalanine, then the disorder manifests itself with skin and hair depigmentation, fits and mental retardation. Treatment involves a low phenylalanine diet until the child is at least 8 years old. When affected females themselves become pregnant, the special diet must be resumed to avoid the toxic metabolites damaging the developing fetus.

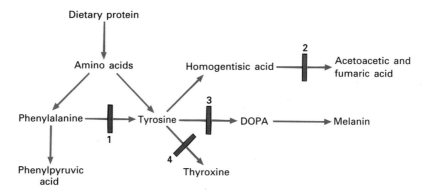

Fig. 7.1 Inborn errors of metabolism in the phenylalanine/tyrosine pathway

1. Phenylketonuria. Lack of phenylalanine hydroxylase blocks conversion of phenylalanine to tyrosine; phenylalanine and phenylpyruvic acid appear in the urine. **2. Alkaptonuria.** Lack of homogentisic acid oxidase causes accumulation of homogentisic acid. **3. Albinism.** Lack of the enzyme tyrosinase prevents conversion of tyrosine via DOPA to melanin. **4. Familial hypothyroidism.** Deficiency of any one of several enzymes impairs iodination of tyrosine in the formation of thyroid hormone.

Alkaptonuria

This rare autosomal recessive deficiency of *homogentisic acid oxidase* (Fig. 7.1) is a good example of an inborn metabolic error that does not produce serious effects until adult life. The condition is sometimes recognised from the observation that the patient's urine darkens on standing; the sweat may also be black! Homogentisic acid accumulates in connective tissues, principally cartilage, where the darkening is called *ochronosis*. This accumulation causes joint damage. The underlying condition cannot be treated; treatment is symptomatic only.

Homocystinuria

Like most other inherited disorders of metabolism, homocystinuria is an autosomal recessive disorder. It is characterised by a deficiency of *cystathionine synthetase*, an enzyme required for the conversion of homocystine via homocysteine to cystathionine. Homocysteine and methionine, its precursor, accumulate in the blood. Homocystine also accumulates, interfering with the cross-linking of collagen and elastic fibres. The ultimate effect resembles Marfan's syndrome (see p. 142), but with the addition of mental retardation and fits.

Storage disorders

Inborn metabolic defects result in storage disorders if an enzyme deficiency prevents the normal conversion of a macromolecule (e.g. glycogen or gangliosides) into its smaller subunits (e.g. glucose or fatty acids) (Table 7.1). The macromolecule accumulates within the cells that normally harbour it, swelling their cytoplasm (Fig. 7.2) and causing organ enlargement and deformities. This situation is harmful to the patient because the swelling of cells often impairs their function, or that of their immediate neighbours due to pressure effects, and because of conditions resulting from deficiency of the smaller subunits (e.g. hypoglycaemia in the case of glycogen storage disorders).

Disorders of cell membrane transport

Inborn metabolic errors can lead to impairment of the specific transport of substances across cell membranes. Examples include:

* *cystic fibrosis* — affecting exocrine secretions
* *cystinuria* — affecting renal tubules and resulting in renal stones
* *disaccharidase deficiency* — preventing absorption of lactose, maltose and sucrose from the gut
* *nephrogenic diabetes insipidus* — due to insensitivity of renal tubules to antidiuretic hormone (ADH).

Cystic fibrosis

Cystic fibrosis, formerly also called mucoviscidosis or fibrocystic disease of the pancreas, is the commonest serious inherited metabolic disorder; it is, however, much commoner in Caucasians than in other races. The autosomal recessive abnormal gene is carried by

Table 7.1   Examples of inborn errors of metabolism resulting in storage disorders

Type of disease/examples	Deficiency	Consequences
Glycogenoses	Debranching enzyme	Hepatomegaly Hypoglycaemia Cardiac failure Muscle cramps
McCardle's syndrome	Muscle phosphorylase	
von Gierke's disease	Glucose-6-phosphate dehydrogenase	
Pompe's disease	Acid maltase	
Mucopolysaccharidoses	Lysosomal hydrolase	Hepatosplenomegaly Skeletal deformity Mental deterioration
Hurler's syndrome	α-L-iduronidase	
Hunter's syndrome	Iduronate sulphate sulphatase	
Sphingolipidoses	Lysosomal enzyme	Variable hepatosplenomegaly Neurological problems
Gaucher's disease	Glucocerebrosidase	
Niemann–Pick disease	Sphingomyelinase	

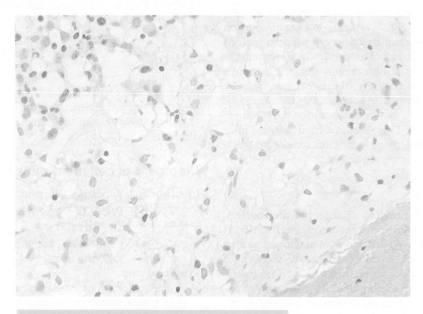

Fig. 7.2   Gaucher's disease affecting bone marrow

Macrophages distended with gangliosides have displaced much of the haemopoietic tissue, thereby causing anaemia.

approximately 1 in 20 Caucasians and the condition affects approximately 1 in 2000 births. The defective gene has been localised to chromosome 7 and ultimately results in abnormal water and electrolyte transport across cell membranes.

Cystic fibrosis transmembrane conductance regulator (CFTR)

The commonest abnormality in the CFTR gene is a deletion resulting in a missing phenylalanine molecule. The defective CFTR is unresponsive to cyclic-

AMP control, and transport of chloride ions and water across epithelial cell membranes is impaired (Fig. 7.3).

Clinicopathological features

Cystic fibrosis is characterised by mucous secretions of abnormally high viscosity. The abnormal mucus plugs exocrine ducts, causing parenchymal damage to the affected organs. The clinical manifestations are:

- meconium ileus in neonates
- failure to thrive in infancy
- recurrent bronchopulmonary infections
- bronchiectasis
- chronic pancreatitis, sometimes accompanied by diabetes mellitus due to islet damage
- malabsorption due to defective pancreatic secretions
- infertility in males.

Diagnosis

The diagnosis can be confirmed by measuring the sodium concentration in the sweat; in affected children it is usually greater than 70 mmol/l. Pregnancies at risk can be screened by prenatal testing of chorionic villus biopsy tissue for the defective CFTR gene.

Treatment

Treatment includes vigorous physiotherapy to drain the abnormal secretions from the respiratory passages, and oral replacement of pancreatic enzymes.

Porphyrias

The porphyrias, transmitted as autosomal dominant disorders, are due to defective synthesis of haem, an iron–porphyrin complex, the oxygen-carrying moiety of haemoglobin. Haem is synthesised from 5-aminolaevulinic acid. The different types of porphyrin accumulate due to inherited defects in this synthetic pathway (Fig. 7.4).

Clinicopathological features

Accumulation of porphyrins can cause clinical syndromes characterised by:

- acute abdominal pain
- acute psychiatric disturbance
- peripheral neuropathy
- photosensitivity (in some porphyrias only)
- hepatic damage (in some porphyrias only).

The pain and psychiatric disturbances are episodic.

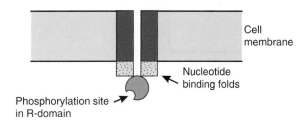

A

NORMAL

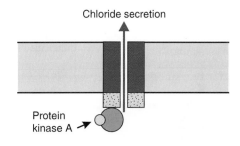

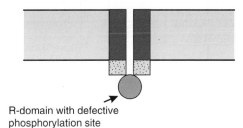

B

CYSTIC FIBROSIS

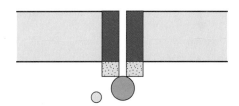

Fig. 7.3 Defective chloride secretion in cystic fibrosis

The normal CFTR is a transmembrane molecule with intracytoplasmic nucleotide binding folds and a phosphorylation site on the R-domain. **A.** In normal cells, interaction of the R-domain with protein kinase A results in opening of the channel and chloride secretion. **B.** In cystic fibrosis, a common defect prevents phosphorylation of the R-domain with the result that chloride secretion is impaired.

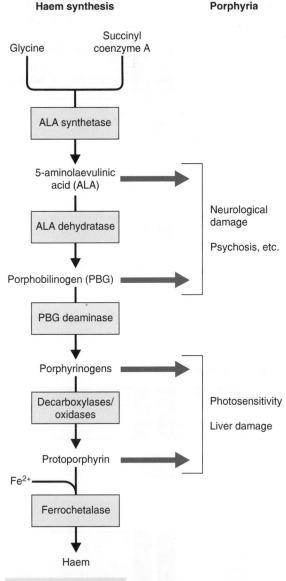

Haem synthesis   **Porphyria**

Fig. 7.4 Porphyrias

Enzyme deficiencies in the pathway of synthesis of haem from glycine and succinyl coenzyme A through 5-aminolaevulinic acid result in the accumulation of toxic intermediate metabolites. Removal of product inhibition due to deficient synthesis of haem enhances the formation of intermediate metabolites. Accumulation of 5-aminolaevulinic acid or porphobilinogen tends to be associated with neurological damage and psychiatric symptoms. Accumulation of porphyrinogens, of which there are several types (uro-, copro-, proto-), tends to be associated with photosensitivity.

During the acute attacks, the patient's urine contains excess 5-aminolaevulinic acid and porphobilinogen. These can be detected by adding an equal volume of

Ehrlich's reagent (paradimethyl aminobenzaldehyde in hydrochloric acid) and two volumes of chloroform; after shaking, the chloroform separates out and any colour remaining in the aqueous layer denotes a positive test.

Acute attacks of porphyria can be precipitated by some drugs, alcohol and hormonal changes (e.g. during the menstrual cycle). The most frequently incriminated drugs include barbiturates, sulphonamides, oral contraceptives and anticonvulsants; these should therefore be avoided.

The skin lesions are characterised by severe blistering, exacerbated by light exposure, and subsequent scarring. This photosensitivity is a distressing feature, but it has led to the beneficial use of injected porphyrins in the treatment of tumours by phototherapy with laser light.

Disorders of connective tissue metabolism

Most inherited disorders of connective tissue metabolism affect collagen or elastic tissue. Examples include:

- *osteogenesis imperfecta*
- *Marfan's syndrome*
- *Ehlers–Danlos syndrome*
- *pseudoxanthoma elasticum*
- *cutis laxa*.

Osteogenesis imperfecta

Osteogenesis imperfecta is the name given to a group of disorders in which there is an inborn error of type I collagen synthesis (see Ch. 25). Type I collagen is most abundant in bone, so the principal manifestation is skeletal weakness resulting in deformities and a susceptibility to fractures; the other names for this condition are 'fragilitas ossium' and 'brittle bone disease'. The teeth are also affected and the sclerae of the eyes are abnormally thin, causing them to appear blue. It occurs in dominantly and recessively inherited forms with varying degrees of severity.

Marfan's syndrome

Marfan's syndrome is a combination of unusually tall stature, long arm span, dislocation of the lenses of the eyes, aortic and mitral valve incompetence, and weakness of the aortic media predisposing to dissecting aneurysms (Ch. 13). The inherited biochemical defect has not yet been well characterised, but recent evidence suggests a defect of fibrillin, a constituent of elastic fibres.

ACQUIRED METABOLIC DISORDERS

Many diseases result in metabolic abnormalities. In others the metabolic disturbance is the primary event. For example, renal diseases almost always result in metabolic changes that reflect the kidneys' importance in water and electrolyte homeostasis. In contrast, a disease like gout is often due to a primary metabolic disorder that may secondarily damage the kidneys. This section deals with metabolic abnormalities as both consequences and causes of disease. Acquired metabolic disorders frequently cause systemic problems affecting many organs. For example, diabetes mellitus is associated with microvascular damage in the retinas, nerves, kidneys and other organs; electrolyte imbalance compromises the function of cells in all tissues.

Diabetes mellitus

▶ Multifactorial aetiology: genetic and environmental factors
▶ Relative or absolute insufficiency of insulin, causing hyperglycaemia
▶ Insulin-dependent and non-insulin-dependent groups
▶ Long-term complications include atheroma, renal damage, microangiopathy, neuropathy

Diabetes mellitus is a group of diseases characterised by impaired glucose homeostasis resulting from a relative or absolute insufficiency of insulin. Insulin insufficiency causes hyperglycaemia and glycosuria. Diabetes is covered in some detail in Chapter 17, but a brief account is relevant here.

The aetiology is multifactorial; although the disorder is acquired, there is an element of genetic predisposition particularly in insulin-dependent (type 1) diabetes. Diabetes mellitus is subclassified into primary and secondary types. Primary diabetes is much more common than diabetes secondary to other diseases.

Primary diabetes mellitus

Primary diabetes mellitus (DM) is subdivided into:

- insulin-dependent (IDDM) or type 1
- non-insulin-dependent (NIDDM) or type 2.

Juvenile-onset diabetes, usually manifesting itself before the age of 20 years, is almost always of IDDM type. There is an inherited predisposition associated with HLA-DR3 and HLA-DR4. There is reliable evidence that the initiating event is viral infection of the insulin-producing β-cells of the islets of Langerhans, precipitating their immune destruction.

Diabetes mellitus developing in adults (over 25 years of age) is most likely to be NIDDM type. It is associated with an acquired resistance to insulin. There is no HLA association, but there is a familial tendency to develop the disease. The affected patients are often, but not always, obese.

Secondary diabetes mellitus

Diabetes may be secondary to:

- chronic pancreatitis (Ch. 16)
- haemochromatosis (Ch. 16)
- acromegaly (Ch. 17)
- Cushing's syndrome (Ch. 17).

Complications of diabetes mellitus

Good control of blood sugar levels reduces the risk of complications. Nevertheless, many diabetics develop complications of their disease. These are covered in more detail in the relevant chapters, but a summary is given here:

- accelerated development of atheroma
- glomerular damage leading to nephrotic syndrome and renal failure
- microangiopathy, causing nerve damage and retinal damage
- increased susceptibility to infections
- cataracts
- diabetic ketoacidosis
- hyperosmolar diabetic coma.

To this list should be added hypoglycaemia which is a frequent and troublesome complication of insulin therapy in IDDM.

There are two possible biochemical explanations for the tissue damage that results from long-term diabetes mellitus:

- *Glycosylation.* The high blood sugar encourages binding of glucose to many proteins; this can be irreversible. This glycosylation often impairs the function of the proteins. The level of glycated haemoglobin is commonly used as a way of monitoring blood sugar control.
- *Polyol pathway.* Tissues containing aldose reductase (e.g. nerves, kidneys and the lenses of the eyes) are able to metabolise the high glucose levels into sorbitol and fructose. The products of this polyol pathway accumulate in the affected tissues, causing osmotic swelling and cell damage.

Gout

> ▶ Multifactorial disorder characterised by high blood uric acid levels
> ▶ Urate crystal deposition causes skin nodules (tophi), joint damage, renal damage and stones

Gout is a common disorder resulting from high blood uric acid levels. Uric acid is a breakdown product of the body's purine (nucleic acid) metabolism (Fig. 7.5), but a small proportion comes from the diet. Most uric acid is excreted by the kidneys. In the blood, most uric acid is in the form of monosodium urate. In patients with gout, the monosodium urate concentration may be very high, forming a supersaturated solution, thus risking urate crystal deposition in tissues causing:

- tophi (subcutaneous nodular deposits of urate crystals)
- synovitis and arthritis (Ch. 25)
- renal disease and calculi (Ch. 21).

Gout occurs more commonly in men than in

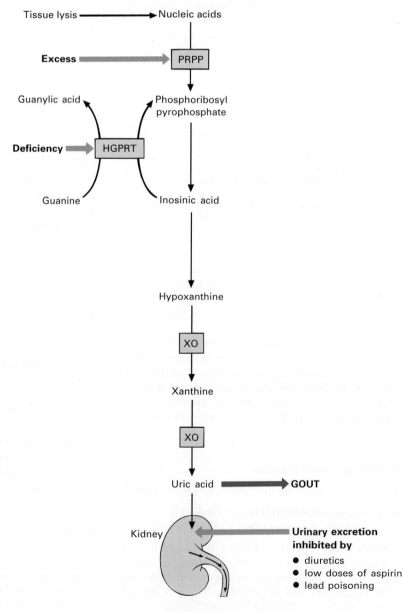

Fig. 7.5 Pathogenesis of gout

The metabolic pathway shows the synthesis of uric acid from nucleic acids. Primary gout can arise from an inherited (X-linked) deficiency of hypoxanthine guanine phosphoribosyl transferase (HGPRT) or excessive activity of 5-phosphoribosyl-1-pyrophosphate (PRPP). Secondary gout results either from increased tissue lysis (e.g. due to tumour chemotherapy) liberating excess nucleic acids or from inhibition of the urinary excretion of uric acid. Xanthine oxidase (XO) is inhibited by allopurinol, an effective long-term remedy for gout.

women, and is rare before puberty. A rare form of gout in children — *Lesch–Nyhan syndrome* — is due to a complete deficiency of the enzyme HGPRT (hypoxanthine guanine phosphoribosyl transferase) (Fig. 7.5) and is associated with mental deficiency and a bizarre tendency to self-mutilation.

Aetiology

Like diabetes mellitus, the aetiology of gout is multi-factorial. There is a genetic component, but the operation of other factors justifies the inclusion of gout under the heading of acquired disorders. Aetiological factors include:

- gender (male>female)
- family history
- diet (meat, alcohol)
- socio-economic status (high>low)
- body size (large>small).

Some of these factors may, of course, be interdependent. Accordingly, gout can be subdivided into *primary gout*, due to some genetic abnormality of purine metabolism, or *secondary gout*, due to increased liberation of nucleic acids from necrotic tissue or decreased urinary excretion of uric acid.

Clinicopathological features

The clinical features of gout are due to urate crystal deposition in various tissues (Fig. 7.6). In joints, a painful acute arthritis results from phagocytosis of the crystals by neutrophil polymorphs, in turn causing release of lysosomal enzymes along with the indigestible crystals, thus accelerating and perpetuating a cyclical inflammatory reaction. The first metatarsophalangeal joint is typically affected.

Water homeostasis

> ► Abnormal water homeostasis may result in excess, depletion or redistribution
> ► Excess may be due to overload, oedema or inappropriate renal tubular reabsorption
> ► Dehydration is most commonly due to gastrointestinal loss (e.g. gastroenteritis)
> ► Oedema results from redistribution of water into the extravascular compartment

Water and electrolyte homeostasis is tightly controlled by various hormones, including antidiuretic hormone (ADH), aldosterone and atrial natriuretic peptide, acting upon selective reabsorption in the renal tubules (Ch. 21). The process is influenced by the dietary intake of water and electrolytes (in food

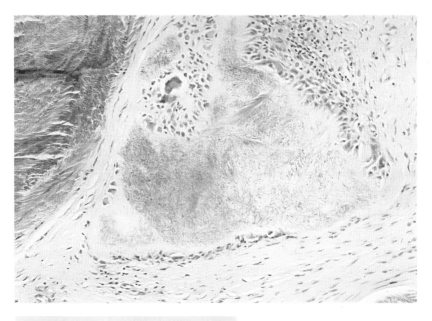

Fig. 7.6 Urate crystal deposition in gout

Aggregates of needle-shaped crystals have elicited an inflammatory and fibrous reaction.

or drinking in response to thirst or social purposes) and the adjustments necessary to cope with disease or adverse environmental conditions.

Many diseases result in problems of water and electrolyte homeostasis. Disturbances can also occur in post-operative patients receiving fluids and nutrition parenterally. Fortunately, any changes are fairly easy to monitor and control by making adjustments to the fluid and electrolyte intake.

Water is constantly lost from the body—in urine, in faeces, in exhaled gas from the lungs, and from the skin. The replenishment of body water is controlled by a combination of the satisfaction of the sensation of thirst and the regulation of the renal tubular reabsorption of water mediated by ADH.

Water excess

Excessive body water may occur in patients with extensive oedema or if there is inappropriate production of ADH (e.g. as occurs with some lung tumours) or if the body sodium concentration increases due to excessive tubular reabsorption (for example, due to an aldosterone-secreting tumour of the adrenal cortex). Water overload can be caused iatrogenically by excessive parenteral infusion of fluids in patients with impaired renal function; this can be avoided by carefully monitoring fluid input and output.

Dehydration

Dehydration results from either excessive water loss or inadequate intake or a combination of both. Inadequate water intake is a common problem in regions of the world affected by drought and famine.

Excessive water loss can be due to:

- vomiting and diarrhoea
- extensive burns
- excessive sweating (fever, exercise, hot climates)
- diabetes insipidus (failure to produce ADH)
- nephrogenic diabetes insipidus (renal tubular insensitivity to ADH)
- diuresis (e.g. osmotic loss accompanying the glycosuria of diabetes mellitus).

Dehydration is recognised clinically by a dry mouth, inelastic skin and, in extreme cases, sunken eyes. The blood haematocrit (proportion of the blood volume occupied by cells) will be elevated, causing an increase in whole blood viscosity. This results in a sluggish circulation and consequent impairment of the function of many organs.

The plasma sodium and urea concentrations are typically elevated, reflecting haemoconcentration and impaired renal function.

Oedema and serous effusions

- ▶ Oedema is excess water in tissues
- ▶ Oedema and serous effusions have similar pathogeneses
- ▶ May be due to increased vascular permeability, venous or lymphatic obstruction, or reduced plasma oncotic pressure

Oedema is an excess of fluid in the intercellular compartment of a tissue. A serous effusion is an excess of fluid in a serous or coelomic cavity (e.g. peritoneal cavity, pleural cavity). The main ingredient of the fluid is always *water*. Oedema and serous effusions share common pathogeneses.

Oedema is recognised clinically by diffuse swelling of the affected tissue. If the oedema is subcutaneous, the affected area shows pitting; i.e. if the skin is indented firmly with the fingers, an impression of the fingers is left transiently on the surface. There is, therefore, usually little difficulty in diagnosing subcutaneous oedema. Oedema of internal organs may be evident during surgery because they are swollen and, when incised, clear or slightly opalescent fluid exudes from the cut surfaces. Pulmonary oedema gives a characteristic appearance of increased radioopacity on a plain chest X-ray and can be heard, through a stethoscope, as crepitations on inspiration.

Oedema, irrespective of its cause, has serious consequences in certain organs. For example, *pulmonary oedema* fluid fills the alveoli and reduces the effective lung volume available for respiration; the patient becomes breathless (dyspnoeic) and, if the oedema is severe, cyanosed. *Cerebral oedema* is an ominous development because it occurs within the rigid confines of the cranial cavity; compression of the brain against the falx cerebri, the tentorial membranes or the base of the skull leads to herniation of brain tissue, possibly causing irreversible and fatal damage. Cerebral oedema can be diagnosed clinically by finding *papilloedema* (oedema of the optic disc) on ophthalmoscopy.

Oedema and serous effusions are due to either:

- excessive leakage of fluid from blood vessels into the extravascular spaces
- impaired reabsorption of fluid from tissues or serous cavities.

Oedema is classified into four pathogenetic categories (Fig. 7.7):

A. Normal

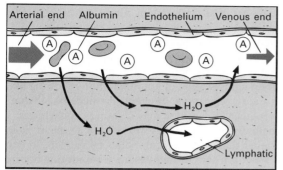

B. Inflammatory oedema

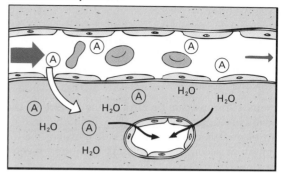

C. Venous oedema

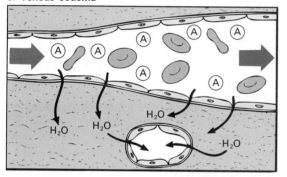

D. Lymphatic oedema

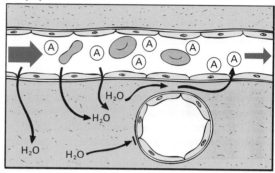

E. Hypoalbuminaemic oedema

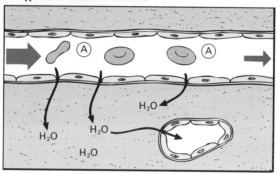

Fig. 7.7 Pathogenesis of oedema

A. Normal. Hydrostatic blood pressure forces water out of capillaries at the arterial end, but the plasma oncotic pressure attributable to albumin sucks water back into capillary beds at the venous end. A small amount of water drains from the tissues through lymphatic channels. **B.** Inflammatory oedema. Gaps between endothelial cells allow water and albumin (and other plasma constituents) to escape from the capillary bed. There is increased lymphatic drainage, but this cannot cope with all the water released into the tissues and oedema results. **C.** Venous oedema. Increased venous pressure (e.g. from heart failure, venous obstruction due to thrombus) causes passive dilatation and congestion of the capillary bed. Increased venous pressure exceeds that of plasma oncotic pressure and so water remains in the tissues. **D.** Lymphatic oedema. Lymphatic obstruction (e.g. by tumour deposits, filarial parasites) prevents drainage of water from tissues.
E. Hypoalbuminaemic oedema. Low plasma albumin concentration reduces the plasma oncotic pressure so that water cannot be sucked back into the capillary bed at the venous end.

- inflammatory: due to increased vascular permeability
- venous: due to increased intravenous pressure
- lymphatic: due to obstruction of lymphatic drainage
- hypoalbuminaemic: due to reduced plasma oncotic pressure.

Serous effusions can be attributable to any of the above causes, but in addition there is another important diagnostic category: neoplastic effusions due to primary or secondary neoplasms (tumours) involving serous cavities (Ch. 11).

Inflammatory oedema

Oedema is a feature of acute inflammation (Ch. 10). In acutely inflamed tissues there is increased vascular (mainly venular) permeability due to the separation of endothelial cells under the influence of chemical mediators. Fluid with a high protein content leaks out of the permeable vessels into the inflamed tissue causing it to swell. This is beneficial, because the proteins in the oedema fluid assist in defeating the cause of the inflammation. For example:

- albumin increases the oncotic pressure of the extravascular fluid, causing water to be imbibed, thus diluting any toxins
- fibrinogen polymerises to form a fibrin mesh which helps to contain the damage
- immunoglobulins and complement specifically destroy bacteria or neutralise toxins.

In addition to the fluid component, the extravasate contains numerous neutrophil polymorphs.

Tissues affected by inflammatory oedema are characterised by the other features of acute inflammation, such as pain and redness.

Venous oedema

Oedema results from increased intravenous pressure because this pressure opposes the plasma oncotic pressure, largely due to the presence of albumin, that draws fluid back into the circulation at the venous end of capillary beds. Increased intravenous pressure results from either *heart failure* or impairment of blood flow due to *venous obstruction* by a thrombus or extrinsic compression. The affected tissues are often intensely congested due to engorgement by venous blood under increased pressure. In heart failure, there is also *pulmonary congestion with oedema* and so-called *passive venous congestion of the liver.*

Venous oedema is seen most commonly in dependent parts of the body, notably the legs; indeed, it is not unusual for mild degrees of venous oedema to occur at the ankles and feet of normal people who have sat in aircraft on long intercontinental flights — immobilisation impairs venous return. The fluid in venous oedema has a low protein content.

Oedema of just one leg is almost always due to venous obstruction by a thrombus. This is a common complication of immobilisation following major surgery or trauma. Bilateral leg oedema, if due to venous causes (there may be other explanations, see below), is more likely to be due to heart failure rather than venous thrombotic obstruction. In either case it is a serious manifestation prompting immediate attention to the underlying condition.

Lymphatic oedema

Some fluid normally leaves capillary beds and drains into adjacent lymphatic channels to return eventually to the circulation through the thoracic duct. If the lymphatic channels are obstructed, the fluid remains trapped in the tissues and oedema results.

Causes of lymphatic oedema include blockage of lymphatic flow by filarial parasites (Ch. 3) or by tumour metastases (Ch. 11), or as a complication of surgical removal of lymph nodes. Blockage of inguinal lymphatics by filarial parasites frequently causes gross oedema of the legs and, in males, the scrotum; the resulting deformity is called *elephantiasis*. Blockage of lymphatic drainage from the small intestine, usually because of tumour involvement, causes *malabsorption* of fats and fat-soluble substances. Blockage of lymphatic drainage at the level of the thoracic duct, or at least close to it, causes *chylous effusions* in the pleural and peritoneal cavities; the fluid is densely opalescent due to the presence of numerous tiny fat globules (chyle).

Fortunately, oedema due to surgical removal of lymph nodes is now a rare event. It used to be a complication of radical mastectomy for breast cancer, but surgical treatment for this tumour now tends to be more conservative.

Hypoalbuminaemic oedema

A low plasma albumin concentration results in oedema because of the reduction in plasma oncotic pressure; thus, fluid cannot be drawn back into the venous end of capillary beds and it remains in the tissues. Causes of hypoalbuminaemia are:

- protein malnutrition (as in kwashiorkor)
- liver failure (reduced albumin synthesis)
- nephrotic syndrome (excessive albumin loss in urine)
- protein-losing enteropathy (a variety of diseases are responsible).

Hypoalbuminaemia as the cause of oedema can be verified easily by measuring the albumin concentration in serum. The underlying cause is then investigated and, if possible, treated. Infusions of albumin will have a beneficial, but temporary, effect.

Ascites and pleural effusions
Ascites is an excess of fluid in the peritoneal cavity. It is one of the five general causes of a distended abdomen: the complete alliterative list is — fluid, fat, faeces (constipation or obstruction), fetus, flatus (gas in the bowel).

Ascites and pleural effusions may be due to any of the above causes of oedema. However, the increased vascular permeability causing inflammatory oedema and effusions may also be induced by tumours. Thus, tumour cells growing within the cavities or on their serous linings cause excessive leakage of fluid. Serous effusions may be a presenting feature of cancer or they may complicate a previously diagnosed case. The fluid has a high protein content, and cytological examination to look for abnormal cells often enables the diagnosis to be made.

Serous effusions may be divided into *transudates* and *exudates* by their protein content. Transudates have a protein concentration of less than 2 g/100 ml, whereas the concentration in exudates is higher. Involvement by tumour is the most important cause of an exudate.

Electrolyte homeostasis

Sodium and potassium homeostasis

> ▶ Sodium may be retained excessively by the body due to action of inappropriately high levels of mineralocorticoid hormones acting on renal tubular reabsorption
> ▶ Sodium may be lost excessively in urine, due to impaired renal tubular reabsorption, or in sweat
> ▶ Potassium may accumulate excessively in the body if there is extensive tissue necrosis or renal failure
> ▶ High serum potassium level is a medical emergency because of risk of cardiac arrest
> ▶ Potassium may be lost excessively in severe vomiting and diarrhoea

Of all the electrolytes in plasma, sodium and potassium are among the most abundant and the most likely to be affected by pathological processes (Table 7.2).

Hypernatraemia
Hypernatraemia (high serum sodium) may occur in conditions in which there is excessive mineralocorticoid (such as aldosterone) production acting on renal tubular reabsorption; Conn's syndrome, due to an adrenal adenoma of the zona glomerulosa cells, is a typical example. The increased total body sodium content may be concealed by a commensurate increase in body water content in an attempt to sustain a normal plasma osmolarity; the serum sodium concentration may therefore underestimate the increase in total body sodium.

Table 7.2 Common abnormalities of serum electrolytes		
Abnormality	Causes	Consequences
Hypernatraemia (i.e. high sodium)	Renal failure Cushing's syndrome Conn's syndrome	Compensatory increased blood volume Oedema
Hyponatraemia (i.e. low sodium)	Addison's disease Excessive diuretic therapy	Reduced blood volume Hypotension
Hyperkalaemia (i.e. high potassium)	Renal failure Acidosis Extensive tissue necrosis	Risk of cardiac arrest
Hypokalaemia (i.e. low potassium)	Vomiting Diarrhoea Diuretic therapy Alkalosis Cushing's syndrome Conn's syndrome	Weakness Cardiac dysrhythmias Metabolic alkalosis
The abnormalities listed often do not occur in isolation and may be associated with other electrolyte changes		

Hyponatraemia

Hyponatraemia (low serum sodium) is a logical consequence of impaired renal tubular reabsorption of sodium. This occurs in Addison's disease of the adrenal glands due to loss of the aldosterone-producing zona glomerulosa cortical cells. Sodium is the electrolyte most likely to be lost selectively in severe sweating in hot climates or during physical exertion such as marathon running; the syndrome of 'heat exhaustion' is due mainly to a combination of dehydration and hyponatraemia. Falsely low serum sodium concentrations may be found in hyperlipidaemic states; the sodium concentration in the aqueous phase of the serum is actually normal but the lipid contributes to the total volume of serum assayed.

Hyperkalaemia

Potassium is more abundant within cells than in extracellular fluids, so relatively small changes in plasma concentration can underestimate possibly larger changes in intracellular concentrations. Furthermore, extensive tissue necrosis can liberate large quantities of potassium into the plasma, causing the concentration to reach dangerously high levels. The commonest cause is renal failure causing decreased urinary potassium excretion. Severe hyperkalaemia (>c.6.5 mmol/l) is a serious medical emergency demanding prompt treatment because of the risk of cardiac arrest. Moderate hyperkalaemia is relatively asymptomatic, emphasising the importance of regular biochemical monitoring to avoid sudden fatal complications.

Hypokalaemia

Hypokalaemia (low serum potassium) has many causes (Table 7.2). It is often accompanied by a metabolic alkalosis due to hydrogen ion shift into the intracellular compartment. Clinically, it presents with muscular weakness and cardiac dysrhythmias.

Vomiting and diarrhoea result in combined loss of water, sodium and potassium. Superimposed on this may be alkalosis from vomiting due to loss of hydrogen ions, or acidosis from diarrhoea due to loss of alkaline intestinal secretions.

Calcium homeostasis

Serum calcium levels are regulated by the vitamin D metabolite — 1,25-dihydroxyvitamin D — and by parathyroid hormone (PTH). The precise role of calcitonin in man is uncertain, but it has a serum-calcium-lowering effect when administered to patients with hypercalcaemia; however, patients with the calcitonin-producing medullary carcinoma of the thyroid (Ch. 17) do not present with hypocalcaemia.

Hypercalcaemia

Acute hypercalcaemia causes fits, vomiting and polyuria. Persistent hypercalcaemia additionally results in 'metastatic' calcification (see p. 158) of tissues and urinary calculi. Causes of hypercalcaemia include:

- primary hyperparathyroidism (Ch. 17)
- hypervitaminosis D
- extensive skeletal metastases
- PTH-like secretion from tumours.

Primary hyperparathyroidism is most commonly due to an adenoma of the parathyroid glands. The excessive and uncontrolled PTH secretion enhances the absorption of calcium and the osteoclastic erosion of bone, thus releasing calcium.

Hypercalcaemia due to neoplasms of other organs is seen most commonly with breast cancer. In the absence of extensive skeletal metastases, this is attributed to a PTH-like hormone secreted by the tumour cells.

Hypocalcaemia

Hypocalcaemia causes neuromuscular hypersensitivity manifested by *tetany*. This condition can be corrected rapidly by giving calcium gluconate intravenously. The commonest cause of acute hypocalcaemia is accidental damage to or removal of parathyroid glands during thyroid surgery. Low serum calcium levels resulting from renal disease or intestinal malabsorption are rapidly corrected, in a patient with intact parathyroid glands, by stimulation of PTH secretion. This eventually causes hyperplasia of the parathyroid glands (secondary hyperparathyroidism) and weakening of the skeleton due to excessive osteoclastic resorption under the influence of PTH.

Tetany also results from respiratory alkalosis, often in patients with hysterical hyperventilation who excessively eliminate carbon dioxide, due to a reduction in the ionised calcium concentration as the pH rises.

Acid–base homeostasis

> ► Body has innate tendency to acidification
> ► Buffers (bicarbonate/carbonic acid, proteins) have limited capacity
> ► Acidosis or alkalosis may be due to respiratory or metabolic causes
> ► Body attempts to restore pH by varying rate of respiration or by adjusting renal tubular function

Metabolic pathways are intolerant of pH deviations. The extracellular pH is tightly controlled at an approximate value of 7.4, but the intracellular pH is marginally lower and varies within an even narrower range. Acidic deviation outside the normal plasma pH range is sensed by chemoreceptors at the carotid bifurcations (carotid bodies), in the aortic arch and in the medulla of the brain.

The body has an innate tendency towards acidification due to production of:

- carbon dioxide from aerobic respiration
- lactic acid from glycolysis
- fatty acids from lipolysis.

This acidic tendency is counteracted by basic (alkaline) buffers (bicarbonate, proteins) in the first instance, but these have limited capacity. Acid–base balance in the plasma is ultimately regulated by:

- elimination of carbon dioxide by exhalation
- renal excretion of hydrogen ions
- metabolism of fatty and lactic acids
- replenishment of bicarbonate ions.

Acidosis and alkalosis

Deviations outside the normal pH range are called acidosis (low pH) and alkalosis (high pH). Either deviation may be further classified as *respiratory* (due to insufficient or excessive elimination of carbon dioxide from the lungs) or *metabolic* (due to non-respiratory causes). Thus there are four possible combinations:

- respiratory acidosis
- metabolic acidosis
- respiratory alkalosis
- metabolic alkalosis.

The causes of these abnormalities of acid–base balance are shown in Table 7.3. The role of normal respiration and respiratory tract diseases in influencing acid–base balance is discussed in Chapter 14.

Respiratory acidosis
Respiratory acidosis can be corrected by increased renal tubular reabsorption of bicarbonate ions (which are alkaline) or by increased urinary loss of hydrogen ions (which are acidic). By either mechanism, the pH is not corrected as promptly as it can be in metabolic acidosis by immediate stimulation of hyperventilation.

Table 7.3 Features of respiratory and metabolic acidosis and alkalosis

Abnormality	Condition	pH	$Paco_2$	HCO_3	Consequences
Acidosis					
Acute respiratory	Asthma Pneumonia Respiratory impairment	↓	↑	N	CO_2 is retained
Chronic respiratory	Emphysema	N	↑	↑↑	Renal retention of HCO_3 normalises plasma pH
Acute metabolic	Diabetic ketoacidosis	↓	N	↓	H^+ ions retained
Chronic metabolic	Cardiac arrest Renal failure	N	↓	↓	Hyperventilation normalises plasma pH by accelerating loss of CO_2
Alkalosis					
Acute respiratory	Hysterical hyperventilation	↑	↓	N	Accelerated loss of CO_2 Reduced ionised Ca^{2+} causes tetany
Chronic respiratory	Diffuse pulmonary fibrosis	N	↓	↓↓	pH normalised by increased renal HCO_3 excretion
Acute metabolic	Excess bicarbonate administration	↑	N	↑	Direct effect of HCO_3
Chronic metabolic	Persistent vomiting	↑	N	↑↑	Ineffective attempts to normalise pH by increased urinary loss of HCO_3 and respiratory retention of CO_2 by hypoventilation

In chronic cases, the consequences reflect the body's attempts to normalise plasma pH.
$Paco_2$ = partial arterial pressure of carbon dioxide; HCO_3 = bicarbonate; CO_2 = carbon dioxide; H^+ = hydrogen ions; Ca^{2+} = calcium ions; N = normal.

Metabolic acidosis

Metabolic acidosis stimulates hyperventilation, often with deep sighing respiratory excursions (Kussmaul respiration), in order to blow off carbon dioxide and thereby maintain the equilibrium of the bicarbonate/carbonic acid ratio, restoring the pH to neutrality.

Respiratory alkalosis

Respiratory alkalosis is always due to hyperventilation, causing excessive elimination of carbon dioxide (which is acid in solution as carbonic acid). There is limited scope for correction by increasing the urinary loss of bicarbonate ions.

Metabolic alkalosis

Metabolic alkalosis is more difficult to correct naturally because the vitally important hypoxic drive to respiration overrides the extent to which carbon dioxide can be conserved by hypoventilation.

METABOLIC CONSEQUENCES OF MALNUTRITION

Malnutrition, a serious medical and socio-economic problem, may be a consequence or a cause of disease. Diseases and conditions commonly complicated by malnutrition include:

- anorexia nervosa
- carcinoma of the oesophagus or stomach
- post-operative states
- dementia.

This section concentrates on the clinicopathological consequences of malnutrition. Malnutrition may be:

- protein–energy malnutrition
- vitamin deficiencies
- a combination of both.

Protein–energy malnutrition

> ▶ Kwashiorkor: severe wasting is concealed by oedema
> ▶ Marasmus: severe wasting
> ▶ Both may be complicated by infections, parasitic infestations and vitamin deficiencies
> ▶ Cachexia: profound wasting often occurring terminally in cancer patients

Protein–energy malnutrition results from the frequent combination of insufficient protein, carbohy-

drate and fat in the diet. Carbohydrate and fat together account for approximately 90% of the energy content of a typical healthy diet. Protein alone cannot replace the necessary energy yield from fats and carbohydrates.

Protein–energy malnutrition frequently co-exists with infections. The infections may exacerbate the deficiency, thus exposing the malnourished state, or they may complicate the deficiency because of impaired body defence mechanisms. In children prolonged malnutrition leads to stunted development due to retardation of linear growth. A shorter period of malnutrition produces body wasting.

Malnutrition in children

Severe malnutrition in children results in two clinical conditions (Fig. 7.8):

- kwashiorkor
- marasmus.

It is not entirely certain what factors prompt which condition to develop in a malnourished child, and some cases show features of both conditions. These conditions often co-exist with infections, parasitic infestations, and vitamin deficiencies.

Kwashiorkor

Kwashiorkor is characterised by oedema which may be very extensive and so belie the extreme wasting of the underlying tissues. The skin is scaly and the hair loses its natural colour. The condition often develops when a child is weaned off breast milk, but without the compensation of adequate dietary protein.

The serum albumin is low and this accounts for the oedema due to reduced plasma oncotic pressure. Hypokalaemia and hyponatraemia are common. The liver is enlarged due to severe fatty change; this occurs because the lack of protein thwarts the production of lipoprotein.

Marasmus

Marasmus is characterised by severe emaciation rather than oedema. The skin is wrinkled and head hair is lost. The serum albumin is usually within the normal range, but hypokalaemia and hyponatraemia are common.

Cachexia

Cachexia is a state of severe debilitation associated with profound weight loss. It is seen in malnutrition (marasmus is akin to cachexia), but the term is most widely associated with the profound weight loss suf-

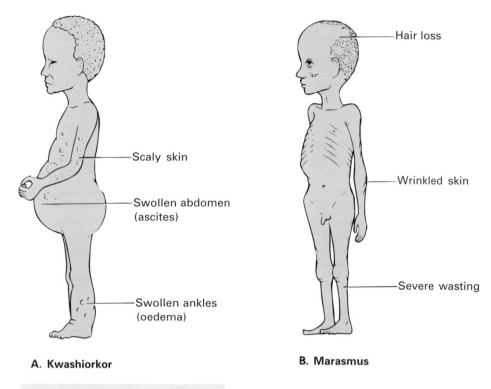

Scaly skin

Swollen abdomen (ascites)

Swollen ankles (oedema)

Hair loss

Wrinkled skin

Severe wasting

A. Kwashiorkor

B. Marasmus

Fig. 7.8   Kwashiorkor and marasmus

Malnutrition in both cases leads to severe wasting. **A.** This is concealed to some extent in kwashiorkor by the oedema and ascites. **B.** It is obvious in marasmus.

fered by patients with cancer. When the tumour involves the gastrointestinal tract, the explanation for the cachexia is often obvious. However, weight loss can be a very early manifestation of cancer and is a particularly common feature of carcinoma of the lung; in this instance, it may be due to factors causing increased protein catabolism as the patient's food intake may be still within normal limits. Among several factors postulated to be responsible for the increased catabolic state in cachexia is *tumour necrosis factor*, a peptide secreted by tumour tissue.

Vitamin deficiencies

▶ Multiple vitamin deficiencies may occur in severe malnutrition
▶ Each vitamin deficiency is associated with specific consequences

Deficiencies of vitamins — so named by Casimir Funk (1884–1967) because he believed (mistakenly) that they were all vital amines — produce more specific abnormalities (Table 7.4) than those encountered in protein–energy malnutrition. This is because of their involvement in specific metabolic pathways. A detailed account of all vitamin deficiencies would be largely irrelevant. However, some are worthy of comment here, because either they are relatively frequent or the consequences are profound.

Thiamine (B₁) deficiency

Thiamine deficiency impairs glycolytic metabolism and affects the nervous system and the heart. The classical deficiency state is called *beri-beri* (from the Sinhalese word 'beri' meaning weakness). This state is characterised by peripheral neuropathy and, in some cases, cardiac failure.

Alcoholism is a common predisposing cause in countries such as the UK, where it is often associated with an inadequate diet. Alcoholics with thiamine deficiency can develop two central nervous system syndromes:

- *Korsakoff's psychosis* — characterised by confusion, confabulation and amnesia

Table 7.4 Vitamin deficiency states

Vitamin	Dietary sources	Consequence of deficiency
A	β-carotene in carrots, etc. Vitamin A in fish, eggs, liver, margarine	Night blindness, xerophthalmia, mucosal infections
B₁ (thiamine)	Cereals, milk, eggs, fruit, yeast extract	Beri-beri, neuropathy, cardiac failure, Korsakoff's psychosis, Wernicke's encephalopathy
B₂ (riboflavine)	Cereals, milk, eggs, fruit, liver	Mucosal fissuring
B₆ (pyridoxine)	Cereals, meat, fish, milk	Confusion, glossitis, neuropathy, sideroblastic anaemia
B₁₂ (cobalamin)	Meat, fish, eggs, cheese	Megaloblastic anaemia, subacute combined degeneration of the spinal cord
Niacin (nicotinic acid)	Meat, milk, eggs, peas, beans, yeast extract	Pellagra, dermatitis, diarrhoea, dementia
Folate	Green vegetables, fruit	Megaloblastic anaemia, mouth ulcers, villous atrophy of small gut
C (ascorbic acid)	Citrus fruits, green vegetables	Scurvy, lassitude, swollen bleeding gums, bruising and bleeding
D	Milk, fish, eggs, liver	Rickets (in childhood), osteomalacia (in adults)
E	Cereals, eggs, vegetable oils	Neuropathy, anaemia
K	Vegetables, liver	Blood coagulation defects

- *Wernicke's encephalopathy*—characterised by confusion, nystagmus and aphasia.

Folate and vitamin B₁₂ deficiency

Folate and vitamin B₁₂ (cobalamin) are essential for DNA synthesis. Deficiency of either impairs cellular regeneration; the effects are seen most severely in haemopoietic tissues, resulting in megaloblastic changes and macrocytic anaemia (Ch. 23). In addition, vitamin B₁₂ deficiency also causes subacute combined degeneration of the spinal cord (Ch. 26).

Folate deficiency may result from:

- dietary insufficiency (principal source is fresh vegetables)
- intestinal malabsorption (e.g. coeliac disease—Ch. 15)
- increased utilisation (e.g. pregnancy, tumour growth)
- anti-folate drugs (e.g. methotrexate).

Vitamin B₁₂ deficiency may result from:

- autoimmune gastritis resulting in loss of intrinsic factor, thus causing pernicious anaemia
- surgical removal of the stomach (e.g. gastric cancer)
- disease of the terminal ileum, the site of absorption (e.g. Crohn's disease—Ch. 15)
- blind loops of bowel in which there is bacterial overgrowth
- infestation with *Diphyllobothrium latum*, a parasitic worm.

Vitamin C deficiency

Vitamin C deficiency is now most common in elderly people and in chronic alcoholics whose diet is often lacking in fresh fruit and vegetables. The vitamin (ascorbic acid) is essential principally for collagen synthesis: it is necessary for the production of chondroitin sulphate and hydroxyproline from proline. Minor degrees of deficiency may be responsible for lassitude and an unusual susceptibility to bruising. Severe deficiency causes *scurvy*, a condition characterised by swollen, bleeding gums, hyperkeratosis of hair follicles, and petechial skin haemorrhages.

Vitamin D deficiency

Vitamin D is derived either from the diet (milk, fish, etc.) as ergocalciferol (D₂) or from the action of ultraviolet light on 7-dehydrocholesterol (D₃) to form cholecalciferol in the skin. The intermediate precursors are activated by hydroxylation sequentially in the liver and kidneys to give 1,25-

dihydroxy-cholecalciferol, a steroid hormone. Hydroxylation in the kidney is stimulated by parathyroid hormone and hypocalcaemia. An apparent deficiency can therefore result from:

- lack of dietary vitamin D with inadequate sunlight
- intestinal malabsorption of fat (vitamin D is fat-soluble)
- impaired hydroxylation due to hepatic or renal disease.

People of races with deeply pigmented skin rely more heavily on dietary vitamin D when they migrate to countries that enjoy less sunlight than do their native lands.

Vitamin D is vital for normal calcium homeostasis. Its action resembles that of parathyroid hormone, ultimately causing elevation of the serum calcium concentration. It does so by:

- promotion of the absorption of calcium (and phosphate to a lesser extent) from the gut
- increased osteoclastic resorption of bone and mobilisation of calcium.

In children, lack of vitamin D impairs mineralisation of the growing skeleton, thus causing *rickets*. In adults, vitamin D deficiency results in *osteomalacia* (Ch. 25). However, the pathogenesis of rickets and osteomalacia is identical; the two conditions are different clinical manifestations of vitamin D deficiency occurring at different stages of skeletal development.

Vitamin K deficiency

Vitamin K is essential for the synthesis of blood-clotting factors. It is involved in the carboxylation of glutamic acid residues on factors II, VII, IX and X. The principal dietary sources are vegetables, leguminous plants and liver. Deficiency may result from:

- lack of dietary vitamin K
- intestinal malabsorption of fat (vitamin K is fat-soluble).

The commonest situation leading to dietary insufficiency is found in neonates on breast milk deficient in vitamin K.

Bruising and an abnormal bleeding tendency are the clinical manifestations of vitamin K deficiency. This occurs not only in the circumstances outlined above, but also in patients with liver failure in whom there is impaired hepatic synthesis of the vitamin K-dependent clotting factors; this can be corrected by giving large doses of vitamin K. It is essential to check the prothrombin time before performing a liver biopsy or any surgery on a patient with suspected liver disease.

TRACE ELEMENTS AND DISEASE

Trace elements are those present at an arbitrarily defined low concentration in a given situation. Some trace elements in man are of vital importance, despite the meagre quantities found in the human body. Trace elements cause disease when the body levels are higher or lower than normal, depending on the specific biological effects of the element.

Many elements, such as iron, cannot be regarded as trace elements because of their abundance in the body; nevertheless, diseases can result from either a deficiency or an excess (anaemia and haemosiderosis respectively in the case of iron).

Diseases associated with trace element abnormalities are summarised in Table 7.5. Sometimes the association is weak and only circumstantial. For example, a study in the UK showed that the death rate from cardiovascular diseases is higher in places with soft drinking water, possibly partially accounting for the higher incidence of deaths from ischaemic heart disease in Scotland. There is, however, insufficient evidence to justify adding hardening agents to water to reverse this trend.

In many instances the link between trace element abnormalities and disease is incontrovertible. A complete survey is not possible, but some examples of well-documented associations will be summarised.

Table 7.5	Trace elements and disease	
Element	Abnormality	Consequences
Zinc	Deficiency	Impaired wound healing Acrodermatitis enteropathica
Selenium	Deficiency	Cardiac failure Hepatic necrosis
Mercury	Excess	Neuropathy
Lead	Excess	Neuropathy Anaemia
Aluminium	Excess	Bone changes Encephalopathy
Copper	Excess	Hepatic damage Basal ganglia damage (i.e. Wilson's disease)
Iodine	Deficiency	Goitre
Cobalt	Excess	Cardiomyopathy

Mercury

The average human body contains only 13 mg of mercury. The safe daily intake is <50 μg.

Mercury has been used in dental amalgams for filling tooth cavities since 1818. Although doubts have been expressed about its safety, metallic mercury and mercury-containing dental amalgams are insoluble in saliva and are, therefore, not absorbed to an appreciable extent. Dentists must, of course, exercise caution in the handling of mercury to minimise the risk of cumulative occupational exposure.

Mercury is neurotoxic. Chronic poisoning also results in a characteristic blue line on the gums. Perhaps the best-known (but fictitious) case is that of the Mad Hatter in *Alice in Wonderland*; hatmakers used mercuric nitrate for making felt out of animal fur! In the 1950s at Minamata, Japan, there was serious water pollution with methyl mercury causing at least 50 deaths and many more cases of permanent neurological disability.

Despite its known toxicity, mercury has been used therapeutically, though not to any great effect. It was a popular, though ineffectual, remedy for syphilis; this gave rise to the adage 'A night with Venus; a lifetime on Mercury'! More recently, pharmaceutical preparations containing mercury were advocated for treating childhood ailments such as measles, teething and diarrhoea. One such preparation containing calomel (mercurous chloride) was sold as a teething powder. It was not until 1942 that it was first suggested to be the cause of 'pink disease', a distressing condition affecting infants and young children, formerly of unknown aetiology. Many authorities doubted the link, but eventually the case was proven and the powder was withdrawn.

Lead

Much effort is being made in many countries to reduce environmental contamination by lead. The human body contains approximately 120 mg of lead and the daily intake should not exceed 500 μg. Excessive ingestion or inhalation can result from contaminated food, water or air; the main sources in the UK appear to be old lead piping in water supplies, and tetra-ethyl and tetra-methyl lead added to petrol as anti-knocking agents. Old plumbing is gradually being replaced and the use of unleaded petrol is increasing.

Toxic effects of lead include central and peripheral nervous system damage, renal damage and sideroblastic anaemia (Ch. 23). It has been alleged that lead exposure may be responsible for mental retardation in children, but it has been difficult to dissociate this from the other consequences of socio-economic deprivation prevalent in the urban environments contaminated with lead.

Aluminium

Aluminium is one of the most abundant elements in the Earth's crust, but only traces are found in the normal human body. Toxic quantities can enter the body in a variety of ways. Aluminium is present in variable concentrations in water supplies and it is used therapeutically in the form of aluminium hydroxide as an antacid. Aluminium is also used in some cooking utensils, from which it can be leached under acid conditions. Aluminium powder has also been used for the treatment of pneumoconiosis, a chronic lung disorder due to the inhalation of toxic or allergenic dusts (Ch. 14).

Aluminium has been incriminated in the development of skeletal abnormalities and encephalopathy in patients on regular haemodialysis for chronic renal failure. In such cases, aluminium has been found deposited on mineralisation fronts in the skeleton, where it may interfere with bone turnover. Dialysis encephalopathy, first reported in 1972, is characterised by progressive dementia, epileptic fits and tremors. In 1976, dialysis encephalopathy was shown to be associated with an abnormally high aluminium concentration in brain tissue obtained from autopsies on affected patients. This finding led to investigations for a possible link between aluminium and dialysis bone disease and, by 1978, the association was virtually proven.

Aluminium is often detectable in the brain lesions in Alzheimer's disease, a relatively common neurodegenerative disorder, but evidence that it is an aetiological factor is very weak.

Copper

Copper is essential for the function of several enzymes (e.g. superoxide dismutase). Copper deficiency appears to be rare. Some people with arthritis claim to derive benefit, undoubtedly psychological, from wearing copper bracelets, though the only observable change is a green discoloration of the underlying skin.

Wilson's disease is the most important disorder of copper metabolism. This is inherited as an autosomal recessive condition in which copper accumulates in the liver (Fig. 7.9), basal ganglia of the brain, kidneys and eyes. The brown ring of copper deposition around the corneal limbus—the Kayser–Fleischer ring—is absolutely diagnostic.

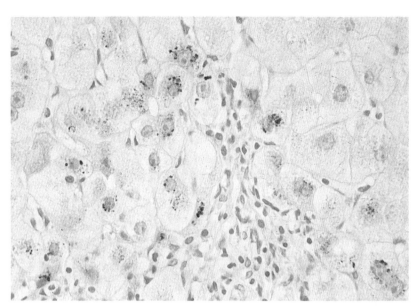

Fig. 7.9   Copper in liver

Liver biopsy, stained for copper (dark granules), showing excessive copper in periportal liver cells. No stainable copper would be present in a normal liver. Copper accumulates in the liver in Wilson's disease and in patients with chronic obstructive jaundice (e.g. primary biliary cirrhosis).

Serum caeruloplasmin levels are usually low. In the liver, the copper accumulation is associated with chronic hepatitis frequently culminating in cirrhosis (Ch. 16). The neurological changes are seriously disabling. Although Wilson's disease is rare, it is absolutely vital to consider the diagnosis in any patient presenting with chronic liver disease and neurological signs. D-penicillamine, a chelating agent, has revolutionised the treatment of Wilson's disease, but it is to little avail if the liver and brain have already been irreversibly damaged.

Iodine

The human body contains only 15–20 mg of iodine, most of which is in the thyroid gland. Iodine is almost unique among elements in having just one known role in the human body: it is essential for the synthesis of thyroxine.

Ingestion of modestly excessive quantities of iodine (as potassium iodide, for example) has no serious adverse consequences. Indeed, large stocks of potassium iodide tablets are kept in the vicinity of nuclear power stations for use in the event of accidental release of radioactive iodine, a cause of thyroid cancer. The potassium iodide competes with the smaller amounts of radioactive iodine for uptake by the thyroid gland.

Iodine deficiency results in goitre (enlargement of the thyroid gland, Ch. 17). Goitre was prevalent in regions where the water and solid food lacked an adequate iodine content, usually in mountainous regions (hence, for example, 'Derbyshire neck'). Maternal iodine deficiency during pregnancy causes cretinism in neonates, characterised by mental retardation and stunted growth. These problems have been eliminated in many countries by the addition of iodides and iodates to table salt.

TISSUE DEPOSITIONS

Tissues, especially connective tissues, can become altered as a result of deposition of calcium salts or of some other abnormal material such as amyloid.

Calcification

▶ Dystrophic calcification in previously damaged tissues
▶ 'Metastatic' calcification due to hypercalcaemia
▶ Pathological calcification may be radiologically evident and diagnostically useful
▶ Resulting hardening of tissues may lead to malfunction

Although calcium ions are vital for the normal function of all cells, precipitates of calcium salts are normally found only in bones, otoliths and teeth. In disease states, however, tissues can become hardened by deposits of calcium salts; this process is called calcification. Calcification may be:

- dystrophic
- 'metastatic'.

'Metastatic' calcification must not be confused with the process of metastasis of tumours. It is an entirely separate condition. In the context of calcification, 'metastatic' only means widespread.

Dystrophic calcification

Calcification is said to be dystrophic if it occurs in tissue already affected by disease. In these cases the serum calcium is normal. The calcification is due to local precipitation of insoluble calcium salts. Common examples are:

- atheromatous plaques
- congenitally bicuspid aortic valves
- calcification of mitral valve ring
- old tuberculous lesions
- fat necrosis
- breast lesions
- calcinosis cutis.

The calcified lesions will often be detectable on a plain X-ray as opacities or, if detected at surgery, will feel extremely hard. Dystrophic calcification does not usually have any special consequences for the patient, with the notable exception of calcification of a congenitally bicuspid aortic valve. A bicuspid aortic valve can function quite normally, but when it becomes calcified, a common event in the elderly, the valve cusps become thick and rigid; this causes stenosis, incompetence and, ultimately, cardiac fail-ure (Ch. 13). The biochemical basis of dystrophic calcification is uncertain except in the instance of fat necrosis, a common result of trauma to adipose tissue or of acute pancreatitis (Ch. 16); the liberated fatty acids bind calcium to form insoluble calcium soaps (Fig. 7.10) sometimes causing hypocalcaemia and tetany.

The presence of dystrophic calcification in breast lesions, particularly some carcinomas, is one of the abnormalities looked for by radiologists in the interpretation of mammograms (X-rays of the breasts) when screening for breast cancer (Fig. 7.11).

A few tumours contain minute concentric lamellated calcified bodies. These are called *psammoma bodies* and are commonly found in:

- meningiomas (Ch. 26)
- papillary carcinomas of thyroid (Ch. 17)
- papillary ovarian carcinomas (Ch. 19).

Psammoma bodies assist the histopathologist in correctly identifying the type of tumour, but their pathogenesis is unknown.

'Metastatic' calcification

Metastatic calcification is much less common than dystrophic calcification and occurs as a result of hypercalcaemia. Calcification may be widespread and occurs in otherwise normal tissues. Frequent causes are:

- hyperparathyroidism
- hypercalcaemia of malignancy.

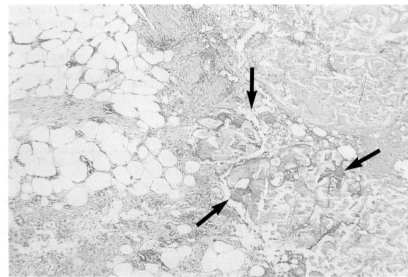

Fig. 7.10 Dystrophic calcification in fat necrosis

Adipose tissue from the abdominal wall of a patient with acute pancreatitis. Leakage of lipases from the inflamed pancreas digests the fat, and the resulting fatty acids bind calcium to form insoluble soaps. The calcification is seen as blue-staining (haematoxyphilic) material (arrows).

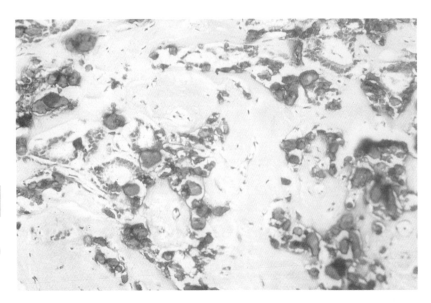

Fig. 7.11 Microcalcification in breast carcinoma

Small particles of dystrophic calcification are common in breast carcinomas. This aids the detection of breast carcinomas by mammography, because the calcification is opaque to X-rays.

In hyperparathyroidism, an adenoma or, less often, a diffuse hyperplasia of the parathyroid glands secretes excess quantities of parathyroid hormone; this liberates calcium from the bone, resulting in hypercalcaemia. In some patients with malignant neoplasms, hypercalcaemia results from either the secretion of a parathyroid hormone-like substance or extensive bone erosion due to skeletal metastases.

In this condition the calcium salts are precipitated on to connective tissue fibres (e.g. collagen, elastin).

Amyloid

> ▶ Extracellular material with affinity for Congo red or Sirius red dyes
> ▶ Composed of immunoglobulin light chains, serum amyloid protein A, peptide hormones, pre-albumin, etc.
> ▶ Systemic amyloidosis may be due to a plasma cell neoplasm (e.g. myeloma) or to a chronic inflammatory disorder
> ▶ Localised amyloid deposits occur in some peptide-hormone-producing tumours
> ▶ Amyloid often impairs the function of the organ in which it is deposited
> ▶ Heart failure and nephrotic syndrome are common complications

Amyloid (meaning starch-like from the Greek 'amylon') is the name given to a group of proteins or glycoproteins which, when deposited in tissues, share the following properties:

- β-pleated sheet molecular configuration with an affinity for certain dyes (e.g. Congo or Sirius red; Fig. 7.12)
- fibrillar ultrastructure (Fig. 7.13)
- presence of a glycoprotein of the pentraxin family (amyloid P protein)
- extracellular location, often on basement membranes
- resistance to removal by natural processes
- a tendency to cause the affected tissue to become hardened and waxy.

Small asymptomatic deposits of amyloid are not uncommon in the spleen, brain, heart and joints of elderly people.

Classification of amyloid

Amyloid can be classified according to:

- chemical composition
- tissue distribution
- aetiology.

All these are equally legitimate and complementary methods of classification. The chemical composition often correlates with the clinical classification (Table 7.6); it can, therefore, be helpful diagnostically and lead to the discovery of the aetiology in an individual case.

Clinically, however, amyloidosis presents with organ involvement which is either:

- systemic (Fig. 7.14)
- localised.

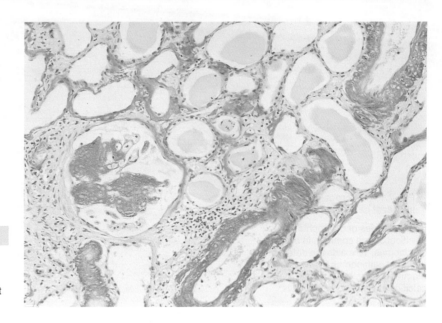

Fig. 7.12 Renal amyloidosis

Renal biopsy stained to show amyloid (red). The amyloid is deposited in the glomeruli, blood vessel walls and tubular basement membranes.

Systemic amyloidosis

In systemic amyloidosis the material is deposited in a wide variety of organs; virtually no organ is exempt. Clinical features suggesting amyloidosis include generalised diffuse organ enlargement (e.g. hepatomegaly, splenomegaly, macroglossia) and evidence of organ dysfunction (e.g. heart failure, proteinuria).

Table 7.6 Classification of amyloid substances

Clinical classification of amyloidosis	Amyloid substance
Myeloma-associated (primary)	AL (immunoglobulin light chains or fragments)
Reactive (secondary)	AA (serum amyloid protein A, an acute phase reactant)
Senile	AS (prealbumin)
Haemodialysis-associated	AH (β_2-microglobulin)
Hereditary and familial neuropathic familial Mediterranean fever	AF (prealbumin) AA
Medullary carcinoma of thyroid	AF (calcitonin or precursor or subunits thereof)

In addition to those amyloid substances listed, all amyloid deposits also contain amyloid P glycoprotein as a common constituent.

Systemic amyloidosis is further classified according to its aetiology:

- myeloma-associated
- reactive (secondary)
- senile
- haemodialysis-associated
- hereditary.

Myeloma-associated amyloidosis

The amyloid substance in myeloma-associated amyloidosis is *AL amyloid*—immunoglobulin light chains.

A *myeloma* is a plasma cell tumour, often multiple, arising in bone marrow and causing extensive bone erosion. It produces excessive quantities of immunoglobulin of a single class (e.g. IgG) with a uniform light chain (e.g. kappa). The light chain forms the amyloid material. The amyloid is deposited in many organs—heart, liver, kidneys, spleen, etc.—but shows a predilection for the connective tissues within these organs.

In some cases, myeloma-associated amyloidosis is called *primary amyloidosis* because of the absence of any clinically obvious myeloma. However, in these cases it is due to a clinically occult plasma cell tumour, with little bone erosion to declare itself, and is accompanied by the presence of a monoclonal immunoglobulin band on serum electrophoresis; this is referred to as a benign *monoclonal gammopathy*.

Amyloidosis is a serious complication of myeloma, making a further contribution to the ill health of the patient.

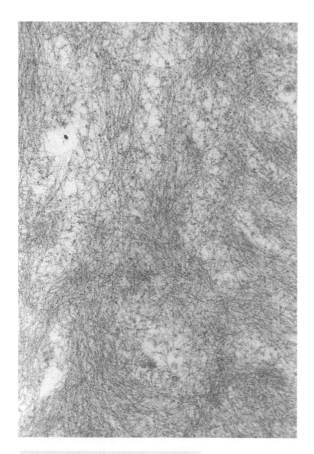

Fig. 7.13   Amyloid ultrastructure

Amyloid substances are characterised by a fibrillar appearance on electron microscopy.

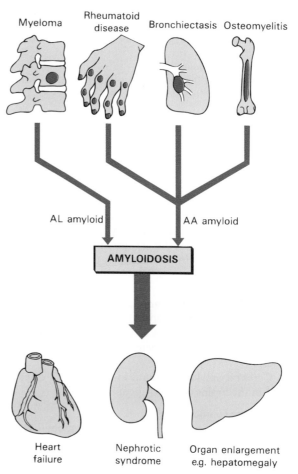

Fig. 7.14   Common causes and consequences of amyloidosis

Reactive (secondary) amyloidosis

The amyloid substance in reactive or secondary amyloidosis is *AA amyloid*, derived from serum amyloid protein A.

Serum amyloid protein A, synthesised in the liver, is an acute phase reactant protein, one of several so called because the serum concentrations rise in response to the presence of a variety of diseases.

Reactive amyloidosis, by definition, always has a predisposing cause; this is invariably a chronic inflammatory disorder. Chronic inflammatory disorders frequently predisposing to secondary amyloidosis are:

- rheumatoid disease
- bronchiectasis
- osteomyelitis.

The amyloid in reactive amyloidosis shows the same tendency to widespread deposition as in myeloma-associated amyloidosis, but it has a predilection for the liver, spleen and kidneys (Fig. 7.13).

Senile amyloidosis

Minute deposits of amyloid, usually derived from serum prealbumin, may be found in the heart and in the walls of blood vessels in many organs of elderly people. However, only in a few cases do they result in significant signs or symptoms.

Haemodialysis-associated amyloidosis

The association of amyloidosis with long-term haemodialysis for chronic renal failure has been recognised only recently. The clinical manifestations include arthropathy and carpal tunnel syndrome. In a few cases there is much more extensive involvement of other organs. The amyloid material deposited in the affected tissues appears to be β_2-microglobulin.

Hereditary amyloidosis
Hereditary and familial forms of amyloid deposition are rare and include:

- familial Mediterranean fever
- Portuguese nephropathy
- neuropathic forms.

Localised amyloidosis

Amyloid material is often found in the stroma of tumours producing peptide hormones. It is particularly characteristic of medullary carcinoma of the thyroid, a tumour of the calcitonin-producing interfollicular C-cells. In this instance, the amyloid contains calcitonin-precursor molecules arranged in a β-pleated sheet configuration.

Localised deposits of amyloid may be found, without any obvious predisposing cause, in virtually any organ; this is, however, a rare occurrence. The skin, lungs and urinary tract seem to be the most frequent sites.

Cerebral amyloid is found in Alzheimer's disease and in the brains of elderly people in:

- neuritic (senile) plaques
- the walls of small arteries (amyloid angiopathy).

Clinical effects and diagnosis

The clinical manifestations of amyloidosis are:

- nephrotic syndrome, eventually renal failure
- hepatosplenomegaly

- cardiac failure due to restricted myocardial movement
- macroglossia
- purpura
- carpal tunnel syndrome
- factor X deficiency (in AL amyloid).

Amyloidosis may be detected on clinical examination because of enlargement of various organs, especially the liver and spleen. As the kidneys are often involved and the amyloid is deposited in glomerular basement membranes, altering their filtration properties, the patients often have proteinuria; in severe cases the proteinuria can result in nephrotic syndrome (Ch. 21). The diagnosis is best confirmed by biopsy of the rectal mucosa, commonly involved in cases of systemic amyloidosis; this procedure is relatively safe and painless. The amyloid in the biopsy can be stained histologically using Congo red or Sirius red dyes. When examined using one fixed and one rotating polarising filter in the light path on either side of the section, the red colour changes to green (dichroism); this is very specific for amyloid. Using special techniques it may be possible to characterise the amyloid substance more precisely to determine its origin and to identify thereby the underlying cause.

Localised amyloid in a tumour is of no clinical consequence other than serving to assist the histopathologist in correctly identifying the tumour as, for example, a medullary carcinoma of the thyroid.

A solitary amyloid deposit is of clinical significance either because it mimics a tumour (e.g. on a plain chest X-ray) or because it compresses a vital structure (e.g. a ureter).

FURTHER READING

Cohen A S, Connors L H 1987 The pathogenesis and biochemistry of amyloidosis. Journal of Pathology 151: 1–10

Lenihan J 1988 The crumbs of creation: trace elements in history, medicine, industry, crime and folklore. Adam Hilger, Bristol

Stanbury R B, Wyngarden J B, Fredrickson D S, Goldstein J L 1983 The metabolic basis of inherited disease. McGraw-Hill, New York

Whitby L G, Smith A F, Beckett G J 1988 Lecture notes on clinical chemistry, 4th edn. Blackwell, Oxford

8

Ischaemia, infarction and shock

A. Thrombosis

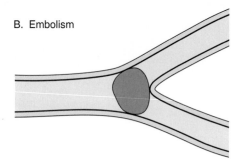

E. Compression

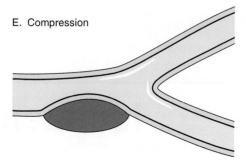

B. Embolism

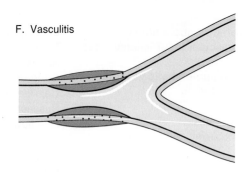

F. Vasculitis

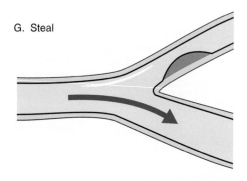

C. Spasm

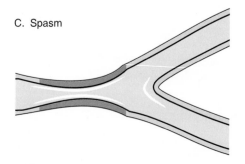

G. Steal

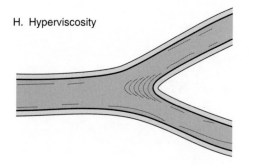

D. Atheroma

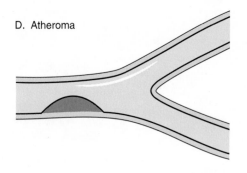

H. Hyperviscosity

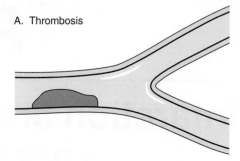

Thrombo-embolic phenomena are major causes of morbidity and mortality in the UK and other developed countries. The majority of readers (and authors) of this book will die of events somewhere along the sequence described in this chapter. Common and serious disorders in which thrombo-embolic mechanisms participate include:

- myocardial infarction
- cerebral infarction
- pulmonary embolism.

However, no organ is exempt from the harmful consequences of an impaired blood supply, although some (e.g. brain, myocardium), because of their nutritional requirements, are more vulnerable than others.

Ischaemia is the result of impaired vascular perfusion, depriving the affected tissue of vital nutrients, especially oxygen. The effects on the tissue can be reversible, but this depends on:

- the duration of the ischaemic period — brief ischaemic episodes may be recoverable
- the metabolic demands of the tissue — cardiac myocytes and cerebral neurones are the most vulnerable.

Infarction is death (necrosis) of tissue as a result of ischaemia. Infarction is irreversible, but tissues vary in their ability to repair and replace the loss. Infarction usually results from thrombo-embolic phenomena completely occluding the artery supplying the affected tissue.

Fig. 8.1   Vascular lesions causing ischaemia

A. Thrombosis: initiated by either abnormal flow (e.g. stasis, turbulence) or damage to vessel wall (e.g. denudation of endothelial lining) or abnormal blood constituents. **B. Embolism. C. Spasm:** due to contraction of smooth muscle in media of vessel, for example due to lack of NO from endothelium. **D. Atheroma:** occurs only in arteries and may in turn be complicated by thrombosis and embolism. **E. Compression:** veins are more susceptible because of their thinner walls and lower intraluminal pressure. **F. Vasculitis:** inflammation of vessel wall narrows lumen and may be complicated by superimposed thrombosis. **G. Vascular steal:** for example, an artery may be narrowed by atheroma but flow is still sufficient to maintain viability of perfused territory; however, flow may be compromised by increased demands of a neighbouring territory. **H. Hyperviscosity:** increased viscosity, in for example hypergammaglobulinaemia resulting from myeloma, causes impaired flow and predisposes to thrombosis.

Shock (pathophysiological rather than psychological) is a state of circulatory collapse resulting in impaired tissue perfusion. Ischaemia, infarction and shock are, therefore, interrelated phenomena. The cellular responses to impaired nutrition are summarised in Chapter 6.

Although the most common causes of ischaemia and infarction are thrombo-embolic phenomena, vascular insufficiency can result also from other causes (Fig. 8.1).

NON-THROMBO-EMBOLIC VASCULAR INSUFFICIENCY

Vascular flow can be impeded by abnormalities other than thrombo-embolic phenomena.

In arteries, the commonest lesion is *atheroma*, which in turn may be complicated by thrombo-embolism. In medium-sized arteries, atheromatous plaques (Ch. 13) often narrow the lumen causing ischaemia and sometimes atrophy of tissues in the hypoperfused territory. Serious consequences include the symptom of angina due to myocardial ischaemia, often heralding the development of irreversible infarction, and hypertension due to renal artery narrowing and hypoperfusion of a kidney which responds physiologically by increased renin secretion.

Transient arterial narrowing can result from *spasm* of the smooth muscle in the vessel wall. This can be due to a decrease in nitric oxide (*endothelium-derived relaxing factor*) production by the vascular endothelium due to cellular injury or loss. Spasm of coronary arteries can lead to angina and both may be relieved by glyceryl trinitrate. Arterial spasm is also responsible for the transient ischaemia of the fingers in Raynaud's phenomenon.

Blood vessels can be partially or totally occluded by *external compression*. This is done intentionally during surgery by ligation to prevent haemorrhage from severed vessels, although the results can be disastrous if, accidentally, the wrong vessel is tied off! Because of their thin walls and low intraluminal pressure, veins are more susceptible to occlusion by external compression. This occurs commonly in strangulated hernias, testicular torsion and torsion of ovaries containing cysts or tumours.

'Steal' syndromes occur when blood is diverted ('stolen') from a vital territory. This results when, proximal to an area of atheromatous narrowing insufficient on its own to produce ischaemia, the arterial stream is diverted along another branch vessel to meet the increased demands of a competing territory or lesion; the territory supplied by the atheromatous vessel then becomes ischaemic. This is a relatively uncommon cause of ischaemia, but often the most challenging diagnostically.

Ischaemia at the arteriolar, capillary and venular level can result from *increased whole blood viscosity*. Viscosity effects contribute relatively little to the flow characteristics of blood in vessels of large calibre, but in small vessels they are a major factor. Hyperviscosity of blood can occur in myeloma, a tumour of plasma cells, as a result of the abnormally high concentration of gammaglobulin in the plasma and rouleaux formation by red cells.

THROMBO-EMBOLIC VASCULAR OCCLUSION

Clot

When blood stagnates due to the cessation of the pumping action of the heart, or if blood is allowed to stand in a bottle or test tube, then the clotting process is set in motion. A complex series of enzymatic steps (see Ch. 23) is activated, resulting in the formation of a fibrin meshwork that entraps the cells into a solid but elastic clot. When this process occurs in the body after death, the red cells tend to settle out before the clot forms, so that these post-mortem clots have two layers: a lower, deep red layer (resembling redcurrant jelly) and an upper, clearer layer (resembling chicken fat), with platelets evenly distributed throughout. Since these clots have formed within the body and represent the blood content of the vessel during life, they are moulded to the shape of the vessels in which they have formed. Some time after death, the various blood cells and the cells of the vessel wall begin to release their hydrolytic enzymes and the clot is dissolved.

The sequence of enzymatic reactions involved in the clotting cascade and abnormalities of this system are discussed in Chapter 23.

Thrombosis

> ▶ A thrombus is a solid mass of blood constituents formed within the vascular system
> ▶ Predisposing factors (Virchow's triad): abnormalities of the vessel wall; abnormalities of blood flow; abnormalities of the blood constituents
> ▶ Arterial thrombosis is most commonly superimposed on atheroma
> ▶ Venous thrombosis is most commonly due to stasis
> ▶ Clinical consequences include: arterial thrombosis (tissue infarction distally); venous thrombosis (oedema, due to impaired venous drainage), and embolism

A thrombus is a solidification of blood contents that forms within the vascular system during life and is therefore different in concept from a clot. Its mode of formation, its structure and its appearance are all different to those of a clot and the two should never be confused.

Role of platelets

The mechanism for closing small gaps in vessel walls brought about by trauma involves the platelets. Platelets are smaller than red blood cells, rather angular in appearance and have no nucleus. They are derived from large, multinucleated cells in the bone marrow called megakaryocytes. Although platelets have no nucleus, they are highly structured internally and contain a variety of organelles, some of which are specific to them. As well as mitochondria and the various cytoskeletal elements found in most cells, platelets also contain alpha granules and dense granules. The *alpha granules* contain several substances involved in the process of platelet adhesion to damaged vessel walls (fibrinogen, fibronectin, platelet growth factor and an antiheparin as well as less well defined substances), and the *dense granules* contain substances such as adenosine diphosphate (ADP) which causes platelets to aggregate.

Platelets are activated and the contents of their granules are released when the platelets come into contact with collagen, as may be found in damaged vessel walls, or with polymerising fibrin. The platelets change shape and extend pseudopodia; their granules release their contents and the platelets form a mass that covers the vessel wall defect until the endothelial cells have regenerated and repaired the vessel permanently. However, if this process is activated within an intact vessel, it results in a thrombus.

Thrombus formation

There are three predisposing situations that may result in thrombus formation. These were described originally by Virchow and are known as *Virchow's triad*. The three factors are:

- changes in the intimal *surface* of the vessel
- changes in the pattern of blood *flow*
- changes in the blood *constituents*.

Not all three are needed for thrombosis to occur, but any one of them may result in thrombosis in a particular case.

If we consider the sequence of events involved in the formation of thrombus on the basis of an atheromatous plaque (Ch. 13), this will serve as a very good example of the factors listed by Virchow.

Arterial thrombosis
In its earliest phase the atheromatous plaque may consist of a slightly raised fatty streak on the intimal surface of any artery, such as the aorta (Fig. 8.2). With time, the plaque enlarges and becomes sufficiently raised to protrude into the lumen and cause a degree of *turbulence* in the blood flow. This turbulence eventually causes *loss of intimal cells*, and the denuded plaque surface is presented to the blood cells, including the platelets. The turbulence itself will predispose to *fibrin deposition* and to *platelet clumping* and the bare luminal surface of the vessel will have collagen exposed and platelets will settle on this surface. Thus we have two of the factors described in Virchow's triad operating in an atheromatous plaque. If this plaque exists in the aorta of a smoker or someone with a high cholesterol and high levels of low density lipoprotein — common risk factors for atheroma — then the third of Virchow's factors is introduced, since these changes in blood constituents are well known to predispose to thrombus formation. This process, once begun, may be self-perpetuating since it has been shown that platelet-derived growth factor, which is contained in the alpha granules, causes proliferation of arterial smooth muscle cells, which are an important constituent of the atheromatous plaque.

Thus, the first layer of the thrombus is a platelet layer. Formation of this layer in turn causes the precipitation of a fibrin meshwork in which red cells are

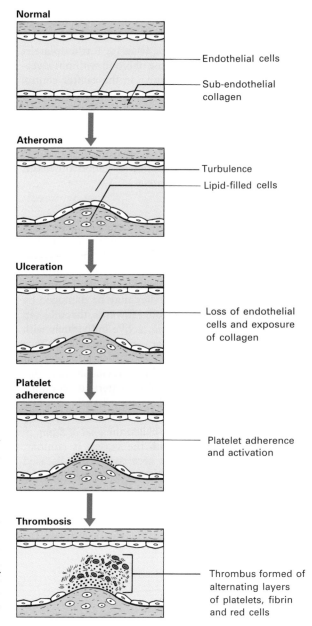

Normal

Endothelial cells

Sub-endothelial collagen

Atheroma

Turbulence

Lipid-filled cells

Ulceration

Loss of endothelial cells and exposure of collagen

Platelet adherence

Platelet adherence and activation

Thrombosis

Thrombus formed of alternating layers of platelets, fibrin and red cells

Fig. 8.2 Thrombosis

Thrombosis is exemplified by its occurrence on an atheromatous plaque, a particularly common event. Important steps in this sequence include: loss of endothelial cells and exposure of the underlying collagen; platelet adherence and activation; partial or complete arterial occlusion by the multilayered thrombus.

trapped and a layer of this meshwork is developed on top of the platelet layer. This complex structure now protrudes even further into the lumen, causing more turbulence and forming the basis for further platelet deposition. The normal flow of blood within the vessels is laminar; the cells move in the swifter central lane and the plasma runs along the walls. Therefore, the greatest degree of turbulence occurs at the downstream side of arterial thrombi, as the blood passes over the thrombus, and on the upstream side of venous thrombi for the same reason. Thrombi will therefore grow in the direction of blood flow; this process is known as *propagation*.

Venous thrombosis

In veins, however, the blood pressure is lower than in arteries and atheroma does not occur; so what initiates venous thrombus formation? Most venous thrombi seem to begin at valves. Valves naturally produce a degree of turbulence since they protrude into the vessel lumen and they may be damaged by trauma, stasis, and occlusion. However, thrombi can also form in veins of young, active individuals with no predisposing factors that can be identified. Once they begin, the thrombi grow by successive deposition in the manner described previously and this process may produce a highly patterned, coralline growth (Fig. 8.3). The alternating bands of white platelets and red blood cells in thrombi were first described by Zahn and are called the *lines of Zahn*.

Since normal flow within the vessels is laminar, most of the blood cells are kept away from diseased walls or from damaged vein valves. However, if the blood pressure is allowed to fall during surgery or following a myocardial infarction, then flow is slower through the vessels and thrombosis becomes a likely

event. Similarly, the venous return from the legs is very reliant upon calf muscle contraction and relaxation which massages the veins and, because of the valves, tends to return the blood heartwards. So, if elderly subjects are immobilised for any reason, they become at great risk from the formation of deep leg vein thromboses. The frequency with which deep vein thrombosis is found to occur following surgery is directly related to the enthusiasm with which it is sought (e.g. by the pathologist at postmortem examination) and the sensitivity of the methods used to demonstrate it. Postmortem studies on unselected medical and surgical patients show significant deep vein thrombosis in 34% of the former and 60% of the latter regardless of the cause of death.

When a vein becomes thrombosed it evokes an inflammatory reaction, a phenomenon known as *thrombophlebitis*; the opposite process also occurs — a vein that is inflamed will often thrombose and this is known as *phlebothrombosis*. The end effect is the same, a thrombosed and inflamed vein, but clearly if there is a predisposing cause then the cause needs to be recognised and treated.

Clinical effects

The effects of thrombosis are apparent only if the thrombus is sufficiently large to significantly affect the flow of blood. Arterial thrombosis results in loss of pulses distal to the thrombus and all the signs of impaired blood supply: the area becomes cold, pale, painful and eventually the tissue dies and gangrene results. In venous thromboses, 95% of which occur in leg veins, the area becomes tender, swollen and reddened, since blood is still carried to the site by the arteries but cannot be drained away by the veins.

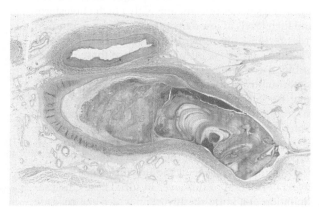

Fig. 8.3 Venous thrombus

Histological section showing the characteristic laminated or coralline structure of a thrombus.

The tenderness is due to developing ischaemia in the vein wall initially, but there is also general ischaemic pain as the circulation worsens.

Phlegmasia alba dolens (white painful leg) occurs with relatively slow thrombosis in the ileofemoral veins and is seen most commonly in medical patients or following pregnancy. The leg becomes white, swollen and painful and, if untreated, progresses over 2–6 weeks to a chronic cold, aching, oedematous limb that requires elastic stockings since the venous system within the limb is permanently disrupted.

Phlegmasia cerulea dolens (blue painful leg) is due to acute massive ileofemoral venous thrombosis and the pain is sharp enough to cause the patients great distress. Shock may develop and some degree of gangrene within the limb is common.

Thrombophlebitis migrans occurs in previously healthy veins in any area of the body. The thromboses appear and disappear, changing site all the time, and the condition may persist for months or even years. It is extremely ominous and usually indicates the presence of visceral cancer, commonly of the pancreas. The mechanism remains obscure.

Strokes may be due to the formation of thrombus in a cerebral vessel although they may be also the result of haemorrhage or embolism (Ch. 26).

Myocardial infarction is often associated with thrombus formation in coronary arteries and is responsible for numerous sudden deaths (Ch. 13).

Fate of thrombi

Various fates await the newly-formed thrombus (Fig. 8.4). In the best scenario it may resolve; the various degradative processes available to the body may dissolve it and clear it away completely. It is not known what proportion of thrombi follow this course, but the total number is likely to be large. A second possibility is that the thrombus may become *organised* into a scar by the invasion of macrophages which clear away the thrombus, as fibroblasts replace it with collagen, occasionally leaving a mural nodule or web that narrows the vessel lumen. A third possibility is that the intimal cells of the vessel in which the thrombus lies may proliferate, and small sprouts of capillaries may grow into the thrombus and later fuse to form larger vessels. In this way the original occlusion may become *recanalised* and the vessel patent again. Another common result is that the thrombus affects some vital centre and causes death before either the body or the clinicians can make an effective response; this event is very common. Finally, fragments of the thrombus may break off into the circulation, a process known as *embolism*.

Embolism

> ▶ An embolus is a mass of material in the vascular system able to become lodged within a vessel and block its lumen
> ▶ Most emboli are derived from thrombi
> ▶ Other types of embolic material include: atheromatous plaque material, vegetations on heart valves (infective endocarditis), fragments of tumour (causing metastases), amniotic fluid, gas and fat
> ▶ Most common occurrence is pulmonary embolism from deep leg vein thrombosis

An embolus is a mass of material in the vascular system able to lodge in a vessel and block its lumen. The material may have arisen within the body or have been introduced from outside. The material may be solid, liquid or gaseous. The end results of embolism are more dependent upon the final resting place of the embolic material than on its nature. Emboli travel in the circulation, passing through the vascular tree until they reach a vessel whose diameter is small enough to prevent their further passage. The clinical effects will therefore depend upon the territory supplied by that vessel and the presence or absence of an alternative (collateral) circulation to that area. The most frequent source of embolic material is a thrombus formed in any area of the circulatory system, but other sources of embolic material should not be disregarded. Over 90% of major emboli are derived from thrombi so we will first consider the principal clinical syndromes associated with this situation and then briefly mention other forms of embolism.

Pulmonary embolism

Around 95% of venous thrombosis occurs in leg veins; the majority of the rest occur in pelvic veins and a very few occur in the intracranial venous sinuses. Therefore, most emboli from such thrombi will arrive in the pulmonary circulation — *pulmonary embolism*. The only possibility for such emboli to arrive in the arterial side of the circulation is if there is an arterial/venous communication such as a perfo-

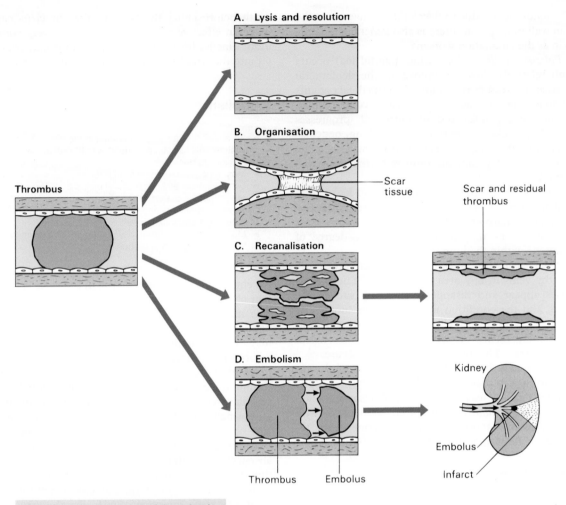

Fig. 8.4 Consequences of thrombosis

A. Lysis of the thrombus and complete restitution of normal structure usually can occur only when the thrombus is relatively small and is dependent upon fibrinolytic activity (e.g. plasmin). **B.** The thrombus may be replaced by scar tissue which contracts and obliterates the lumen; the blood bypasses the occluded vessel through collateral channels. **C.** Recanalisation occurs by the ingrowth of new vessels which eventually join up to restore blood flow, at least partially. **D.** Embolism caused by fragmentation of the thrombus and resulting in infarction at a distant site.

rated septum in the heart (paradoxical embolus), but this event is exceptionally rare.

The effects of pulmonary emboli depend upon their size. Small emboli may occur unnoticed and be lysed within the lung or they may become organised and cause some permanent, though small, respiratory deficiency. Such a respiratory deficiency may only come to light with the eventual accumulation of damage from many such tiny embolic events. The accumulation of such damage over a long period

may be the cause of so-called 'idiopathic' *pulmonary hypertension* (Ch. 14).

A second class of pulmonary emboli may be large enough to cause *acute respiratory and cardiac problems* that may resolve slowly with or without treatment. The main symptoms are chest pain and shortness of breath due to the effective loss of the area of lung supplied by the occluded vessel; the area may even become infarcted (see p. 173). This occlusion puts some strain on the heart which is evident on the

ECG as right heart strain with deep S waves in lead 1 and the presence of Q waves and inverted T waves in lead 3 (S1, Q3, T3). This ECG pattern is one of the few that a pathologist will look for in the case notes before performing an autopsy on a patient suspected of having had a pulmonary embolus in life; without these findings the embolus is unlikely to have caused death. Although many patients recover from such episodes, their lung function is impaired and, of course, they are at risk from further emboli from the same source. Consequently, they require symptomatic therapy for the embolus as well as treatment for the causative thrombus.

The third class of pulmonary emboli are massive and result in *sudden death*. These are usually long thrombi derived from leg veins and have the shape of the vessels in which they arose, rather than that of the vessels in which they are found at postmortem examination. They are often impacted across the bifurcation of one of the major pulmonary arteries as a 'saddle embolus', a descriptive term for their appearance. As with all thrombi, even if they have undergone embolisation, they retain the appearance of a thrombus with lines of Zahn and a granular, friable consistency. This consistency is distinct from the elastic, 'chicken fat and redcurrant jelly' appearance of postmortem clots.

Systemic embolism

Systemic emboli arise in the arterial system and again their effects are due to their size and to the vessel in which they finally lodge. The thrombi from which they come generally form in the heart or on atheromatous plaque (Fig. 8.5). In the heart, thrombi may form on areas of cardiac muscle which has died as a result of myocardial infarction, since these areas will have lost their normal endothelial lining and will expose the underlying collagen to the circulating platelets. These areas of dead myocardium will also be adynamic and will disrupt the normal blood flow within the heart, creating turbulence and predisposing to thrombus formation at that site.

Another common cause of thrombosis within the heart is the presence of atrial fibrillation. This ineffectual movement of the atria causes blood to stagnate in the atrial appendages and thrombosis to occur. When the normal heart rhythm is re-established the atrial thrombus may be fragmented and emboli broken off.

Emboli from the heart are usually derived from thrombi on the left side of the circulation. These emboli may travel to the brain causing cerebrovascular incidents such as transient ischaemic attacks or strokes, or they may travel to any of the viscera, or to the limbs.

Large emboli may lodge at the bifurcation of the aorta as a saddle embolus cutting off the blood supply to the lower limbs, a situation that requires rapid diagnosis if the embolus is to be removed before the changes in the limbs become irreversible. Smaller emboli may lodge in smaller vessels nearer the periphery and cause gangrene of the digits. Small emboli may travel into the kidneys or spleen and be relatively asymptomatic, even when they cause the death of the area of tissue distal to their site of impaction; such ischaemic scars are not uncommon findings at autopsy with no clinical history to lead one to suspect that such events had been occurring.

More dramatic consequences develop as a result of emboli travelling to the intestine, often passing down the superior mesenteric artery; this impaction can cause death of whole sections of small bowel, which unlike kidneys or spleen depends upon the whole organ to be intact in order to function. The death of even a small area of bowel means perforation and peritonitis, whereas the death of a small area of kidney or spleen means only a small scar.

Vegetations on the heart valves are an important source of emboli. Most seriously, in *infective endocarditis* the vegetations consist of micro-organisms, usually bacteria, and are extremely friable. Marantic vegetations, consisting of platelets and fibrin, occur on the heart valves of patients who are severely debilitated, for example by cancer; these vegetations are often firmly adherent and are less likely to embolise.

Embolic atheroma
Fragments of atheromatous plaque may embolise and these are frequently seen in the lower limbs of arteriopathic patients. The precise cause of such ischaemic toes is rarely investigated thoroughly enough to be diagnosed. The embolic fragments may be recognised in histological preparations by the cigar-shaped clefts left behind when the cholesterol crystals dissolve out during histological processing.

Platelet emboli
Since the early stages of atheroma involve mainly platelet deposition, emboli from early lesions may be composed solely of platelets. In general these are

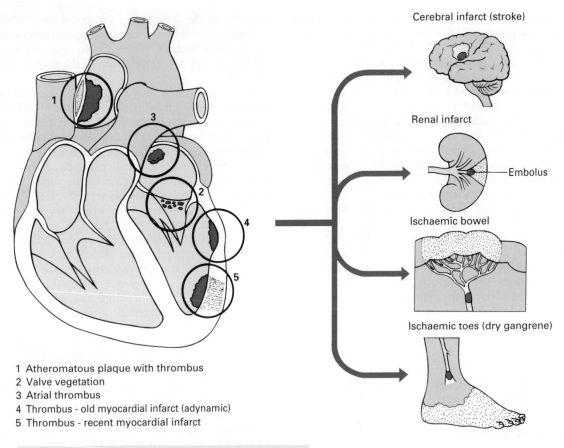

Cerebral infarct (stroke)

Renal infarct

Embolus

Ischaemic bowel

Ischaemic toes (dry gangrene)

1 Atheromatous plaque with thrombus
2 Valve vegetation
3 Atrial thrombus
4 Thrombus - old myocardial infarct (adynamic)
5 Thrombus - recent myocardial infarct

Fig. 8.5 Origins and effects of systemic arterial emboli

Systemic arterial emboli almost invariably originate from the left side of the heart or from major arteries. Infarction or gangrene are the usual consequences.

very tiny emboli and do not present with severe clinical signs. The exception is in the brain where even small emboli manifest with striking clinical symptoms and signs. A stroke which lasts less than 24 hours and which is associated with complete clinical recovery is termed a *transient ischaemic attack* (TIA); although these show complete resolution, they are risk markers for subsequent major strokes. While many TIAs are thought to be due to platelet emboli there is some evidence that in some cases they may also be caused by arterial spasm.

Infective emboli
Infected lesions within the blood stream, in particular the vegetations on diseased heart valves

(Ch. 13), may break off and lodge in small vessels in the usual way. But here, the usual effects of emboli are compounded by the infective agent present and this agent may weaken the wall of the vessel, causing the development of a mycotic aneurysm. (Mycotic is a misnomer since the infective agent is usually bacterial and not fungal.)

Fat embolism
Fat embolism usually arises following some severe trauma with fracture to long bones. Fat from the bone marrow is released into the circulation and comes to lodge in various organs. A similar situation arises in severe burns and in extensive soft tissue injury. Much of the circulating fat enters the lungs

and this indicates that it must travel by way of the venous system. However, fat globules are fluid and so small that many also enter the systemic arterial circulation, causing confusion or coma, renal impairment and skin petechiae. It has also been suggested that systemic effects of trauma, particularly burns, can cause changes in the stability of fat held in micellar suspension, resulting in free fat appearing in the circulation. This fat could then travel in the circulation in exactly the same way as a true fat embolism. Some degree of fat embolism probably occurs in most cases of long bone injury but it is generally asymptomatic.

Gas embolism

There are various causes of embolic events involving gas; several are iatrogenic. The classic form is *Caisson disease*, experienced by divers when they are transferred too rapidly from high to low pressure environments. At high pressure, increased volumes of gas dissolve in the blood and during rapid decompression these come out as bubbles. In the case of air, the oxygen and carbon dioxide redissolve but the nitrogen bubbles remain and enter bones and joints, causing the pains of the 'bends', or they lodge in the lungs causing the respiratory problems of the 'chokes'.

The other causes of gas embolism are mainly surgical when some vessel is opened to the air. This also occurs in suicide attempts when the neck veins are cut, or accidentally when patients are disconnected from intravenous lines and air enters. The 'secret murders' by air injection so favoured by thriller writers are rare, since the volume of air needed to cause death in this fashion is around 100 ml.

The pathological signs of this condition at autopsy include visible bubbles in the vessels such as those of the meninges, and sometimes a frothy ball of fibrin and air in the right side of the heart occluding one of the valves.

Amniotic embolism

With the vastly increased pressures in the uterus during delivery, the head engages and the pressure is transferred to the amniotic fluid which may be forced into the maternal uterine veins. These amniotic fluid emboli travel in the circulation and lodge in the lungs, causing respiratory distress like other pulmonary emboli. They can be recognised histologically since they contain the shed skin cells of the infant.

Tumour embolism

Tumour emboli are mainly small and break off as tumours which penetrate vessels (see Ch. 11). They do not usually cause immediate physical problems in the way that other emboli do, but this mechanism is a major route of dissemination of malignancies through the body (metastasis).

Embolism of foreign matter

Particles of foreign matter may contaminate fluids injected intravenously. This is rare when such fluids are injected for medical reasons, but talc, etc. is a common contaminant of fluids injected by intravenous drug abusers. The foreign particles elicit a granulomatous reaction in the organs in which they lodge.

INFARCTION

> ▶ Ischaemic death (necrosis) of tissue
> ▶ Infarcts elicit an inflammatory reaction
> ▶ Gangrene is infarction of mixed tissues in bulk (e.g. gut wall, part of a limb)
> ▶ In some tissues, ischaemic necrosis may result from impaired vascular flow short of total cessation

Infarction is ischaemic death of tissue within the living body. This means that death of tissue from other causes, such as toxins or trauma, is not infarction but is simply necrosis, which is the general term for death of tissue within the living organism. Only death of tissue due to restricted blood supply is infarction. The word infarction means 'stuffed full' and reflects the fact that the first types of infarction that were recognised were those in which the blockage was venous and the arterial supply continued to pump blood into the organ when the outlet was blocked. A similar effect may be seen in those cases where a second blood supply is present and, although the arterial inflow is blocked, blood still enters the organ from this second supply; a good example of this is the lung, which has both pulmonary and bronchial arterial supplies. In the past, pathologists classically divided infarcts into grey and red infarcts, but these merely represent stages in the same process; not all infarcts in the same organ go through these stages, so the division is pointless.

Reperfusion injury

Many of the tissue effects of ischaemic injury para-doxically seem to occur not during the ischaemic episode but when perfusion is re-established. This is not as illogical as it may seem because much of this damage is oxygen dependent and the only way for oxygen to get to the site is by blood flow. When the blood flow returns to an area of tissue that has been ischaemic it encounters tissue where transport mechanisms across the cell membrane have been disrupted to a variable extent and, in particular, where calcium transport out of the cell and from organelles such as mitochondria is impaired. This appears to be the trigger for the activation of oxygen-dependent free radical systems that begin the clear-ing away of dead cells which we recognise as a part of reperfusion injury. At the same time polymorphs and macrophages enter the area and begin to clear away debris and themselves import their own intrinsic oxygen free radicals into the area. Experimentally, reperfusion injury can be prevented with anti-oxidants but this only has a small effect on the ultimate amount of tissue loss. What we see here is another example of an adaptive process (clearing up of dead and damaged cells) which produces deleterious effects (scarring) and which can be marginally modified pharmacologically.

Appearance of infarcts

The appearance of infarcted areas depends upon the time that has elapsed between the infarct occurring and the lesion coming to the attention of the pathologist (Fig. 8.6). If the tissue is examined within 24 hours of the infarct there will be no direct evidence of the event. Between 24 and 48 hours the dead tissue is beginning to evoke a response from the surrounding living tissues and inflammatory cells can be seen moving into the infarcted area. In rou-tine histological sections stained with haematoxylin and eosin the cytoplasm contains proteins, which stain pink, and RNA which stains blue. In normal tissue, the cytoplasm therefore has a slightly purple tinge and in areas that have been dead a few hours the RNA is broken down and the cytoplasm becomes bright pink. It should be borne in mind that all histological sections of tissue are 'dead' and that what we are looking at is the consequence of the

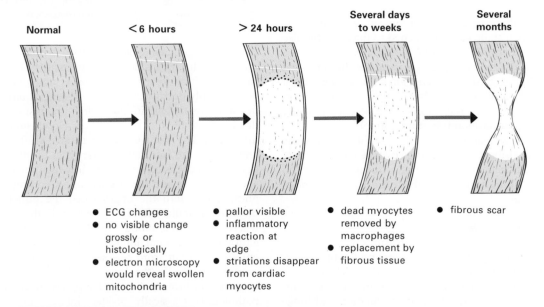

Normal   **<6 hours**   **>24 hours**   **Several days to weeks**   **Several months**

- ECG changes
- no visible change grossly or histologically
- electron microscopy would reveal swollen mitochondria

- pallor visible
- inflammatory reaction at edge
- striations disappear from cardiac myocytes

- dead myocytes removed by macrophages
- replacement by fibrous tissue

- fibrous scar

Fig. 8.6 Evolution of an infarct

This is typified by a myocardial infarct in which naked-eye abnormalities are rarely evident until many hours have elapsed. The dead tissue elicits an inflammatory reaction, characteristically neutrophil polymorphs and, later, macrophages. Unless complications intervene, the infarct heals by fibrosis.

time that has elapsed between the infarcted tissue dying and the rest of the tissue being killed by being dropped into formalin or some other fixative.

If the infarcted tissue has stayed in the living patient for some days before being removed (by biopsy or autopsy) then the degradative processes of the body in the form of macrophages and polymorphs will have begun to clear away the dead tissue, which will consequently have an amorphous, acellular appearance apart from the numerous inflammatory cells. At this stage, the tissue is at its weakest; myocardial infarction patients who have survived the acute episode 10 days previously may suddenly die with rupture of the healing infarct and consequent haemopericardium and cardiac tamponade (Ch. 13). The gross appearance of the tissue at this time is very variable; if small blood vessels in the vicinity have also become ischaemic they may die and blood will escape into the infarct, giving it a patchy or confluent red appearance. On the other hand, there may be no bleeding into the area, in which case it remains pale with a red hyperaemic rim, and grows progressively paler as healing takes place.

If the patients survive this danger period the damaged tissue either regenerates or repairs itself with the formation of a scar (Ch. 6). Such a scar is apparent as a grey, contracted area consisting of collagenous fibrous tissue. A scar solves the tissue deficit in the sense that the organ is intact and the hole is mended, but the scarred area is no longer functional; a healed myocardial infarct is adynamic and can be the site of further problems for the patient. In the heart, this may take the form of an aneurysm as the scar is subjected to cyclic pressure loads and becomes stretched without any ability to contract again.

The overall shape of infarcts depends upon the territory of perfusion of the occluded blood supply; some classical appearances are the wedge-shaped infarcts seen in the lung and the triangular infarcts (conical in three dimensions) seen in the kidneys at autopsy. Other scarred infarcts such as those in the spleen (Fig. 8.7) are less predictable since the blood supply is less regular and marked overlaps of vascular territories occur, and because the soft tissue distorts as the scar contracts. In the brain the dead tissue is cleared away so efficiently that a fluid-filled cyst is often all that remains (Ch. 26).

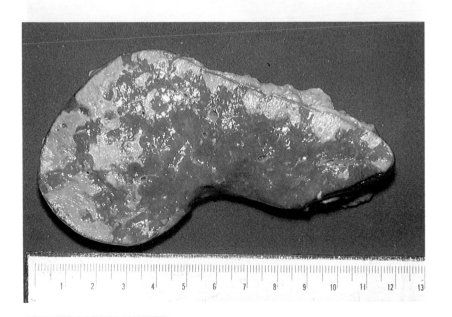

Fig. 8.7 Splenic infarcts

Note the pallor of the infarcts; this is characteristic of coagulative necrosis.

Gangrene

When whole areas of a limb or a region of the gut have their arterial supply cut off and large areas of mixed tissues die in bulk, such a process is termed gangrene. Two types of gangrene are recognised:

- Dry gangrene—where the tissue dies and becomes mummified and healing occurs above it, so that eventually the dead area drops off (Fig. 8.8). This is a sterile process, and is the common fate of gangrenous toes in the diabetic.
- Wet gangrene—where bacterial infection supervenes as a secondary complication; in this case the gangrene spreads proximally and the patient dies of overwhelming sepsis.

Another mechanism that results in gangrene is torsion: the gut may twist on a lax mesentery, or an ovary or testis may twist on its pedicle, occluding the venous return. The organ swells and the oedema further compresses the drainage. The arteries continue to pump blood into the organ, but ischaemia supervenes and infarction develops.

Gas gangrene results from infection of ischaemic tissue by gas-producing anaerobic bacteria such as *Clostridium perfringens*.

Capillary ischaemia

In frostbite, the capillaries are damaged in exposed areas and contract so severely that the area they normally supply becomes ischaemic and dies. Exposure to cold without freezing causes capillary contraction followed by a fixed dilatation; this is the mechanism of damage in 'trench foot' and related conditions.

Capillaries may also be blocked by parasites, by abnormal cells in sickle cell disease or by abnormal proteins that precipitate in the cold (cryoglobulinaemia) and these phenomena also lead to local ischaemia and infarction.

The balance of thrombotic and thrombolytic mechanisms is delicate; this balance may be secondarily disturbed by several different disease processes and, unfortunately, by some therapeutic interventions. In such cases, thrombosis may become activated without effective counterbalance, with the result that minute thrombi may form throughout the

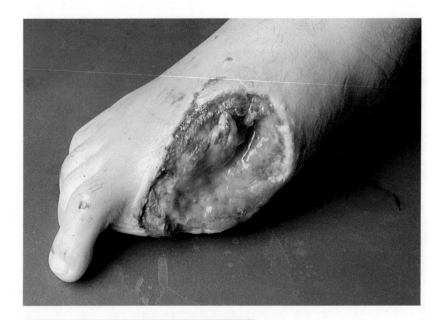

Fig. 8.8   Auto-amputation due to gangrene

The toe became gangrenous due to arterial occlusion. It detached spontaneously, leaving tissue exposed to the threat of infection, thus emphasising the advantages of surgical amputation with wound closure.

body and, consequently, bleeding may occur at multiple sites due to consumption of clotting factors; this phenomenon is called *disseminated intravascular coagulation* or *DIC* (Fig. 8.9). It occurs as a complication of many disease states such as cancer or infection (Ch. 23).

Susceptibility to ischaemia

Different tissues show differing susceptibility to ischaemia for a variety of reasons. Some tissues have only one arterial supply and if this is blocked there is no possibility of collateral supplies taking over; one such 'end artery' situation is the retinal artery and thrombosis of this artery leads inevitably to blindness. Tissues also vary in the degree of ischaemia that they can tolerate, commonly as a function of differing metabolic needs; even within a tissue, different areas have different susceptibilities. Within the heart the sub-endocardial zone is at a watershed between the coronary supply from the outside and the diffusion zone from blood within the chambers. If the coronary arteries are narrowed by the presence of atheroma, these patients are at great risk of developing sub-endocardial infarctions if their systemic blood pressure drops for any reason. Consequently,

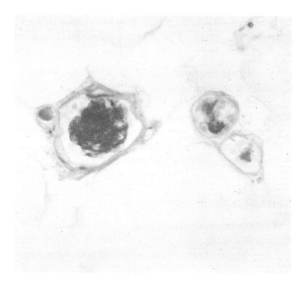

Fig. 8.9 Disseminated intravascular coagulation

In this condition, small vessels are occluded by minute thrombi (stained red in this histological section), causing scattered ischaemic lesions in many organs.

such patients may develop the complications of sub-endocardial infarction following trauma, surgery or toxic shock from infections.

Low-flow infarction

In some tissues, infarction may be due to impaired blood flow (or oxygenation) rather than an absolute cessation of flow. Tissues that are especially vulnerable to low-flow infarction include:

- 'watershed' areas
- tissues perfused by a portal vasculature
- tissues distal to pathological arterial stenoses
- metabolically active tissues.

'Watershed' areas

Tissue at the interface between the adjacent territory of two arteries is prone to infarction if there is an impairment of blood or oxygen supply. The tissue is normally situated precariously on the fringes of the territories perfused by the arteries, with no collateral circulation to provide blood from alternative vessels.

Examples include:

- the splenic flexure of the colon; this is situated at the interface between the territories of the superior and inferior mesenteric arteries
- regions of the cerebral hemispheres at the interface between the territories of the major cerebral arteries
- the deep myocardium between the sub-endocardial myocardium (oxygenated directly from blood in the ventricles) and that which is perfused by the coronary arteries.

Patients who are severely shocked and hypotensive may develop ischaemic lesions in these sites.

Portal vasculature

Some tissues are perfused by blood which has already passed through one set of capillaries; this vascular arrangement is described as portal. Therefore, there is normally a drop in intravascular pressure across the first set of capillaries, rendering the tissue perfused by the second set of capillaries vulnerable to ischaemic injury.

Examples include:

- the anterior pituitary, which is perfused by blood

that has already perfused the median eminence of the hypothalamus

- the renal tubular epithelium, which is perfused by blood issuing from the glomerular capillaries
- some parts of the exocrine pancreas, which are perfused by blood that has already perfused islets of Langerhans in the vicinity.

These patterns of vascular microanatomy account for the pituitary infarction, renal tubular necrosis and acute pancreatitis that may occur in severely shocked patients.

Arterial stenoses

Atheromatous narrowing or stenosis of arteries may be of insufficient severity to cause infarction distally in normotensive individuals. However, if the blood pressure and, therefore, blood flow falls, the tissue distal to the arterial stenosis may become infarcted. Thus, patients who become severely shocked may develop ischaemic changes in various organs without there being any sign of *total* vascular occlusion.

Transient arterial spasm can also cause infarction in vulnerable tissues such as the brain and heart.

Infarction and metabolic activity

Cells with large metabolic requirements are exceptionally vulnerable to ischaemic damage and infarction. Cerebral neurones are the most at risk; irreversible damage occurs within a few minutes of cessation of blood flow and oxygenation. Cardiac myocytes also have a considerable requirement for oxygen and other nutrients; they may be irreversibly damaged if the coronary arteries, which may be narrowed by atheroma, cannot supply these requirements during tachycardia associated with exertion.

SHOCK

The word 'shock' has different meanings in different contexts. In the emotional context, which almost all of us experience to varying degrees, it means a severe psychological reaction to an event for which we were unprepared. Another meaning is the unpleasant and often painful sensation experienced when high voltage electricity flows through the body. These meanings of the word 'shock' are not relevant here, but

they can be a source of great confusion when talking to patients.

Shock as a pathological process is characterised by profound circulatory failure resulting in life-threatening hypoperfusion of vital organs. Compensatory mechanisms maintain blood pressure until they too are defeated, resulting in hypotension. Shock may be classified as:

- cardiogenic — commonly due to myocardial infarction
- hypovolaemic — due to reduction in the *effective* circulating blood volume.

In the early stages the arterial networks in many vital organs can compensate to some extent. For example, by a process of autoregulation, the cerebral arteries dilate when blood pressure is reduced, so that the cerebral vascular resistance falls and a normal rate of flow is maintained. In other tissues, with less vital functions, there is compensatory vasoconstriction in order to increase peripheral vascular resistance and thus maintain the effective blood pressure supplying vital organs; this increased vascular tone is mediated by adrenergic mechanisms and by the effects of angiotension.

If the compensatory mechanisms fail and hypotension ensues, various tissues will be vulnerable to ischaemic injury. This is an extremely serious clinical problem which, depending on the primary cause, is frequently fatal. The clinicopathological consequences include:

- irreversible neuronal injury
- renal failure due to acute tubular necrosis
- acute pancreatitis
- risk of cerebral infarction in 'watershed' areas between the adjacent territories of cerebral arteries.
- infarction distal to any pathological arterial narrowing, usually atheromatous.

Cardiogenic shock

The commonest cause of cardiogenic shock is acute myocardial infarction. Death of part of the left ventricular myocardium reduces the heart's functional capacity and, even at rest, the left ventricular stroke volume is reduced. If shock proceeds to the hypotensive phase, it should only be corrected with extreme caution; by artificially increasing the blood pressure, additional strain will be placed on the myocardium with the risk of catastrophic failure.

Hypovolaemic shock

Hypovolaemic shock is characterised by loss of effective circulating blood volume. This may be due to:

- haemorrhage, internally or externally
- generalised increased vascular permeability and/or dilatation.

The pathogenesis of shock resulting from haemorrhage is logical. Internal or external bleeding, for example due to traumatic rupture of an internal organ or accidental severing of a major vessel, causes a reduction in the normal blood volume. Blood pressure is initially maintained by compensatory mechanisms, some of which enable the condition to be suspected clinically; symptoms and signs include a cold, clammy skin and a high pulse rate.

Shock due to generalised increased vascular permeability and/or dilatation can occur as a result of:

- neurogenic mechanisms (e.g. spinal cord injury)
- anaphylactic reactions
- extensive burns
- bacterial toxaemia.

In these situations there are varying degrees of vasodilatation and increased vascular permeability. Blood pools in the dilated vessels and, if there is endothelial damage (for example in severe burns or bacterial toxaemia), fluid leaks from the vessels into the extravascular compartment, causing a profound reduction in the effective circulating blood volume. Examples mediated by bacterial toxins include (see Ch. 3):

- the *toxic shock syndrome*, first described as a serious consequence of prolonged retention of a tampon which then became infected with staphylococci
- *Gram-negative septicaemia*, due to serious infection with endotoxin-producing bacteria.

Other vascular effects of bacterial toxaemia

The bacterial toxins have not only a hypotensive effect, but they also activate the complement and blood coagulation cascades. The latter may lead to *disseminated intravascular coagulation* (DIC) (Ch. 23). In this condition, which may also be precipitated by the release of tissue thromboplastins from necrotic tissue, fibrin is deposited on endothelial surfaces of blood vessels, thus interfering with trans-endothelial flow of nutrients. The fibrin may also form a mesh across the lumen of small blood vessels resulting in:

- haemolysis due to mechanical injury to circulating erythrocytes
- microinfarcts
- thrombocytopenia due to fibrin-induced platelet aggregation.

The fibrinolytic activity of endothelial cells can cope with small amounts of fibrin deposition; DIC results when the rate of fibrin deposition exceeds the rate of fibrinolysis. DIC is diagnosed by its multisystem clinical features, by the frequent accompaniments of haemolysis and thrombocytopenia, by the haemorrhagic tendency due to consumption of coagulation factors (*consumption coagulopathy*), and by finding fibrin degradation products.

FURTHER READING

Cotton D W K, Thrombosis, embolism and infarction. Videotape available from the Audiovisual & Television Centre, University of Sheffield, Sheffield
Dewar M S, Greaves M 1990 Coagulation failure. Care of the Critically Ill 6: 19–23

Greaves M, Preston F E 1991 Clinical and laboratory aspects of thrombophilia. In: Potter L (ed) Recent advances in blood coagulation 5. Churchill Livingstone, Edinburgh, pp. 119–140

Hypovolaemic shock

FURTHER READING

9

Immunology and immunopathology

DEFENCE AGAINST INFECTION

> ▶ Non-specific mechanisms include the skin barrier, lysozyme in some secretions, ciliary motion in respiratory tract, and colonisation by harmless bacteria
> ▶ Specific mechanisms are those of immunity
> ▶ Immunity is characterised by specificity and memory

Our environment contains numerous potential microbial invaders (e.g. bacteria, viruses). Fortunately, the healthy body is able to resist infection by the organisms through non-specific (innate) and specific (inducible) mechanisms.

Innate immunity

Many non-specific mechanisms prevent invasion of the body by micro-organisms. They include:

- *Mechanical factors* — for example, the intact skin and the epithelium of mucous membranes are normally impermeable to microbial invasion. Additionally, movement can reject microbes, as in reflexes like coughing, sneezing and vomiting, together with constant movement such as the beating of cilia in the respiratory tract and peristalsis in the gut.
- *Humoral factors* — for example: lysozyme in tears, nasal secretions, saliva and intestinal fluids; sebum released by sebaceous glands in the skin; gastric acidity and vaginal acidity (produced by commensal bacteria); complement and interferons; can all either kill or inhibit the growth of micro-organisms.
- *Cellular factors* — polymorphonuclear leukocytes and macrophages phagocytose and destroy micro-organisms. Mast cells and basophils produce soluble mediators of the inflammatory response. A subpopulation of lymphocytes called natural killer (NK) cells kill infected tissue cells in a non-specific manner.

Immunity is a term reserved for the *specific* response of the immune system. Immunity to infections either develops following exposure to the causative organism or can be induced artificially by *immunisation* prior to the risk of exposure.

ESSENTIAL FEATURES OF THE IMMUNE SYSTEM

The immune system has four essential features:

- specificity
- diversity
- memory
- recruitment of other defence systems.

Specificity

Immune responses in mammals have specificity for one particular antigen; usually there is no cross-reaction with other, closely related antigens, even when the chemical difference between the two antigens amounts to only a comparatively minor alteration in molecular structure. An example is the ability of the immune system to distinguish between different blood group antigens.

Diversity

The immune system is likely to encounter many different antigens during the life of the individual. It therefore follows that it must have considerable diversity of response. This diversity is partly inherited and partly acquired during maturation of the immune system.

Memory

When an antigen reacts with a clone of immunologically competent cells with specificity for the antigen, there is expansion of the clone as well as adaptation of the cells to give the highest possible specificity for the antigen. During this process, memory cells are generated so that, if the antigen is introduced a second time, the immune response will be more rapid and specific. This is the basis for all active immunisation procedures.

Recruitment of other defence systems

Recognition of foreign material by the immune system does not, by itself, usually result in destruction of the material. The cells of the immune system release chemical messengers (such as cytokines, p. 201) which recruit and activate other cells (such as polymorphs, macrophages and mast cells) or chemical systems (such as complement, p. 190, the amines, Ch. 10; kinins, Ch. 10; and lysosomal enzymes) to destroy the foreign material.

ANTIGENS

An antigen is any substance capable of inducing an immune response (in which case it is also called an *immunogen*); this response may include the formation of specific antibodies or primed T-cells. To be more precise, an antigen is also a substance which reacts with antibodies or primed T-cells irrespective of its ability to generate them. Most antigens are large molecules (of molecular weight over 1000). Smaller molecules do not usually provoke an immune response unless bound to a large *carrier molecule*. The smallest topographical structure on the surface of a large molecule recognisable by the immune system is termed a *hapten, epitope* or *antigenic determinant*.

The immune system can respond to an antigen in two ways:

- by cell-mediated immunity (CMI)
- by humoral immunity (the production of antibodies).

CELLULAR COMPONENTS OF THE IMMUNE RESPONSE

> ▶ Cell-mediated immunity is attributable to T-lymphocytes
> ▶ Humoral immunity is attributable to antibody (immunoglobulin) produced by plasma cells derived from B-lymphocytes
> ▶ T-lymphocytes can help and suppress B-lymphocyte activity

Both CMI and humoral immunity are dependent upon specifically responsive *lymphocytes* which recognise and react to the presented antigen. During development, lymphocytes become *committed*, that is, capable of recognising only one antigenic determinant. Thus, the presentation of one antigen stimulates only the relevant committed lymphocytes.

The lymphocytes responsible for CMI are called *T-lymphocytes* (thymus-dependent), because they or their precursors mature in the specialised environment of the thymus; from there they migrate out into the peripheral lymphoid tissues. T-lymphocytes have antigen receptors on their surface and, on recognising an antigen, they proliferate to produce a clone of *specifically primed* T-lymphocytes.

The lymphocytes responsible for antibody production (humoral immunity) are called *B-lymphocytes*.

This is because, in birds, they mature in a gut-associated organ called the *bursa of Fabricius*. There is no such structure in man, but the gut-associated lymphoid tissue is believed to perform a similar function. When stimulated by an antigen to which it is reactive, the B-lymphocyte proliferates to give a clone of cells all capable of reacting with the antigen. Some of these B-lymphocytes differentiate into *plasma cells* which are lymphocytes specially adapted for the manufacture and secretion of immunoglobulins.

Some of the specifically reactive T- or B-lymphocytes are long-lived and persist as *memory cells*. These cells are responsible for the increased rapidity and specificity of the *secondary immune response*, which occurs if the same antigen is encountered again.

Some T-cells co-operate with B-cells to assist them in the production of antibody: these are called *helper T-cells*. Others suppress the production of antibody and are called *suppressor T-cells*: these appear to exert a regulatory function over the immune system.

HUMORAL IMMUNITY

> ▶ Immunoglobulins (Ig) are produced by plasma cells
> ▶ Immunoglobulin molecules comprise light chains (either κ or λ) and heavy chains (γ, μ, α, δ, ε)
> ▶ Molecules can be enzymatically separated into antigen-binding fragment (Fab) and crystallisable (Fc) fragment; some leukocytes have receptors for Fc

Humoral immunity is immunity dependent on the production of immunoglobulins and their actions.

Antibodies are *immunoglobulin* (Ig) plasma proteins (sometimes called gamma globulins because of their mobility on a plasma electrophoresis strip). Their ultimate biological effect, by binding to antigen, includes:

- the *lysis* of bacteria
- *neutralisation* of toxins
- *opsonisation* of foreign material to promote engulfment by phagocytic cells
- antibody-dependent cell-mediated *cytotoxicity* (ADCC).

The word opsonisation is derived from a Greek word meaning 'to prepare for the table'; it is the surface coating of particles by complement to promote engulfment by phagocytic cells which have cell surface receptors for complement.

Antibody production

Antibodies are produced by plasma cells in the

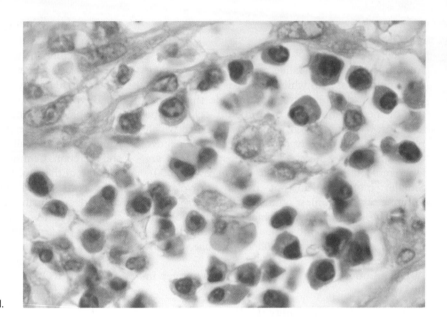

Fig. 9.1   Plasma cells

The nuclei are eccentrically placed.

lymph nodes, bone marrow and spleen. The cells are ovoid with an eccentrically placed nucleus. The cytoplasm is rather basophilic, and electron microscopy reveals abundant rough endoplasmic reticulum, correlating with its production of proteins for export (Fig. 9.1). One plasma cell produces antibody of one class reactive with only one antigen.

The basic structural unit of any immunoglobulin is shown in Figure 9.2. It consists of two pairs of identical polypeptide chains. The larger pair — the *heavy chains* — have about twice the molecular weight of the smaller pair — the *light chains*. If the molecule is digested by the enzyme papain, it cleaves into two Fab (fragment antigen-binding) fragments, which contain the antigen binding sites, and one Fc (fragment crystallisable) fragment. The Fc fragment of certain immunoglobulin classes has a role in complement activation.

There are five *classes* of immunoglobulin: IgG, IgM, IgA, IgD and IgE, characterised by the different structures of their heavy chains, which are called by the Greek letters γ, μ, α, δ and ε respectively. There are only two types of light chains, called κ (kappa) or λ (lambda), and each Ig molecule has only one or the other type of light chain.

The antigen binding site of an Ig molecule is at the N-terminal end of the Fab polypeptide chains. This area has been shown, by amino acid sequencing, to contain hypervariable regions which account for the variations in tertiary structure of the antigen binding site, and the consequent range in specificities. These variations are enabled by *gene rearrangement*, which is

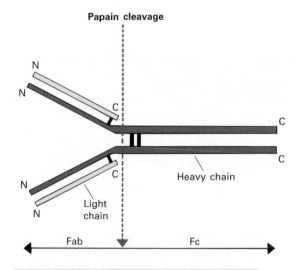

Papain cleavage

Fig. 9.2   The basic immunoglobulin structure

The two identical light chains and two identical heavy chains are held together by disulphide bonds. (Fab = fragment antigen binding; Fc = fragment crystallisable.)

also responsible for the variability of T-cell antigen receptors (see p. 187).

Some of the properties of the different classes of immunoglobulins are summarised in Table 9.1.

Immunoglobulin G

IgG is the most abundant immunoglobulin in the plasma and extracellular fluid. It can cross the pla-

Table 9.1   Properties of the different immunoglobulin classes

Ig class	Structure	Serum concentrations (gl⁻¹)	Molecular weight	Antigen binding sites	Complement activation	Antibody activity and properties
IgG		5–15	150 000	2	Yes	Cytotoxic. Neutralising. Can cross placenta. Characteristic of secondary immune response
IgA		1.5–5	320 000 as dimer	4	By the alternative pathway	Secreted locally in tears, saliva, mucus. Dimers of Ig joined by a J chain
IgM		0.5–1.5	900 000 as pentamer	10	Yes	Pentameric. Activates complement readily. Good agglutinator. Characteristic of primary immune response
IgE	Mast cell	$2–4.5 \times 10^{-7}$	200 000	2	No	Largely bound to mast cells and to basophils. Anaphylactic hypersensitivity and immune responses to parasites
IgD	B-lymphocyte	0–0.5	185 000	2	No	Function largely unknown. Possibly a lymphocyte surface antigen receptor

centa, and is therefore important in the passive transfer of immunity to the fetus. It is capable of neutralising toxins and may be cytolytic through the activation of complement. Polymorphs and macrophages have surface receptors for the Fc fragment of IgG; thus binding of IgG to particulate antigen promotes adhesion of these cells and subsequent phagocytosis of the antigen.

Immunoglobulin A

IgA is secreted locally by plasma cells in the respiratory passages, salivary and lacrimal glands and the intestinal mucosa. It is an important constituent of breast milk. It is secreted as a dimer of two Ig molecules joined by a J (junction) chain. Coupled to a 'transport piece', it is secreted at these sites, where it has a local defensive function. It can activate complement by the alternative pathway.

Immunoglobulin M

IgM is formed by J chains into pentamers of Ig molecules and these attain the very high molecular weight of 900 000. The large molecular size prevents it from leaving the plasma, except when permitted by increased vascular permeability in inflammatory lesions. As it has ten antigen-combining sites, it has good agglutinating and complement-fixing properties. It is the first class of antibody to be formed in

immune responses, and is characteristic of the primary immune response (first encounter with antigen); IgG is typically produced in large amounts in the secondary immune response.

Immunoglobulin E

IgE binds selectively to mast cells and to basophils by its Fc fragment. The binding of antigen to its Fab fragment triggers release of histamine and other substances important in anaphylactic type hypersensitivity.

Immunoglobulin D

The function of IgD is largely unknown, but it may act as an antigen receptor on the lymphocyte surface.

CELL-MEDIATED IMMUNITY

- ▶ T-lymphocytes are dependent upon the thymus gland for their development
- ▶ Helper T-lymphocytes recognise foreign antigens, secrete lymphokines, and help B-lymphocytes to produce a humoral response
- ▶ Suppressor/cytotoxic T-lymphocytes suppress B-lymphocytes and also destroy virus-infected cells

Cell-mediated immunity (CMI) is immunity dependent on the production of specifically primed immune cells and their actions.

T-lymphocytes

The essential role of the T-lymphocyte in cell-mediated immunity (CMI) is apparent from neonatal thymectomy experiments in animals, and from a congenital thymic deficiency in humans (p. 218). In the absence of T-lymphocytes, the host cannot mount cell-mediated immune responses; there may also be some impairment of humoral immunity.

Immature lymphocytes ('prothymocytes') reach the thymus via the blood, and mature in the specialised environment of the thymic epithelium into various types of T-lymphocytes. There is evidence that this differentiation is stimulated by various locally produced hormones, collectively termed 'thymic lymphopoietic hormone'. This process reaches its peak during fetal and early neonatal life; in later life the thymus atrophies, but still continues to export T-lymphocytes. These stages of differentiation are shown in Figure 9.3.

T-lymphocytes cannot usually be distinguished from B-lymphocytes by ordinary light microscopy (Fig. 9.4). Originally, T-lymphocytes were identified by their ability, empirically, to form 'rosettes' in suspensions by binding to sheep red blood cells; B-lymphocytes were recognised by immunofluorescence techniques to detect their surface immunoglobulin. The availability of *monoclonal antibodies* to cell surface markers or antigens of lymphocytes has made it possible to distinguish not only T-lymphocytes from B-lymphocytes, but also between different subtypes of T-lymphocyte. The cell surface antigens are designated *cluster of differentiation (CD) antigens*; their nomenclature is agreed by international consensus. Usually, the monoclonal antibodies are applied to frozen sections of fresh (unfixed) tissue, and their binding detected by an enzymatic reaction (Figs 9.5 and 9.6).

There are two main subsets of T-lymphocytes which can be distinguished by their CD antigens using monoclonal antibodies, or by their functional activity:

- helper T-lymphocytes (CD4)
- suppressor/cytotoxic T-lymphocytes (CD8).

The majority of T-cells express CD4 or CD8, but never both. CD antigens on T-cells have many different functions, but their primary role appears to be to direct T-cells to recognise foreign antigens when complexed with different classes of major histocompatibility (MHC) molecules.

Helper T-lymphocytes

Helper T-lymphocytes recognise foreign antigens in conjunction with class II HLA antigens (p. 209). When stimulated by antigens, they proliferate and transform into T-immunoblasts, which eventually differentiate into small T-lymphocytes responsive to the antigen.

On encountering antigen, helper T-lymphocytes release chemical messengers called *cytokines* (p. 201) which regulate the proliferation of other lymphocytes, cause an acute inflammatory reaction and immobilise macrophages in the area. They 'help'

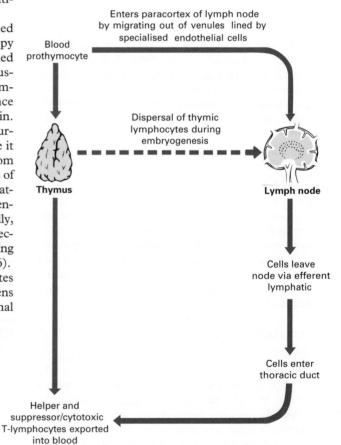

Blood prothymocyte

Enters paracortex of lymph node by migrating out of venules lined by specialised endothelial cells

Dispersal of thymic lymphocytes during embryogenesis

Thymus

Lymph node

Cells leave node via efferent lymphatic

Cells enter thoracic duct

Helper and suppressor/cytotoxic T-lymphocytes exported into blood

---

Fig. 9.3   The two pathways of T-lymphocyte differentiation

This takes place in either the thymus or the paracortex ('T-dependent zone') of lymph nodes.

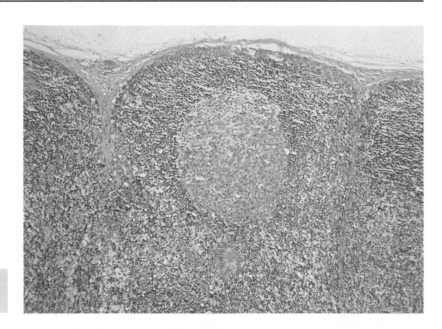

Fig. 9.4 Lymphoid follicle in a lymph node, surrounded by paracortex

B-lymphocytes to produce a humoral (antibody) immune response by 'presenting' antigens to B-lymphocytes in such a way as to stimulate them, and by the release of chemical messengers. Helper T-lymphocytes may be recognised by certain specific cell-surface antigens, detected by monoclonal antibodies.

There is evidence that, for some responses, antigen has to be presented to T-cells in association with various intercellular adhesion molecules (ICAMs) which are present on macrophages and other cell types.

Suppressor/cytotoxic T-lymphocytes

The other major subset of T-lymphocytes, recognised similarly by their cell-surface antigens, are called suppressor/cytotoxic T-lymphocytes. These T-lymphocytes have a *suppressive* effect on B-lymphocytes and have a central role in regulation of the immune response. They are important in the prevention of autoimmune disease. A further activity of this subset of lymphocytes is recognition and destruction of cells infected by viruses which express viral-coded antigen on their surface — hence the term *cytotoxic* T-lymphocytes.

T-cell receptors and immune recognition

The commonest T-cell receptor for antigens each consists of two cross-linked chains (α and β) on the cell surface. The α- and β-chains each have a constant region near the cell membrane and an outer variable region. The variable region offers considerable diversity necessary for the recognition of a wide range of possible antigens. A minority population (5%) of mature T-cells expresses a different receptor comprising γ and δ chains; this receptor's function is currently unclear. The CD3 antigen, which is associated with the T-cell antigen receptor, is widely used to recognise mature T-cells in diagnostic and investigative pathology.

Gene rearrangements and antigen specificities

The mechanism responsible for the expression of a wide range of permutations in the variable region of the receptor is gene rearrangement. The same mechanism is responsible for antibody diversity in B-cells; indeed, there is a significant degree of homology between the structure of T-cell receptors and immunoglobulin molecules.

Gene rearrangement involves the excision, splicing and post-transcriptional modification of segments of 4 gene regions:

- *V* or *variable* region
- *C* or *constant* region
- *D* or *diversity* region
- *J* or *joining* region.

This results in the synthesis of numerous V-D-J-C

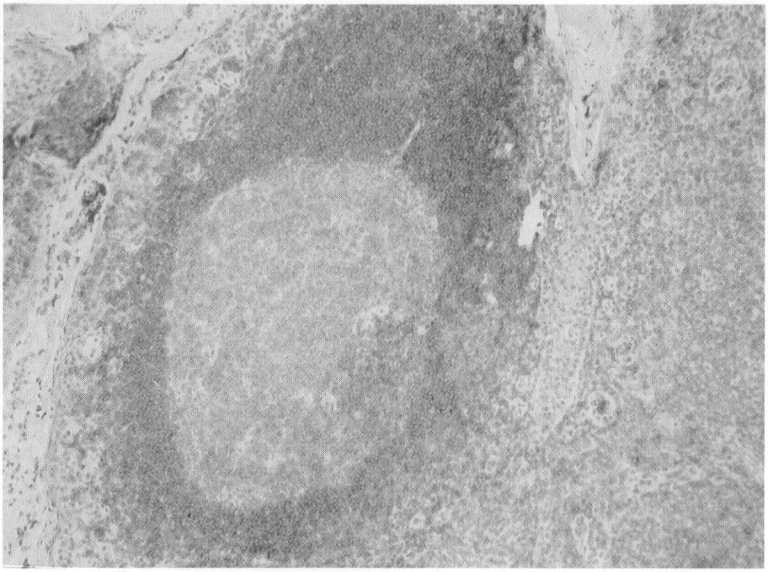

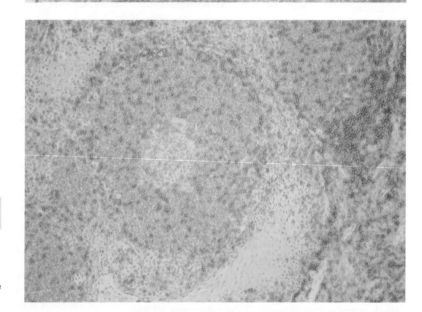

Fig. 9.5   A lymphoid follicle stained by a monoclonal antibody (anti-CD20) which reacts with B-cells

The cells of the follicle and its mantle zone are stained.

Fig. 9.6   Immunohistochemical identification of T-cells

The section (adjacent to that in Fig. 9.5) is stained by a monoclonal antibody (anti-CD3) which reacts with T-cells. Cells of the paracortex are stained and there are few T-cells in the follicle.

RNA molecules each encoding for T-cell receptor chains with different antigen specificities.

Macrophages

Macrophages have a central role in CMI (Fig. 9.7). Once they have phagocytosed particulate antigens, they sometimes re-secrete the antigen or present it on their cell surface, thereby presenting antigens to other cells of the immune system. They thus have a similar role to that of Langerhans' cells (p. 201), the antigen-presenting cells of the epidermis.

Macrophages also act as effector cells of the immune response by phagocytosing micro-organisms, especially if these have been coated with IgG, or with IgM and the C3b component of complement (p. 190).

CHANGES IN LYMPH NODES DURING THE IMMUNE RESPONSE

The cellular interactions in the immune response, outlined above, take place in the lymph nodes, ton-

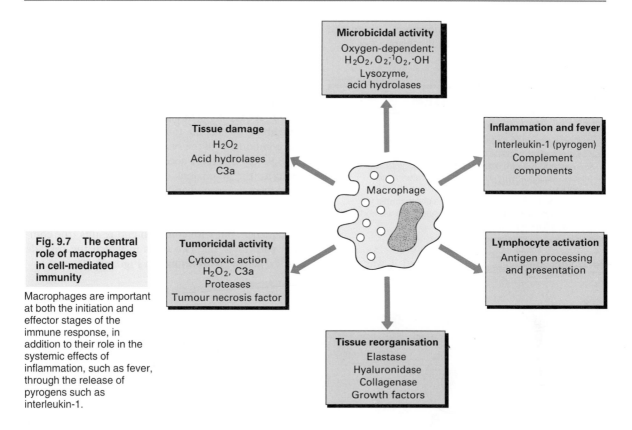

Microbicidal activity
Oxygen-dependent:
$H_2O_2, O_2^-, {}^1O_2, \cdot OH$
Lysozyme,
acid hydrolases

Tissue damage
H_2O_2
Acid hydrolases
C3a

Inflammation and fever
Interleukin-1 (pyrogen)
Complement
components

Macrophage

Fig. 9.7 The central role of macrophages in cell-mediated immunity

Macrophages are important at both the initiation and effector stages of the immune response, in addition to their role in the systemic effects of inflammation, such as fever, through the release of pyrogens such as interleukin-1.

Tumoricidal activity
Cytotoxic action
H_2O_2, C3a
Proteases
Tumour necrosis factor

Lymphocyte activation
Antigen processing
and presentation

Tissue reorganisation
Elastase
Hyaluronidase
Collagenase
Growth factors

sils, gut-associated lymphoid tissues (Peyer's patches) and in the peri-arteriolar lymphoid sheaths and lymphoid nodules (Malpighian bodies) of the spleen.

The structure of a lymph node is shown in Figure 9.8. Lymph enters the node via the afferent lymphatics to reach the marginal sinus. Beneath the sinus is the cortex, which contains nodules of tightly packed lymphocytes called *follicles*; these contain proliferation foci called *germinal centres*. The follicles contain mainly B-lymphocytes (Fig. 9.5) and outside the follicle there is a rim, or *mantle zone* of pre-follicular B-lymphocytes. Towards the *hilum* of the node there are *medullary cords* packed with plasma cells and lymphocytes; the intervening *sinuses* are lined by histiocytes.

When the node is subjected to antigenic stimulation, the structural changes reflect the type of immune response being mounted. In B-lymphocyte-mediated (humoral) immune responses, for example to bacterial antigens, the follicles become hyperplastic with mitoses in their germinal centres. In T-lymphocyte-mediated CMI, there is expansion of the paracortex, which contains many large T-cells. Drainage of particulate antigen into the node, and the presence of certain tumours in the zone of lymph drainage to

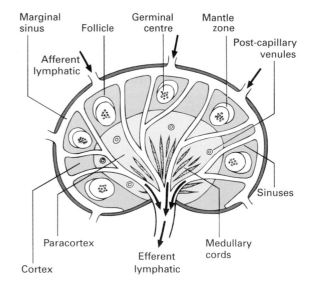

Marginal sinus · Follicle · Germinal centre · Mantle zone · Post-capillary venules · Afferent lymphatic · Sinuses · Paracortex · Cortex · Efferent lymphatic · Medullary cords

Fig. 9.8 Structure of a normal lymph node

The locations of T- and B-lymphocytes are illustrated in Figures 9.4–9.6. The paracortex contains venules lined by plump endothelial cells. Some circulating T-lymphocytes migrate out of these venules into the paracortex.

189

the node, results in sinus histiocytosis, where the medullary sinuses become packed by histiocytes.

THE COMPLEMENT SYSTEM

► Complement is a group of substances functioning as an enzymatic cascade
► Cascade may be activated by immunoglobulins (classical pathway) or by bacteria (alternative pathway)
► End products of the cascade are chemotactic for leukocytes, enhance bacterial phagocytosis, and lyse cell membranes

Soon after antibodies were discovered it was found

that their ability to inactivate micro-organisms was dependent on a system of proteins which complemented the activity of antibodies, hence the term *complement*. The chief ways in which the complement system participates in the immune response are shown in Figure 9.9. The proteins of the complement system are mostly synthesised in the liver, and comprise about 10% of the total plasma protein. The protein components of the system are termed C1,4,2,3,5, 6,7,8,9. C4 occupies second place in the sequence owing to the anomalous order in which the components were discovered and named. C1 is a complex of three components; they function as an enzymatic cascade which can be activated at two main points along its sequence, but with common end results (the common pathway). The two ways in which the cascade may be activated are shown in Figure 9.10.

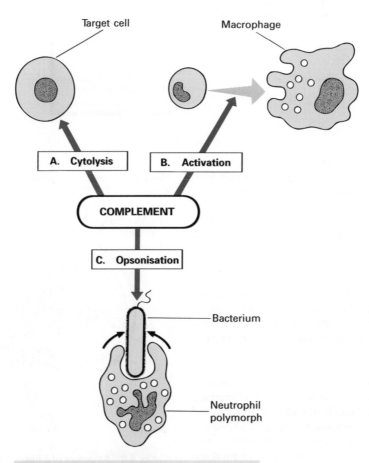

Fig. 9.9 The major biological functions of the complement system

A. Cytolysis of target cells. **B.** Activation of macrophages. **C.** Opsonisation, facilitating the phagocytosis of bacteria by neutrophil polymorphs.

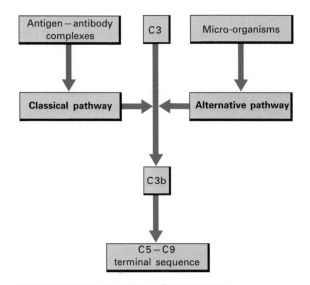

Fig. 9.10   The classical and alternative complement pathways

The classical pathway is activated by antigen–antibody complexes, while the alternative pathway is activated by lipopolysaccharide cell wall materials of various bacteria. Both result in conversion of C3 to C3b, triggering a common sequence generating active products.

Classical pathway

The classical pathway is activated by:

- antigen–antibody complexes containing IgG or IgM
- viruses
- bacterial products.

Activation occurs when one of the three components comprising C1 binds to the activating agent (Fig. 9.11). Activated C1 then activates C4 and C2; C2 binds to a fragment of C4 called C4b which in turn activates it. The resulting complex of C4b2a is the *classical-pathway converting enzyme* which cleaves C3 to yield C3a and a larger fragment which binds covalently to the activating agent. The complex C4b2a3b acts as an enzyme which cleaves C5 into C5a and C5b, a larger fragment, which binds briefly to the surface of the activating agent, thus acting as a focus for the sequential binding of C6, C7, C8, and C9 to form the C5b–9 *membrane attack complex*. Electron microscopy reveals this complex to be cylindrical; it penetrates cell membranes, disrupting them and causing cell lysis.

Alternative pathway

The alternative pathway is activated by micro-organ-

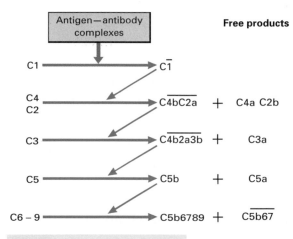

Fig. 9.11   The classical pathway

The classical pathway results from the action of antigen–antibody complexes on C1.

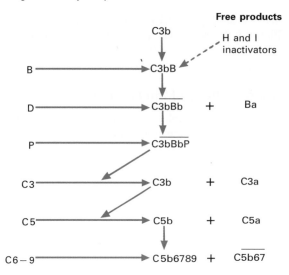

Fig. 9.12   The alternative pathway

C3b is continuously generated by hydrolysis of C3; however, it is usually inactivated by factors such as H and I. Bacterial endotoxins and IgA immune complexes stabilise C3b, leading to progression of the cascade. Factors B, D and P (properdin) are required where shown.

isms including bacteria (Fig. 9.12). There is no involvement of C1, C2, or C4. The C3b required for the initiation of the subsequent cascade is provided by the continuous slow lysis of C3. The resulting C3b binds factor B resulting in the complex C3bB which is then stabilised by the protein *properdin* (P) which binds to C3b. The complex C3bBP is called *properdin-stabilised alternative pathway C3 convertase* which activates C3 and C5 to stimulate formation of the *membrane attack complex*; this is assembled as in the classical pathway.

Role of C3b

Conversion of C3 to C3b is at the junction between both the classical and alternative sequences and the terminal sequence of the complement cascade. C3b therefore has a pivotal role not only in initiating the terminal sequence, but also because it promotes adhesion between neutrophils and macrophages (which have membrane receptors for C3b) and antibody-coated target cells.

Biological actions of complement

The biological activities of complement are mediated by the free products of the cascades shown in Figures 9.11 and 9.12, and by the end product C5b6789. These biological activities are summarised in Figure 9.13. The functions shown in Figure 9.9. are of central importance in the acute inflammatory response (Ch. 10) and in types II and III hypersensitivity (pp. 195–197).

Abnormalities of the complement system

Deficiency of complement components illustrates the importance of the system in defence against disease. For example, defects in the classical pathway result in frequent infections. Deficiency of the late components of the sequence, such as C5–8, results in disseminated infections with Neisseria organisms. Hereditary deficiency of C1-INH, an inhibitory factor, causes hereditary angio-oedema. Complement is also important in the clearance of immune complexes, and defects of components of the classical pathway result in immune complex glomerulonephritis (Ch. 21).

HYPERSENSITIVITY REACTIONS

> ► Severe and harmful immunological reactions
> ► *Type I:* binding of antigen to IgE antibody on surface of mast cells causes release of histamine, etc.
> ► *Type II:* antigen on cell (e.g. bacteria) surface binds antibody, prompting lysis by either defensive cells or end products of complement cascade
> ► *Type III:* antigen combines with antibody to form immune complexes which activate complement
> ► *Type IV:* T-lymphocytes produce a delayed (>12 hours) response to antigen
> ► *Stimulatory hypersensitivity* stimulates activity of target cell (e.g. effect of LATS on thyroid in Graves' disease)

Hypersensitivity is a state of altered immunological responsiveness in which an excessively severe and harmful immune reaction occurs on exposure to an antigen. The reaction is brought about through either humoral immunity (antibodies) or CMI (sensitised T-lymphocytes); products of the reaction lead to lesions which can range from local inflammation to generalised shock, including possibly fatal circulatory collapse.

In many instances, hypersensitivity reactions are provoked by *foreign antigens* such as pollens, moulds, food substances and drugs. However, in some instances, the offending antigen is a bodily constituent; hypersensitivity to antigens of the host's own body is known as *autoimmune disease* (p. 204). The widespread development of allogeneic organ transplantation has meant that a special instance of hypersensitivity, *transplant rejection* (p. 211), is more commonly seen.

Hypersensitivity reactions are traditionally classified by the *Gell and Coombs classification* which is based on the type of immunological mechanisms involved in the response. Hypersensitivity reactions all involve mechanisms seen in normal immune responses; it is their extent or occurrence in inappropriate circumstances which causes harm.

Type I (anaphylactic or 'immediate type') hypersensitivity

Type I hypersensitivity is an immediate immune reaction, occurring within minutes of exposure to the causative antigen.

The commonest examples of type I hypersensitivity are hay fever, childhood eczema and extrinsic asthma. The tendency to develop this type of reaction is found in about one-tenth of the population and is termed *atopy*. For example, in hay fever, the commonest manifestation of atopy, exposure to minute quantities of allergens such as grass pollen leads to acute inflammation in the conjunctival and nasal mucosae. Besides these local reactions, in rare instances, entry of traces of an allergen into the body causes acute systemic anaphylaxis characterised by circulatory collapse, dyspnoea and convulsions, sometimes leading to death. The allergen may be a systemically administered drug, such as penicillin, or radiological contrast media, or the venom of a snake or insect.

Diagnosis

Diagnosis of type I hypersensitivity is usually made by the demonstration of a relationship between

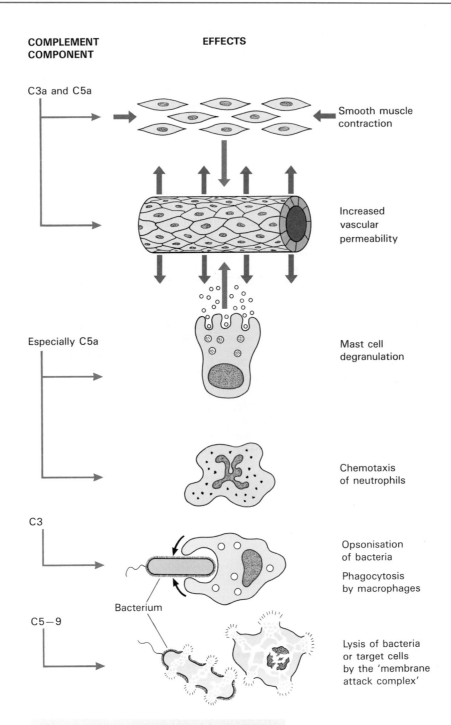

COMPLEMENT COMPONENT

EFFECTS

C3a and C5a

Smooth muscle contraction

Increased vascular permeability

Especially C5a

Mast cell degranulation

Chemotaxis of neutrophils

C3

Opsonisation of bacteria

Phagocytosis by macrophages

Bacterium

C5−9

Lysis of bacteria or target cells by the 'membrane attack complex'

Fig. 9.13 The biological effects of complement

exposure to a particular environmental antigen and onset of symptoms in a carefully taken clinical history. If it is necessary to confirm which particular allergen is responsible for the hypersensitivity, provocation tests may be performed. The commonest examples of these are skin tests, in which a dilute solution of the suspected antigen is placed on the skin, which is pricked to allow entry of the antigen. If the test antigen is the source of the patient's hypersensitivity, a local wheal and flare reaction occurs within a few minutes; this is immediate type hypersensitivity. Typically, atopic individuals show such hypersensitivity to general environmental antigens. Occasionally, when it is essential to identify the allergen causing the symptoms of extrinsic asthma, the patient is challenged by inhalation of the suspected antigen, and is monitored for bronchial constriction responses. All such tests are carried out under close medical supervision to control any unduly severe reactions.

Further tests may include the measurement of serum IgE levels, which are elevated in atopy, and the radio-allergo-sorbent test (RAST). This is a type of radio-immunoassay, in which the levels of IgE class antibodies to suspected allergens can be measured. Such in vitro tests avoid the risks associated with the in vivo provocation tests.

Mechanism

IgE class antibodies with affinity specific for the provoking allergen, sometimes known as *reaginic antibodies* or *reagin*, are central to type I hypersensitivity. They have long been suspected of being responsible for this type of hypersensitivity, following transfer experiments in which injection of serum from an atopic individual into a normal individual caused temporary transfer of the atopic tendencies into the recipient. A modern example of this phenomenon is occasionally seen in blood transfusion. If blood from an atopic donor is transfused into a non-atopic recipient, the recipient may transiently develop the full range of hypersensitivities which the donor displayed.

The reaginic IgE binds by its Fc component (Fig. 9.14) to mast cells and basophil leukocytes, which have specific surface receptors for this class of immunoglobulin. Both cell types contain basophilic cytoplasmic granules which consist of stored histamine and other vasoactive compounds. These cells are commonly situated close to small blood vessels. Basophil leukocytes differ from mast cells by being motile.

The binding of relevant antigen to the IgE molecules attached to the cell surface causes cross-linking of the IgE molecules, which appears to be the stimulus to the cell to release its stored granules. These intracellular events are triggered by a rise in the intracellular messenger, cyclic-AMP (cAMP).

The mast cell degranulation reaction results in local release of the vasoactive compounds stored in the granules:

- histamine
- eosinophil chemotactic factors.

Other compounds, the 'slow reacting substances of anaphylaxis', are synthesised by the cell and also released. They comprise:

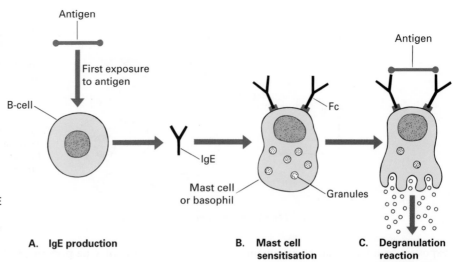

Fig. 9.14   Type I hypersensitivity

A. The antigen stimulates B-cells to produce IgE. **B.** IgE binds to mast cells or basophils via its Fc fragment, causing them to be 'sensitised'. **C.** Further exposure to antigen causes cross-linking of bound IgE on mast cells, resulting in degranulaton.

A.   IgE production

B.   Mast cell sensitisation

C.   Degranulation reaction

Chemical mediators induce hay fever, eczema, asthma

- prostaglandins
- leukotrienes
- thromboxanes
- platelet activation factors.

The combined effect of these compounds is to produce the vasodilatation, increased vascular permeability, oedema and ingress of eosinophils typical of the local atopic response. In the case of asthma, they also cause hypersecretion by the bronchial mucous glands and bronchospasm (Ch. 14).

Many features of the local atopic response, such as vasodilatation and oedema, are similar to those seen in the acute inflammatory response. However, while neutrophil polymorphs are the chief infiltrating cells of acute inflammation, eosinophil polymorphs are characteristic of atopic reactions. While tissue damage, and even necrosis, may be seen in acute inflammation, these are not a feature of the atopic response.

Acute systemic anaphylaxis

In acute systemic anaphylaxis, the most serious manifestation of atopy, entry of the allergen into the circulating plasma causes degranulation of IgE-coated basophils with release into the circulation of chemical mediators (p. 194). Arachidonic acid metabolites are the most important chemical mediators in this setting. Mast cells may also be activated by entry of antigen into the tissues. Generalised peripheral vasodilatation causes hypotension with shock, while contraction of bronchial smooth muscle results in dyspnoea. The skin may show a widespread urticarial reaction. Death may result from circulatory collapse.

Modification of the atopic response

Medical therapy has been directed to all stages of the atopic response. For example, mast cells may be stabilised and prevented from degranulating by glucocorticoids and drugs such as disodium cromoglycate, which is thought to act by inhibiting the transmembrane influx of calcium ions needed to trigger degranulation. Anti-histamine drugs may antagonise the products of sensitised mast cells. Occasionally, hyposensitisation is attempted. In this therapy, small doses of the offending antigen are given subcutaneously and may result in production of classes of immunoglobulin other than IgE; these may then bind with the offending antigen to prevent it from reaching sensitised mast cells. Such treatments carry the risk of producing severe hypersensitivity reactions.

Individual susceptibility to atopic responses

Genetic factors must predispose to the atopic tendency since there is evidence that it is familial. Individuals in families prone to atopy tend to have higher circulating IgE levels; thus it appears that the IgE responses are genetically determined. Further evidence for genetic determination of atopy comes from its association with certain HLA types.

There is some evidence that atopic individuals may have defective secretion of IgA on to the mucous membranes. It is suggested that this may allow ingress of environmental antigens to cause hypersensitivity.

Regulation of the immune response by T-cells may be important in preventing atopy. For example, children with the rare inherited T-cell defect in Wiskott–Aldrich syndrome frequently become atopic.

Type II (cytotoxic) hypersensitivity

The characteristic feature of type II hypersensitivity is damage to cells by binding of specific antibodies to antigens on the cell surface. The damage to the cell does not usually result primarily from binding of the antibody; it is dependent on the help of other lymphocytes or macrophages or on the complement system.

The commonest examples of cytotoxic hypersensitivity involve cells of the blood, but cells of other tissues may be involved.

Cytotoxic antibodies to blood cells

The best-known example of cytotoxic antibody development to blood cells is *autoimmune haemolytic anaemia*, in which auto-antibodies of the IgG or IgM class develop to antigens on the red cell surface (Ch. 23). Such antibodies may be detected in the Coombs' (antiglobulin) test (Fig. 9.15). Once coated by IgG, red cells become bound to macrophages because they have receptors for the Fc fragments of immunoglobulins. This results in phagocytic destruction of the red cells. IgM antibodies, which are powerful agglutinins, may agglutinate red cells in the red pulp of the spleen, resulting in cellular destruction. IgM may also activate complement, resulting in cellular lysis or promoting binding to macrophages. (For the actions of complement, see p. 193.)

In *idiopathic thrombocytopenic purpura*, antibodies develop to surface antigens on the platelets, resulting in their destruction, especially in the spleen.

In many instances, cytotoxic auto-antibodies to surface antigens on red cells are produced sponta-

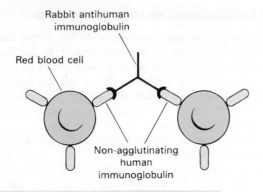

Fig. 9.15   The Coombs' (antiglobulin) test

Human immunoglobulins bound to red cells do not cause agglutination, but addition of rabbit antihuman immunoglobulin agglutinates the coated red cells.

neously. However, sometimes a drug or its metabolite may bind firmly to the cell surface to give a highly immunogenic epitope. For example, a metabolite of benzyl penicillin binds to the red cell membrane, and some individuals develop cytotoxic IgG class antibodies to this, resulting in the destruction of red cells, especially in the spleen. In other instances, drugs may promote the development of auto-antibodies to cell surface antigens unrelated to the drug molecule; for example, the antihypertensive drug alpha-methyldopa occasionally promoted the development of cytotoxic auto-antibodies to rhesus blood group antigens.

Naturally occurring antibodies to blood group antigens A and B are of IgM class. If, for example, an individual of blood group B is given group A blood by mistake, the naturally occurring antibody causes complement-mediated lysis of the donated cells. Other systems of blood group antigens, besides the ABO system, may cause similar problems. One such system is the rhesus (Rh) system.

Rhesus system
If an Rh-negative woman is pregnant with an Rh-positive fetus, then during delivery, obstetric manipulations or abortion there may be transfer of fetal red cells into the maternal circulation. This causes the development of IgG class antibodies to Rh antigens. If the woman has a subsequent pregnancy with an Rh-positive fetus, these IgG antibodies may cross the placenta to enter the fetal circulation. Lysis of the fetal red cells results in anaemia, cardiac failure (hydrops fetalis) and neonatal jaundice through the release of bilirubin. It is generally possible to prevent Rh-negative mothers from developing Rh antibodies

by injecting them with Rh antibody within 48 hours of the birth of an Rh-incompatible child. These probably serve to destroy any fetal red cells which enter her circulation before they can stimulate antibody production.

Auto-antibodies to other tissues

Antibodies to tissue elements are found in a wide variety of diseases. For example, in *Goodpasture's syndrome* (Ch. 21), an auto-antibody develops to both glomerular capillary basement membrane, and that of alveolar capillaries in the lung. This results in local complement activation at these sites, causing pulmonary haemorrhages and glomerulonephritis.

In *myasthenia gravis*, antibodies develop to acetylcholine receptors on skeletal muscle causing weakness (Ch. 26).

An example of the development of auto-antibodies to an intracellular antigen is *systemic lupus erythematosus* (SLE), in which antibodies develop to a range of antigens found in the nucleus. This is one of the so-called non-organ-specific autoimmune diseases.

In some instances, the binding of auto-antibody of IgG class to cell surface antigens is believed to stimulate certain lymphocytes with cytotoxic properties, sometimes called K-cells, to destroy the sensitised cell. This mechanism, called antibody-dependent lymphocyte cytotoxicity, may be involved in Hashimoto's thyroiditis (Ch. 17).

Type II hypersensitivity is summarised in Figure 9.16.

Type III (immune complex) hypersensitivity

Type III hypersensitivity is due to the formation of antigen–antibody complexes, which may activate complement and hence produce tissue injury.

Immune complexes result from the reaction of antibody, usually of IgG or IgM class, with antigen, with subsequent activation of complement. The three main circumstances in which immune complexes are formed are shown in Table 9.2.

Persistent infection. In some persistent infections, such as infective endocarditis (Ch. 13) due to organisms such as alpha-haemolytic streptococci, parasitic infections such as malaria, or viral hepatitis, immune complexes are formed which contain antigens from the infecting organism. These immune complexes may become deposited in the tissues.

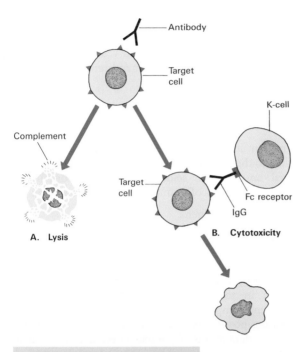

Fig. 9.16 Type II hypersensitivity

Antibodies develop to surface antigen of the individual's own cells. **A.** The binding of such antibodies may lead to complement-mediated lysis. **B.** Alternatively it may lead to cytotoxicity by K-cells.

Table 9.2 The three types of immune complex disease

Type	Antigen	Site of immune complex deposition
Infections	Exogenous: part of organism or a synthesised product	Site of infections Blood vessels Glomeruli
Inhaled allergens	Exogenous: organic dust	Lungs
Autoimmune	Endogenous: self-antigen	Blood vessels Joints Glomeruli

Autoimmune disease. Sometimes, the offending antigen is a self-antigen, as in systemic lupus erythematosus (SLE), where immune complexes of various nuclear antigens with IgG may be formed in large amounts, exceeding the capacity of the mononuclear phagocytic system to dispose of them.

Extrinsic disease. Immune complexes may be formed locally at the point of entry of an environmental antigen into the body, most commonly in the lung as in extrinsic allergic alveolitis (Ch. 14). For example, farmers sometimes develop IgG antibodies to inhaled spores from moulds growing in hay. Subsequent inhalation of the spores results in immune complex formation in the alveolar walls, resulting in an acute inflammatory response called 'farmer's lung'. This response is different from extrinsic asthma, which involves IgE bound to mast cells.

Experimental immune complex disease

Nicholas Maurice Arthus developed an experimental model for local immune complex disease in 1902. Animals were repeatedly injected with doses of foreign antigen until they developed high levels of IgG class antibodies. Further subcutaneous injection of the antigen resulted in severe oedema and haemorrhage at the injection site.

Immune complex deposition in the walls of venules results in activation of complement, yielding reaction products such as C3a and C5a which are known as *anaphylatoxins*. These cause acute inflammation, are chemotactic for neutrophils, and release histamine from mast cells. The neutrophil polymorphs, in phagocytosing the immune complexes, release their lysosomal enzymes, resulting in tissue damage (Fig. 9.17). Vascular thrombosis may also occur.

A similar response, the *Arthus reaction*, was seen in man when antisera raised in animals were injected to neutralise bacterial toxins in tetanus and diphtheria. The animal proteins were highly immunogenic, resulting in an IgG antibody response. This reaction is now rarely seen because purified specific human immunoglobulin is preferred.

Disease due to circulating immune complexes may be produced in animals by the single injection of a large amount of antigen. At first, antigen is present in excess over the concentration of antibody. This results in the formation of small, soluble immune complexes which are not easily phagocytosed and which persist in the circulation. As the concentration of free antigen continues to fall and the concentration of antibody rises, the stage is reached where immune complexes are formed 'at equivalence' (at the same molar concentrations of both antigen and antibody). These complexes are

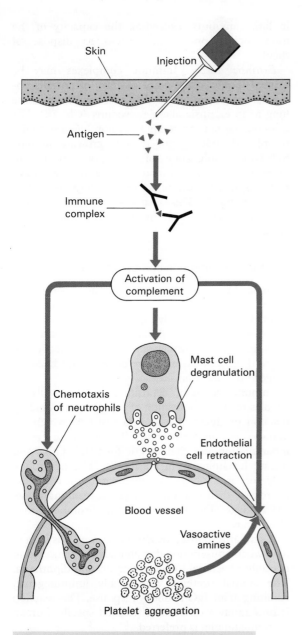

Fig. 9.17 Mechanisms of the Arthus reaction

Intradermal injection of antigens results in local immune complex formation, with activation of complement. Complement C3a and C5a components cause endothelial cell retraction, mast cell degranulation, and chemotaxis of neutrophil polymorphs. Immune complexes also induce platelet aggregation and release of vasoactive amines.

large and readily phagocytosed, being cleared away by the reticulo-endothelial system (Fig. 9.18). However, soluble immune complexes, still present in the circulation, result in complement activation and an increase in vascular permeability, and may be deposited in the walls of blood vessels, especially in the glomerular basement membrane, resulting in glomerulonephritis (Ch. 21).

Clinical immune complex disease

In man, immune complex disease is rarely attributable to the injection of foreign antigens now that animal antisera are seldom used. The commonest antigenic causes of immune complex disease are:

- microbial antigens
- self-antigens in autoimmune disease
- drugs.

For example, a sore throat due to beta-haemolytic streptococci of certain types may be followed by deposition in the glomerular basement membrane of immune complexes containing streptococcal antigens, causing post-streptococcal acute diffuse proliferative glomerulonephritis. A similar effect may be seen in chronic infections, such as malaria, syphilis and leprosy. Drugs may also be immunogenic, causing similar renal damage through immune complex deposition.

Certain forms of arteritis, such as polyarteritis nodosa (Fig. 9.19; see also Ch. 13), are believed to be due to immune complex deposition in the arterial wall; in a small proportion of cases the offending antigen is hepatitis B surface antigen. The possible mechanisms of vascular damage in immune complex disease are shown in Figure 9.20.

Immune complex deposition is also important in autoimmune diseases. In rheumatoid arthritis (Ch. 25), IgM antibodies develop to the Fc fragment of IgG, especially when it is already bound to antigen. The resulting immune complexes may cause local tissue injury by activating complement and, rarely, vasculitis. In SLE immune complexes between antibodies and various antigens from the cell nucleus may cause damage to various tissues, notably the kidneys and skin.

Type IV (delayed type) hypersensitivity

Type IV (delayed type) hypersensitivity was classified by Gell and Coombs in 1963 as any hypersensitivity reaction which takes more than 12 hours to develop. It is now known that the common factor shared by delayed type hypersensitivity (DTH) responses is involvement of specifically primed T-lymphocytes, and that humoral immunity (the antibody response) is not involved. This was demon-

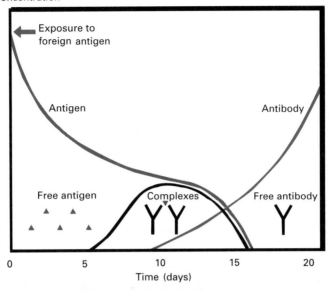

Fig. 9.18 Experimental serum sickness

Immune complexes are formed when antigen concentration is falling and antibody production is commencing. These may be deposited in the walls of arteries and in the glomerular basement membrane, where they activate complement causing inflammation.

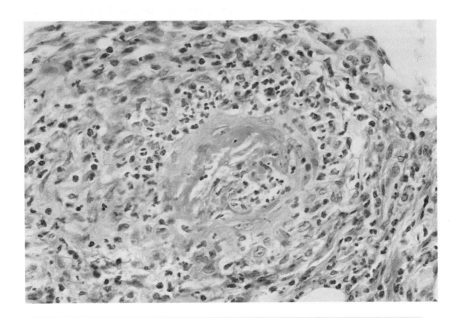

Fig. 9.19 Immune complex deposition in arterial wall in polyarteritis nodosa

The artery shows infiltration of all layers of the wall by inflammatory cells, including neutrophil polymorphs, and the thrombosis of its lumen. This is an early stage of involvement by polyarteritis nodosa.

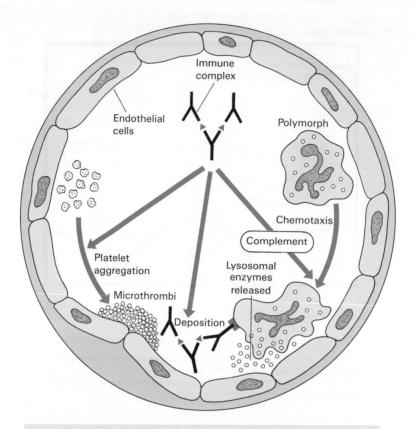

Fig. 9.20   Steps in vascular damage by immune complex deposition

Immune complexes in the vessel wall cause platelet aggregation (microthrombi) and activate complement. Polymorphs brought in by chemotaxis release their lysosomal enzymes, compounding the vessel wall damage.

strated originally in animals: transfer of T-lymphocytes from one animal to another caused the recipient to develop DTH, but transfer of serum had no such effect.

DTH is involved in the normal cell-mediated immune response to viruses, fungi and certain bacteria, notably mycobacteria. Local tissue damage is the unwanted side-effect of this otherwise protective immune response.

DTH responses may also develop to transplanted organs, to self-antigens which have become altered by foreign haptens, and to various environmental antigens. All of these are unwanted effects of the immune response. However, there is evidence that T-lymphocyte-mediated immune responses may also occur to antigens on the surface of tumour cells. The extent to which such responses may be useful in combating tumour growth is the subject of intensive investigation.

Cellular reaction

The best-known example of DTH is the tuberculin reaction. If a small amount of purified protein derivative (PPD) of tubercle bacilli is injected intradermally (Mantoux or Heaf test) in non-immune individuals, there is no effect. However, in individuals with cell-mediated immunity to tubercle bacilli, either as a result of previous tuberculous infection or immunisation with BCG (bacille Calmette–Guérin, a live, but non-virulent, strain of *Mycobacterium bovis*), an area of reddening and induration develops after 12–24 hours.

The dermis of the reaction site becomes infiltrated by lymphocytes and macrophages around small blood vessels, with oedema and vascular dilatation. In contrast to the situation in the acute inflammatory response, polymorphs are rare. In some naturally occurring DTH responses, notably those to mycobacteria and some fungi, macrophages may undergo terminal differentiation into epithelioid cells (characteristic of granulomatous inflammation; Ch. 10) or to multinucleate giant cells. The inter-relationships of monocytes, macrophages, epithelioid cells and giant cells are shown in Chapter 10.

Granulomatous hypersensitivity
Granulomatous hypersensitivity is the form of T-cell-mediated immunity most likely to produce disease. The usual cause is the ingestion by macrophages of antigenic materials which they are unable to destroy. Examples include mycobacteria such as *M. tuberculosis* and *M. leprae*, inorganic antigens such as zirconium, inert minerals such as silica, and locally produced immune complexes in extrinsic allergic alveolitis. In the systemic granulomatous disease, sarcoidosis (Chs 10 and 14), the stimulus to granuloma formation is unknown.

A *granuloma* is defined as a collection of epithelioid histiocytes. These epithelioid cells are larger than their parent macrophages and have eosinophilic cytoplasm. Electron microscopy shows them to have increased endoplasmic reticulum but few phagolysosomes, unlike activated macrophages. The reason for this adaptation is not understood. In addition to the formation of epithelioid cells, macrophages may differentiate into multinucleate giant cells. This is especially seen in the reaction to *M. tuberculosis*,

where cells with a peripheral crescent of nuclei (Langhans' giant cells) form (Fig. 9.21).

Mechanism

The interaction of specifically primed T-lymphocytes with antigen is central to the DTH response (Fig. 9.22). It is not known how such primed T-cells leave the circulation to reach the site of antigen accumulation in the tissues. It may be that only a very small number of primed T-cells need to reach the antigen, perhaps through random circulation, to trigger the response. Generally, helper T-lymphocytes do not react with free antigen, recognising antigens only when presented in conjunction with class II HLA molecules (p. 209). Such HLA molecules are present on the surface of the so-called *antigen-presenting cells* which include macrophages and a specialised cell with dendritic processes in the epidermis, called the *Langerhans' cell* (Fig. 9.23; not to be confused with the Langhans' giant cell). This reaction stimulates the helper T-cells to secrete a range of compounds, collectively termed *cytokines*, which activate cytotoxic and suppressor T-cells and recruit macrophages into the area (Fig. 9.22). The effects of some of the known cytokines are summarised in Table 9.3.

There are other important chemical mediators of the DTH response in addition to the cytokines; these include the many factors secreted by

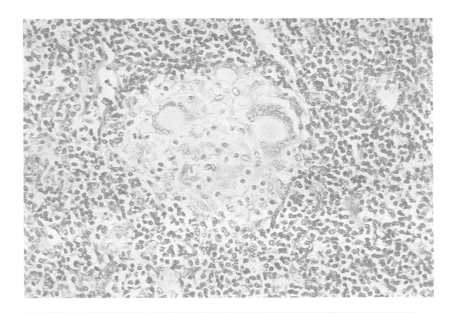

Fig. 9.21 A granuloma in a tuberculous lymph node, containing Langhans' giant cells

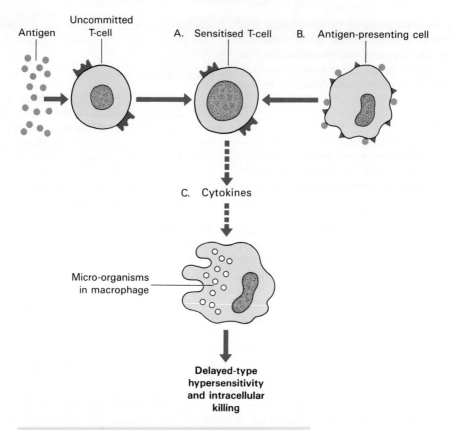

Fig. 9.22   Mechanisms of delayed type hypersensitivity

A. T-cells become sensitised and are induced to proliferate by the presence of foreign antigen. **B.** This antigen is presented by an antigen-presenting cell to the T-cell in the context of the host's class II HLA antigens. **C.** Cytokines are released, with the effects shown in Table 9.3.

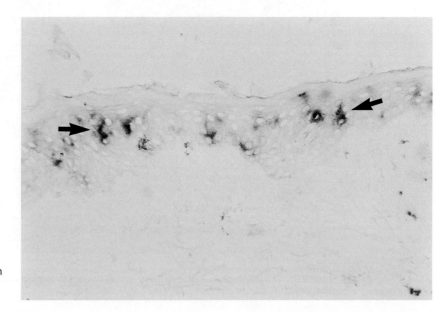

Fig. 9.23   Langerhans' cells

Epidermis stained by the immunoperoxidase method for CD1. The cells with dendritic cytoplasmic processes high up in the epidermis (arrows) are Langerhans' cells.

Table 9.3 Some important cytokines and their effects		
Cytokine	Cell of origin	Known functions
Interferon α/β	Macrophages/fibroblasts	Antiviral Activates NK cells and macrophages Enhances class II HLA expression
Interferon γ	Activated T-cells NK cells	Activates macrophages Induces class II HLA expression Antiviral
Interleukin (IL) 1	Macrophages Thymic epithelium NK cells	Stimulates T-cells and B-cell growth Endogenous pyrogen
IL-2	Helper T-cells	Stimulates T-cell growth and differentiation, B-cell growth and NK cell activation
IL-3	Helper T-cells	Marrow stem cell growth
IL-4	Helper T-cells	B-cell and T-cell growth Enhances IgE production
IL-5	Helper T-cells	B-cell growth and differentiation Enhances IgA production
IL-6	Activated T-cells, fibroblasts, macrophages and keratinocytes	B-cell differentiation Endogenous pyrogen
IL-7	Bone marrow stromal cells	Early T-cell and B-cell growth
IL-8	Macrophages, fibroblasts, endothelial cells and keratinocytes	Chemo-attraction of neutrophils and T-cells Activation of T-cells
Tumour necrosis factor (TNF) α	Macrophages, activated T-cells and NK cells	Inflammatory effects similar to IL-1 Inhibits neoplastic cell growth Induces class I HLA expression Stimulates angiogenesis
TNF β	Helper T-cells	Similar to TNF α

macrophages (cytokines). One important cytokine is interleukin-1, which promotes the release of the acute phase reactants by the liver, increases the proliferation of T-cells and acts on the hypothalamic thermoregulatory centre to induce fever. It is thus responsible for some of the systemic symptoms of DTH.

Contact dermatitis

Some chemicals in the environment are too small to act as antigens. However, if they bind to a protein molecule in the host they may become immunogenic, thus acting as a 'hapten'. Several instances of this are found in dermatology, contact dermatitis being a specific example of DTH.

Relatively simple chemicals may be absorbed by the skin and, acting as a *hapten–protein complex*, stimulate a cell-mediated immune response via the Langerhans' cells. Chemicals known to do this include nickel (present in jewellery and clothing-fasteners), chromium salts, formaldehyde, cyanoacrylate adhesives, photographic developers, and

substances from the primula plant. Subsequent exposure to the antigen induces lymphocytic infiltration around dermal blood vessels, together with dermal and epidermal oedema leading to vesicle formation. The histological appearance of contact dermatitis is shown in Figure 9.24.

Stimulatory hypersensitivity

The original classification of hypersensitivity reactions provided no heading for the type now known as stimulatory hypersensitivity, of which there is only one example in clinical medicine. In the autoimmune disease *Graves' thyroiditis* (Ch. 17) an IgG class auto-antibody is formed to thyroid epithelial cells. The binding of this antibody, 'long-acting thyroid stimulator' (LATS), has a similar effect on the thyroid epithelial cell to that of the binding of thyroid stimulating hormone to its receptor: the cell is activated into secreting thyroxine. Patients with this disorder thus develop thyrotoxicosis. The binding of an auto-antibody to cell-surface antigens is the same

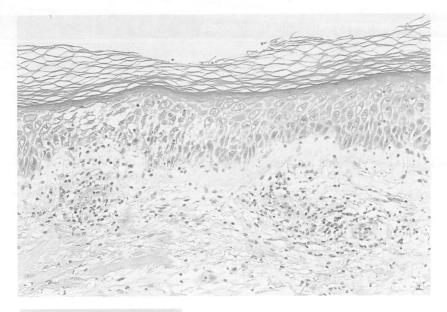

Fig. 9.24   Contact dermatitis
There is epidermal spongiosis, and a lymphocytic infiltrate surrounds dermal blood vessels.

mechanism as that of type II hypersensitivity, but in the case of Graves' thyroiditis this has, paradoxically, a stimulatory rather than cytotoxic effect.

Hypersensitivity and the normal immune response

All of the hypersensitivity reactions described above are merely excessive or inappropriate activities of the normal immune response. Table 9.4 summarises the mechanisms involved and shows how each can have desirable (normal) or undesirable (hypersensitivity) effects.

AUTOIMMUNE DISEASE

> ▶ Tissue damage due to immune reactions with self-antigens
> ▶ May be humoral or cell-mediated
> ▶ Examples include Hashimoto's disease of the thyroid, rheumatoid disease, and some haemolytic anaemias
> ▶ Female preponderance

An autoimmune disease is one in which the immune system, through either humoral (antibody) or cell-mediated immunity, leads to tissue damage by react-ing with self-antigens. The diversity of antigen recognition in the immune system is so large that it is capable of recognising self-antigens and of reacting against these. In the normal individual, however, although recognition of self-antigens by clones of lymphocytes does occur, a harmful autoimmune response is kept at bay by active control mechanisms within the immune system (p. 208). Autoimmune disease results when these control mechanisms break down.

Auto-antibodies

Auto-immunisation appears to occur quite common-ly, since many individuals have low concentrations of circulating antibodies to the DNA of nuclei, to gastric parietal cells and to thyroglobulin. However, high concentrations of such auto-antibodies are strongly associated with clinical disease. For example, patients with high concentrations of antibodies to thyroglobulin and to thyroid epithelial cells commonly have hypothyroidism due to Hashimoto's thyroiditis (Ch. 17).

In some cases, microbial infection tricks the immune system into producing antibodies which cross-react with self-antigens. For example, *Streptococcus pyogenes* contains certain antigens which are similar to antigens in the normal myocardium. Thus defensive antibodies raised to infecting strepto-cocci may cross-react with the myocardium causing rheumatic fever (Ch. 13).

Table 9.4 Comparison of the desirable and undesirable effects of immunity

Mechanism	Immune reactant	Desirable effects	Undesirable effects
Anaphylactic	IgE antibody	Increases vascular permeability allowing antibodies, complement and defensive cells to enter tissues; expels gut parasites	Type I hypersensitivity: hay fever; extrinsic asthma; anaphylaxis
Cytotoxic	IgM or IgG antibody	Kills bacteria	Type II hypersensitivity: haemolytic anaemias; blood transfusion reactions
Immune complex	IgG antibody	Mobilises polymorphs to site of infection	Type III hypersensitivity: glomerulonephritis; vasculitis
Cell-mediated	T-lymphocytes	Destroy organisms such as viruses; kill infected cells; isolate organisms such as *M. tuberculosis*, even though it is not killed	Type IV hypersensitivity: graft rejection; tuberculosis; leprosy; sarcoidosis

Cell-mediated autoimmunity

There is evidence from in vitro tests that clones of T-lymphocytes exist which recognise self-antigens in certain autoimmune diseases. It thus appears that cell-mediated immunity may be involved in the tissue damage in diseases such as juvenile-onset diabetes mellitus (Ch. 17), in which lymphocytes accumulate in the islets of Langerhans at the onset of the disease.

The range of autoimmune disease

If the immune system reacts against an antigen which is present in only one organ (for example thyroxine, which is present only in the thyroid) then it follows that the disease produced will be specific for that organ, i.e. it is *organ-specific*. In many cases, however, the immunising self-antigen is a constituent of many, or even all, tissues (for example nuclear DNA in systemic lupus erythematosus). In this case, damage is not specific for any organ and multiple tissues may be damaged—hence the term non-organ-specific autoimmune disease. If immune complexes are formed in the reaction with self-antigens, the resulting type III hypersensitivity will cause damage in the renal glomeruli, skin, synovium and arterial walls. Since these generalised lesions are most apparent in the connective tissues, some of the non-organ-specific autoimmune diseases are termed 'connective tissue diseases'. The two categories of autoimmune disease are contrasted in Figure 9.25.

Organ-specific autoimmune diseases

In organ-specific autoimmune conditions, the target tissue is destroyed by type II (cytotoxic) hypersensitivity, or antibody-dependent lymphocyte toxicity.

The affected tissue shows eventual loss of the target cells, fibrosis, and infiltration by lymphocytes and plasma cells. Some of the plasma cells are producing the auto-antibody locally. The best-known example of such destruction is Hashimoto's thyroiditis (Ch. 17). The thyroid is the site of two related autoimmune diseases: Graves' thyroiditis (Ch. 17), in which stimulatory type hypersensitivity leads to thyrotoxicosis, may occasionally evolve into Hashimoto's thyroiditis. The main examples of organ-specific autoimmune disease are shown in Figure 9.25.

Thomas Addison (1793–1860) described two autoimmune diseases before the aetiology of either was known. In Addisonian pernicious anaemia, antibodies develop to an antigen associated with the microvilli of the canalicular system of gastric parietal cells and to intrinsic factor itself. The result is achlorhydria caused by chronic gastritis due to parietal cell destruction, with failure to absorb vitamin B_{12} in the absence of intrinsic factor.

Two notable features of the organ-specific autoimmune diseases are:

- many of them affect endocrine tissues
- there is a tendency of the diseases to be associated with each other; thus, patients with pernicious anaemia very commonly also have autoimmune thyroid disease.

There is some debate as to whether the development of an auto-antibody is the primary event in all cases, or whether destruction of some of the cells of an endocrine gland, for example by viral infection, results in auto-sensitisation. It has been suggested that Type I (juvenile-onset) diabetes mellitus may follow Coxsackie or mumps viral infection in this way.

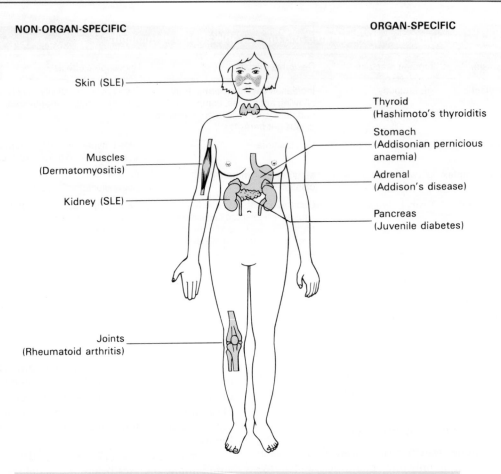

NON-ORGAN-SPECIFIC

ORGAN-SPECIFIC

Skin (SLE)

Muscles
(Dermatomyositis)

Kidney (SLE)

Joints
(Rheumatoid arthritis)

Thyroid
(Hashimoto's thyroiditis)

Stomach
(Addisonian pernicious
anaemia)

Adrenal
(Addison's disease)

Pancreas
(Juvenile diabetes)

Fig. 9.25   Comparison of organ-specific and non-organ-specific autoimmune diseases

Non-organ-specific autoimmune diseases: 'connective tissue' diseases

Rheumatoid disease

Rheumatoid disease is the commonest 'connective tissue' disease and an important cause of disability. Although its main feature is a destructive polyarthritis (Ch. 25) characterised by infiltration of the synovium by lymphocytes, plasma cells and macrophages, the disease has multisystem effects (Fig. 9.26). Rheumatoid 'disease' is thus a better term than rheumatoid 'arthritis', emphasising as it does this multisystem involvement.

The serum of most patients contains rheumatoid factors, immunoglobulins (normally IgM, but sometimes (IgG) which react with the Fc fragment of the host's own IgG once it has bound to antigen. These are assayed in the 'latex test', which measures the agglutinating titre of patient's serum for latex beads coated with IgG. This replaces the Rose–Waaler test, in which sheep red cells coated with IgG were agglutinated.

The rheumatoid factors thus bind to IgG, forming immune complexes which are formed locally in, or deposited in, the synovium. This gives rise to a type III hypersensitivity response with complement activation, resulting in tissue damage. Deposition of the immune complexes at other sites (for example, arterial walls) accounts for some of the systemic effects of the disease. There is also evidence that cell-mediated immunity may be involved in rheumatoid disease.

An important systemic complication of the continuing inflammation occurring in this disease is the development of secondary amyloidosis, which commonly leads to renal failure (Chs 7 and 21).

Systemic lupus erythematosus

The multisystem disease, systemic lupus erythematosus (SLE), causes lesions in the skin (Ch. 24),

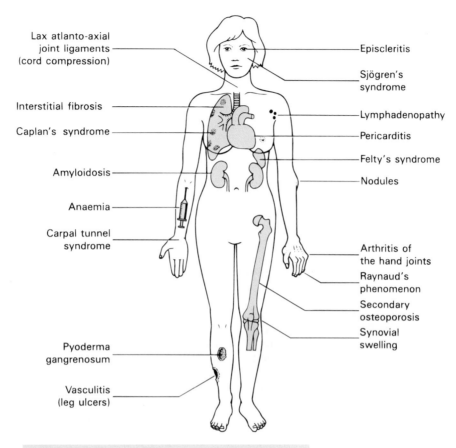

Fig. 9.26   The systemic effects of rheumatoid disease

These are mediated chiefly by immune complex deposition with secondary complement activation. Amyloidosis may be secondary to the continuing chronic inflammation.

joints (Ch. 25), renal glomeruli (Ch. 21), blood vessel walls and other sites. It is characterised by the development of auto-antibodies known as *antinuclear antibodies*. These react with various constituents of the nucleus, including DNA. The antibodies are not cytotoxic, and probably do not damage normal cells. However, when cells break down, nuclear antigens are released and these form circulating immune complexes (type III hypersensitivity) with the auto-antibodies. The deposition of these immune complexes in small blood vessel walls, especially near the renal glomerular basement membrane, accounts for the diverse effects of the disease. Auto-antibodies to DNA and other nuclear antigens are usually detected in the indirect immunofluorescence test.

Other autoimmune diseases

There is evidence that the bile duct destruction char-

acteristic of primary biliary cirrhosis (Ch. 16) is caused by autoimmunity, while antibodies to constituents of hepatocytes are found in the lupoid type of chronic active hepatitis and in progressing alcoholic cirrhosis.

In some diseases, auto-antibodies develop to extracellular antigen: for example, in bullous pemphigoid, one of the skin blistering diseases (Ch. 24), antibody develops to the epidermal basement membrane.

Aetiopathogenesis of autoimmune disease

Autoimmune disease may arise for a number of different reasons:

- defective suppression mechanisms
- increased or abnormal antigenic stimulation

- enhanced immunogenicity of self-antigens
- antigen presentation by class II HLA molecules
- HLA antigen type.

Defective suppression mechanisms

Tolerance to self-antigens was originally thought to be brought about by destruction of clones of T- and B-cells reactive to 'self'-antigens in the fetus — the 'forbidden clone' hypothesis. However, there is now evidence from in vitro experiments that such clones do exist, but are controlled by active suppression mechanisms. Central to these mechanisms are the suppressor T-lymphocytes, which appear capable both of recognising self-antigens, and of specifically suppressing helper T-lymphocytes and B-lymphocyte reactivity to self-antigens.

For example, in SLE there is evidence of thymic dysfunction, and suppressor T-cell activity has been shown to be defective. The association of myasthenia gravis with thymic hyperplasia and thymic tumours suggests some modifications in T-cell control mechanisms in this disease. In certain types of liver disease, such as primary biliary cirrhosis, anti-mitochondrial antibodies are commonly present in the serum, but the role of these in the pathogenesis of the disease is not known.

Abnormal antigenic stimulation

In other instances, the immune system appears to be normal, but subject to increased or abnormal antigenic stimulation. For example, antigens in certain sites (the 'immunologically privileged sites') appear to be hidden from the immune system. Such sites include the eye, parts of the central nervous system and the testis. Not only are there no clones of helper T-lymphocytes or B-lymphocytes reactive to antigens at these sites, but there are also no primed suppressor T-lymphocytes to identify antigens in these sites as self-antigens. Thus, for example, following a penetrating testicular injury or the rupture of an epididymal cyst, agglutinating auto-antibodies may develop to spermatozoa, resulting in sterility. Particularly serious are perforating injuries to the eye; not only is the injured eye under threat, but there may also be autoimmune destruction of the non-injured eye (sympathetic ophthalmitis; Ch. 26).

Enhanced immunogenicity of self-antigens

In some autoimmune diseases, self-antigens appear to have been modified or rendered more immunogenic by chemicals, such as drugs. An example is the antihypertensive drug, methyldopa, which stimulates antibody production to rhesus blood group antigens on red cells.

Antigen presentation

The context in which antigens are presented to the immune system may be important in determining whether reactivity to the antigen develops. Helper T-cells can recognise antigens only in association with class II HLA molecules, and the majority of cells do not express these. There is now increasing evidence that cells of some target tissues in autoimmune diseases express class II HLA molecules (HLA-DR antigens) on their surface, thus enabling helper T-cells to respond to antigens in their vicinity.

Associations with HLA antigens

Certain HLA antigen types (Ch. 3) are associated with an increased risk of developing autoimmune disease. This could be because certain HLA antigens are themselves similar to various environmental antigens, exposure to which then results in autoimmunity to an HLA antigen. Alternatively, certain HLA haplotypes could be linked to genes regulating the immune response, so that the defects resulting in autoimmunity would be genetically determined.

IMMUNOLOGY OF ORGAN TRANSPLANTATION

▶ Rejection can be minimised by matching ABO blood groups and HLA antigens
▶ Class I HLA antigens (loci A, B and C) are expressed on all nucleated cells
▶ Class II HLA antigens (locus D) are expressed only on B-lymphocytes and antigen-presenting cells
▶ Graft rejection may be humoral or cell-mediated
▶ Grafted bone marrow may cause graft-versus-host disease if not matched

The basic immunology of organ transplant rejection was established in 1943 by Gibson and Medawar. Skin grafts between allogeneic (unrelated) mice were rejected 10–20 days after grafting, while those transplanted between syngeneic animals (inbred strains) were permanently accepted. However, if mice were injected at birth with cells from an allogeneic animal, they were then found to accept permanently skin grafts from that donor animal; in other words, immunological tolerance had been induced. If the tolerant animal was then injected with lymphocytes from a mouse which had previously rejected a graft from the allogeneic strain, the tolerance was overcome and the graft promptly rejected. Thus, the immune system displays memory and specificity in transplant rejection, and these attributes lie in the lymphocytes. The terminology of clinical and experimental organ transplantation is summarised in Table 9.5.

Skin grafting to replace areas of epidermis lost through burns or trauma is a long-established practice. Such grafts are usually autografts, and rejection does not occur. However, in the developing science of renal transplantation, rejection can be a major problem and cross-matching of the donor to the recipient, determining that the cell surface antigens

of the donor are as similar as possible to those of the recipient, is important. The organs currently being transplanted and the extent of tissue cross-matching are shown in Table 9.6.

Tissue typing and the HLA system

In humans, the *major histocompatibility complex* (MHC) is a series of genes on chromosome six which code for various antigens most readily detected on the surface of leukocytes, and hence called *human leukocyte antigens* (HLA). Closely linked to these genes is a family of genes controlling immune responses. All nucleated cells express HLA-A, -B and -C antigens (Fig. 9.27), but HLA-D and -DR antigens (sometimes called class II HLA antigens)

Table 9.5 Terminology of organ transplantation

Relationship between donor and recipient	Terminology		
	Genetic	Antibody and antigen	Transplant
Same animal	—	Auto-antibody Self-antigen	Autograft
Identical/inbred strain	Syngeneic or isogeneic	—	Isograft
Unrelated animal, same species	Allogeneic	Iso-antibody Iso-antigen	Allograft
Different species	Xenogeneic or heterogeneic	Hetero-antibody Hetero-antigen	Xenograft

Table 9.6 Current status of clinical organ transplantation

Organ	Uses	Cross-matching requirements
Kidney	In renal failure, to avoid chronic haemodialysis	ABO-matching essential; HLA-matching advantageous
Skin	Burns and trauma	Usually an autograft, and therefore perfectly matched
Bone marrow	Treatment of leukaemia and lymphoma (after whole body irradiation) and storage diseases	HLA-matched to avoid graft-versus-host disease
Liver	Treatment of primary liver cancer, biliary atresia, primary biliary cirrhosis, etc.	HLA-matching not required
Heart	Treatment of intractable cardiac failure	Few donors, therefore HLA-matching not required; however survival is inversely proportional to number of HLA-mismatches
Lungs	Primary pulmonary hypertension (heart usually transplanted also)	Not HLA-matched
Islets of Langerhans	Experimental treatment for diabetes mellitus	
Cornea	Replacement of opaque cornea	Immunologically privileged site requiring no tissue matching
Bone	Orthopaedic reconstructions	No matching used; even if grafted bone dies it acts as a scaffold for ingrowth of host tissue

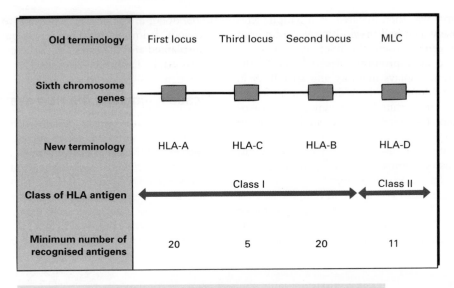

Fig. 9.27   Genetic map of the human major histocompatibility complex

MLC = mixed lymphocyte culture, the mechanism whereby class II HLA antigens are detected.

are normally expressed only on B-cells and antigen-presenting cells.

HLA antisera are obtained from recipients of previous blood transfusions or tissue transplants, or are produced artificially as monoclonal antibodies. The typing antibody and complement are mixed with cells of the individual to be typed. If these cells express the corresponding iso-antigen, they are lysed.

Tissue-typing for the HLA antigens, although desirable, is not carried out for transplants of all types of organ. For example, the rarity of heart, lung and liver donors means that cross-matching in these cases is restricted to the ABO blood group system.

Failure to cross-match for blood group substances results in hyperacute graft rejection (Table 9.7).

Functions of the HLA system

The existence of the MHC was discovered by observations on the fate of experimental organ grafts in laboratory animals. The human analogue, the HLA system, has been characterised by using antibodies in sera from transplantation and transfusion recipients. Although HLA-matching between donor and recipient is important to minimise the risk of graft rejection, the *natural* function of the HLA system is to enable T-cells to interact more specifically with

Table 9.7 Types of transplant rejection* classified by time course			
Type of rejection	Time course	Effector mechanism	Mechanism
Hyperacute	Within minutes	Ab	Preformed cytotoxic antibodies to donor antigens, especially blood group substances
Accelerated	2–4 days	CMI ± Ab	Previous sensitisation to donor HLA antigens, e.g. previous graft(s)
Acute	7–21 days	CMI ± Ab	CMI response to donor antigens
Chronic	After 3 months	CMI ± Ab	Breakdown of tolerance

*Only in hyperacute rejection is graft damage due primarily to antibody (Ab); the other types of rejection are due mainly to cell-mediated immunity (CMI).

other host cells by a process known as *dual recognition*. Class I and class II substances have different roles in this process.

Cytotoxic T-cells recognise and eliminate host cells bearing foreign antigens (e.g. viral products) and class I HLA substances (HLA-A, -B, and -C) on their surfaces. Cytotoxic T-cells would be ineffective against free virus particles, but the dual recognition of adjacent viral antigen and class I HLA substances on the surface of virus-infected cells restricts the cytotoxic effects of T-cells.

Class II HLA substances (HLA-DR, -DP and -DQ) on antigen-presenting cells enable their recognition by helper T-cells which then interact with B-cells and plasma cells to induce specific antibody synthesis; class II HLA substances are present on antigen-presenting cells and B-cells. Class II HLA substances on antigen-presenting cells bearing foreign antigens protect them selectively from recognition and elimination by cytotoxic T-cells. This requirement for the juxtaposition of foreign antigen and class II substances is another example of the importance of dual recognition in immune responses.

Graft rejection

Different tissues vary in their ability to provoke an immune response from the recipient. For example, the bone marrow and skin appear to be highly immunogenic, while failure of liver transplants is more often through technical problems than immunological rejection.

The terminology of transplant rejection is summarised in Table 9.7. Hyperacute rejection, characterised by vascular thromboses, necrosis and polymorphonuclear infiltration, is rarely seen in clinical practice due to the practice of ABO cross-matching, but the other types of rejection are a major clinical problem. Accelerated rejection may be seen in sensitised patients who have received previous grafts, while acute and chronic rejection are primary immune responses to the donor antigens.

In the context of the kidney, rejection via cell-mediated immunity has two main histological components. There is interstitial infiltration by lymphocytes (many are T-cells) and macrophages, together with vascular damage including arterial intimal swelling and disruption of the internal elastic lamina.

The action of cell-mediated immunity in transplant rejection is shown in Figure 9.28. The action of antibodies in transplant rejection is variable. In some instances (for example, hyperacute rejection) they are cytotoxic, while in others they may bind to HLA antigens, thus masking them from recognition by T-lymphocytes (graft enhancement). The factors which favour prolonged graft survival (taking renal transplants as a specific example) are:

- ABO compatibility
- good class II HLA cross-match (especially identical sibling)
- previous blood transfusion (induces tolerance).

Factors impairing graft survival include:

- drug side-effects
- infection
- recurrence of the disease which originally necessitated transplantation.

Immunosuppression

Some form of immunosuppressive therapy is usually needed in all grafts other than autografts. The commonest form of immunosuppression is non-specific in effect (it makes the whole immune system less responsive) and is an iatrogenic form of acquired immunodeficiency. Such therapeutic methods include: immunosuppressive drugs, including steroids and azathioprine; cytotoxic drugs, such as cyclophosphamide; lymphoid irradiation; and the relatively new drug, cyclosporin A. This drug is a major advance in immunosuppressive therapy because it shows selective cytotoxicity for antigen-primed T-cells, thus disrupting cell-mediated immunity against the graft. All non-specific immunosuppressive treatments make the patient prone to serious infection. Sometimes this is by opportunistic pathogens, agents which are normally of low virulence in the immunocompetent individual (Ch. 3 and Figs 9.29 and 9.30).

Graft-versus-host disease

The typical recipient of a bone marrow transplant has severe immunodeficiency, either as a consequence of the disease necessitating transplant (e.g. leukaemia), or as a result of cytotoxic drugs or radiotherapy. Transplanted bone marrow is immunocompetent, containing viable T-lymphocytes which may stimulate a severe, and sometimes fatal, immune response against the host's antigens — 'graft-versus-host' (GVH) disease. The clinical features of GVH disease include diarrhoea due to malabsorption, a characteristic dermatitis, destruction of blood cells, and cholestatic liver disease.

The risk of GVH disease can be reduced by careful HLA cross-matching, and by selective destruction of T-lymphocytes in the graft using monoclonal antibodies.

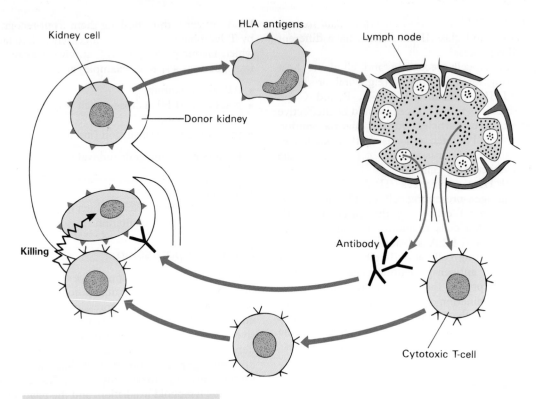

Fig. 9.28   Renal transplant rejection

HLA antigens from the graft are conveyed by macrophages to the lymph node, stimulating both cell-mediated and humoral immunity against the graft.

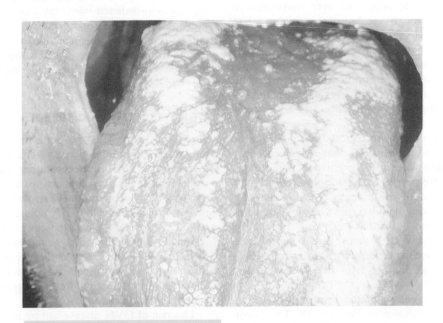

Fig. 9.29   Candidiasis of the tongue

Infection by *Candida albicans* does not extend beyond the mucous membranes, unless there is immunosuppression.

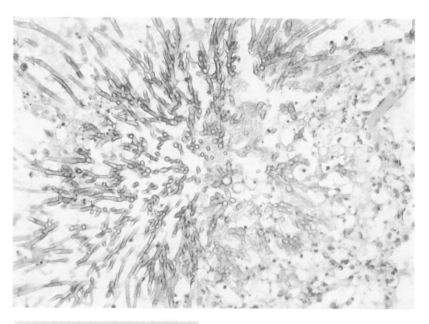

Fig. 9.30   Systemic aspergillosis

High-power histology of the lung of a patient dying from systemic aspergillosis due to immunosuppressive treatment for a renal transplant. The periodic acid–Schiff (PAS) stain shows the branching hyphae of *Aspergillus fumigatus*.

IMMUNE RESPONSE TO TUMOURS

▶ Clinical importance of anti-tumour immune responses is controversial
▶ Lymphocytic infiltration of tumours is associated with better prognosis
▶ Tumour immunotherapy regimes include monoclonal antibodies, lymphokine (cytokine) activated killer cells, and interferon

There is plentiful histological evidence to suggest that the host mounts a cellular response to tumours. At the invasive edge of tumours, the surrounding stroma often contains an infiltrate of lymphocytes and macrophages. For example, medullary carcinoma of the breast is typically surrounded by masses of lymphocytes (Fig. 9.31), seminoma of the testis often contains many lymphocytes, and malignant melanomas of the skin are commonly surrounded by a cellular infiltrate. Lymph nodes draining tumour sites show a variety of tissue reactions suggestive of antigenic stimulation, including follicular hyperplasia and sinus histiocytosis.

Lymphocytic infiltration in human tumours has prognostic significance and may correlate with improved survival in carcinoma of the breast, stomach, colon and rectum. Some studies have shown a correlation between the presence of sinus histiocytosis in lymph nodes draining the breast, and a better prognosis. Less clear evidence for the role of the immune system in defending the host against tumours comes from well-documented reports of total or partial tumour regression. For example, in patients with disseminated malignant melanoma it is sometimes impossible to find the primary tumour, implying that it has regressed. Whether these events are mediated wholly through the immune system is not known.

The advent of monoclonal antibodies, which enable different classes of lymphocytes to be demonstrated immunohistochemically in tissue sections, has revolutionised the study of the host's cellular response to tumours. Cellular infiltrates around tumours often contain a predominance of T-lymphocytes, including the helper and suppressor/cytotoxic subsets. The natural killer (NK) cell, a class of lymphocyte which possesses the ability, at least in vitro, to kill tumour cells without prior antigenic stimulation, has been detected in these infiltrates. The in vivo function of NK cells is not known.

The presence of Langerhans' cells, the dendritic antigen-presenting cells of the normal epidermis, has been demonstrated in certain epithelial tumours. It is postulated that these cells may be able to pick up

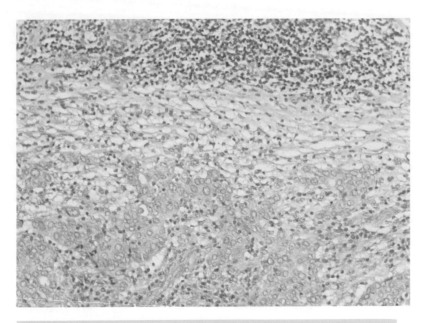

Fig. 9.31 Medullary carcinoma of the breast (bottom) with a surrounding lymphocytic infiltrate (top)

tumour antigens and carry them to regional lymph nodes, presenting them, together with class II HLA antigens, to T-lymphocytes.

The cellular interactions which have been proposed as mechanisms of tumour cell killing are shown in Figure 9.32. These interactions depend on the production, by T-lymphocytes, of cytokines (p. 203).

Are tumour cells antigenic?

There is experimental evidence that tumour cells express the HLA and blood group antigens of the host, although sometimes at reduced concentrations. However, a tumour cell can be recognised by the host as distinct from the normal tissues only if it expresses new antigens.

Several human tumours express the so-called *oncofetal antigens*. These are immunologically detectable substances which are expressed by normal populations of cells in the developing fetus, but are not usually expressed by cells in the adult. The reappearance of these 'antigens' is an example of the 'cellular anarchy' of tumour cells. Examples include *alpha-fetoprotein*, which may be produced by hepatocellular carcinoma, and *carcinoembryonic antigen* which may be expressed by various adenocarcinomas, but there is no evidence that these induce a useful immune response in the host.

In experimental tumours in animals, a class of cell surface antigens called *tumour associated transplantation antigens* (TATAs) has been discovered. These antigens cause rejection of transplanted tumour cells in a pre-immunised syngeneic host, and appear to be unique for the individual experimentally produced tumour. Antigens of this class may be the most important immunogens responsible for the host's immune response to tumour.

Immunological surveillance against tumours

Macfarlane Burnet suggested that T-lymphocytes monitor the host's cells and react against any which have developed novel surface antigens. In this way, clones of potentially malignant cells would be destroyed. There is evidence favouring immunological surveillance in tumours. Patients with congenital and acquired immunodeficiency states have a high risk of malignant tumour development, and the range of tumours is different from that seen in otherwise normal individuals. For example, renal transplant recipients, commonly treated by long-term immunosuppression, have a greatly increased incidence of non-Hodgkin's lymphoma; this may arise in sites such as the brain, which is a most unusual site for such lesions in normal individuals.

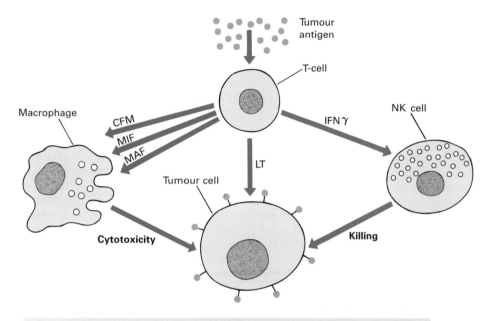

Fig. 9.32   Proposed mechanisms of cellular co-operation in tumour cell killing

Tumour antigens stimulate T-cells to release: interferon γ (IFN γ) which stimulates natural killer (NK) cells to divide; lymphotoxin (LT), which acts directly on tumour cells; and chemotactic factor for macrophages (CFM), macrophage-activating factor (MAF), and migration inhibition factor (MIF), increasing the number of macrophages in the area.

Various skin tumours also have an increased incidence.

Kaposi's sarcoma is an exceedingly rare tumour in the general population, yet commonly develops in patients with venereally transmitted acquired immunodeficiency syndrome (AIDS), in which defects in cell-mediated immunity are prominent.

These findings could suggest that some normally operating surveillance mechanism, which destroys mutant clones of cells before spread can occur, has broken down. However, caution is needed in interpreting the observations, because some immunosuppressive agents, such as radiotherapy and the alkylating agents, are oncogenic in their own right.

Immunosuppressed patients are known to be prone to chronic viral infection, and some viruses (hepatitis B virus, Epstein–Barr virus, human papilloma viruses and herpes virus) have proven oncogenic properties. This may be an important cause of the increased risk of malignancy in the immunocompromised.

Tumour evasion of the host's immune response

Despite the many immune mechanisms known to be active against tumour cells, the natural history of most cancers, if not surgically ablated, is one of relentless progression culminating in death.

The immunogenicity of some tumours appears to be reduced by shedding or endocytosis of antigens, or masking them with mucin substances. Tumour antigens free in the circulation may block antigen recognition sites. Alternatively, antibodies to tumour antigens may bind to these antigens on the cell surface, masking them from T-cell receptors. Antigen–antibody complex could bind to T-cells, blocking their tumour-recognition mechanisms. Alternatively, a growing tumour, by initially presenting only a very small antigen load, may induce tolerance to itself.

Immunotherapy

Early attempts at non-specific immunotherapy, such as the administration of BCG at a skin site draining to the axillary lymph nodes in patients with mammary carcinoma, have been disappointing. However, a number of approaches currently being developed are more promising.

Monoclonal antibodies

The development of monoclonal antibodies offers

exciting potential for specific immunotherapy. It is possible to generate large quantities of monoclonal antibodies to tumour antigens. Cytotoxic agents may be chemically bound to the antibodies, thus ensuring their delivery to the target cell.

Cytokine-activated killer (CAK) cell therapy

In cytokine-activated killer cell therapy, an experimental treatment, patients are first subjected to leukapheresis (the white cells are extracted from their blood using a special centrifuge), and the harvested lymphocytes are then cultured for several days with interleukin-2 (IL-2) to induce cytotoxic cells. These autologous cells are then returned to the patient intravenously together with high doses of IL-2. Early results suggest that reduction in apparent tumour bulk occurs with some renal cell carcinomas (hypernephromas), melanomas and colorectal tumours; sarcomas appear unresponsive.

Interferon therapy

Most studies of interferon therapy to date have used interferon α. The most encouraging responses have been with the rare, hairy cell leukaemia and with mycosis fungoides, a T-cell lymphoma of the skin. Responses have also been reported with renal cell carcinomas, melanomas, colorectal tumours, lymphomas and Kaposi's sarcoma. The mechanism of action is unknown but could include:

- direct antiproliferative action on tumour cells
- activation of natural killer cells and/or macrophages
- increased expression of class I HLA antigens on tumour cells.

IMMUNODEFICIENCY

▶ Presents with abnormal susceptibility to infections
▶ Primary deficiencies are due to congenital defects of B- or T-lymphocyte function or both
▶ Secondary deficiencies are due to causes such as malnutrition, immunosuppressive drugs, AIDS, etc.

Immunodeficiency presents clinically as an abnormal tendency to develop infections, many of which are due to organisms which would not be pathogenic in the healthy individual; these are termed *opportunistic infections*. The commonest infections encountered depend on whether the main defect is in

T-cells, B-cells or phagocytic cells such as neutrophil polymorphs (Table 9.8). Additionally, in AIDS, which is a special instance of T-cell defect, a characteristic constellation of opportunistic infections occurs, some of which may have been acquired by the same route as the HIV virus (e.g. venereally). Immunodeficiency should be suspected in any patient who develops infections by organisms which are not pathogenic in the normal individual ('opportunistic pathogens'). Such infections include *Pneumocystis carinii* pneumonia (Fig. 9.33), cytomegalovirus infection, or infection by atypical mycobacteria. Organisms which normally cause only superficial infections may produce systemic infection in the immunocompromised, for example fungi such as *Candida* (Fig. 9.29), *Aspergillus* (Fig. 9.30) and *Mucor*. Hence any unusually extensive infection by a common infective agent should be viewed with suspicion.

Table 9.8   Association between opportunistic infections and category of immunodeficiency

Immunodeficiency state	Opportunistic infections
T-cell deficiency	*Pneumocystis carinii* pneumonia *Toxoplasma gondii* Mucosal candidiasis *Cryptococcus neoformans* *Histoplasma capsulatum* *Coccidioides immitis* Mycobacteria Salmonella Nocardia Legionella Viruses, e.g. cytomegalovirus, JC, papova
B-cell deficiency	*Streptococcus pneumoniae* *Haemophilus influenzae* Shigella
Neutropenia	Invasive fungal infections: candida, aspergillus, mucor *Staphylococcus albus* *Streptococcus faecalis* Various Gram-negative bacteria: e.g. *Pseudomonas*
AIDS	Cytomegalovirus *Pneumocystis carinii* pneumonia *Cryptococcus neoformans* *Histoplasma capsulatum* *Coccidioides immitis* *Toxoplasma gondii* *Isospora belli* *Mycobacterium avium intracellulare* Salmonella

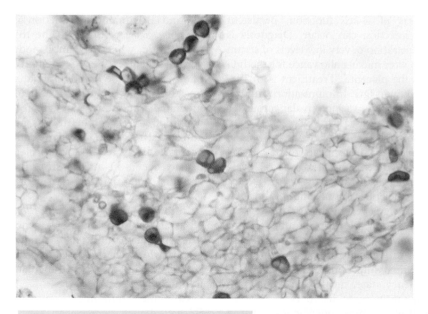

Fig. 9.33 *Pneumocystis carinii* pneumonia

A foamy exudate fills the alveoli. The methenamine silver stain shows the organisms as black spheres.

Immunodeficiency may be classified into two major types:

- deficiencies of non-specific resistance
- deficiencies in specific immune responsiveness.

Deficiencies of non-specific resistance include defects of neutrophil function, abnormalities of the complement system, and systemic diseases such as diabetes mellitus. In addition, there may be local impairment of resistance to infection in an otherwise normal patient, for example in a gangrenous limb.

Deficiencies in specific immune responsiveness are usually classified as:

- *primary immunodeficiencies*, which usually present in infancy and are often genetically mediated
- *secondary immunodeficiencies*, which are usually acquired later in life and are secondary to some other disease.

Further classification is based on whether cell-mediated immunity or immunoglobulin production is chiefly affected.

Primary immunodeficiencies

Primary immunodeficiencies are congenital immuno-deficiencies not resulting from any other disease state. They comprise:

- defect mainly in B-lymphocyte function
  — Bruton-type agammaglobulinaemia
  — transient hypogammaglobulinaemia
- defect mainly in T-lymphocyte function
  — Di George syndrome
- defects of both B- and T-lymphocytes
  — severe combined immunodeficiency
  — ataxia telangiectasia
  — Wiskott–Aldrich syndrome.

Defects mainly of B-lymphocyte function

The *Bruton type of agammaglobulinaemia* is the leading example of immunodeficiency due to defective B-lymphocyte function. It is transmitted as an X-linked recessive genetic defect and is first noticed in infancy in males. Pre-B-cells fail to differentiate into B-lymphocytes. Germinal centres are absent from the lymph nodes, the tissues do not contain plasma cells, and B-lymphocytes are virtually absent from the blood. Circulating levels of IgG, IgM and IgA are negligible. Immunisation procedures have no effect, and there are repeated severe infections with pyogenic bacteria once initial protection by placentally transferred maternal IgG has been lost. Pneumococcal and meningococcal septicaemias, alimentary infections by *Giardia lamblia* and various opportunistic infections occur commonly. While viral infections are less of a problem in defects of B-cell function, persistent hepatitis B virus infection can occur. Diagnosis is based upon demonstration of very low levels of serum IgG, IgM and IgA after making allowance for the IgG transferred across the placenta. Treatment is by life-long injections of human IgG. Immunisation with live organisms (e.g. Sabin polio vaccine) is dangerous, as this may produce virulent disease.

A less serious form of B-cell deficiency is *transient hypogammaglobulinaemia*; this appears to be a delay in maturation of the B-cell system, as it is relatively common in premature infants of both sexes. Immunoglobulin deficiency is usually limited to IgG, and the defect usually recovers by the age of 3 years.

One of the commonest selective immunodeficiencies is IgA deficiency. The lack of IgA in exocrine secretions exposes the patient to repetitive and persistent gastrointestinal infections. Paradoxically in an immune deficiency state, there is an association with allergies and autoimmune disorders.

Some patients with immunodeficiency have a reduced concentration of all classes of immunoglobulin. This is *common variable immunodeficiency*, a combined defect of T-helper cells and B-lymphocytes.

Defects mainly of T-lymphocyte function

The leading example of defective T-lymphocyte function is the *Di George syndrome*, a rare defect in development of the third and fourth branchial arches resulting in an almost complete absence of the thymus and the parathyroid glands. The condition appears to arise sporadically, and there is no clear mode of inheritance. Apart from the hypocalcaemic problems of hypoparathyroidism, affected infants have decreased circulating levels of lymphocytes, especially of T-lymphocytes. Lymph nodes show a selective lack of paracortical (T-cell) areas. Immunoglobulin levels are usually normal, but specific immunoglobulin production to some antigens is reduced, probably because of a lack of helper T-cell activity. Infection with pyogenic bacteria is not a feature of this condition. However, patients develop severe infections with fungi, viruses and opportunistic pathogens such as *Pneumocystis carinii*; cell-mediated immunity is known to be essential in defence against these agents. In its severest form, the condition is fatal, but transplantation of thymic tissue from a well cross-matched donor offers some hope of a cure.

Combined defects of T- and B-lymphocyte function

The most serious example of a combined defect of T- and B-lymphocyte function is *severe combined immunodeficiency* (SCID). The thymus in SCID is hypoplastic, while the lymph nodes show defective germinal centres. Very few circulating lymphocytes of any type can be found, circulating immunoglobulin levels may be nearly undetectable and cell-mediated immunity is greatly reduced. The condition may be inherited as an X-linked or an autosomal recessive disorder. Immunisation by live agents is likely to produce virulent disease. Death usually occurs in infancy from multiple infections, although bone marrow transplantation has effected cure in some cases.

In the rare condition *ataxia telangiectasia* (inherited as an autosomal recessive gene), apart from the cerebellar ataxia and telangiectatic lesions of blood vessels which characterise the syndrome, there are combined defects of cell-mediated and humoral immunity.

Combined immunodeficiency is also seen in the *Wiskott–Aldrich syndrome*, an X-linked genetic defect in which there are platelet function defects, T-lymphocyte defects, and immunoglobulin deficiency, especially of IgA. Affected children show atopic eczema and recurrent infections, particularly otitis media.

Secondary immunodeficiencies

Immunodeficiency may be acquired secondary to various disease processes or drug effects. Examples include:

- protein deficiency
- haematological or advanced malignancy
- acute infection
- chronic renal failure
- immunosuppressive drug therapy, cancer therapy
- splenectomy
- radiotherapy
- sarcoidosis
- AIDS.

The commonest cause of secondary immunodeficiency worldwide is *protein deficiency* due to malnutrition, which causes defects in cell-mediated immunity. Similar effects may be seen in the cachectic state of disseminated cancer, where defects of both T- and B-cell function may be observed.

The *haematological malignancies* such as leukaemias and lymphomas cause severe acquired immunodeficiency states, because the normal cell populations of the marrow and lymph nodes are replaced by neoplastic cells which do not function normally.

Acute viral infections may depress immunological

responsiveness: for example patients with infectious mononucleosis due to Epstein–Barr virus are prone to develop other infections. Similarly, overwhelming *bacterial infections* may disturb immune functions. An example is the reactivation of cold sores (due to Herpes simplex type I virus) during pneumococcal pneumonia.

Patients with *chronic renal failure*, even when treated by regular dialysis, develop combined acquired immunodeficiencies, probably due to toxic effects of accumulated metabolites.

In Western countries, many cases of acquired immunodeficiency are *iatrogenic*, for example due to steroid or other immunosuppressive drug therapy following organ transplantation, or following cytotoxic or radiotherapy for treatment of malignant disease.

Splenectomy, which is sometimes carried out as a staging procedure for Hodgkin's lymphoma or following traumatic splenic rupture, leads to a characteristic immunodeficiency state in which patients are susceptible to infection by pyogenic bacteria, especially pneumococcal septicaemia.

Acquired immune deficiency syndrome (AIDS)

Since 1980, an increasing number of cases of the newly defined acquired immune deficiency syndrome (AIDS) have occurred, initially in the United States of America. The syndrome was first described in homosexuals, intravenous drug abusers, Haitians and haemophiliacs. While the prevalence in Western countries continues to increase, disturbing evidence is becoming available about its endemic nature in some 'Third-world' countries including those in Africa.

AIDS is characterised by a profound defect in cell-mediated immunity, with lymphopenia and diminished T-lymphocyte responses.

The circumstances in which AIDS develops point to some parenterally transmitted infective agent, present in various body fluids, as the cause. In 1984, Gallo and colleagues isolated human T-lymphocytotrophic virus III (HTLV III) from patients with AIDS. The virus has since been renamed human immunodeficiency virus (HIV). Antibodies to HIV have been detected in virtually all patients wth AIDS, and in a large proportion of population groups known to be at risk of AIDS.

Transmission of HIV

Since the initial description of the syndrome, the natural history of AIDS has been changing: it is becoming less confined to homosexuals and more prominent in the heterosexual population, having the same epidemiology as other sexually transmitted diseases.

HIV may also be transmitted by blood and blood products, hence its prevalence in haemophiliacs who receive pooled clotting factor VIII concentrates. The development of screening tests for antibodies to HIV in potential blood donors is a major advance in the prevention of transmission through blood products.

HIV has been demonstrated in other body fluids including semen, tears and saliva. This has major implications for the handling of patients who have AIDS or are carrying HIV, and for the conduct of autopsy examinations on victims of the disease.

Clinicopathological features

HIV infection may be clinically silent, or may present in a variety of ways. Some patients, on developing antibodies to HIV, develop the *acute seroconversion illness* characterised by symptoms resembling glandular fever, possibly associated with acute encephalopathy and acute myelopathy. Other patients chronically infected with HIV develop haematological cytopenias, minor opportunistic skin infections and lymphadenopathy. The lymphadenopathy seen in chronic HIV infection is termed *persistent generalised lymphadenopathy* (PGL). This is defined as enlarged nodes at least 10 mm in diameter in two or more (non-contiguous) extrainguinal sites persisting for at least 3 months in the absence of any current illness or medication known to cause enlarged nodes.

A proportion of patients go on to develop *AIDS-related complex*, which is characterised by constitutional symptoms and abnormal laboratory tests of immunological competence falling short of AIDS. The onset of overt AIDS is usually signalled by the development of multiple opportunistic infections, which may include *Pneumocystis carinii* pneumonia, cytomegalovirus infections, cerebral toxoplasmosis, atypical mycobacterial infections, systemic fungal infections and parasitic infestations of the gastrointestinal tract. About one-third of patients develop an otherwise rare sarcoma, possibly of vascular endothelial cells, called Kaposi's sarcoma. Before the recognition of AIDS, Kaposi's sarcoma was virtually confined to the southern European countries, being most common in Italians and Jews, and to central Africa. The prognosis for AIDS patients is very poor; about 90% die within two years of diagnosis.

The development of HIV infection does not necessarily lead to clinical AIDS, but why the syndrome develops in only some infected individuals is not known.

Pathogenesis

Cell-borne rather than free virus is thought to be the main source of infection. This explains the virtual confinement of infectiveness to parenteral and venereal transmission. There follows an acute virus infection with spread primarily to lymphoid tissues and peripheral blood leukocytes. HIV attaches to cell receptors, of which there are at least four types; these include:

- the CD4 molecule on helper T-cells
- galactosyl ceramide on brain and bowel cells
- Fc receptors
- complement receptors.

After viral fusion with the cell, the nucleocapsid enters the cell and viral replication commences. Initially, however, the replication rate is suppressed by intracellular factors and by cellular immunity mediated by CD8-bearing suppressor/cytotoxic T-cells, enhanced by dominant helper T-cell subset 1 responses.

In those individuals progressing to AIDS, there then follows a gradual loss of helper T-cell function and numbers, with a switch to the helper T-cell subset 2 which produces cytokines such as IL-10, known to inhibit the CD8-bearing lymphocytes' anti-HIV responses.

Increased release of virus results in increased numbers of HIV-infected cells. With the enhanced replication of the virus, the frequency of viral mutations (which occur up to 10 mutations per replication cycle) increases, eventually leading to more pathogenic strains. The ensuing catastrophic loss of CD4-bearing lymphocytes and their function then leads to overt AIDS.

Prospect of vaccines

The genetic and antigenic variability of HIV (a second virus, HIV2, has been isolated in parts of Africa) are the key factors impeding development of a vaccine. However, experimental simian immunodeficiency virus and HIV vaccines have been shown to induce protective immunity in macaques and chimpanzees. The challenge in the development of a successful vaccine is the production of *group specific* neutralising antibodies and/or cell-mediated immunity, rather than a *strain specific* response.

Safety and immunogenicity human trials (phases 1 and 2) of 12 candidate vaccines tested in HIV-negative human volunteers have shown that they are well tolerated and induce neutralising antibody and cell-mediated responses. There are currently no data on their potential clinical benefit.

FURTHER READING

Black C M, Welsh K I 1986 Clinical immunology. In: Read A E, Barritt D W, Langton-Hewer R L (eds) Modern medicine: a textbook for students. Churchill Livingstone, Edinburgh, pp 139–157

Brenner M K 1986 Annual review: clinical immunology. Hospital Update 12: 431–440

Cavallo M G, Pozzilli P, Thorpe R 1994 Cytokines and autoimmunity. Clinical and Experimental Immunology 96: 1–7

Chapel H, Heaney M 1993 Essentals of clinical immunology. 3rd edn Blackwell, Oxford

Dick H M, Powis S H 1987 HLA and disease: possible mechanisms. In: Anthony P P, MacSween R N M (eds) Recent advances in histopathology 13. Churchill Livingstone, Edinburgh, pp 1–12

Erber W N 1990 Human leucocyte differentiation antigens: review of CD nomenclature. Pathology 22: 61–69

Esparza J, Osmanov S 1993 The development and evaluation of HIV vaccines. Current Opinion on Infectious Diseases 6: 218–229

Foulis A K 1986 Class II major histocompatibility complex and organ specific autoimmunity in man. Journal of Pathology 150: 5–12

French M A H 1986 Acquired immunodeficiency. Update 32: 193–204

Levy J A 1993 HIV pathogenesis and long term survival. AIDS 7: 1401–1410

McLean A R 1993 The balance of power between HIV and the immune system. Trends in Microbiology 1: 9–13

Millard P R, Chapel H M 1987 Immunodeficiency states including AIDS. In: Anthony P P, MacSween R N M (eds) Recent advances in histopathology 13. Churchill Livingstone, Edinburgh, pp 129–158

Millard P R, Esiri M 1992 The pathology of AIDS: an update. In: Anthony P P, MacSween R N M (eds) Recent advances in histopathology 15. Churchill Livingstone, Edinburgh, pp 67–92

Paul W E, Seder R A 1994 Lymphocyte responses and cytokines. Cell 76: 241–251

Roitt I M 1994 Essential immunology, 8th edn. Blackwell Scientific Publications, Oxford

Roitt I M, Brostoff J, Male D K 1989 Immunology, 2nd edn. Churchill Livingstone, Edinburgh

Scott D W, Dawson J R 1985 Key facts in immunology. Churchill Livingstone, Edinburgh

Underwood J C E, Rooney N 1985 Immunopathology of tumors. In: Hancock B W, Ward A M (eds) Immunological aspects of cancer. Martinus Nijhoff, Boston, pp 179–191

Zaleski M B 1991 Cell surface molecules in the regulation of immune responsiveness. Immunological Investigations 20: 103–131

10

Inflammation

Inflammation is the local physiological response to tissue injury. It is not, in itself, a disease, but is usually a manifestation of disease. Inflammation may have beneficial effects, such as the destruction of invading micro-organisms and the walling-off of an abscess cavity, thus preventing spread of infection. Equally, it may produce disease; for example, an abscess in the brain would act as a space-occupying lesion compressing vital surrounding structures, or fibrosis resulting from chronic inflammation may distort the tissues and permanently alter their function.

Inflammation is usually classified according to its time course as:

- *acute inflammation* — the initial and often transient series of tissue reactions to injury
- *chronic inflammation* — the subsequent and often prolonged tissue reactions following the initial response (p. 236).

The two main types of inflammation are also characterised by differences in the cell types taking part in the inflammatory response.

ACUTE INFLAMMATION

> ▶ Initial reaction of tissue to injury
> ▶ Vascular phase: dilatation and increased permeability
> ▶ Exudative phase: fluid and cells escape from permeable venules
> ▶ Neutrophil polymorph is the characteristic cell
> ▶ Outcome may be resolution, suppuration (e.g. abscess), organisation, or progression to chronic inflammation

Acute inflammation is the initial tissue reaction to a wide range of injurious agents; it may last from a few hours to a few days. The process is usually described by the suffix '-itis', preceded by the name of the organ or tissues involved. Thus, acute inflammation of the meninges is called meningitis. The acute inflammatory response is similar whatever the causative agent.

Causes of acute inflammation

The principal causes of acute inflammation are:

- microbial infections, e.g. pyogenic bacteria, viruses
- hypersensitivity reactions, e.g. parasites, tubercle bacilli
- physical agents, e.g. trauma, ionising irradiation, heat, cold

- chemicals, e.g. corrosives, acids, alkalis, reducing agents, bacterial toxins
- tissue necrosis, e.g. ischaemic infarction.

Microbial infections

One of the commonest causes of inflammation is microbial infection. Viruses lead to death of individual cells by intracellular multiplication. Bacteria release specific exotoxins — chemicals synthesised by them which specifically initiate inflammation — or endotoxins, which are associated with their cell walls. Additionally, some organisms cause immunologically-mediated inflammation through hypersensitivity reactions (Ch. 9). Parasitic infections and tuberculous inflammation are instances where hypersensitivity is important.

Hypersensitivity reactions

A hypersensitivity reaction occurs when an altered state of immunological responsiveness causes an inappropriate or excessive immune reaction which damages the tissues. The types of reaction are classified in Chapter 9 but all have cellular or chemical mediators similar to those involved in inflammation.

Physical agents

Tissue damage leading to inflammation may occur through physical trauma, ultraviolet or other ionising radiation, burns or excessive cooling ('frostbite').

Irritant and corrosive chemicals

Corrosive chemicals (acids, alkalis, oxidising agents) provoke inflammation through gross tissue damage. However, infecting agents may release specific chemical irritants which lead directly to inflammation.

Tissue necrosis

Death of tissues from lack of oxygen or nutrients resulting from inadequate blood flow (infarction, see Ch. 8) is a potent inflammatory stimulus. The edge of a recent infarct often shows an acute inflammatory response.

Essential macroscopic appearances of acute inflammation

The essential physical characteristics of acute inflammation were formulated by Celsus (30 BC–

38 AD) using the Latin words rubor, calor, tumor and dolor. Loss of function is also characteristic.

Redness (rubor)

An acutely inflamed tissue appears red, for example skin affected by sunburn, cellulitis due to bacterial infection or acute conjunctivitis. This is due to dilatation of small blood vessels within the damaged area (Fig. 10.1).

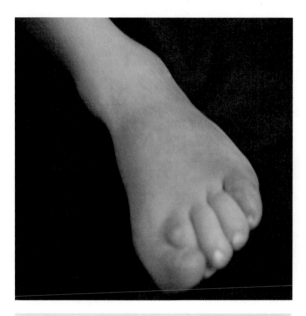

Fig. 10.1 Redness (erythema) of the skin of the left foot due to cellulitis

Heat (calor)

Increase in temperature is seen only in peripheral parts of the body, such as the skin. It is due to increased blood flow (hyperaemia) through the region, resulting in vascular dilatation and the delivery of warm blood to the area. Systemic fever, which results from some of the chemical mediators of inflammation, also contributes to the local temperature.

Swelling (tumor)

Swelling results from oedema — the accumulation of fluid in the extravascular space as part of the fluid exudate — and, to a much lesser extent, from the physical mass of the inflammatory cells migrating into the area (Fig. 10.2).

Pain (dolor)

For the patient, pain is one of the best-known features of acute inflammation. It results partly from the stretching and distortion of tissues due to inflammatory oedema and, in particular, from pus under pressure in an abscess cavity. Some of the chemical mediators of acute inflammation, including bradykinin, the prostaglandins and serotonin, are known to induce pain.

Loss of function

Loss of function, a well-known consequence of inflammation, was added by Virchow (1821–1902) to the list of features drawn up by Celsus. Movement of an inflamed area is consciously and reflexly inhib-

Fig. 10.2 Early acute appendicitis

The appendix is swollen due to oedema, the surface is covered by fibrinous exudate, and there is vascular dilatation.

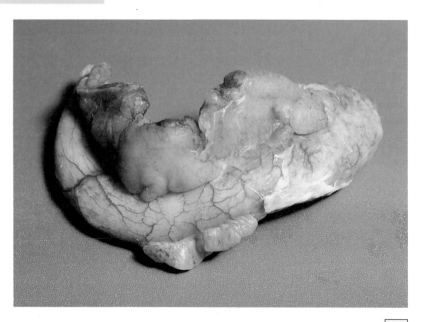

ited by pain, while severe swelling may physically immobilise the tissues.

Early stages of acute inflammation

In the early stages, oedema fluid, fibrin and neutrophil polymorphs accumulate in the extracellular spaces of the damaged tissue. The presence of the cellular component, the *neutrophil polymorph*, is essential for a histological diagnosis of acute inflammation. The acute inflammatory response involves three processes:

• changes in vessel calibre and, consequently, flow
• increased vascular permeability and formation of the fluid exudate
• formation of the cellular exudate — emigration of the neutrophil polymorphs into the extravascular space.

Changes in vessel calibre

The microcirculation consists of the network of small capillaries lying between arterioles, which have a thick muscular wall, and thin-walled venules. Capillaries have no smooth muscle in their walls to control their calibre, and are so narrow that red blood cells must past through them in single file. The smooth muscle of arteriolar walls forms precapillary sphincters which regulate blood flow through the capillary bed. Flow through the capillaries is intermittent, and some form preferential channels for flow while others are usually shut down (Fig. 10.3).

In blood vessels larger than capillaries, blood cells flow mainly in the centre of the lumen (axial flow), while the area near the vessel wall carries only plasma (plasmatic zone). This feature of normal blood flow keeps blood cells away from the vessel wall.

Changes in the microcirculation occur as a physiological response; for example, there is hyperaemia in exercising muscle and active endocrine glands. The changes following injury which make up the vascular component of the acute inflammatory reaction were described by Lewis in 1927 as 'the triple response to injury': a flush, a flare and a wheal. If a blunt instrument is drawn firmly across the skin, the following sequential changes take place:

• A momentary white line follows the stroke. This is due to arteriolar vasoconstriction, the smooth muscle of arterioles contracting as a direct response to injury.
• *The flush:* a dull red line follows due to capillary dilatation.
• *The flare:* a red, irregular, surrounding zone then

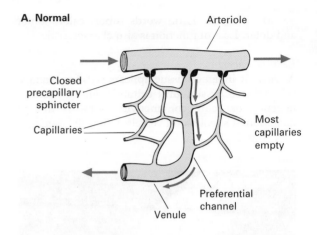

A. Normal

Arteriole

Closed precapillary sphincter

Capillaries

Most capillaries empty

Preferential channel

Venule

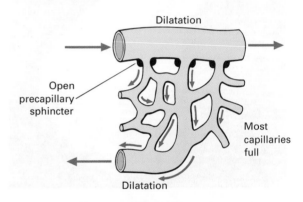

B. Acute inflammation

Dilatation

Open precapillary sphincter

Most capillaries full

Dilatation

Fig. 10.3 Vascular dilatation in acute inflammation

A. Normally, most of the capillary bed is closed down by precapillary sphincters. **B.** In acute inflammation, the sphincters open, causing blood to flow through all capillaries.

develops, due to arteriolar dilatation. Both nervous and chemical factors are involved in these vascular changes.
• *The wheal:* a zone of oedema develops due to fluid exudation into the extravascular space.

The initial phase of arteriolar constriction is transient, and probably of little importance in acute inflammation. The subsequent phase of vasodilatation (active hyperaemia) may last from 15 minutes to several hours, depending upon the severity of the injury. There is experimental evidence that blood flow to the injured area may increase up to ten-fold.

As blood flow begins to slow again, blood cells begin to flow nearer to the vessel wall, in the plasmatic zone rather than the axial stream. This allows 'pavementing' of leukocytes (their adhesion to the vascular epithelium) to occur, which is the first step in leukocyte emigration into the extravascular space.

The slowing of blood flow which follows the phase of hyperaemia is due to increased vascular permeability, allowing plasma to escape into the tissues while blood cells are retained within the vessels. The blood viscosity is therefore increased.

Increased vascular permeability

Small blood vessels are lined by a single layer of endothelial cells. In some tissues, these form a complete layer of uniform thickness around the vessel wall, while in other tissues there are areas of endothelial cell thinning, known as fenestrations. The walls of small blood vessels act as a microfilter, allowing the passage of water and solutes but blocking that of large molecules and cells. Oxygen, carbon dioxide and some nutrients transfer across the wall by diffusion, but the main transfer of fluid and solutes is by ultrafiltration, as described by Starling. The high colloid osmotic pressure inside the vessel, due to plasma proteins, favours fluid return to the vascular compartment. Under normal circumstances, high hydrostatic pressure at the arteriolar end of capillaries forces fluid out into the extravascular space, but this fluid returns into the capillaries at their venous end, where hydrostatic pressure is low (Fig. 10.4). In acute inflammation, however, not only is capillary hydrostatic pressure increased, but there is also escape of plasma proteins into the extravascular space, increasing the colloid osmotic pressure there. Consequently, much more fluid leaves the vessels than is returned to them. The net

A. Normal

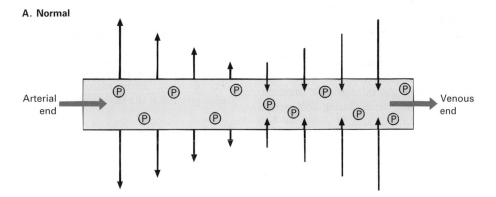

B. Acute inflammation

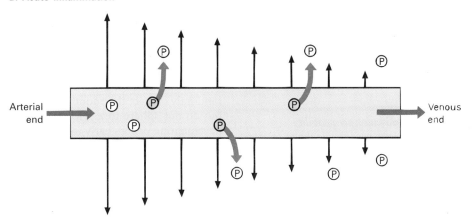

Fig. 10.4   Ultrafiltration of fluid across the small blood vessel wall

A. Normally, fluid leaving and entering the vessel is in equilibrium. **B.** In acute inflammation, there is a net loss of fluid together with plasma protein molecules (P) into the extracellular space, resulting in oedema.

escape of protein-rich fluid is called *exudation*; hence, the fluid is called the *fluid exudate*.

Features of the fluid exudate
The increased vascular permeability means that large molecules, such as proteins, can escape from vessels. Hence, the exudate fluid has a high protein content of up to 50 g/l. The proteins present include immunoglobulins, which may be important in the destruction of invading micro-organisms, and coagulation factors, including fibrinogen, which result in fibrin deposition on contact with the extravascular tissues. Hence, acutely inflamed organ surfaces are commonly covered by fibrin: the *fibrinous exudate*. There is a considerable turnover of the inflammatory exudate; it is constantly drained away by local lymphatic channels to be replaced by new exudate.

Ultrastructural basis of increased vascular permeability
The ultrastructural basis of increased vascular permeability was originally determined using an experimental model in which histamine, one of the chemical mediators of increased vascular permeability, was injected under the skin. This caused transient leakage of plasma proteins into the extravascular space. Electron microscopic examination of venules and small veins during this period showed that gaps of 0.1–0.4 μm in diameter had appeared between endothelial cells. These gaps allowed the leakage of injected particles, such as carbon, into the tissues. The endothelial cells are not damaged during this process. They contain contractile proteins such as actin, which, when stimulated by the chemical mediators of acute inflammation, cause contraction of the endothelial cells, pulling open the transient pores. The leakage induced by chemical mediators, such as histamine, is confined to venules and small veins. Although fluid is lost by ultrafiltration from capillaries, there is no evidence that they too become more permeable in acute inflammation.

Other causes of increased vascular permeability
In addition to the transient vascular leakage caused by some inflammatory stimuli, certain other stimuli, e.g. heat, cold, ultraviolet light and X-rays, bacterial toxins and corrosive chemicals, cause delayed prolonged leakage. In these circumstances, there is direct injury to endothelial cells in several types of vessels within the damaged area (Table 10.1).

Tissue sensitivity to chemical mediators
The relative importance of chemical mediators and of direct vascular injury in causing increased vascu-

Table 10.1 Causes of increased vascular permeability

Time course	Mechanisms
Immediate transient	Chemical mediators, e.g. histamine
Immediate sustained	Severe direct vascular injury, e.g. trauma
Delayed prolonged	Endothelial cell injury, e.g. X-rays, bacterial toxins

lar permeability varies according to the type of tissue. For example, vessels in the central nervous system are relatively insensitive to the chemical mediators, while those in the skin, conjunctiva and bronchial mucosa are exquisitely sensitive to agents such as histamine.

Formation of the cellular exudate

The accumulation of *neutrophil polymorphs* within the extracellular space is the diagnostic histological feature of acute inflammation. The stages whereby leukocytes reach the tissues are shown in Figure 10.5.

Margination of neutrophils
In the normal circulation, cells are confined to the central (axial) stream in blood vessels, and do not flow in the peripheral (plasmatic) zone near to the endothelium. However, loss of intravascular fluid and increase in plasma viscosity with slowing of flow at the site of acute inflammation allow neutrophils to flow in this plasmatic zone.

Adhesion of neutrophils
The adhesion of neutrophils to the vascular endothelium which occurs at sites of acute inflammation is termed 'pavementing' of neutrophils. Neutrophils randomly contact the endothelium in normal tissues, but do not adhere to it. However, at sites of injury, pavementing occurs early in the acute inflammatory response and appears to be a specific process occurring independently of the eventual slowing of blood flow. The phenomenon is seen only in venules.

Increased leukocyte adhesion results from interaction between *adhesion molecules* on leukocyte and endothelial surfaces. Leukocyte surface adhesion molecule expression is increased by:

- complement component C5a
- leukotriene B4
- tumour necrosis factor.

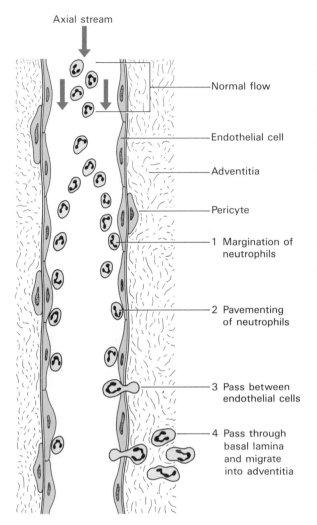

Axial stream

Normal flow

Endothelial cell

Adventitia

Pericyte

1 Margination of neutrophils

2 Pavementing of neutrophils

3 Pass between endothelial cells

4 Pass through basal lamina and migrate into adventitia

Fig. 10.5 Steps in neutrophil polymorph emigration

(1) Neutrophils marginate into the plasmatic zone; (2) adhere to endothelial cells; (3) pass between endothelial cells; and (4) pass through the basal lamina and migrate into the adventitia.

Endothelial cell expression of endothelial–leukocyte adhesion molecule-1 (ELAM-1) and intercellular adhesion molecule-1 (ICAM-1), to which the leukocytes' surface adhesion molecules bond, is increased by:

- interleukin-1
- endotoxins
- tumour necrosis factor.

In this way, a variety of chemical inflammatory mediators promote leukocyte–endothelial adhesion

as a prelude to leukocyte emigration.

Neutrophil emigration
Leukocytes migrate by active amoeboid movement through the walls of venules and small veins, but do not commonly exit from capillaries. Electron microscopy shows that neutrophil and eosinophil polymorphs and macrophages can insert pseudopodia between endothelial cells, migrate through the gap so created between the endothelial cells, and then on through the basal lamina into the vessel wall. The defect appears to be self-sealing, and the endothelial cells are not damaged by this process.

Diapedesis
Red cells may also escape from vessels, but in this case the process is passive and depends on hydrostatic pressure forcing the red cells out. The process is called diapedesis, and the presence of large numbers of red cells in the extravascular space implies severe vascular injury, such as a tear in the vessel wall.

Later stages of acute inflammation

Chemotaxis of neutrophils

It has long been known from in vitro experiments that neutrophil polymorphs are attracted towards certain chemical substances in solution—a process called chemotaxis. Time-lapse cine photography shows apparently purposeful migration of neutrophils along a concentration gradient. Compounds which appear chemotactic for neutrophils in vitro include certain complement components, cytokines and products produced by neutrophils themselves. It is not known whether chemotaxis is important in vivo. Neutrophils may possibly arrive at sites of injury by random movement, and then be trapped there by immobilising factors (a process analogous to the trapping of macrophages at sites of delayed type hypersensitivity by migration inhibitory factor; Ch. 9).

Chemical mediators of acute inflammation

The spread of the acute inflammatory response following injury to a small area of tissue suggests that chemical substances are released from injured tissues, spreading outwards into uninjured areas. These chemicals, called *endogenous chemical mediators*, cause:

- vasodilatation
- emigration of neutrophils
- chemotaxis
- increased vascular permeability.

Chemical mediators released from cells

Histamine. This is the best-known chemical mediator in acute inflammation. It causes vascular dilatation and the immediate transient phase of increased vascular permeability. It is stored in mast cells, basophil and eosinophil leukocytes, and platelets. Histamine release from these sites (for example, mast cell degranulation) is stimulated by complement components C3a and C5a, and by lysosomal proteins released from neutrophils.

Lysosomal compounds. These are released from neutrophils and include cationic proteins, which may increase vascular permeability, and neutral proteases, which may activate complement.

Prostaglandins. These are a group of long-chain fatty acids derived from arachidonic acid and synthesised by many cell types. Some prostaglandins potentiate the increase in vascular permeability caused by other compounds. Others include platelet aggregation (prostaglandin I_2 is inhibitory while prostaglandin A_2 is stimulatory). Part of the anti-inflammatory activity of drugs such as aspirin and the non-steroidal anti-inflammatory drugs is attributable to inhibition of one of the enzymes involved in prostaglandin synthesis.

Leukotrienes. These are also synthesised from arachidonic acid, especially in neutrophils, and appear to have vasoactive properties. SRS-A (slow reacting substance of anaphylaxis), involved in type I hypersensitivity (Ch. 9), is a mixture of leukotrienes.

5-hydroxytryptamine (serotonin). This is present in high concentration in mast cells and platelets. It is a potent vasoconstrictor.

Cytokines. This family of chemical messengers released by lymphocytes is described in Chapter 9. Apart from their major role in type IV hypersensitivity, cytokines may also have vasoactive or chemotactic properties.

Plasma factors

The plasma contains four enzymatic cascade systems — complement, the kinins, the coagulation factors and the fibrinolytic system — which are inter-related and produce various inflammatory mediators.

Complement system. The complement system is a cascade system of enzymatic proteins (Ch. 9). It can be activated during the acute inflammatory reaction in various ways:

- In tissue necrosis, enzymes capable of activating complement are released from dying cells.
- During infection, the formation of antigen–antibody complexes can activate

complement via the *classical pathway*, while the endotoxins of Gram-negative bacteria activate complement via the *alternative pathway* (Ch. 9).
- Products of the kinin, coagulation and fibrinolytic systems can activate complement.

The products of complement activation most important in acute inflammation include:

- C5a: chemotactic for neutrophils; increases vascular permeability; releases histamine from mast cells
- C3a: similar properties to those of C5a, but less active
- C567: chemotactic for neutrophils
- C56789: cytolytic activity
- C4b, 2a, 3b: opsonisation of bacteria (facilitates phagocytosis by macrophages).

Kinin system. The kinins are peptides of 9–11 amino acids; the most important vascular permeability factor is bradykinin. The kinin system is activated by coagulation factor XII (Fig. 10.6). Bradykinin is also a chemical mediator of the pain which is a cardinal feature of acute inflammation.

Coagulation system. The coagulation system (Ch. 23) is responsible for the conversion of soluble fibrinogen into fibrin, a major component of the acute inflammatory exudate.

Coagulation factor XII (the Hageman factor), once activated by contact with extracellular materials such as basal lamina, and various proteolytic enzymes of bacterial origin, can activate the coagulation, kinin and fibrinolytic systems. The inter-relationships of these systems are shown in Figure 10.7.

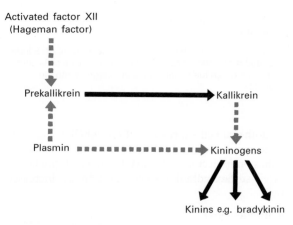

Fig. 10.6   The kinin system

Activated factor XII and plasmin activate the conversion of prekallikrein to kallikrein. This stimulates the conversion of kininogens to kinins, such as bradykinin.

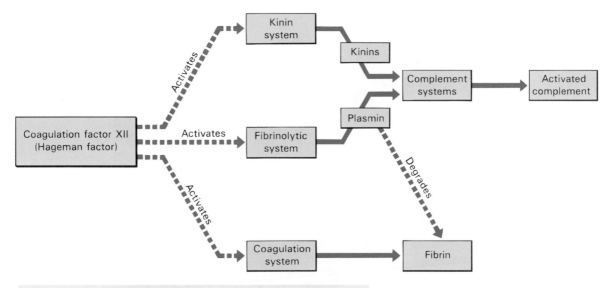

Fig. 10.7   Interactions between the systems of chemical mediators

Coagulation factor XII activates the kinin, fibrinolytic and coagulation systems. The complement system is in turn activated.

Fibrinolytic system. Plasmin is responsible for the lysis of fibrin into fibrin degradation products, which may have local effects on vascular permeability.

Table 10.2 summarises the chemical mediators involved in the three main stages of acute inflammation.

Role of the lymphatics

Terminal lymphatics are blind-ended, endothelium-lined tubes present in most tissues in similar numbers to capillaries. The terminal lymphatics drain into collecting lymphatics which have valves and so propel lymph passively, aided by contraction of neighbouring muscles, to the lymph nodes. The basal lamina of lymphatic endothelium is incomplete, and the junctions between the cells are simpler and less robust than those between capillary endothelial cells. Hence, gaps tend to open up passively between the lymphatic endothelial cells, allowing large protein molecules to enter.

In acute inflammation, the lymphatic channels become dilated as they drain away the oedema fluid of the inflammatory exudate. This drainage tends to limit the extent of oedema in the tissues. The ability of the lymphatics to carry large molecules and some particulate matter is important in the immune response to infecting agents; antigens are carried to the regional lymph nodes for recognition by lymphocytes (Ch. 9).

Role of the neutrophil polymorph

The neutrophil polymorph is the characteristic cell of the acute inflammatory infiltrate (Fig. 10.8). The actions of this cell will now be considered.

Movement

Contraction of cytoplasmic microtubules and gel/sol changes in cytoplasmic fluidity bring about amoeboid movement. These active mechanisms are

Table 10.2 Endogenous chemical mediators of the acute inflammatory response	
Stages of acute inflammatory response	Chemical mediators
Vascular dilatation	Histamine Prostaglandins Complement components C3a and C5a
Increased vascular permeability	Transient phase — histamine Prolonged phase — possibly kinins potentiated by prostaglandins
Emigration of leukocytes	Complement components — C5a Leukotrienes Cationic proteins of neutrophils

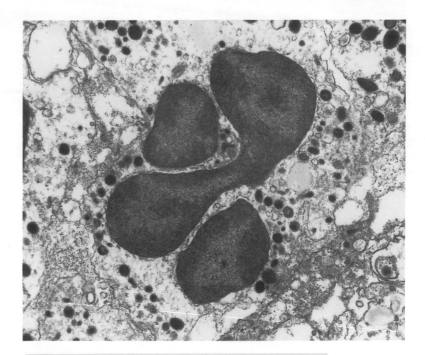

Fig. 10.8   Electron micrograph of a neutrophil polymorph

The nucleus is polylobate and the cytoplasm shows dense granules which contain myeloperoxidase and other enzymes (x 12 500).

dependent upon calcium ions and are controlled by intracellular concentrations of cyclic nucleotides. The movement shows a directional response (chemotaxis) to the various chemicals of acute inflammation.

Adhesion to micro-organisms
Micro-organisms are *opsonised* (from the Greek word meaning 'to prepare for the table'), or rendered more amenable to phagocytosis either by immuno-globulins or by complement components. Bacterial lipopolysaccharides activate complement via the alternative pathway (Ch. 9), generating component C3b which has opsonising properties. In addition, if antibody binds to bacterial antigens, this can activate complement via the classical pathway, also generat-ing C3b. In the immune individual, the binding of immunoglobulins to micro-organisms by their Fab components leaves the Fc component (Ch. 9) exposed. Neutrophils have surface receptors for the Fc fragment of immunoglobulins, and consequently bind to the micro-organisms prior to ingestion.

Phagocytosis
The process whereby cells (such as neutrophil poly-morphs and macrophages) ingest solid particles is termed phagocytosis. The first step in phagocytosis is adhesion of the particle to be phagocytosed to the cell surface. This is facilitated by opsonisation. The phagocyte then ingests the attached particle by send-ing out pseudopodia around it. These meet and fuse so that the particle lies in a phagocytic vacuole (also called a phagosome) bounded by cell membrane. Lysosomes, membrane-bound packets containing the toxic compounds described below, then fuse with phagosomes to form phagolysosomes. It is within these that intracellular killing of micro-organ-isms occurs.

Intracellular killing of micro-organisms
Neutrophil polymorphs are highly specialised cells, containing noxious microbicidal agents, some of which are similar to household bleach. The microbi-cidal agents may be classified as:

• those which are oxygen-dependent
• those which are oxygen-independent.

Oxygen-dependent mechanisms. The neutrophils produce hydrogen peroxide which reacts with myeloperoxidase in the cytoplasmic granules

(Fig. 10.8) in the presence of halide, such as Cl⁻, to produce a potent microbicidal agent. Other products of oxygen reduction also contribute to the killing, such as peroxide anions (O_2^-), hydroxyl radicals (•OH) and singlet oxygen $(^1O_2)$.

Oxygen-independent mechanisms. These include lysozyme (muramidase), lactoferrin which chelates iron required for bacterial growth, cationic proteins, and the low pH inside phagocytic vacuoles.

Release of lysosomal products

Release of lysosomal products from the cell damages local tissues by proteolysis by enzymes such as elastase and collagenase, activates coagulation factor XII, and attracts other leukocytes into the area. Some of the compounds released increase vascular permeability, while others are pyrogens, producing systemic fever by acting on the hypothalamus.

Special macroscopic appearances of acute inflammation

The cardinal signs of acute inflammation are modified according to the tissue involved and the type of agent provoking the inflammation. Several descriptive terms are used for the appearances.

Serous inflammation

In serous inflammation, there is abundant protein-rich fluid exudate with a relatively low cellular content. Examples include inflammation of the serous cavities, such as peritonitis, and inflammation of a synovial joint, acute synovitis. Vascular dilatation may be apparent to the naked eye, the serous surfaces appearing injected (Fig. 10.2), i.e. having dilated, blood-laden vessels on the surface (like the appearance of the conjunctiva in 'blood-shot' eyes).

Catarrhal inflammation

When mucus hypersecretion accompanies acute inflammation of a mucous membrane, the appearance is described as catarrhal. The common cold is a good example.

Fibrinous inflammation

When the inflammatory exudate contains plentiful fibrinogen, this polymerises into a thick fibrin coating. This is often seen in acute pericarditis and gives the parietal and visceral pericardium a 'bread and butter' appearance.

Haemorrhagic inflammation

Haemorrhagic inflammation indicates severe vascular injury or depletion of coagulation factors. This occurs in acute pancreatitis due to proteolytic destruction of vascular walls, and in meningococcal septicaemia due to disseminated intravascular coagulation.

Suppurative (purulent) inflammation

The terms 'suppurative' and 'purulent' denote the production of pus, which consists of dying and degenerate neutrophils, infecting organisms and liquefied tissues. The pus may become walled-off by granulation tissue or fibrous tissue to produce an *abscess* (a localised collection of pus in a tissue). If a hollow viscus fills with pus, this is called an *empyema*, for example, empyema of the gallbladder (Fig. 10.9) or of the appendix (Fig. 10.10).

Membranous inflammation

In acute membranous inflammation, an epithelium becomes coated by fibrin, desquamated epithelial cells and inflammatory cells. An example is the grey

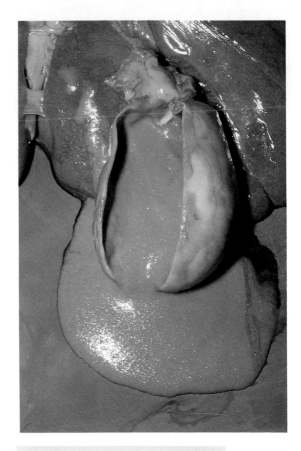

Fig. 10.9 Empyema of the gallbladder

The gallbladder lumen is filled with pus.

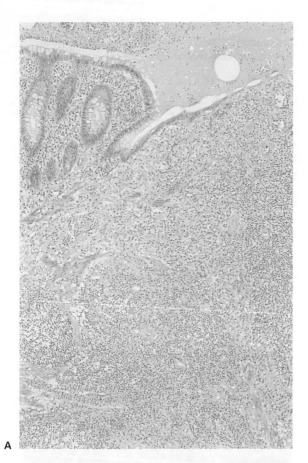

A

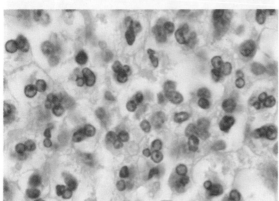

B

Fig. 10.10   Empyema of the appendix

A. The appendix lumen is filled with pus, there is focal mucosal ulceration, and the appendicular wall and meso-appendix (bottom) are thickened due to an acute inflammatory exudate.
B. Pus in the lumen of the appendix. Pus consists of living and degenerate neutrophil polymorphs together with liquefied tissue debris.

membrane seen in pharyngitis or laryngitis due to *Corynebacterium diphtheriae.*

Pseudomembranous inflammation
The term 'pseudomembranous' describes superficial mucosal ulceration with an overlying slough of disrupted mucosa, fibrin, mucus and inflammatory cells. This is seen in pseudomembranous colitis due to *Clostridium difficile* colonisation of the bowel, usually following broad-spectrum antibiotic treatment (Ch. 15).

Necrotising (gangrenous) inflammation
High tissue pressure due to oedema may lead to vascular occlusion and thrombosis, which may result in widespread septic necrosis of the organ. The combination of necrosis and bacterial putrefaction is *gangrene*. Gangrenous appendicitis is a good example.

Effects of acute inflammation

Acute inflammation has local and systemic effects, both of which may be harmful or beneficial. The local effects are usually clearly beneficial, for example the destruction of invading micro-organisms; but at other times they appear to serve no obvious function, or may even be positively harmful.

Beneficial effects

Both the fluid and cellular exudates may have useful effects. Beneficial effects of the fluid exudate are:

- *Dilution of toxins,* such as those produced by bacteria, allows them to be carried away in lymphatics.
- *Entry of antibodies,* due to increased vascular permeability into the extravascular space, where they may lead either to lysis of micro-organisms, through the participation of complement, or to their phagocytosis by opsonisation. Antibodies are also important in neutralisation of toxins.
- *Transport of drugs* such as antibiotics to the site where bacteria are multiplying.
- *Fibrin formation* (Fig. 10.11) from exuded fibrinogen may impede the movement of micro-organisms, trapping them and so facilitating phagocytosis.
- *Delivery of nutrients and oxygen,* essential for cells such as neutrophils which have high metabolic activity, is aided by increased fluid flow through the area.
- *Stimulation of immune response* by drainage of this fluid exudate into the lymphatics allows particulate and soluble antigens to reach the local

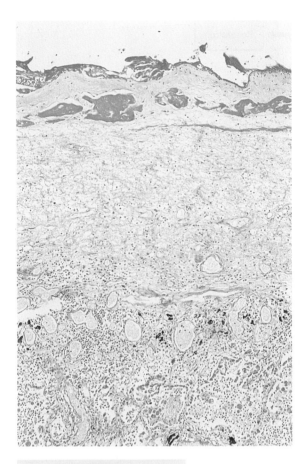

Fig. 10.11 Fibrinous exudate

Histology of the fibrinous exudate (dark-stained material)
adherent to the pleura in acute lobar pneumonia.

lymph nodes where they may stimulate the
immune response.

The role of neutrophils in the cellular exudate has
already been discussed. They have a life-span of only
1–3 days and must be constantly replaced. Most die
locally, but some leave the site via the lymphatics.
Blood *monocytes* also arrive at the site and, on leaving
the blood vessels, transform into *macrophages*,
becoming more metabolically active, motile and
phagocytic. Phagocytosis of micro-organisms is
enhanced by *opsonisation* by antibodies or by complement. In most acute inflammatory reactions,
macrophages play a lesser role in phagocytosis compared with that of neutrophil polymorphs. They
appear late in the response and are usually responsible for clearing away tissue debris and damaged
cells.

Both neutrophils and macrophages may discharge

their lysosomal enzymes into the extracellular fluid
by exocytosis, or the entire cell contents may be
released when the cells die. Release of these enzymes
assists in the *digestion of the inflammatory exudate*.

Harmful effects

The release of lysosomal enzymes by inflammatory
cells may also have harmful effects:

- *Digestion of normal tissues.* Enzymes such as
  collagenases and proteases may digest normal
  tissues, resulting in their destruction. This may
  result particularly in vascular damage, for example
  in type III hypersensitivity reactions (Ch. 9) and in
  some types of glomerulonephritis (Ch. 21).
- *Swelling.* The swelling of acutely inflamed tissues
  may be harmful: for example, in children the
  swelling of the epiglottis in acute epiglottitis due
  to *Haemophilus influenzae* infection may obstruct
  the airway, resulting in death. Inflammatory
  swelling is especially serious when it occurs in an
  enclosed space such as the cranial cavity. Thus,
  acute meningitis or a cerebral abscess may *raise
  intracranial pressure* to the point where blood flow
  into the brain is impaired, resulting in ischaemic
  damage, or may force the cerebral hemispheres
  against the tentorial orifice and the cerebellum into
  the foramen magnum (pressure coning; Ch. 26).
- *Inappropriate inflammatory response.* Sometimes,
  acute inflammatory responses appear
  inappropriate, such as those which occur in type I
  hypersensitivity reactions (e.g. hay fever; Ch. 9)
  where the provoking environmental antigen (e.g.
  pollen) otherwise poses no threat to the individual.
  Such allergic inflammatory responses may be life-
  threatening, for example extrinsic asthma.

Sequelae of acute inflammation

The sequelae of acute inflammation depend upon
the type of tissue involved and the amount of tissue
destruction, which depend in turn upon the nature
of the injurious agent. The possible outcomes of
acute inflammation are shown in Figure 10.12.

Resolution

The term resolution means the complete restoration
of the tissues to normal after an episode of acute
inflammation. The conditions which favour resolution are:

- minimal cell death and tissue damage
- occurrence in an organ or tissue which has

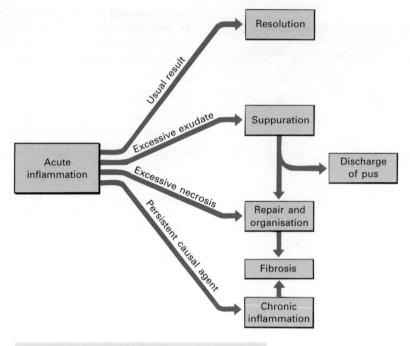

Fig. 10.12   The sequelae of acute inflammation

Resolution is the usual event, unless any of the adverse factors shown exist.

regenerative capacity (e.g. the liver) rather than in one which cannot regenerate (e.g. the central nervous system)

- rapid destruction of the causal agent (e.g. phagocytosis of bacteria)
- rapid removal of fluid and debris by good local vascular drainage.

A good example of an acute inflammatory condition which usually resolves completely is acute lobar pneumonia (Ch. 14). The alveoli become filled with acute inflammatory exudate containing fibrin, bacteria and neutrophil polymorphs. The alveolar walls are thin and have many capillaries (for gas exchange) and lymphatic channels. The sequence of events leading to resolution is usually:

- phagocytosis of bacteria (e.g. pneumococci) by neutrophils and intracellular killing
- fibrinolysis
- phagocytosis of debris, especially by macrophages, and carriage through lymphatics to the hilar lymph nodes
- disappearance of vascular dilatation.

Following this, the lung parenchyma would appear histologically normal.

Suppuration

Suppuration is the formation of pus, a mixture of living, dying and dead neutrophils and bacteria, cellular debris and sometimes globules of lipid. The causative stimulus must be fairly persistent and is virtually always an infective agent, usually pyogenic bacteria (e.g. *Staphylococcus aureus, Streptococcus pyogenes, Neisseria* species or coliform organisms). Once pus begins to accumulate in a tissue, it becomes surrounded by a 'pyogenic membrane' consisting of sprouting capillaries, neutrophils and occasional fibroblasts. Such a collection of pus is called an *abscess*, and bacteria within the abscess cavity are relatively inaccessible to antibodies and to antibiotic drugs (thus, for example, acute osteomyelitis, an abscess in the bone marrow cavity, is notoriously difficult to treat).

Abscess
An abscess (for example, a boil) usually 'points', then bursts; the abscess cavity collapses and is obliterated by organisation and fibrosis, leaving a small scar. Sometimes, surgical incision and drainage is necessary to eliminate the abscess.

If an abscess forms inside a hollow viscus (e.g. the

gallbladder) the mucosal layers of the outflow tract of the viscus may become fused together by fibrin, resulting in an empyema (Fig. 10.9).

Such deep-seated abscesses sometimes discharge their pus along a *sinus tract* (an abnormal connection, lined by granulation tissue, between the abscess and the skin or a mucosal surface). If this results in an abnormal passage connecting two mucosal surfaces or one mucosal surface to the skin surface, it is referred to as a *fistula*. Sinuses occur particularly when foreign body materials are present, which are indigestible by macrophages and which favour continuing suppuration. The only treatment for this type of condition is surgical elimination of the foreign body material.

The fibrous walls of longstanding abscesses may become complicated by *dystrophic calcification* (Ch. 7).

Organisation

Organisation of tissues is their replacement by granulation tissue. The circumstances favouring this outcome are when:

- large amounts of fibrin are formed, which cannot be removed completely by fibrinolytic enzymes from the plasma or from neutrophil polymorphs
- substantial volumes of tissue become necrotic or if the dead tissue (e.g. fibrous tissue) is not easily digested
- exudate and debris cannot be removed or discharged.

During organisation, new capillaries grow into the inert material (inflammatory exudate), macrophages migrate into the zone and fibroblasts proliferate, resulting in *fibrosis*. A good example of this is seen in the pleural space following acute lobar pneumonia. Resolution usually occurs in the lung parenchyma, but very extensive fibrinous exudate fills the pleural cavity (Fig. 10.11). The fibrin is not easily removed and consequently capillaries grow into the fibrin, accompanied by macrophages and fibroblasts (the exudate becomes 'organised'). Eventually, fibrous adhesion occurs between the parietal and visceral pleura (Fig. 10.13).

Progression to chronic inflammation

If the agent causing acute inflammation is not removed, the acute inflammation may progress to the chronic stage. In addition to organisation of the tissue just described, the character of the cellular exudate changes, with lymphocytes, plasma cells and macrophages (sometimes including multinucleate

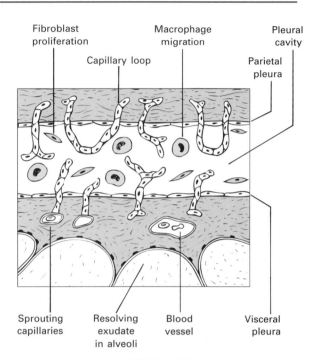

Fig. 10.13 Organisation of the fibrinous pleural exudate

Capillary loops are growing into the exudate, accompanied by fibroblasts and capillaries.

giant cells) replacing the neutrophil polymorphs (Fig. 10.14). Often, however, chronic inflammation occurs as a primary event, there being no preceding period of acute inflammation.

Systemic effects of inflammation

Apart from the local features of acute and chronic inflammation described above, an inflammatory focus produces systemic effects.

Pyrexia
Polymorphs and macrophages produce compounds known as *endogenous pyrogens* which act on the hypothalamus to set the thermoregulatory mechanisms at a higher temperature. Release of endogenous pyrogen is stimulated by phagocytosis, endotoxins and immune complexes.

Constitutional symptoms
Constitutional symptoms include malaise, anorexia and nausea.

Weight loss
Weight loss, due to negative nitrogen balance, is

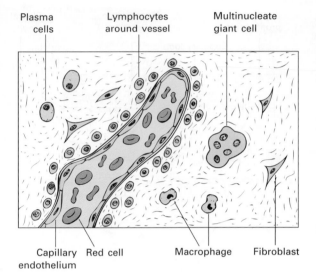

Plasma cells · Lymphocytes around vessel · Multinucleate giant cell

Capillary endothelium · Red cell · Macrophage · Fibroblast

Fig. 10.14   The cells involved in chronic inflammation

Neutrophil polymorphs have disappeared from the site, and mononuclear cells such as lymphocytes and macrophages are prominent. Some specialised lymphocytes called plasma cells are present; these produce immunoglobins. Some of the macrophages may become multinucleate giant cells. Fibroblasts migrate into the area and lay down collagen.

common when there is extensive chronic inflammation. For this reason, tuberculosis used to be called 'consumption'.

Reactive hyperplasia of the reticulo-endothelial system
Local or systemic lymph node enlargement commonly accompanies inflammation, while splenomegaly is found in certain specific infections (e.g. malaria, infectious mononucleosis).

Haematological changes
    Increased erythrocyte sedimentation rate. An increased erythrocyte sedimentation rate is a non-specific finding in many types of inflammation.
    Leukocytosis. Neutrophilia occurs in pyogenic infections and tissue destruction; eosinophilia in allergic disorders and parasitic infection; lymphocytosis in chronic infection (e.g. tuberculosis), many viral infections and in whooping cough; and monocytosis occurs in infectious mononucleosis and certain bacterial infections (e.g. tuberculosis, typhoid).
    Anaemia. This may result from blood loss in the inflammatory exudate (e.g. in ulcerative colitis), haemolysis (due to bacterial toxins), and 'the anaemia of chronic disorders' due to toxic depression of the bone marrow.

Amyloidosis
Longstanding chronic inflammation (for example, in rheumatoid arthritis, tuberculosis and bronchiectasis), by elevating serum amyloid A protein (SAA), may cause amyloid to be deposited in various tissues resulting in *secondary (reactive) amyloidosis* (Ch. 7).

CHRONIC INFLAMMATION

▶ Lymphocytes, plasma cells and macrophages predominate
▶ Usually primary, but may follow recurrent acute inflammation
▶ Granulomatous inflammation is a specific type of chronic inflammation
▶ A granuloma is an aggregate of epithelioid histiocytes
▶ May be complicated by secondary (reactive) amyloidosis

The word 'chronic' applied to any process implies that the process has extended over a long period of time. This is usually the case in chronic inflammation, but here the term 'chronic' takes on a much more specific meaning, in that the type of cellular reaction differs from that seen in acute inflammation. Chronic inflammation may be defined as an inflammatory process in which lymphocytes, plasma cells and macrophages predominate, and which is usually accompanied by the formation of granulation tissue, resulting in fibrosis. Chronic inflammation is usually primary, sometimes called chronic inflammation *ab initio*, but does occasionally follow acute inflammation.

Causes of chronic inflammation

Primary chronic inflammation

In most cases of chronic inflammation, the inflammatory response has all the histological features of chronic inflammation from the onset, and there is no initial phase of acute inflammation. Some examples of primary chronic inflammation are listed in Table 10.3.

Transplant rejection
Cellular rejection of, for example, renal transplants involves chronic inflammatory cell infiltration.

Progression from acute inflammation

Most cases of acute inflammation do not develop

Table 10.3 Some examples of primary chronic inflammation	
Cause of inflammation	Example
Resistance of infective agent to phagocytosis and intracellular killing	Tuberculosis, leprosy, brucellosis, viral infections
Foreign body reactions	Endogenous materials, e.g. necrotic adipose tissue, bone, uric acid crystals Exogenous materials, e.g. silica, asbestos fibres, suture materials, implanted prostheses
Some autoimmune diseases	Organ-specific disease, e.g. Hashimoto's thyroiditis, chronic gastritis of pernicious anaemia Non-organ-specific autoimmune disease, e.g. rheumatoid arthritis Contact hypersensitivity reactions, e.g. self-antigens altered by nickel
Specific diseases of unknown aetiology	Chronic inflammatory bowel disease, e.g. ulcerative colitis
Primary granulomatous diseases	Crohn's disease, sarcoidosis, reactions to beryllium

into the chronic form, but resolve completely. The commonest variety of acute inflammation to progress to chronic inflammation is the suppurative type. If the pus forms an abscess cavity which is deep-seated, and drainage is delayed or inadequate, then by the time that drainage occurs the abscess will have developed thick walls composed of granulation and fibrous tissues. The rigid walls of the abscess cavity therefore fail to come together after drainage, and the stagnating pus within the cavity becomes organised by the ingrowth of granulation tissue, eventually to be replaced by a fibrous scar.

Good examples of such chronic abscesses include: an abscess in the bone marrow cavity (osteomyelitis), which is notoriously difficult to eradicate; and empyema thoracis which has been inadequately drained.

Another feature which favours progression to chronic inflammation is the presence of indigestible material. This may be keratin from a ruptured epidermal cyst, or fragments of necrotic bone as in the sequestrum of chronic osteomyelitis (Ch. 25). These materials are relatively inert, and are resistant to the action of lysosomal enzymes. The most indigestible forms of material are inert foreign body materials:

for example, some types of surgical suture, wood, metal or glass implanted into a wound, or deliberately implanted prostheses such as artificial joints. It is not known why the presence of foreign body materials gives rise to chronic suppuration, but it is a well-established fact that suppuration will not cease without surgical removal of the material.

Foreign bodies have in common the tendency to provoke a special type of chronic inflammation called 'granulomatous inflammation' (p. 241), and to cause macrophages to form multinucleate giant cells called 'foreign body giant cells' (Fig. 10.21B; p. 245).

Recurrent episodes of acute inflammation

Recurring cycles of acute inflammation and healing eventually result in the clinicopathological entity of chronic inflammation. The best example of this is chronic cholecystitis, normally due to the presence of gallstones (Ch. 16); multiple recurrent episodes of acute inflammation lead to replacement of the gallbladder wall muscle by fibrous tissue and the predominant cell type becomes the lymphocyte rather than the neutrophil polymorph.

Macroscopic appearances of chronic inflammation

The commonest appearances of chronic inflammation are:

- *chronic ulcer*, such as a chronic peptic ulcer of the stomach with breach of the mucosa, a base lined by granulation tissue and with fibrous tissue extending through the muscle layers of the wall (Fig. 10.15)
- *chronic abscess cavity*, for example osteomyelitis, empyema thoracis
- *thickening of the wall of a hollow viscus* by fibrous tissue in the presence of a chronic inflammatory cell infiltrate, for example Crohn's disease, chronic cholecystitis (Fig. 10.16)
- *granulomatous inflammation*, perhaps with caseous necrosis as in chronic fibrocaseous tuberculosis of the lung
- *fibrosis*, which may become the most prominent feature of the chronic inflammatory reaction when most of the chronic inflammatory cell infiltrate has subsided. This is commonly seen in chronic cholecystitis, 'hour-glass contracture' of the stomach, where fibrosis distorts the gastric wall and may even lead to acquired pyloric stenosis, and in the strictures which characterise Crohn's disease (Ch. 15).

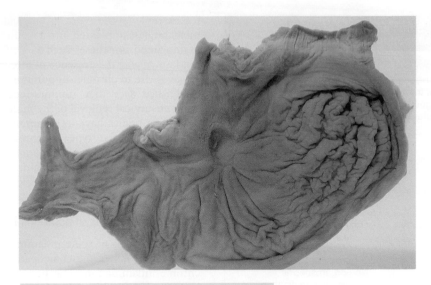

Fig. 10.15 Chronic peptic ulcer of the stomach

Continuing tissue destruction and repair cause replacement of the gastric wall muscle layers by fibrous tissue. As the fibrous tissue contracts, permanent distortion of the gastric shape may result.

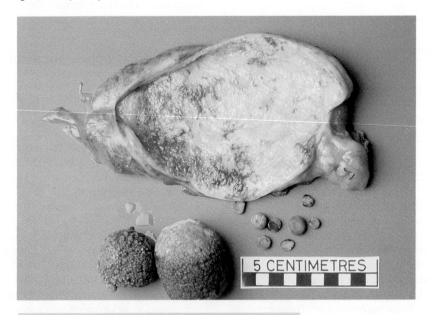

Fig. 10.16 Gallbladder showing chronic cholecystitis

The wall is greatly thickened by fibrous tissue. One of the gallstones was impacted in Hartmann's pouch, a saccular dilatation at the gallbladder neck.

Microscopic features of chronic inflammation

The cellular infiltrate consists characteristically of lymphocytes, plasma cells and macrophages. A few eosinophil polymorphs may be present, but neutrophil polymorphs are scarce. Some of the macrophages may form multinucleate giant cells. Exudation of fluid is not a prominent feature, but there may be production of new fibrous tissue from granulation tissue (Figs 10.15–17). There may be evidence of continuing destruction of tissue at the same time as tissue regeneration and repair. Tissue necrosis may be a prominent feature, especially in granulomatous conditions such as tuberculosis. It is not usually possible to predict the causative factor from the histological appearances in chronic inflammation.

Paracrine stimulation of connective tissue proliferation

Healing involves regeneration and migration of spe-cialised cells, while the predominant features in repair are angiogenesis followed by fibroblast prolif-eration and collagen synthesis. These processes are regulated by low molecular weight proteins called *growth factors* which bind to specific receptors on cell membranes and trigger a series of events culminat-ing in cell proliferation (Table 10.4).

Cellular co-operation in chronic inflammation

The lymphocytic tissue infiltrate contains two main types of lymphocyte (described more fully in Ch. 9).

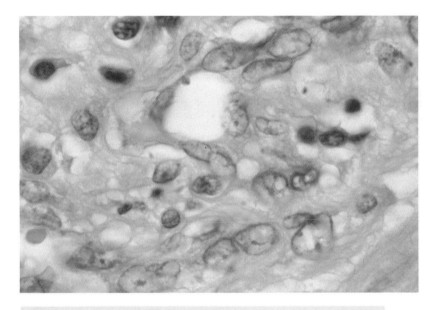

Fig. 10.17 Chronic inflammation at the edge of a chronic peptic ulcer
Ingrowing capillaries are surrounded by mononuclear cells and fibroblasts.

Table 10.4 Growth factors involved in healing and repair associated with inflammation

Growth factor	Abbreviation	Function
Epidermal growth factor	EGF	Regeneration of epithelial cells
Transforming growth factor α	TGF α	Regeneration of epithelial cells
Transforming growth factor β	TGF β	Stimulates fibroblast proliferation and collagen synthesis Controls epithelial regeneration
Platelet-derived growth factor	PDGF	Mitogenic and chemotactic for fibroblasts and smooth muscle cells
Fibroblast growth factors	FGF	Stimulates fibroblast proliferation, angiogenesis and epithelial cell regeneration
Insulin-like growth factor-1	IGF-1	Synergistic effect with other growth factors
Tumour necrosis factor	TNF	Stimulates angiogenesis

B-lymphocytes, on contact with antigen, become progressively transformed into plasma cells, which are cells specially adapted for the production of antibodies. The other main type of lymphocyte, the T-lymphocyte, is responsible for cell-mediated immunity. On contact with antigen, T-lymphocytes produce a range of soluble factors called cytokines, which have a number of important activities.

- *Recruitment of macrophages into the area.* It is thought that macrophages are recruited into the area mainly via factors such as migration inhibition factor (MIF) which trap macrophages in the tissue. Macrophage activation factors (MAF) stimulate macrophage phagocytosis and killing of bacteria.
- *Production of inflammatory mediators.* T-lymphocytes produce a number of inflammatory mediators, including cytokines, chemotactic factors for neutrophils, and factors which increase vascular permeability.
- *Recruitment of other lymphocytes.* Interleukins stimulate other lymphocytes to divide and confer

on other lymphocytes the ability to mount cell-mediated immune responses to a variety of antigens. T-lymphocytes also co-operate with B-lymphocytes, assisting them in recognising antigens.

- *Destruction of target cells.* Factors, such as perforins (Ch. 6), are produced which destroy other cells by damaging their cell membranes.
- *Interferon production.* Interferon γ, produced by activated T-cells, has antiviral properties and, in turn, activates macrophages. Interferons α and β, produced by macrophages and fibroblasts, have antiviral properties and activate natural killer (NK) cells and macrophages.

These pathways of cellular co-operation are summarised in Figure 10.18.

Macrophages in chronic inflammation

Macrophages are relatively large cells, up to 30 μm in diameter, which move by amoeboid motion

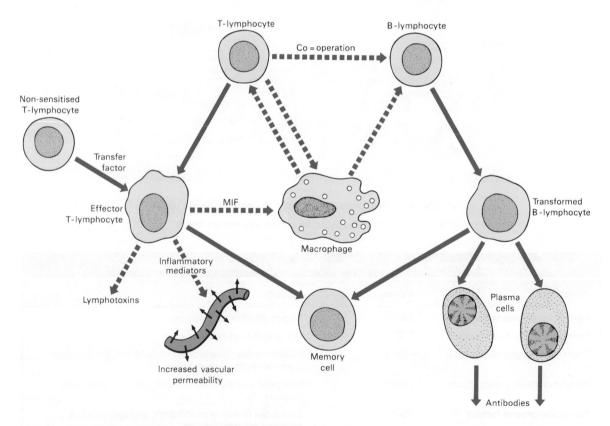

Fig. 10.18   Cellular co-operation in chronic inflammation

Solid arrows show pathways of cellular differentiation. Dotted arrows show intercellular communication. (MIF = migration inhibition factors.)

through the tissues. They respond to certain chemotactic stimuli (possibly cytokines and antigen–antibody complexes) and have considerable phagocytic capabilities for the ingestion of micro-organisms and cell debris. When neutrophil polymorphs ingest micro-organisms, they usually bring about their own destruction and thus have a limited life-span of up to about three days. Macrophages can ingest a wider range of materials than can polymorphs and, being long-lived, they can harbour viable organisms if they are not able to kill them by their lysosomal enzymes. Examples of organisms which can survive inside macrophages include mycobacteria, such as *Mycobacterium tuberculosis* and *Mycobacterium leprae*, and organisms such as *Histoplasma capsulatum*. When macrophages participate in the delayed type hypersensitivity response (Ch. 9) to these types of organism, they often die in the process, contributing to the large areas of necrosis by release of their lysosomal enzymes.

Macrophages in inflamed tissues are derived from blood monocytes which have migrated out of vessels and have become transformed in the tissues. They are thus part of the *mononuclear phagocyte system* (Fig. 10.19). This system is in turn part of the *reticuloendothelial system* which refers not only to the phagocytic cells, but also to interdigitating reticulum cells of lymph nodes and the endothelial cells in lymphoid organs.

The mononuclear phagocyte system, shown in Figure 10.19, is now known to include macrophages, fixed tissue histiocytes in many organs and, probably, the osteoclasts of bone. All are derived from monocytes which in turn are derived from a haemopoietic stem cell in the bone marrow.

The 'activation' of macrophages as they migrate into an area of inflammation involves an increase in size, protein synthesis, mobility, phagocytic activity and content of lysosomal enzymes. Electron microscopy reveals that the cells have a roughened cell membrane bearing filopodia, while the cytoplasm contains numerous dense bodies—phagolysosomes (formed by the fusion of lysosomes with phagocytic vacuoles).

Macrophages produce a range of important cytokines, including interferons α and β, interleukins 1, 6 and 8, and tumour necrosis factor (TNF) α (see Ch. 9).

Specialised forms of macrophages and granulomatous inflammation

A *granuloma* is an aggregate of epithelioid histiocytes (Fig. 10.20).

Epithelioid histiocytes

Named for their vague histological resemblance to

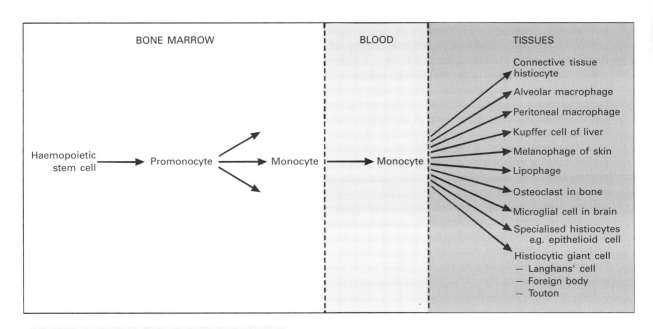

Fig. 10.19 The mononuclear phagocyte system

All of the differentiated cell types on the right are derived from blood monocytes.

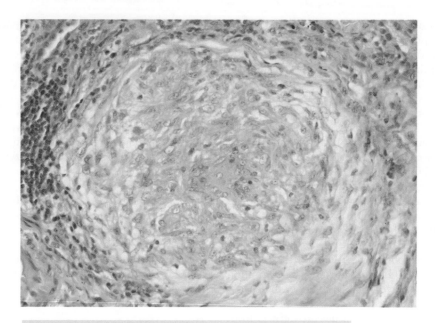

Fig. 10.20   A granuloma: a collection of epithelioid histiocytes

This example is from a case of sarcoidosis involving the liver.

epithelial cells, epithelioid histiocytes have large vesicular nuclei, plentiful eosinophilic cytoplasm and are often rather elongated. They tend to be arranged in clusters. They have little phagocytic activity, but appear to be adapted to a secretory function. The full range, or purpose, of their secretory products is not known, although one product is *angiotensin converting enzyme*. Measurement of the activity of this enzyme in the blood can act as a marker for systemic granulomatous disease, such as sarcoidosis.

The appearance of granulomas may be augmented by the presence of caseous necrosis (as in tuberculosis) or by the conversion of some of the histiocytes into multinucleate giant cells (Fig. 10.21). A common feature of many of the stimuli which induce granulomatous inflammation is indigestibility of particulate matter by macrophages. In other conditions, such as the systemic granulomatous condition *sarcoidosis*, there appear to be far-reaching derangements in immune responsiveness favouring granulomatous inflammation. In other instances, small traces of elements such as beryllium induce granuloma formation, but the way in which they induce the inflammation is unknown. Some of the commoner granulomatous conditions are shown in Table 10. 5.

Histiocytic giant cells

Histiocytic giant cells tend to form where particulate

Table 10.5 Causes of granulomatous disease	
Cause	**Example**
Specific infections	Mycobacteria, e.g. tuberculosis, leprosy, atypical mycobacteria Many types of fungi Parasites, larvae, eggs and worms Syphilis
Foreign bodies	Endogenous, e.g. keratin, necrotic bone, cholesterol crystals, sodium urate Exogenous, e.g. talc, silica, suture materials, oils, silicone
Specific chemicals	Beryllium
Drugs	Hepatic granulomas due to allopurinol, phenylbutazone, sulphonamides
Unknown	Crohn's disease Sarcoidosis Wegener's granulomatosis

matter which is indigestible by macrophages accumulates, for example inert minerals such as silica, or bacteria such as tubercle bacilli which have cell walls containing mycolic acids and waxes which resist enzymatic digestion. The multinucleate giant cells,

Fig. 10.21   Giant cells

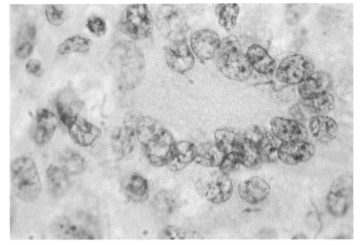

A. Langhans' giant cell. Multiple nuclei are arranged in a horseshoe shape at one pole of the cell. This example is in a tuberculous lymph node.

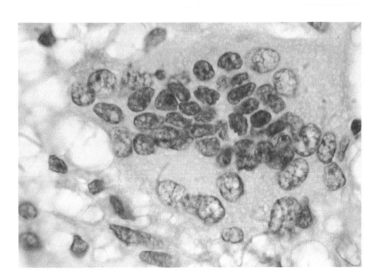

B. Foreign body giant cell. Multiple nuclei are scattered randomly throughout the cytoplasm of this giant cell from the site of a surgical incision sutured with synthetic material.

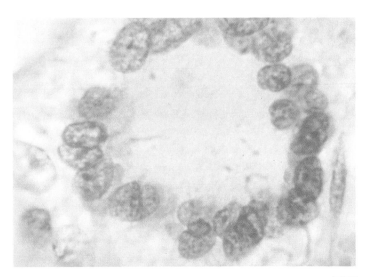

C. Touton giant cell. The multiple nuclei are arranged in a ring, surrounded by clear lipid-containing cytoplasm. This is from a cutaneous xanthoma.

which may contain over 100 nuclei, are thought to develop 'by accident' when two or more macrophages attempt simultaneously to engulf the same particle; their cell membranes fuse and the cells unite. The multinucleate giant cells resulting have little phagocytic activity and no known function. They are given specific names according to their microscopic appearance.

Langhans' giant cells

Langhans' giant cells have a horseshoe arrangement of peripheral nuclei at one pole of the cell (Fig. 10.21A) and are characteristically seen in tuberculosis, although they may be seen in other granulomatous conditions. (They must not be confused with Langerhans' cells, the dendritic antigen-presenting cells of the epidermis; Ch. 9.)

Foreign-body giant cells

So-called 'foreign-body giant cells' are large cells with nuclei randomly scattered throughout their cytoplasm (Fig. 10.21B). They are characteristically seen in relation to particulate foreign-body material.

Touton giant cells

Touton giant cells have a central ring of nuclei while the peripheral cytoplasm is clear due to accumulated lipid (Fig. 10.21C). They are seen at sites of adipose tissue breakdown and in xanthomas (tumour-like aggregates of lipid-laden macrophages).

Although giant cells are commonly seen in granulomas, they do not constitute a defining feature. Solitary giant cells in the absence of epithelioid histiocytes do not constitute a granuloma.

FURTHER READING

Adams D O 1976 The granulomatous inflammatory response. American Journal of Pathology 84: 163–192

Allison A C 1978 Lysosomes in pathology. In: Anthony P P, Woolf N (eds) Recent advances in histopathology 10. Churchill Livingstone, Edinburgh, pp 69–90

Cohen M S 1994 Molecular events in the activation of human neutrophils for microbial killing. Clinical Infectious Diseases 18 (suppl 2): 170–179

Fantone J C, Ward P A 1985 Polymorphonuclear leucocyte-mediated cell and tissue injury: oxygen metabolites and their relations to human disease. Human Pathology 16: 973–978

Fossum S, Ford WL 1983 The organisation of cell populations within lymph nodes. Histopathology 9: 469–499

Hurley J V 1983 Acute inflammation, 2nd edn. Churchill Livingstone, Edinburgh

Nelson D S 1976 Immunobiology of the macrophage. Academic Press, London

Roitt M, Brostoff J, Male D K 1985 Immunology. Churchill Livingstone, Edinburgh

Wilkinson P C 1982 Chemotaxis and inflammation, 2nd edn. Churchill Livingstone, Edinburgh

Zweifach B W 1973–74. The inflammatory process. Academic Press, New York

11

Carcinogenesis and neoplasia

GENERAL CHARACTERISTICS OF NEOPLASMS (TUMOURS)

▶ Tumours result from genetic alterations (e.g. mutations) in cells, resulting in abnormal (neoplastic) growth persisting in the absence of the initiating causes
▶ Malignant (invasive) tumours develop in approximately 25% of individuals
▶ Incidence increases with age
▶ Structure comprises neoplastic cells and connective tissue stroma of which the vascular supply is essential for growth

Definitions

The word *tumour* means literally an abnormal swelling. However, in the language of modern medicine, the word has a much more specific meaning. *A tumour (neoplasm) is a lesion resulting from the autonomous or relatively autonomous abnormal growth of cells which persists after the initiating stimulus has been removed.*

Tumours can result from the *neoplastic transformation* of any nucleated cell in the body, although some cell types are more prone to tumour formation than others; the transformed cells are called *neoplastic cells*. By transformation involving a series of *genetic alterations* (e.g. mutations), cells escape permanently from normal growth regulatory mechanisms. The neoplastic cells in tumours designated *malignant* possess additional potentially lethal abnormal characteristics enabling them to *invade* and to *metastasise*, or spread, to other tissues.

Neoplastic cells grow to form abnormal swellings, but this is not the only cause of abnormal swellings. Swellings or organ enlargement can also result from inflammation, hypertrophy or hyperplasia.

The term *neoplasm* (new growth) is synonymous with the medical meaning of the word tumour and is often used in preference because it is less ambiguous and not quite so alarming when overheard by patients. *Cancer* is a word used more in the public arena than in medicine; it has emotive connotations and generally refers to a *malignant* tumour or neoplasm.

Incidence of tumours

Malignant neoplasms—those that invade and spread and are therefore of greater clinical importance—develop in approximately 25% of the population in the UK. The individual risk increases with age, but

tumours can occur even in infancy (Fig. 11.1). The mortality rate is high, despite modern therapy, so that cancer accounts for about one-fifth of all deaths in developed countries. However, the mortality rate varies considerably between specific tumour types.

The relative incidence by diagnosis and death of various common types of cancer is shown in Table 11.1. Lung cancer is the most frequent single malignant neoplasm in the UK and USA, and its importance is compounded by the extremely poor prognosis. In other countries other cancers are more common, and these differences often provide important aetiological clues.

For various reasons most epidemiological data on cancer incidence probably underestimate the true incidence. Not all tumours become clinically evident and, unless a thorough autopsy is performed, may never be detected. For example, autopsy surveys have revealed a higher than expected incidence of occult carcinoma of the prostate in elderly men, although these often minute lesions are probably of little clinical consequence. Cancer incidence may also be underestimated due to a failure of detection or diagnosis in countries and communities with poor health care.

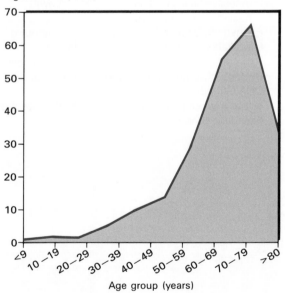

Cancer registrations ('000)

Age group (years)

Fig. 11.1   Cancer registration in different age groups in the UK, 1984

Cancer occurs at all ages but is most common over the age of 50 years. The declining incidence in the very elderly is partly due to the reduced population size.

Table 11.1 Tumour incidence and mortality in the United Kingdom.
Ten highest ranking tumours are listed in order of incidence and mortality (based on annual data from 1985–89 and published by Cancer Research Campaign, 1991)

Incidence ranking (total cancer cases 253 110)		Mortality ranking (total cancer deaths 163 770)	
Males (total cancer cases 119 960)	**Females** (total cancer cases 133 150)	**Males** (total cancer deaths 84 710)	**Females** (total cancer deaths 79 060)
Lung 24%	Breast 19%	Lung 32%	Breast 20%
Skin 12%	Skin 9%	Prostate 10%	Lung 16%
Prostate 9%	Lung 9%	Stomach 7%	Colon 9%
Bladder 6%	Colon 7%	Colon 7%	Ovary 6%
Colon 6%	Ovary 4%	Rectum 4%	Stomach 5%
Stomach 6%	Stomach 4%	Bladder 4%	Pancreas 5%
Rectum 5%	Rectum 3%	Oesophagus 4%	Rectum 4%
Pancreas 3%	Cervix 3%	Pancreas 4%	Oesophagus 3%
Oesophagus 2%	Uterus 3%	Leukaemia 3%	Cervix 3%
Leukaemia 2%	Pancreas 2%	Brain 2%	Leukaemia 2%

Structure of tumours

Solid tumours consist of *neoplastic cells* and *stroma* (see below and Fig. 11.2). The neoplastic cell population reproduces to a variable extent the growth pattern and synthetic activity of the parent cell of origin. Depending on its functional resemblance to the parent tissue, it continues to synthesise and secrete cell products such as collagen, mucin or keratin; these often accumulate within the tumour where they are recognisable histologically. Other cell products may be secreted into the blood where they can be detected by other methods.

Stroma

The neoplastic cell population is embedded in and

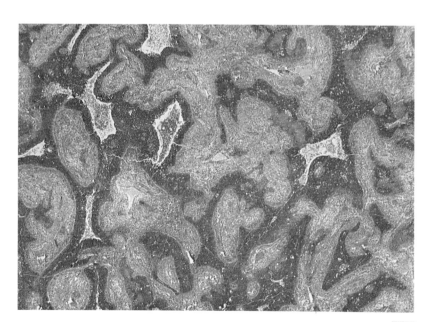

Fig. 11.2 Tumour cells and stroma

Histology of an invasive squamous cell carcinoma of the cervix showing the darkly-staining tumour cells embedded in a lighter-staining connective tissue stroma.

supported by a connective tissue framework called the stroma (from the Greek word meaning a mattress), which provides mechanical support and nutrition to the neoplastic cells. The process of stroma formation is called a *desmoplastic reaction* and may be due to induction of connective tissue proliferation by growth factors in the immediate tumour environment.

Tumour stroma always contains blood vessels which perfuse the tumour (Fig. 11.3); this vascular proliferation is thought to be induced by angiogenic factors produced by the tumour cells. The growth of a tumour is dependent upon its ability to induce blood vessels to perfuse it, for unless it becomes permeated by a vascular supply its growth will be limited by the ability of nutrients to diffuse into it, and the tumour cells will cease growing when the nodule has attained a diameter of no more than 1–2 mm (Fig. 11.4).

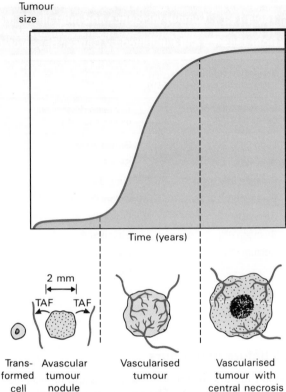

Fig. 11.4 Tumour angiogenesis

Neoplastic transformation of a single cell results in the growth of a tumour nodule, limited by the ability of nutrients to diffuse into it to a diameter of 1–2 mm. Production of tumour angiogenic factors (TAF) stimulates the proliferation and ingrowth of blood vessels, enabling tumour growth to be supported by perfusion. Eventually, the tumour outgrows its blood supply, and areas of necrosis appear resulting in slower growth.

Fibroblasts offer some mechanical support for the tumour cells and may in addition have nutritive properties. Stromal myofibroblasts are often abundant, particularly in carcinomas of the breast; their contractility is responsible for the puckering and retraction of adjacent structures.

The stroma often contains a lymphocytic infiltrate of variable density; this may reflect a host immune reaction to the tumour (Ch. 9), a hypothesis supported by the observation that patients whose tumours are densely infiltrated by lymphocytes tend to have a better prognosis.

Tumour shape and correlation with behaviour

The gross appearance of a tumour on a surface (e.g. gastrointestinal mucosa) may be described as sessile,

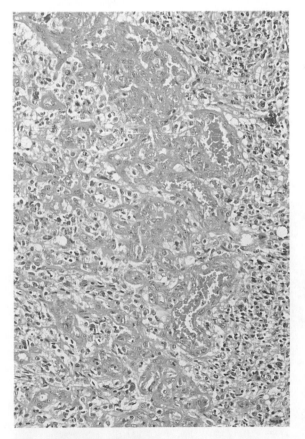

Fig. 11.3 Vascular stroma

Histology of an astrocytoma in the brain in which the stroma consists of numerous small blood vessels.

generally benign, i.e. unlikely to spread beyond the tissue of origin (Fig. 11.6), whereas ulceration is more commonly associated with aggressive behav-

iour (Fig. 11.7).

Ulcerated tumours can often be distinguished from non-neoplastic ulcers, such as peptic ulcers in the stomach, because the former tend to have heaped-up or rolled edges.

The shape of connective tissue neoplasms can be misleading. Although circumscription by a clearly defined border is one of the characteristics of benign tumours, some malignant connective tissue tumours are also well circumscribed.

Tumours are usually firmer than the surrounding tissue, causing a palpable lump in accessible sites such as the breasts. Extremely hard tumours are often referred to as 'scirrhous'. Softer lesions are sometimes called 'medullary'; they occur in the thyroid and breasts.

The cut surfaces of malignant tumours are often variegated due to areas of necrosis and degene-

Sessile

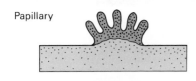

Pedunculated polyp

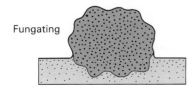

Papillary

Fungating

Ulcerated

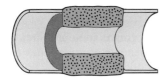

Annular

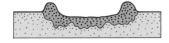

Fig. 11.5 Tumour shapes

Sessile, polypoid and papillary tumours are usually benign. Fungating, ulcerated or annular tumours are more likely to be malignant. Annular tumours encircling a tubular structure (e.g. intestine) are common in the large bowel, where they often cause intestinal obstruction.

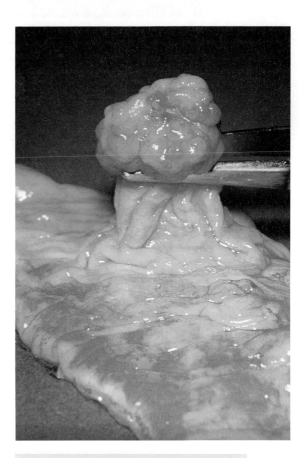

Fig. 11.6 Adenomatous polyp of the colon

This common lesion has a clearly visible stalk enabling relatively easy removal by endoscopy. Although benign, these lesions are precursors of adenocarcinoma of the large bowel.

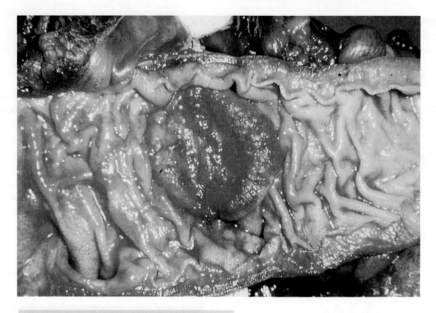

Fig. 11.7   Adenocarcinoma of the colon
The lesion has an ulcerated surface and invades the underlying bowel wall.

ration, but some, such as lymphomas and seminomas, appear uniformly bland.

CLASSIFICATION OF TUMOURS

> ▶ Behavioural classification: benign or malignant
> ▶ Histogenetic classification: cell of origin
> ▶ Precise classification of individual tumours is important for planning treatment

Tumours are classified according to their *behaviour* and *histogenesis* (cell of origin).

Behavioural classification

The behavioural classification divides tumours into:

- benign
- malignant.

The principal pathological criteria for classifying a tumour as benign or malignant are summarised in Table 11.2. Some tumours, such as some ovarian tumours, defy precise behavioural classification, because their histology is intermediate between that associated with benign and malignant tumours; these are often referred to as 'borderline' tumours.

Benign tumours

> ▶ Non-invasive and remain localised
> ▶ Slow growth rate
> ▶ Close histological resemblance to parent tissue

Benign tumours remain localised. They are slowly growing lesions which do not invade the surrounding tissues or spread to other sites in the body.

When a benign tumour arises in an epithelial or mucosal surface, the tumour grows away from the surface, because it cannot invade, often forming a *polyp* which may be either pedunculated (stalked) or sessile; this non-invasive outward direction of growth creates an *exophytic* lesion (Fig. 11.8). Benign tumours in solid organs are typically well circumscribed, often surrounded by a fibrous capsule. Histologically, benign tumours closely resemble the parent cell or tissue.

Although benign tumours are, by definition, confined to their site of origin, they may cause clinical problems due to:

- pressure on adjacent tissues (e.g. benign meningeal tumour causing epilepsy)
- obstruction to the flow of fluid (e.g. benign epithelial tumour blocking a duct)
- production of a hormone (e.g. benign thyroid tumour causing thyrotoxicosis)

Table 11.2 Principal characteristics of benign and malignant tumours

Feature	Benign	Malignant
Growth rate	Slow	Relatively rapid
Mitotic activity	Low	High
Histological resemblance to normal tissue	Good	Variable, often poor
Nuclear morphology	Often normal	Usually hyperchromatic, irregular outline, multiple nucleoli and pleomorphic
Invasion	No	Yes
Metastases	Never	Frequent
Border	Often circumscribed or encapsulated	Often poorly defined or irregular
Necrosis	Rare	Common
Ulceration	Rare	Common on skin or mucosal surfaces
Direction of growth on skin or mucosal surfaces	Often exophytic	Often endophytic

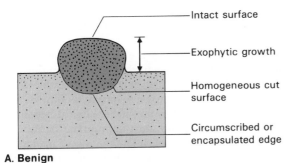

Intact surface
Exophytic growth
Homogeneous cut surface
Circumscribed or encapsulated edge

A. Benign

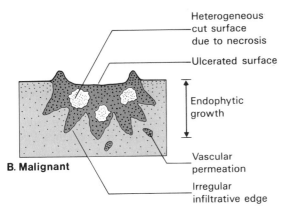

Heterogeneous cut surface due to necrosis
Ulcerated surface
Endophytic growth
Vascular permeation
Irregular infiltrative edge

B. Malignant

Fig. 11.8 Benign and malignant tumours growing on surfaces (e.g. skin, bowel wall), showing the principal differences in their gross appearances.

- obstruction to the flow of fluid (e.g. benign epithelial tumour blocking a duct)
- production of a hormone (e.g. benign thyroid tumour causing thyrotoxicosis)
- transformation into a malignant neoplasm (e.g. adenomatous polyp progressing to an adenocarcinoma)
- anxiety (because the patient fears that the lesion may be something more sinister).

Malignant tumours

- ▶ Invasive and thus capable of spreading directly or by metastasis
- ▶ Relatively rapid growth rate
- ▶ Variable histological resemblance to the parent tissue

Malignant tumours are, by definition, invasive. They are typically rapidly growing and poorly circumscribed. Histologically, they resemble the parent cell or tissue to a lesser extent than do benign tumours. Malignant tumours encroach on and destroy the adjacent tissues (Fig. 11.8), enabling the neoplastic cells to penetrate the walls of blood vessels and lymphatic channels and thereby disseminate to other sites. This important process is called *metastasis* and the resulting secondary tumours are called *metastases* (see p. 286). Patients with widespread metastases are often said to have *carcinomatosis*.

Not all tumours categorised as malignant exhibit metastatic behaviour. For example, basal cell carcinoma of the skin (rodent ulcer) rarely forms metastases, yet is regarded as malignant because it is highly invasive and destructive.

Malignant tumours on epithelial or mucosal surfaces may form a protrusion in the early stages, but eventually invade the underlying tissue; this invasive inward direction of growth gives rise to an *endophytic* tumour. Ulceration is common.

Malignant tumours in solid organs tend to be

poorly circumscribed, sometimes throwing out strands of neoplastic tissue into the adjacent normal structures; it is from the resemblance of the cut surface of these lesions to a crab (Latin: *cancer*) that the disease gets its name. Malignant tumours often show *central necrosis* because of defective vascular perfusion.

The considerable morbidity and mortality associated with malignant tumours may be due to:

- pressure on and destruction of adjacent tissue
- formation of secondary tumours (metastases)
- blood loss from ulcerated surfaces
- obstruction of flow (e.g. malignant tumour of the colon causing intestinal obstruction)
- production of a hormone (e.g. ACTH and ADH from some lung tumours)
- other paraneoplastic effects causing weight loss and debility
- anxiety and pain.

Histogenetic classification

> ► Classification by cell of origin
> ► Histologically determined
> ► Degree of histological resemblance to parent tissue allows tumours to be graded
> ► Histological grade correlates with clinical behaviour

Histogenesis — the specific cell of origin of an individual tumour — is determined by histopathological examination and specifies the tumour *type*. This is eventually incorporated in the name given to the tumour (e.g. squamous cell carcinoma).

Histogenetic classification includes numerous subdivisions, but the major categories of origin are:

- from epithelial cells
- from connective tissues
- from lymphoid and haemopoietic organs.

Although some general differences exist between the main groups of malignant tumours (Table 11.3), individual lesions have to be more precisely categorised both in clinical practice and for epidemiological purposes. It is inadequate to label the patient's tumour as merely having an epithelial or connective tissue origin; efforts must be made to determine the precise cell type. The classification of individual tumours is vitally important. It is dependent upon thorough histological examination of the tumour, sometimes using special techniques like electron microscopy and immunocytochemistry to detect subtle features that betray its provenance.

Table 11.3 Principal characteristics of carcinomas and sarcomas

Feature	Carcinoma	Sarcoma
Origin	Epithelium	Connective tissues
Behaviour	Malignant	Malignant
Frequency	Common	Relatively rare
Preferred route of metastasis	Lymph	Blood
In situ phase	Yes	No
Age group	Usually over 50 years	Usually below 50 years

Differentiation

The term *differentiation* means the degree to which the tumour resembles histologically its cell or tissue of origin; it determines the tumour *grade*. Benign tumours are not usually further classified in this way because they nearly always closely resemble their parent tissue and because a description of the degree of differentiation offers no further clinical benefit in terms of dictating the most appropriate treatment. However, the degree of differentiation of malignant tumours is clinically useful both because it correlates strongly with patient survival (prognosis), and because it often indicates the most appropriate treatment. Thus, malignant tumours are usually graded either as well, moderately or poorly differentiated or numerically, often by strict criteria, as grade 1, grade 2 or grade 3.

A well-differentiated tumour more closely resembles the parent tissue than does a poorly differentiated tumour, while moderately differentiated tumours are intermediate between these two extremes. Poorly differentiated tumours are more aggressive than well-differentiated tumours.

A few tumours are so poorly differentiated that they lack easily recognisable histogenetic features. There may even be great difficulty in deciding whether they are carcinomas or lymphomas, for example, although immunocytochemistry and electron microscopy often enable a distinction to be made. Tumours defying precise histogenetic classification are often referred to as 'anaplastic', or by some purely descriptive term such as 'spindle cell' or 'small round cell' tumour. Fortunately, advances in diagnostic histopathology have resulted in considerably fewer unclassifiable tumours and these descriptive terms are rapidly becoming obsolete.

NOMENCLATURE OF TUMOURS

> ▶ All have the suffix '-oma'
> ▶ Benign epithelial tumours are either papillomas or adenomas
> ▶ Benign connective tissue tumours have a prefix denoting the cell of origin
> ▶ Malignant epithelial tumours are carcinomas
> ▶ Malignant connective tissue tumours are sarcomas

Tumours justify separate names because, although they are all manifestations of the same disease process, each separately named tumour has its own characteristics in terms of cause, appearance and behaviour. Accurate diagnosis and naming of tumours is essential so that patients can be optimally treated. A tumour that defies accurate classification is designated *anaplastic*; such tumours are always malignant.

The specific name of an individual tumour invariably ends in the suffix '-oma'. However, relics of this suffix's former wider usage remain, as in 'granuloma', an inflammatory aggregate of epithelioid macrophages, 'tuberculoma', the large fibrocaseating lesion of tuberculosis, and 'mycetoma', a fungal mass populating a lung cavity; these are *not* neoplasms.

There are exceptions to the rules of nomenclature that follow and these are a potential source of misunderstanding. For example, the words 'melanoma' and 'lymphoma' are both commonly used to refer to malignant tumours of melanocytes and lymphoid cells respectively, even though, from the rules of tumour nomenclature, these terms can be mistakenly interpreted as meaning benign lesions. To avoid confusion, which could be clinically disastrous, their names are often preceded by the word 'malignant'. Similarly, a 'myeloma' is a malignant neoplasm of plasma cells.

The suffix for neoplastic disorders of blood cells is '-aemia', as in leukaemia; but again, exceptions exist. For example, anaemia is not a neoplastic disorder.

Detailed descriptions of individual tumours are, in most instances, included in the relevant systems chapters. Examples of tumour nomenclature are given below and, for reference, in Table 11.4.

Epithelial tumours

Epithelial tumours are named histogenetically according to their specific epithelial type and behaviourally as benign or malignant.

Benign epithelial tumours

Benign epithelial tumours are either:

- papillomas
- adenomas.

A *papilloma* is a benign tumour of non-glandular or non-secretory epithelium, such as transitional or stratified squamous epithelium (Fig. 11.9). An *adenoma* is a benign tumour of glandular or secretory epithelium (Fig. 11.10). The name of a papilloma or adenoma is incomplete unless prefixed by the name of the specific epithelial cell type or glandular origin; examples include squamous cell papilloma, transitional cell papilloma, colonic adenoma and thyroid adenoma.

Table 11.4	**Examples of tumour nomenclature**	
Type	Benign	Malignant
Epithelial		
Squamous cell	Squamous cell papilloma	Squamous cell carcinoma
Transitional	Transitional cell papilloma	Transitional cell carcinoma
Basal cell	Basal cell papilloma	Basal cell carcinoma
Glandular	Adenoma (e.g. thyroid adenoma)	Adenocarcinoma (e.g. adenocarcinoma of breast)
Mesenchymal		
Smooth muscle	Leiomyoma	Leiomyosarcoma
Striated muscle	Rhabdomyoma	Rhabdomyosarcoma
Adipose tissue	Lipoma	Liposarcoma
Blood vessels	Angioma	Angiosarcoma
Bone	Osteoma	Osteosarcoma
Cartilage	Chondroma	Chondrosarcoma
Mesothelium	Benign mesothelioma	Malignant mesothelioma
Synovium	Synovioma	Synovial sarcoma

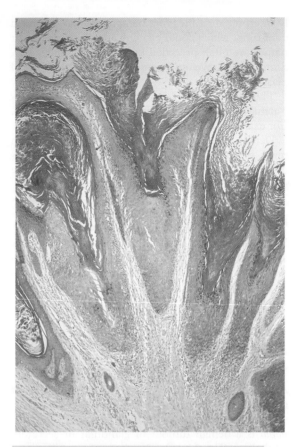

Fig. 11.9 Histology of a benign tumour of non-secretory epithelium: squamous cell papilloma

The tumour is non-invasive and grows outwards from the skin surface (i.e. it is exophytic). The tumour cells closely resemble those of the normal epidermis. This benign tumour is commonly caused by a human papilloma virus.

Malignant epithelial tumours

Malignant tumours of epithelium are always called *carcinomas*. Carcinomas of non-glandular epithelium are always prefixed by the name of the epithelial cell type; examples include squamous cell carcinoma and transitional cell carcinoma. Malignant tumours of glandular epithelium are always designated *adenocarcinomas*, coupled with the name of the tissue of origin; examples include adenocarcinoma of the breast, adenocarcinoma of the prostate and adenocarcinoma of the stomach.

Carcinomas should be further categorised according to their degree of differentiation: their resemblance to the tissue of origin (Fig. 11.11).

Carcinoma in situ

The term *carcinoma in situ* refers to an epithelial neo-plasm exhibiting all the cellular features associated with malignancy, but which has not yet invaded through the epithelial basement membrane separating it from potential routes of metastasis—blood vessels and lymphatics (Fig. 11.12). It is only at this very early stage that excision of a carcinoma will guarantee a cure. Detection of carcinomas at the in situ stage, or of their precursor lesions, is the aim of population screening programmes for cervical, breast and some other carcinomas. The phase of in situ growth may last for several years before invasion commences.

Carcinoma in situ may be preceded by a phase of *dysplasia*, in which the epithelium shows disordered differentiation short of frank neoplasia. Some dysplastic lesions are almost certainly reversible. As there are other applications of the word 'dysplasia' as well as some difficulty in reliably distinguishing between carcinoma in situ and dysplasia in biopsies, the term is now less favoured. The term '*intraepithelial neoplasia*', as in cervical intraepithelial neoplasia (CIN), is used to embrace both carcinoma in situ and the precursor lesions formerly known as dysplasia.

Connective tissue and other mesenchymal tumours

Tumours of connective and other mesenchymal tissues are, like epithelial tumours, named according to their cell of origin and their behavioural classification.

Benign connective tissue and mesenchymal tumours

Benign mesenchymal tumours are named after the cell or tissue of origin suffixed by '-oma', as follows:

- *lipoma*: benign tumour of the lipocytes of adipose tissue
- *rhabdomyoma*: benign tumour of striated muscle
- *leiomyoma*: benign tumour of smooth muscle cells
- *chondroma*: benign tumour of cartilage
- *osteoma*: benign tumour of bone
- *angioma*: benign vascular tumour.

Malignant connective tissue and mesenchymal tumours

Malignant tumours of mesenchyme are always designated *sarcomas*, prefixed by the name that describes the cell or tissue of origin. Examples include:

- *liposarcoma*: malignant tumour of lipocytes
- *rhabdomyosarcoma*: malignant tumour of striated muscle

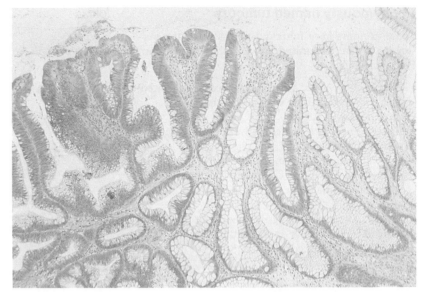

Fig. 11.10 Histology of a benign tumour of secretory epithelium: adenoma of the colon

The tumour grows into the lumen of the bowel on a stalk to form a polyp. The tumour cells closely resemble those of the normal colonic epithelium and contain mucin within their cytoplasm.

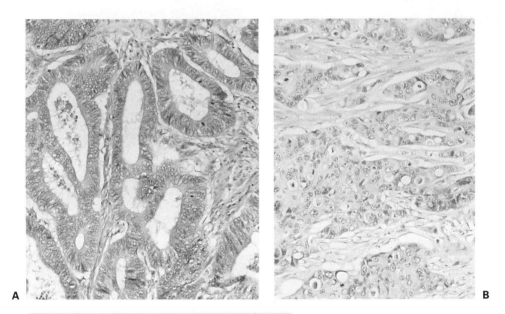

A

B

Fig. 11.11 Histological grading of differentiation

A. Well-differentiated adenocarcinoma of the colon characterised by glandular structures similar to those in normal mucosa.
B. Poorly differentiated adenocarcinoma of the colon characterised by a more solid growth pattern with little evidence of gland formation.

- *leiomyosarcoma*: malignant tumour of smooth muscle
- *chondrosarcoma*: malignant tumour of cartilage
- *osteosarcoma*: malignant tumour of bone
- *angiosarcoma*: malignant vascular tumour.

As with carcinomas, sarcomas can be further categorised according to their grade or degree of differentiation (Fig. 11.13).

Eponymously named tumours

Some tumours have inherited the name of the person who first recognised or described the lesion. Examples include:

- *Burkitt's lymphoma*: a B-cell lymphoma associated with the Epstein–Barr virus and endemic in certain parts of Africa
- *Ewing's sarcoma*: a malignant tumour of bone of uncertain histogenesis
- *Grawitz tumour*: a carcinoma of renal tubular epithelium, now more commonly called renal adenocarcinoma or clear-cell carcinoma of the kidney
- *Kaposi's sarcoma*: a malignant neoplasm possibly derived from vascular endothelium, now commonly associated with AIDS.

Miscellaneous tumours

Most tumours can be categorised according to the scheme of nomenclature already described. There are, however, important exceptions.

Teratomas

A teratoma is a neoplasm formed of cells representing all three germ cell layers: ectoderm, mesoderm and endoderm. In their benign form, these cellular types are often easily recognised; the tumour may contain teeth and hair, and, on histology, respiratory epithelium, cartilage, muscle, neural tissue, etc. In their malignant form, these representatives of ectoderm, mesoderm and endoderm will be less easily identifiable.

Teratomas are of germ cell origin. They occur most often in the gonads, where germ cells are abundant. Although all cells in the body contain the same genetic information, it is perhaps in the germ cells that this information is in the least repressed state and is therefore capable of programming such divergent lines of differentiation. Supporting evidence for a germ cell origin for teratomas comes from karyotypic analysis of their sex chromosome content. Teratomas in the female are always XX, whereas only 50% of those in the male are XX and the remainder XY; this correlates with the sex chromosome distribution in the germ cells of the two sexes.

Ovarian teratomas are almost always benign and cystic; in the testis, they are almost always malignant and relatively solid. As germ cells in the embryo originate at a site remote from the developing gonads,

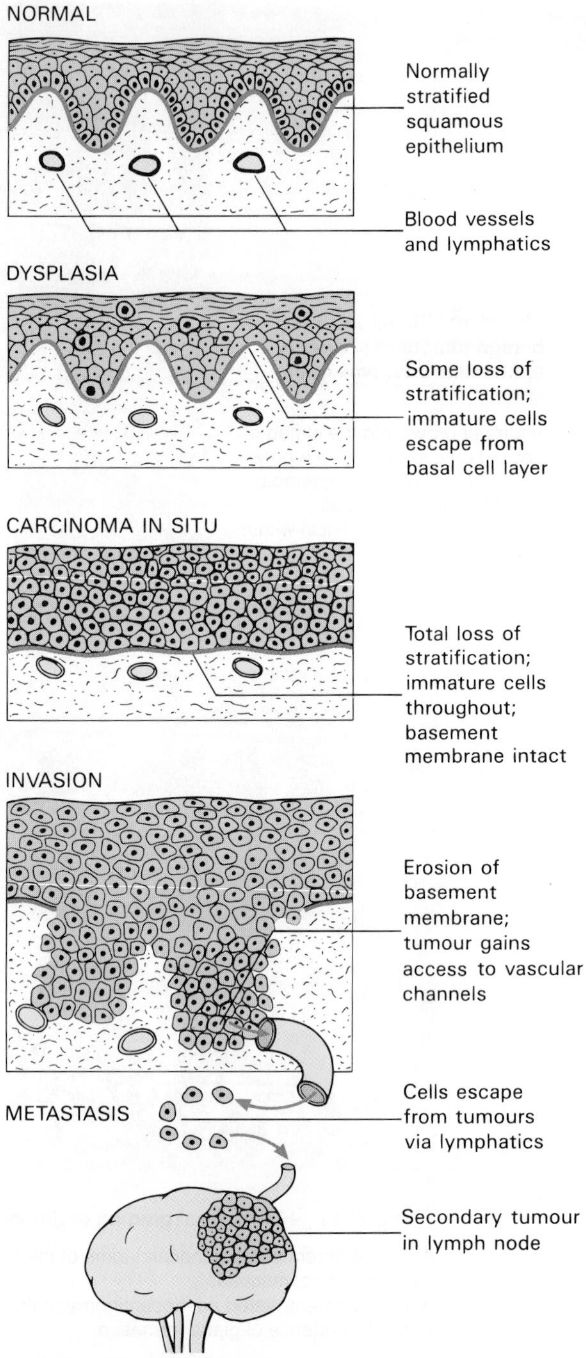

NORMAL
Normally stratified squamous epithelium

Blood vessels and lymphatics

DYSPLASIA
Some loss of stratification; immature cells escape from basal cell layer

CARCINOMA IN SITU
Total loss of stratification; immature cells throughout; basement membrane intact

INVASION
Erosion of basement membrane; tumour gains access to vascular channels

METASTASIS
Cells escape from tumours via lymphatics

Secondary tumour in lymph node

Fig. 11.12   Evolution of an invasive squamous cell carcinoma from the precursor lesions of dysplasia and carcinoma in situ (usually grouped together as intraepithelial neoplasia)

Note that the tumour cells cannot reach routes of metastasis such as blood vessels and lymphatics until the basement membrane has been breached.

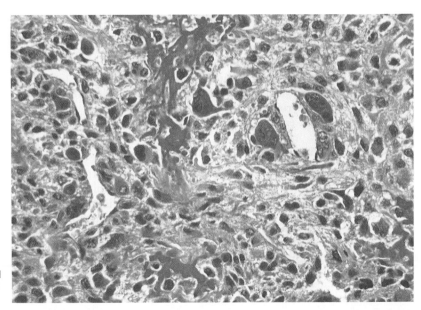

Fig. 11.13 Osteosarcoma
Histology showing pleomorphic tumour cells sufficiently differentiated to produce the osteoid lying between them.

teratomas arise occasionally elsewhere in the body, usually in the midline, possibly from germ cells that have been arrested in their migration. These extragonadal sites for teratomas include the mediastinum and sacro-coccygeal region.

Embryonal tumours: the 'blastomas'

Some types of tumour occur almost exclusively in the very young, usually in those below 5 years of age, and bear a histological resemblance to the embryonic form of the organ in which they arise. Examples include:

- *retinoblastoma*, which arises in the eye and for which there is an inherited predisposition
- *nephroblastoma* or *Wilms' tumour*, which arises in the kidney
- *neuroblastoma*, which arises in the adrenal medulla or nerve ganglia and occasionally 'matures' into a harmless benign ganglioneuroma
- *hepatoblastoma*, which arises in the liver.

Mixed tumours

Mixed tumours show a characteristic combination of cell types. The best example is the mixed parotid tumour (pleomorphic salivary adenoma); this consists of glands embedded in a cartilaginous or mucinous matrix derived from the myoepithelial cells of the gland. Another common mixed tumour is the fibroadenoma of the breast, a lobular tumour con-

sisting of epithelium-lined glands or clefts in a loose fibrous tissue matrix.

The occurrence of mixed tumours in an individual organ can sometimes be predicted from its embryology. This is illustrated by the Müllerian tract tumours that occur in the female genital tract; these often contain a mixture of carcinomatous and sarcomatous elements reflecting the intrinsic capacity of the tissue for divergent differentiation.

A tumour may also have a mixed appearance because of metaplasia within it. For example, transitional cell carcinomas of the bladder sometimes exhibit foci of glandular or squamous differentiation.

APUDomas and carcinoid tumours

APUD (*a*mine content and/or *p*recursor *u*ptake and *d*ecarboxylation) is the acronym used to describe the cells of the diffuse endocrine system, such as the calcitonin-producing 'C' cells of the thyroid gland, the cells of the islets of Langerhans, and the argentaffin and argyrophil cells of the lungs and the gastrointestinal tract. The APUD acronym describes their histochemical properties, which correlate both with these cells' ability to synthesise peptide hormones and with their content of either 5-hydroxytryptamine or 5-hydroxytryptophan. Tumours derived from these cells are called collectively *APUDomas*.

The name of those APUDomas containing or secreting a specific peptide hormone is usually derived from the name of the hormone, together with the suffix '-oma'. For example, the insulin-producing tumour originating from the β-cells of the islets of Langerhans is called an insulinoma. There are exceptions: for example, the calcitonin-producing tumour of the thyroid gland is called a 'medullary carcinoma of the thyroid gland' because it was described as a specific entity before its true histogenesis was known.

APUDomas of the gut and respiratory tract that do not produce any known peptide hormone are called *carcinoid tumours*. The appendix is the commonest site, but, here, these tumours are usually an incidental finding of little clinical significance. Carcinoids arising elsewhere (the small bowel is the next commonest site) often metastasise to mesenteric lymph nodes and the liver. Extensive metastases lead to the carcinoid syndrome (tachycardia, sweating, skin flushing, anxiety and diarrhoea) due to excessive production of 5-hydroxytryptamine and prostaglandins.

Many APUDomas are functionally active, and clinical syndromes often result from excessive secretion of their products (Table 11.5).

APUDomas often pursue an indolent course, growing relatively slowly and metastasising late. Their behaviour cannot always be predicted from their histological features.

Some individuals have an inherited familial predisposition to develop APUDomas; they are said to have a multiple endocrine neoplasia (MEN) syndrome.

Carcinosarcomas

Carcinosarcomas are very rare tumours which appear to consist of separate carcinomatous and sarcomatous components. Some may arise from carcinogenic events simultaneously affecting adjacent epithelial and mesenchymal cells. Others may be the result of collision of a coincidentally arising carcinoma and sarcoma.

Hamartomas

A hamartoma is a tumour-like lesion, the growth of which is co-ordinated with the individual; it lacks the autonomy of a true neoplasm. Hamartomas are always benign and usually consist of two or more mature cell types normally found in the organ in which the lesion arises. A common example occurs in the lung, where a hamartoma typically consists of a mixture of cartilage and bronchial-type epithelium (the so-called 'adenochondroma'; see Ch. 14). Pigmented naevi or 'moles' (Ch. 24) may also be considered as hamartomatous lesions. Their clinical importance is:

- hamartomas may be mistaken for malignant neoplasms, on a chest X-ray for example
- hamartomas are sometimes associated with clinical syndromes, as, for example, in tuberous sclerosis (Ch. 26).

Cysts

A cyst is a fluid-filled space lined by epithelium. Cysts are not necessarily tumours or neoplasms but, because they may have local effects similar to those produced by true tumours, it is pertinent to consider them here. Common types of cysts are:

- *congenital* (e.g. branchial and thyroglossal cysts) due to embryological defects
- *neoplastic* (e.g. cystadenoma, cystadenocarcinoma, cystic teratoma)
- *parasitic* (e.g. hydatid cysts due to *Echinococcus granulosus*)
- *retention* (e.g. epidermoid and pilar cysts of the skin)
- *implantation* (e.g. as a result of surgical or accidental implantation of epidermis).

The only type of cyst whose aetiology merits its inclusion within this chapter is the neoplastic cyst. This is seen most commonly in the ovary, where it may be either a benign cystic teratoma, filled with sebaceous material, or a cystadenoma or cystadenocarcinoma, each of which may be filled with either serous fluid or mucus depending on the secretory properties of the lining epithelium.

Table 11.5 Some APUDomas and their associated clinical syndromes	
APUDoma	Clinical syndrome
Insulinoma	Episodes of hypoglycaemia
Gastrinoma	Extensive peptic ulceration of the upper gut (Zollinger–Ellison syndrome)
Phaeochromocytoma	Paroxysmal hypertension
Carcinoid	If metastases are present, flushing, palpitations and pulmonary valve stenosis

BIOLOGY OF TUMOUR CELLS

> ▶ No single biological feature is unique to neoplastic cells
> ▶ Neoplastic cells are relatively or absolutely autonomous, unresponsive to extracellular growth control
> ▶ Neoplastic cells frequently have quantitative and qualitative abnormalities of DNA
> ▶ Tumour products include fetal substances and unexpected hormones

Contrary to past claims and an enduring hope, there is no therapeutically exploitable single feature unique to neoplastic cells other than the general property of relative or absolute growth autonomy. Many of the other features have normal counterparts: mitotic activity is a feature also of regenerating cells; placental trophoblast is invasive; and the nucleated cells of the blood and lymph wander freely around the body, settling in other sites.

One of the many difficulties in studying tumours is their genetic instability, leading to the formation of many clones with divergent properties within one tumour. This is often reflected in the histology which may show a heterogeneous growth pattern, some areas appearing better differentiated than others. Clinically, this instability and consequent heterogeneity is important because it enables some tumours to resist chemotherapy; consequently, many chemotherapeutic regimes employ a combination of agents administered simultaneously or sequentially.

DNA of tumour cells

Tumour cells have abnormal nuclear DNA. The total amount of DNA per cell commonly exceeds that of the normal diploid (2N) population. This is evident in histological sections as *nuclear hyperchromaticism*. The amount of DNA may appear to increase in exact multiples of the diploid state (polyploidy) such as tetraploid (4N) and octaploid (8N); alternatively there may be aneuploidy, the presence of inexact multiples of DNA per cell.

Aneuploidy and *polyploidy* are associated with increased tumour aggressiveness and are recognisable in histological sections as variations in nuclear size and staining (*pleomorphism*).

At a chromosomal level these abnormalities of DNA are associated with the presence of additional chromosomes and often with chromosomal translocations. A very few of these *karyotypic abnormalities*

have a regular association with specific tumours; the best known and one of the most consistent is the association of the Philadelphia chromosome with chronic myeloid leukaemia.

Genetic abnormalities are being discovered with increasing frequency in tumours. Some of these may be relatively late events, epiphenomena with no central role in the cancer process. However, others may be of fundamental importance, appearing at an early stage in the development of the tumour. Abnormalities of oncogenes and tumour suppressor genes are of considerable interest in this regard because of their involvement in carcinogenesis (see p. 276).

Mitotic and apoptotic activity

Malignant tumours frequently appear to exhibit more mitotic activity than the corresponding normal cell population. In histological sections, mitoses are abundant, and mitotic figures are often grossly abnormal showing tripolar and other bizarre arrangements. It is likely that these aberrant mitoses are incapable of proceeding to completion. Cellular proliferation can be estimated by mitosis counting, DNA measurements and determination of the frequency of expression of cell-cycle associated proteins (e.g. Ki-67 antigen, proliferating cell nuclear antigen). Prognostic information can be derived from these estimations: higher frequencies of cellular proliferation are associated with a worse prognosis.

Perhaps as important as the increased mitotic activity is cell loss in tumours through ischaemic and apoptotic necrosis; the latter is a common finding in slow-growing tumours with a high mitotic rate (e.g. basal cell carcinoma of the skin). The net growth rate of a tumour is the balance between cellular proliferation and loss.

Metabolic abnormalities

Although tumour cells show a tendency towards *anaerobic glycolysis*, there are no metabolic abnormalities entirely specific to the neoplastic process. The known metabolic abnormalities of tumour cells are simply discordant with the normal physiological state of the tissue or host.

The surface of tumour cells is abnormal. Tumour cells have a greater *negative surface charge* than do normal cells, and are also less cohesive. In epithelial neoplasms, poor cellular cohesion is also due to a reduction in specialised intercellular junctions such as desmosomes. These changes may explain the ease with which malignant tumour cells spread through tissues and detach themselves to populate distant organs (see p. 284).

Tumour cells may retain the capacity to synthesise and secrete products characteristic of the normal cell type from which they are derived, often doing so in an excessive and uncontrolled manner. In addition, tumours often show evidence of *gene derepression*. All somatic cells contain the same genetic information, but only a small proportion of the genome is transcribed into RNA and translated into protein in any normal cell. Most genes are repressed, and only those required for the function of the particular cell are selectively expressed. However, in many tumour cells, some genes become *derepressed*, resulting in the inappropriate synthesis of unexpected substances.

Tumour products

The major types of tumour product are:

- substances appropriate to their cell of origin (e.g. keratin from a squamous cell carcinoma, steroid hormones from an adrenocortical adenoma)
- substances inappropriate or unexpected for their cell of origin (e.g. ACTH and ADH from oat cell carcinomas of the lung)
- fetal reversion substances (e.g. carcinoembryonic antigen from adenocarcinomas of the gastrointestinal tract, alpha-fetoprotein from liver cell carcinomas and testicular teratomas)
- substances required for growth and invasion (e.g. autocrine growth factors, angiogenic factors, collagenases).

Some tumour products are useful as markers for diagnosis or follow-up (Table 11.6). They can be detected in histological sections or their concentrations measured in the blood. Rising blood levels suggest the presence of tumour; falling levels indicate a sustained response to therapy (Fig. 11.14).

Growth factors, hormones and their receptors

Neoplastic cells sustain their growth either by producing growth factors for which they already have receptors, or by producing receptors for growth factors already present in the cellular environment. This process is known as *autocrine control* (see p. 282). Many oncogenes, frequently found to be abnormally expressed in neoplastic cells, encode for some growth factors, their receptors, or closely related molecules.

The autonomy of neoplastic cells is often relative rather than absolute. For example, approximately two-thirds of breast carcinomas retain the capacity to synthesise oestrogen receptors; these tumours are better differentiated than receptor-negative breast carcinomas and they have a better prognosis. Furthermore, if women with oestrogen-receptor-positive breast carcinomas are given tamoxifen (a drug which blocks the receptor) or have their ovaries removed surgically (which removes the major source of oestrogens) they survive longer than women with receptor-positive tumours who have not been treated in these ways.

Table 11.6 Commonly used tumour markers

Tumour	Marker	Comment
Myeloma	Monoclonal immunoglobulin Bence Jones protein	In blood Immunoglobulin light chain (kappa or lambda) in urine
Liver cell carcinoma	Alpha-fetoprotein (AFP)	Also associated with testicular teratoma
Gastrointestinal adenocarcinomas	Carcinoembryonic antigen (CEA)	False positives occur in some non-neoplastic conditions
APUDomas (other than carcinoids and phaeochromocytomas)	Peptide hormones (e.g. insulin, gastrin)	Excessive hormone production may have clinical effects
Phaeochromocytoma	Vanillyl mandelic acid (VMA)	Metabolite of catecholamines in urine
Carcinoid	5-hydroxyindole-acetic acid (5-HIAA)	Metabolite of 5-hydroxytryptamine (5-HT) in urine
Choriocarcinoma	Human chorionic gonadotrophin (hCG)	In blood or urine
Malignant teratoma	AFP hCG	In blood In blood or urine

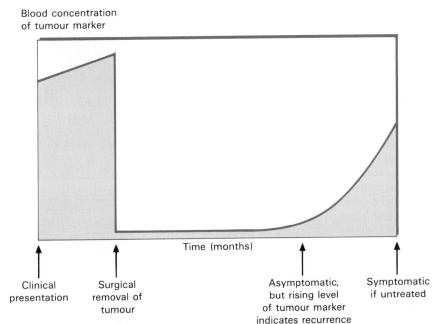

Blood concentration
of tumour marker

Time (months)

Clinical
presentation

Surgical
removal of
tumour

Asymptomatic,
but rising level
of tumour marker
indicates recurrence

Symptomatic
if untreated

Fig. 11.14 Use of tumour markers to monitor clinical progress

Abnormally high levels of the marker can be used to detect tumours before they become symptomatic, either by screening a population at risk or, as in the example shown here, by regular monitoring to detect early recurrences. The events shown here could take place over a total period of 12 months.

CARCINOGENESIS

Carcinogenesis is the process which results in the transformation of normal cells to neoplastic cells by causing permanent genetic alterations or mutations.

Tumours arise from single cells that have become transformed by cumulative mutational events. Spontaneous mutations during normal DNA replication are probably common, but many are rectified by repair mechanisms. The probability of neoplastic transformation increases with the number of cell divisions experienced by a cell; this may explain why the incidence of cancer increases with age. Exposure to carcinogens increases the probability of specific mutational events.

Carcinogenesis embraces the causation of all tumours, but, because malignant tumours are much more serious, most epidemiological, clinical and experimental observations have been concentrated on them. Indeed, *carcinogenesis* strictly applies to the causation only of malignant tumours (cancers), whereas *oncogenesis* includes the causation of all tumours, benign and malignant. The principles of carcinogenesis can be used to elucidate the mechanisms that distinguish benign from malignant tumours.

A *carcinogen* is an agent known or suspected to participate in the causation of tumours. Such agents are said to be *carcinogenic* (cancer causing) or *oncogenic* (tumour causing). The ultimate site of action of all carcinogens is the DNA in which genes are encoded. Carcinogens are therefore also *mutagenic*. Very often more than one carcinogen is necessary to produce tumours from normal tissues and cells, and there is good evidence that the process occurs in several discrete steps; this is the *multistep hypothesis*.

Once started, the process does not require the continued presence of the carcinogen. It is rather a 'hit-and-run' situation and evidence of the specific causative agent(s) is not usually found in the eventual tumours. Exceptions include some suspected carcinogenic viruses, genetic material of which persists in the resulting tumours, and some insoluble substances, such as thorium dioxide and asbestos, which cannot be eliminated from the tissues. The 'hit-and-run' character of carcinogenesis is one of several reasons why carcinogens have proved so elusive.

Recent research has considerably improved our knowledge and understanding of the molecular basis of carcinogenesis. Genetic alterations are absolutely fundamental to the carcinogenic process. The central role of these genetic abnormalities will be considered in detail after the different classes of carcinogen have been described.

Identification of carcinogens

> ► Most cancers are attributed to environmental causes
> ► Laboratory testing can identify some carcinogens
> ► Some carcinogens can be suspected from epidemiological studies
> ► Many carcinogens require co-factors
> ► Long latent interval between exposure and detection of the consequent tumour hampers identification

Most tumours are thought to result from an environmental cause, though there is increasing evidence, in some tumours, of an inherited or constitutional risk. It has been estimated that approximately 85% of the cancer risk is due to environmental agents.

Ethics prohibit the testing of suspected carcinogens in humans, so that much of our knowledge of carcinogenesis in man is derived from indirect or circumstantial evidence. Identification is hampered both by the complexity of the human environment, which makes it difficult to isolate a single causative factor from the many possible candidates, and by the very long time interval between exposure to a carcinogen and the appearance of signs and symptoms leading to the diagnosis of the tumour; this *latent interval* may be two or three decades.

Carcinogens may be identified from:

- epidemiological studies
- assessment of occupational risks
- direct accidental exposure
- carcinogenic effects in laboratory animals
- transforming effects on cell cultures
- mutagenicity testing in bacteria.

Epidemiological evidence

Some types of cancer are more common in certain countries, regions or communities within them than others (Fig. 11.15). Epidemiology has proved to be a fruitful source of information about the causes of tumours. Tumour incidence is more important than mortality data in this regard, because only a proportion of tumours prove fatal and the precise cause of deaths may not be well documented. It is thus essential to survey populations thoroughly for tumour incidence; in countries with well-developed health services, investigators can usually rely on diagnostic records and cancer registries, but elsewhere it may be necessary to visit and examine the population under study. Variations in tumour incidence may genuinely be due to environmental factors, but the data must first be standardised to eliminate the effect of, for example, any differences in the age distribu-

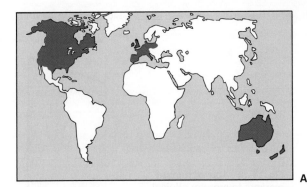

A

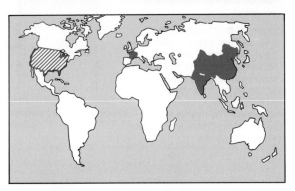

■ High-incidence country

▨ High-incidence community

B

Fig. 11.15 World map showing countries in which there is a relatively high incidence of specific types of cancer

A. Colorectal cancer. **B.** Oesophageal cancer. Low-incidence countries may conceal high-incidence regions or communities; for example, oesophageal carcinoma is relatively common among blacks in the USA (hatched area). Note that colorectal cancer is much commoner in countries whose inhabitants eat a more refined diet. Dietary associations with oesophageal cancer are less well defined.

tion. The long latent period between exposure to a carcinogen and the appearance of the tumour means that it is necessary to consider also the effect of population movement. This effect can be used to distinguish between racial (hereditary) and environmental factors in determining cancer incidence in migrants.

Having found a high tumour incidence in a population, it is then necessary to compare lifestyle, diet and occupational risks with those of a low tumour-incidence control population, so that specific causative associations can be identified.

The following examples illustrate how carcinogens can be identified in this way.

Hepatocellular carcinoma

In countries such as the United Kingdom or the USA, hepatocellular carcinoma is a relatively uncommon tumour and, when it does occur, it is usually associated with cirrhosis. However, the worldwide incidence of hepatocellular carcinoma is high, and in some countries it is the most common tumour (Ch. 16). Epidemiology reveals two factors which may be involved in the high prevalence in endemic areas: *mycotoxins* and *hepatitis viruses B and C*.

There is a positive correlation between the incidence of hepatocellular carcinoma in different regions of Uganda and the frequency with which food samples in those regions are found to be contaminated with aflatoxins. Aflatoxins are mycotoxins produced by the fungus *Aspergillus flavus*, and are a highly carcinogenic group of compounds. The fungus grows on food stored in humid conditions in the high-incidence areas. However, the situation is not clear-cut, because of the prevalence of hepatitis B virus in the area. There is a high incidence of point mutations of specific codons in p53, a tumour suppressor gene, in hepatocellular carcinomas associated epidemiologically with aflatoxins.

There is a strong correlation between the incidence of hepatitis B and C virus infection and hepatocellular carcinoma in many countries. Suspicion that hepatitis B virus may be oncogenic (tumour-causing) is reinforced by the discovery, in such cases, of a copy of the viral genome incorporated within the genome of the liver cancer cells.

Oesophageal carcinoma

The very high incidence of oesophageal carcinoma in China and in the Caspian littoral region of Iran has been intensively studied by epidemiologists. Several factors have been implicated, including the dyes used in carpet making, nitrates in the soil, abrasives in the diet, and opium dross, but no single aetiological factor has yet emerged from these studies.

One of the most informative natural experiments on the causation of oesophageal carcinoma took place in China when it was decided to build a reservoir in the Linhsien area. People living in this district were known to have a very high incidence of oesophageal carcinoma as, remarkably, did their domestic chickens. A dietary factor was suspected because the chickens were usually fed with their owner's waste food. The reservoir displaced these people to Fanhsien where they continued to have a high incidence of oesophageal carcinoma. They left their chickens behind and re-stocked with a local strain in which oesophageal carcinoma was uncommon. However, fed with the table-scraps and waste food from their new owners, the local strain subsequently developed a high incidence of oesophageal carcinoma. A dietary factor is thus clearly implicated, but this remains to be identified precisely.

Occupational and behavioural risks

Certain types of cancer are, or have been, more common in people engaged in specific activities. The discovery in a given community of a link between a higher risk of developing a cancer and the person's occupation helps to separate general environmental causes of carcinogenesis from those that are probably specific to an individual person or group in the community.

Scrotal carcinoma

Percival Pott is credited with the first observation, in 1777, linking a particular tumour with a specific occupation. He noticed a high incidence of carcinoma of the scrotal skin in men who were or had been chimney sweeps, and postulated that the soot was responsible. It was not until 150 years later that the specific carcinogen, a polycyclic aromatic hydrocarbon, was identified.

Lung carcinoma

Lung carcinoma is a major public health problem in many countries. In the United Kingdom, approximately 35 000 deaths are attributed to this cause annually; the actual incidence is only marginally higher because this form of cancer has an extremely poor prognosis. The unarguable association with cigarette smoking was established by meticulous epidemiological research. The problem, a common one for epidemiologists, was that people who smoke are commonly exposed to many other possible risks: they tend to live in cities, inhale atmospheric pollutants from cars, domestic fires and industry, be fond of alcoholic drinks, etc. However, careful analysis of environmental factors showed that cigarette smoking correlated most strongly with the incidence of lung carcinoma. There is an almost linear dose–response relationship between the number of cigarettes smoked daily and the risk of developing lung cancer (Fig. 11.16). Furthermore, the incidence of lung carcinoma has declined in those groups of people, such as British male doctors, whose tobacco consumption has fallen substantially.

Carcinoma of the cervix

The observation that carcinoma of the cervix is commonest amongst prostitutes and an extreme rarity in celibate nuns, suggested that the disease may be due to a venereally transmitted agent. The risk of carcinoma of the cervix is strongly associated with sexual intercourse, in particular with the number of partners and thus the risk of exposure to a possible carcinogenic agent conveyed by the male. For some years, smegma from beneath the male prepuce was considered to be the culprit, because of the apparently higher incidence of cervical carcinoma among the spouses and sexual partners of uncircumcised males. However, more discriminating epidemiology indicates that sexual promiscuity is most strongly correlated with the risk; the number of partners and age at first intercourse are particularly incriminated. Further research suggested herpes simplex virus 2 as the most likely cause, but it now appears that the herpes virus antibodies found more commonly in the serum of women with cancer of the cervix simply reflect a higher incidence of previous genital herpes viral infection in this group, rather than a causal relationship. Evidence favouring a human papillomavirus (HPV) is more compelling because the viral DNA can be found incorporated into DNA extracted from many cervical carcinomas. This group of viruses are known to be capable of causing human epithelial cell proliferations, in that they cause the common viral wart. Smoking is an aetiological co-factor for carcinoma of the cervix.

Bladder carcinoma

In the 1890s, epidemiologists noted a higher than expected incidence of bladder cancer among men employed in the aniline dye and rubber industries. Further analysis led to the identification of β-naphthylamine as the causative agent. Although stringent precautions are now taken to minimise the risk, people working in these industries are regularly screened for bladder cancer by cytological examination of their urine and, if bladder cancer occurs, the patient is entitled to compensation on the assumption that the disease has been acquired occupationally.

Direct evidence

It is fortunately a rare event for someone to be knowingly exposed to a single agent which causes cancer. Sadly, such happenings are often the adverse result of diagnostic or therapeutic medical intervention, but we must not overlook the opportunity to learn much from them.

Thorotrast

Thorotrast was a colloidal suspension of thorium dioxide widely used in many countries during

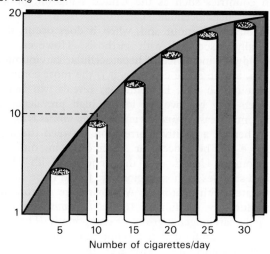

Relative risk of lung cancer

Number of cigarettes/day

Fig. 11.16 Approximate dose–response relationship between cigarette consumption and the relative risk of developing lung cancer

Smoking at the rate of 10 cigarettes per day increases the risk of developing lung cancer tenfold. (1 = non-smoker.)

1930–1950 as a contrast medium in diagnostic radiology. When it was first introduced for medical use two potentially hazardous properties of Thorotrast were known: thorium dioxide is naturally radioactive, emitting alpha-radiation and possessing an extremely long half-life of 1.39×10^{10} years; the colloidal suspension is rapidly and irreversibly taken up by the body's phagocytic cells, such as those lining the vascular sinusoids in the liver and the spleen (Fig. 11.17). Despite these potential hazards, Thorotrast proved such a good contrast medium, particularly for angiography, that its popularity was assured. However, in 1947 the first report was published of a patient who developed angiosarcoma of the liver after Thorotrast administration. As other cases were recognised Thorotrast was withdrawn from use. Nevertheless, this unfortunate episode has given us an opportunity to learn about and confirm the carcinogenic effects of alpha-radiation.

Thyroid carcinoma and radiation in children

The thyroid gland is vulnerable to the carcinogenic effects of external irradiation and of the radioactive isotopes of iodine (the latter are concentrated by the thyroid gland in the synthesis of thyroid hormone). For example, in April 1986 a nuclear reactor exploded at Chernobyl in Ukraine, releasing a large quanti-

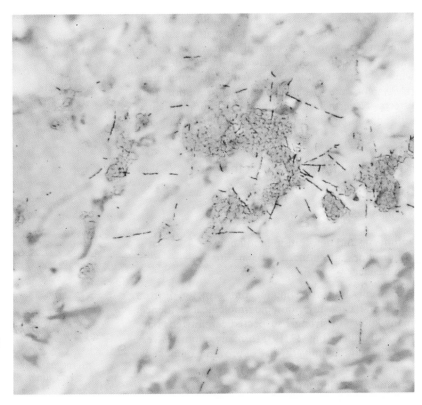

Fig. 11.17 Autoradiograph of a section of liver from a man who died from hepatic angiosarcoma several decades after carotid angiography with Thorotrast

Black lines of silver in the developed photographic emulsion mark the trails of alpha particles from the insoluble colloidal thorium dioxide in the underlying section.

ty of radioactive material into the atmosphere. The material released included radioactive iodine. After a four-year latent interval, there has been a dramatic increase in the incidence of thyroid carcinoma in children in Ukraine (Fig. 11.18). To minimise this risk, non-radioactive iodine is usually given to people immediately after any accidental exposure to radioactive iodine to compete with the latter for uptake by the thyroid gland.

Experimental observations

Carcinogens are not united by any common physical or chemical properties; it is therefore considered necessary to screen all new drugs, food additives and potential environmental pollutants in non-human systems before they are introduced for human use. Three types of test system for carcinogenic or mutagenic activity are employed:

- laboratory animals in which the incidence of tumours is monitored
- cell and tissue cultures in which growth-transforming effects are sought
- bacterial cultures for mutagenicity testing (Ames test).

None of these is a perfect test system; animals and isolated cell cultures often metabolise the agent under test in a way that differs from normal human metabolic pathways, and mutagenicity in bacterial

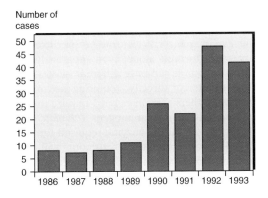

Fig. 11.18 Rising incidence of thyroid carcinoma in children (0–14 years) in Ukraine

Thyroid carcinoma in children is relatively uncommon, but since the nuclear reactor explosion in 1986 at Chernobyl there has been a significantly increased incidence. An increased incidence may also occur in adults, but after a longer latent interval.

DNA may not correspond to carcinogenicity. In addition, the dynamics of these test systems are very different from that of clinical cancer; cancer in humans is a chronic process often lasting decades, whereas tests for carcinogenic activity in experimental systems are usually seeking more immediate effects. Nevertheless, despite these limitations, it is still appropriate to investigate possible carcinogens in this way.

Known or suspected carcinogens

The main classes of carcinogenic agent are:

- chemicals
- viruses
- ionising and non-ionising radiation
- hormones, mycotoxins and parasites
- miscellaneous agents.

As a result of direct testing for mutagenicity, or from accidental exposures or epidemiological evidence, many known or strongly suspected carcinogens have been identified (Fig. 11.19). In many countries very strict legislation limits the use of proven carcinogens.

Chemical carcinogens

> ▶ No common structural features
> ▶ Most require metabolic conversion into active carcinogens
> ▶ Major classes include polycyclic aromatic hydrocarbons, aromatic amines, nitrosamines, azo dyes, alkylating agents

Many chemical carcinogens have now been identified. The main categories are shown in Table 11.7.

The carcinogenic risk cannot be predicted from the structural formula alone; even apparently closely related compounds can have different effects.

Some agents act directly, requiring no metabolic conversion. Others *(procarcinogens)* require metabolic conversion into active carcinogens *(ultimate carcinogens)* (Fig. 11.20). If the enzyme required for conversion is ubiquitous within tissues, tumours will occur at the site of contact or entry; for example, polycyclic aromatic hydrocarbons induce skin tumours if painted on to the skin, or lung cancer if inhaled in tobacco smoke. Other agents require metabolic conversion by enzymes confined to certain organs, and thus often induce tumours remote from the site of entry; for example, aromatic amines require hydroxylation in the liver before expressing their carcinogenic effects. In a few instances the carcinogen is synthesised in the body from ingredients in the diet; thus, carcinogenic

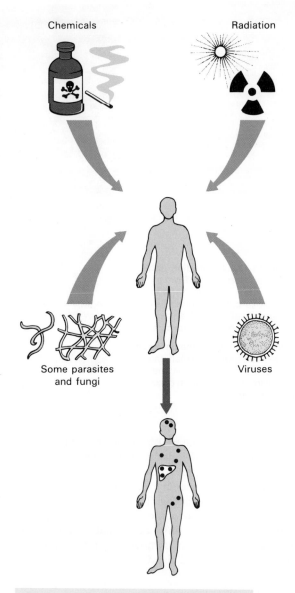

Fig. 11.19   Major categories of carcinogens

nitrosamines are synthesised by gut bacteria utilising dietary nitrates and nitrites.

Polycyclic aromatic hydrocarbons
Polycyclic aromatic hydrocarbons were the first chemical carcinogens to be intensively studied. In 1917, Yamagiwa and Itchikawa in Japan reported that skin tumours could be induced in rabbits by painting their skin with tar. Tar was a suspected carcinogen because of the high incidence of skin cancer among tar-workers, particularly on the hands, which

Table 11.7   Examples of proven or suspected chemical carcinogens and the tumours with which they are associated

Chemical	Tumour	Comments
Polycyclic aromatic hydrocarbons e.g. 3,4-benzpyrene	Lung cancer Skin cancer	Strong link with smoking Following repeated exposure to mineral oils
Aromatic amines e.g. β-naphthylamine	Bladder cancer	In rubber and dye workers
Nitrosamines	Gut cancers	Proven in animals
Azo dyes e.g. 2-acetylaminofluorene	Bladder and liver cancer	Proven in animals
Alkylating agents e.g. cyclophosphamide	Leukaemia	Small risk in humans
Other organic chemicals e.g. vinyl chloride	Liver angiosarcoma	Used in PVC manufacture
Arsenical compounds	Skin cancer	No longer a common event

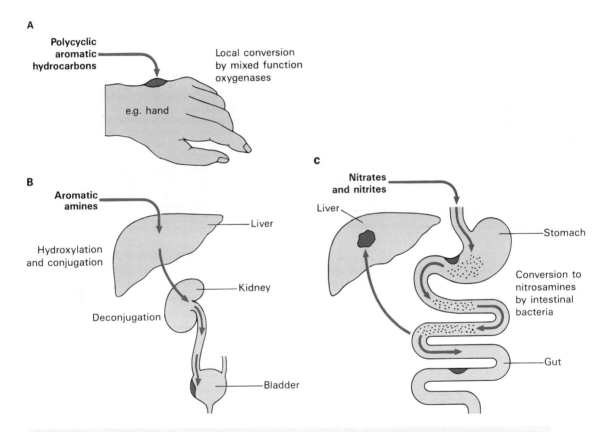

Fig. 11.20   Summary of some metabolic pathways for conversion of chemical procarcinogens into the active ultimate carcinogens

A. Polycyclic aromatic hydrocarbons. **B.** Aromatic amines. **C.** Nitrates and nitrites. (See text for details.)

were frequently in contact with it. In the 1930s in London, Cook and Kennaway fractionated tar and attributed the carcinogenic effect to the polycyclic aromatic hydrocarbons. Like many chemicals implicated in the development of cancer, these are procarcinogens, requiring metabolic conversion by hydroxylation to form ultimate carcinogens. In this case, the carcinogenic effect is invariably at the site of contact because the hydroxylating enzymes (e.g. aryl carbohydrate hydroxylase) are ubiquitous in human tissues and readily induced in susceptible individuals. However, if the substance is absorbed into the body, this may lead to a risk of cancer at sites remote from the point of initial contact; there is, for example, an increased incidence of bladder cancer in tobacco smokers.

The tumour most commonly associated with exposure to polycyclic aromatic hydrocarbons is carcinoma of the lung. This tumour is much more common in smokers than in non-smokers and the risk to an individual or group parallels the quantity of tobacco consumed. Tobacco smoke contains many candidates for carcinogenic activity, the most important is probably 3,4-benzpyrene. Tobacco is also chewed in some countries, and there it is associated with a risk of carcinoma of the mouth.

Aromatic amines

The high incidence of bladder carcinoma in workers in the dye and rubber industries has now been attributed to β-naphthylamine. Unlike the polycyclic aromatic hydrocarbons, this substance has no local carcinogenic effect. It requires conversion by hydroxylation in the liver into the active carcinogenic metabolite, 1-hydroxy-2-naphthylamine. However, the carcinogenic effect is masked immediately by conjugation with glucuronic acid in the liver. Bladder cancer results because the conjugated metabolite is excreted in the urine and deconjugated in the urinary tract by the enzyme glucuronidase, thus exposing the urothelium to the active carcinogen.

Nitrosamines

While ultimate proof of a causal relationship with human cancers is lacking, there is epidemiological evidence linking carcinomas of the gastrointestinal tract to dietary nitrates and nitrites. Nitrates are used widely as fertilisers, and are eventually washed by the rain into rivers and underground water tables where they can contaminate drinking water. In addition, both nitrates and nitrites are used as food additives. Although these radicals are not in themselves carcinogenic, they are readily metabolised by commensal bacteria within the gut and converted to carcinogenic nitrosamines by combination with secondary amines and amides. Direct proof of a major role in carcinogenesis in man is still awaited, but these substances are potent carcinogens in laboratory animals and it is unlikely that man would be exempt from this effect.

Azo dyes

The carcinogenic potential of azo dyes, derivatives of aromatic amines, was recognised at an early stage and their use has thus been severely restricted. In laboratory animals, dimethylaminoazobenzene—otherwise known as 'butter yellow' because it was once used to impart a tasteful yellow colour to margarine—causes liver cancer.

Alkylating agents

Many categories of chemical carcinogen, including polycyclic hydrocarbons, have alkylation as the ultimate common pathway, so it is not surprising that alkylating agents themselves can be carcinogenic. Alkylating agents bind directly to DNA, the ultimate site of action of all carcinogens. Nitrogen mustard is a well-known example, but these agents are not otherwise widely implicated as a major cause of human cancer.

Oncogenic viruses

▶ Clusters of cancer cases in space and time suggest a viral aetiology
▶ Tumours associated with viruses tend to be more common in youth
▶ Immunosuppression favours viral oncogenesis
▶ Viruses implicated in human carcinogenesis include Epstein–Barr virus (Burkitt's lymphoma) and human papillomaviruses (cancer of the cervix)
▶ Oncogenic DNA viral genome is directly incorporated into host cell DNA
▶ Oncogenic RNA viral genome is transcribed into DNA by reverse transcriptase prior to incorporation (oncogenic retrovirus)

Viruses were first implicated as carcinogenic agents through the experiments of Rous (in 1911) and Shope (in 1932) who studied fowl sarcomas and rabbit skin tumours respectively. They showed that it was possible to transmit the tumours from one animal to another, in the manner of an infectious disease; tumours could be induced by injecting a cell-free filtrate of each tumour. The only possible transmissible agent was considered to be a virus, as the pores of the filter were too fine to permit the passage of bacteria or whole tumour cells. Since these experiments, some other postulated transmissible causes of cancer have subsequently been shown to be viruses. A good example is the 'Bittner milk factor' associated with the high incidence of mammary cancer in certain strains of mice, which has been discovered to be an RNA virus which is oncogenic in the oestrogenic milieu of female mice of strains with the appropriate genetic constitution.

Relatively few human tumours are thought to be associated with viruses (Table 11.8). However, the study of oncogenic retroviruses in laboratory animals has had a seminal effect on our understanding of the molecular basis of tumour development and

Table 11.8	Oncogenic viruses implicated in human tumours	
Virus	**Tumour**	**Comments**
Human papillomavirus	Common wart (squamous cell papilloma) Cervical carcinoma	Benign, spontaneously regressing lesion Strong association with HPV types 16 and 18
Epstein–Barr virus	Burkitt's lymphoma Nasopharyngeal cancer	Requires a co-factor, probably malaria In China and Africa
Hepatitis B virus	Hepatocellular carcinoma	Strong association

has led to the discovery of *oncogenes* (Fig. 11.21 and Table 11.12).

Human tumours for which a viral aetiology has been proposed or proven include:

- carcinoma of the cervix (human papillomaviruses)
- Burkitt's lymphoma (Epstein–Barr virus)
- nasopharyngeal carcinoma (Epstein–Barr virus)
- hepatocellular carcinoma (hepatitis B virus)
- T-cell leukaemia/lymphoma in Japan and the Caribbean (RNA retrovirus).

Human papillomaviruses

Human papillomaviruses (HPV), of which there are many subtypes, are known to cause the common wart (squamous cell papilloma). This lesion occurs most commonly on the hand, a frequent site of physical contact enabling transmission between individuals, and the virus is abundant within the abnormal cells of the lesion. The often florid anogenital warts are also due to HPV, raising the possibility that other genital epithelial neoplasms may also be attributable to this cause. Evidence is also accumulating to suggest involvement of HPV in squamous neoplasia of the upper respiratory and digestive tracts.

Epidemiological evidence strongly favours a venereally transmitted agent as a cause of cancer of the cervix; this is discussed in more detail in Chapter 19.

Epstein–Barr virus

The Epstein–Barr (EB) virus was discovered first in cell cultures from Burkitt's lymphoma, a B-cell lymphoma endemic in certain regions of Africa and occurring only sporadically elsewhere. Early hopes that EB virus was the sole cause of Burkitt's lymphoma were dashed when it was discovered, following the accidental infection of a laboratory worker, that infection by the virus on its own causes infectious mononucleosis, a common, benign lymphoproliferative disorder which remits spontaneously in

most cases. Clearly a co-factor is involved in the pathogenesis of Burkitt's lymphoma; epidemiological evidence suggests that this is malaria.

EB virus is also implicated in the causation of nasopharyngeal carcinoma in the Far East, where there is a relatively high incidence of this tumour.

Radiant energy

> ► Ultraviolet light is a major cause of skin cancer
> ► Exposure to ionising radiation is associated with an increased risk of cancer of many sites, including leukaemia

Ultraviolet light

Skin cancer is more common on parts of the body regularly exposed to sunlight, and ultraviolet light (UVL) is now considered to be a major causal factor, UVB more so than UVA. Skin cancer is less common in people with naturally pigmented skin, as the melanin has a protective effect; it is more common in fair-skinned people, particularly those who get sunburnt easily, living in sunny climates (e.g. Australia).

Most types of skin cancer are associated with UVL exposure, but the risk is particularly high for malignant melanoma and basal cell carcinoma ('rodent ulcer'). This risk is greatly increased in patients with *xeroderma pigmentosum*, a rare congenital deficiency of DNA repair enzymes, in whom numerous skin cancers occur due to unrepaired damage to the DNA of the skin cells induced by UVL.

Ionising radiation

The carcinogenic effects of radiation are long-term and must be distinguished from the more immediate, dose-related, acute effects such as skin erythema and, more seriously, bone marrow aplasia (see Ch. 6).

Evidence that relatively high doses of ionising radiation are carcinogenic is indisputable and comes

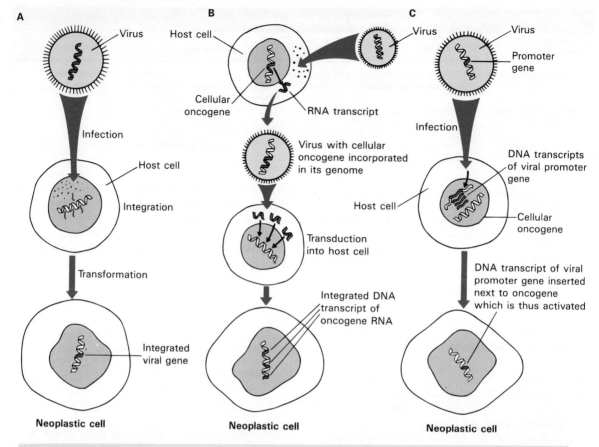

Fig. 11.21 Simplified mechanisms of integration of oncogenic viral genes, or DNA transcripts, into the host cell DNA

A. Oncogenic DNA virus: the viral genome is integrated into host cell DNA; neoplastic transformation is a postulated consequence. **B.** 'Acute' transforming oncogenic RNA virus: transduction into the host cell of an RNA transcript of a cellular oncogene picked up from another cell. **C.** 'Slow' transforming oncogenic RNA virus: insertion of a viral promoter gene next to a cellular oncogene. In both **B** and **C**, DNA transcripts are made from the RNA conveyed by the virus using the enzyme reverse transcriptase and, in contrast to cellular oncogenes, they lack introns.

from many sources. The carcinogenic effect of low levels of radiation continues to be a matter of great public concern because of the debate over the safety of nuclear power sources. Exposure to some ionising radiation from cosmic and other natural sources (background radiation) is inescapable; however, linear extrapolation of the low-dose risk from the quantifiable carcinogenic risk from higher levels of radiation is generally conceded to exaggerate the problem.

An increased incidence of cancer following exposure to ionising radiation has been witnessed since the earliest work with radioactive materials. Before protective measures were introduced there was a well-recognised increased incidence of leukaemia in

radiology workers, and of skin cancer in those who regularly placed their hands in X-ray beams. The therapeutic use of radiation, often without adequate justification (e.g. radiation of the thymus gland in children with miscellaneous ailments; see Chapter 6), has resulted in cancers. Radiation from military sources, such as in Hiroshima and Nagasaki in 1945, continues to result in a high incidence of certain tumours. Industrial exposure to radiation includes the risk of carcinoma of the lung associated with the mining of radioactive uranium. There has been a dramatic increase in the incidence of thyroid cancer in children near Chernobyl in Russia, the site of a nuclear accident in 1986 (see p. 264).

Some tissues are more vulnerable than others to

the carcinogenic effects of ionising radiation, and specific risks are associated with particular radioactive elements if they are concentrated in specific tissues; for example, radioactive iodine concentrated in the thyroid gland. Tissues which appear particularly sensitive to the carcinogenic effects of ionising radiation include thyroid, breast, bone and haemopoietic tissue.

Biological agents

Most cancers attributable to environmental causes follow exposure to some extrinsic physical or chemical agent not normally produced by, or found in, biological systems such as living cells. However, even some compounds naturally occurring in the human body (e.g. oestrogens) have a role in carcinogenesis. Cancer may also result from infection with other living organisms (e.g. some parasites) or from the ingestion of food contaminated with the metabolic products of other organisms (e.g. mycotoxins).

Hormones

It is somewhat surprising that substances occurring naturally in the body and indispensable for normal bodily functions should be implicated as at least cofactors in carcinogenesis. For example, oestrogens can be shown experimentally to promote the formation of mammary and endometrial carcinomas; the association between breast carcinoma and oral contraceptives containing oestrogens remains unproven. Androgenic and anabolic steroids are known to induce hepatocellular tumours in humans, and oestrogenic steroids may make pre-existing lesions (e.g. adenomas and focal nodular hyperplasia) abnormally vascular, thus causing otherwise asymptomatic lesions to present clinically.

Mycotoxins

Mycotoxins are toxic substances produced by fungi. Those having the greatest relevance in human carcinogenesis are the aflatoxins produced by *Aspergillus flavus*. Aflatoxins, particularly aflatoxin B_1, are among the most potent carcinogens and have been specifically linked to the high incidence of hepatocellular carcinoma in certain parts of Africa (Ch. 16).

Parasites

There is good evidence, both epidemiological and direct, to implicate at least two parasites, *Schistosoma* and *Clonorchis sinensis*, in the causation of human cancer. In both cases, there is a high incidence of the tumour in infested areas, and the parasites can often be found actually within or in the immediate vicinity of the tumour.

Schistosoma is strongly implicated in the high incidence of bladder carcinoma, usually of squamous cell type, in areas where infestation with the parasite (schistosomiasis) is rife, such as Egypt. The ova of the parasite can often be found in the affected tissue.

Clonorchis sinensis, the Chinese liver fluke, dwells in the bile ducts where it induces an inflammatory reaction, epithelial hyperplasia and sometimes eventually adenocarcinoma of the bile ducts (cholangiocarcinoma). There is a high incidence of this tumour in parts of the Far East and other fluke-infested areas.

Miscellaneous carcinogens

In contrast to radiation, chemicals and viruses, which ultimately damage or bind to DNA, there are a number of miscellaneous carcinogens whose mechanism of action is not well understood, despite their proven association with cancer.

Asbestos

Inhalation of asbestos fibres results in various lesions: asbestosis, pleural plaques, mesothelioma and carcinoma of the lung (Fig. 11.22). Of the two neoplastic consequences, the association with mesothelioma is the more specific because this tumour is exceptionally rare in the absence of asbestos exposure. The pleura is the most frequent site for mesothelioma, but the association with asbestos is just as strong for peritoneal mesothe-

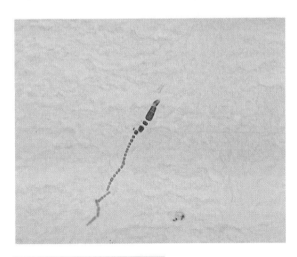

Fig. 11.22 Asbestos body

In a section of a carcinoma of the lung associated with industrial exposure, the asbestos body consists of an asbestos fibre encrusted with beads of haemosiderin.

lioma. There is also an association with carcinoma of the lung which is enhanced by cigarette smoking.

Metals

Some metals are associated with a cancer risk, particularly in industrial situations. For example, exposure to compounds containing nickel leads to a risk of carcinoma of the mucosa lining the nasal cavities and of the lung.

Host factors in carcinogenesis

In addition to the extrinsic or environmental factors in carcinogenesis, there are also several important host factors which influence the cancer risk. These are:

- race
- diet
- constitutional factors (gender, inherited risks, etc.)
- premalignant lesions and conditions
- transplacental exposure.

Race

The precise role of race in determining an individual's risk of developing specific types of cancer is complicated by the fact that racial differences often coincide with differences of place of residence, diet and habit. While in some instances the link is obvious—for example, skin cancer is uncommon in blacks because the melanin in their skin protects them from the carcinogenic effects of ultraviolet sunlight—apparent racial differences are often explicable in terms of habit or cultural practices. Thus, oral cancer is relatively common in India and South-East Asia; but this is not associated directly with race, rather with tobacco or betel chewing and the remarkable habit of 'reverse smoking' in which the burning end of the cigarette is habitually placed in the mouth!

The relative contributions of race and environment to the incidence of cancer can be deduced from comparing the incidence in racial groups who have migrated to other countries. For example, cancer of the stomach is relatively uncommon in Africa, but the incidence in North American blacks of African descent approximates to the higher risk in the white population.

Diet

Dietary factors may be linked to cancer risk because:

- the diet may contain procarcinogens or carcinogens

- the diet may lack protective factors
- intestinal transit time may alter exposure of gut mucosa to carcinogens in diet.

There is a possible positive correlation between dietary fat and the risk of breast and colorectal cancer; alcohol appears to be a risk factor for breast cancer; and there is experimental evidence to suggest that a low protein diet has a protective effect against certain chemical carcinogens by reducing the levels of mixed function oxygenases in the liver. Dietary fibre appears to be protective for colorectal cancer by promoting more rapid intestinal transit; any carcinogens in the bowel contents therefore remain in contact with the mucosa for a shorter time.

Constitutional factors

Inherited predisposition

Some individuals inherit an increased risk of developing certain tumours (Table 11.9). There is, for example, an inherited predisposition to breast cancer; a woman whose mother and one sister have developed breast cancer has a 50% probability of developing one herself. A gene responsible for this inherited risk (BRCA1 on chromosome 17) has been identified. Sometimes the inherited risk is well defined, as in the condition xeroderma pigmentosum, a deficiency of DNA repair enzymes. Polyposis coli is an autosomal dominant inherited predisposition to develop multiple adenomatous polyps of the large bowel; consequently there is an increased risk of carcinoma of the colon and rectum arising in these polyps. Retinoblastoma, a malignant tumour of the eye in children, is familial and often bilateral in approximately one-third of cases; in these patients there is usually an abnormality of chromosome 13.

Age

The incidence of cancer increases with age. There are several possible explanations: the cumulative risk of exposure to carcinogens with increasing age; the long latent interval between exposure to the initiating carcinogenic agent and the clinical appearance of the resulting tumour means that there is inevitably a tendency for most tumours to begin to appear only after a few decades of life have elapsed; accumulating genetic lesions (mutations) may render the ageing cell more sensitive to carcinogenic effects. Finally, it may be that incipient tumours developing in young individuals are recognised and eliminated by some innate defence system, such as natural killer cells, and that this protective effect is lost with age.

Table 11.9 Examples of inherited cancer risks

Inherited disorder	Tumour(s)	Comment
Multiple endocrine neoplasia (MEN) syndromes	Endocrine tumours, e.g. phaeochromocytoma, medullary carcinoma of the thyroid, parathyroid adenoma	Several types (MEN I, II, etc.) attributed to RET gene on chromosome 10 and others on chromosome 11
Xeroderma pigmentosum	Skin cancers, e.g. basal cell carcinoma, melanoma	Deficiency of DNA repair enzymes
Familial polyposis coli	Colorectal carcinoma	Preceded by numerous adenomatous polyps; autosomal dominant APC gene on chromosome 5
von Hippel–Lindau syndrome	Cerebellar haemangioblastoma, phaeochromocytoma, hypernephroma	
Li–Fraumeni syndrome	Breast carcinoma, soft-tissue sarcomas	Autosomal dominant inheritance associated with abnormalities on chromosomes 13 (Rb1 gene), 11 and 17 (p53 gene)
Retinoblastoma	Retinoblastoma (frequently bilateral)	Inherited allelic loss of one inhibitory Rb1 gene on chromosome 13
Familial breast carcinoma	Breast carcinoma Ovarian carcinoma (Prostatic carcinoma in male family members)	Attributed to mutated BRCA1 gene on chromosome 17

Gender

Breast cancer is at least 200 times commoner in women than in men. This is probably due to the greater mammary epithelial volume and to the promoting effects of oestrogens in females. It is more common in women who are nulliparous or who have not breast fed their children, and those who have experienced an early menarche and/or late menopause. The precise pathophysiological explanation for these observations has not yet been fully characterised, but endocrine factors are undoubtedly important.

Associations with gender occur in other cancers, but these are more often due to, for example, smoking habits, than to hormonal factors.

Premalignant lesions and conditions

A *premalignant lesion* is an identifiable local abnormality associated with an increased risk of a malignant tumour developing at that site. Examples include adenomatous polyps of the colon and rectum, and epithelial dysplasias in various sites, notably the cervix. Studies of these lesions reinforce the multistep theory of carcinogenesis (Fig. 11.23); it may be that these lesions represent the growth of partially transformed cells which have not yet achieved full neoplastic status.

A *premalignant condition* is one which is associated with an increased risk of malignant tumours. In chronic ulcerative colitis, for example, there is an increased risk of colorectal cancer and this can be predicted by seeking the premalignant lesion (in this case dysplasia) in rectal biopsies. Sometimes congenital abnormalities predispose to cancer; the undescended testis is, for example, more prone to neoplasms than the normally located organ.

It is vitally important to identify patients with premalignant lesions and conditions so that they can be followed up carefully, and tumours detected at an early stage when they are more amenable to potentially curative treatment (Table 11.10). This is the

Table 11.10 Examples of premalignant lesions and conditions

Lesion/condition	Cancer risk
Premalignant lesion	
Adenomatous polyp of colorectum	Colorectal adenocarcinoma
Cervical epithelial dysplasia	Carcinoma of the cervix
Mammary ductal epithelial hyperplasia	Carcinoma of the breast
Premalignant condition	
Hepatic cirrhosis	Hepatocellular carcinoma
Xeroderma pigmentosum	Skin cancer
Ulcerative colitis	Colorectal adenocarcinoma Bile duct carcinoma

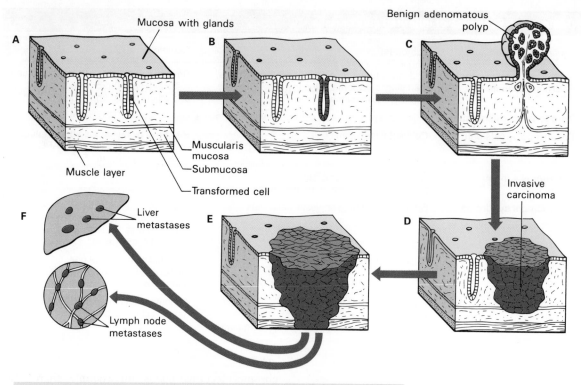

Fig. 11.23   Carcinoma of the large bowel as a model of tumour progression

A. A single epithelial cell within a mucosal gland becomes transformed into a tumour cell by carcinogenic events. **B.** The abnormal cell proliferates to produce a clone of cells populating one gland. **C.** Further proliferation results in the formation of a benign, non-invasive polyp (adenoma) protruding from the mucosal surface. **D.** The transformed cells become invasive as a result of further genetic changes; the lesion is now regarded as malignant (carcinoma). **E.** The malignant cells invade blood vessels and lymphatics, and are carried to the liver and lymph nodes, respectively, to form secondary tumours (metastases) (**F**).

principle of the population screening programmes for carcinoma of the cervix.

Transplacental carcinogenesis

In the 1940s some pregnant women with threatened miscarriages were treated with diethylstilbestrol, a synthetic oestrogenic compound, in an attempt to avert the fetus being aborted. The female progeny of those pregnancies which went successfully to full term were later discovered to have a high incidence of vaginal adenocarcinoma, an otherwise rare tumour, in early adult life. This is an example of transplacental carcinogenesis; the carcinogen, presumably diethylstilbestrol, was administered to the mother, but the carcinogenic effect was exhibited only in the child resulting from the pregnancy, when she reached young adulthood.

CELLULAR AND MOLECULAR EVENTS IN CARCINOGENESIS

▶ Multistep process
▶ May require initiating and promoting agents
▶ Growth persists in the absence of the causative agents
▶ Genetic alterations of oncogenes and tumour suppressor genes

Having considered the various types of carcinogen, we can now turn our attention to the way in which these agents actually transform normal cells into neoplastic cells, capable of autonomous growth and, in malignant neoplasms, of invasion and metastasis.

Experimental observations

Evidence for a *multistep theory* of carcinogenesis is derived mostly from observations on the effects of chemical agents on laboratory animals.

Latency

Part of the reason for the long latent interval between exposure to a carcinogen and clinical recognition of the tumour is the fact that tumours result from the clonal proliferation of single cells; it takes an appreciable time for this transformed single cell to grow into a nodule of cells large enough to cause signs and symptoms. However, another important factor is that, with the possible exceptions of ionising radiation and of some fast-transforming oncogenic retroviruses, the change from a normal cell into a growing and potentially lethal neoplasm is thought to entail more than one event.

Initiation and promotion

Experimental carcinogenesis has revealed two major steps in the transformation of cells from normal to neoplastic: initiation and promotion. *Initiation* is the event that actually induces the lesion in the cell's genome that bestows neoplastic potential. *Promotion* is the event stimulating clonal proliferation of the initiated transformed cell. The most frequently cited example of this two-step process is the effect of successive applications of methylcholanthrene and croton oil on mouse skin. A single application of methylcholanthrene only results in a tumour if it is followed by repeated painting of the site with non-carcinogenic croton oil; methylcholanthrene is the initiator inducing lesions in the DNA of the target cell; croton oil promotes the growth of the initiated cell (Fig.11.24).

Such experiments cannot, of course, be performed in man. However, a possible counterpart to the initiated cell of experimental carcinogenesis is provided by the lesions of epithelial dysplasia seen commonly, for example, in the cervix and in large bowel mucosa affected by chronic ulcerative colitis; in both instances there is a significant risk of progression to frank carcinoma, possibly by an event paralleling promotion in experimental carcinogenesis.

Many tumours probably arise without the need for external promoters. A promoting effect probably results from further random mutational genetic abnormalities co-operating with those resulting from the initiating agent.

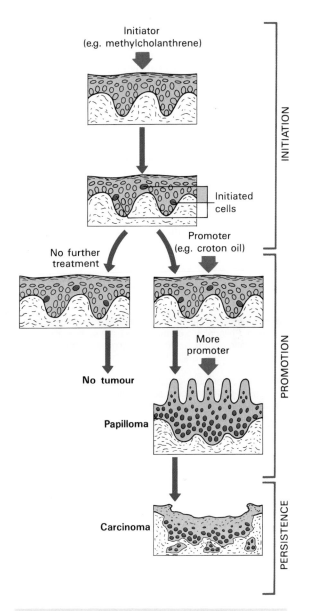

.Fig. 11.24   Initiation, promotion and persistence, as illustrated by the multiple steps involved in experimental chemical carcinogenesis in the epidermis

Latency is represented by the time interval between exposure to the initiating agent and the growth of a detectable neoplasm. (See text for details)

Persistence

The stage of persistence is reached when the clonal proliferation of the tumour cells no longer requires the presence of initiators or promoters, and the tumour cells are exhibiting autonomous growth. Earlier events have altered the expression of genes (cellular or proto-oncogenes) causing them to function inappropriately and thus enabling the cells to grow by autocrine stimulation (p. 282). Later stages in the process involve the induction of vascular ingrowth into the tumour through the action of tumour angiogenic factors, so that its further enlargement can be sustained by perfusion with nutrients; and, if the tumour is malignant, the formation of secondary tumours by the process of *metastasis*. The formation of secondary tumours does not, of course, necessitate a recapitulation of the earlier stages of carcinogenesis; they form from the growth of cells from the primary tumour which have already been transformed.

Genetic abnormalities in tumours

▶ Chromosomal abnormalities, sometimes consistent (e.g. Philadelphia chromosome), are common
▶ Oncogenes, genes directing cell growth and differentiation, are abnormally expressed in many tumours
▶ Inherited or mutational loss of tumour suppressor genes permits tumour development
▶ Oncogene expression results in autocrine growth stimulation

Chromosomal abnormalities

Until quite recently the only technique for examining the genome of cells was chromosomal (karyotypic) analysis. This involves culturing the cells in the presence of colchicine, which blocks formation of the mitotic spindle and arrests mitosis in metaphase. On exposure to a hypotonic medium, the osmotic shock causes the cells to explode and spill their chromosomes on to the surface of a glass slide where they can be stained, counted and examined in detail. Unfortunately, at this relatively crude level of analysis in molecular terms, very few recurring patterns of chromosomal abnormality have been found in tumours. Abnormalities such as additional chromosomes and translocation of part of one chromosome to another are very common, but few are constant even among a single tumour type (Table 11.11). One of the few exceptions is the Philadelphia chromosome; this is one of the most consistent chromosomal abnormalities yet discovered, and is commonly found in chronic myeloid (granulocytic) leukaemia. More recently, however, chromosomes have been studied by in situ hybridisation, a technique that enables determination of the number and location of specific DNA sequences (Fig. 11.25).

Genetic mechanisms in carcinogenesis

There are two genetic mechanisms leading to tumour growth (Fig. 11.26):

• loss or inactivation of recessive inhibitory genes — *tumour suppressor genes*
• enhanced or abnormal expression of dominant stimulatory genes—*oncogenes*.

Both mechanisms operate in most tumours, but loss or inactivation of tumour suppressor genes explains inherited predispositions to the development of tumours.

A single genetic alteration is probably not sufficient for tumour development; the transformation of a normal cell into a neoplastic lineage requires a series of genetic alterations. These genetic alterations are inherited by the daughter cells.

Table 11.11	Examples of non-random chromosomal abnormalities in neoplastic diseases	
Neoplasm	Chromosomal abnormality	Comment
Burkitt's lymphoma	Translocation of c-*myc* oncogene from chromosome 8 to an immunoglobulin gene locus on chromosome 14	Results in expression of c-*myc* gene
Chronic myeloid leukaemia	Translocation involving chromosomes 9 and 22 (Philadelphia chromosome)	Results in fusion of c-*abl* and *bcr* genes; *bcr-abl* protein has tyrosine kinase activity
Follicle centre cell lymphoma	Translocation involving chromosomes 14 and 18	Results in expression of *bcl*-2 gene inhibiting apoptosis
Ewing's tumour Peripheral neuroectodermal tumour	Translocation involving chromosomes 11 and 22	Distinguishes these tumours from neuroblastoma, which they may resemble histologically

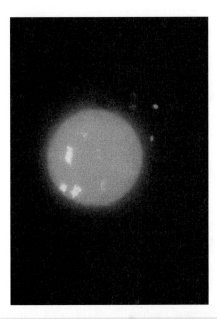

Fig. 11.25   Chromosomal abnormality revealed by FISH

Three X chromosomes revealed by FISH (fluorescent in situ hybridisation) in the nucleus of a lymphoma cell probed with complementary DNA labelled with a fluorescent dye. FISH enables chromosomal abnormalities to be detected in intact tumour cell nuclei. (Courtesy of Dr M Goyns, Sheffield)

Tumour suppressor genes

Clues to the existence of inhibitory genes came from observations on the behaviour of transformed cells that were fused with untransformed cells; the resulting hybrid cells behaved like untransformed cells until specific chromosomes bearing the inhibitory genes were lost, causing the cells to revert to their transformed state. The existence of inhibitory genes

was also postulated by Alfred Knudson in 1971. Using a statistical approach to familial cancer incidence he formulated a *two-hit hypothesis*.

Rb gene

The first inhibitory gene to have been well characterised is the Rb1 gene associated with retinoblastomas. Retinoblastomas are malignant tumours derived from the retina; they occur almost exclusively in children. In some cases they are hereditary, occurring bilaterally and also in some of the patient's siblings. In other cases they are sporadic, occurring unilaterally and without any familial associations. Individuals with hereditary retinoblastomas show a germline deletion on chromosome 13, corresponding to the known site of the Rb1 gene. Therefore, only one further mutational loss of the paired gene in the target retinal cell is required for the tumour to develop. Sporadic retinoblastoma cases have a normal chromosome 13 and therefore require two mutational losses before the tumour can develop (Fig. 11.27).

p53 gene

The tumour suppressor gene p53, situated on the short arm of chromosome 17, is the most frequently mutated and extensively studied in human cancer. The normal functions of p53 are to enable:

- repair of damaged DNA before S-phase in the cell cycle by arresting the cell cycle in G_1 until the damage is repaired
- apoptotic cell death if there is extensive DNA damage.

The p53 levels rise in cells which have sustained DNA damage, until either the damage is repaired or the cell undergoes apoptosis. This prevents propaga-

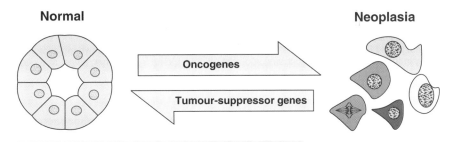

Fig. 11.26   Oncogenes and tumour suppressor genes

Abnormal expression of oncogenes drives normal cells towards the neoplastic state. Loss of tumour suppressor gene function permits neoplastic transformation as a result of oncogene expression.

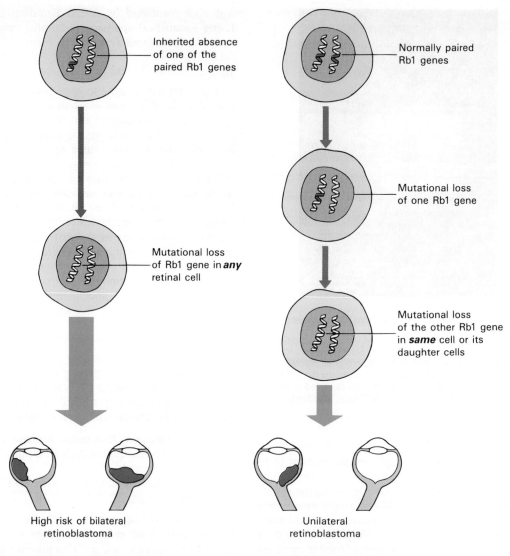

A. INHERITED RETINOBLASTOMA

B. SPORADIC RETINOBLASTOMA

Fig. 11.27   Loss of tumour inhibitory genes (anti-oncogenes) and inherited retinoblastoma

Loss of the inhibitory genes permits tumour development. **A.** Individuals with an inherited predisposition to develop retinoblastoma are born with absence of one of the normally paired Rb1 suppressor genes; only one further mutational loss of the remaining Rb1 gene is required for retinoblastomas to develop. **B.** Normal individuals with paired Rb1 genes have a low incidence of retinoblastoma, because two mutational losses have to occur in the same cell or its daughters; sporadic retinoblastoma is, therefore, a very rare event.

tion of possibly mutated genes. This important function of p53 results in it being called 'the guardian of the genome'.

p53 can lose its normal function by a variety of mechanisms:

- *mutations* which either render the gene unreadable (non-sense mutations) or encode for a defective protein (mis-sense mutations)
- *complexes* of normal p53 and mutant p53 (in heterozygous individuals or cells) inactivating the function of the normal allele
- binding of normal p53 protein to proteins

encoded by *oncogenic DNA viruses* (e.g. human papillomavirus, polyomaviruses).

These events have major implications. Cells with damaged DNA, possibly with mutated oncogenes, undergo mitotic replication rather than apoptotic death (Fig. 11.28). Also, cytotoxic chemotherapy against the tumour may be less effective if the cells fail to respond by apoptosis.

Inherited germline (present in all cells) mutations of p53 occur in the rare *Li–Fraumeni syndrome*. Affected individuals have an inherited predisposition to a wide range of tumours. At birth they are heterozygous for the defective gene (only very rarely are the maternal and paternal alleles both defective). Eventually, the normal allele is itself lost or mutated *(loss of heterozygosity)* in a

variety of cells, thus enabling their neoplastic transformation.

Oncogenes

Oncogenes are genes governing the neoplastic behaviour of cells. Originally proposed as a hypothesis, oncogenes were 'discovered' as a result of studies of oncogenic RNA retroviruses. These are RNA viruses which have the ability to transfer their genome, or parts of it, to the genome of the cells they infect. Normally the transfer of genomic information is in the opposite direction: DNA sequences are transcribed into RNA, which then determines the amino acid sequence of a peptide or protein. However, retroviruses contain an enzyme, *reverse transcriptase*, which

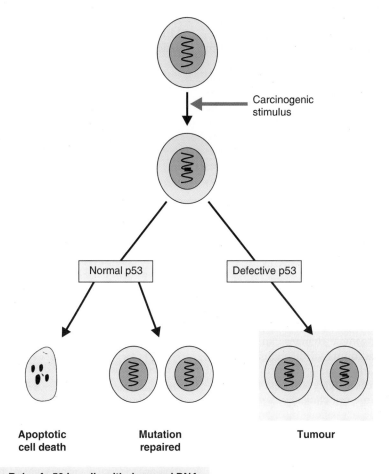

Fig. 11.28   Role of p53 in cells with damaged DNA

In the presence of normal p53, cells with a mutation resulting from a potentially carcinogenic stimulus are arrested in G_1 of the cell cycle until either the mutation is repaired or, if the damage is severe, apoptosis occurs. If the p53 is defective, as a result of mutation or binding, the cells proceed to S-phase and the mutation is propagated to daughter cells, possibly eventually leading to a tumour.

enables the viral RNA to be transcribed into complementary DNA which is then incorporated into the infected cell's genome. In the case of oncogenic retroviruses, these genes were called *oncogenes*.

The next major discovery was of the presence of DNA sequences identical to viral oncogenes (*v*-oncogenes) in the genome of normal cells (cellular or proto-oncogenes). However, in normal cells these oncogenes are present at the frequency of only one copy per haploid genome, and their transcription is tightly controlled as required for cell growth and differentiation.

They are present in the genome of even the most primitive protozoa and metazoa; this high degree of evolutionary conservation is usually associated with a function indispensable to normal life. The result of much research now leads us to conclude that these cellular oncogenes are essential for normal cell and tissue growth and differentiation particularly during embryogenesis and healing. It is when they are aberrant or inappropriately expressed that they result in the growth of a tumour.

At least 60 oncogenes have now been identified. Some sceptics argue that alterations in the expression of oncogenes are relatively late events in the development of tumours, postulating that they are a consequence rather than a cause of transformation. Experimental evidence, however, suggests otherwise. Normal or partially transformed cell cultures can be fully transformed by the addition of DNA bearing oncogenes, a process known as *transfection*. Alternatively, oncogenic (or carcinogenic) retroviruses can transform cells by transferring oncogenes from another cell, a process known as *transduction*.

Experiments with cell cultures and transgenic mice show that some oncogenes, notably *myc* and *ras*, have well-characterised effects corresponding to the early stages of tumourigenesis (Fig. 11.29). Mutant *ras* genes have also been detected in some of the early lesions of neoplasia. Nevertheless, there is no doubt that further genetic changes can take place in tumour cells; this accounts for the cellular heterogeneity seen particularly in malignant tumours, and may result in the increased aggressiveness of a malignant tumour often witnessed clinically.

Oncogenes can be classified into five groups according to the function of the gene product (oncoprotein):

- *nuclear-binding oncoproteins* involved in the regulation of cellular proliferation (e.g. *myc*)
- *tyrosine kinase activity* (e.g. *src*)
- *growth factors* (e.g. *sis* coding for platelet derived growth factor)

- *receptors for growth factors* (e.g. *erb*B coding for epidermal growth factor receptor)
- *cyclic nucleotide binding activity* (e.g. *ras* and GTP) disrupting intracellular signalling.

Abnormalities of oncogene expression are of crucial relevance to the growth and behaviour of tumour cells.

Abnormalities of oncogene expression in tumours
Oncogene expression can become altered to result in either:

- normal quantities of the oncoprotein molecule altered by mutation in such a way that it is abnormally active
- normal oncoprotein produced in excessive quantities because of gene amplification or enhanced transcription.

Mutant oncoproteins may have less or greater biological activity than the normal molecule. This can

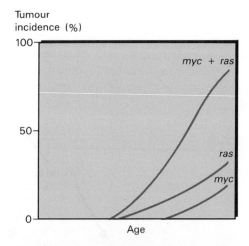

Fig. 11.29   Experimental evidence for the role of oncogenes in tumour development

Transgenic mice with either *myc* or *ras* oncogenes coupled to promoter/enhancer sequences—and thus producing abnormally high concentrations of the respective oncoprotein—were monitored, and the incidence of tumours recorded. Note that both *myc* and *ras* are associated with tumour development, otherwise a relatively rare event in normal mice. Transgenic mice expressing both oncogenes show an incidence of tumours greater than the summation of the effects of *myc* or *ras* alone. However, even with the combined expression of both oncogenes, there is a delay in the appearance of tumours and only a few cells are transformed; this suggests the necessity for further mutations, as yet uncharacterised.

have profound effects on receptor function and intracellular signalling. For example, the mutant protein product of the *ras* oncogene family is a hyperactive protein acting on cyclic nucleotides (GTP); the oncoprotein binds GTP and has GTPase activity.

Increased expression of oncogenes has been found in many tumours. The mechanisms are summarised in Figure 11.30.

Increased expression may be detected by:

- the presence of more of the oncogene product *(oncoprotein)* within or on the cells
- increased production of mRNA transcripts of the oncogene
- increased numbers of copies of the oncogene in the genome.

Increased numbers of copies result from infection by a retrovirus, which causes reverse transcription of its RNA and insertion of *multiple copies* of the resulting DNA into the DNA of the host cell genome.

This property of retroviruses is well documented experimentally, but is probably not a major cause of human cancer. A more common example in humans is DNA amplification resulting in multiple gene copies, such as in the *myc* family of oncogenes in neuroblastoma; this can be recognised in chromosome preparations from tumour cells by the presence of *homogeneously staining regions* and *double minute chromosomes*. *Increased transcription* can occur if the oncogene, not normally transcribed in the genome, is moved to another part of the genome where active transcription is occurring. This is often evident from the karyotype; part of one chromosome which is known to bear an oncogene may be translo-

cated to another chromosome where a gene known to be actively transcribed is situated. Specific examples include:

- translocation of the c-*abl* gene from chromosome 9 to chromosome 22, an event which results in the formation of the Philadelphia chromosome and expression of a *bcr-abl* fusion gene product in chronic myeloid leukaemia

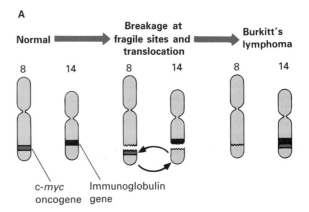

A

Normal ➡ Breakage at fragile sites and translocation ➡ Burkitt's lymphoma

8   14   8   14   8   14

c-*myc* oncogene   Immunoglobulin gene

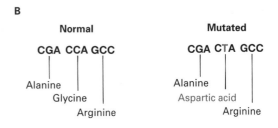

B

Normal	Mutated
CGA CCA GCC	CGA CTA GCC
Alanine	Alanine
Glycine	Aspartic acid
Arginine	Arginine

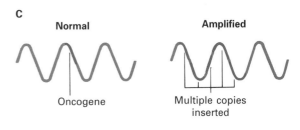

C

Normal   Amplified

Oncogene   Multiple copies inserted

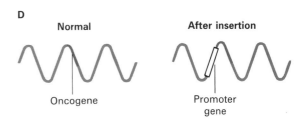

D

Normal   After insertion

Oncogene   Promoter gene

Fig. 11.30 Mechanisms of oncogene activation

A. Translocation of an oncogene from an untranscribed site to a position adjacent to an actively transcribed gene; e.g. simplified chromosomal translocation in Burkitt's lymphoma, in which the c-*myc* oncogene is often translocated from chromosome 8, its normal location, to chromosome 14, where it is placed adjacent to one of the immunoglobulin genes and is thus inappropriately transcribed. **B.** Point mutation (in this case in codon 12 of the *ras* oncogene), in which the substitution of a single base in the oncogene is translated into an amino acid substitution in the oncoprotein causing it to be hyperactive. **C.** Amplification by the insertion of multiple copies of the oncogene (in this case, c-*myc* in neuroblastoma), resulting in cellular proliferation stimulated by excessive quantities of the oncoprotein. **D.** Increased oncogene expression by gene insertion (*insertional mutagenesis*) resulting in proximity of an oncogene to a promoter or enhancing gene; this is one mechanism of retroviral carcinogenesis.

- translocation of the c-*myc* oncogene from chromosome 8 to chromosome 14, where its expression is assured by juxtaposition with one of the immunoglobulin genes which will be actively transcribed in the B-cell which is the origin of Burkitt's lymphoma.

Alternatively, the cellular oncogene may undergo a *point mutation* resulting in a gene product, such as a protein kinase, with increased or inappropriate activity.

Effects of oncogene products in tumour growth
Cell cultures transformed by carcinogens, and showing increased or mutant oncogene expression, exhibit a variety of changes corresponding to the abnormal behaviour and appearance of tumour cells in vivo:

- independence of the requirement for extrinsic growth factors
- production of tumours when injected into immunotolerant animals
- production of plasminogen activator and proteases to assist invasion
- reduced cell cohesiveness, thus assisting metastasis
- immortalisation
- an increase in plasma membrane and cellular motility
- growth to higher cell densities
- abnormal cellular orientation.

Autocrine growth stimulation
Oncogene products play an important role in cellular growth and differentiation (Table 11.12). By their expression in inappropriate circumstances a cell can become autonomous, proliferating without the usual requirement for external signals (Fig. 11.31). For example, an oncogene product may be a receptor for a growth factor (Ch. 5) already normally produced by that cell; the cell then responds to stimulation by

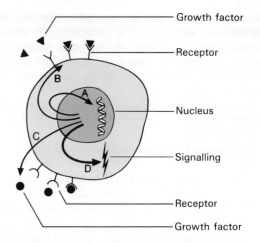

Fig. 11.31   Self-stimulation of neoplastic cell proliferation mediated by oncoproteins

A = Direct stimulation of DNA synthesis by an oncoprotein which binds to DNA. B = Synthesis of receptors (Y) for a growth factor (▼) already present in the extracellular environment. C = Synthesis of a growth factor (●), receptors for which (Y) are normally present on the cell.
D = Interference with intracellular signalling between the cell membrane and the nucleus.

its own growth factor. Alternatively, the oncogene product may be a growth factor for which the cell already normally bears a specific receptor. In both cases the result is *autocrine stimulation of growth*.

Other oncogene products act directly within the nucleus to stimulate mitosis or on intracytoplasmic second messengers, such as cyclic nucleotides, thus modulating *intracellular signalling*.

Interaction of carcinogens with oncogenes and tumour suppressor genes

The neoplastic behaviour of tumour cells persists after withdrawal of carcinogenic stimuli and this behaviour is passed on to subsequent cellular gener-

Table 11.12	Examples of oncogenes and the apparent function of their oncoprotein products	
Oncogene	Function of oncoprotein	Abbreviated from
abl	Protein-tyrosine kinase activity	Abelson mouse leukaemia
myc	Binds to DNA, directly stimulating synthesis	Myelocytomatosis
sis	Growth factor (platelet derived growth factor)	Simian sarcoma
erbB	Receptor for epidermal growth factor	Avian erythroblastosis (also *erbA*)
ras	Acts on intracellular signalling (cyclic nucleotides)	Rat sarcoma

ations through mitotic divisions; it is therefore concluded that the lesion responsible for neoplastic behaviour is within the genome. This has led to a search for the final common pathway through which the very diverse range of known carcinogens acts — a search for the molecular lesion within the genome that is the end result of carcinogenesis.

Ultimately, the metabolism of chemical carcinogens results in the formation of DNA adducts, but the mere presence of adducts is insufficient for tumours to develop. Further molecular alterations, such as mutations, during DNA replication, and clonal expansion of the mutated cells are required before a tumour results. The formation of adducts can be reversed by virtue of their innate instability, or by DNA repair enzymes; their effect may also be minimised by dilution with new DNA through normal replication.

The selectivity of a carcinogenic metabolite for a particular nucleotide is thought to explain the site-specific mutations induced in oncogenes that can result in their abnormal expression. For example, several chemical carcinogens have been shown experimentally to result in single base substitutions in codons 12 and 61 of the *ras* oncogene, leading to the synthesis of a hyperactive mutant protein. Site-specific mutations of p53 are reported to be present in hepatocellular carcinomas associated with aflatoxin exposure.

The mutational effects of ionising radiation are probably random throughout the genome, but when they occur in oncogenes or tumour suppressor genes the cells harbouring the mutant genes have a selective growth advantage, eventually resulting in tumours.

The role of viruses in tumour induction can be attributed directly to the genetic material within them and its incorporation within the host cell.

Epigenetic control of tumour growth

Current evidence favours the *genetic theory* of carcinogenesis, that tumours result only from induced or congenital genetic abnormalities which dictate the aberrant behaviour of the cells. Experimental evidence favouring the *epigenetic theory* — that the behaviour of tumour cells results from the expression of deregulated or abnormally controlled *non-mutated genes* — does not necessarily imply that the primary carcinogenic event is epigenetic; it simply shows that, in some instances, the neoplastic behaviour of tumour cells can be influenced by epigenetic factors. Indeed, a recent observation indicates that, in some lesions at least, there may be an epigenetic

influence. If the cells of a malignant teratoma are injected into an early mouse embryo, the neoplastic cells differentiate normally and no tumour develops. In other words, the otherwise autonomous growth and incompletely differentiated state of this particular malignant neoplasm can be corrected by an epigenetic influence.

BEHAVIOUR OF TUMOURS

The clinical effects of tumours are determined by the biological behaviour of the neoplastic cells within them. Their most important property, in malignant tumours, is the ability to invade and metastasise.

Invasion and metastasis

> ▶ Invasion is the most important sole criterion for malignancy
> ▶ Invasion is due to abnormal cell motility, reduced cellular cohesion, and production of proteolytic enzymes
> ▶ Metastasis is the process of formation of distant secondary tumours
> ▶ Common routes of metastasis include lymphatic channels, blood vessels, and through body cavities

Invasion and metastasis merit detailed consideration because they are responsible for most of the lethal consequences of tumours. They also determine the most appropriate treatment. There is no point in simply removing the tumour itself. In most instances the tumour should be removed in continuity with a wide margin of apparently normal tissue, to ensure that the plane of resection is clear of the invasive edge of the tumour; the regional lymph nodes may also be resected. Incomplete local removal of a tumour may result in a local recurrence because the original plane of resection transected the invasive edge of the lesion.

Tumours should be manipulated with care during clinical examination or surgical removal, to minimise the risk of pumping tumour cells into blood and lymphatic channels. A ligature is therefore often tied around the vascular pedicle at an early stage in the surgical removal of a tumour.

Invasion

The invasiveness of malignant neoplasms is determined by the properties of the neoplastic cells within them. Factors influencing tumour invasion are:

- abnormal or increased cellular motility
- secretion of proteolytic enzymes
- decreased cellular adhesion.

Cellular motility is abnormal in that the cells are not only more motile than their normal counterparts (which may not move at all), but also show loss of the normal mechanism that arrests or reverses normal cellular migration: contact inhibition of migration.

Proteinases and inhibitors

Matrix metalloproteinases are among the most important proteinases in neoplastic invasion. These enzymes are secreted by malignant neoplastic cells, enabling them to digest the surrounding connective tissue. There are three families:

- *interstitial collagenases* — degrade types I, II and III collagen
- *gelatinases* — degrade type IV collagen and gelatin
- *stromelysins* — degrade type IV collagen and proteoglycans.

These enzymes are counteracted by *tissue inhibitors of metalloproteinases* (TIMPs). The net effect is determined by the balance between metalloproteinases and their inhibitors. It may be possible to limit the invasiveness of tumour cells by artificially increasing the level of inhibitory activity.

Invasion often occurs along tissue planes offering less resistance to tumour growth, such as perineural spaces and, of course, vascular lumina. Other tissues are extremely resistant to neoplastic invasion, such as cartilage and the fibrocartilage of intervertebral discs.

Clinicopathological significance

Invasion is the single most important criterion of malignancy. Metastasis is a consequence, and thus a manifestation, of invasion. In epithelial tumours, invasion is relatively easy to recognise because the basement membrane serves as a clear line of demarcation between the tissue boundaries (Fig. 11.12). In connective tissue tumours, invasion is less easy to recognise unless there is clear evidence of vascular or lymphatic permeation; other histological features, such as mitotic activity, are usually taken into consideration for prognostic purposes.

Invasion within epithelium is known as *pagetoid infiltration*; it is named after Paget's disease of the nipple, which is due to infiltration of the epidermis of the nipple by tumour cells from a ductal carcinoma in the underlying breast. This route of infiltration can also occur with a few other epithelial malignancies.

Metastasis

Metastasis is the process whereby malignant tumours spread from their site of origin (the *primary tumour*) to form other tumours (*secondary tumours*) at distant sites. The total tumour burden resulting from this process can be very great indeed, and the total mass of the secondary tumours invariably exceeds that of the primary lesion; it is not uncommon at autopsy to find a liver weighing several kilograms more than normal, laden with metastases. The word *carcinomatosis* is used to denote extensive metastatic disease.

Sometimes, metastases can be the presenting clinical feature. Bone pain or fractures due to skeletal metastases can be a manifestation of a clinically occult internal malignancy. Palpable lymph nodes, due to metastatic involvement, may appear before the signs and symptoms of the primary tumour.

The metastatic cascade

Neoplastic cells must successfully complete a cascade of events before forming a metastatic tumour (Fig. 11.32). Only a proportion of the neoplastic cells in a malignant tumour may have the full repertoire of properties necessary for completion of the cascade. Many tumours studied experimentally in animals consist of metastatic and non-metastatic clones, and metastatic tumours in humans often appear histologically less well differentiated than the primary lesion, suggesting that there is clonal evolution of the metastatic phenotype. There is experimental evidence for the inactivation of 'anti-metastatic' genes ('metastogenes'), such as nm23, in neoplastic cells capable of metastasis, but their precise role in the metastatic cascade is uncertain.

The sequential steps involved in the metastatic cascade are:

1. *detachment* of tumour cells from their neighbours
2. *invasion* of the surrounding connective tissue to reach conduits for metastasis (blood and lymphatic vessels)
3. *intravasation* into the lumen of vessels
4. *evasion* of host defence mechanisms, such as natural killer cells in the blood
5. *adherence* to endothelium at remote location
6. *extravasation* of the cells from the vessel lumen into the surrounding tissue.

On reaching the site of metastasis there is a recapitulation of the events that were required to form the primary tumour. The tumour cells must proliferate and, if they are to grow to form a nodule larger than

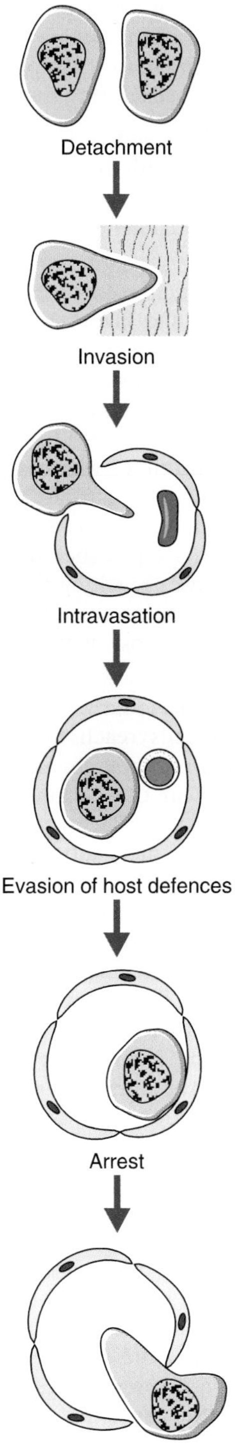

Process	Possible mediators	Consequence

Detachment

- Loss of surface adhesion molecules (e.g. cadherins)

Migration of individual cells enabled

Invasion

- Metalloproteinases
- Up regulation of integrin expression
- Down regulation of tissue inhibitors of metalloproteinases

Erosion of tissue boundaries

Intravasation

- Metalloproteinases
- Down regulation of tissue inhibitors of metalloproteinases

Access to vascular routes of dissemination

Evasion of host defences

- Reduced expression of MHC class 1 antigen
- Shedding of ICAM-1 blocks T-cell receptor

Survival against host defences

Arrest

- Binding of CD44 to endothelial ligand

Arrest of movement by adhesion to endothelium

Extravasation

- Integrins
- Laminin receptor

Colonisation of site of metastasis

Fig. 11.32 Metastatic cascade

The spread of tumour cells from the site of origin, the primary tumour, to form secondary tumours in other locations requires completion of a logical sequence of events mediated by tumour–host interactions.

a few millimetres in diameter, the ingrowth of blood vessels must be elicited by angiogenic factors.

Alterations in cell adhesion molecules are important at several points in the metastatic cascade; these affect cell–cell and cell–substrate adhesion. Studies on experimental and human tumours show that reduced expression of *cadherins*, which are involved in adhesion between epithelial cells, correlates positively with invasive and metastatic behaviour. Increased expression of *integrins* appears to be important for the invasive migration of neoplastic cells into connective tissues.

Routes of metastasis

The routes of metastasis are (Fig. 11.33):

- *haematogenous*, by the blood stream, to form secondary tumours in organs perfused by blood which has drained from a tumour
- *lymphatic*, to form secondary tumours in the regional lymph nodes

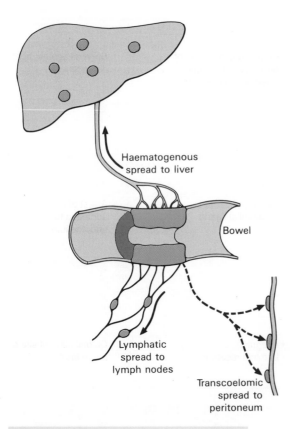

Fig. 11.33 Routes of metastasis exemplified by a carcinoma of the bowel.

- *transcoelomic*, in pleural, pericardial and peritoneal cavities where this invariably results in a neoplastic effusion
- *implantation*, for example by accidental spillage of tumour cells during the course of surgery.

Carcinomas tend to favour lymphatic spread, while sarcomas favour haematogenous spread. However, exceptions to these tendencies are common, and carcinomas often generate blood-borne metastases.

Haematogenous metastasis

Bone is a site favoured by haematogenous metastases from five carcinomas—lung, breast, kidney, thyroid and prostate. Other organs commonly involved by haematogenous metastases are lung, liver and brain (Fig. 11.34). The metastases are frequently multiple, whereas primary tumours arising in the affected organs are usually solitary. Curiously, tumours rarely metastasise to skeletal muscle or to the spleen, despite their lavish blood supply.

Metastases reaching the surface of the liver often have a central depression ('umbilication') as a consequence of necrosis within the tumour nodule.

Lymphatic metastasis

Tumour cells reach the lymph node through the afferent lymphatic channel. The tumour cells settle and grow in the periphery of the node, gradually extending to replace it (Fig. 11.35). Lymph nodes involved by metastatic tumours are usually firmer and larger than normal. Groups of involved lymph nodes may be matted together by both tumour tissue and the connective tissue reaction to it. Lymph node metastases often interrupt lymphatic flow, thus causing oedema in the territory that they drain.

Clinically, it is necessary to be cautious in interpreting the significance of enlarged lymph nodes draining tumours because the enlargement could simply be due to reactive changes.

Transcoelomic metastasis

The peritoneal, pleural and pericardial cavities are common sites of transcoelomic metastasis, which results in an effusion of fluid into the cavity. The fluid is rich in protein (i.e. it is an exudate) and may contain fibrin. The fluid also contains the neoplastic cells causing the effusion, and cytological examination of the aspirated fluid is very important in diagnosing the cause of effusions into body cavities (Fig. 11.36). The tumour cells often grow as nodules on the mesothelial surface of the cavity.

Peritoneal effusions (ascites) may be due to involvement by any abdominal tumour, but pri-

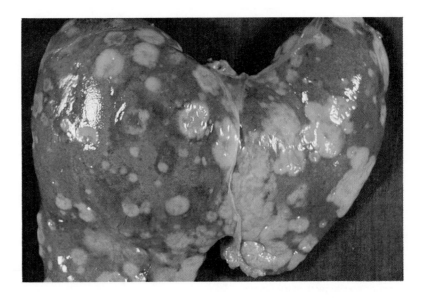

Fig. 11.34   Liver metastases

Liver from an autopsy on a patient who died from carcinomatosis due to carcinoma of the breast.

maries within the ovaries are particularly common. Pleural and pericardial effusions are common consequences of carcinomas of the breasts and lungs.

Clinical effects of tumours

> ▶ Local effects due to compression, invasion, ulceration or destruction of adjacent structures
> ▶ Metabolic effects due to appropriate or unexpected neoplastic cell products
> ▶ Effects due to metastases if tumour is malignant

The clinical effects of tumours are attributable to their location, their cell of origin and their behaviour. The effects may be local, or occur at some distance from the tumour.

Local effects

Tumours exert local effects through *compression* and *displacement* of adjacent tissues and, if malignant, through their *destruction* by actual invasion. These effects can be clinically inconsequential if the organ is large relative to the size of the tumour or if no vital structure is threatened. However, even benign tumours can have life-threatening effects on neighbouring structures; for example, a functionally inactive adenoma of the pituitary gland may obliterate the adjacent functioning pituitary tissue, such is the confined space in which the gland sits, resulting in hypopituitarism.

Malignant neoplasms obviously have more serious local effects because they *invade* and destroy local

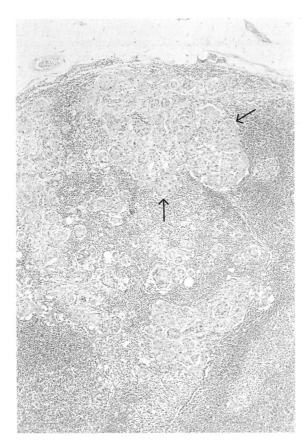

Fig. 11.35   Lymph node metastasis

The lymph node is partly replaced by a deposit of metastatic adenocarcinoma (arrowed) from a primary in the stomach.

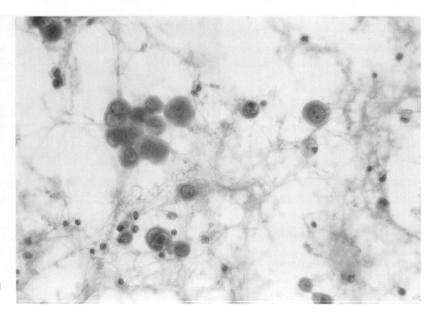

Fig. 11.36   Ascites due to carcinoma

The fluid has been aspirated and centrifuged to concentrate the cells onto a slide where they are then stained. The carcinoma cells are clumped and larger than the normal mesothelial and inflammatory cells.

structures. This may be fatal if a vital structure is eroded, for example a pulmonary artery by a carcinoma of the lung. In the case of basal cell carcinoma of the skin ('rodent ulcer'), its local effects are sufficient to justify the label 'carcinoma' because, although the tumour rarely metastasises, its invasiveness can be very disfiguring.

Malignant tumours on mucosal surfaces are often ulcerated. Blood can ooze from these lesions; this blood loss can be occult in the case of gastrointestinal tumours and this is a very important cause of *anaemia*. Ulcerated surfaces also expose the patient to the risk of infection.

Metabolic effects

The metabolic effects of tumours can be subdivided into those specific to individual tumours and those of a general nature.

Tumour-type specific effects
Well-differentiated endocrine tumours often retain the functional properties of the parent tissue. Since such tumours are relatively autonomous and because the total number of functioning cells often greatly exceeds that in the normal organ, clinical effects are common. For example:

- thyrotoxicosis may result from a thyroid adenoma
- Cushing's syndrome may result from an adrenocortical adenoma
- hyperparathyroidism may result from a parathyroid adenoma.

Sometimes the metabolic consequences of a tumour are unexpected or inappropriate, at least in the light of our current knowledge; for example, oat cell (small cell) carcinomas of the lung commonly secrete ACTH and ADH, although this rarely gives rise to clinically significant consequences.

Other specific tumour-associated phenomena have no metabolic consequences but are nevertheless probably mediated by humoral factors. The most common example is finger-clubbing and hypertrophic osteoarthropathy in patients with carcinoma of the lung.

Non-specific metabolic effects
Disseminated malignant tumours are commonly associated with profound weight loss despite apparently adequate nutrition. The catabolic clinical state of a cancer patient with severe weight loss and debility is known as *cachexia* and is thought to be mediated by tumour-derived humoral factors that interfere with protein metabolism. Cachexia can also occur quite early in the course of the disease, notably in patients with carcinoma of the lung. Weight loss can, of course, also be due to interference with nutrition because of, for example, oesophageal obstruction, severe pain or depressive illness.

Neuropathies and *myopathies* are associated with the presence of malignant neoplasms, particularly with carcinoma of the lung. A tendency to *venous thrombosis* is associated with mucus-producing adenocarcinomas, notably of the pancreas. *Glomerular injury* can result from deposition of immune complexes in which one of the ingredients is tumour antigen (Ch. 9).

Prognosis

Malignant tumours have a variable prognosis (Table 11.13). This is determined partly by the innate characteristics of the tumour cells (e.g. growth rate, invasiveness), and partly by the effectiveness of modern cancer therapy for individual types of tumour.

Prognostic indices

One of the major efforts in histopathology continues to be the search for features that more accurately predict the likely behaviour of individual tumours. It is insufficient merely to diagnose a tumour as malignant and to identify its origin. The patient's treatment is guided by the most accurate determination of:

- tumour type (e.g. melanoma, squamous cell carcinoma, leiomyosarcoma)
- grade or degree of differentiation
- stage or extent of spread
- stromal features such as lymphocytic infiltration.

It is also important to determine whether the presenting lesion is a primary tumour or a metastasis. This can be difficult. There may be little point in performing radical surgery for a tumour if it is a metastasis, and the primary tumour and perhaps other metastases are left unattended.

Tumour type
The tumour type is usually determined from the growth pattern of the tumour and its relationship to the surrounding structures from which an origin may be evident. Thus, a gland-forming neoplasm in the breast is most likely to be a primary adenocarcinoma of the breast, particularly if carcinoma cells are also present within the original breast ducts near the tumour (intraduct carcinoma). A squamous cell carcinoma is often recognisable from the production of keratin, and it may be in continuity with adjacent squamous epithelium that may show carcinoma in situ.

Some types of tumour need to be subclassified because variants with differing behaviour exist. Malignant lymphomas, for example, are subclassified into Hodgkin's and non-Hodgkin's lymphoma, each of which is then further subclassified by detailed appraisal of the histology (Ch. 22).

Electron microscopy or immunohistology may be necessary to type tumours that do not have obvious differentiated features detectable on routine light microscopy.

Tumour grade
The grade of a tumour is an assessment of its degree of malignancy or aggressiveness. This can be inferred from its histology. The most important features contributing to the assessment of tumour grade are:

- mitotic activity
- nuclear size and pleomorphism
- degree of resemblance to the normal tissue (i.e. differentiation).

Grading systems have been devised for many types of tumour, and most involve an assessment of the above features. Tumours are often heterogeneous, and the grading should be performed on what appears to be the least differentiated area as this is likely to contain the most aggressive clone or clones of tumour cells.

Tumour stage
The stage of a tumour is the extent of spread. This is determined by histopathological examination of the resected tumour and by clinical assessment of the patient, often involving imaging techniques. Perhaps the best-known staging system is that devised

---

Table 11.13   Prognosis of some different types of solid malignant tumour, based on experience of responses to treatment in the UK

Prognostic category		
Good	**Intermediate**	**Poor**
Seminoma of testis	Carcinomas of breast, colon, rectum, larynx, uterus, bladder and kidney	Carcinomas of lung, pancreas, stomach, oesophagus and liver
Basal cell carcinoma of skin	Malignant melanoma	Mesothelioma
	Teratoma of testis	
	Osteosarcoma	

A good prognosis implies a greater than 80% 5-year survival; poor prognosis implies a less than 20% 5-year survival. Prognosis in individual cases is, of course, influenced by tumour grade and stage at presentation.

by Cuthbert Dukes for colorectal carcinomas (see Ch. 15):

- Dukes' A: invasion into, but not through, the bowel wall
- Dukes' B: invasion through the bowel wall but without lymph node metastases
- Dukes' C: involvement of the local lymph nodes
- Dukes' D (a stage added by some surgeons): hepatic metastases present.

The most generally applicable staging system is the TNM system (Fig. 11.37):

- 'T' refers to the primary tumour and is suffixed by a number that denotes tumour size or local anatomical extent. The number varies according to the organ harbouring the tumour.
- 'N' refers to lymph node status and is suffixed by a number denoting the number of lymph nodes or groups of lymph nodes containing metastases.
- 'M' refers to the anatomical extent of distant metastases.

For example, a T1 breast carcinoma is equal to, or less than, 20 mm in diameter; large numbers denote large tumours. N0 denotes no nodal metastases, N1 one or few nodal metastases, and N2 many nodal metastases. M0 denotes an absence of metastases, and M1 and greater denotes increasing numbers of metastases.

Stromal features

Many surveys have shown that tumours showing infiltration of their stroma by lymphocytes and other defensive or immune cells have a better prognosis than tumours lacking such infiltrates (Ch. 9). However, it has to be admitted that the prognostic effect is often rather weak and that stromal features have less clinical value than do accurate typing, grading and staging of tumours. Nevertheless, the observation is of interest and has prompted much research into treating tumours by immunological methods.

Tumour dormancy

After surgical removal, radiotherapy and/or chemotherapy there may be no clinically detectable tumour remaining in a patient. This does not mean that the tumour has been completely eradicated, however, as minute deposits can evade detection by even the most sophisticated imaging techniques. These occult tumour foci can remain clinically dormant for perhaps several years before their regrowth

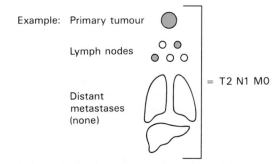

Fig. 11.37 Summary of TNM system for staging of tumours

This system is just one of many in current use.

causes signs and symptoms. For this reason, it is virtually impossible to speak of a cancer patient as being 'cured', and prognosis can be given only in terms of the probability of survival or the length of the disease-free interval. The prognostic information derived from tumour type, grade and stage is used to predict the patient's chances of surviving, say, 5 years.

EARLY DETECTION OF CANCER

It should be evident from the above description of the pathology, biology and clinical aspects of tumours that their prevention and early diagnosis are just as important as treatment in determining the outcome of the disease. Preventive measures can be planned from the results of epidemiological studies that identify specific risks. The success of early diagnosis relies upon finding tumours at a curable stage before they have had a chance to spread from their site of origin. This is best achieved by screening asymptomatic people, concentrating on those at greatest risk, in the hope of detecting very early lesions. In many countries there are active screening programmes for cervical and breast cancer.

Cervical intraepithelial neoplasia (CIN) can be detected by exfoliative cytology of the cervix. Cells are scraped from the cervix, smeared on to glass slides, stained, and then examined by a cytologist trained to detect abnormalities. Breast cancer can be detected at an early stage by regular screening by mammography (X-ray imaging of the breast), followed by diagnosis by fine-needle aspiration cytology or biopsy.

While these approaches work in theory, in practice the benefit may be less than anticipated. This is partly because some people are reluctant to be screened; those that do volunteer may not be from the socio-economic groups most at risk, particularly in the case of cancer of the cervix. Furthermore, early detection may not significantly affect the overall mortality from the screened cancer, but merely cause individuals premature anxiety about a disease that would not have become symptomatic for a few more years. Finally, it is not certain that all of the early cancers detected by screening would have progressed to more serious lesions within the otherwise natural lifetime of the individual concerned.

However, despite these doubts, screening for early cancers is likely to be a major area of progress in the next few decades. The successful prevention and early detection of cancer are highly dependent on public education targeted at those groups most at risk and on adequate financial investment.

FURTHER READING

Alberts B et al 1989 Molecular biology of the cell, 2nd edn. Garland, New York, pp 1187–1218

Bock G, Whelan J (eds) 1988 Metastasis. Ciba Foundation Symposium 141. Wiley, Chichester

Brusted T, Langmark F, Reitan J B 1990 Radiation and cancer risk. Taylor & Francis, London

Cavanee W K, White R L 1995 The genetic basis of cancer. Scientific American, March 1995: 50–57

Henson D E, Albores-Saavedra J 1986 The pathology of incipient neoplasia. W B Saunders, Philadelphia

International Agency for Research on Cancer 1987 Cancer incidence in five continents, vol 5. IARC, Lyon

Luderer A A, Weetall H H 1986 The human oncogenic viruses: molecular analysis and diagnosis. Humana, Clifton, New Jersey

Ponder B A J (ed) 1994 Genetics of malignant disease. British Medical Bulletin 50: 517–752

Rabbitts T H 1994 Chromosomal translocations in human cancer. Nature 372: 143–149

Sikora K, Evan G, Watson J V 1991 The cancer cell. British Medical Bulletin 47: 1–243

Yuspa S H, Poirier M C 1988 Chemical carcinogenesis: from animal models to molecular mechanisms in one decade. Advances in Cancer Research 50: 25

12

Ageing and death

Ageing and death are linked phenomena; as people age their death becomes more likely until, in extreme old age, we begin to be more surprised by continued life than by the occurrence of death. In general we believe that the older an object is the more likely it is that some disaster will overtake it; old cars break down, old buildings fall down, many old trees have to be cut down. But this is not a universal phenomenon; unicellular animals that reproduce by asexual division, in a sense live for ever. Every amoeba alive today is in direct line of cytoplasmic and nuclear descent from the very first amoeba that ever lived. The single cells of multicellular animals do not behave like this. Some, such as neurones or heart muscle cells, stop dividing at around the time of birth and, if one dies, it is not replaced. Even those cells that can reproduce in the human body do so less efficiently with the passage of time and it is a common clinical observation that elderly subjects show slower wound healing. There is even experimental evidence to support this. If cells from young animals are cultured they seem to be capable of about fifty cell divisions, but cells from older individuals are capable of progressively fewer cell divisions.

AGEING

Let us consider some of the clinical features of old age. It is often said that we are as old as our arteries, suggesting that arterial disease, which certainly increases with old age, is the cause of all the clinical signs of old age. Arterial degeneration, particularly atherosclerosis, is the commonest cause of debility and death in developed countries (Ch. 2). It would seem logical to think that many diseases might also have their roots in a progressively diminishing supply of oxygen and nutrients. However, in routine autopsies it is not uncommon to see people who have apparently died of 'old age' without significant arterial disease, which shows that at least some cases of ageing are not due to arterial problems even though this is commonly associated with ageing. It is also true that in many developing societies the aged population is not particularly afflicted by atherosclerosis and yet such individuals show all of the classic bodily features of old age; no matter which society you study it is generally possible to distinguish the older from the younger individuals. There is a significant difference between the diseases that patients die with and the diseases that they die from, but it is a difference that is often very difficult to establish scientifically.

Theories of ageing

▶ Hypotheses include inbuilt genetic mechanisms (clonal senescence) and 'wear and tear' (replication senescence)
▶ Ageing is influenced by genetic and environmental factors
▶ Replicative life-span of untransformed cells is limited (Hayflick limit)
▶ Cumulative free radical mediated intracellular injury may be important

Basically there are two main groups of ageing theories: *inbuilt genetic* mechanisms and environmental *'wear and tear'* mechanisms. There are data to support either theory but like the nature/nurture arguments in other areas of biology, such as the development of intelligence or of sexual orientation, the two possibilities are not mutually exclusive.

Inbuilt genetic mechanisms (clonal senescence theory)

Common experience supports the idea that there is an inbuilt 'allotted life-span' for humans and other animals. For instance, each animal species seems to have a characteristic *natural life expectancy* ranging from one day for a mayfly to well over one hundred years for various amphibia; not all individuals reach this — under natural conditions prevailing in the wild it may be that no individual reaches this natural limit because of the effects of predators, accidents and disease, or the younger individuals may actively drive out or kill an aged member of the group or more passively neglect them when they are no longer useful or economically viable. If animals are kept under ideal conditions it does appear that they age and die at around the same time; barring accidents, there is a characteristic life-span. Most human cultures reflect this in their belief that there is a natural age at which to die (around 'three score years and ten', though modern estimates would put it around 75) and that there are natural phases in life: infancy, adolescence, adulthood and ageing.

Evidence for genetic factors
From a scientific point of view, few would deny that the processes of embryogenesis, infancy, adolescence and maturity are genetically programmed, although the individual experience of these stages in life may be very highly modified by environmental conditions; the current estimate is that the more complex and variable features such as behaviour are about 60% genetic and 40% environmental. The

process of ageing seems to have a genetic component: members of the same family tend to live to the same sort of age and they age at the same sort of rate, leaving aside accident and disease. The actual inherited mechanism(s) that is responsible for the genetic component of ageing is still unclear but it is worth noting that longevity appears to be inherited through the female line and that all mammalian mitochondria come from the egg and none are transmitted via the sperm. Cell culture experiments suggest that some gene(s) affecting ageing are carried on chromosome 1, but, again, the way in which they influence ageing is unclear. There are also some remarkable 'natural experiments' in which some human subjects with rare genetic conditions (progerias) such as Werner's syndrome show premature ageing and die of old-age diseases such as advanced atheroma whilst still chronologically in their teens or early adulthood. Similarly, Down's syndrome patients generally age more rapidly than the rest of the population and it has been found that their fibroblasts are capable of fewer cell divisions in culture than those from age-matched controls. But this is far from being final proof that ageing is genetic; it shows us only that some features of ageing can be affected by genetic mechanisms. On the other hand, these conditions may be true models of the ageing process in which the gene(s) for ageing is amplified or expressed early.

Interaction with environmental factors
Social correlations with ageing and death are more difficult to interpret. It is well known that most diseases are more common in people from lower socio-economic groups and that people in these groups show ageing changes and die earlier than age- and sex-matched people from higher socio-economic groups. The most immediate interpretation of these phenomena is that people in these groups are disadvantaged in terms of diet, housing and social welfare generally. A good 'social experiment' that supports this idea is the decline in tuberculosis with improved social conditions which long preceded the introduction of antibiotics and the resurgence of the disease amongst the new poor in the UK. This is by no means proven, however—a genetic interpretation could explain the data just as well; this is a politically sensitive area and there are great social dangers involved in the casual and uncritical acceptance of either model.

Wear and tear (replication senescence)

The 'wear and tear' theories suggest that the normal loss of cells due to the vicissitudes of daily life and the accumulation of sublethal damage in cells lead eventually to system failure of sufficient magnitude that the whole organism succumbs; this theory provides a good explanation of why it is that cardiac and central nervous system failure are such common causes of death since the functionally important cells in these crucial tissues have no ability to regenerate. This theory ultimately depends upon a statistical view of ageing, suggesting that we are all exposed to roughly the same amount of wear and tear and therefore have a narrow range of life expectancy that appears to give us a characteristic life-span; it is hard to reconcile this with the one-day life-span of the mayfly and its relatives (but of course humans *may* be unique).

The various cellular and subcellular mechanisms that have been suggested as the cause of this sort of error accumulation include:

- protein cross-linking
- DNA cross-linking
- true mutations in DNA making essential genes unavailable or functionally altered
- damage to mitochondria
- other defects in oxygen and nutrient utilisation.

Role of free radicals
The common pathway resulting in cellular deterioration is currently thought to be the generation of highly reactive molecular species called 'free radicals' (Ch. 6). Free radicals are created in neutrophils and macrophages, under carefully controlled conditions, to kill ingested infective organisms; if they are generated accidentally elsewhere there are numerous enzymatic and quenching processes in cells to dispose of them before they can do harm. However, the greater the exposure to free radical generating environmental processes (such as toxins in the diet, ionising radiation, etc.) the greater the chance that some damage will occur; these insults will accumulate until they become visible as the ageing process. The power of this theory lies not only in the mechanical analogy of wear and tear in machines but also in the way that it parallels our concepts of the role of free radicals in some forms of carcinogenesis, particularly by those involving radiant energy (Ch. 11).

Defective repair
Natural experiments lend support to the wear and tear model. There are mechanisms in the cell that deal with damage, particularly DNA damage. These DNA repair mechanisms are numerous but very few deficiency states are well known; the best characterised of these is *xeroderma pigmentosum*. In this con-

dition young children who are exposed to sunlight develop skin atrophy and numerous skin tumours that are usually characteristic of elderly subjects with a long history of chronic sun exposure. This condition suggests that there are at least some mechanisms that hold many of the manifestations of ageing at bay; it is certainly possible that these mechanisms themselves could be susceptible to wear and tear, thus paving the way for more general decline.

Living systems are distinguished from most mechanical systems by their ability to regenerate. If the gastric mucosa is damaged, as it is every day by the simple process of eating, then unspecialised reserve cells at the base of the crypts divide and one of the progeny differentiates to become a new crypt cell; this mechanism is common to most tissues. But the *Hayflick phenomenon* suggests that most cells have the capacity for only a limited number of divisions (unlike cancer cells which seem to be immortal) and that this is under genetic control. Therefore in the final analysis *replicative* senescence seems to be dependent upon some form of *clonal* senescence, and the modifications to the cell during its lifetime act upon an intrinsic life-span program (Fig. 12.1).

Telomeric shortening
At the tip of each chromosome, there is a non-coding tandemly repetitive DNA sequence; this is the *telomere*. These telomeric sequences are not fully copied during DNA synthesis prior to mitosis. As a result, a single-stranded tail of DNA is left at the tip of each chromosome; this is excised and, with each cell division, the telomeres are shortened. Eventually the telomeres are so short that DNA polymerase is unable to engage in the subtelomeric start positions for transcription and the cell is then incapable of further replication. In human cells, it is only in germ cells and in embryos that telomeres are replicated by the enzyme telomerase.

Telomeric shortening could explain the replication ('Hayflick') limit of cells. This is supported by the finding that telomeric length decreases with the age of the individual from which the chromosomes are obtained. In progeria, there is premature telomeric shortening. Furthermore, short telomeres permit chromosomal fusion, and this correlates with the higher incidence of karyotypic aberrations in cells from elderly individuals and in senescent cells in culture.

Clinopathological features of ageing

> ► Some features associated with ageing are merely accompaniments; others are directly involved in the ageing process
> ► Every organ changes with age, often with progressive functional impairment
> ► Multiple pathology is common in the elderly

The chronological age of a human subject can often be estimated to within a decade or so on the basis of physical appearances alone. This is true at all ages

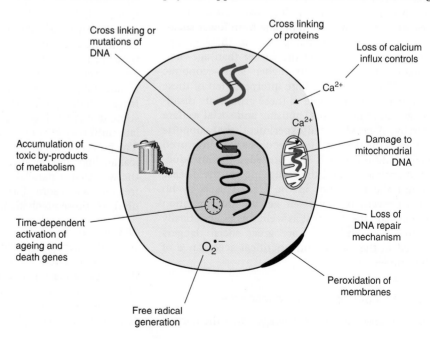

Fig. 12.1 Suggested cellular mechanisms of ageing and death

There is direct or circumstantial evidence supporting each of the mechanisms illustrated. Some mechanisms interact with others; for example, free radicals may be responsible for DNA mutations.

Cross linking or mutations of DNA

Cross linking of proteins

Loss of calcium influx controls

Ca^{2+}

Ca^{2+}

Accumulation of toxic by-products of metabolism

Damage to mitochondrial DNA

Time-dependent activation of ageing and death genes

Loss of DNA repair mechanism

$O_2^{\bullet -}$

Peroxidation of membranes

Free radical generation

and is certainly true in the elderly. The processes of development merge into the processes of ageing interrupted only by a period of maximum biological capacity commonly referred to as maturity. In most mammals maturity is the period of maximum reproductive capacity and is also the period of greatest prowess in the various 'pecking orders' and other social hierarchies that permit the transmission of an individual's genetic characteristics. As old age supervenes, this complex biological peak or prime begins to deteriorate and the chances of transmitting various genetic combinations decrease. The situation is a little complicated in the human in that the accumulation of wealth in males and the manipulation of fertility in females can modify this decline, but these exceptions are rare and do not affect the general rule.

One of the consequences of a cessation of reproductive capacity in the elderly is that diseases with a genetic component whose expression in a young adult might result in negative selection pressure have no such effect; such diseases therefore become preponderant in the elderly. For instance, a disease with a genetic component that proves lethal before or during the reproductive phase would impair the reproductive potential of that individual and the trait would eventually die out apart from new mutations; this obviously does not affect those diseases which only become manifest in old age since these individuals will already have reproduced and passed on the defective gene(s).

There are also other situations in which diseases may be associated with old age but are not related to the causes of old age. Any individual who has lived for 60 years has had more opportunities for accidents than an individual who has only lived for ten years so far, but this does not mean that accidents are part of the ageing process, although elderly individuals may be more prone to accidents because of failing eyesight, increased fragility of bones or decreasing mental acuity. So we should attempt to distinguish between the *process* of ageing and *accompaniments* of ageing, and this proves very difficult to do (Fig. 12.2).

Ageing of skin

At a fairly gross level the elderly are identifiable from

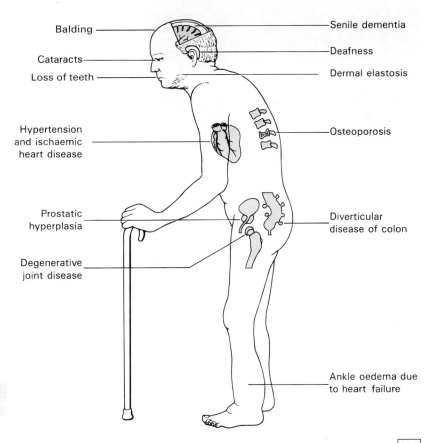

Balding
Cataracts
Loss of teeth
Hypertension and ischaemic heart disease
Prostatic hyperplasia
Degenerative joint disease

Senile dementia
Deafness
Dermal elastosis
Osteoporosis
Diverticular disease of colon
Ankle oedema due to heart failure

Fig. 12.2 Multiple pathology in the elderly

A typical case.

their wrinkled skin, loss of hair and sagging facial muscles (Fig. 12.3). Often the skin is also fragile, loses its youthful elastic recoil and is prone to bruising. Histologically the skin contains less collagen and less elastin, and what is still present is abnormal (Fig. 12.4), as judged by its biochemical properties. Both of these proteins are produced by fibroblasts so it is tempting to wonder whether fibroblasts alter with ageing. Research carried out on fibroblasts in culture has shown that cells cultured from young individuals are capable of more cell divisions (about 50 in total) than are cells derived from elderly individuals. It looks, therefore, as though there is a clear decline in cellular function with age that appears to be built into the genetics of the cell.

However, it is not enough to concentrate on the obvious; as in all clinical assessments we must consider the whole patient. If we make a full assessment of the skin we will see that the wrinkling that we took to be a cardinal sign of ageing is most pronounced on the sun-exposed areas of the skin; those areas that have remained covered for most of the patient's life

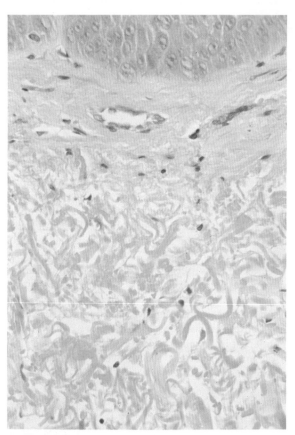

Fig. 12.4   Elastosis in skin

Skin biopsy from the face of an elderly man showing masses of thick homogeneous fibres in the dermis resulting from chronic damage to the dermal collagen by sunlight.

look decades 'younger' by this criterion. So, what are we to conclude? Is ageing an environmental phenomenon induced by sunlight? It seems unlikely since it is hard to believe that the diffuse, multiorgan phenomena that we associate with ageing could all be produced by exposing the skin to ultraviolet light.

Osteoarticular ageing

Elderly individuals are often stooped and susceptible to fractures, particularly of the femoral neck. Many post-menopausal women and elderly men have some degree of osteopenia or bone loss. In most cases this is due to *osteoporosis* (see Ch. 25), in which the bone matrix is normally mineralised but the trabeculae in particular are thinned; this results in fractures from relatively minor trauma and even in spontaneous fractures, commonly of the vertebral bodies leading

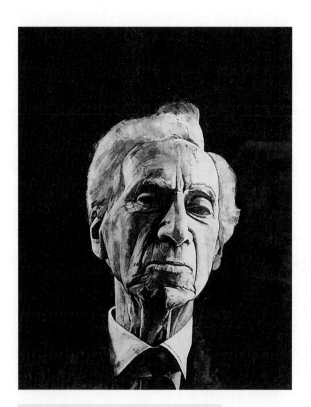

Fig. 12.3   Bertrand Russell in old age

The processes of ageing do not run synchronously. Bertrand Russell was very active intellectually into his tenth decade. (Painting by Barry Fantoni)

to a stooped posture (so-called 'Dowager's hump'). This would appear to be a clear indication that spontaneous deterioration in hormonal function (ovarian function in the case of post-menopausal women) leads to a classic ageing phenomenon; this is often treated with hormone replacement therapy (HRT). However, it is now becoming clear that the development of osteoporosis in old age is much more common in those who were inactive or who had diets low in calcium or vitamin D in youth, and epidemiological evidence is accumulating that many classic features of old age are controlled in this way by things that happen during the youth of the individual: an example which has been known for many years is the development of valvular heart disease in the elderly due to episodes of rheumatic fever in youth (see Ch. 13).

Impaired immunity

The relative immune paresis of old age can result in the recurrence of infections that were contracted many years before and which have never been cleared from the body but have lain dormant. Tuberculosis may erupt again in the elderly, particularly if they become immune-suppressed due to the development of cancer or due to the therapy for cancer, both of which may be immunosuppressive. If *Mycobacterium tuberculosis* organisms are present, tuberculosis can also arise as a spontaneous expression of progressive decline in the immune system which has been holding the disease in check, often for many years. Similarly, the chickenpox (varicella) virus can emerge from its hiding place in nerve ganglia and appear as shingles (herpes zoster) whenever the immune system is suppressed, whether by disease, chemotherapy or just old age.

The ageing of the immune system results in a partial loss of the ability to resist new infections and to continue to control old ones, but there is a paradoxical increase in autoimmune diseases with advancing age. Several possible explanations might be advanced for this: perhaps the processes that maintain immune self-tolerance age quicker than immune system; autoimmune diseases often follow damage to the tissue concerned and the elderly have had more time to accumulate damage; autoimmune diseases often follow on infections and we know that the elderly are more prone to infection. The mechanisms are discussed in Chapter 9.

Brown atrophy

Many body organs in the elderly are reduced in size (atrophy, Ch. 5) and are abnormally brown; this condition is 'brown atrophy'. The heart and liver are affected commonly. The atrophy is due to senile involution. The brown appearance is caused by excessive amounts of lipofuscin, a granular brown intracellular pigment (Fig. 12.5), often referred to as 'wear-and-tear' pigment because of its supposed association with excessive usage of an organ. The mere presence of excess lipofuscin does not appear to interfere with the function of the affected organ.

Cardiovascular changes

In the developed world the major cause of death in adults is the various deteriorations in the cardiovascular system, particularly heart attacks and strokes (see Ch. 13). So common is this that we begin to believe that this is the final common pathway of ageing and death. In the developing world, however,

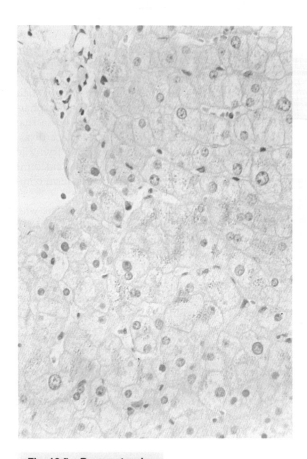

Fig. 12.5 Brown atrophy

Liver histology from an elderly person showing numerous brown perinuclear granules of lipofuscin in the liver cells. The liver was also unusually small due to senile atrophy.

these diseases are rare, although they are becoming more common as Western lifestyles and affluence spread; although a smaller percentage of the population survive into old age, those that do still show the classical features of senescence. Postmortem series show that in Western society most people die with the features of cardiovascular disease, but otherwise identical people in both the developed and developing world die without these features and with no obvious causes for death other than that they are old.

A very common concomitant of ageing is a progressive increase in blood pressure — *idiopathic hypertension*. This is an interesting condition because the initial pathological event appears to be a permanent increase in small vessel resistance; the hypertension is a 'physiological' attempt to overcome this and to maintain the essential perfusion pressure to peripheral tissues. Unfortunately the increased blood pressure has detrimental effects in larger vessels, such as increased atheroma with increased damage to cardiovascular function — this produces the age-associated major causes of death in Western societies. A significant clinical problem arises from this situation since it is tempting to treat hypertension because of its known association with disease. However, elderly patients need at least part of their hypertension to maintain effective perfusion; pharmacologically lowering their blood pressure to that of a healthy young adult is likely to produce disastrous effects on the end organs that one is trying to protect. The treatment of idiopathic hypertension is a delicate balance of short-term and long-term clinical advantages and disadvantages.

Atheroma itself is a disease which we associate with increasing age, but the war in Vietnam provided the opportunity to perform numerous autopsies on young American adult males; these autopsies revealed fatty streaks in the aorta in many young, otherwise healthy individuals dying from trauma. This again provides evidence that the diseases of old age have unexpected roots in youth and young adulthood.

Fate of permanent cells

Neurological function often declines with age; although a part of this can be attributed to decreased cardiovascular function, many subjects show specific deteriorations and accumulations peculiar to the brain (see Ch. 26). Nerve cells, like myocardial cells, are post-mitotic. There are no reserve cells and so damage to both brain and heart tissue is permanent. The advantage of this is that nerve cells and cardiomyocytes rarely give rise to tumours in the adult; brain tumours in the adult are derived from the vari-

ous connective tissue cells of the brain or are secondary deposits from cancers elsewhere in the body. It seems strange that such cells cannot replicate, especially since this inability results in so much clinical damage, but both organs rely upon highly ordered complex electrical activity and it may be that replicating cells within such a system would create more problems than they could solve.

Neoplastic diseases

Most neoplasms are commoner in old age but some, such as neuroblastoma and retinoblastoma, occur only in children. Other tumours may have a biphasic distribution, such as osteosarcoma in which there is a peak incidence in adolescence and a second peak in old age (see Ch. 25), but the tumours arising in adolescents appear spontaneous whereas those arising in old age almost always occur on the basis of longstanding disease (such as osteomyelitis, malunion of a fracture or Paget's disease) and it seems probable that these are two different tumours that are just impossible to separate morphologically. A similar situation applies with malignant melanoma of the skin; the peak incidence of melanoma on the legs of women and the backs of men (the commonest sites for melanoma) occurs around the third decade, but another type of malignant melanoma occurs on the face of the elderly (lentigo maligna melanoma). This curious age distribution appears to be related to episodic and severe sun exposure in the younger group, but to chronic long-term exposure in the elderly.

These observations suggest the interesting possibility that at least some tumours arise on a background of chronic tissue damage that seems to require many years of exposure to produce a cancer. Examples include smoking and bronchial carcinoma in which the risk increases regularly with dose of the carcinogens (number of cigarettes smoked) and the length of time that this exposure is continued; some cancers arise in longstanding venous ulcers on the legs of the elderly, so-called Marjolin ulcers (see Ch. 24).

DEATH

► Modes of death differ according to the ultimate cause
► Causes of death are categorised as natural (due to disease) or unnatural (due to accident, homicide, etc.)
► Sudden infant death syndrome requires thorough investigation to exclude determinable causes

Most definitions of death are, in general, rather unsatisfactory; the United Nations Statistic defines death as the permanent disappearance of all signs of life, but this presupposes that we have a useful and clear definition of life, which is far from being the case. One of the prime characteristics of living systems is that they are able to maintain homeostasis in the presence of quite extreme fluctuations in the environment; our core body temperature, the concentration of ions in cells, the circulation of the blood and the level of oxygenation of tissues are all kept constant within a tight range that we recognise as physiological. Other factors within the body may vary but we can see these as attempts to bring the body back into a normal range; shivering generates heat in cold situations, sweating causes heat to be lost in hot situations — the end effect is to return the individual to the normal physiological state. Sometimes these mechanisms are overwhelmed, as in hypothermia or in heat-stroke, but we immediately recognise these situations as pathological. If the body cannot return these functions to normal then vital homeostatic control has been permanently lost and death supervenes. This is true at the level of the whole organism (death of the individual) and at the cellular level (cell death, apoptosis). In some cases death of a large group of cells (such as heart cells or brain cells) may result in death of the individual, but death of a single cell by apoptosis cannot, by itself, result in death of the whole organism.

Even though many genetically controlled factors seem to contribute to ageing and death, they do not seem to be synchronous; one individual may be physically very fit and yet develop pre-senile dementia, whilst another may continue to dominate some intellectual field despite being physically severely incapacitated by old age. Others may be crippled by osteoarthritic disease (an age-associated condition) and yet show no deterioration in any other system. It seems that although ageing occurs (at least potentially) in all tissues the final collapse and dissolution is not due to *orchestrated* deterioration but to the effects of one of the systems reaching a critical and catastrophic point; this then becomes the cause of death (Table 12.1).

Dying and death

Dying and death must be carefully distinguished. This is not just an interesting academic point — it also concerns many patients. People will often make the distinction by saying that they are not afraid of death, but they are afraid of dying because this may be painful, undignified or distressing to their rela-

Table 12.1	Common modes of death	
Mode of death	Common causes	Clinical manifestations
Cardiac arrest or dysrhythmia	Ischaemic heart disease	Sudden and often unexpected death
	Pulmonary embolism	Sudden death after period of immobilisation causing deep vein thrombosis
Shock	Haemorrhage	Profound hypotension and tachycardia
	Toxaemia due to infection	Hypotension, tachycardia and pyrexia
Respiratory failure	Emphysema, pneumonia, asthma	Cyanosis, tachypnoea
Stroke	Raised intracranial pressure (e.g. tumour, bleeding)	Localised neurological defects, coma
	Cerebral infarction	
Renal failure	Chronic renal disease	Low renal output, high blood urea and creatinine
Liver failure	Acute hepatitis, decompensated cirrhosis, paracetamol poisoning	Jaundice, coma, bleeding

tives. Religion, the existence of God and life after death are matters of personal belief, but may have great significance for many patients and doctors and may provide some comfort. Also the relationship between dying and death is by no means automatic: someone killed in a road traffic accident was not necessarily dying immediately beforehand; someone with a ruptured aortic aneurysm is certainly dying but in some instances may be saved and not die.

Clinical features of death

The collapsed elderly patient with no clinical history poses a significant problem. There are no obvious signs of life and preliminary resuscitation attempts have not altered the patient's state. The ECG shows no complexes. There is no rigor mortis (postmortem muscular spasm) and there is no obvious wound of sufficient severity to suggest a cause of death. Is the patient dead? In practical terms there is a sequence of tests that most doctors will use because they know that any one test is fallible. They will look for so-called 'vital' signs:

- respiration (both by observation and aided by the stethoscope)
- pulses (at the wrist, in the neck, in the groins)
- responses to progressively greater pain stimuli
- stagnation in the circulation in the form of 'beading' of blood in the arteries.

In the absence of all such vital signs they will still consider the possibility of hypothermia and deep drug comas as well as more obscure conditions. If there is doubt early on and if there are no contraindications (such as obvious advanced cancer) then they may try more active resuscitation techniques involving direct electrical stimulation of the heart or intravenous drugs for the same purpose. If none of these manoeuvres is effective then most doctors will be satisfied and willing to declare the subject dead. Can they still be wrong? Unfortunately in very rare cases the answer is 'yes'.

The practical importance of accurately establishing the presence of death (or absence of life) is brought into sharp focus by the needs of transplant surgery; there are strict criteria for deeming a patient to be dead under these circumstances:

1. The pupils are fixed in diameter and do not respond to sharp changes in the intensity of incident light.
2. There is no corneal reflex.
3. The vestibulo-ocular reflexes are absent.
4. No motor responses within the cranial nerve distribution can be elicited by adequate stimulation of any somatic area.
5. There is no gag reflex or reflex response to bronchial stimulation by a suction catheter passed down the trachea.
6. No respiratory movements occur when the patient is disconnected from the mechanical ventilator for long enough to ensure that the arterial CO_2 level rises above the threshold for stimulation of respiration.

It is important to recognise that factors such as body temperature and the presence of drugs in the body can modify these circumstances. For practical purposes the application of these tests is restricted to expert doctors with a suitable level of expertise, in the presence of another, independent, doctor who must not be part of the transplant team.

All this serves to underline the difficulty in defining death and in satisfactorily demonstrating it. The definition of death that describes it as the 'permanent loss of all signs of life' is doubtless true, but it depends upon the term 'permanent' — in clinical situations this is often the crucial central issue. It is obviously very unpleasant for all concerned to make a mistake over this issue and it is clinically unacceptable to allow someone to progress from a deep but reversible hypothermic coma to the permanence of death. The problem has been brought into even sharper focus by organ donation for transplants where the interests of establishing death with certainty and the need to harvest the tissues in as viable a condition as possible may come into conflict.

Biological mechanisms of death

Sometimes death is sudden and results from damage that exceeds the body's ability to restore homeostasis. Such situations are common in severe trauma or in cases of system failure of massive dimensions such as total coronary artery occlusion or massive cerebral haemorrhage. In many other cases the immediately pre-terminal state is either coma or shock (Ch. 8). In the case of *shock* many of the measured features are aberrant biochemical states, such as ketoacidosis, that are themselves the pathological event which, if uncorrected, may go on to cause death. Many other features are bodily mechanisms that have been called into play in an attempt to limit or reverse the damage; these include the adrenergic surge leading to vasoconstriction, increased heart rate and redirection of blood flow away from non-essential sites, together within incidental effects such as sweating, that characterise shock, exemplified by the classic cold, sweaty, 'shut down' patient with a rapid pulse. If these adjustments prove inadequate and effective medical intervention is not available then the patient will progress to death. Under such circumstances it is important to work with the bodily processes which are attempting to restore a normal physiological state and not to try to correct them just because they are abnormal and do not look nice.

Blood loss is a particular variant of hypovolaemic shock; here the main thrust of therapy is to identify and treat the cause while returning the circulating volume to normal. Hypovolaemic shock may also be due to infection by bacteria producing toxins which damage vascular endothelium, resulting in vascular dilatation and increased permeability and fluid loss.

Cardiogenic shock produces relative hypovolaemia by failure of the heart to pump an adequate volume into the vessels; simply increasing the circulating volume would convert the signs of acute cardiac failure into those of chronic cardiac failure. In anaphylactic shock the basis of treatment is to withdraw the precipitating cause and to give therapy aimed at reducing the symptoms. Neurogenic shock is often induced by partial abortion where some products of conception are stuck in the uterine os; treatment consists of removing these as rapidly as possible. The principal point is that treatment should be directed at the specific form and cause of shock in order to prevent its progression to death.

Causes of death

Natural causes

The accurate recording of the causes of death is crucial to our understanding of disease in society (see Ch. 2), but what exactly caused death in a particular situation is not always easy to determine. Though many people die with widespread cancer and their deaths are quite validly recorded as being due to that cancer, it is by no means always clear what it was about the cancer that killed them. For instance, if someone is said to have died of bronchial carcinoma it is always possible to find a case in which another patient died at a much later stage with a far greater load of cancer, so the volume of disease per se cannot explain why it can kill some people and not others. In such cases we commonly fall back on rather diffuse explanations involving one person's 'resistance' or 'strength' compared to another, but the differences can be huge. It is well known that cancers produce various substances that have body-wide effects, such as cachexin (tumour necrosis factor alpha) and there are many other interleukins that may play a role in the disturbed metabolism of many cancer patients. Tumours may also produce various hormones, resulting in paraneoplastic syndromes (Ch. 11). Thus it is entirely possible that many cancer deaths are mechanistically metabolic deaths. Careful examination of the heart in advanced cancer cases reveals a surprising number of occult deposits of metastatic tumours, and terminal dysrhythmias probably account for a significant number of cancer deaths.

Unnatural causes

Death due to disease and old age is generally classified as 'death from natural causes', but the doctor is faced with a wide variety of deaths that cannot be considered 'natural' and also with many deaths in which a mixture of natural and unnatural causes have combined. Obvious unnatural causes include

suicide, *murder* and *accidents*; less clear are suicides by the mentally ill and accidents caused by natural disease, such as a car crash resulting from a heart attack. From the point of view of the law and the issuing of death certificates a death is natural if caused by natural disease or old age and is accidental if the accident would not have occurred in the absence of the disease. These kinds of decision are a matter for the medico-legal authorities, as is the decision whether a death is suicide or murder.

All deaths in which there is an element of doubt must be referred to the appropriate legal officer (for example, the Coroner in England and Wales or the Procurator Fiscal in Scotland). The doctor's role in these cases is to offer a medical opinion as to the ultimate cause of death. The motivation is a matter for the legal agencies; a doctor may decide that death was due to hanging or paracetamol overdose, but he or she cannot say whether or not this was accident, suicide or murder. This is particularly fortunate in those cases where the significance of the deceased's actions is in doubt; it is reasonable for a doctor to say that the cause of death was lung cancer due to cigarette smoking and to leave the decision about apportioning responsibilities to the courts.

Within the category of unnatural death we still need to be careful in our interpretation of what caused death. Pressure on the neck can cause death and it may appear to be clear from the circumstances that death was due to hanging or to strangulation. However, pressure on the neck can kill in a variety of ways: mild pressure may be enough to occlude venous return and the subject will die with a congested appearance, swollen protruding tongue and petechial haemorrhages in the eyes; firmer pressure may occlude arterial supply to the brain and the congested features will be much less marked, although the death will still be due to cerebral ischaemia; yet stronger pressure may occlude the trachea, usually breaking the hyoid bone, and death will be due to asphyxia; sudden pressure on the neck may result in instant death by vaso-vagal inhibition with no physical features of congestion at all. In comparison to this, judicial hanging was directed towards dislocation of the atlanto-axial joint with disruption of the transverse ligament and spinal cord.

Sudden infant death syndrome

The cause of deaths assigned to this category, together with the less well known adult variant, remains obscure. The syndrome occurs in young children in all social classes and no common factor has been detected. It may be a collection of disparate and as yet unrecognised disease states, possibly related to the infant's social condition, or it is still possible that it is an aberrant early expression of a 'death gene'. In spite of a vast amount of research many cases remain an unexplained tragedy. The term 'sudden infant death syndrome' is used only when an exhaustive postmortem examination fails to reveal an identifiable cause of death.

Terminal events

In many cases of terminal states that have been studied it seems that perturbations of the central nervous system are the final common pathway leading to irreversibility. Curiously, similar changes are found in elderly patients who are otherwise fit; a sudden decrease in intellectual ability often precedes spontaneous natural death, a situation referred to as the 'terminal drop'. Perhaps it is not so surprising that a highly complex organism such as the human body should be so crucially dependent upon its coordinating and control system that we should come to use this system to determine death and to find that its disruption so closely precedes that final human step.

Pathology of bed rest

Terminally ill patients are often confined to bed. However, prolonged bed rest is not without complications; some are serious. Most complications can be prevented by careful nursing and active physiotherapy.

Decubitus ulcers (bed sores)
Decubitus ulcers occur over pressure points, such as the sacrum and heels in a patient lying supine. They are due to ischaemic necrosis of the skin caused by compression of the vascular network. Emaciated patients are especially liable to develop decubitus ulcers because there is less subcutaneous fat to diffuse the pressure over bony prominences.

The skin first appears gangrenous and then sloughs to expose a raw base of connective tissue. The resulting ulcer frequently becomes infected and may lead to septicaemia.

Decubitus ulcers can be prevented by regularly turning the patient and by using special mattresses. Comatose or severely debilitated patients require highly skilled nursing care to prevent this complication.

Venous thrombosis
Venous return of blood from the legs results from the movement of the surrounding muscles combined with the effect of valves. Immobilised patients commonly develop deep leg vein thrombosis because of venous stasis; this has two consequences:

- venous oedema of the leg
- risk of pulmonary embolism.

The latter is an ominous event causing either pulmonary infarction or even sudden death (Ch. 8).

Leg vein thrombosis can be prevented by anticoagulation in cases at risk and by physiotherapy

Osteoporosis and muscle wasting
Osteoporosis is a condition in which there is a reduction in bone mass (Ch. 25). Patients confined to bed for prolonged periods inevitably lose some bone mass. It also occurs in astronauts in the weightless environment of space. Osteoporosis not only weakens the skeleton, but also liberates much calcium, leading to hypercalciuria and a risk of renal stone formation.

Skeletal muscle mass reduces in immobilised or bed-ridden patients. This mass can be restored when the patient recovers, but physiotherapy may be necessary to accelerate the process.

Hypostatic pneumonia
Patients lying supine in bed have a reduced respiratory excursion and, if severely ill, may have reduced cough reflexes. Furthermore, the posterior regions of the lungs become congested with blood and alveolar oedema can occur. These events combine to predispose the patient to develop a form of bronchopneumonia (Ch. 14) known as hypostatic pneumonia. Hypostatic pneumonia is a serious complication requiring vigorous physiotherapy and antibiotics, unless the patient has some otherwise incurable disease.

FURTHER READING

Cotton D W K 1995 Death; the individual. Progress in Pathology 1: 1–11
Cotton D W K 1989 Death (video). Sheffield University Television, University of Sheffield, Sheffield
Gonzalez-Crussi F 1987 Three forms of sudden death. Picador

Hayflick L 1994 How and why we age. Ballantine
Holliday R 1995 Understanding ageing. Cambridge University Press
Steel M 1995 Telomerase that shapes our ends. Lancet 354: 935–936

Part 3

SYSTEMATIC PATHOLOGY

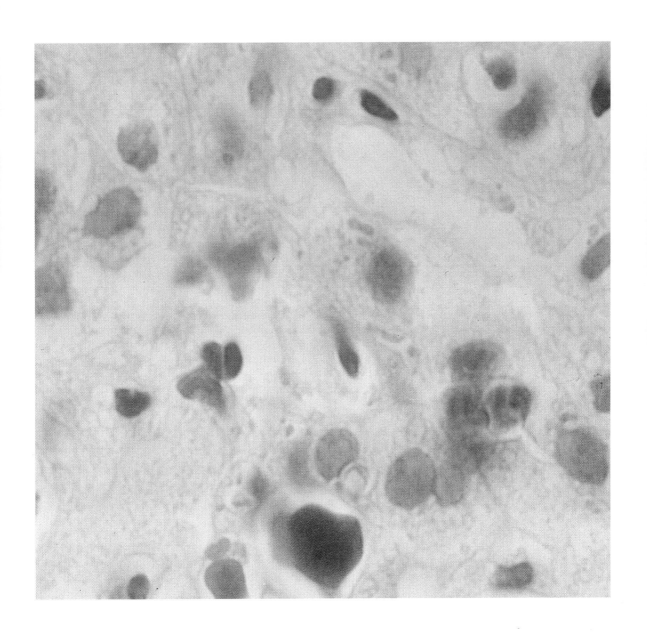

13

Cardiovascular system

Cardiovascular disorders are now the leading cause of death in most Western societies (Ch. 2). In England and Wales ischaemic heart disease currently accounts for 27%, and cerebral vascular disorders for 13%, of all deaths.

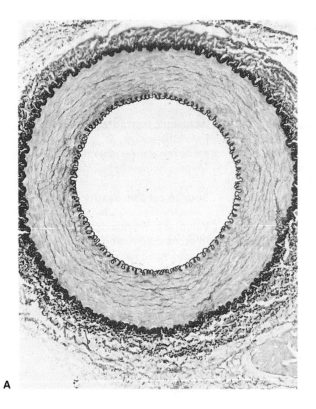

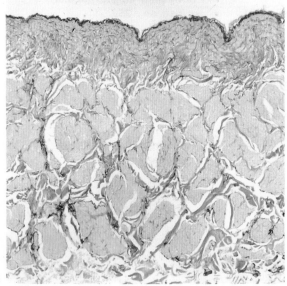

A

B

DISEASES OF THE ARTERIES AND OTHER VESSELS

Atherosclerosis is the commonest and most important vascular disease, but many other vascular disorders are recognised.

Normal arterial structure

In all parts of the arterial system, three anatomical layers can be distinguished. The innermost, the *intima*, is composed of a single layer of endothelium with a thin supporting framework of connective tissue. The internal elastic lamina separates the intima from the middle layer, the *media* (Fig. 13.1). The aortic media is particularly rich in elastic tissue, but in most medium-sized arteries, such as the coronary arteries, smooth muscle predominates. The outermost layer, the *adventitia*, is fibrous connective tissue. Small blood vessels, the vasa vasorum, enter from the adventitial aspect and supply much of the media. The intima and innermost media receive nutrients by direct diffusion from the vascular lumen.

AGE-RELATED VASCULAR CHANGES

A variety of ageing changes occur in the aorta, arteries and arterioles. Although there is considerable individual variation, changes are usually inconsequential before 40, and most common after 70 years of age. The most important changes are:

- progressive fibrous thickening of the intima
- fibrosis and scarring of the muscular or elastic media
- the accumulation of mucopolysaccharide-rich ground substance
- fragmentation of the elastic laminae.

The net effect of these changes is to reduce both the strength and elasticity of the vessel wall. Progressive dilatation is a common ageing phenomenon in both the aorta and the coronary arteries. In the ascending

Fig. 13.1 Structure of blood vessels

A. A muscular artery from a young child. The intima is extremely thin. **B.** Renal vein from a 72-year-old man. Elastic lamellae are indistinct and there is some intimal fibrosis (red coloration). The underlying muscle bundles (pale yellow) are not arranged as regularly as in arteries.

aorta this can lead to stretching of the aortic valve ring and aortic incompetence. Dilatation of the arch and thoracic aorta produces the characteristic 'unfolding' seen in chest X-rays (Fig. 13.2).

The age-related changes that occur in muscular arteries are usually termed *arteriosclerosis*. Even arterioles can be affected. Characteristic alterations include smooth muscle hypertrophy and the apparent reduplication of the internal elastic laminae by extra layers of collagen. There is often marked intimal fibrosis and this further reduces the diameter of the vessel (Fig. 13.3). Arteriosclerosis contributes to the high frequency of cardiac, cerebral, colonic and renal ischaemia in the elderly population. The clinical effects become most apparent when the cardiovascular system is further stressed by haemorrhage, major surgery, infection or shock.

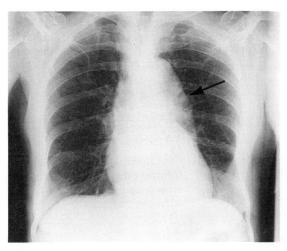

A The prominent bulge (arrow) of the dilated arch and descending aorta.

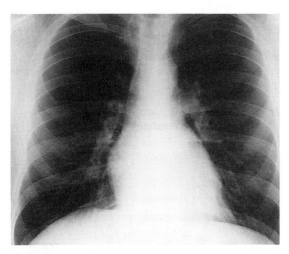

B Normal X-ray for comparison.

Fig. 13.2 Unfolding aorta

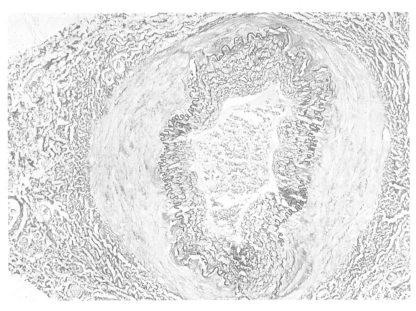

Fig. 13.3 Artery from a 70-year-old man

Note the numerous concentric layers of fibrous intimal thickening.

ATHEROSCLEROSIS

▶ Affects large and medium-sized arteries
▶ Lesions comprise fatty streaks, fibrolipid plaques and complicated lesions
▶ Risk factors include increasing age, male gender, hypertension, smoking and diabetes
▶ Associated with increased levels of LDL-cholesterol, Lp(a), fibrinogen and factor VII and reduced levels of HDL-cholesterol
▶ Major cause of organ ischaemia (e.g. myocardial infarction)

Atherosclerosis is a degenerative disease of large and medium-sized arteries, characterised by lipid deposition and fibrosis. Its frequency has increased dramatically during the past 50 years. In some countries, notably the United States, the incidence of the disease appears to have peaked and, indeed, is now declining. However, in the United Kingdom and several other European countries, atherosclerosis, or at least its complications, continues to increase. The aorta and large and medium-sized arteries are most affected and a wide range of clinical disorders results (Fig. 13.4).

Aetiology

One of the most striking features of atherosclerosis is the wide variation in the severity and distribution of lesions between individuals, even within the same population groups. Pathologists have argued for

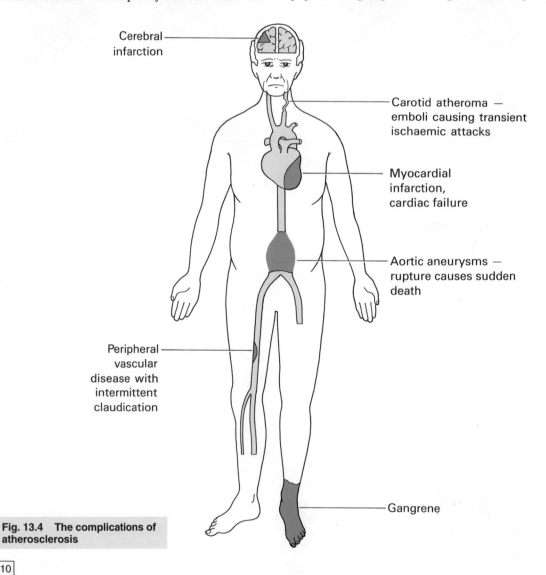

Fig. 13.4 The complications of atherosclerosis

Cerebral infarction

Carotid atheroma — emboli causing transient ischaemic attacks

Myocardial infarction, cardiac failure

Aortic aneurysms — rupture causes sudden death

Peripheral vascular disease with intermittent claudication

Gangrene

Pathological basis of cardiovascular signs and symptoms	
Sign or symptom	Pathological basis
Angina	Myocardial ischaemia due to spasm, atheroma or thrombosis of coronary arteries
Abnormal blood pressure	
• hypertension	Either 'essential' (primary, idiopathic) due to as yet undefined genetic and environmental factors, or secondary to a disease resulting in increased levels of hormones with hypertensive effects
• hypotension	Reduction of actual or effective circulating blood volume
Abnormal heart sounds	
• murmurs	Turbulence of blood flow through stenotic or incompetent valves
• friction rub	Pericarditis
• indistinct sounds	Pericardial effusion
Abnormal ECG	
• altered waveform	Disturbed myocardial depolarisation/repolarisation commonly due to ischaemia or infarction
• altered rhythm	Disturbed conduction of electrical activity due to, for example, disease affecting conducting tissue or causing appearance of foci of ectopic electrical activity
Abnormal pulse	Disordered heart rhythm or arterial flow
Raised jugular venous pressure	Increased central venous pressure due to right or congestive cardiac failure
Oedema	If due to vascular disease, attributable to raised venous pressure (e.g. in cardiac failure or venous thrombosis) exceeding plasma oncotic pressure
Dyspnoea	Pulmonary oedema due to left ventricular failure or mitral stenosis
Cyanosis	Partial bypass of pulmonary circulation or acquired impairment of circulation or oxygenation
Raised serum creatine phosphokinase or lactate dehydrogenase	Release of cardiac enzymes into blood due to myocardial infarction
	(contd)

Pathological basis of cardiovascular signs and symptoms (*continued*)	
Sign or symptom	Pathological basis
Joint pains	Synovial inflammation in rheumatic fever
Skin lesions	
• leg ulcers	Impaired arterial or venous flow
• gangrene	Interruption of arterial supply
• splinter haemorrhages (under nails)	Microemboli from infective endocarditis
• purpuric rash	Microhaemorrhages in skin due to vasculitis
Hemiplegia	Cerebral artery occlusion by thrombus or embolus
Visual impairment	Cranial (giant cell) arteritis Hypertensive retinopathy
Sudden collapse	Vaso-vagal syncope Severe dysrhythmia (e.g. ventricular fibrillation) due to myocardial infarction

more than a century about the cause of atheroma. Many factors increase the risk of an individual developing severe or premature atheroma, but some patients who present with clinical disease have no obvious risk factors. The incidence of atherosclerosis increases with *age*. Significant disease in females is unusual before the menopause. *Hypertension, raised LDL-cholesterol levels* and *diabetes* are important risk factors in both sexes, while *cigarette smoking* is of more significance in younger males. Less important risk factors include *obesity*, a *sedentary lifestyle* and *low socio-economic status*.

Morphology

The three major types of atheromatous lesion are:

- fatty streak
- fibrolipid plaque
- complicated lesion.

Fatty streaks are linear elevations composed of lipid-filled histiocytes and are most obvious in the thoracic aorta and coronary arteries. They have been identified in all population groups that have been studied in detail. It is likely that, in patients predisposed to atherosclerosis by genetic or environmental factors, they progress to fibrolipid plaques and complicated

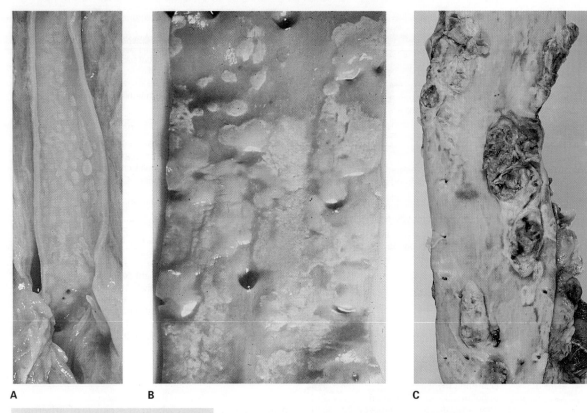

A   B   C

Fig. 13.5   Lesions of atherosclerosis

A. Multiple fatty streaks in the carotid artery of a 39-year-old male. **B.** Large fibrolipid plaques in the abdominal aorta of a 64-year-old male with extensive atherosclerosis. **C.** Complicated aortic atherosclerosis in a 73-year-old female.

lesions (Fig. 13.5). Fatty streaks and fibrolipid plaques have little clinical significance. It is the progressive enlargement of these lesions which leads to the obstruction of the lumen of arteries.

Important complications of atherosclerosis are:

- haemorrhage into plaques
- plaque rupture or fissuring
- thrombus formation
- aneurysm formation.

Rupture of the endothelial covering (plaque fissuring) with exposure of underlying collagen is a stimulus to thrombus formation, as well as permitting the seepage of blood from the lumen into the plaque itself. The importance of haemorrhage and thrombus formation as factors responsible for complications of atherosclerosis cannot be overemphasised. For example, coronary arteriography performed within hours of acute myocardial infarction usually demonstrates total occlusion of the coronary artery supplying the affected tissue.

Furthermore, careful dissection of the coronary arteries in patients dying with established myocardial infarcts reveals coronary arterial thrombi in the vast majority of cases.

Very little is known of the mechanisms which influence where and when plaques develop. Careful studies of postmortem material have shown that these lesions often occur close to arterial bifurcations, sites at which turbulent blood flow normally occurs. Plaques that are rich in lipid or protrude into the lumen eccentrically are at particular risk of rupture.

Pathogenesis

Despite the development of many imaging techniques, it is difficult to follow the progression of atherosclerosis in individual patients. For this reason, much of the information on the evolution of atheromatous plaques comes from studies in animals

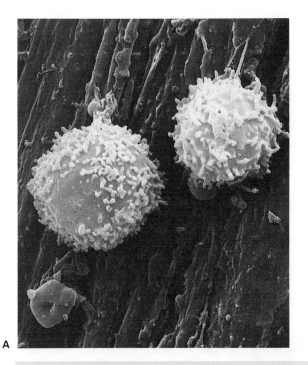

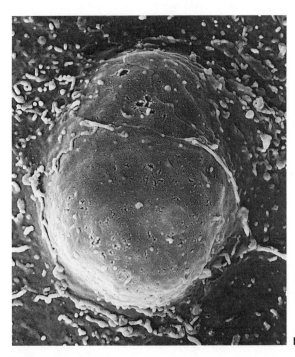

A   B

Fig. 13.6   Scanning electron micrographs of the aortic intima

A. Two macrophages adhering to the surface of the endothelium. **B.** A small elevation of the aortic endothelium produced by an underlying macrophage.

which develop atherosclerosis either spontaneously or following high-fat or cholesterol-supplemented diets. Electron microscopy has demonstrated a variety of changes in the early stages of disease (Fig. 13.6). In sites predisposed to atherosclerosis, macrophages can be seen entering and leaving the arterial wall between endothelial cells. In certain circumstances, the gap between endothelial cells may be widened, and there may be focal or transient areas of endothelial cell loss. The accumulation of lipid-laden macrophages in the subendothelial zone is one of the earliest features of the disease. The molecular mechanisms which allow macrophages to adhere to the endothelium are similar to those that occur in acute inflammation (Ch. 10) but are not as clearly understood. Endothelial cells overlying atheromatous plaques show enhanced expression of some cell adhesion molecules, including ICAM-1 and E-selectin. This may be one mechanism by which inflammatory cells accumulate in plaques. A more advanced atheromatous plaque contains a mixture of macrophages, lymphocytes and smooth muscle cells, and is usually capped by a layer of fibrous tissue (Fig. 13.7).

Growth factors, particularly platelet-derived growth factor (PDGF), stimulate the proliferation of intimal smooth muscle cells (myointimal cells) and their subsequent synthesis of collagen, elastin and mucopolysaccharide. PDGF is secreted by a large number of cells of connective tissue origin, by macrophages and by endothelium. Experiments in tissue culture have shown that it binds rapidly to smooth muscle cells and fibroblasts, and induces a rapid increase in DNA synthesis and subsequent cell division.

Some abnormalities follow quite trivial endothelial injury and, even in the absence of definite endothelial necrosis, platelet aggregation is a common event. Haemodynamic stress around arterial bifurcations may damage the vascular endothelium and predispose to platelet deposition. The subsequent release of growth factors such as PDGF may have a role in stimulating the proliferation and secretory activity of underlying smooth muscle cells. The interactions that occur between macrophages, platelets and vascular endothelium, and their influence on the secretion of growth factors and cytokines and the expression of adhesion molecules are under intensive study.

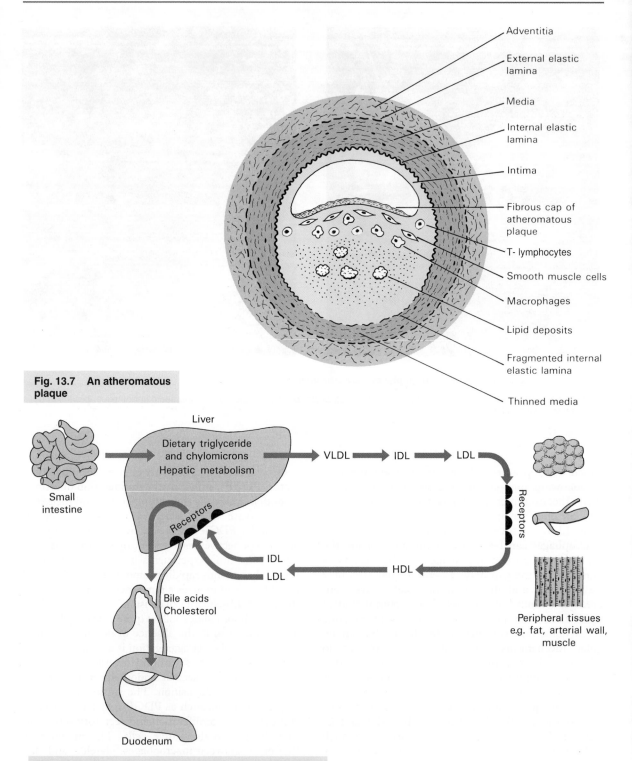

Fig. 13.7   An atheromatous plaque

Adventitia
External elastic lamina
Media
Internal elastic lamina
Intima
Fibrous cap of atheromatous plaque
T- lymphocytes
Smooth muscle cells
Macrophages
Lipid deposits
Fragmented internal elastic lamina
Thinned media

Liver
Dietary triglyceride and chylomicrons
Hepatic metabolism
VLDL → IDL → LDL
Small intestine
Receptors
IDL
LDL
HDL
Bile acids
Cholesterol
Duodenum
Receptors
Peripheral tissues e.g. fat, arterial wall, muscle

Fig. 13.8   The major pathways of lipoprotein metabolism

VLDL = very-low-density lipoprotein; IDL = intermediate-density lipoprotein; LDL = low-density lipoprotein; HDL = high-density lipoprotein

Lipoproteins and atherosclerosis

In the middle of the 19th century Rudolph Virchow, the father of modern cellular pathology, stressed that lipid was an important constituent of atheromatous lesions. It is now clear that raised levels of certain types of lipoprotein substantially increase the risk of atherosclerosis in individual patients. Intensive efforts are therefore being made to unravel the extraordinarily complex pathways of lipoprotein metabolism. Figure 13.8 is a much simplified summary of the major pathways involved.

Low-density-lipoprotein (LDL)-cholesterol
An increased blood level of low-density-lipoprotein (LDL)-cholesterol is the commonest and most important abnormality which predisposes to atherosclerosis. LDL-cholesterol levels are influenced by both genetic and environmental factors. In large population surveys the level of LDL-cholesterol can be closely correlated with the death rate from coronary heart disease.

Nutritional studies have attempted to identify dietary factors that influence serum cholesterol levels and, therefore, the incidence of atherosclerotic disease. These studies are expensive, difficult to organise and complete, and are often heavily criticised. The increased risk of coronary heart disease in the United Kingdom and many other Northern European countries has been associated with diets high in saturated fat. In Mediterranean communities, a much lower proportion of energy is obtained from saturated fat, and coronary heart disease death rates are much lower. Dietary cholesterol consumption has comparatively little influence on plasma cholesterol levels.

The most compelling evidence of the importance of LDL-cholesterol comes from studies of patients and animals who have a complete or partial lack of cell membrane receptors for LDL. Many different cells possess receptors which recognise the apoprotein moiety of the LDL particle. The molecular structure of the LDL receptor has now been determined, and the mechanisms that control its synthesis and transfer to the cell surface are largely understood. In approximately 1 in 500 Caucasians the numbers of functional receptors expressed at the cell's surface are markedly reduced. Although there are many different molecular abnormalities responsible for this, the majority are inherited as autosomal dominant characteristics. Serum LDL-cholesterol values are markedly increased (over 8 mmol/l) in heterozygous patients, most of whom develop coronary heart disease in their forties or fifties (Fig. 13.9). The rare patients who are homozygous for this deficiency (approximately 1 per

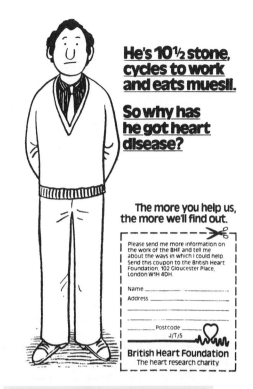

Fig. 13.9 Aetiology of atherosclerosis
The gentleman in this advertisement may well have heterozygous familial hypercholesterolaemia. Alternatively he may have hypertension. Blood pressure and cholesterol should be measured in all middle-aged men.

million) usually die from coronary artery atheroma in infancy or their teens.

The exact mechanism by which an elevated LDL-cholesterol accelerates atherosclerosis is uncertain. High circulating cholesterol levels may increase the endothelial membrane cholesterol content, causing increased membrane 'viscosity'; this decreases the malleability of endothelial cells and predisposes them to damage. Other investigators have suggested that, when LDL is oxidised by macrophages in the arterial wall, the free radicals generated can damage smooth muscle cells or the overlying endothelium. Furthemore, chronic hypercholesterolaemia may induce the secretion of abnormal amounts of growth factors, such as PDGF, by endothelium.

High-density-lipoprotein (HDL)-cholesterol
High-density lipoprotein (HDL) is involved in the transport of cholesterol from peripheral tissues to the liver. There is strong epidemiological evidence that

high levels of HDL-cholesterol are associated with a reduced risk of heart disease due to coronary artery atheroma. Detailed investigations are under way to determine precisely which subcategories of HDL, and which apoprotein moieties, are most important in this respect.

Triglycerides

Hypertriglyceridaemia is a weaker risk factor for atherosclerosis, but some inherited abnormalities of lipid metabolism are associated with increased levels of both cholesterol and triglyceride.

Other pathogenetic factors

Histological studies of atheromatous lesions in both man and animals have shown that fibrin and platelets are important constituents of early lesions. Any change that predisposes to platelet aggregation and blood coagulation would have important influences on the formation of atheromatous lesions and the development of acute coronary syndromes such as unstable angina and acute myocardial infarction. There is now strong evidence that increased levels of *blood coagulation factor VII* are associated with an increased risk of ischaemic heart disease.

The earliest changes in thrombus formation include platelet activation following adhesion to subendothelial collagen. Some of the biochemical and structural changes associated with platelet activation have been unravelled. Agents that stimulate platelet activation include collagen, thrombin, thromboxane A_2 (TXA_2), adenosine diphosphate and noradrenaline. It is now clear that these act as agonists, stimulating glycoprotein receptors on the platelet membrane. The most carefully studied of these is an integrin named *platelet glycoprotein IIb/IIIa*. Low doses of aspirin are given to many patients with clinical evidence of atheromatous disease and have undoubted beneficial effects. Aspirin appears to be a specific inhibitor of thromboxane A_2 mediated platelet activation. The search is on for other methods of inhibiting the glycoprotein IIb/IIIa receptor and these are likely to be among the first 'anti-integrins' to be used in patients. A modified monoclonal antibody to the IIb/IIIa receptor has been developed and appears to be effective clinically. Increased bleeding is the major complication.

Early atheromatous lesions are derived from a monoclonal proliferation of smooth muscle cells. This suggests that a single cell, or clone of cells, may have been induced to grow by a protein which stim-ulates abnormal and uncontrolled proliferation (a 'mutagen'). In this way, atheromatous lesions have been likened to small benign tumours. Although this is an attractive theory, no growth factor, proto-oncogene or exogenous mutagen has been identified that might act in this way.

Treatment and prevention

Once the underlying pathology of a disease is understood, it should be possible to devise logical methods of treatment and prevention. Now that the overwhelming importance of increased lipid levels in atherosclerosis has been established, large trials have been conducted to determine whether the incidence of atheroma and its complications can be reduced by lowering blood lipid levels, particularly that of LDL-cholesterol. Most studies have concentrated on male patients with a serum cholesterol level greater than 9 mmol/l. Both drugs and low-fat diets have been used, and in most studies a substantial reduction in blood cholesterol levels was achieved. In each of the major studies some reduction in the incidence of symptomatic ischaemic heart disease resulted. In the first instance patients with high serum cholesterol levels should lower their cholesterol by dietary means and eliminate, or at least control, additional risk factors such as smoking or high blood pressure. A variety of drugs are available for patients with persistent elevations of LDL-cholesterol.

Meanwhile, biochemists are continuing to unravel the pathways of lipoprotein metabolism, and pharmacologists to search for safer and more effective drugs to lower serum LDL-cholesterol levels. One group of compounds inhibits the enzyme β-hydroxyl-β-methylglutaryl-CoA (HMGCoA) reductase, which catalyses the conversion of acetate to cholesterol in the liver. As a result, intrahepatic cholesterol concentrations fall, more LDL receptors are expressed on the surface of liver cells, and the serum LDL-cholesterol is reduced. Another drug, cholestyramine, is not absorbed from the gut but binds bile acids, preventing their reabsorption. A feedback mechanism then operates to increase hepatic conversion of cholesterol to bile acids, with a resulting increase in LDL receptor formation. The mechanism by which fibrates (e.g. clofibrate and gemfibrozil) reduce LDL and elevate HDL levels is uncertain, but a large Finnish study has demonstrated their effectiveness in reducing the incidence of coronary heart disease. There is now little doubt that reduction in serum cholesterol levels is beneficial in patients who have already had a myocardial infarct ('secondary prevention').

Table 13.1 Clinical effects of aneurysms		
Type of aneurysm	Site	Clinical effects
Atherosclerotic	Lower abdominal aorta and iliac arteries	Pulsatile abdominal mass Lower limb ischaemia Rupture, with massive retroperitoneal haemorrhage
Aortic dissection	Aorta and major branches	Loss of peripheral pulses (e.g. radials) Haemopericardium External rupture (retroperitoneal haemorrhage) Re-entry from dissected media to lumen causing 'double-barrelled' aorta
Berry	Circle of Willis	Subarachnoid haemorrhage
Micro-aneurysms (Charcot–Bouchard)	Intracerebral capillaries	Intracerebral haemorrhage, associated with hypertension
Syphilitic	Ascending and arch of aorta	Aortic incompetence
Mycotic (infective)	Root of aorta (direct extension from aortic valve endocarditis) Any vessel	Thrombosis or rupture, causing cerebral infarction or haemorrhage

ANEURYSMS

- ▶ Localised, permanent, abnormal dilatation of a blood vessel
- ▶ *Atherosclerotic.* Usually occur in the abdominal aorta; rupture causes retroperitoneal haemorrhage
- ▶ *Dissecting.* Usually occur in the thoracic aorta; dissection along the media causes vascular occlusion and haemopericardium
- ▶ *Berry.* Occur in the circle of Willis; rupture causes subarachnoid haemorrhage
- ▶ *Capillary micro-aneurysms.* May be intracerebral (in hypertension), causing cerebral haemorrhage, or retinal (in diabetes), causing diabetic retinopathy
- ▶ *Syphilitic.* Usually occur in the thoracic aorta
- ▶ *Mycotic.* Rather rare; commonest in the cerebral arteries

An aneurysm is a localised permanent dilatation of part of the vascular tree. (A 'false aneurysm' is a blood-filled space due to an organised haematoma following vascular rupture, often traumatic; it is not strictly an aneurysm). Permanent dilatation implies that the vessel wall has been weakened. The clinical and pathological features of aneurysms are summarised in Table 13.1.

Atherosclerotic abdominal aortic aneurysms

Atherosclerotic abdominal aortic aneurysms commonly develop in elderly patients and often rupture into the retroperitoneal space (Fig. 13.10). The only effective treatment is surgical, but in the future some may be managed by the percutaneous insertion of supportive stents. Aneurysms of the proximal and

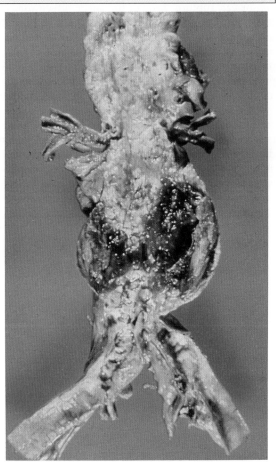

Fig. 13.10 Ruptured atherosclerotic aneurysm
Abundant thrombus is adherent to the intimal surface. The location of the aneurysm is typical—between the origins of the renal and iliac arteries.

thoracic aorta are much less common, and are seldom the result of atherosclerosis alone. There is usually a pronounced loss of elastic tissue and fibrosis of the media. This is due to ischaemia of the muscle of the aortic media, and release of macrophage enzymes causing fragmentation of elastic fibres. These changes are secondary to the intimal atheroma, and reflect the importance of inflammatory reactions (possibly due to autoimmune responses to damaged arterial tissue) in the pathogenesis of atherosclerotic aortic aneurysms.

Aortic dissection (dissecting aneurysms)

In aortic dissection, blood is forced through a tear in the aortic intima to create a blood-filled space in the aortic media (Fig. 13.11). This can track back into the pericardial cavity causing a fatal *haemopericardium*, or can rupture through the aortic adventitia. In occasional cases the track re-enters the main lumen to create a 'double-barrelled' aorta. The underlying pathology is poorly understood, but there is always pronounced degeneration of the aortic media. The principal degenerative change is called '*cystic medial necrosis*', a misnomer because the lesions are neither cystic nor necrotic; rather, there is mucinous degeneration and elastic fibre fragmentation. This change is seen typically in *Marfan's syndrome*, a congenital disorder of the expression of a glycoprotein, *fibrillin*, closely associated with elastin fibres. More commonly, however, dissecting aneurysms occur in elderly individuals. Many patients are also hypertensive. In some cases the intimal 'entry' tears are around atheromatous plaques, but in most cases they involve disease-free parts of the aorta. Without treatment, the mortality from dissecting aneurysm is at least 50% at 48 hours, and 90% within one week. The immediate aim of treatment is to contain the propagating haematoma by reducing arterial pressure. Surgical repair is now feasible in some patients.

'Berry' aneurysms

In the so-called 'berry' aneurysms in the circle of Willis, the normal muscular arterial wall is replaced by fibrous tissues. The lesions arise at points of branching on the circle of Willis, and are more common in young hypertensive patients. The important complication is *subarachnoid haemorrhage*.

Capillary micro-aneurysms

Capillary micro-aneurysms (Charcot–Bouchard aneurysms) are associated with both hypertension and diabetic vascular disease (p. 324). In hypertension, they are particularly common in branches of the middle cerebral artery, particularly the lenticulostriate. They are thought to be the precursors of primary hypertensive intracerebral haemorrhage, which characteristically occurs in the basal ganglia, cerebellum or brainstem.

Syphilitic aneurysms

Tertiary syphilis is now rare in the developed world but was previously a common cause of proximal aortic aneurysms. They rarely rupture but frequently

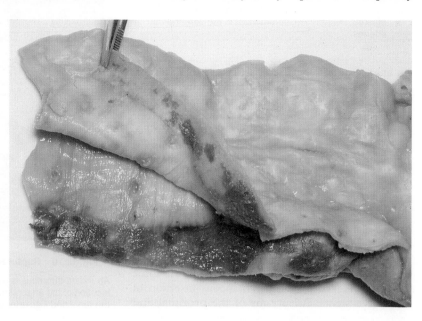

Fig. 13.11 Aortic dissection

The innermost portion of the aortic wall has been peeled away to reveal the underlying haemorrhagic tract.

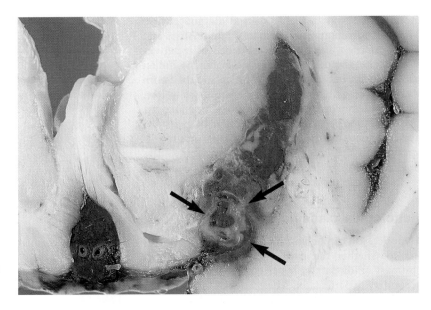

Fig. 13.12 Mycotic aneurysm in brain

This patient had infective endocarditis. A mycotic aneurysm (arrows) has ruptured. There is haemorrhage into the basal ganglia which has extended into the subarachnoid space.

produce aortic incompetence. The aneurysm is due to ischaemic damage to the media, causing fibrosis and loss of elasticity, secondary to inflammation and narrowing of the vasa vasorum.

Mycotic aneurysms

Mycotic aneurysms are the result of weakening of the arterial wall, secondary to bacterial or fungal infection. The organisms are thought to reach the arterial wall via the blood stream and enter the media via the vasa vasorum. Lesions are commonest in the cerebral arteries (Fig. 13.12) but almost any area can be affected. Bacterial endocarditis is the commonest underlying infection.

HYPERTENSION

▶ Classified aetiologically into essential (primary) hypertension, in which there is no evident cause, and secondary hypertension
▶ Secondary hypertension may be due to renal disease, adrenal cortical and medullary tumours, aortic coarctation or steroid therapy
▶ Further classified dynamically into benign hypertension, in which there is gradual organ damage, and malignant hypertension, in which there is severe and often acute renal, retinal and cerebral damage

Definition

Hypertension is the commonest cause of cardiac fail-

ure in many societies and a major risk factor for atherosclerosis. Furthermore, it is a major risk factor for cerebral haemorrhage, another leading cause of death worldwide. There is no universally agreed definition of hypertension, but most authorities would accept that a sustained resting blood pressure of more than 160/95 mmHg is definite hypertension. Furthermore, this would be categorised as:

- *mild* when the diastolic pressure is between 95 and 104 mmHg
- *moderate* at 105–114 mmHg
- *severe* at pressure above 115 mmHg.

Borderline hypertension encompasses the range 140/90 to 160/95 mmHg. The diagnosis of an individual patient as hypertensive can be fraught with difficulties. Single blood pressure readings are often spuriously high, and great care must be taken to ensure that the blood pressure is accurately recorded with an inflatable cuff of appropriate size and shape.

Epidemiology

Hypertension is a serious cause of morbidity and mortality.

The incidence of hypertension varies markedly in different countries. In most, but not all, communities, blood pressure tends to rise with age. There is good evidence that high blood pressure is heritable, although the precise genetic pattern is uncertain. Blood pressures of parents and their natural children are correlated, whereas those of parents and adopted children are not. The correlation of blood pressures in monozygotic twins is higher than in dizygotic twins. Many black communities, both in Western Africa and North America, have a high incidence of hypertension, whereas values tend to be lower on the Indian subcontinent. In certain parts of Africa and the South Pacific, average blood pressures are unusually low. Many epidemiological studies have confirmed a positive correlation between body weight and both systolic and diastolic blood pressure. This association is strongest in the young and middle-aged, but is less predictable in the elderly. Hypertensive patients who lose weight can reduce their blood pressure.

Aetiological classification

Hypertension can be classified aetiologically according to whether the cause is unknown — essential (primary or idiopathic) hypertension—or is known— secondary hypertension. Most cases of hypertension are classified as 'essential', but the possibility of an underlying cause should always be considered.

Essential hypertension

Up to 90% of patients who present with elevated blood pressure will have no obvious cause for their hypertension and are therefore said to have essential or primary hypertension (Table 13.2).

Detailed clinical and physiological investigations in patients with essential hypertension indicate that it is not a single entity, and that several different mechanisms may be responsible. The key feature in all patients with established hypertension is an increase in total peripheral vascular resistance. The pathophysiological mechanisms currently under scrutiny involve:

- sodium homeostasis
- the sympathetic nervous system
- the renin–angiotensin–aldosterone system.

Sodium homeostasis
Impaired renal sodium excretion may be one of the first changes in the development of hypertension. Sodium retention is followed by an expansion of blood volume and a subsequent increase in cardiac output. Peripheral autoregulation increases peripheral vascular resistance and eventually leads to hypertension. In patients with essential hypertension, sodium–potassium transport in both red and white cells is abnormal. Furthermore, plasma from hypertensive patients can affect sodium–potassium transport in the white cells of normotensive individuals. It has been proposed that patients with diminished sodium excretory capacity have a circulating

Table 13.2 Pathogenesis of systemic hypertension

Aetiological classification	Causes
Essential (primary) hypertension	Unknown, but probably multifactorial involving: • Genetic susceptibility • Excessive sympathetic nervous system activity • Abnormalities of Na/K membrane transport • High salt intake • Abnormalities in renin–angiotensin–aldosterone system
Secondary hypertension	Renal disease: • Chronic renal failure Renal artery stenosis • Acute glomerulonephritis Endocrine causes: • Adrenal tumours (cortical or medullary) • Cushing's syndrome Coarctation of aorta Drugs, e.g. corticosteroids, oral contraceptives

substance that inhibits sodium transport in the kidney and elsewhere. Total body sodium levels are positively correlated with blood pressure in some hypertensive patients, but not in normotensive controls. Most healthy adults show little variation in blood pressure over a wide range of salt intakes. Some hypertensives appear to be 'salt-sensitive', but the nature of the underlying defect is not known. It is postulated that increased sodium leakage into cells of the arterial wall may also increase the intracellular calcium content. This in turn increases resting vascular tone and hence peripheral vascular resistance.

The sympathetic nervous system
Blood pressure is a function of total peripheral resistance and cardiac output; both of these are, to some extent, under the control of the sympathetic nervous system. When compared with controls, patients with essential hypertension have higher blood pressures at any given level of circulating plasma catecholamines, suggesting an underlying hypersensitivity to these agents. The circulating levels of catecholamines are highly variable and can be influenced by age, sodium intake, posture, stress and exercise. Nevertheless, young hypertensives tend to have higher resting plasma noradrenaline levels than age-matched, normotensive controls.

The renin–angiotensin–aldosterone system

Renin is released from the juxtaglomerular apparatus of the kidney, diffusing into the blood via the efferent arterioles (Ch. 17). It then acts on a plasma globulin, variously called 'renin substrate' or angiotensinogen, to release angiotensin I. This is in turn converted to angiotensin II by angiotensin converting enzyme (ACE). Angiotensin II is a powerful vasoconstrictor and is therefore capable of inducing hypertension. However, only a small proportion of patients with essential hypertension have raised plasma renin levels, and there is no simple correlation between plasma renin activity and the pathogenesis of hypertension. There is some evidence that angiotensin can stimulate the sympathetic nervous system centrally, and many patients with essential hypertension respond to treatment with ACE inhibitors (e.g. captopril and enalapril maleate), which inhibit the enzyme converting angiotensin I to angiotensin II.

Several therapeutic trials have shown that ACE inhibitors given soon after an acute myocardial infarct decrease mortality, perhaps by preventing myocardial dilatation. Recently, variations or mutations in the genes coding for angiotensinogen, angiotensin converting enzyme and some of the receptors for angiotensin II have been linked with hypertension. Polymorphisms of the ACE gene have also been associated with acute myocardial infarction and with unexplained cardiac hypertrophy in normotensive patients. The precise mechanism by which these genetic variations produce structural or pathophysiological changes is unknown.

Secondary hypertension

Hypertension may result from several underlying conditions:

- renal hypertension
- endocrine causes
- coarctation of the aorta
- drug therapy.

Renal hypertension

Some forms of acute, and all forms of chronic, renal disease can be associated with hypertension. The two chief mechanisms involved are:

- renin-dependent hypertension
- salt and water overload.

The possibility of renal disease should be considered in all patients with hypertension. In a few cases, a focal stenosis of one renal artery, as a result of atheroma or fibromuscular dysplasia of the renal artery, is responsible for unilateral renal ischaemia and hyper-reninism.

Surgical treatment can be curative in selected patients. Patients in terminal renal failure are extremely sensitive to changes in salt and water balance. Hypertension in these patients can often be managed by restriction of salt and water intake and by careful dialysis.

Endocrine causes

The hypersecretion of corticosteroids in Cushing's syndrome is associated with systemic hypertension. Similarly, adrenal tumours which secrete aldosterone (Conn's syndrome) or catecholamines (phaeochromocytoma) can cause hypertension. However, these are found in less than 1% of all hypertensive patients.

Coarctation of the aorta

Systemic hypertension is one of the commonest features in coarctation. Raised blood pressure will be detected in either arm, but not in the legs. The femoral pulse is often delayed relative to the radial. Death usually results from cardiac failure, hypertensive cerebral haemorrhage or dissecting aneurysm.

Drug therapy

Corticosteroids, many types of contraceptive pill and some non-steroidal anti-inflammatory drugs can induce hypertension.

Pathological classification

Hypertension is classified also according to the clinicopathological consequences of the blood pressure elevation. *Benign* hypertension is indolent, often asymptomatic and discovered only during a medical examination for insurance purposes. *Malignant* hypertension is a serious condition necessitating prompt treatment to minimise organ damage or the risk of sudden death from cerebral haemorrhage.

Benign hypertension

The increased peripheral vascular resistance and cardiac workload associated with hypertension produce left ventricular hypertrophy. During life this can be detected electrocardiographically, and at postmortem there is often substantial, concentric thickening of the left ventricle. With the development of congestive cardiac failure, the hypertrophy can be obscured by left ventricular dilatation. Some patients with hypertension also have coronary arterial atherosclerosis and evidence of consequent ischaemic heart disease.

Longstanding hypertension produces generalised disease of arterioles and small arteries (p. 323), in addition to enhancing the development of atherosclerosis. The changes are most easily appreciated in the retina during life, and in the kidneys at autopsy. Medium-sized renal arteries and renal arterioles show marked *intimal proliferation* and *hyalinisation of the muscular media*. This produces focal areas of ischaemia with scarring, loss of tubules and periglomerular fibrosis. The cortical surfaces are finely granular.

A number of other disorders are accelerated or, indeed, precipitated by hypertension. These include:

- spontaneous intracerebral haemorrhage
- aortic dissection (dissecting aneurysm)
- subarachnoid haemorrhage due to rupture of berry aneurysms.

Malignant hypertension

Malignant hypertension is a clinical and pathological syndrome. The characteristic features are a markedly raised diastolic blood pressure, usually over 130–140 mmHg, and progressive renal disease. Renal vascular changes are prominent, and there is usually evidence of acute haemorrhage and papilloedema (Fig. 13.13). Malignant hypertension can occur in previously fit individuals, often black males in their third or fourth decade. However, most cases occur in patients with evidence of previous benign hypertension; this is sometimes termed *accelerated hypertension*.

The consequences of malignant hypertension are:

- cardiac failure with left ventricular hypertrophy and dilatation
- blurred vision due to papilloedema and retinal haemorrhages
- haematuria and renal failure due to fibrinoid necrosis of glomeruli
- severe headache and cerebral haemorrhage.

The characteristic histological lesion of malignant hypertension is *fibrinoid necrosis* of small arteries and arterioles (Fig. 13.14). The kidney is frequently affected and some degree of renal dysfunction is inevitable. Occasionally there is massive proteinuria, and renal failure develops. Acute left ventricular failure can occur, and severe headache and blurring of vision with papilloedema are characteristic.

Pulmonary hypertension

The pathophysiological mechanisms associated with pulmonary hypertension are summarised in Table 13.3.

When pulmonary hypertension develops rapidly (following acute left ventricular failure, for example), there is massive transudation of fluid from the pulmonary capillaries into the pulmonary interstitial space and alveoli. This causes the characteristic clinical picture of acute and distressing shortness of breath and expectoration of lightly bloodstained, watery fluid. In chronic pulmonary hypertension, the pulmonary arteries develop a progressive series of reactive changes. These include muscular hypertrophy, intimal fibrosis and dilatation. There are repeated episodes of haemorrhage into the alveolar spaces, which contain haemosiderin (iron pigment)-laden macrophages.

Vascular and systemic effects

Vascular changes
Hypertension accelerates atherosclerosis, but the lesions have the same histological appearances and

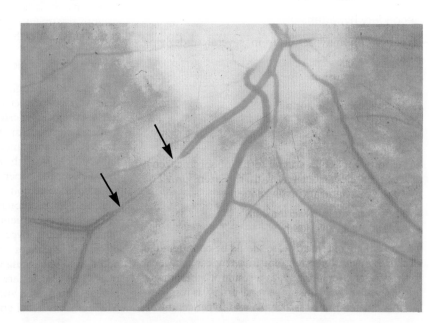

Fig. 13.13 Hypertensive fundus

This ocular fundus from a patient with hypertension shows arteriolar narrowing (arrowed).

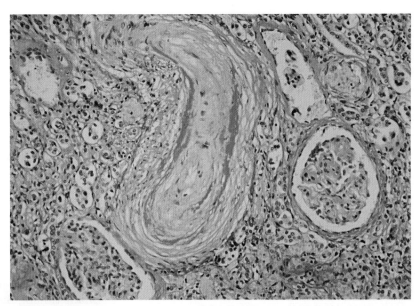

Fig. 13.14 Malignant hypertension

There is fibrinoid necrosis (red) in the wall of a medium-sized renal artery.

Table 13.3 Pathological causes and physiological changes in pulmonary hypertension

Cause	Pathophysiology
Acute or chronic left ventricular failure	Raised left ventricular pressure →raised venous pressure
Mitral stenosis	Raised left atrial pressure→raised pulmonary venous pressure
Chronic bronchitis and emphysema	Hypoxia→pulmonary vasoconstriction→raised pulmonary venous pressure
Emphysema	Loss of pulmonary tissue→ reduced vascular bed
Recurrent pulmonary emboli	Reduction in pulmonary vascular bed available for perfusion
Primary pulmonary hypertension	Cause of raised pulmonary pressure unknown

distribution as in normotensive subjects. However, hypertension also causes thickening of the media of muscular arteries. This is the result of hyperplasia of smooth muscle cells and collagen deposition close to the internal elastic laminae. In contrast to atherosclerosis, which affects larger arteries, it is the smaller arteries and arterioles which are especially affected in hypertension (Fig. 13.15).

Hypertension increases the normal flow of protein into the vessel wall and the amount of high molecular weight protein, such as fibrinogen, that passes through the junctions between endothelial cells,

resulting in protein deposition. These deposits are called '*hyaline*' in benign and '*fibrinoid*' in malignant hypertension. Hyaline change is a common degenerative feature of many ageing arteries, and refers to the homogeneous appearance of the vessel wall, due to the insudation of plasma proteins. Fibrinoid change is a combination of fibrin with necrosis of the vessel wall. There is no evidence that an immunological reaction is involved in hypertensive vascular disease.

Heart
Hypertension accelerates atherosclerosis, thus *ischaemic heart disease* is a frequent complication. A large, ongoing longitudinal population study in Framingham, Massachusetts, has shown hypertension to be the major cause of cardiac failure in previously fit subjects. The left ventricle undergoes hypertrophy and may 'outgrow' its blood supply, particularly if there is associated coronary atherosclerosis. Patients with hypertensive *left ventricular hypertrophy* are more liable to *spontaneous arrhythmias* than normal subjects.

Nervous system
Intracerebral haemorrhage is a frequent cause of death in hypertension. There is good evidence that effective control of blood pressure reduces the risk of hypertensive cerebral haemorrhage.

Kidneys
The degree of renal damage due to glomerular sclerosis or necrosis varies considerably from patient to patient. *Proteinuria* is a common complication of benign hypertension, while *renal failure* is a characteristic of the malignant phase.

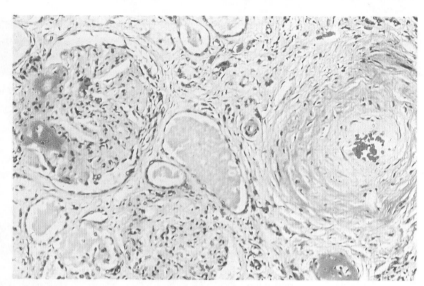

Fig. 13.15   Kidney in longstanding hypertension and diabetes

Note the pronounced thickening of the small renal artery on the right. The glomerulus on the left shows hyalinisation of both the afferent and efferent renal arterioles; this is a characteristic feature of diabetic renal vascular disease.

DIABETIC VASCULAR DISEASE

▶ Lesions include premature atherosclerosis, and microangiopathy causing damage to kidneys, nerves and retina
▶ Complications include gangrene, renal failure and blindness
▶ Effective control of diabetes reduces the incidence of renal, and perhaps retinal, disease.

Patients with diabetes, particularly juvenile-onset insulin-dependent diabetes, may develop three forms of vascular disease.

Atherosclerosis. Both males and females develop premature, and sometimes severe, atherosclerosis. Even diabetic pre-menopausal females can develop substantial atheroma.

Hypertensive vascular disease. This is a frequent complication, especially when there is diabetic renal disease (Ch. 21).

Capillary microangiopathy. This is the most important and characteristic change in diabetes. The alterations are found throughout the systemic circulation and can be viewed directly in the retina (Fig. 13.16). Small arterioles and capillaries are affected and there is both basement membrane thickening and intimal fibrosis. Although thickened,

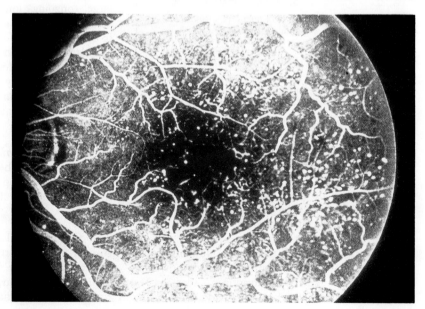

Fig. 13.16   A fluorescein angiogram of the eye of a diabetic patient

Note the numerous, small, dot-like capillary micro-aneurysms.

the basement membranes are unusually permeable, and there is increased passive transudation of protein. In the eye, protein leakage stimulates a fibrous and vascular response, which damages the complex neural network of the retina. Some degree of diabetic retinal disease is inevitable in longstanding diabetes, but only a minority of patients become blind. Intimal thickening of renal arterioles and microaneurysm formation in the glomerular capillaries are the underlying causes of diabetic renal disease (Fig. 13.15). Proteinuria is the first indication of this.

IMMUNOLOGICAL VASCULAR DISORDERS

> ▶ Mechanism is usually immune complex formation and complement activation
> ▶ Specific types include polyarteritis nodosa, Wegener's granulomatosis, systemic lupus erythematosus and Henoch–Schönlein purpura
> ▶ Multisystem disorders but with a predilection for highly vascular tissue such as skin, renal glomerulus, synovium and eye

Pathogenesis

An immunological vascular disorder is the suspected underlying cause in several distinctive clinical diseases. Clinical and experimental studies suggest that the underlying pathology is a deposition of complexes of antigen and antibody in the vessel wall. Immune complexes are not inherently harmful, but if they lodge in tissues and activate complement they incite an acute inflammatory reaction and trigger the coagulation system. Much of our current knowledge of immune complex vasculitis is derived from experiments in which animals have been injected with antigen or antigen–antibody complexes; only intermediate-sized complexes localise in the walls of arteries, arterioles and venules. Very low molecular weight complexes are able to circulate harmlessly, while large complexes are phagocytosed by macrophages in the reticulo-endothelial system. Other factors, such as increased arterial pressure and local vascular turbulence, have a bearing on where complexes lodge. Repeated minor trauma may be the reason that the lesions of some vascular disorders develop on the extensor surfaces of the arms and in the buttocks (Fig. 13.17). Venous stasis may account for the fact that some examples of vasculitis are particularly prominent in the lower leg.

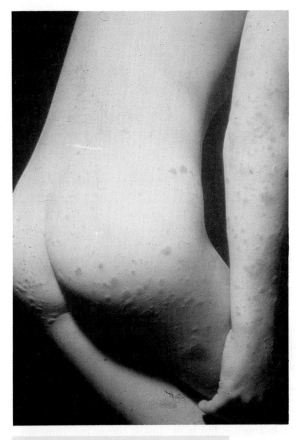

Fig. 13.17   Henoch–Schönlein purpura

Note that the lesions in this 20-year-old man are most prominent on the buttocks and elbows, sites of everyday trauma.

Clinicopathological features

In most immune-complex vascular disorders the pathological changes in the vessels are broadly similar. A dense infiltrate of acute and chronic inflammatory cells is usually present, and immunological techniques often demonstrate abnormal deposits of immunoglobulin and complement in the intima and media (Fig. 13.18). The antigen should be demonstrable in the same position, but its exact nature is usually uncertain.

The patterns of disease in immunological vascular disorders are largely a result of the size of the vessel affected. In disorders such as *polyarteritis nodosa* and *Wegener's granulomatosis*, large muscular vessels are involved and there is usually dense associated inflammation. In contrast, in *Henoch–Schönlein purpura*, inflammation of capillaries and venules leads to a purpuric rash. The major clinical and pathological features of some common immunological vascular disorders are summarised in Table 13.4.

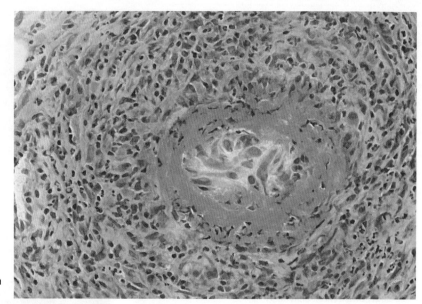

Fig. 13.18 Polyarteritis nodosa

Fibrinoid necrosis and heavy inflammatory cell infiltration in a medium-sized artery in a patient with polyarteritis nodosa.

A skin rash is one of the commonest presenting features of *acute vasculitis* (Fig. 13.19), and is sometimes closely related to treatment with a particular drug, or injection of a radiological contrast medium. In these circumstances that foreign substance probably acts as a hapten in the induction of an immunological reaction. Many forms of vasculitis are self-limiting, but their clinical course can sometimes be shortened by anti-inflammatory drugs, such as steroids. In polyarteritis nodosa, rheumatoid vasculitis and Wegener's granulomatosis the prognosis is often poor, but cytotoxic drugs, such as cyclophosphamide, may induce clinical remissions.

Complications

Complications of vasculitis include thrombosis with resulting ischaemia or infarction. Multiple sites are usually involved simultaneously; it is suspected that complexes lodge in areas which have a high blood flow per unit mass of tissue, for example:

- renal glomeruli
- skin
- synovium
- choroid of the eye.

In many patients with these disorders there are increased levels of circulating immune complexes,

Table 13.4 Clinical and pathological features of immunological vascular diseases

Disease	Clinical features	Vessels involved	Antigenic component of immune complexes	Auto-antibodies
Polyarteritis nodosa	Microinfarcts and haemorrhages from aneurysms	Muscular arteries	HBsAg in a few cases	None
Rheumatoid vasculitis	Arthritis Cutaneous vasculitis	Aorta, arteries and arterioles	DNA in some cases	Anti-DNA Rheumatoid factor
Wegener's granulomatosis	Destructive nasal lesions Lung and renal lesions	Arteries, arterioles and venules	Not known	Anti-neutrophil cytoplasmic antibody (ANCA)
Systemic lupus erythematosus	Skin rash Renal disease	Arterioles and capillaries	DNA and RNA in some cases	Anti-DNA
Henoch–Schönlein purpura	Characteristic skin rash	Capillaries and venules	Not known	None

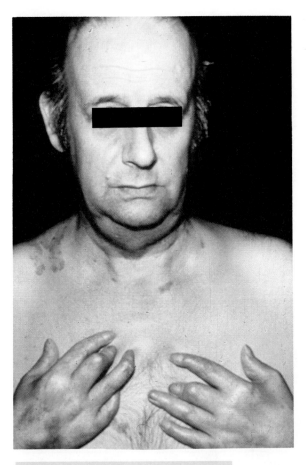

Fig. 13.19 Chronic rheumatoid disease

The haemorrhagic lesions around the neck and anterior chest of this 62-year-old man are the result of an acute vasculitis.

and the complement concentrations may be low, particularly when the disease is active. Auto-antibodies are present in some patients (see Table 13.4). Some are directed against components of vascular endothelial cells (anti-neutrophil cytoplasmic antibodies—ANCA) and have disease specificity.

VASCULAR DISEASES OF UNKNOWN AETIOLOGY

Scleroderma (systemic sclerosis)

The vascular changes of scleroderma (systemic sclerosis) are similar to those of benign or malignant hypertension, but only 25% of the patients are hypertensive. Muscular arteries and arterioles are narrowed by newly formed layers of collagen and mucopolysaccharide (Ch. 25). The cause of this curious disorder is unknown. There may be an underlying abnormality of collagen synthesis which affects not only arteries but also the subcutaneous tissues of the extremities and gastrointestinal tract. The most characteristic clinical feature is progressive subcutaneous fibrosis, which leads to marked tightening of the skin of the arms and hands. There is no effective treatment.

Cranial (giant cell) arteritis

Cranial (giant cell) arteritis was first recognised by Sir Jonathan Hutchinson, who in 1890 described an 80-year-old retired hospital porter who was prevented from wearing his hat by tender and inflamed temporal arteries. Although the arteries of the head and neck are most frequently involved, almost any part of the arterial system can be affected. If the disease affects the ophthalmic or posterior ciliary arteries, blindness can result.

In florid clinical cases the superficial temporal artery is hard, tender and pulseless, and the patient complains of a severe headache. The ESR is usually high, generally >50 mm/h. Microscopically there is marked intimal thickening and oedema, and a dense, sometimes granulomatous, chronic inflammatory and giant cell reaction with phagocytosis of fragmented elastic fibres (Fig. 13.20). The clinical diagnosis can often be confirmed by biopsy, but this is not always positive; focal involvement of the superficial temporal artery is the probable reason for these negative biopsies.

The cause of cranial arteritis is unknown and there is little evidence that it is of immunological origin. In up to 50% of cases, it is associated with polymyalgia rheumatica. Almost all cases of cranial arteritis respond well to steroid therapy and, in severe cases, prompt treatment can prevent blindness.

Pulseless (Takayasu's) disease

Pulseless, or Takayasu's, disease is a rare inflammatory disorder of the aorta and its proximal branches. Most patients are young or middle-aged females, who present with hypertension or ischaemic symptoms in the arms. Renal arterial involvement can cause hypertension. Characteristically, there is a severe necrotising inflammation with some similarities to cranial arteritis. Unfortunately, only a proportion of these patients respond to treatment, either with steroids or other agents, and the outlook is much worse than in cranial arteritis. Few patients make a complete recovery, and the associated hypertension may be difficult to control.

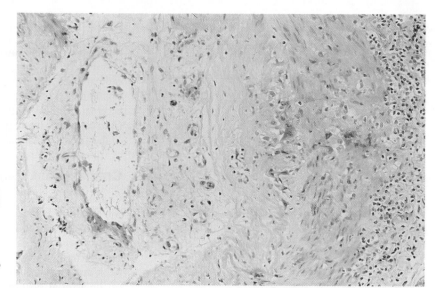

Fig. 13.20 Cranial arteritis

This biopsy of a superficial temporal artery shows marked intimal thickening and a dense mononuclear and giant cell infiltrate. The lumen is restricted to a tiny slit.

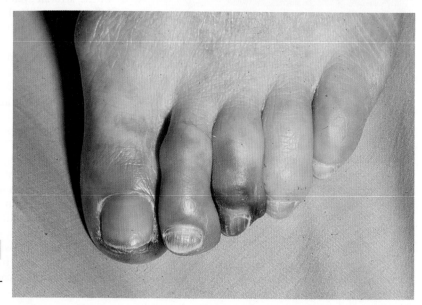

Fig. 13.21 Buerger's disease

The toes are gangrenous. After nine months, this patient required a below-knee amputation.

Buerger's disease

Buerger's disease (thrombo-angiitis obliterans) is a rare disease more strongly associated with smoking than any other vascular disorder. Most patients are male, and Jews are affected twice as commonly as non-Jews. The clinical picture is very distinctive. Peripheral gangrene develops in the fingers and toes, but the changes are progressive and serial amputations are often required (Fig. 13.21).

Pathological alterations are less specific. Small arteries in the arms and lower leg are mainly involved and show marked intimal fibrosis, thrombus formation with evidence of recanalisation, and peri-arteritis with adventitial tissue changes affecting adjacent veins and nerves. Apart from the striking association with heavy smoking, little is known of its cause.

RADIATION VASCULAR DISEASE

Some pathological change is almost inevitable in any tissue which has been irradiated. The most prominent chronic reactions in vascular tissue are intimal thickening of arteries and arterioles, and dilatation of capillaries and venules. Following radiation there is a substantial reduction of the capillary vascular bed, and this inevitably produces ischaemia and subsequent fibrosis. Strictures in the large and small intestines sometimes follow radiotherapy for carcinoma of the cervix. Patients with lymphoma or other tumours who receive mediastinal radiotherapy frequently, develop pericarditis, but damage to small myocardial vessels may produce patchy interstitial fibrosis, and proximal coronary arteries occasionally develop premature atherosclerosis.

DISEASES OF VEINS

Normal venous structure

Like arteries, veins have an intima, media and adventitia (Fig. 13.1B). There is no definite internal elastic lamina and as in arteries the thickness of the intima increases with age (phlebosclerosis). Small veins have only a thin muscular wall but in larger channels, such as the saphenous vein, and the inferior vena cava, there are coarse bundles of irregular muscle, partially organised into longitudinal and circular layers.

Venous thrombosis

Any condition which impedes normal venous return predisposes to thrombosis (Ch. 8). Common predisposing causes include:

- immobility (e.g. in severe cardiac failure, post-operative phase, bed rest, leg fractures)
- malignant neoplasia
- pregnancy and childbirth
- oestrogen therapy (e.g. oral contraceptives, therapy for carcinoma of prostate)
- haematological disorders (e.g. polycythaemia, antithrombin III deficiency, dehydration producing increased blood viscosity)
- intravenous cannulae.

The veins of the lower abdomen, pelvis and legs are most frequently affected. Thrombi often form in the deep veins of the leg when patients are immobilised in bed, for example after a fracture or surgical operation (where the risk is exacerbated by a rise in coagulation factors and platelets) or during a serious illness. There is evidence that anticoagulant drugs reduce the incidence of post-operative deep venous thrombosis, but their beneficial effects must be weighed against the increased danger of post-operative haemorrhage.

In haematological disorders, such as polycythaemia, and in some patients with malignant tumours, the blood is hypercoagulable and venous thrombosis is common. Inherited disorders enhancing coagulation have been described in the last 10 years (see Ch. 23). In the distinctive clinical syndrome of *thrombophlebitis migrans*, superficial venous thrombi form and resolve in different subcutaneous sites. A proportion of these patients have malignant tumours.

Varicosities

Tortuous and distended ('varicose') veins or *varices* are a common clinical problem. There is often associated ulceration, usually on the medial aspect of the ankle and lower leg (Fig. 13.22). There are both superficial and deep venous plexuses in the lower limb, connected by perforating veins. The return of blood from the deep veins is aided by the normal contraction of the calf and thigh muscles. If the valves in the perforating veins become incompetent, blood can be forced from the deep to the superficial venous plexuses; this is a major factor in the development of varicosities. The exact cause of varicose

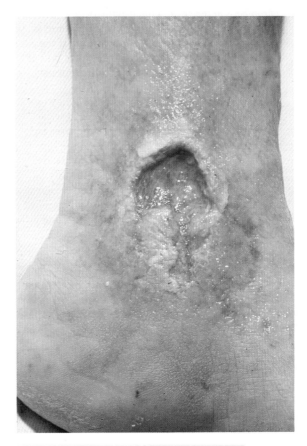

Fig. 13.22 Venous ulceration of the ankle

This is a common complication of varicose veins.

ulceration is uncertain, but impaired venous return with resulting stasis, lower limb oedema and fibrin deposition around small capillaries and veins have been implicated. In many cases, there has been a previous deep leg vein thrombosis. Some ulcers heal after surgical treatment of varicose veins.

Varices frequently develop close to the oesophago-gastric junction in portal hypertension due to, for example, hepatic cirrhosis (Ch. 16).

COMPLICATIONS IN VESSELS USED AS ARTERIAL BYPASSES

Surgical operations in which atheromatous coronary or lower limb arteries are bypassed with the internal mammary artery or a length of saphenous vein are now common. Although these procedures are often successful in restoring distal blood flow, complications can occur. The two most important are:

- *Thrombosis of the graft.* This usually occurs within days or weeks of the operative procedure and is often related to technical complications. If the graft is either too long or too short, blood flow is not optimal and this predisposes to thrombosis. Thrombus can also form at the surgical anastomosis. If the distal part is grafted on to a narrowed segment of artery, the blood flow, or 'run-off', is impeded, and this predisposes to thrombosis.
- *Atherosclerotic lesions.* Veins subjected to arterial pressure develop intimal thickening and this progresses in time to produce lesions indistinguishable from atherosclerosis. This process is particularly marked in veins used as coronary bypass grafts. This may lead to recurrent ischaemic heart disease, even necessitating replacement of the original graft.

Prosthetic vessels made of various types of cloth can be used to repair lower abdominal aortic aneurysms or to bypass iliac or femoral arteries. Although these grafts do not develop true atherosclerosis, a fibrous pseudo-intima develops. Thrombosis may also occur.

Many new techniques have been developed to treat occlusive vascular disease. Some involve balloon dilatation (angioplasty) from within the vascular lumen. Atheromatous material can be excised surgically (endarterectomy) and carotid disease is often treated in this way. Thrombosis and restenosis are important pathological complications of these procedures.

DISEASES OF LYMPHATICS

Normal lymphatic structure

The largest lymphatic vessels, such as the thoracic duct, resemble veins. They are lined by endothelium and have a well-defined muscular wall. In contrast the most peripheral lymphatics begin as closed sacs, lined by a single layer of endothelium and supported by thin strands of collagen. They have valves which give them a beaded appearance.

Lymphatic involvement in disease

Frequently lymphatics provide the channels by which malignant tumours can spread from the primary site to the regional lymph nodes (Ch. 11). In acute inflammation the flow of lymph is markedly increased and, occasionally, lymphatic vessels draining such an area become secondarily inflamed. In infestations with filarial parasites, lymphatic channels are obstructed and marked swelling results; the skin become thickened and boggy ('elephantiasis').

TUMOURS OF BLOOD VESSELS

Benign tumours

Haemangiomas are common benign tumours of small capillaries (Fig. 13.23). They are particularly common on the face and scalp area of infants, and frequently regress. In adults they can occur on almost any part of the skin. On the lips and fingers they are frequently inflamed and are usually known as *pyogenic granulomas*; they are probably reactive lesions rather than true neoplasms.

A *glomus tumour* is a distinctive, benign, but sometimes exquisitely painful, blood-vessel neoplasm which generally arises in the finger or nail bed. It may develop from some component of the arteriovenous anastomosis that is particularly frequent in these sites.

Arterio-venous malformations are not strictly true tumours. They are most common in the cerebral and cerebellar hemispheres and in the lungs. The possibility of an arterio-venous malformation should be considered in any young person who presents with cerebral haemorrhage.

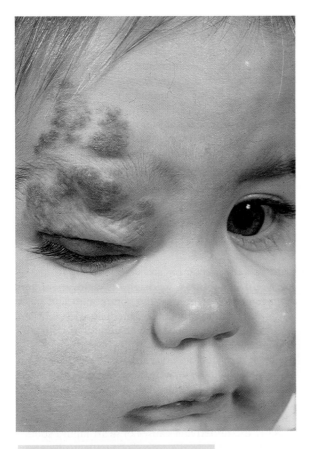

Fig. 13.23   Haemangioma in a child

Although these lesions in this 18-month-old child are unsightly, they are benign and often regress.

Malignant tumours

Angiosarcoma is rare, but has a notoriously aggressive behaviour. The lesion is composed of masses of interconnecting vascular channels lined by a pleomorphic endothelium. Lesions most commonly develop in the soft tissues of the lower limbs, and the head and neck of elderly individuals.

Kaposi's sarcoma, originally described by a Hungarian dermatologist, is a common malignant tumour in black Africans. Its precise cell of origin is uncertain but may well be lymphatic endothelium. In both blacks and whites, Kaposi's sarcoma is one of the tumours which develops in patients with venereally-transmitted acquired immune deficiency syndrome (AIDS) and is currently attributed to human herpes virus 8.

NORMAL STRUCTURE AND FUNCTION OF THE HEART

The heart is a muscular pump divided on each side into two chambers — an *atrium* and a *ventricle* — each separated by a *valve*, tricuspid on the right, mitral on the left. The embryogenesis of these chambers and valves is covered in the section on 'Congenital cardiovascular disease' (p. 352), where it is of immediate relevance. The inner wall of the cardiac chambers and the surface of the valve cusps is lined by a layer of endothelial cells — the *endocardium*. The bulk of the chamber wall — the *myocardium* — comprises a network of striated muscle cells, each separated by an intercalated disc. The heart is invested by patches of adipose tissue and a layer of mesothelium — the *epicardium*. This layer of mesothelium forms the visceral aspect of the *pericardial sac* which normally contains a small volume of clear fluid to lubricate the surfaces during cardiac contraction.

Venous blood from the systemic circulation drains into the right atrium which contracts during *diastole* to force the blood through the *tricuspid valve* into the right ventricle. During *systole* the right ventricle contracts, expelling the blood through the *pulmonary valve* and into the pulmonary circulation. A synchronous sequence of events takes place on the left side: the pulmonary veins drain oxygenated blood into the *left atrium*; in diastole the blood is forced through the *mitral valve*; in systole the left ventricle contracts to expel blood through the *aortic valve* into the aorta. The atria on each side are of similar dimensions, but the myocardium of the left ventricle is much thicker than that of the right ventricle; this is commensurate with the relative systolic blood pressure in the aorta and pulmonary artery trunk.

The regular and co-ordinated contraction of the myocardium is determined by the pacemaker cells in the *sino-atrial (SA)* and *atrio-ventricular (AV) nodes*; the action potentials propagate through the *bundle of His* and *Purkinje network*. The electrical activity of the heart can be monitored on the skin surface by electrocardiography (ECG); the P wave corresponds to atrial contraction; the QRS complex reflects propagation of the action potential into the ventricles and their subsequent contraction; and the T wave is due to repolarisation of the myocardium.

Myocardial cell contraction and relaxation is brought about by changes in the concentration of cytosolic calcium. The cyclical contraction of the heart is initiated by the spontaneous depolarisation of the pacemaker cells in the SA node during diastole. The contraction rate, however, is modulated by the autonomic nervous system: β-adrenergic receptors permit the heart rate to be accelerated by sympathetic stimulation; the vagus nerve through its parasympathetic effects, mediated by acetylcholine, slows the heart rate.

The myocardium is supplied by the *coronary arteries* originating from the root of the aorta just above the aortic valve cusps. The right coronary artery usually supplies the right ventricle, the posterior part of the interventricular septum, and part of the posterior wall of the left ventricle. The left coronary artery, via its principal branches—the anterior descending and the circumflex arteries—supplies the anterior part of the interventricular septum and most of the left ventricular myocardium. It is not unusual, however, to find that one artery is dominant, supplying a larger territory than usual. Blood flow through the coronary arteries is maximal during diastole when the ventricular myocardium is relaxed.

In life, cardiac structure can be assessed by a variety of invasive and non-invasive techniques. Chest X-rays provide a general guide to cardiac and aortic size. Echocardiography, coupled with Doppler techniques, gives a detailed view of individual chambers and in particular the contractile function of the ventricular cavities, the appearances of the individual valves and the direction of blood flow through them. More detailed images are obtained by passing a transducer into the oesophagus or stomach—*transoesophageal echocardiography*. At present the detailed anatomy of the coronary artery tree can be analysed only by injecting radio-opaque contrast medium into the coronary arterial orifices—*coronary arteriography*. Computerised tomographic scans (CT scans) and nuclear magnetic resonance imaging (MRI) are increasingly used by cardiac radiologists and can provide detailed images of individual chambers and the aortic lumen and wall.

The cardiac myocytes are permanent cells; if some die, as in myocardial infarction, the others cannot regenerate to replace those that are lost and the defect is repaired by fibrosis. Similarly, in either hypertension or narrowing of the ventricular outflow tracts, the myocardium of the appropriate chamber becomes correspondingly thicker due to hypertrophy rather than hyperplasia.

Part of the right atrial wall produces a peptide hormone—*atrial natriuretic peptide* (ANP)—that acts on renal tubular epithelium to enhance the urinary excretion of sodium.

Although the heart is vulnerable to ischaemia, it is usually unerringly reliable and robust. For example,

assuming an average heart rate of 80 per minute, the cardiac pump completes approximately 42 million contraction/relaxation cycles per annum! In response to increased demand, such as exercise, the rate can be increased rapidly by β-adrenergic effects. The stroke volume, normally about 65 ml, can be increased in response to increased diastolic ventricular filling and myocardial fibre stretching (Starling's law of the heart). However, with a sustained increase in workload (e.g. hypertension, aortic or pulmonary stenosis), the ventricular myocardium becomes thickened by hypertrophy.

CARDIAC FAILURE

Cardiac failure complicates virtually all forms of severe cardiac disease; its diagnosis, assessment and management are amongst the commonest and most important problems in clinical medicine. Established cardiac failure has a poor prognosis with median survival rates of about three years.

The clinical features of cardiac failure depend on many factors. These include the age of the patient, the exact underlying pathological changes in the heart, the rapidity with which they develop, and the presence or absence of disease in other systems. Wherever possible the underlying causes of heart failure should be identified early in the course of a patient's illness.

Pathophysiology

Cardiac failure exists when the heart is unable to pump blood at the rate required for normal metabolism. The exact underlying biochemical and structural abnormalities in cardiac failure are imperfectly understood. A single mechanism is unlikely to be responsible in all cases. Despite the wide range of drugs now available the outlook for patients with established heart failure is poor. Current research aims to define the normal and abnormal distribution of molecules which affect myocardial contractility. These include angiotensin converting enzyme, angiotensinogen and its various receptors, and certain forms of nitric oxide synthase. Attempts have already been made to modify the expression of some of these molecules by gene therapy.

In the early stages of heart failure the pumping action of the heart may be maintained by compensatory mechanisms such as increased ventricular filling (*increased preload*). The clinical diagnosis of early, compensated heart failure is very difficult and there is no laboratory test which is helpful in this regard. Eventually cardiac hypertrophy and/or dilatation develops and the symptom complex of congestive heart failure develops.

Acute and chronic failure

The clinical features of heart failure depend on the rapidity with which the underlying pathological changes develop. For example, severe acute failure can occur within minutes of an acute myocardial infarct. Typically, the patient presents with sudden severe shortness of breath and marked pulmonary oedema. In contrast, valvular defects, such as mitral stenosis and some forms of mitral incompetence, may develop over a period of years and the patient may describe only a very gradual worsening of symptoms. Not infrequently, chronic congestive heart failure develops after an episode of acute failure, for example after a myocardial infarct.

Right and left heart failure

Because the right and left ventricles share an interventricular septum and function together in a closed circuit, it is inevitable that the failure of one ventricular chamber is followed by a failure of the other. Nevertheless, in the early stages of cardiac failure, the clinical signs and symptoms may appear 'one sided'. The immediate consequence of left heart failure is pulmonary congestion and oedema. In contrast, right heart failure may produce prominent systemic venous congestion, raised jugular venous pressure and enlargement of the liver. In congestive cardiac failure, there is both right and left ventricular failure and a complex combination of systemic and pulmonary signs.

Low and high output failure

In most patients with heart failure, cardiac output fails to increase, or may even decline during exercise, and eventually it is decreased even at rest. This is low output failure and is the direct consequence of the inability of the heart to pump normally. Some patients may develop pulmonary congestion and oedema when the total cardiac output and ejection fraction of the left ventricle is normal or even increased. This is sometimes termed *high output failure*. The causes of this include an increase in blood volume, for example during pregnancy, from accumulation of excess salt and water due to salt-retaining steroids or renal failure. It is also associated with an abnormally increased venous return and/or decreased peripheral resistance, for example in hyperthyroidism, cirrhosis and severe anaemia.

Causes of cardiac failure

The principal causes of heart failure are:

- ischaemic heart disease
- systemic hypertension
- valvular heart disease
- congenital heart disease.

Ischaemic heart disease, systemic hypertension and valvular heart disease, either singly or in combination, are responsible for the vast majority of clinical cases of cardiac failure. Only when these have been excluded should other less common causes be considered. Ischaemia, hypertension and most valvular defects initially present with signs and symptoms such as shortness of breath, fatigue and pulmonary oedema, indicating left heart failure. In many patients, right heart failure follows as an inevitable consequence of failure of the opposite ventricle. In about 15% of cases the initial presentation is with pure right-sided failure. When this is secondary to diseases of the lung, such as chronic bronchitis and emphysema, it is termed *cor pulmonale*. Mitral stenosis is another cause of right ventricular failure.

Clinicopathological features

The major symptoms and signs of of heart failure—shortness of breath, pulmonary oedema, systemic venous congestion and oedema—have a clear pathological basis. Not all patients will have all of these changes and it is important to recognise that symptoms in children and the very elderly may be slightly different.

Dyspnoea

Except after exercise, breathing is normally automatic and effortless. Dyspnoea is the subjective symptom of shortness of breath or difficulty in breathing and is usually the first symptom of heart failure. In left heart failure there is an increase in both the blood and water content of the lungs, and this must be at the expense of the air volume. Intense dyspnoea follows acute left ventricular failure, for example after acute myocardial infarction. The abrupt rise in pulmonary venous pressure causes massive transudation of fluid from the capillaries into the interstitial tissues of the lung, the alveoli and terminal alveoli; crackles can be heard with a stethoscope, especially in the dependent parts of the lungs.

Shortness of breath while lying flat (orthopnoea) and paroxysmal nocturnal dyspnoea are characteristic signs of left ventricular failure. The basis of orthopnoea is the increased venous return from the legs and gastrointestinal veins to the lungs that results from

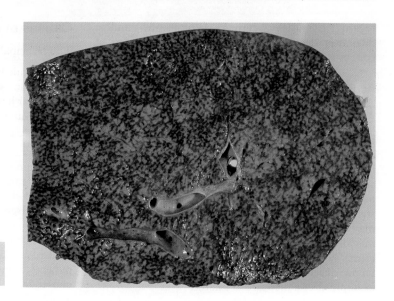

Fig. 13.24   A congested 'nutmeg' liver from a patient with severe congestive heart failure

lying flat. In paroxysmal nocturnal dyspnoea there is a sudden and urgent shortness of breath during sleep, probably because of progressive pulmonary venous congestion.

Increased pulmonary venous pressure and chronic heart failure causes recurrent episodes of alveolar haemorrhage. Some patients in heart failure cough up rusty brown or obviously bloodstained sputum. The rusty colour is the result of haemosiderin-laden macrophages.

Systemic venous congestion and oedema

Fluid retention by the kidney is a compensatory mechanism in cardiac failure. This produces an increased venous return, an increase in ventricular preload and 'volume overloading' of the ventricles. Veins are the reservoir for an increased blood volume and in established heart failure there is widespread congestion of the systemic veins. Distention of the superficial jugular vein in the semi-erect position is one of the earliest signs of this. In congestive heart failure, the liver is enlarged as a direct consequence of engorgement of the centrilobular veins and hepatic sinusoids. The associated ischaemia causes fatty change in hepatocytes (Fig. 13.24). In prolonged cardiac failure, liver function tests can be abnormal, and slight increases in serum bilirubin and transaminases are not uncommon. Dilatation of the left ventricle may be a prominent radiological and echocardiographic feature (Fig. 13.25).

A variety of factors contribute to the accumulation of fluid in subcutaneous tissues and in the pleural, pericardial and peritoneal cavities. A hydrothorax is a

pleural effusion composed of transudated fluid of low protein content. It is a common feature of congestive cardiac failure, but is rare in uncomplicated right heart failure. High systemic venous pressure is not only responsible for the increased transudation of fluid from pleural capillaries, but also impairs drainage from the lymphatics and the thoracic duct. Large pleural effusions also contribute to the dysp-

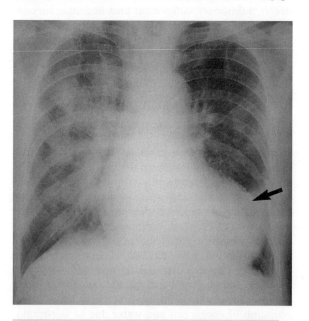

Fig. 13.25   Chest X-ray in congestive heart failure

Note the marked dilatation of the heart (arrow), as compared with the normal chest X-ray in Figure 13.2B, and the increased opacity of the lungs due to congestion and oedema.

noea of heart failure. Pericardial and peritoneal effusions (ascites) are features of severe congestive failure.

Other symptoms

Heart failure is a common cause of 'pre-renal' renal failure. Proteinuria is common but is rarely severe.

Non-specific symptoms frequently seen in advanced heart failure include nausea and vomiting, lethargy, headache and difficulty in sleeping. These are loosely attributed to congestion in the large venous beds of the intestine and to reduced cerebral blood flow. These symptoms are prominent in elderly patients.

ISCHAEMIC HEART DISEASE

> ▶ A common cause of cardiac failure
> ▶ Usually due to coronary artery atheroma
> ▶ Myocardial lesions include ischaemic fibrosis and acute infarction
> ▶ Most frequent cause of death in Western societies

Pathophysiology

Under normal conditions, the blood flow in coronary arteries is closely matched to the metabolic demands of cardiac muscle. Ischaemic heart disease results when the blood supply becomes insufficient, because:

- either the blood supply itself is impaired or
- the myocardium becomes hypertrophic and makes a greater demand on the blood supply.

Coronary blood flow is normally independent of aortic pressure. An efficient autoregulatory mechanism exists to control the blood flow through the coronary vascular bed. When an obstruction develops in a major coronary artery, usually because of atherosclerosis, coronary blood flow is initially preserved, because peripheral resistance distal to the obstruction is reduced. When the vessel lumen is more than 75% occluded, ischaemia develops, particularly if the coronary collateral circulation is poorly developed. Cardiac muscle is extremely active metabolically, and mitochondria constitute over 30% of the volume of individual fibres. Aerobic metabolism is essential, as there are very poor reserves of high-energy phosphates. Cardiac muscle death occurs when tissue adenosine triphosphate (ATP) levels are very low and when anaerobic glycolysis has virtually ceased. As with other tissues, the precise cause of death is uncertain, but lethal cardiac muscle injuries are associated with membrane damage and the sudden entry of calcium into the cell cytoplasm. After brief periods of ischaemia cardiac

blood flow can be re-established. However, after a critical interval 'reperfusion' is impossible, probably as a result of swelling of capillary endothelial cells.

The sub-endocardial layers of the myocardium are at particular risk from ischaemia. Even though there is a well-developed sub-endocardial plexus of blood vessels, flow in this part of the myocardium is restricted to diastole. Blood vessels are collapsible tubes and are susceptible to compression when tension within the myocardial wall increases. This tension is greatest when the ventricles are dilated, especially in the sub-endocardial layer.

Atherosclerosis accounts for the vast majority of coronary artery disease and is most marked in the proximal (epicardial) parts of the coronary arteries. The intramural branches may show slight intimal thickening, but are generally free of true atherosclerosis. Ischaemia is produced by:

- progressive atherosclerotic stenosis
- atherosclerosis with superimposed thrombosis
- haemorrhage into the intima beneath and around atherosclerotic plaques.

Some cases of ischaemic heart disease result from narrowing of the openings (ostia) of coronary arteries. In the past this was usually the result of syphilis, but is now usually atherosclerotic in origin. Occasionally emboli lodge in coronary arteries, usually as a result of infective endocarditis or calcific disease of the aortic valve. Other coronary artery diseases, such as polyarteritis nodosa, are extremely rare.

Ischaemic heart disease can also result from low coronary arterial perfusion. Shock, especially as a result of haemorrhage, is a frequent cause of this. Severe aortic valve disease, either stenosis or incompetence, can also impair coronary blood flow. Some patients with severe anaemia can develop symptoms of ischaemic heart disease.

Acute myocardial infarction

> ▶ Necrosis of heart muscle, usually left ventricular, is usually due to coronary artery atheroma with superimposed thrombus or plaque haemorrhage
> ▶ Necrosis is followed by inflammatory infiltration and fibrous repair
> ▶ Enzymes released from necrotic muscle into blood, and leukocytosis, are useful diagnostically
> ▶ Complications include arrhythmias, cardiac failure, mitral incompetence, myocardial rupture leading to haemopericardium, mural thrombus leading to embolism, and cardiac aneurysm

A myocardial infarct is an area of necrosis of heart muscle resulting from a sudden, absolute or relative, reduction in the coronary blood supply. The commonest precipitating cause is thrombosis superimposed on, or haemorrhage within, an atheromatous plaque in an epicardial coronary artery.

Clinical features

The most frequent symptom of acute myocardial infarction is severe chest pain. This often develops suddenly but may build up gradually, and generally lasts for several hours. Pain is usually accompanied by profuse sweating, nausea and vomiting. Many patients give a previous history of angina or of non-specific chest pain in the weeks before the acute event. In at least 10% of patients, myocardial infarction is painless or 'silent'; this is particularly true in the elderly.

Morphology

The location and size of the infarct depend on:

- the site of the coronary artery occlusion
- the anatomical pattern of blood supply
- the presence or absence of an anastomotic circulation within the coronary arterial tree.

In clinical practice the ECG changes give a good guide to the area of myocardium which is infarcted (Fig. 13.26).

When coronary angiograms are performed in patients with typical symptoms and signs of acute myocardial infarction, a complete obstruction of a major coronary artery can be demonstrated in up to 90% of cases within 3–4 hours of the initial episode of pain (Fig. 13.27). At later intervals fewer patients have complete obstructions, suggesting that coronary artery spasm may also be involved. Coronary artery thrombi may dissolve ('lyse'), and this may account for the much lower incidence of coronary thrombi observed when careful autopsies are performed on patients dying of myocardial infarcts. Aspirin and activators of the plasminogen system, such as streptokinase or alteplase, are now used routinely in acute myocardial infarction; given within 24 hours they reduce mortality by about 25%.

The macroscopic and microscopic changes of myocardial infarcts follow a predictable sequence (Table 13.5). The chief features are necrosis, inflammatory cell infiltration and, as cardiac muscle cannot regenerate, repair by fibrous tissue (Figs 13.28 and 13.29). The extensive necrosis of cardiac muscle is associated with the release of cardiac enzymes into the circulation. A predictable pattern of enzyme elevation develops after myocardial infarction. Most patients show a transient leukocytosis in the first 1–3 days, but the value rarely exceeds $15 \times 10^9/l$.

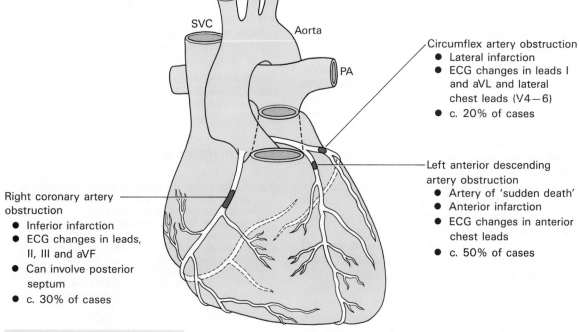

Circumflex artery obstruction
- Lateral infarction
- ECG changes in leads I and aVL and lateral chest leads (V4–6)
- c. 20% of cases

Left anterior descending artery obstruction
- Artery of 'sudden death'
- Anterior infarction
- ECG changes in anterior chest leads
- c. 50% of cases

Right coronary artery obstruction
- Inferior infarction
- ECG changes in leads, II, III and aVF
- Can involve posterior septum
- c. 30% of cases

Fig. 13.26 Myocardial infarction

Obstruction of each major coronary artery results in infarction of specific areas of the myocardium.

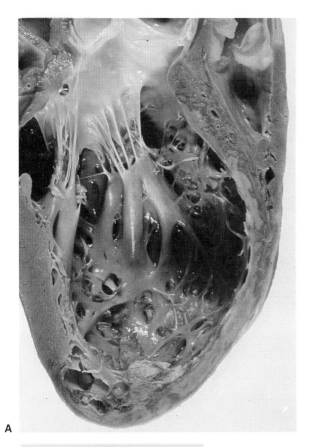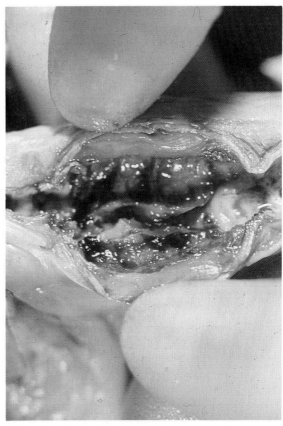

A   B

Fig. 13.27   Myocardial infarction

A. Note the pale and focally haemorrhagic appearance of the infarcted muscle (lower left). There is adherent mural thrombus.
B. An occlusive thrombus overlies an atheromatous plaque in the right coronary artery of this patient.

Table 13.5   Macroscopic and microscopic features of myocardial infarcts

Time after onset of clinical symptoms	Macroscopic changes	Microscopic changes
Up to 18 hours	None	None
24–48 hours	Pale oedematous muscle	Oedema, acute inflammatory cell infiltration, necrosis of myocytes
3–4 days	Yellow rubbery centre with haemorrhagic border	Obvious necrosis and inflammation; early granulation tissue
1–3 weeks	Infarcted area paler and thinner than unaffected ventricle	Granulation tissue, then progressive fibrosis
3–6 weeks	Silvery scar becoming tough and white	Dense fibrosis

Sub-endocardial infarcts

The microanatomy of the arterial and arteriolar supply of the left ventricular myocardium is complex. Almost all of the left ventricular muscle is supplied by perforating branches arising from the arteries on the epicardial surface of the heart. Not surprisingly,

the heart muscle most distant from these, the sub-endocardial zone, is most at risk of ischaemia. In almost all myocardial infarcts there is sub-endocardial necrosis. In some patients the necrosis is confined to the sub-endocardial zone and characteristically there are ST or T wave changes, without

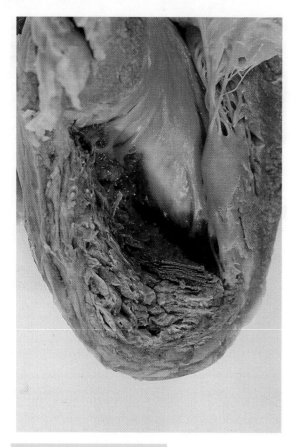

Fig. 13.28 Mural thrombus

Many layers of thrombus have formed on the infarcted myocardium. This can fragment and embolise.

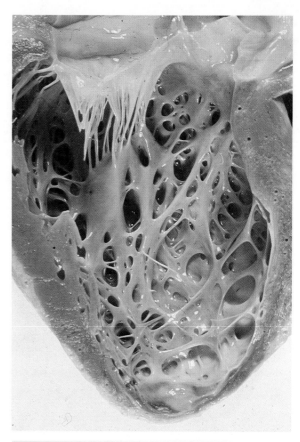

Fig. 13.29 Healed myocardial infarction

Note that the ventricular wall is very thin at the apex of the heart where there is a white fibrous scar.

associated Q waves (sub-endocardial or non-Q-wave infarcts). These are less specific changes and the diagnosis should be based also on the clinical pattern of chest pain and the demonstration of a leukocytosis or raised levels of serum enzymes. Sub-endocardial infarcts have a good initial prognosis and the incidence of cardiac failure and death is less than with transmural infarcts. However, the risk of subsequent arrhythmias and reinfarction is greater with sub-endothelial cardiac infarcts and they cannot therefore be viewed as insignificant clinical events.

Complications

The complications of myocardial infarction are listed in Table 13.6.

Early detection and prompt treatment of complications is important in the management of patients with myocardial infarction. Cardiac arrhythmias, sometimes leading to ventricular fibrillation and sudden death, are frequent in the first 24–48 hours after the initial infarct. Pericarditis, mitral incompetence and cardiac failure are the important complications in the first week after infarction. Later complications include embolism from mural thrombus formation, and the development of ventricular aneurysms. As with all patients who are immobilised, there is a substantial risk of deep venous thrombosis and the possibility of subsequent pulmonary embolism. Prolonged bed rest is not essential for cases of uncomplicated myocardial infarction, and early mobilisation has done much to reduce the incidence of post-infarction pulmonary embolism.

Chronic ischaemic heart disease

Clinical features

Angina is one of the commonest clinical features of patients with a long history of ischaemic heart disease.

Table 13.6 Complications of myocardial infarcts		
Complication	Interval	Mechanism
Sudden death	Usually within hours	Often ventricular fibrillation
Arrhythmias	First few days	
Persistent pain	12 hours–few days	Progressive myocardial necrosis (extension of infarct)
Angina	Immediate or delayed (weeks)	Ischaemia of non-infarcted cardiac muscle
Cardiac failure	Variable	Ventricular dysfunction following muscle necrosis Arrhythmias
Mitral incompetence	First few days	Papillary muscle dysfunction, necrosis or rupture
Pericarditis	2–4 days	Transmural infarct with inflammation of pericardium
Cardiac rupture (ventricular wall, septum or papillary muscle)	3–5 days	Weakening of wall following muscle necrosis and acute inflammation
Mural thrombosis	One week or more	Abnormal endothelial surface following infarction
Ventricular aneurysm	Four weeks or more	Stretching of newly formed collagenous scar tissue
Dressler's syndrome (chest pain, fever, effusions)	Weeks–few months	Autoimmune
Pulmonary emboli	One week or more	Deep venous thrombosis in lower limbs

A history of chest pain, induced by exercise and relieved by rest, should be sought in any patient in whom ischaemic heart disease is suspected. Impaired left ventricular function, following one or more previous episodes of myocardial infarction, may result in left ventricular and, ultimately, congestive cardiac failure.

Morphology

Most patients with a definite clinical history of angina have extensive coronary arterial atheroma. Typically, two or three of the major coronary arteries have patches of stenosis in which the lumen is reduced to less than 75% of its normal cross-sectional area (Fig. 13.30). Paradoxically some patients with a typical clinical history of angina have relatively normal coronary angiograms. It may be that the recurrent episodes of coronary spasm are responsible for pain in these patients: this is sometimes called 'variant angina'.

Postmortem examinations on patients with a long history of ischaemic heart disease frequently demonstrate areas of healed myocardial infarction, dilatation of the left ventricle, and other changes related to chronic heart failure such as peripheral oedema, pleural and peritoneal effusions, and pulmonary oedema and congestion.

SUDDEN CARDIAC DEATH

The sudden, unexpected death of a previously fit person is an all too common tragedy in the community. General practitioners, junior hospital doctors and the police are commonly involved, and a medicolegal autopsy may be ordered. In the vast majority of cases, the cause is directly or indirectly related to the cardiovascular system.

Aetiology

Acute cardiac failure as a result of ischaemic heart disease is one of the commonest diagnoses made by pathologists in cases of sudden unexpected death. In many cases, significant narrowing of one or more coronary arteries is identified. When detailed radiological and histological studies are made in patients dying within six hours of the onset of ischaemic symptoms, a coronary thrombosis can be found in approximately 75% of cases. At this stage, however, there will be no associated macroscopic or histological evidence of recent myocardial infarction. Other common causes of sudden death include ruptured or dissecting aneurysms of the aorta and pulmonary emboli. Aortic stenosis is a frequent cause of Stokes–Adams ('drop') attacks and can also lead to sudden death; acute coronary insufficiency is the probable mechanism (Fig. 13.31).

Prevention

Ventricular fibrillation is often the immediate cause of death in patients with acute ischaemic heart disease.

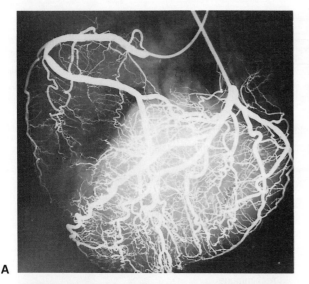

A

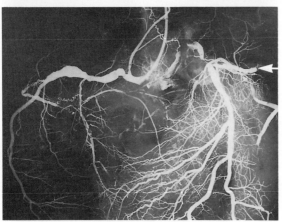

B

Fig. 13.30 Coronary angiograms

A. Normal; note the widely patent right coronary artery, upper left. **B.** The contours of the right coronary are irregular and there is a complete obstruction of the circumflex branch (arrow).

Many ambulance crews now carry a portable defibrillator and administer DC shock to appropriate patients en route to hospital. There is some evidence from community studies that prompt cardio-pulmonary resuscitation can prevent death in such circumstances.

Pulmonary embolism causes many tragic deaths, sometimes in previously fit patients in the post-operative period. Early mobilisation helps to minimise the risk of deep venous thrombosis. Anticoagulant therapy reduces the incidence of venous thrombosis and subsequent embolism, and patients at high risk of developing venous thrombi are sometimes treated prophylactically.

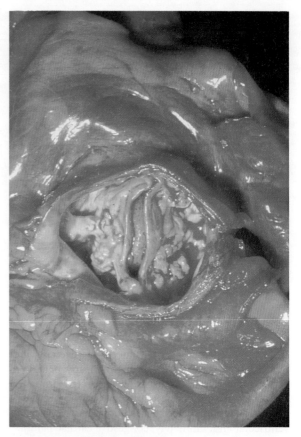

Fig. 13.31 Aortic stenosis

This 58-year-old male died suddenly. Note that the valve is bicuspid and nodular due to heavy calcification.

VALVULAR HEART DISEASE

The normal function of cardiac valves is to prevent retrograde flow of blood between the atria and ventricles, and between the ventricles and the aorta or pulmonary artery. Heart sounds are produced by the vibration of blood as valves close. The first heart sound is the result of the closure of the mitral valve and, to a lesser extent, the tricuspid valve, early in systole. In the same way, the second heart sound results from aortic and pulmonary valve closure. In many healthy children and adults, the aortic valve closes shortly before the pulmonary valve, leading to a double or 'split' second sound.

Pathological problems result from:

● *valvular stenosis*, in which valves become thickened or calcified and obstruct the normal flow of blood into a chamber or vessel

- *valvular incompetence* (also called regurgitation or insufficiency), in which valves lose their normal function as valves and fail to prevent the reflux of blood after contraction of an individual cardiac chamber
- *vegetations*, in which the valve leaflets bear either infective or thrombotic nodules that can fragment and embolise.

The main pathological causes of valvular heart disease are:

- rheumatic valvular disease
- calcific aortic valve disease
- age-related degenerative changes.

Rheumatic valvular disease

> ▶ Antistreptococcal antibodies postulated to cross-react with myocardial tissue antigens
> ▶ Causes valvulitis (usually left-sided), myocarditis (Aschoff bodies) and pericarditis (fibrinous exudate)
> ▶ Valvular stenosis and/or incompetence are long-term complications
> ▶ Predisposes to infective endocarditis

Rheumatic valvular disease results from rheumatic fever, a condition which can occur 2–3 weeks after a streptococcal, upper respiratory tract infection. Recurrent attacks are typical, usually in children between 5 and 15 years of age. The disease was once common in the developed world but is now most frequently seen in parts of Central Africa, in the Middle East and in India. Rheumatic fever is associated with poor nutrition and overcrowding. It is a self-limiting disease which affects:

- the *heart*: pericarditis, myocarditis and endocarditis
- the *joints*: flitting polyarthritis
- the *skin*: subcutaneous nodules and skin rashes (erythema marginatum)
- the *arteries*: arteritis.

The chief pathological features are:

- oedema of connective tissue
- fibrinoid degeneration of collagen
- small aggregates of lymphocytes and macrophages (Aschoff bodies)
- fibrosis.

Bacterial cultures of the heart, joints and other tissues are sterile, but there is serological evidence of a streptococcal infection. Antibodies to streptococcal polysaccharides are substantially elevated (antistreptolysin O titre, ASOT). The precise mechanism responsible is not fully understood, but it is likely that antibodies

to streptococci may also cross-react with some component of cardiac muscle. Repeated attacks of rheumatic fever lead to progressive fibrosis, affecting both the endocardium and the valves (Fig. 13.32). The mitral valve is most commonly affected (c. 90% of all cases), sometimes with the aortic valve (c. 40% of cases). Fibrosis, calcification and fusion of the mitral leaflets produce mitral stenosis. In addition to this, rigid and immobile mitral cusps can cause incompetence because of ineffective closure. Similarly, aortic stenosis and incompetence can follow rheumatic involvement of the aortic valve.

Calcific aortic valve disease

Calcific aortic valve disease is increasing in importance as the incidence of rheumatic heart disease declines, at least in Western countries. Severe calcific disease produces rigid cusps and results in aortic stenosis. This causes progressive and substantial left ventricular hypertrophy. Coronary blood flow may become inadequate, particularly if there is associated coronary atheroma. Most elderly patients with calcific aortic valve disease have pure aortic stenosis, whereas in rheumatic heart disease there is sometimes aortic incompetence and the mitral valve is also usually involved. The pathological processes responsible for calcification of the aortic valve, largely a disorder of the elderly, are unknown. Approximately 1% of the population have a bicuspid, rather than a tricuspid, aortic valve; these valves are particularly liable to calcification, sometimes at a relatively young age (Fig. 13.31).

Other causes of valvular disease

Many patients, particularly those with mitral incompetence and aortic incompetence, have no previous history of rheumatic fever and clearly do not have calcific valvular disease. Some cases of aortic incompetence can be attributed to the progressive dilatation of the aortic valve ring which occurs with ageing. The valve leaflets become small in relation to the enlarged cross-sectional area of the aortic root, and aortic incompetence develops. Pulmonary valve or tricuspid valve stenosis can occur in the carcinoid syndrome (Ch. 15).

Clinicopathological features

The clinicopathological effects of aortic and mitral valve lesions are shown in Table 13.7. Modern imaging techniques such as echocardiography can be used to visualise the movement of the valve cusps; vegetations may also be seen. Doppler techniques

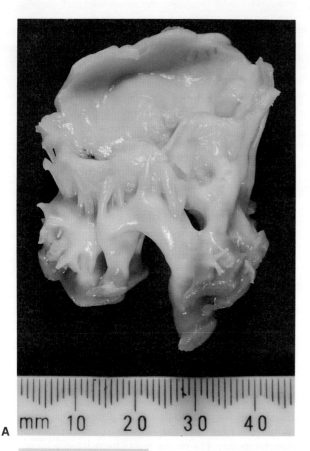

can measure the rate of blood flow through the valves and the pressure gradients across them.

Mitral incompetence

Mitral incompetence is one of the commonest valvular lesions and is sometimes referred to as mitral insufficiency or regurgitation. A minor degree of incompetence is often seen in patients who have some papillary muscle fibrosis after myocardial infarction or who have a dilated mitral valve annulus in association with left ventricular failure. This is often well tolerated and may produce few clinical symptoms. Left atrial pressure is considerably lower than that of the aorta, so blood regurgitates through the mitral valve immediately after the start of ventricular contraction. By the time the aortic valve has opened, as much as a quarter of the stroke volume may already have entered the left atrium. There is usually a loud pansystolic murmur and a third heart sound may be heard. Most patients are in sinus rhythm, unless there is co-existent rheumatic valvular or ischaemic heart disease.

Acute mitral incompetence is usually the result of papillary muscle rupture in myocardial infarction (Fig. 13.33). Most patients go into cardiogenic shock and will die within 48 hours. Surgical replacement of the valve can be life-saving, but the associated mortality is inevitably high.

Mucoid degeneration of the mitral valve is a common finding at postmortem and is seen in at least 15% of patients over the age of 70. The valves have a floppy or billowed appearance (Fig. 13.34) and prolapse towards the left atrium during ventricular contraction;

Fig. 13.32   Rheumatic valvular disease

A. Thickening and fusion of the chordae tendineae and mitral valve leaflets. This patient had longstanding mitral stenosis, and a successful mitral valve replacement was performed.
B. This heavily calcified aortic valve was replaced surgically.

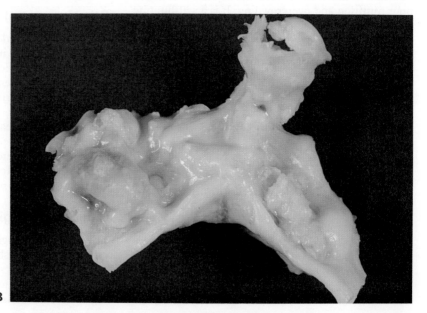

Table 13.7   Pathological causes and clinical features of mitral and aortic valvular lesions

Valvular lesion	Pathological cause	Clinical features
Mitral stenosis	Rheumatic fever	Pulmonary hypertension, left atrial and right ventricular hypertrophy Opening snap and diastolic murmur
Mitral incompetence	Rheumatic fever Dilatation of mitral valve annulus Papillary muscle fibrosis and dysfunction Mucoid degeneration of valve cusps (mitral valve prolapse)	Variable haemodynamic effects Pansystolic murmur Mid-systolic click and late systolic murmur in mitral prolapse
Aortic stenosis	Calcific degeneration Rheumatic fever	Ejection systolic murmur Left ventricular hypertrophy Angina, syncope, left ventricular failure or sudden death
Aortic incompetence	Rheumatic fever Dilatation of aortic root (age-related or syphilitic) Some rheumatological disorders (e.g. rheumatoid arthritis, ankylosing spondylitis)	Diastolic murmur Wide pulse pressure, collapsing pulse, angina, left ventricular failure

this is easily seen on echocardiography. Classical clinical signs are a mid-systolic click and a late systolic murmur. Pathologically there is thickening of the cusps, the result of fibrosis and increased mucopolysaccharide deposition. In severe disease there are abnormal stresses on the mitral valve apparatus and this predisposes to rupture of chordae tendineae when there is severe associated mitral incompetence and mitral valve replacement is indicated.

Mitral stenosis

The primary abnormality in mitral stenosis is mechanical obstruction to emptying of the left atrium.

The normal cross-sectional area of the mitral valve annulus is about 5 cm^2, and signs and symptoms of mitral stenosis result when this is reduced to 1 cm^2 or less. In mitral regurgitation and aortic valve disease the primary haemodynamic abnormality is in the left ventricle, but in mitral stenosis left ventricular function can be normal. Mitral stenosis causes poor emptying of the left atrium, increased pulmonary venous pressure, pulmonary hypertension and right ventricular hypertrophy, dilatation and failure. *Atrial fibrillation* often complicates mitral stenosis due to rheumatic valvulitis. Other causes of atrial fibrillation include ischaemic heart disease, thyrotoxicosis and cardiac surgery; some cases are idiopathic. Ineffective

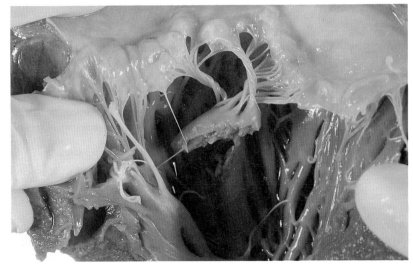

Fig. 13.33   Acute mitral incompetence

The mitral valve has become acutely incompetent due to infarction and rupture of a papillary muscle.

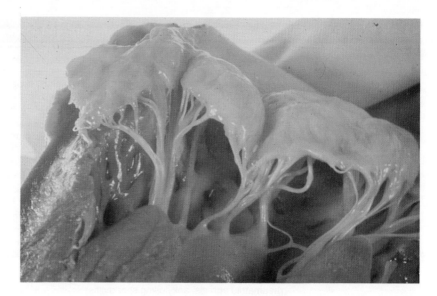

Fig. 13.34 Mucoid degeneration of the mitral valve

Note the marked billowing of the cusps.

atrial contraction leads to stastis and thrombus formation within the atrial appendages; these are a potential source of systemic thrombo-emboli.

Aortic stenosis

Unsuspected aortic stenosis is a frequent postmortem finding. The lesion can be present for many years and produce few, if any, clinical symptoms. The major features of aortic stenosis are syncope (abrupt episodes of faintness), angina and left ventricular failure. Typically, cardiac output is well maintained until late in the course of the disease and, at autopsy, there is often massive left ventricular hypertrophy. The systolic murmur typical of aortic stenosis begins well after the first heart sound, and ends before the second. It reaches a peak of intensity in mid- or late systole. Older patients should be carefully screened for aortic stenosis. Aortic valve replacement is a successful surgical procedure, even in the very elderly.

Aortic incompetence

In aortic incompetence, blood flows back from the aorta into the left ventricle producing an increased end diastolic volume. This causes an increased stroke volume, systolic hypertension and a wide pulse pressure, producing the typical 'collapsing' or 'water-hammer' pulse. A diastolic murmur is characteristic, but systolic ejection murmurs can result from the large stroke volume, and mitral diastolic murmurs from impairment of normal mitral opening by the regurgitant aortic stream. Left ventricular failure is a feature

of severe aortic incompetence. Mild aortic incompetence is sometimes detected in healthy subjects, some of whom have bicuspid valves, and in some rheumatological disorders (Ch. 25).

Tricuspid and pulmonary valve disease

Disorders of the aortic and mitral valve produce far more substantial symptoms than disorders affecting the valves of the right side of the heart.

Many patients with cardiac failure develop tricuspid incompetence, but this may not produce clinical symptoms. The absence of an effective tricuspid valve alters the pattern of the jugular venous pulse during systole. The pulmonary valve is seldom affected by acquired disease, but pulmonary stenosis can occur as an isolated congenital lesion or as part of a complex of malformations such as Fallot's tetralogy. Pulmonary stenosis can be treated surgically or by percutaneous dilatation with a balloon catheter.

Infective endocarditis

Infective endocarditis is an acute or chronic disease resulting from infection of a focal area of the endocardium. A heart valve is usually involved, but the process may affect the mural endocardium of the atrium or ventricle, or a congenital defect such as a patent ductus arteriosus or coarctation of the aorta.

Aetiology

Endocarditis is categorised according to the causative organism. Except in special circumstances, these originate from the normal flora of the body surfaces, liberated into the blood stream in a variety of different ways.

Oropharynx

Endocarditis is most commonly caused by bacteria with 'sticky surfaces', that is those with pili or well-developed capsules. These include streptococci, especially *Streptococcus viridans,* which form a major part of the normal microbial flora of the oropharynx. Dental procedures, including descaling of teeth and minor fillings, instrumentation of the upper respiratory tract or even aggressive chewing, release small showers of organisms into the blood stream.

Skin

Various staphylococci and yeasts such as *Candida* are normally present on skin surfaces. These can be introduced into the blood stream by insertion of cannulae or simple venepuncture. Sometimes, they are directly implanted from the surgeon's skin if a glove is punctured during an operation.

Gastrointestinal and urinary tracts

Streptoccus faecalis is normally present in the large intestine and can cause urinary tract infections. During cystoscopy or prostatectomy, organisms may be disseminated into the blood stream and initiate endocarditis.

Many of these organisms are normally unable to invade healthy tissue. In order to survive in the blood stream, they must be resistant to the killing action of antibody and complement. For this reason Gram-positive bacteria, which have a thick layer of rigid mucopeptide protecting the cell membrane, are the usual causes of endocarditis.

Morphology

The characteristic lesion of infective endocarditis is the *vegetation.* This can vary in size from a small nodule to a large friable mass that can all but occlude the valve orifice (Fig. 13.35). Almost all vegetations occur on valve leaflets or chordae tendineae. Occasionally, congenital defects such as patent ductus arteriosus, coarctation or an arteriovenous fistula can be involved. Surprisingly, vegetations never occur on atheromatous plaques in the aorta; the marked surface irregularities of the latter should make these ideal sites for a vegetation to develop, and why this does not occur is a mystery. Experimental work suggests that vegetations form in areas where there is flow across a high pressure gradient, as in an incompetent valve.

In the course of septicaemia, virulent bacteria, such as *Staphylococcus aureus,* are thought to invade normal endocardial tissue. However, less virulent organisms, such as some streptococci, can infect the endocardium only at the sites of pre-existing damage (Fig. 13.35). Important diseases which predispose to endocarditis include:

- mitral and aortic valvular disease following rheumatic fever
- degenerative, atherosclerotic or syphilitic valve disease
- congenital defects
- prosthetic heart valves (see below).

The probable sequence of events in the formation of a vegetation is shown in Figure 13.36.

Endocarditis in unusual hosts

Patients with prosthetic heart valves

Up to 2–3% of patients with artificial heart valves develop endocarditis (Fig. 13.37). Surface irregularity associated with the cloth covering of the prosthesis or the anchoring sutures provides the initial nidus for thrombus formation. Staphylococci account for at least 50% of cases. Many of these are coagulase-negative.

The commonest initial presenting symptom is postoperative fever. When residual wound sepsis and pulmonary or urinary tract infections have been excluded, prosthetic valve endocarditis should be seriously considered. Repeated blood cultures are an essential part of management. Despite medical and surgical treatment, the mortality can be as high as 70%. In some patients, prosthetic valve endocarditis develops weeks or months after the operation, and this possibility should always be considered in a pyrexial patient who has had a previous valve replacement. Improved cloth covering on the valves, non-wettable sutures and anti-coagulation have all been used in an attempt to reduce the incidence of post-operative endocarditis.

The elderly

In the pre-antibiotic era, infective endocarditis was rare in elderly people. It is now far commoner, and if the trend continues endocarditis will eventually become a disease of the geriatric age group. Calcific valve disease is the most frequent pathology. Predisposing factors include genito-urinary infection, diabetes, tooth extraction, pressure sores and surgical procedures. It appears that virulent organisms such as *Staphylococcus aureus* may be more frequent as the infecting organisms in elderly patients. Complications also appear to be more common than in younger patients. Presenting signs and symptoms are often atypical because of other co-existing disease processes, such as respiratory tract infection and cardiac failure.

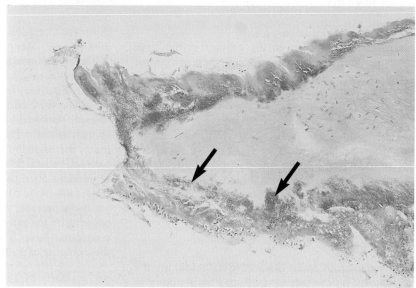

Fig. 13.35 Infective endocarditis

A. A friable vegetation attached to the base of the mitral valve. There is a small perforation of the mitral valve cusp (arrow).
B. A photomicrograph of the vegetation. Clusters of bacteria are arrowed. In this patient the causative organism was *Staphylococcus aureus*.

Drug addicts

Infective endocarditis in drug addicts has increased in all Western societies. The skin is the most common source of micro-organisms; most cases are due to *Staphylococcus aureus* or *Staphylococcus epidermidis*, and fungi such as *Candida*. The bacteraemia has various causes:

- The drug preparation, and the water used to dilute it, can contain virulent micro-organisms that enter the circulation by direct inoculation.
- Bacterial cellulitis may occur at the sites of injection. If drugs are then injected through the inflamed skin, bacteraemia will result.
- If the cellulitis is extensive, thrombophlebitis will develop and this in itself can lead directly to bacteraemia.

Very few intravenous drug abusers presenting with their first episode of endocarditis have previously damaged heart valves. Perhaps the repeated intravenous injection of 'foreign' material damages the endocardial surfaces producing abnormal (roughened) areas. These become sites of platelet aggrega-

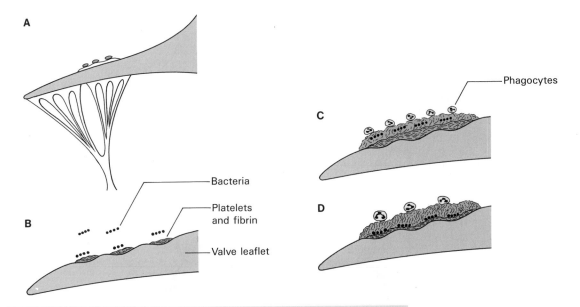

Fig. 13.36 Formation of vegetation on a valve leaflet in infective endocarditis

A. A focal area of abnormality on the endocardium of a valve leaflet is covered with tiny deposits of platelets and fibrin; this is in effect the beginnings of a thrombus. **B.** Circulating micro-organisms (released into the blood stream under any of the circumstances described in the text) colonise the platelet thrombus. **C** and **D.** When sufficient bacteria have settled, further blankets of platelets and fibrin are laid down. The bacteria proliferate slowly to form colonies occupying a relatively superficial position in the vegetation. They are separated from the blood stream by a thin layer of fibrinous material. This layer prevents the phagocytes reaching the bacteria, but is not a significant barrier to the diffusion of nutrients from the blood stream.

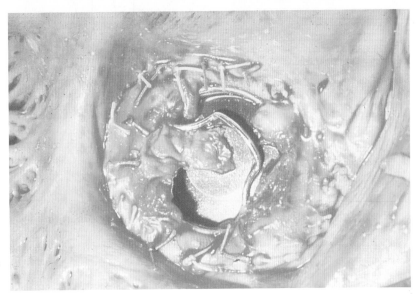

Fig. 13.37 Prosthetic valve endocarditis

The large vegetations impaired valve movement in this patient who died of acute mitral stenosis.

tion and therefore the development of vegetations. This may account for the high incidence of tricuspid valvular involvement in drug addicts, as this valve is closest to the injection site.

Vegetations in drug addicts are often large, particularly in fungal endocarditis. As infection primarily involves the right side of the heart, vegetations can embolise to the lungs. Endocarditis must be suspected

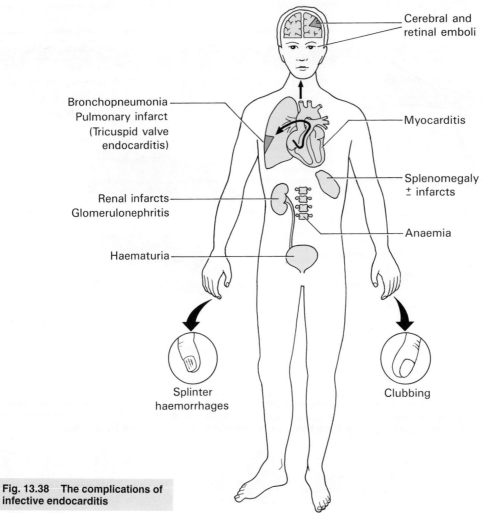

Fig. 13.38   The complications of infective endocarditis

See text for details.

in any drug addict presenting with signs or symptoms of pneumonia, pulmonary embolism or infarction.

Complications

The complications of endocarditis are summarised in Figure 13.38.

Local effects
All but the smallest vegetations have some effect on valvular function, and many cause *valvular incompetence*. A heart murmur is one of the most important physical signs of infective endocarditis. As the vegetations enlarge, valve cusps can perforate or chordae tendineae rupture. This is one cause of death in endocarditis and is now one of the indications for valvular replacement. *Myocarditis* is an important complication of endocarditis; the inflammation

probably spreads directly from the valve leaflet to involve the annulus and adjacent myocardium. Vegetations can embolise to coronary arteries but this is extremely uncommon.

Systemic effects
Fever, weight loss, malaise and splenomegaly are common findings in infective endocarditis and can be attributed to the persistent bacteraemia. Parts of the vegetations may break away from the heart valves and lodge in many different sites; the spleen, kidney and brain are those most frequently involved. Small *emboli* produce tiny haemorrhagic lesions, essentially small infarcts, in the skin, mucous membranes and retina. Linear haemorrhages beneath the tips of the nails (splinter hemorrhages, Fig. 13.39) are frequent in infective endocarditis, but equally can follow everyday trauma. *Clubbing* (Fig. 13.40) is another

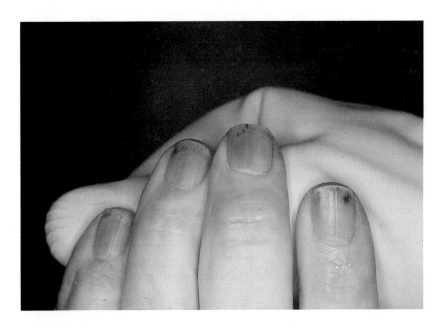

Fig. 13.39 Splinter haemorrhages in infective endocarditis

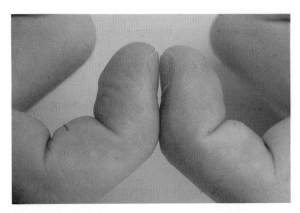

A. Normal nail beds.

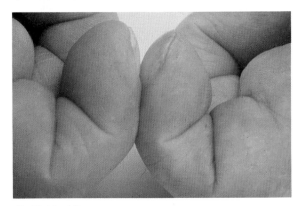

B. Clubbed fingers.

Fig. 13.40 Clubbing in infective endocarditis

common clinical feature; its cause is unknown. It is also known as Shamroth's sign after the physician who described the changes in his own fingers while suffering from endocarditis.

A focal segmental *glomerulonephritis* can be seen in infective endocarditis. This is almost certainly the result of immune complex deposition in glomeruli (Ch. 21). The antigen is probably derived from the micro-organism and the antibody produced by the host in response to it. Some other manifestations of infective endocarditis, such as Osler's nodes in the ·fingers, may be the result of an *immune complex arteritis* in the soft tissues.

Diagnosis, treatment and prevention

Laboratory investigations

It is important to isolate the causative organism from the blood stream. This not only establishes the diagnosis but indicates which antibiotic or combination of drugs is needed to destroy the infecting organism.

In taking blood cultures, it is essential to prevent skin and airborne bacteria contaminating the blood sample. Particular care should be taken to sterilise the skin overlying the vein, using a strong antiseptic such as chlorhexidine in 70% ethanol. Up to one-quarter of blood cultures grow skin bacteria, and this can lead to erroneous diagnoses and inappropriate treatment. Release of bacteria from vegetations is probably episodic and the numbers released may be small. Multiple blood cultures should be taken each day, perhaps for two or even three days. In practice, patients are often so ill that treatment must be started as soon as the diagnosis is suspected clinically, and certainly before the results of blood culture are available. In many patients with good evidence of endocarditis, blood cultures are negative. Failure to recover the causative organism can be due to:

- 'walling off' of bacteria within the fibrinous masses of the vegetation
- antibiotic treatment before blood cultures were taken; where there is serious clinical doubt it may be justified to stop treatment temporarily and then take blood cultures
- occasional unusual organisms, such as rickettsiae causing 'Q' fever, which will not grow in the usual culture medium; in these cases a diagnosis may be established by the pattern of serial antibody tests.

Echocardiography is now an essential investigation in infective endocarditis, not only to identify vegetations at the initial presentation but also to determine how their size changes with treatment (Fig. 13.41).

Treatment
Before the introduction of penicillin in the early 1940s, virtually all patients with bacterial endocarditis died, even when the causative bacteria were relatively non-pathogenic organisms, such as some streptococci. Gram-positive bacteria are not easily lysed by complement; they are killed by phagocytosis, and opsonisation with antibody or complement is usually required for this. The avascular structure of the vegetation prevents the invasion of large num-

bers of phagocytes, and because of this it is essential to sterilise the heart valve with antibiotics. The antibiotics chosen must kill the bacteria, not just inhibit their growth. An antibiotic of the penicillin or cephalosporin group combined with gentamicin is one of the most popular treatments. Even 'bacteriocidal' antibiotics only kill growing organisms, and in a vegetation bacteria grow very slowly. For this reason, treatment must be continued for many weeks.

Prevention
Any patient with valvular heart disease is at risk of developing endocarditis as a result of bacteraemia associated with even the most minor surgical or dental procedure. It is therefore essential that the blood contains a high concentration of bacteriocidal antibiotics immediately before and during these procedures. The aim is to kill bacteria in the blood stream before they settle on the heart valve. Endocarditis still has an appreciable mortality, and the importance of these prophylactic measures cannot be overemphasised. Tragically, cases of endocarditis still occur in previously fit individuals not given appropriate antibiotic cover during minor procedures.

Non-infective endocarditis

Small thrombotic vegetations can occur on the closure lines of valve cusps in patients severely debilitated by serious systemic disease. These are called *marantic vegetations.*

Thrombotic vegetations can occur also in

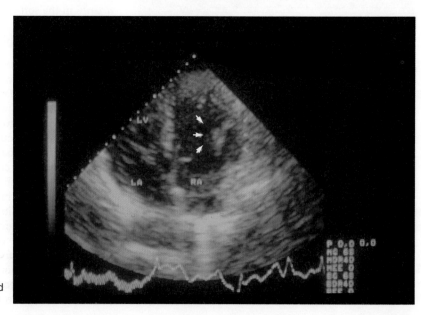

Fig. 13.41 Echocardiographic appearance of valve vegetations

In this case these are on the tricuspid valve (arrowed).

Libman–Sacks endocarditis complicating some cases of systemic lupus erythematosus.

In both conditions the thrombotic material can fragment and cause embolic phenomena.

PERICARDITIS AND MYOCARDITIS

Pericarditis

In pericarditis, there is an inflammatory reaction involving the visceral and/or parietal pericardial layers. There are many causes (Table 13.8) but the commonest are acute, non-specific (viral) pericarditis, myocardial infarction, and uraemia.

Acute pericarditis

In acute pericarditis there is invariably a fibrinous exudate on the pericardial surfaces with associated acute inflammation (Fig. 13.42). In many cases, there is an exudate of serous fluid (pericardial effu-

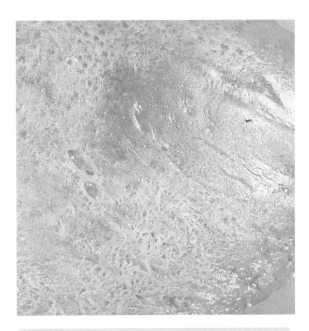

Fig. 13.42   Acute fibrinous pericarditis in a patient with uraemia

This appearance is sometimes called 'bread-and-butter' pericarditis.

Table 13.8 Clinical causes and pathological forms of pericarditis	
Clinical causes	Pathology
Acute non-specific or acute viral pericarditis	Acute fibrinous pericarditis
Myocardial infarction	Initially acute fibrinous, and later fibrous, pericardial adhesions
Uraemia	Acute fibrinous reaction
Carcinomatous pericarditis	Secondary neoplastic deposits (often from bronchus) Serous or haemorrhagic effusion
Connective tissue disease (e.g. rheumatic fever or rheumatoid arthritis)	Fibrinous pericarditis
Bacterial pericarditis	Acute purulent or fibrino-purulent reaction
Tuberculosis	Fibrous or calcific pericarditis, sometimes causing constrictive pericarditis
Post-cardiac surgery	Acute fibrinous reaction
Post-myocardial infarction (Dressler's syndrome)	Autoimmune

sion) and this may become haemorrhagic. Common viral causes include coxsackievirus A and B, herpes simplex and influenza. Bacterial pericarditis results either from direct spread from an intrathoracic focus or from a blood stream infection.

Chronic pericarditis

Chronic pericarditis is a feature of connective tissue diseases such as rheumatoid arthritis, and of tuberculosis. In many cases an effusion develops and there is marked fibrous thickening of the pericardial layers. Many patients with a previous history of myocardial infarction have areas of old pericardial fibrosis, the result of healing of previous acute pericarditis.

Clinicopathological features

Typically, patients with pericarditis complain of chest pain which may be either sharp or dull and aching. Young patients who present with acute non-specific or viral pericarditis often have severe chest pain which can be confused with acute myocardial infarction. Severe pain is uncommon in other forms of pericarditis. A pericardial friction rub is a characteristic feature of acute fibrinous pericarditis, but it may be transient and variable in its intensity. Pericardial effusions of less than 50 ml are usually undetectable clinically. With large effusions, the area of cardiac dullness to percussion is increased and the heart sound may be diminished. Large effusions may interfere with diastolic filling of the heart and produce cardiac tamponade. The jugular venous pressure is raised, and there is an exaggerated variation in pulse pressure during inspiration and expiration (pulsus paradoxus). Chronic constrictive pericarditis may also seriously impair cardiac function, and surgical excision of the densely fibrotic pericardium may improve cardiac output. In some cases, there is associated calcification of the pericardium which may be seen on chest X-rays, particularly lateral views (Fig. 13.43).

Myocarditis

Pathogenesis

The chief causes of inflammation of the myocardium are:

- viral infections, e.g. coxsackie groups A and B,

influenza, echovirus, Epstein–Barr virus (infectious mononucleosis), HIV
- bacterial infections, e.g. diphtheria, leptospirosis, meningococcus
- parasitic infections, e.g. trypanosomiasis (sleeping sickness), Chagas' disease
- ionising radiation
- drugs, e.g. adriamycin, doxorubicin.

Coxsackie B virus is the commonest *known* infectious cause of pericarditis and myocarditis in Western Europe and North America. The diagnosis is suggested by rising titres of specific antibodies in the serum. Many other viruses have been implicated. Diphtheria has not been eradicated from developing countries and cardiac failure is a frequent cause of death; an exotoxin inhibits protein synthesis in cardiac muscle. Myocarditis can complicate infective endocarditis and in some cases myocardial abscesses form around valve rings.

Clinicopathological features

In most patients myocarditis is a self-limiting condition with only mild pleuritic chest pain. Fatalities are relatively uncommon (Fig. 13.44). In some patients cardiac failure develops and coronary angiography may be performed to exclude coronary artery disease. An endomyocardial biopsy may be performed at the same time and may show lymphocytic infiltration and myocyte necrosis. However, even in the most typical clinical cases the proportion of positive biopsies is very small. Anti-inflammatory drugs are generally used in severe myocarditis but there is no definite evidence that they are effective.

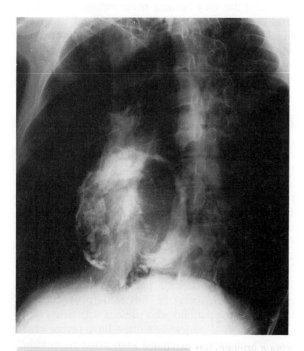

Fig. 13.43 Calcific pericarditis

Lateral chest X-ray from a patient with constrictive pericarditis with calcification due to tuberculosis.

CONGENITAL CARDIOVASCULAR DISEASE

- ▶ Relatively common and the usual cause of heart failure in children
- ▶ Haemodynamic consequences vary according to the location and nature of anomaly
- ▶ Multiple anomalies occur (e.g. Fallot's tetralogy)
- ▶ Many patients can be treated or palliated surgically

Aetiology

Congenital cardiovascular disease is the result of a structural or functional abnormality of the cardiovascular system at birth. In the vast majority of cases, the structural defects can be attributed to a

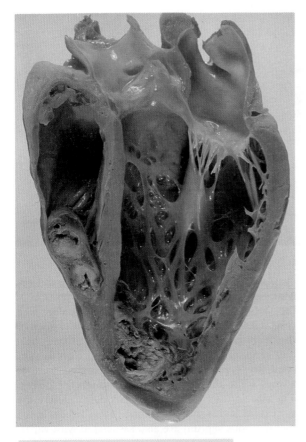

Fig. 13.44 Coxsackievirus myocarditis

This heart is from a 19-year-old female who was fit six months before her death. Note the marked thinning of the right ventricular wall and the areas of adherent mural thrombus.

specific disturbance of normal embryological development.

The incidence of congenital heart disease (CHD) is around 8 per 1000 live births and is much higher if bicuspid aortic valves are included. In about one-third of cases critical illness develops early in life. Associated extracardiac abnormalities occur in about a quarter of infants with CHD. In Down's syndrome, for example, there is a high incidence of atrial or ventricular septal defect, or a patent ductus arteriosus.

In at least 80% of cases the cause of congenital heart disease is unknown. Environmental factors, such as maternal viral infections (especially rubella), chronic maternal alcohol abuse and drugs such as thalidomide, are all clearly related to CHD. These factors are of greatest importance between the fourth and ninth weeks after conception. During this

period, the common atrial and ventricular chambers are divided by septa, the cardiac valves develop and the primitive truncus arteriosus divides into the aorta and pulmonary artery. The incidence of CHD is somewhat increased in the children of mothers with insulin-dependent diabetes or phenylketonuria. There is a weak but definite family incidence of congenital cardiovascular disorders, but generally only one of a pair of monozygotic twins is affected. The risk of a congenital heart lesion in the siblings of affected individuals varies with the nature of the defect, for example from 2% for coarctation of the aorta to over 4% for ventricular septal defects. When two or more members of a family are affected, the risk appears to be substantially higher and, in these instances, genetic counselling is advisable. Nevertheless, the distribution of defects does not generally follow any obvious pattern of Mendelian inheritance.

Clinicopathological features

Some of the most prominent clinical and pathological features of CHD are:

- poor feeding, failure to thrive and impaired growth
- respiratory disease or tachypnoea
- cyanosis
- clubbing
- polycythaemia
- cardiac failure
- pulmonary hypertension
- infective endocarditis.

Most children below one year of age who present with cardiac failure have a structural abnormality of the cardiovascular system. The severity of cardiac failure and the presence or absence of additional signs, such as cyanosis, depend on the precise structural abnormalities. Echocardiography and cardiac catheterisation now permit a detailed understanding of disordered anatomy before cardiac surgery.

Individual cardiac disorders

Atrial septal defects (ASD)

Between the fourth and seventh weeks of fetal life two distinct flaps of tissue develop to divide the common cavity into the left and right atria. The first, the *septum primum*, has two defects but these are normally covered when the second partition, the *septum secundum*, grows upwards from the atrioventricular ring. The higher of these defects, the *ostium secun-*

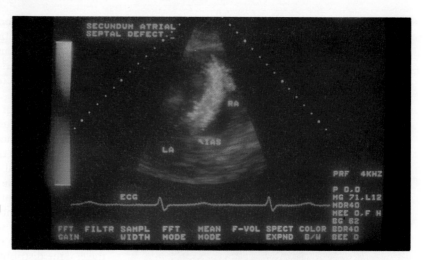

Fig. 13.45   Atrial septal defect

This combined ultrasound and colour Doppler image shows abnormal blood flow through an atrial septal defect. (RA = right atrium; LA = left atrium; IAS = septal defect).

dum, is covered by a flap of the septum secundum. In fetal life this acts as a flap valve allowing blood entering the right atrium from the systemic veins to bypass the lungs by flowing into the left atrium. When the pulmonary circulation is established it closes and in most cases the two layers of the flap fuse together. In many children and some adults a probe can be passed between the layers, the so-called *'probe patent' foramen ovale*. A defect in this area is the usual form of atrial septal defect (Fig. 13.45). Less common types of ASD are related to defects low in the interatrial septum, close to the atrioventricular ring. There may be associated abnormalities in the mitral valve, and surgical repair is more complex. Other abnormalities are associated with defects in the development of the pulmonary veins or the coronary sinus.

Atrial septal defects make up approximately 10% of all congenital abnormalities of the heart. They are often asymptomatic, although, in the past, many untreated patients developed signs of right heart failure in the third and fourth decades. A diastolic rumbling murmur, due to increased flow across the tricuspid valve, may be heard and, because of delayed closure of the pulmonary valve, there is often wide splitting of the second heart sound. The right ventricle is compliant and easily dilates to accommodate the increased pulmonary blood flow, but right ventricular hypertrophy and pulmonary hypertension inevitably develop. Surgical closure is therefore indicated, ideally early in childhood.

Ventricular septal defects

Ventricular septal defects account for approximately 25% of all cases of congenital heart disease in infan-

cy. A variety of anatomical forms are recognised. Many involve the membranous (fibrous) portion of the septum, close to the atrioventricular ring (Fig. 13.46). A few are present towards the apex of the heart in the muscular portion of the interventricular septum. As the left ventricular pressure is substantially greater than that in the right, there is always some shunting of blood through the defect. The size and site of the ventricular defect determine the extent of this shunt. In some cases, defects in the membranous septum are also associated with valvular abnormalities, particularly aortic incompetence, and this influences the clinical presentation.

The most prominent physical sign of ventricular septal defect is a loud pansystolic murmur, often with an associated thrill. Defects may become smaller, or even close completely, as a child grows. Large defects will lead to cardiac failure; because of this, and the risk of infective endocarditis, surgical closure is usually considered.

Patent ductus arteriosus

In fetal life, the pulmonary vascular resistance is high and the right heart pressure exceeds that of the left. Consequently there is a flow from the right to the left atrium through the foramen ovale, and from the pulmonary artery to the aorta via the ductus arteriosus. At birth, the pulmonary vascular resistance declines dramatically, and the ductus arteriosus closes within the first few days of life. If the ductus remains open (patent), there is an abnormal shunt of blood from the *aorta to the pulmonary artery*. This increases both pulmonary arterial and left heart blood flow, but the right atrium and ventricle are virtually unaffected (Fig. 13.47).

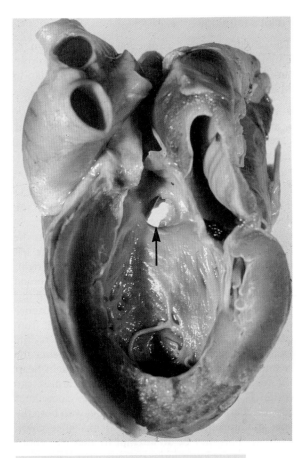

Fig. 13.46   A ventricular defect high in the interventricular septum

Lesions such as these (arrowed) should be treated surgically.

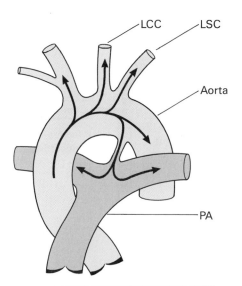

Fig. 13.47   Diagram of circulation in patent ductus arteriosus

(PA = pulmonary artery; LCC = left common carotid artery; LSC = left subclavian artery).

As in ventricular septal defects the symptoms are proportional to the size of the left-to-right shunt. A continuous 'machinery' murmur is characteristic, and is loudest at the time of the second heart sound. If the shunt is large, a left ventricular impulse ('heave') is usually present. If a patent ductus does not close spontaneously, surgical treatment is indicated. Pre-operative studies are necessary to exclude unusual anomalies, such as incomplete separation of the aortic and pulmonary trunks (aorto-pulmonary window).

Coarctation of the aorta

A congenital localised constriction in the diameter of the aorta is known as a 'coarctation'. This defect accounts for up to 5% of all forms of congenital cardiovascular disease and is substantially more common in males. Coarctations are divided into two broad categories—the *adult* type and the *infantile* (or *fetal*) type—differing anatomically and in their clinical presentation.

Adult type
In the adult form of coarctation the narrowing occurs just distal to the ductus arteriosus, which is usually closed. In a proportion of cases there are associated aortic valve abnormalities, usually a congenitally bicuspid valve.

The signs and symptoms are largely dependent on the degree of constriction (Fig. 13.48). If this is severe, a collateral circulation develops to increase blood flow to the lower part of the body. This process involves branches of the intercostal arteries, which become dilated and tortuous. In time, the enlarged vessels may erode portions of the rib producing 'notching' on chest X-ray. The most characteristic clinical finding is hypertension in the upper limbs, with a much lower pressure in vessels distal to the coarctation. The intensity of the femoral pulse is often much reduced. The abnormal blood flow through the coarcted segment may produce a systolic murmur, best heard in the posterior chest.

Some patients with coarctation are asymptomatic and may survive to old age. However, most die prematurely, usually as a result of:

* *congestive heart failure* following prolonged hypertension

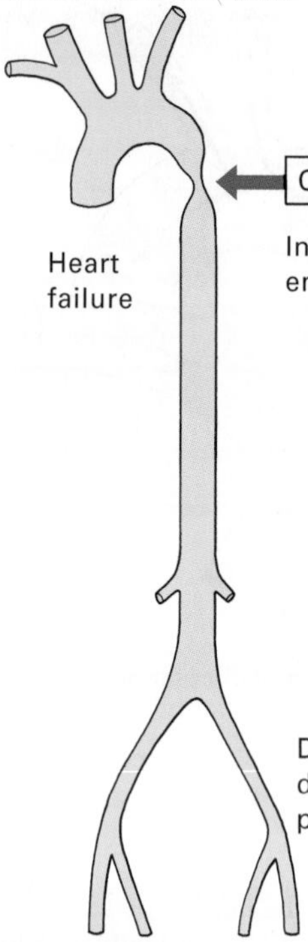

Hypertension in upper limbs,
cerebrovascular accidents

Coarctation

Heart
failure

Infective
endocarditis

Diminished and
delayed femoral
pulses

Fig. 13.48   Coarctation of the aorta

Clinical features.

- *intracerebral haemorrhage*
- *bacterial endocarditis*, either at the site of aortic constriction or, less commonly, in association with a bicuspid aortic valve
- *rupture of a dissecting aneurysm*. This is substantially more common in patients with both hypertension and bicuspid aortic valves. The exact pathogenesis is uncertain (p. 317).

In view of these complications, and the shortened life-span of many patients, surgical treatment is usually indicated.

Infantile (fetal) type
A less common form of coarctation, the infantile or fetal type, involves the aorta distal to the left subclavian artery, but proximal to the ductus arteriosus. The narrowing is often marked, and systemic circulation to the lower part of the body may depend on a right-to-left shunt through a persistently patent ductus arteriosus. In this type of coarctation, pulmonary pressure is elevated and right ventricular hypertrophy develops early in life, or even in utero. Early surgical treatment is indicated.

Fallot's tetralogy

The combination of congenital defects known as Fallot's tetralogy was first described in the 19th century by Etienne-Louis Arthur Fallot, a physician in Marseilles. The four components are:

- ventricular septal defect
- an enlarged aorta which 'overrides' the defect and receives blood from both the right and left ventricles
- stenosis of pulmonary valve
- associated right ventricular hypertrophy.

The major underlying embryological defect is in the development of the interventricular septum.

The clinical features are often characteristic. As the aorta receives both oxygenated blood from the left ventricle and deoxygenated blood from the right, cyanosis develops. Pulmonary stenosis restricts blood flow from the right ventricle into the lungs and, if this is severe, survival is only possible if the ductus arteriosus remains open. The systolic murmurs result from either the ventricular septal defect, or, if severe, the pulmonary stenosis. As in all hypoxic patients the haemoglobin concentration is increased. Right heart failure is inevitable and bacterial endocarditis can ensue. Dyspnoeic children with Fallot's sometimes adopt a characteristic squatting posture, with both the knee and hip joint sharply bent, or sit in a 'knee–chest' position. This may be an attempt to increase venous return from the lower limbs or, more speculatively, to reduce peripheral arterial perfusion, thereby increasing the flow across the ductus arteriosus or ventricular septal defect to the right side of the circulation. Before the advent of surgical treatment (Fig. 13.49), most patients died well before adult life.

Congenital valvular abnormalities

The only common and significant congenital valvular defect is a bicuspid aortic valve. The vast majority of these are asymptomatic, and the valve is neither incompetent nor stenotic. However, the risk of aortic stenosis in adult life is substantially increased (Fig. 13.31) and there is a strong association with dissection of the aorta. Occasional cases of congenital aortic or pulmonary stenosis do occur, but tricuspid and mitral stenosis as isolated congenital lesions are uncommon. Small defects (fenestrations) are frequently observed at autopsy, usually in aortic valves, but have no functional significance.

Transposition of the great vessels

These are complex abnormalities which present

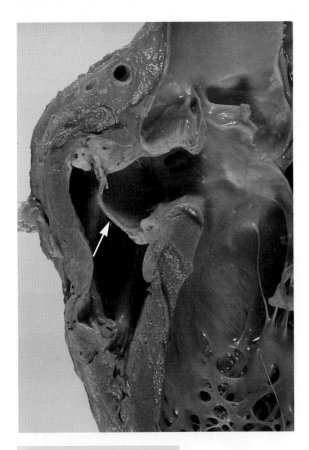

Fig. 13.49 Fallot's tetralogy

A partial surgical correction was made many years before this patient's death. The ventricular defect has been closed with a fabric patch (arrowed).

the length and distribution of the terminal parts of the right artery. Similarly, the coronary arterial ostia are occasionally malpositioned, but these cause no obvious clinical effects. However, sometimes one, or even both, of the coronary arteries arise from the pulmonary artery, and the myocardium is therefore wholly or partially perfused with deoxygenated blood. Myocardial ischaemia and cardiac failure are then inevitable.

UNUSUAL CARDIAC DISEASES

Most cases of cardiac failure can be attributed to ischaemic heart disease, hypertension, valvular disorders, congenital defects or lung disease. Only when these have been excluded are unusual causes considered. The term *cardiomyopathy* is often loosely applied to these disorders, but strictly speaking this term should be restricted to disorders of completely unknown cause or clinical association, i.e. *idiopathic* or *primary cardiomyopathy*. In addition, expressions such as alcoholic or amyloid cardiomyopathy are sometimes used to describe cardiac disease in patients with a known systemic disorder which affects the heart.

Unusual disorders of known cause or association

Multisystem diseases

Cardiac changes are often present in association with multisystem disease. In *sarcoidosis* and *rheumatoid disease*, for example, granulomatous lesions can develop in the heart, and, if they involve the conduction pathways, arrhythmias or heart block can develop. In some forms of *amyloidosis* (Ch. 7), the heart is involved. At autopsy, the cardiac muscle has a characteristic glassy brown appearance and, if deposits are extensive, cardiac failure develops. Massive cardiac hypertrophy is a feature of *acromegaly*, and cardiac failure is the usual cause of death in these patients.

Major cardiac abnormalities are well recognised in both thyrotoxicosis and myxoedema. In severe *thyrotoxicosis*, the increase in the metabolic rate necessitates an increased cardiac output and peripheral blood flow. Occasionally, this may in itself precipitate 'high output' cardiac failure. More frequently, thyrotoxicosis unmasks subclinical coronary or hypertensive heart disease. Atrial fibrillation is particularly common in elderly patients with thyrotoxicosis.

early in life and require prompt surgery. There are several different forms but in the most important the aorta drains the right ventricle and the pulmonary artery the left. This creates two closed circulations. Post-natal life is only possible if these mix via an atrial or ventricular septal defect or a patent ductus arteriosus. A complete surgical correction is often possible, usually by 'switching' the pulmonary artery and aorta at their origin from the heart.

Coronary arterial abnormalities

There is considerable variation in the normal anatomy of the major coronary vessels and this is usually of no clinical importance. For example, the circumflex branch of the left coronary artery is sometimes small and there is a corresponding increase in

Most patients with *myxoedema* have an enlarged cardiac outline on chest X-ray. This may be due to left ventricular dilatation or pericardial effusion; these can be distinguished by echocardiography. Characteristically, there is a bradycardia, low voltage ECG and decreased cardiac output. There are usually no specific pathological findings either macroscopically or microscopically. The response to thyroid hormone therapy is often excellent, but angina, and even myocardial infarction, can be precipitated with anything but the smallest doses.

Alcoholism

Cardiac failure is not uncommon in chronic alcoholism. In some cases it can be attributed to common disorders such as coronary artery disease or hypertension. However, in a proportion of patients, no specific cause is determined and 'alcoholic cardiomyopathy' is diagnosed. In these patients the macroscopic and microscopic findings are identical to those of other forms of idiopathic cardiomyopathy, and there is some debate as to the exact role of heavy alcohol consumption.

Pregnancy

Substantial circulatory changes occur in pregnancy, most notably an increase in circulating blood volume. Cardiac failure may become apparent for the first time during pregnancy, especially in patients with valvular disorders. Hypertension is one of the cardinal signs of pre-eclampsia but, while cardiac failure and pulmonary oedema can develop in the full syndrome, the disorder is not primarily cardiac in origin (Ch. 19). A characteristic form of cardiomyopathy (discussed below) occasionally develops in the post-partum period.

Iatrogenic disease

Iatrogenic ('doctor-induced') cardiac disease is now of some importance because of the increasing use of cytotoxic drugs and of radiotherapy in the treatment of mediastinal tumours. Radiotherapy causes patchy areas of interstitial fibrosis in the myocardium (probably as a result of direct damage to small capillaries) and pericarditis. Some degree of cardiac muscle cell necrosis is a frequent result of treatment with cytotoxic drugs, such as adriamycin and doxorubicin, which interfere with DNA and RNA replication and protein synthesis.

Idiopathic cardiomyopathies

The diagnosis of cardiomyopathy should be made only when all other causes of cardiac failure, such as hypertension, ischaemic heart disease, valvular and congenital heart disease have been excluded. There is growing evidence that many cases of cardiomyopathy in children and young adults have a genetic basis.

Congestive (dilated) cardiomyopathy

The incidence of this disorder in Europe and North America is 2–8 cases per 100 000 per year. The median age at presentation is about 50 years but young adults are commonly affected. Typically, the coronary arteries are patent but the ventricles are dilated and hypertrophied (Fig. 13.50). There may

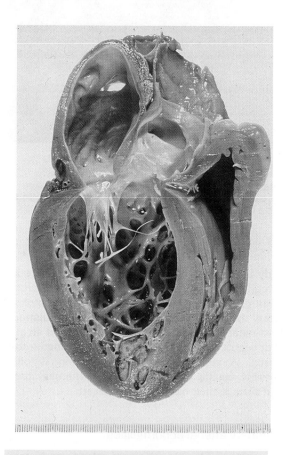

Fig. 13.50   Dilated (congestive) cardiomyopathy

There is marked hypertrophy of both the left and right ventricles. Note the adherent mural thrombus at the apex of the left ventricle. No underlying cause was determined in this patient.

be adherent mural thrombi and histological evidence of interstitial fibrosis and hypertrophy of muscle fibres. Some cases of viral myocarditis appear to progress to dilated cardiomyopathy but there is no firm evidence of viral infection in the majority of cases. The pathological features of chronic alcoholic heart disease and dilated cardiomyopathy are similar. The outlook in dilated cardiomyopathy is poor and only 50–60% of patients survive two years. It is essential to investigate these patients in the hope of identifying a treatable disorder such as coronary artery or aortic valve disease. Young patients with dilated cardiomyopathy are often considered for cardiac transplantation.

Hypertrophic (obstructive) cardiomyopathy

The clinical, echocardiographic and pathological features in hypertrophic cardiomyopathy are often

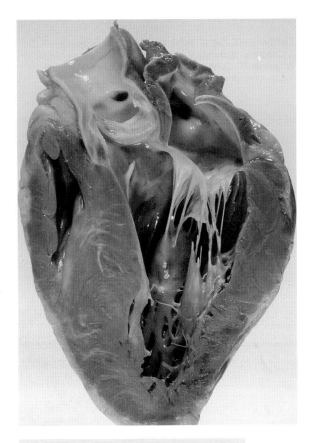

Fig. 13.51 Hypertrophic cardiomyopathy

The patient was a 24-year-old male who died suddenly. Note the marked and asymmetrical enlargement of the interventricular septum.

characteristic (Fig. 13.51). The chief feature is massive left ventricular hypertrophy, usually most marked in the interventricular septum close to the aortic outflow tract.

Patients present with a variety of signs or symptoms but atrial fibrillation, ventricular arrhythmias and sudden death are the most important complications.

Some cases are familial and chromosomal abnormalities can be identified in up to 50% of patients. Point mutations have been studied in the gene on chromosome 14 which codes for the beta chain of cardiac muscle myosin. It is likely that the exact nature of the amino acid substitution influences the course of the disease. Small amounts of the mRNA for cardiac myosin are expressed ectopically in leukocytes. This can be amplified by PCR techniques and screened for mutations. This has important implications because echocardiographic changes may develop over a period of years and there is evidence that treatment with beta blockers or calcium channel blocking agents may improve prognosis. A variety of other genetic abnormalities have been detected in young patients with cardiomyopathy. Some relate to fatty acid oxidation, mitochondrial oxidative phosphorylation or the cardiac-specific expression of the dystrophin gene. At least three other genes have been implicated in hypertrophic cardiomyopathy and their products include the structural proteins troponin T and α-tropomyosin. In the future it is likely that many forms of cardiomyopathy will be classified and treated on the basis of the exact underlying genetic abnormality.

Other cardiomyopathies

Other forms of cardiomyopathy have been described, usually in specific clinical settings.

Puerperal cardiomyopathy occurs in the last months of pregnancy, or within six months of delivery. There is no history of pre-existing cardiac disease and the clinical outcome is variable. In some cases, cardiac failure resolves completely, although recurrence in subsequent pregnancies is likely.

Endomyocardial fibrosis is a curious form of myocardial disease found in the tropics, chiefly in Uganda and the Sudan. The cause is unknown, but there is marked fibrosis of the inner parts of the myocardium, and mural thrombi are common. In some patients with severe cardiac failure, there is a prominent persistent peripheral blood eosinophilia and evidence of multiple systemic emboli (Löffler's endocarditis). This occurs in both tropical Africa and, sporadically, in the West and is usually fatal. The cause is uncertain.

TUMOURS OF THE HEART AND PERICARDIUM

Primary tumours of the heart and pericardium are extremely rare; only a few cases are seen annually in each regional cardiothoracic centre in the United Kingdom. The *myxoma* is the most frequent primary tumour (25%) and usually arises from the endocardium as a polypoid or pedunculated tumour mass. Three-quarters of myxomas occur in the left atrium, and in almost one-half of all cases there are signs and symptoms of mitral valve disease. The tumours are often friable and can fragment and embolise. Myxomas can be present at almost any age, but are most common in adults. The tumours have a characteristic histological appearance and probably arise from undifferentiated connective tissue cells in the sub-endocardial layers of the heart wall. Other primary tumours include *lipomas*, which are usually found in the interatrial septum. *Rhabdomyomas* arise from cardiac muscle and are often multiple. Many occur in newborn infants and cause stillbirth, or death within the first days of life. Primary malignant tumours of the myocardium include *rhabdomyosarcoma* and *angiosarcoma*.

The commonest primary pericardial tumour is *mesothelioma*. Inevitably, the heart and pericardium are often involved by local extension of primary intrathoracic tumours. Bronchial carcinoma is by far the commonest cause of this.

FURTHER READING

Anderson RH, Becker AE 1992. The heart. Structure in health and disease. Gower Medical Publishing, London

Silver MD 1992 Cardiovascular disease, 2nd edn. Churchill Livingstone, Edinburgh

Souhami RL, Moxham J 1994 Textbook of medicine, 2nd edn. Churchill Livingstone, Edinburgh

Stehbens WE, Lie JT (eds) 1995 Vascular pathology. Chapman and Hall, London

Willerson JT, Cohn JN (eds) 1995 Cardiovascular medicine. Churchill Livingstone, Edinburgh

Respiratory tract

Respiratory disease, particularly lung infections, causes most damage in developing countries where, together with gastrointestinal infections, it accounts for most deaths. However, respiratory disease is also a common cause of death in the industrialised nations. Lung cancer accounts for about 9% of male deaths and about 4% of female deaths in the UK, although the latter figure is rising due to the recent increase in female smokers. All other respiratory diseases account for about 14% of deaths in each sex. There is also considerable morbidity due to respiratory diseases: it is estimated that, in the UK, about 40% of absence from work is the result of such diseases, about 85% of which are transient infections of the upper respiratory tract.

Most respiratory illness is due to environmental factors, especially smoking; genetic factors have a minor role (Table 14.1).

Table 14.1 Major aetiological factors in respiratory disease

Aetiological factor	Disease
Genetic	Cystic fibrosis α_1-Antitrypsin deficiency Some asthma
Environmental Smoking	Lung cancer Chronic bronchitis and emphysema Susceptibility to infection
Air pollution	Chronic bronchitis Susceptibility to infection
Occupation	Pneumoconiosis Asbestosis, mesothelioma and lung cancer
Infection	Influenza Measles Bacterial pneumonias Tuberculosis

NORMAL STRUCTURE AND FUNCTION

The respiratory system extends from the nasal orifices to the periphery of the lung and the surrounding pleural cavity. From the nose to the distal bronchi, the mucosa is lined with mainly pseudo-stratified ciliated columnar epithelium with mucus-secreting goblet cells; this is *respiratory mucosa* (Fig. 14.1). A portion of the larynx is covered with stratified squamous epithelium.

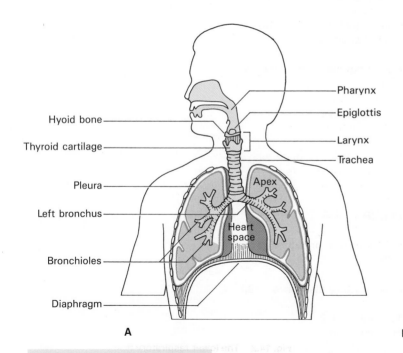

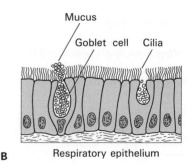

Fig. 14.1 The respiratory system

A. Anatomy of the respiratory tract. **B.** Histology of respiratory epithelium. With the exception of the pharynx, epiglottis and vocal cords, the respiratory tract is lined by specialised ciliated mucus-secreting epithelium.

The co-ordinated rhythmic beating of the cilia in the surface of the respiratory mucosa wafts mucus containing dust particles from the depths of the lung up to the larynx. From there the mucus can be either expectorated or swallowed.

Nasal passages and sinuses

The nasal passages and sinuses are in continuity and are lined with respiratory mucosa. The hairs in the nose trap large particles of foreign material, thereby filtering the air. The air is also warmed and humidified as it passes through the nasal cavity. The middle ear, also lined with respiratory epithelium, connects with the nasal cavity via the Eustachian tube.

Larynx

The larynx connects the trachea to the pharynx. Consisting of a complicated system of cartilages and muscles, it allows air into the trachea, with the epiglottis preventing the passage of food into the lungs, and also produces sound for speaking. Part of the larynx, including the vocal cords and epiglottis, is covered with non-keratinising squamous epithelium similar to that lining the oral cavity, pharynx and oesophagus.

Lungs

The lungs are divided into *lobes*: the right lung has three lobes (upper, middle, lower); the left lung has only two lobes (upper and lower). Each lung is formed of ten anatomically defined *bronchopulmonary segments*. Each segment is supplied by a segmental artery and bronchus, but the veins draining adjacent segments often anastomose before they reach the hilum.

The lungs develop from an outpouching of the anterior wall of the primitive foregut at about the fifth week of development. From this tube, two lateral outgrowths appear which eventually form the right and left lungs. These outgrowths are surrounded by mesenchyme from which forms the connective tissue of the respiratory tree. Thus the lungs, like the gastrointestinal tract, develop from endoderm, and developmental abnormalities such as cysts can therefore be lined by either respiratory or gastrointestinal mucosa. The larynx forms at the proximal end of the trachea and is partially lined with squamous epithelium.

The *lower respiratory tract* consists of the trachea, bronchi, bronchioles, alveolar ducts and alveoli (Fig. 14.2). The structure of each portion differs (Table 14.2).

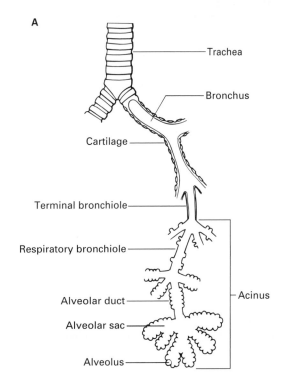

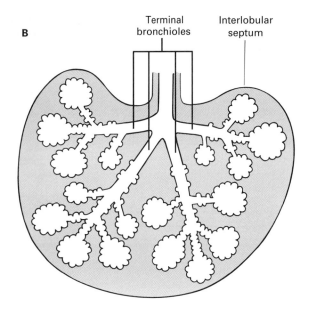

Fig. 14.2 The lower respiratory tract

A. Structure and nomenclature of the lower respiratory tract. **B.** Schematic detail of a lobule. Different diseases affect different parts of the tract.

Table 14.2 Structure of the respiratory tree	
Part of respiratory tract	Structure
Trachea	Anterior C-shaped plates of cartilage with posterior smooth muscle. Mucous glands
Bronchi	Discontinuous foci of cartilage with smooth muscle. Mucous glands
Bronchioles	No cartilage or submucosal mucous glands. Clara cells secreting proteinaceous fluid. Ciliated epithelium
Alveolar duct Alveoli	Flat epithelium. No glands. No cilia Type I and II pneumocytes

The *respiratory tree* is designed to transport clean, humidified air into distal airways and alveoli, where the waste product of metabolism (CO_2) is exchanged for O_2.

Bronchioles branch until they form terminal bronchioles less than 2 mm in diameter. The respiratory system distal to the terminal bronchiole is called the *acinus* or *terminal respiratory unit*, where gas exchange occurs. Small airways, defined as having an internal diameter of less than 2 mm, consist of terminal and respiratory bronchioles. Respiratory bronchioles are involved with gas exchange, having alveoli in their walls. A group of 3–5 respiratory acini is called a *lobule*.

The *alveoli* are lined by flattened type I pneumocytes with occasional type II pneumocytes; the latter are rounded cells with surface microvilli and osmiophilic (affinity for osmium stain) lamellated inclusions in their cytoplasm. Type II cells secrete surfactant, and replicate quickly after injury to alveolar walls. Beneath these alveolar cells lies a basement membrane and some interstitial matrix, including elastin fibres, separating the airspaces from the capillary wall (Fig. 14.3). The structure of the alveolar–capillary membrane permits rapid and efficient diffusion of oxygen and carbon dioxide.

The *pleura* consists of a double layer of fibrous connective tissue lined by mesothelial cells. A thin film of fluid lubricates the two layers, allowing easy movement of the lungs against the thoracic cage wall.

The lungs and pleura are enclosed within the chest by the diaphragm, ribs and intercostal muscles, vertebral column and sternum.

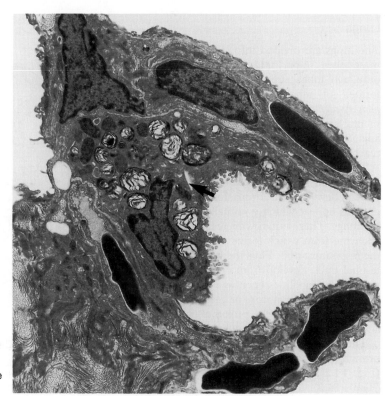

Fig. 14.3 Alveolar wall

Electron micrograph showing a type II pneumocyte (arrow) containing intracytoplasmic lamellated inclusions of surfactant. The remainder of the alveolar surface is lined by thin, flat cytoplasm of type I pneumocytes.

Blood supply and lymphatic drainage

The lungs are perfused by a *dual arterial blood supply*. The trunk of the *pulmonary artery* arises from the right ventricle, splits into main right and left pulmonary arteries and thence follows the airways. The *bronchial arteries* arise from the descending thoracic aorta and supply oxygenated blood to lung parenchyma around the hilum. Pulmonary veins take all the blood from the lungs back to the left atrium. The obvious benefit of a dual blood supply is that, should a pulmonary artery branch become blocked (e.g. due to pulmonary embolism), the structure of the lung can remain intact as it is still supplied with nutrients from the bronchial arteries. However, this rarely happens because most pulmonary infarcts are peripheral whereas bronchial arteries supply only hilar regions.

Pulmonary *veins* course along the interlobular septa with *lymphatics*. The lymphatics drain into the thoracic duct and thence into the left subclavian vein.

Control of respiration

Respiration is controlled by the *respiratory centre* in the medulla oblongata, and the carotid bodies situated at the carotid bifurcations. The medullary centre senses any change in CO_2 concentration in the cerebrospinal fluid, and modifies respiration by nervous stimulation of respiratory muscles and the diaphragm. The partial pressure of O_2 in the blood is monitored by the *carotid bodies*, which can then stimulate the respiratory centre through the glossopharyngeal nerves. Carotid bodies can become hyperplastic in response to chronic arterial hypoxaemia, such as occurs in:

- high altitude dwellers
- pulmonary emphysema
- diffuse pulmonary fibrosis
- kyphoscoliosis with chronic hypoventilation
- Pickwickian syndrome (gross obesity with chronic hypoxaemia).

Gas exchange

Air is drawn into the lungs by contraction of the diaphragm and intercostal muscles, creating a negative intrapleural pressure. On relaxation of these muscles, air is expelled as the lungs contract under the action of gravity and the elasticity in the lung connective tissue. The stiffness of the lungs, or *compliance*, is a measure of change in volume per unit change in pressure, and is therefore a measure of

compressibility; for example, in pulmonary fibrosis the lungs cannot be easily compressed and therefore the compliance is decreased.

Clearly, gas exchange occurs only in alveoli that are both perfused and ventilated. Ventilation of non-perfused alveoli increases the 'dead space', that proportion of inspired air not involved with gas exchange. Perfusion of non-ventilated alveoli leads to physiological right-to-left shunting of non-oxygenated blood as it passes through the pulmonary circulation.

Acid–base balance

Normal acid–base balance in blood is dependent on both efficient alveolar ventilation and perfusion, with consequent successful gas exchange. This leads to the normal partial pressures of O_2 and CO_2 in arterial blood (PaO_2 and $PaCO_2$), and a normal blood pH. Various metabolic disease states lead to disturbances in acid–base balance (Fig. 14.4). If the disease becomes chronic, compensatory mechanisms by both the lungs and kidneys operate in an attempt to restore blood pH (Ch. 7.)

MEASUREMENT OF LUNG CAPACITY AND FUNCTION

In normal quiet respiration under diaphragmatic drive, only a relatively small proportion of the *total lung capacity* (TLC) is inhaled and exhaled; this is the *tidal volume* (TV). TLC is made up of the amount of air totally exhaled after maximum inspiration (the *vital capacity* or VC) and the *residual volume* (RV). TLC, RV, TV and VC are all easily measured in the laboratory using helium dilution techniques.

Pulmonary function tests

In addition to calculating volume parameters, some techniques also assess pulmonary function. *Spirometry* measures the amount of exhaled air per second. The maximum volume of air blown from the lungs within the first second after a previous maximum inspiration is called the *forced expiratory volume* (FEV_1). This figure, highly reproducible in each individual, is governed by the state of major intrathoracic airways (trachea and bronchi). It is also dependent on the patient's age, sex and size; for example, the small lungs of a child obviously cannot expel as much air as those of an adult. The total amount of air expired after maximum inspiration is the *vital capac-*

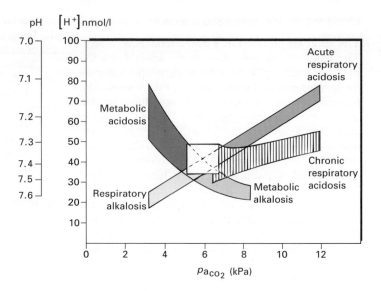

pH [H⁺] nmol/l

Fig. 14.4   Acid–base imbalance

Changes in blood pH can occur as a result of alterations in hydrogen ion and carbon dioxide concentrations. These lead to different states of acidosis and alkalosis.

ity (VC). The ratio FEV_1/VC compensates to a degree for the variability of lung size. It is possible to inhale more rapidly than exhale because, during inspiration, forces on the airways tend to open them further; during expiration, opposite forces tend to close airways and thus restrict airflow. For a given lung volume, the *expiratory flow rate* reaches a peak (PEFR), which is again a measure of airways resistance.

An assessment of the ability of the lungs to exchange gas efficiently can be made by measuring the *transfer factor* for carbon monoxide (T_{CO}). Air containing a known concentration of carbon monoxide is inhaled; the breath is held for 15 seconds and then exhaled. The amount of carbon monoxide absorbed is a measure of pulmonary gas exchange. T_{CO} is dependent on the concentration of blood haemoglobin, which has a strong affinity for carbon monoxide. Diseases that diffusely affect the alveolar–capillary membrane (such as any diffuse pulmonary fibrosis) will result in a low T_{CO}.

Obstructive and restrictive defects

There are two major groups of patients in whom the above pulmonary function tests are of great value: those with *obstructive defects* (e.g. asthma) and those with *restrictive defects* (e.g. pulmonary fibrosis). Restrictive diseases are those that restrict normal lung movement during respiration. Both types of lung disease show a contrasting pattern of pulmonary function tests (Table 14.3).

In obstructive airways disease, RV and TLC are

Table 14.3   Respiratory function tests and their diagnostic significance

Test	Diagnostic significance
Peak expiratory flow rate (PEFR)	Reduced with obstructed airways or muscle weakness
Forced expiratory volume in 1 second (FEV_1)	Reduced with obstructed airways, pulmonary fibrosis or oedema, or muscle weakness
Vital capacity (VC)	Reduced with reduction in effective lung volume (fibrosis or oedema), chest wall deformity (kyphoscoliosis), or muscle weakness
Forced expiratory ratio (FEV_1/VC)	Low in obstructive defects Normal or high in restrictive defects
Carbon monoxide transfer (T_{CO})	Reduced in pulmonary fibrosis, oedema, embolism and anaemia

mildly increased due to hyperinflation of the lung distal to diseased airways. Clearly, in asthma, the results of pulmonary function tests will depend on the clinical state of the patient, whether in an acute attack of asthma or in remission.

These tests are of most value in the follow-up of patients. They can also give an indication as to the possible benefits of treatment; for example, observing the improved FEV_1/VC and PEFR after treat-

Pathological basis of respiratory signs and symptoms

Sign or symptom	Pathological basis
Sputum • clear or mucoid	Excess secretion from bronchial mucus glands in, for example, asthma and chronic bronchitis
• purulent	Inflammatory exudate from respiratory tract infection
• with blood	Extravasation of red cells due to cardiac failure, pulmonary infarction or ulceration of respiratory mucosa (e.g. by tumour)
Cough	Physiological reflex response to presence of mucus, exudate, tumour or foreign material
Wheezing • on inspiration	Narrowing of larynx, trachea or proximal bronchi (e.g. by tumour)
• on expiration	Distal bronchial narrowing (e.g. asthma)
Dyspnoea	Decreased oxygen in the blood from impaired alveolar gas exchange, left heart failure or anaemia
Cyanosis	Increased non-oxygenated haemoglobin, e.g. circulatory bypassing of lungs in congenital heart diseases or impaired alveolar gas exchange
Pleuritic pain	Irritation of the pleura due to pulmonary inflammation, infarction or tumour
Pleural effusion • transudate (low protein)	Cardiac failure Hypoalbuminaemia (e.g. cirrhosis, nephrotic syndrome)
• exudate (high protein)	Pleural inflammation Tumour
Clubbing	Often accompanies carcinoma of lung and pulmonary fibrosis, as well as, less commonly, cirrhosis and chronic inflammatory bowel disease
Weight loss	Protein catabolic state induced by chronic inflammatory disease (e.g. tuberculosis) or tumours
Auscultation signs • crackles	Sudden inspirational opening of small airways resisted by fluid or fibrosis *(contd)*

Pathological basis of respiratory signs and symptoms (*continued*)

Sign or symptom	Pathological basis
• wheezes	Generalised or localised airway narrowing
• pleural rub	Pleural surface roughened by exudate
Percussion signs • dullness	Solidification of lung by exudate (pneumonia) or fibrosis Pleural effusion
• hyper-resonance	Increased gas content of thorax due to pneumothorax or emphysema

ment with a bronchodilator would be a measure of the reversibility of the airways obstruction.

RESPIRATORY FAILURE

Respiratory failure can occur as a result of:

- ventilation defects
- perfusion defects, if diffuse or extensive, e.g. cardiac failure or multiple pulmonary emboli
- gas exchange defects, if diffuse and severe, e.g. emphysema or diffuse pulmonary fibrosis.

Ventilation defects may be:

- nervous, e.g. due to narcotics, encephalitis, a space-occupying lesion, poliomyelitis, motor neurone disease, etc.
- mechanical, e.g. due to trauma, kyphoscoliosis, muscle disease, pleural effusion, gross obesity (Pickwickian syndrome).

The effects of respiratory failure include impaired clearance of CO_2 from the lungs, resulting in hypercapnia, and impaired absorption of O_2 from the air, resulting in hypoxaemia. The patient is typically dyspnoeic, cyanosed and lapsing into coma. Hypercapnia (high blood CO_2 concentration) is associated with a bounding pulse and warm, moist extremities.

DISEASES OF INFANCY AND CHILDHOOD

Respiratory diseases of infancy and childhood may arise as a result of either developmental abnormalities or immaturity.

Developmental abnormalities

Developmental abnormalities include:

- tracheo-oesophageal fistula
- congenital diaphragmatic hernia with pulmonary hypoplasia
- bronchogenic and alveolar cysts
- pulmonary sequestration
- congenital lobar emphysema.

Tracheo-oesophageal fistula
Embryologically, the oesophagus and the trachea begin as a single tube; the trachea then buds off to form the pulmonary tree. In a tracheo-oesophageal fistula, the oesophagus ends in a blind pouch; the trachea then usually connects to the stomach via a fistula. On ingestion of food, the upper pouch quickly fills and overflows into the pulmonary tree with choking and coughing, leading to aspiration pneumonia. Treatment is by surgery, usually after a period of feeding via gastrostomy.

Congenital diaphragmatic hernia with pulmonary hypoplasia
This presents as neonatal respiratory distress due to herniation of the stomach and loops of bowel into the thorax; usually the left diaphragm is defective. Surgical correction to normal thoracic and abdominal anatomy is essential at the earliest possible opportunity. However, even after this there is still a considerable mortality from the associated severe pulmonary hypoplasia, usually of the left lung.

Bronchogenic and alveolar cysts
These occur in the lung, lined either by bronchial elements such as cartilage, smooth muscle and ciliated respiratory epithelium (bronchogenic cysts), or by simple flattened alveolar type epithelium (alveolar cysts). Usually, such cysts are asymptomatic, although complications may occur.

Pulmonary sequestration
A sequestered piece of lung is a mass of abnormal lung that does not communicate anatomically with the tracheo-bronchial tree; it is supplied by an anomalous artery, usually from the aorta. Sequestered pieces of lung are found most often around the left lower lobe. Histology shows a multi-lobulated cystic mass with fibrosis and variable inflammation. An endogenous lipid pneumonia may result.

Congenital lobar emphysema
This condition is characterised by overdistension of a lobe due to intermittent bronchial obstruction. Symptoms arise due to pressure effects caused by the massively distended lobe. Usually, the left upper lobe is affected. The pathogenesis is thought to be abnormal bronchial cartilage allowing inspiration of air but not expiration. Extrabronchial compression by enlarged lymph nodes may cause a similar clinical picture. Treatment is surgical removal of the diseased lobe.

Immaturity

Diseases due to immaturity include:

- hyaline membrane disease or idiopathic respiratory distress syndrome
- bronchopulmonary dysplasia.

Hyaline membrane disease or idiopathic respiratory distress syndrome

> ▶ Complication of prematurity (less than 36 weeks' gestation)
> ▶ Due to deficiency of pulmonary surfactant
> ▶ Tachypnoea, dyspnoea, expiratory grunting, cyanosis
> ▶ Diffuse alveolar damage with hyaline membranes
> ▶ Associated with maternal diabetes, multiple pregnancy, caesarean section, amniotic fluid aspiration
> ▶ Many similarities to adult respiratory distress syndrome (ARDS)

Hyaline membrane disease (HMD) is almost always seen in premature infants of birth weight less than 2.5 kg. Infants are usually of less than 36 weeks' gestation, and the incidence of HMD rises as the gestational age decreases. Other associated factors include maternal diabetes, birth by caesarean section, multiple births and difficult deliveries complicated by amniotic fluid aspiration.

Clinical features
After a few hours of relatively normal respiration, symptoms of tachypnoea and dyspnoea with expiratory grunting appear. Cyanosis quickly follows, with worsening respiratory distress. Hypoxaemia refractory to high concentration of inhaled oxygen is one hallmark of the disease, a finding also characteristic of adult respiratory distress syndrome (ARDS).

Pathogenesis

The pathogenesis is thought to be due to a deficiency of surfactant. This is secreted by type II pneumocytes, and normally lines distal airways; it reduces surface tension, thereby allowing airway opening during inspiration. Without normal quantities of surfactant, airways need greater effort to open, leading to respiratory distress.

Morphology

At autopsy the lungs are heavy, purple and solid, and sink in water. Histology shows unopened alveoli with hyaline membranes lining alveolar ducts. Pulmonary lymphatics are dilated. As in ARDS, if the infant survives, resolution follows within the next few days, although pulmonary fibrosis may occur in a minority of cases. Treatment is with oxygen and artificial ventilation.

Bronchopulmonary dysplasia

Bronchopulmonary dysplasia is the term used to describe the picture of lung organisation after HMD. Often, infants have been previously treated with high levels of oxygen, and it is not clear whether bronchopulmonary dysplasia is a separate disorder, solely related to oxygen toxicity, or merely a result of organisation after HMD. Certainly, the features are almost identical to those seen with organisation of ARDS; there is interstitial fibrosis with peribronchial fibrosis, and features of pulmonary hypertension; airways may show extensive squamous metaplasia.

NASAL PASSAGES AND SINUSES

▶ Inflammatory diseases, e.g. rhinitis, are very common
▶ Nasal polyps are either inflammatory or allergic
▶ Malignant tumours are rare

INFLAMMATORY DISORDERS

Rhinitis (the common cold) is caused by many different viruses, especially rhinoviruses, although respiratory syncytial virus (RSV), para-influenza viruses, coronaviruses, coxsackieviruses, echoviruses and bacteria, such as *Haemophilus influenzae*, may also be implicated. Rhinitis may also be caused by inhaled allergens as in 'hay fever'; the inflammatory reaction is mediated via type I and type III hypersensitivity reactions (Chs 9 and 10).

Nasal polyps may result from either chronic infective inflammation or chronic allergic inflammation. They consist of polypoid oedematous masses of connective tissue infiltrated with chronic inflammatory cells, especially plasma cells; eosinophils may be numerous if allergy is the cause.

Sinusitis is inflammation of the paranasal sinuses; it may be acute or chronic. If the drainage orifice is blocked by inflamed swollen mucosa, an abscess may follow. Cranial osteomyelitis, meningitis or cerebral abscess may then result from sinusitis by direct extension.

TUMOURS

Tumours of the nasal passages and sinuses are uncommon. They may be:

- benign: haemangioma, squamous papilloma, juvenile angiofibroma
- malignant: squamous cell carcinoma, adenocarcinoma, plasmacytoma.

Haemangioma and *squamous papilloma* are benign lesions, the former often presenting with troublesome epistaxis (nosebleeds). Some squamous papillomas may be caused by human papillomavirus.

Juvenile angiofibromas are rare and occur exclusively in males, usually during adolescence. They are extremely vascular, and surgical removal can be difficult. These tumours contain androgen receptors, explaining the male preponderance.

Squamous cell carcinoma may be well differentiated, producing keratin, or very poorly differentiated. The latter may contain many lymphocytes and have been misnamed 'lympho-epitheliomas'. Such tumours are more common in China and the Far East, and evidence suggests Epstein–Barr virus may be involved in its aetiology and pathogenesis.

Adenocarcinoma of the nasal passages and sinuses occurs more frequently in people who have worked in woodwork and furniture industries. These tumours may present clinically up to 40 years after initial exposure.

Plasmacytomas are tumours composed of plasma cells. They can occur as part of multiple myeloma or as isolated lesions without systemic disease.

INFLAMMATORY DISORDERS

Laryngitis may occur in association with viral or bacterial inflammation of trachea and bronchi; this is laryngotracheobronchitis. *Diphtheria* was once a common, and serious, bacterial cause of laryngitis, leading to the formation of a fibrinopurulent membrane that could cause airway obstruction. Now, as a result of immunisation in infancy with diphtheria toxoid, the disease is rare.

Epiglottitis is caused by capsulated forms of *Haemophilus influenzae* type B. The epiglottis becomes inflamed and greatly swollen, leading to airway obstruction (Fig. 14.5). Treatment is by intubation, although, rarely, tracheostomy may be necessary; antibiotics are also given to treat the infection.

Allergic laryngitis occurs after inhalation of an allergen. There may be gross oedema leading to airway obstruction. *Irritative laryngitis* may be due to cigarette smoke or mechanical factors, e.g. endotracheal intubation.

Laryngeal polyps often develop in singers and are thus sometimes referred to as 'singer's nodes'. Even when only a few millimetres in diameter they can alter the character of the voice. They consist of oedematous myxoid connective tissue covered with squamous mucosa with amyloid-like material in the stroma.

TUMOURS

Laryngeal tumours may be:

• benign: papilloma
• malignant: squamous cell carcinoma.

Papilloma may be caused by types of human papillomavirus. Papillomas consist of papillomatous squamous epithelium covering fibrovascular cores of stroma. They may be multiple and recurrent, especially in children, but are usually single in adults. Such papillomas can extend into the trachea and bronchi.

Squamous cell carcinoma of the larynx typically affects males over 40 years of age and is associated with cigarette smoking. There may also be an increased risk in asbestos workers. As in squamous epithelium of the cervix, neoplasia is thought to be preceded by a phase of dysplasia. The dysplasia, especially if low grade, may be reversible on withdrawal of causative factors.

Most laryngeal carcinomas arise on the vocal cords (Fig. 14.6) although they may arise above, in the pyriform fossa, or below, as upper tracheal car-

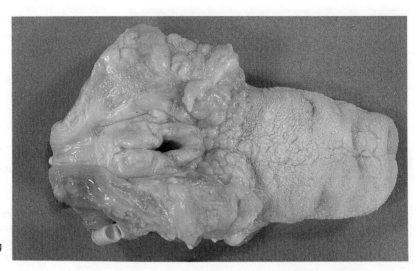

Fig. 14.5 Acute epiglottitis
Gross swelling of the epiglottis leading to respiratory obstruction in a child.

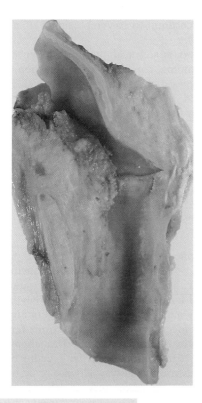

Fig. 14.6   Laryngeal carcinoma
The tumour is protruding into the larynx and invading the underlying tissues.

cinomas. The lesions ulcerate, fungate and invade locally, later causing metastases in regional lymph nodes and beyond. Symptoms are hoarseness of voice and, later, pain, haemoptysis and dysphagia. Treatment is by resection and/or radiotherapy.

THE LUNGS

RESPIRATORY INFECTIONS

The lungs have an exposed internal surface area of approximately 500 m^2. It is therefore not surprising that respiratory infections are relatively common. Countering the threat of pathogens are the defence mechanisms, any abnormality in which will predispose to infection. Such abnormalities include:

- loss or suppression of the cough reflex, e.g. in coma, anaesthesia, neuromuscular disorders, or after surgery
- ciliary defects, e.g. in immotile cilia syndromes, or loss of ciliated cells with squamous metaplasia
- mucus disorders, e.g. excessive viscosity as in cystic fibrosis or chronic bronchitis
- acquired or congenital hypogammaglobulinaemia, e.g. with decreased IgA in the mucus
- immunosuppression, e.g. with loss of B- and/or T-lymphocytes
- macrophage function inhibition, e.g. in people who smoke or are hypoxic
- pulmonary oedema with flooding of the alveoli.

Infections can be classified as *primary*, with no underlying predisposing condition in a healthy individual, or *secondary*, when local or systemic defences are weakened. The latter are by far the most common types of respiratory infection in developed countries, and are becoming yet more important with the spread of AIDS.

Bronchitis

> ▶ Characterised by cough, dyspnoea, tachypnoea, sputum
> ▶ Usually viral
> ▶ Often superimposed on chronic obstructive airways disease

In acute bronchitis, the trachea and larynx are involved as well as the lungs, and the disease is then known as *acute laryngotracheobronchitis* (or 'croup'). The disease is more severe in children, with symptoms of cough, dyspnoea and tachypnoea. Viruses are usually the cause, especially respiratory syncytial virus (RSV), although *Haemophilus influenzae* and *Streptococcus pneumoniae* are frequent bacterial causes. Exacerbations of acute bronchitis are common in chronic obstructive airways disease, and cause a sudden deterioration in pulmonary function with cough and the production of purulent sputum. Acute bronchitis may be caused by direct chemical injury from air pollutants, such as smoke, sulphur dioxide and chlorine.

Chronic bronchitis is a clinical term defined as cough and sputum for 3 months in 2 consecutive years; it is discussed below under chronic obstructive airways disease (p. 383).

Bronchiolitis

▶ Often with bronchopneumonia
▶ Can be primary in infants
▶ Causes dyspnoea and tachypnoea
▶ Usually viral, especially respiratory syncytial virus (RSV)

Primary bronchiolitis is an uncommon respiratory infection caused by viruses, especially RSV, in infants. Symptoms are of acute respiratory distress with dyspnoea and tachypnoea. Most cases resolve within a few days, although a minority may develop bronchopneumonia.

Follicular bronchiolitis with lymphoid aggregates and germinal centres, compressing the airway, can occur in rheumatoid disease.

Bronchiolitis obliterans is characterised by polypoid masses of organising inflammatory exudate and granulation tissue extending from alveoli into bronchioles; it may occur in viral infections, especially RSV, after inhalation of toxic fumes, with extrinsic allergic alveolitis, in pulmonary fibrosis, after aspiration, and with collagen vascular diseases.

Pneumonia

▶ Alveolar inflammation
▶ Protein-rich exudate
▶ Polymorphs and later lymphocytes and macrophages
▶ Lobar or bronchopneumonia

Pneumonia is usually due to infection affecting distal airways, especially alveoli, with the formation of an inflammatory exudate. Pneumonia may be clas-sified according to several criteria (Table 14.4, Fig. 14.7).

The two anatomical patterns, lobar and bronchopneumonia, can result from infection by one of several types of bacteria, some of which have been mentioned above. There are also several other pathogens that cause distinct types of pneumonia.

Bronchopneumonia

▶ Patchy consolidation
▶ Centred on bronchioles or bronchi
▶ Usually in infancy or old age
▶ Usually secondary to pre-existing disease

Bronchopneumonia has a characteristic patchy distribution, centred on inflamed bronchioles and bronchi with subsequent spread to surrounding alveoli (Fig. 14.7). It occurs most commonly in old age, in infancy and in patients with debilitating diseases, such as cancer, cardiac failure, chronic renal failure or cerebrovascular accidents. Bronchopneumonia may also occur in patients with acute bronchitis, chronic obstructive airways disease or cystic fibrosis. Failure to clear respiratory secretions, such as is common in the post-operative period, also predisposes to the development of bronchopneumonia.

Causative organisms may be low-virulence pathogens, especially in an immunosuppressed patient, and as such would not cause similar disease in a young, healthy individual. Typical organisms include staphylococci, streptococci, *Haemophilus influenzae*, coliforms and fungi. Patients often become septicaemic and toxic, with fever and reduced consciousness. The areas of affected lung can be identified clinically by hearing crackles (crepitations) on auscultation.

Table 14.4	Classification of pneumonia	
Criterion	Type	Example/comment
Clinical circumstances	Primary	In an otherwise healthy person
	Secondary	With local or systemic defects in defence
Aetiological agent	Bacterial	*Streptococcus pneumoniae, Staphylococcus aureus, Mycobacterium tuberculosis*, etc.
	Viral	Influenza, measles, etc.
	Fungal	*Cryptococcus, Candida, Aspergillus*, etc.
	Other	*Pneumocystis carinii, Mycoplasma*, aspiration, lipid, eosinophilic
Host reaction	Fibrinous	
	Suppurative	
Anatomical pattern	Bronchopneumonia	
	Lobar pneumonia	

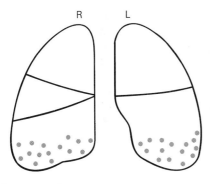

A. Bronchopneumonia

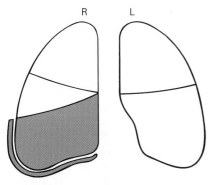

B. Lobar pneumonia

Fig. 14.7 Distribution of lesions in lobar and bronchopneumonia

A. Bronchopneumonia is characterised by focal inflammation centred on the airways; it is often bilateral.
B. Lobar pneumonia is characterised by diffuse inflammation affecting the entire lobe. Pleural exudate is common.

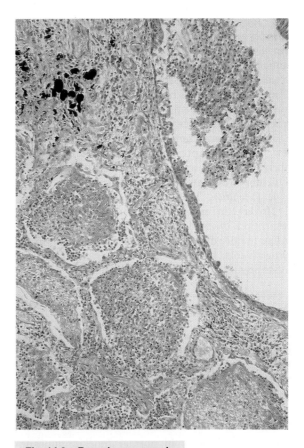

Fig. 14.8 Bronchopneumonia

The bronchiole contains inflammatory cells and the adjacent alveoli are filled with exudate. The black pigment is carbon, a common finding.

Affected areas of the lung tend to be basal and bilateral, and appear focally grey or grey-red at postmortem. The inflamed lung parenchyma can be demonstrated by gently pressing on an affected area; normal lung recoils like a sponge, whilst pneumonic lung offers little resistance. Histology shows typical acute inflammation with exudation (Fig. 14.8). With antibiotics and physiotherapy, the areas of inflammation may resolve, or heal by organisation with scarring.

Lobar pneumonia

▶ Affects a large part, or the entirety of, a lobe
▶ Relatively uncommon in infancy and old age
▶ Affects males more than females
▶ 90% due to *Streptococcus pneumoniae* (pneumococcus)
▶ Cough and fever with purulent or 'rusty' sputum

Pneumococcal pneumonia typically affects otherwise healthy adults between 20 and 50 years of age; however, lobar pneumonia caused by *Klebsiella* typically affects the elderly, diabetics or alcoholics. Symptoms include a cough, fever and production of sputum. The sputum appears purulent and may contain flecks of blood, so-called 'rusty' sputum. Fever can be very high (over 40°C), with rigors. Acute pleuritic chest pain on deep inspiration reflects involvement of the pleura. As the lung becomes consolidated, the chest signs are dullness to percussion with increased whispering pectoriloquy, and bronchial breathing. The dullness recedes with resolution of the exudate.

The pathology of lobar pneumonia is a classic example of acute inflammation, involving four stages:

1. *Congestion*. This first stage lasts for about 24 hours and represents the outpouring of a protein-rich exudate into alveolar spaces, with venous congestion. The lung is heavy, oedematous and red.

2. *Red hepatisation.* In this second stage, which lasts for a few days, there is massive accumulation in the alveolar spaces of polymorphs, together with some lymphocytes and macrophages. Many red cells are also extravasated from the distended capillaries. The overlying pleura bears a fibrinous exudate. The lung is red, solid and airless, with a consistency resembling fresh liver.

3. *Grey hepatisation.* This third stage also lasts a few days and represents further accumulation of fibrin, with destruction of white cells and red cells. The lung is now grey-brown and solid.

4. *Resolution.* This fourth stage occurs at about 8–10 days in untreated cases, and represents the resorption of exudate and enzymatic digestion of inflammatory debris, with preservation of the underlying alveolar wall architecture. Most cases of acute lobar pneumonia resolve in this way.

Special pneumonias

Special pneumonias may be subclassified into those occurring in normal (non-immunosuppressed) hosts, and those occurring in immunosuppressed hosts.

In normal hosts

Special pneumonias in normal (non-immunosuppressed) hosts may be due to:

- viruses, e.g. influenza, RSV, adenovirus and mycoplasma
- Legionnaires' disease.

Viral and mycoplasma pneumonia
The clinical course is varied depending on the extent and severity of the disease. In fatal cases, the lungs appear heavy, red and consolidated as in adult respiratory distress syndrome (ARDS; p. 389). Histology shows interstitial inflammation consisting of lymphocytes, macrophages and plasma cells. Hyaline membranes of fibrinous exudate are prominent (Fig. 14.9). The alveoli may be relatively free of cellular exudate.

Mycoplasma pneumonia tends to cause a more low-grade chronic pneumonia, with interstitial inflammation and fewer hyaline membranes. The chronic nature of the disease may result in organisation of the inflammation and pulmonary fibrosis.

Influenza viruses can cause an acute fulminating pneumonia with pulmonary haemorrhage; the clinical course may be rapidly fatal.

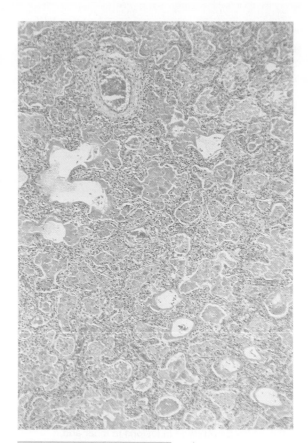

Fig. 14.9   Viral pneumonia

The lung is infiltrated by inflammatory cells and there is deposition of fibrinous exudate within alveoli as pink-stained amorphous material.

Legionnaires' disease
Since the first well-described outbreak in 1976, in a group of American Legion conventioneers, this disease has become increasingly recognised; about 150 cases are reported annually in the United Kingdom. It is caused by a bacillus, *Legionella pneumophila*, transmitted in water droplets from contaminated air humidifiers and water cisterns. Patients may be previously well, although a proportion have an underlying chronic illness, such as heart failure or carcinoma. Symptoms include cough, dyspnoea and chest pain, together with more systemic features, such as myalgia, headache, confusion, nausea, vomiting and diarrhoea. About 10–20% of cases are fatal. At autopsy the lungs are very heavy and consolidated.

In immunosuppressed hosts

When immunosuppression affects a patient, for example in AIDS, the lungs are prone to disease by unusual organisms that are non-pathogenic in non-immunosuppressed individuals; these are known as 'opportunistic' infections. In any immunosuppressed patient, the onset of fever, shortness of breath and cough, together with pulmonary infiltrates, is an ominous event.

Common offending 'opportunistic' agents include:

- *Pneumocystis carinii*
- other fungi, e.g. *Candida, Aspergillus*
- viruses, e.g. cytomegalovirus, measles.

Pneumocystis carinii

Alveoli are filled with a bubbly pink exudate. Round or crescent-shaped organisms are seen using a silver impregnation stain (Ch. 9). There may also be diffuse alveolar damage.

Fungi

Both *Candida* and *Aspergillus* species can cause widespread areas of necrosis (Fig. 14.10). Micro-abscesses contain the characteristic fungal filaments (hyphae; Fig. 14.11).

Viruses

Viral infection may produce diffuse alveolar damage. Characteristic intranuclear inclusions are seen with infections by cytomegalovirus (CMV). Measles pneumonitis produces widespread giant pneumocytes with squamous metaplasia of bronchi and bronchioles.

Non-infective pneumonias

Aspiration pneumonia

Aspiration pneumonia occurs when fluid or food is aspirated into the lung, resulting in consolidation and secondary inflammation. Clinical situations where patients are at risk include sedation, operations, coma, stupor, laryngeal carcinoma and severe debility. The parts of the lung affected vary according to the patient's posture: lying on the back, the affected area is the apical segment of the lower lobe; lying on the right side, the posterior segment of the upper lobe is affected. Often, such areas of aspiration pneumonia contain anaerobic organisms, and a lung abscess containing foul material may ensue.

Lipid pneumonia

Lipid pneumonia may be endogenous, associated with airway obstruction causing distal collections of foamy macrophages and giant cells. This is often seen distal to bronchial carcinoma or an inhaled foreign body. Alternatively, lipid pneumonia may be exogenous, due to aspiration of material containing a high concentration of lipid. Such materials include liquid paraffin or oily nose drops. Vacuoles of lipid are ingested by foreign-body giant cells; there may be some interstitial fibrosis.

Eosinophilic pneumonia

Eosinophilic pneumonia is characterised by numer-

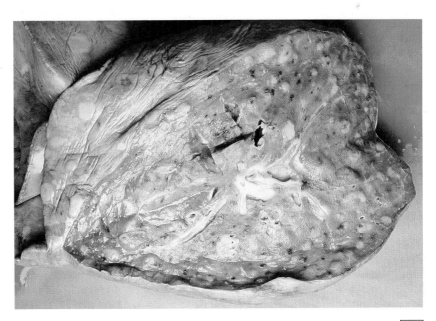

Fig. 14.10 Aspergillus pneumonia

Lung at autopsy showing focal yellow areas of consolidation.

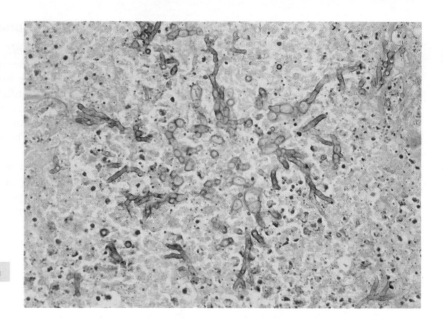

Fig. 14.11 Fungal pneumonia
Numerous fungal hyphae infiltrate
necrotic lung tissue (PAS stain).

ous eosinophils in the interstitium and alveoli. There may be plugging of proximal airways by mucus, as in asthma, or by aspergilli, as in bronchopulmonary aspergillosis. Recurrent bronchial inflammation can lead to destruction of the wall with replacement by granulation tissue and giant cells; this is *bronchocentric granulomatosis*. In addition, eosinophilic pneumonia may be seen when microfilaria migrate through the pulmonary circulation. It may also be idiopathic, associated with blood eosinophilia in Löffler's syndrome.

Pulmonary tuberculosis

> ▶ Lung is commonest site for tuberculosis
> ▶ Chronic alcoholism, diabetes mellitus,
>   immunosuppression, etc. are predisposing
>   conditions
> ▶ Often reactivation of primary or secondary lesion
> ▶ A major cause of death in the developing countries

Pulmonary tuberculosis (TB) is a major cause of death globally, even though there has been a dramatic fall in such deaths in the United Kingdom. The reasons for this enormous decrease are not entirely clear, but probably involve socio-economic factors such as better nutrition, better housing, and a decrease in overcrowding. The advent of successful antituberculous treatment and immunisation using BCG (bacille Calmette–Guérin) has also been of great significance in the campaign against this dis-

ease. TB is, however, the principal cause of HIV-related death in, for example, Africa and the Far East.

Clinicopathological features

Clinical and pathological features of pulmonary tuberculosis are extremely variable, and depend on the extent, stage and activity of the disease (Fig. 14.12). Symptoms may vary from insidious weight loss with night sweats and a mild chronic cough, to rampant bronchopneumonia with fever, dyspnoea and respiratory distress ('galloping consumption'). Most early cases of primary tuberculosis are clinically silent.

Primary tuberculosis
The lungs are usually the initial site of contact between tubercle bacilli and man. The focus of primary infection, which is usually asymptomatic, is called a Ghon complex. The pulmonary lesion is usually about 10 mm in diameter, and consists of a central zone of caseous necrosis surrounded by palisaded epithelioid histiocytes, the occasional Langhans' giant cell, and lymphocytes. Similar granulomas are seen in lymph nodes that drain the affected portion of the lung.

In almost all cases, a primary lesion will organise, leaving a fibrocalcific nodule in the lung, and there will be no clinical sequelae. However, tubercle bacilli may still be present within such scarred foci and may persist as viable organisms for years. In a few

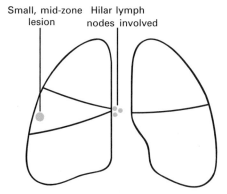

Small, mid-zone lesion   Hilar lymph nodes involved

A. Primary TB

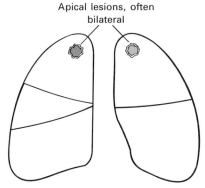

Apical lesions, often bilateral

B. Secondary TB

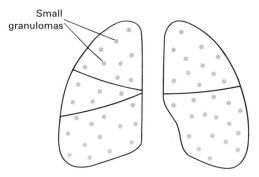

Small granulomas

C. Miliary TB

Fig. 14.12   Types of pulmonary tuberculosis

A. Primary TB produces a small mid-zone lesion with involvement of hilar lymph nodes. **B.** In secondary TB, the lesions are usually apical and often bilateral. **C.** In miliary TB, the lungs and many other organs contain numerous small granulomas.

cases, complications may occur, especially if the individual is immunocompromised.

Secondary tuberculosis
As indicated above, most secondary TB represents

reactivation of old primary infection. These lesions are nearly always located in the lung apices, sometimes bilaterally, and are about 30 mm in diameter at clinical presentation (Fig. 14.13). Histologically, typical granulomas are seen, most having central zones of caseous necrosis (Ch. 10). Progression of the disease depends on the balance between host sensitivity and organism virulence. Most lesions are converted to fibrocalcific scars, a frequent finding in the lungs of elderly people at autopsy. However, as in primary TB, many complications can ensue.

Miliary tuberculosis
Miliary TB may be a consequence of either primary or secondary TB in which there is severe impairment of host resistance. The disease becomes widely disseminated, resulting in numerous small granulomas in many organs. Lesions are commonly found in the lungs, meninges, kidneys, bone marrow and liver, but no organ is exempt. The granulomas often contain numerous mycobacteria, and the Mantoux test is frequently negative (see below). This is an acute medical emergency necessitating prompt treatment with antituberculous chemotherapy if a fatal outcome is to be averted.

Host resistance to tuberculosis and the tuberculin (Mantoux or Heaf) test

A delicate balance exists between the properties of

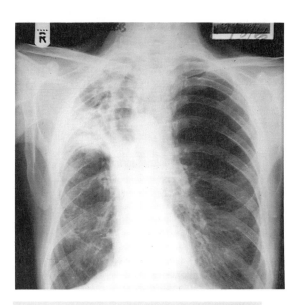

Fig. 14.13   Secondary pulmonary tuberculosis

Chest X-ray showing cavitation and scarring at the apex of the right upper lobe.

the tubercle bacillus and host (man's) resistance. Tuberculosis is the classical infective example of the type IV delayed hypersensitivity reaction (Ch. 9). Killing is mediated by cytotoxic T-lymphocytes, with recruitment of macrophages responding to the secretion of cytokines, such as migration inhibiting factor (MIF), and subsequent macrophage arming. This process takes time; sensitivity to tubercle bacilli becomes detectable only about 2–4 weeks after inoculation. At this time, a challenge with tubercle bacillus antigen (the *Mantoux, Heaf* or *tuberculin test*) will give a positive reaction. Antigenicity and virulence are probably related to the lipid properties of the bacillus cell wall; hence hypersensitivity can usually be induced by immunisation with BCG, a vaccine made from non-virulent tubercle bacilli.

It follows that, in a primary infection, there is no specific hypersensitivity to tubercle bacilli and the inflammatory reaction is relatively mild with little caseous necrosis. In secondary tuberculosis, sensi-

tised T-cells recognise the new threat and, mediated by lymphokines, recruit macrophages to form large granulomas; caseous tissue necrosis is extensive. The disease becomes disseminated when resistance becomes lowered (Fig. 14.14). Nevertheless, even when host resistance is strong, tubercle bacilli remain extremely difficult to eradicate, and may survive and replicate within the same macrophages recruited as their executioners.

VASCULAR DISEASE OF THE LUNGS

Vascular disease of the lungs may be caused by:

- damage to vessel walls, e.g. arteritis
- obstruction, e.g. emboli
- variations in intravascular pressure, e.g. pulmonary arterial or venous hypertension.

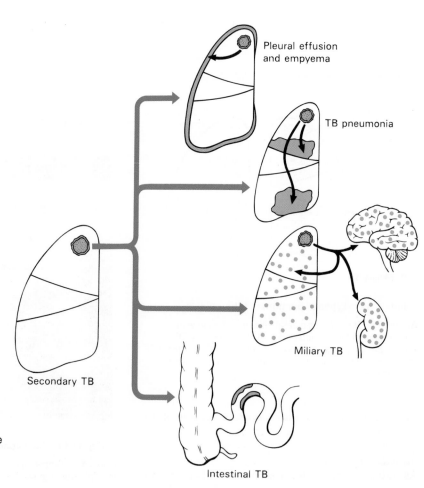

Pleural effusion and empyema

TB pneumonia

Miliary TB

Secondary TB

Intestinal TB

Fig. 14.14 Complications of pulmonary tuberculosis

The most frequent complications are intrapulmonary or pleural spread. Miliary dissemination and intestinal disease are less common.

Damage to vessel walls

> ▶ Arteritis with ischaemia and local necrosis, e.g. Wegener's granulomatosis, Churg–Strauss syndrome
> ▶ Goodpasture's syndrome with anti-glomerular basement membrane antibody

Diseases of the lungs due to vessel wall damage are uncommon. Most are thought to be immunologically mediated, e.g. *Goodpasture's syndrome*; in this disease circulating anti-glomerular basement membrane antibody (Ch. 21) binds to the cross-reacting antigens on the pulmonary basement membrane leading to pulmonary haemorrhage. *Wegener's granulomatosis* is a necrotising vasculitis affecting the lungs, upper respiratory tract and kidneys, with the formation of a necrotising glomerulonephritis (Ch. 21). The aetiology is unknown. Pulmonary involvement is characterised by large areas of necrosis associated with a necrotising granulomatous vasculitis affecting veins and arterioles. *Churg–Strauss syndrome* (allergic angiitis and granulomatosis) may lead to similar necrotising granulomas in the lungs. There is often a history of bronchial asthma. The kidneys and upper respiratory tract are not involved.

Obstruction

> ▶ Due to thrombus, air, fat, cancer cells, epithelial squames in amniotic fluid
> ▶ Blockage may lead to a pulmonary infarct
> ▶ Multiple emboli can cause pulmonary arterial hypertension
> ▶ Risk factors for thrombo-embolism include immobilisation, pregnancy, oral contraceptives, malignancy (especially pancreatic), cardiac failure, and the post-operative recovery phase

Thrombo-embolism
Thrombo-embolism is the commonest pulmonary vascular lesion. Most emboli are thrombotic, originating in veins (Ch. 8): typical sites are the deep pelvic veins or the deep veins of the calf (Fig. 14.15).

Depending on the size, emboli may lodge in various sites in the pulmonary arterial tree. Symptoms will be related to the volume of lung tissue deprived of blood:

- A saddle embolus at the bifurcation of the left and right pulmonary arteries usually causes sudden death or severe chest pain with dyspnoea and shock. Most patients die within a few hours.

- Occlusion of one main pulmonary artery (Fig. 14.16) also frequently leads to death. Alternatively, there may be severe chest pain and shock, mimicking myocardial infarction.
- Occlusion of a lobar or segmental artery causes chest pain and may lead to distal lung infarction, especially in the presence of raised pulmonary venous pressure, as in left ventricular failure or mitral stenosis.
- Multiple small emboli occluding arterioles result in gradual occlusion of the pulmonary arterial bed; this leads to pulmonary arterial hypertension. The effects are discussed below.

Clearly, prevention of deep vein thrombosis is of major importance. Encouragement of improved venous flow in deep leg veins is effected by early ambulation of patients after operations, the use of tight elastic stockings, and leg exercises. Prophylactic anticoagulation is also used in some high-risk patients. Treatment of a major pulmonary embolus includes fibrinolytic agents and even surgical embolectomy. Such heroic measures must be tempered by the fact that patients with a pulmonary embolus have about a 30% chance of developing further emboli. Some patients experiencing repeated pulmonary embolism have an inherited thrombotic tendency (Ch. 23).

Fat emboli
Fat emboli may occlude pulmonary arterioles, leading to breathlessness and sudden death. Such emboli result from fractures of bones containing fatty marrow, or from massive injury to subcutaneous fat. Globules of lipid enter the torn veins and thereby lead to embolism (Fig. 14.17). Marrow tissue may also be seen within pulmonary vessels.

Air emboli
Air emboli occur occasionally during childbirth or with abortion. Bubbles in the circulation can also occur when dissolved nitrogen comes out of solution, for example in divers during rapid decompression (Caisson disease or 'the bends'). These microemboli can cause tiny infarcts in several organs, including muscle, bone, brain and lung.

Amniotic fluid emboli
Amniotic fluid emboli may occur during delivery or abortion. Flakes of keratin and vernix from fetal skin are seen in pulmonary arterioles.

Tumour emboli
Tumour emboli are, of course, very common; this is

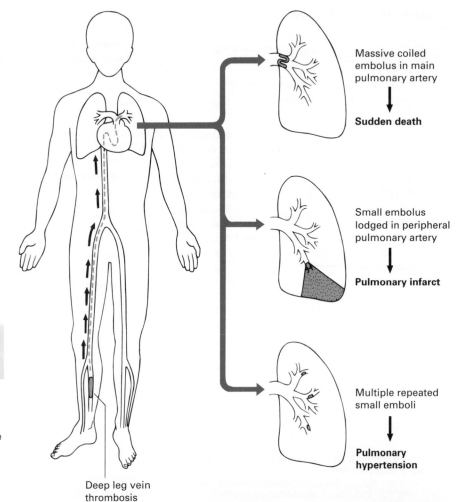

Massive coiled embolus in main pulmonary artery

↓

Sudden death

Small embolus lodged in peripheral pulmonary artery

↓

Pulmonary infarct

Multiple repeated small emboli

↓

Pulmonary hypertension

Deep leg vein thrombosis

**Fig. 14.15
Pathogenesis of pulmonary thrombo-embolism**

The thrombus usually originates from the deep leg veins and, after detachment, becomes lodged in the pulmonary artery vasculature causing sudden death (if massive), pulmonary infarction (if small), or pulmonary hypertension (if small and multiple).

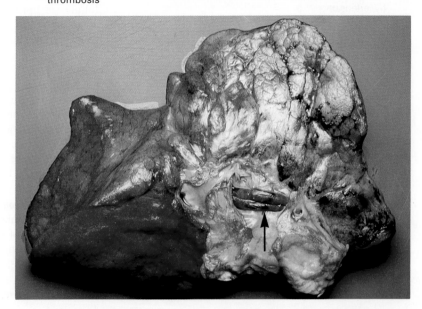

Fig. 14.16   Pulmonary embolism

A massive fatal embolus (arrowed) lodged in a major branch of the pulmonary artery.

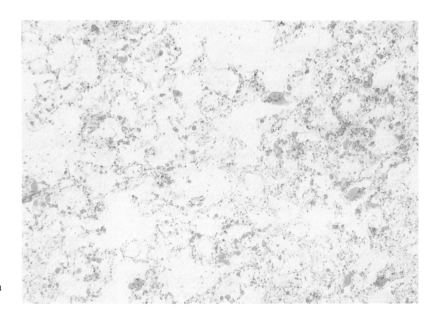

Fig. 14.17   Fat embolism

Lung histology stained to show numerous fat globules (stained orange) in alveolar capillaries from a patient with multiple bone fractures.

an important mechanism in the development of metastases (Ch. 11).

Variations in intravascular pressure

Several disorders are associated with changes in intravascular pressure:

- venous congestion and pulmonary oedema
- pulmonary veno-occlusive disease
- pulmonary hypertension and 'cor pulmonale'
- pulmonary arterial hypertension with a right-to-left shunt.

Venous congestion and pulmonary oedema

Pulmonary oedema can result from:

- increased venous hydrostatic pressure
- injury to the alveolar–capillary wall
- lowered plasma oncotic pressure (a rare cause of pulmonary oedema)
- blockage of lymphatic drainage.

An initial increase in venous hydrostatic pressure leads to pulmonary venous congestion. Common causes are:

- left ventricular failure
- mitral stenosis
- mitral incompetence.

Secondary pulmonary venous hypertension follows, with congestion of alveolar wall capillaries. Fluid is then forced out of the venous circulation into the alveoli to form pulmonary oedema. However, this occurs only after the normal lymphatic drainage capacity has been exceeded; lymphatic flow can increase by about 10-fold before the onset of pulmonary oedema. If lymphatic drainage is blocked, for example by cancer cells, then pulmonary oedema will occur more readily.

The lungs are heavy, congested and wet. Airways contain bubbly fluid. In chronic congestion, recurrent alveolar haemorrhages lead to the accumulation of haemosiderin-laden macrophages (heart-failure cells) with some interstitial fibrosis, so-called 'brown induration of the lung'.

Clinically, there is dyspnoea with a cough, producing bubbly fluid. Auscultation reveals fine crackles in the chest due to air bubbling through numerous fluid-soaked airways. There is respiratory impairment with hypoxaemia. The boggy lungs are prone to secondary infection.

Pulmonary veno-occlusive disease

Pulmonary veno-occlusive disease is rare; it leads to chronic venous congestion with interstitial fibrosis and many haemosiderin-laden macrophages in alveolar spaces. The left heart is normal, and disease is caused by internal thickening and occlusion of pulmonary veins in the septa. The aetiology is largely unknown, although some cases have been reported in association with drugs and radiotherapy. Symptoms are of progressive dyspnoea and 'cor pulmonale'.

Pulmonary hypertension and 'cor pulmonale'

Pulmonary hypertension may be:

- pre-capillary, e.g. pulmonary emboli, left-to-right shunts, primary pulmonary hypertension
- capillary, e.g. fibrosing alveolitis, chronic obstructive airways disease
- post-capillary, e.g. left ventricular failure, mitral stenosis
- chronic hypoxaemia, e.g. Pickwickian syndrome, kyphoscoliosis, poliomyelitis.

All the above mechanisms lead to 'cor pulmonale' or heart failure caused by respiratory disease, which is manifested by pulmonary hypertension and right ventricular hypertrophy.

Pre-capillary pulmonary hypertension may be:

- due to multiple *pulmonary emboli*: numerous tiny emboli block arterioles leading to eventual obliteration of the vascular bed
- due to *left-to-right shunts*, such as cardiac septal defect: blood shunts from the high-pressure left heart to the right heart, causing an increase in its volume and pressure on the pulmonary arterial tree
- primary or of *unknown cause*: this disease tends to affect young women. The cause of primary pulmonary hypertension is uncertain, but may include: ingestion of drugs and toxins (the appetite suppressant, Aminorex, and plant alkaloid, *Crotalaria spectabilis*, are known to cause pulmonary hypertension); overactivity of the sympathetic nervous system leading to vasoconstriction; or 'occult' showers of tiny pulmonary emboli.

Capillary pulmonary hypertension is due to disease in the pulmonary vascular bed. Examples include fibrosing alveolitis, or honeycomb lung from any cause. Severe chronic obstructive airways disease may also cause pulmonary hypertension and 'cor pulmonale'.

Post-capillary pulmonary hypertension is due to high pressure in the pulmonary venous system causing secondary back pressure into the arterial tree. Examples include mitral stenosis, left ventricular failure from any cause, and the rare pulmonary veno-occlusive disease.

Any cause of *chronic hypoxaemia* may lead to pulmonary hypertension, including living at high altitude. The Pickwickian syndrome is characterised by chronic hypoxaemia and pulmonary hypertension caused by poor respiration associated with gross obesity.

Obviously, the gross and microscopic pathology in each instance is determined by the underlying cause.

There are also relatively constant changes seen in the pulmonary arterial tree, including muscular hypertrophy, intimal proliferation, capillary dilatation and necrotising arteritis.

Pulmonary arterial hypertension with right-to-left shunt

In patients with a congenital atrial septal defect (Ch. 13), often asymptomatic, who subsequently develop pulmonary hypertension, the raised right intra-atrial blood pressure causes blood to flow through the defect into the left atrium (right-to-left shunt). This has two important consequences:

- *Paradoxical embolism.* Venous emboli usually impact in the pulmonary arteries. If there is a right-to-left shunt there is a risk of venous emboli bypassing the pulmonary arteries and entering the systemic arterial circulation, thus causing infarcts in the brain, kidneys, spleen, etc.
- *Impaired oxygenation.* Diversion of venous blood through the atrial septal defect from right-to-left causes dilution of the blood in the left atrium with blood that has not been oxygenated by passage through the lungs. This exacerbates the impaired oxygenation that already exists in patients with lung disorders associated with pulmonary hypertension.

OBSTRUCTIVE AIRWAYS DISEASE

Obstructive airways disease falls into two major groups:

- localised
- diffuse.

Localised obstructive airways disease

> ▶ Obstruction by tumour or foreign body
> ▶ Causes distal collapse or over-expansion
> ▶ May be complicated by distal lipid or infective pneumonia
> ▶ Usually normal pulmonary function tests

Localised obstructive airways disease is caused by mechanical factors, for example a foreign body obstructing an airway. The area involved is usually small with little respiratory embarrassment, but tissue damage may occur.

When a bronchus or bronchiole becomes obstructed, the distal lung usually collapses. Numerous lipid-

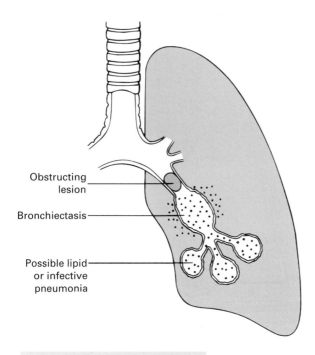

Obstructing lesion

Bronchiectasis

Possible lipid or infective pneumonia

Fig. 14.18   Bronchial obstruction

The obstructing lesion causes a lipid or infective pneumonia in the distal lung and, if unrelieved, distal bronchiectasis.

laden macrophages may fill the alveolar spaces distal to the obstruction with possible secondary infection leading to bronchopneumonia (Fig. 14.18). Bronchiectasis may result if the obstruction is not relieved. Occasionally, the lung distal to an obstruction may become over-expanded, perhaps due to a valve effect caused by the obstruction. The obstruction is usually by a carcinoma or inhaled foreign body.

Clinical symptoms are related to the underlying pathology and to secondary obstructive events. A localised wheeze may be heard over the lesion. Bronchoscopy usually identifies the problem, and the treatment is surgical. Rarely, a foreign body may partially obstruct the trachea; in this situation, there is profound respiratory distress with stridor.

Chronic (diffuse) obstructive airways disease

▶ Reversible and intermittent, or irreversible and persistent
▶ Centred on bronchi and bronchioles
▶ 'Obstructive' pulmonary function tests
▶ Usually many airways involved, therefore a diffuse disease

Chronic (or diffuse) obstructive airways disease is due to reversible or irreversible abnormalities in numerous bronchi and/or bronchioles. There is, therefore, significant respiratory impairment causing chronic airflow limitation and a characteristic obstructive pattern of pulmonary function tests:

- reduced vital capacity (VC)
- reduced FEV_1/VC ratio
- reduced peak expiratory flow rate (PEFR).

The major diseases are:

- chronic bronchitis and emphysema
- asthma
- bronchiectasis.

Chronic bronchitis and emphysema almost always co-exist to some degree. Together they caused over 25 000 deaths in England in 1992, mostly in males. Chronic bronchitis is a *clinical* term defined as chronic cough and sputum for at least 3 months each year for 2 consecutive years. Emphysema is an *anatomical* term defined as permanent enlargement of airspaces distal to the terminal bronchioles, together with destruction of their walls.

Chronic bronchitis

▶ Defined clinically as cough and sputum for 3 months in 2 consecutive years
▶ Mucus hypersecretion with bronchial mucous gland hypertrophy
▶ Respiratory bronchiolitis
▶ Most cases caused by smoking

Aetiology
There is no doubt that chronic bronchitis is almost always entirely due to cigarette smoking. In the United Kingdom, before the Clean Air Act of 1956, urban air pollution was a significant factor. However, the incidence of chronic bronchitis over the last 10 years has remained steady in spite of ever-reducing air pollution; the only change has been a small reduction in male chronic bronchitis, undoubtedly resulting from less cigarette smoking in males.

Clinical factors
Chronic bronchitis typically affects middle-aged men who are heavy smokers. Clinical episodes are associated with recurrent, low-grade bronchial infections caused by bacteria such as *Haemophilus influenzae* and *Streptococcus pneumoniae*, or viruses such as respiratory syncytial virus and adenovirus. Treat-

ment is with antibiotics and physiotherapy and, sometimes, short-term use of oxygen therapy. There may also be a reversible element to the airways obstruction due to local bronchial irritation causing bronchoconstriction; bronchodilators, such as salbutamol, are therefore also used in the treatment of an attack of chronic bronchitis.

In time, the obstructive airways disease becomes progressively more severe and is accompanied by hypercapnia, hypoxaemia and cyanosis. Such patients have been called 'blue bloaters'. 'Pink puffers' are those with more emphysema than bronchial obstruction; they therefore hyperventilate to produce a relatively normal blood gas profile. However, it must be emphasised that most patients have a *mixture* of chronic bronchitis and emphysema, and therefore fall between the above two extremes, showing degrees of hypercapnia, hypoxaemia and hyperventilation. Eventually, right heart failure (cor pulmonale) or respiratory failure ensues.

Morphology

The earliest abnormality in chronic bronchitis is thought to be a respiratory bronchiolitis, affecting airways of less than 2 mm in diameter. This may lead to destruction of the wall and surrounding parenchymal elastin, with the development of centrilobular emphysema. The reduced airway tension and mural weakness, together with mucus plugging, lead to obstructive clinical features. Bronchioles are so numerous that bronchiolar obstruction must be extensive and widespread to give clinical symptoms.

Bronchial abnormalities are mainly mucus hypersecretion with chronic inflammation; these features produce the typical cough and sputum. Irritation and inflammation in the bronchial epithelium can produce squamous metaplasia with loss of ciliated cells. The metaplastic squamous epithelium may become dysplastic from persistent injury by smoking, and may even become malignant (squamous cell carcinoma of bronchus).

Emphysema

> ▶ Defined anatomically as enlargement of alveolar airspaces with destruction of elastin in walls
> ▶ Frequent association with chronic bronchitis

There are various types of emphysema (Fig. 14.19). Although each category has a precise anatomical definition, it must be emphasised that in advanced cases there is usually a *mixed* picture, and an accurate classification in an individual patient is therefore

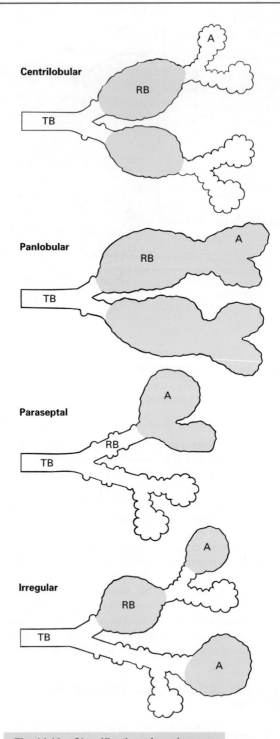

Fig. 14.19 Classification of emphysema

Emphysema is classified according to the pattern of distribution of lesions. These can, to some extent, be correlated with specific aetiological factors, e.g. centrilobular emphysema and cigarette smoke. (TB = terminal bronchiole; RB = respiratory bronchiole; A = alveolus.)

not possible. Suffice to say that all forms of pulmonary emphysema show destruction of distal lung parenchyma (Fig. 14.20).

Centrilobular emphysema

Centrilobular (centriacinar) emphysema involves airspaces in the centre of lobules. This lesion is commonest in men, and is closely associated with cigarette smoking, although mild centrilobular emphysema may be seen in patients with coalworker's pneumoconiosis. The lesions are most common in the upper lobes. As noted above, a respiratory bronchiolitis is also frequently present, together with some large airways disease such as is seen in chronic bronchitis. Dust-laden macrophages and chronic inflammatory cells are often seen in the walls of dilated airways in this type of emphysema. Although the pathogenesis is unknown, it is suggested that respiratory bronchiolitis is the precursor lesion of centrilobular emphysema, with local destruction of airway walls and elastin in adjacent lung parenchyma.

Panlobular emphysema

Panlobular (panacinar) emphysema involves all airspaces distal to the terminal bronchioles. Usually, lower lobes are affected, the bases being most severely involved. Grossly, the lungs appear overdistended and voluminous. The aetiology and pathogenesis of panlobular emphysema is largely unknown. However, 70–80% of patients with α_1-antitrypsin (α_1AT) deficiency in the homozygous state will develop this type of respiratory disease, usually before the age of about 50 years. α_1AT is an acute phase serum protein which inhibits the actions of collagenase, elastase and other proteases, including trypsin. One action of α_1AT is to inhibit enzymes released from dying neutrophils and macrophages. Any stimulus, such as smoking, that leads to increased numbers of inflammatory cells in the lung will lead to alveolar wall destruction (emphysema) in patients with α_1AT deficiency. The enzyme deficiency is inherited as an autosomal dominant trait, and the homozygous deficiency state is said to affect about 1 in 3630 Caucasians; the defect is even rarer in black people.

Paraseptal emphysema

Paraseptal (distal acinar) emphysema involves airspaces at the periphery of the lobules, typically adjacent to pleura. There is often adjacent scarring and fibrosis. The dilated airspaces can become large and, if over 10 mm in diameter, are termed bullous. Upper lobes are more frequently involved.

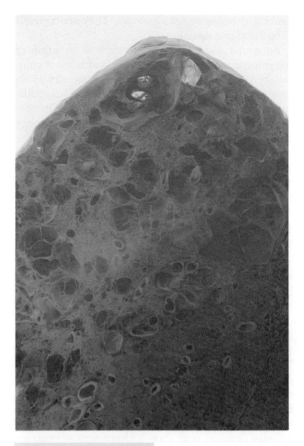

Fig. 14.20 Emphysema

This is severe emphysematous change characterised by large bullae.

Irregular emphysema

Irregular emphysema irregularly involves the respiratory acinus. This type is almost always associated with scarring and there is almost certainly an overlap with paraseptal emphysema. The pathogenesis is thought to be air trapping caused by fibrosis; this irregular pattern of emphysema is therefore commonly present around old healed tuberculous scars at lung apices.

Other pathological types

In addition to the four anatomical types of pulmonary emphysema discussed above, some other categories exist.

Bullous emphysema. This is *not* a separate category of emphysema but refers merely to the presence of balloon-like foci of emphysema over 10 mm in diameter. Cases of emphysema with bullae should, where possible, be classified into one of the four anatomical types discussed above. Bullae are prone to rupture, causing *spontaneous pneumothorax*. They are typically subpleural and apical.

Interstitial emphysema. This refers to inflation of the interstitium of the lung by air, and is most commonly due to traumatic rupture of an airway or spontaneous rupture of an emphysematous bulla. Interstitial emphysema may spread to the mediastinum or subcutis, giving the characteristic spongy crepitus on palpation.

Senile emphysema. This is also a misnomer, as there is no destruction of alveolar walls. Alveolar surface area decreases, and alveolar ductular size increases, progressively after the age of 30 years, leading to the overdistended, apparently voluminous lungs seen at autopsy in aged patients. This process is one of normal senile involution and is not a disease.

Clinical features

About one-third of lung capacity must be destroyed before clinical symptoms of emphysema appear. In cases of 'pure' emphysema without chronic bronchitis, overventilation leads to relatively normal levels of $Pa\text{CO}_2$ and $Pa\text{O}_2$ at rest (so-called 'pink puffers'). The progressive dyspnoea leads to weight loss and right heart failure. Cough and sputum are related to the degree of associated 'chronic bronchitis'. The chest is overinflated and hyper-resonant with loss of the area of cardiac dullness to percussion. Pulmonary function tests show a characteristic obstructive picture with a relatively normal T_{CO}, reflecting the presence of normal alveolar–capillary walls in the remaining lung parenchyma.

In typical cases of 'chronic bronchitis and emphysema', recurrent pulmonary infections are associated with increased dyspnoea and purulent sputum. If respiratory failure accompanies an episode of 'chronic bronchitis', short-term oxygen therapy is used. However, there are grave doubts about the benefits of long-term oxygen therapy in the management of severe obstructive airways disease, as patients needing this treatment are unlikely ever to be free from the cumbersome equipment required.

Asthma

> ▶ Increased irritability of bronchi causes bronchospasm
> ▶ Paroxysmal attacks
> ▶ Overdistended lungs
> ▶ Mucus plugs in bronchi
> ▶ Enlarged bronchial mucous glands

Asthma is defined as increased irritability of the bronchial tree with paroxysmal narrowing of the airways, which may reverse spontaneously or after treatment. Asthma is increasingly common in many countries, but it is a relatively rare cause of death.

There are five major clinical categories of asthma:

- atopic
- non-atopic
- aspirin-induced
- occupational
- allergic bronchopulmonary aspergillosis.

Each type has different predisposing factors, and is mediated in different ways. However, the resulting clinical symptoms and pathology are similar to those seen in atopic asthma. Any important differences are outlined below.

Atopic asthma

Atopic asthma is triggered by a variety of environmental agents, including dust, pollens, foods and animal danders, e.g. faecal pellets from housedust mites. There is often a family history of asthma, hay fever or atopic eczema. Patients with atopic asthma may also suffer from atopic disorders such as hay fever or eczema.

Bronchoconstriction is mediated by a type I hypersensitivity reaction (Ch. 9); bronchoconstriction leads to the clinical effects of wheezing, tachypnoea and dyspnoea (Fig. 14.21). Rarely, symptoms persist for days (status asthmaticus) leading to respiratory failure and even death. Release of histamine and slow-reacting substance of anaphylaxis (SRS-A) leads to bronchoconstriction, increased vascular permeability and mucus hypersecretion. Eosinophil chemotactic factor of anaphylaxis (ECF-A) attracts numerous eosinophils to the bronchial walls.

Platelet activating factor (PAF) leads to the aggregation of platelets with the release of further histamine and 5-hydroxytryptamine (5-HT) from their granules. The results of the hypersensitivity reaction are:

- bronchial obstruction with distal overinflation or atelectasis (collapse)
- mucus plugging of bronchi
- bronchial inflammation
- Curschmann's spirals: whorls of shed epithelium within mucus plugs
- Charcot–Leyden crystals: crystals within aggregates of eosinophils
- mucous gland hypertrophy
- bronchial wall smooth muscle hypertrophy
- thickening of bronchial basement membrane.

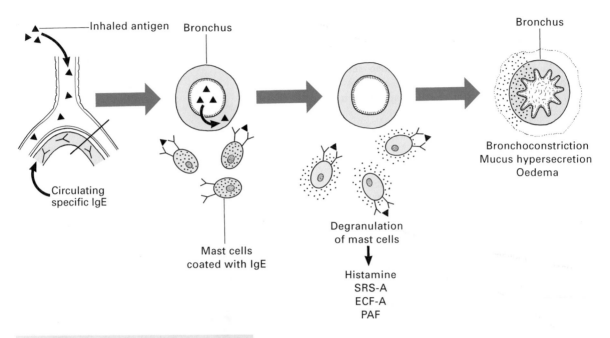

Fig. 14.21   Pathogenesis of allergic asthma

Inhalation of allergen (antigen) causes degranulation of mast cells bearing specific IgE molecules. Release of vasoactive substances from the mast cells causes bronchial constriction, oedema and mucus hypersecretion.

Bronchial inflammation may extend into bronchioles and cause local obstruction, leading to centrilobular emphysema.

Non-atopic asthma
Non-atopic asthma is associated with recurrent respiratory tract infections, especially in chronic bronchitis, and does not appear to be immunologically mediated. Testing for allergens by skin patching is negative. Bronchoconstriction may be due to local irritation in patients with unusually reactive airways.

Aspirin-induced asthma
Patients with this form of asthma may also have recurrent rhinitis with nasal polyps, and skin urticaria. The mechanism of induction of asthma by aspirin is unknown, but may involve locally decreased prostaglandins or increased leukotrienes leading to airway irritability.

Occupational asthma
Occupational asthma is induced by hypersensitivity to an agent inhaled at work. Inhaled agents may act as non-specific stimuli precipitating an asthmatic attack in those with hyper-reactive airways, or they may act as agents capable of inducing asthma and airway hyper-reactivity. There are many different occupationally inhaled agents that can cause asthma. The mechanism of airway reaction is thought to be a combination of type I and type III hypersensitivity (Ch. 9).

In the United Kingdom, if asthma can be proved to be the result of an agent inhaled at work, the patient is entitled to statutory compensation.

Allergic bronchopulmonary aspergillosis
Allergic bronchopulmonary aspergillosis causes asthma and is due to inhalation of spores of the fungus *Aspergillus fumigatus*, inducing an immediate type I and delayed immune complex type III hypersensitivity reaction. Mucus plugs in bronchi contain the hyphae of aspergilli.

Pathogenesis of asthma
As noted above, some forms of asthma are mediated by type I and type III hypersensitivity reactions, yet in others the mechanisms are unknown. One hypothesis that would explain all types of asthma is that patients have bronchial β-receptors relatively insensitive to catecholamines; thus, bronchi are

partially constricted in the non-challenged resting state, and do not dilate well to β-agonists, such as adrenaline. In addition to reacting to specific agents, these hyper-reactive airways also react to non-specific factors, such as cold, exercise and emotional stress. Why this should happen remains unsolved.

Bronchiectasis

> ▶ Results from bronchial obstruction with distal infection and scarring, or severe infection alone
> ▶ Destruction of alveolar walls, especially interstitial elastin, and fibrosis of lung parenchyma
> ▶ Airways then dilate, as surrounding scar tissue (fibrosis) contracts
> ▶ Secondary inflammatory changes lead to further destruction of airways
> ▶ Symptoms are a chronic cough with dyspnoea and production of copious amounts of foul-smelling sputum
> ▶ Complications include pneumonia, lung abscess, emphysema, remote abscesses, amyloid, pulmonary fibrosis and cor pulmonale

Bronchiectasis is characterised by permanent dilatation of bronchi and bronchioles (Fig. 14.22).

Aetiology
Bronchiectasis is almost always associated with bronchial obstruction and severe inflammation. Even in rare congenital abnormalities, such as Kartagener's syndrome (immotile cilia syndrome), the cause of the bronchiectasis is nearly always severe distal inflammation leading to lung fibrosis, then dilatation of airways and damage to their walls.

Clinical features
Usually, the lower lobes are affected, leading to pooling of bronchial secretions with further infection. Symptoms are usually a chronic cough with expectoration of large quantities of foul-smelling sputum, sometimes flecked with blood. Patients may have finger-clubbing. Recurrent respiratory tract infections result from the inability of the patient to clear pooled secretions. Infective processes may remain localised to the bronchi, or spread.

Complications include:

• pneumonia
• empyema
• septicaemia

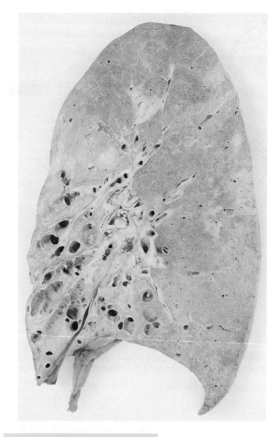

Fig. 14.22 Bronchiectasis
Permanent dilatation of bronchi.

• meningitis
• metastatic abscesses, e.g. in brain
• amyloid formation.

Recurrent infection and inflammation lead to further airway necrosis and destruction of lung tissue. Depending on the extent of disease, cor pulmonale may result. Secondary amyloidosis may occur systemically (Ch. 7).

Morphology
There is dilatation of bronchi and bronchioles, with inflammatory infiltration, especially polymorphs, during acute exacerbations. The inflammation and associated fibrosis extend into the adjacent lung tissue. The dilated bronchi and bronchioles can appear cylindrical, saccular or fusiform; these terms are purely descriptive of the variable morphology and are of no aetiological or prognostic significance.

INTERSTITIAL DISEASES OF THE LUNG

> ▶ Increased tissue in the lung causing increased stiffness and therefore decreased compliance
> ▶ Restrictive lung defect
> ▶ Alveolar–capillary wall is the site of lesion
> ▶ Acute or chronic clinical picture
> ▶ Numerous different causes giving similar ultimate pathology

Interstitial diseases of the lung imply increased amounts of tissue within the lung. Therefore, a chest X-ray will show increased lung density, and the lung will be stiff with reduced compliance. This leads to a restrictive respiratory defect of pulmonary function:

- reduced T_{CO}
- reduced VC
- reduced FEV_1
- relatively normal FEV_1/VC ratio
- relatively normal PEFR.

Diseases may be grouped into acute and chronic categories on the basis of clinical history and histological findings.

Each disorder shows a basic pattern of either acute alveolar injury or chronic pulmonary fibrosis; many diseases also display their own characteristic features, allowing the specific aetiology to be identified.

Acute interstitial diseases

Acute interstitial diseases are characterised by a short history of dyspnoea, tachypnoea and respiratory distress. There is diffuse alveolar damage with alveolar exudation, formation of hyaline membranes and type II pneumocyte hyperplasia. Examples include:

- adult respiratory distress syndrome (ARDS)
- drug and toxin reactions
- radiation pneumonitis
- diffuse intrapulmonary haemorrhage.

Adult respiratory distress syndrome

> ▶ Diffuse alveolar damage with hyaline membranes
> ▶ Many different clinical conditions, all associated with severe injury to alveolar–capillary walls
> ▶ Fatal in 50% of cases
> ▶ Causes acute respiratory distress with tachypnoea, dyspnoea, pulmonary oedema and arterial hypoxaemia refractory to O_2 therapy

Aetiology
Adult respiratory distress syndrome (ARDS) is a medical catastrophe; it can affect people of any age who are victims of:

- shock, e.g. haemorrhagic, cardiogenic, septic, anaphylactic, endotoxic
- trauma, e.g. direct pulmonary trauma, or multisystem trauma
- infections, e.g. viral or bacterial pneumonia
- gas inhalation, e.g. NO_2, SO_2, smoke, Cl_2
- narcotic abuse, e.g. heroin, methadone
- ionising radiation
- gastric aspiration
- disseminated intravascular coagulation
- oxygen toxicity.

ARDS came to prominence during the Vietnam War when it was found that many soldiers were dying of respiratory failure during the first few days of recovery from severe wounds; most had suffered shock from blood loss, but this had been successfully treated by medical officers at the battleground. Clinically, there is respiratory distress with tachypnoea, dyspnoea and hypoxaemia refractory to oxygen therapy.

Pathogenesis
All the clinical situations listed above deliver a massive insult to alveolar–capillary walls, leading to diffuse alveolar damage. In many cases, the exact pathogenesis is unknown; in others, there may be O_2 toxicity, in which damage is thought to be caused by free radicals, such as superoxides and peroxides. Polymorphs are also thought to be important in the pathogenesis, with release of enzymes and activation of complement.

Morphology
In the acute stages the lungs are heavy, oedematous and congested with areas of haemorrhage. Histology shows hyaline membranes lining alveolar ducts and alveoli, together with pulmonary oedema and extravasation of red cells. Resolution occurs via resorption of the oedema, and ingestion of red cells and hyaline ,membranes by alveolar macrophages; there is then regeneration of type II pneumocytes which later differentiate to type I flattened pneumocytes.

Prognosis
About 50% of cases die within the first few days despite intensive therapy. Most of the survivors progress to full recovery with resolution of the inflammation and restoration of the normal alveolar architecture; however, a small number heal by organisation, leading to pulmonary fibrosis.

Drug and toxin reactions

Cytotoxic drugs, such as busulphan and bleomycin, lead to a low-grade alveolitis with healing by interstitial fibrosis and type II pneumocyte hyperplasia; many of the latter have atypical hyperchromatic nuclei with prominent nucleoli. These features are characteristic of lung disease caused by cytotoxic agents.

Paraquat is a potent herbicide acting by release of hydrogen peroxide and the superoxide free radical. It is therefore understandable that ingestion of this toxin leads to diffuse alveolar damage. Pulmonary symptoms occur after about 5–7 days because the drug remains highly concentrated in the lungs for several days after ingestion. Once pulmonary symptoms develop, the condition is rapidly progressive. The pathological findings are very similar to those seen in ARDS, with prominent fibroblastic proliferation in alveolar spaces.

Radiation pneumonitis

The clinical effects of radiation toxicity to the lungs are highly dependent on the dose given (Ch. 6), the volume of lung irradiated and the length of treatment. If heavily exposed, a picture of diffuse alveolar damage is seen. If exposure is less severe and occurs over a longer period, progressive pulmonary fibrosis is seen with the typical restrictive defect of pulmonary function.

Diffuse intrapulmonary haemorrhage

Goodpasture's syndrome is characterised by haemoptysis, haematuria, anaemia and pulmonary infiltrates. Most cases have circulating anti-glomerular basement membrane antibody in their blood. This antibody causes glomerulonephritis, and also acts on alveolar membranes leading to pulmonary haemorrhage.

· *Idiopathic pulmonary haemosiderosis* is a rare condition presenting most often in children. Clinically, patients may present with recurrent episodes of intra-alveolar haemorrhage associated with haemoptysis, cough and dyspnoea; alternatively, they may present with insidious pulmonary fibrosis. The more acute form shows evidence of diffuse alveolar damage, with type II pneumocyte hyperplasia.

Chronic interstitial diseases

Chronic interstitial diseases give a clinical history lasting months or years with slowly increasing respiratory insufficiency, dyspnoea, cough and finger-clubbing. There is interstitial fibrosis, infiltration with lymphocytes and macrophages, and microcyst formation. Examples include:

- fibrosing alveolitis (idiopathic pulmonary fibrosis)
- pneumoconioses
- sarcoidosis
- histiocytosis X
- alveolar lipoproteinosis
- diffuse malignancies
- rheumatoid disease.

Fibrosing alveolitis

> ▶ Progressive chronic pulmonary fibrosis of unknown aetiology
> ▶ Probably arises as a low-grade smouldering 'alveolitis'
> ▶ Progressive dyspnoea and fatigue leading to respiratory failure and/or cor pulmonale
> ▶ Finger- and toe-clubbing
> ▶ Results in end-stage lung fibrosis (honeycomb lung)

Fibrosing alveolitis is a progressive chronic pulmonary fibrosis of unknown aetiology.

Clinical features
Most patients are aged between 45 and 65 years and present with increasing dyspnoea and a dry cough. This progresses to respiratory failure, with or without cor pulmonale, within about 5 years. Fatigue and considerable weight loss may occur, raising the clinical suspicion of malignancy. Examination often shows finger- and toe-clubbing; auscultation of the chest reveals dry crackles, reflecting the opening and closing of fibrotic airspaces. Signs of right ventricular strain or failure may be present.

Pathogenesis
The pathogenesis of fibrosing alveolitis is unknown. Pulmonary function tests give the characteristic restrictive pattern.

Morphology
The lungs show abnormally large and irregular airspaces separated by coarse fibrous septa (honeycomb lung). The subpleural regions of the lower lobes are predominantly affected.

Histology shows interstitial fibrosis with hyperplasia of type II pneumocytes lining airspaces; varying numbers of chronic inflammatory cells are seen. This pattern of histology is known as *usual interstitial pneumonitis*. Alveolar macrophages may be seen in unusually large numbers, with relatively little interstitial fibrosis; this pattern is known as *desquamative interstitial pneumonitis*. Its significance is that some benefit may be gained in treating these patients with corticosteroids. Small airways may be filled with granulation and loose connective tissue, an appearance known as *bronchiolitis obliterans*. It is merely a histological observation and is seen in some other clinical situations, including extrinsic allergic alveolitis, certain viral infections, aspiration pneumonitis and collagen vascular diseases.

Pneumoconioses

> ▶ Lung disease caused by inhaled dusts
> ▶ Dusts may be inorganic (mineral) or organic
> ▶ Reaction may be inert, fibrous, allergic or neoplastic
> ▶ Co-existing disease may aggravate the reaction

When exposed to dust the lung can respond in several ways. Such a reaction may be:

- inert, e.g. simple coal-worker's pneumoconiosis
- fibrous, e.g. progressive massive fibrosis, asbestosis, silicosis
- allergic, e.g. extrinsic allergic alveolitis
- neoplastic, e.g. mesothelioma, lung carcinoma.

The distribution of lung disease depends on the physical properties of each separate type of dust which determine where the particles settle in the lung. Particles of less than 2–3 μm in diameter reach distal alveoli, but larger particles are trapped in the nose or excreted by the mucociliary staircase. Exceptions to this rule are asbestos fibres, some of which may be up to 100 μm long yet can eventually settle in terminal respiratory units. This is because, although very long, asbestos fibres are very thin (about 0.5 μm in diameter).

Dust particles are phagocytosed by alveolar macrophages, which then collect and drain into peribronchiolar lymphatics and thence to hilar lymph nodes. Not surprisingly, lesions caused by dust in the lungs are also often present in the sinuses of hilar lymph nodes. X-ray appearances are related to the degree of associated fibrosis and to the atomic number of the dust involved; for example, tin, with an atomic number of 56, will give a more dense 'abnormal' radiograph than carbon, of atomic number 12, given the same amount of particles inhaled.

Coal-worker's pneumoconiosis
In coal-worker's pneumoconiosis (CWP), coal dust is ingested by alveolar macrophages (dust cells), which then aggregate around bronchioles; the degree

of black pigment in the lung (anthracosis) is related to the amount of inhaled carbon. The consequences of coal-dust inhalation are variable, ranging from trivial to lethal.

Anthracosis is simply the presence of coal-dust pigment in the lung. It is not associated with disability.

Macular CWP consists of focal aggregates of dust-laden macrophages in and around the walls of respiratory bronchioles, pulmonary arterioles and pulmonary veins. Similar cells are seen in lymphatics and hilar lymph nodes. No significant scarring is present, although there is often some local dilatation of respiratory bronchioles representing mild centrilobular emphysema. This may, however, be related to concomitant cigarette smoking, rather than resulting purely from coal-dust inhalation.

Nodular CWP is a progression from the macular stage; nodules less than 10 mm in diameter are seen in a background of more extensive macular CWP. Again, there is no significant scarring and little functional respiratory impairment.

Progressive massive fibrosis (PMF) is represented by large, irregular nodules with scarring (Fig. 14.23); they are greater than 10 mm in diameter and can be massive. These fibrotic black nodules may show central liquefaction and, when cut at autopsy, exude viscid jet-black liquid. They may contract, leading to adjacent irregular emphysema. Large nodules are usually mid-zonal or in upper lobes, and may be bilateral. The associated emphysema is always severe, often with the formation of bullae. Progression of the disease leads to further scarring and lung destruction. Honeycomb lung with respiratory failure, or cor pulmonale, are terminal features.

Caplan's syndrome is characterised by the presence of large pigmented necrobiotic nodules in patients with CWP. This occurs in the presence of severe seropositive rheumatoid disease, although lung nodules may precede the development of systemic features. The nodules may regress.

It is known that in a group of miners working at the same pit for the same length of time, some will develop PMF and die, while others develop little respiratory impairment. The reasons why only some miners develop PMF are unknown. Theories include:

- the amount of concurrently inhaled silica or quartz
- superimposed infection with tubercle bacilli or atypical mycobacteria
- hypersensitivity reactions caused by the death of pulmonary macrophages
- fibrosis mediated by immune complexes.

However, none of these theories is proven, and some

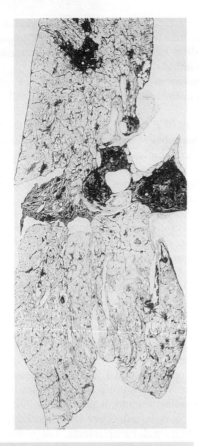

Fig. 14.23 Coal-worker's pneumoconiosis

This transilluminated thin slice of lung shows several large black fibrotic nodules.

investigators believe that the determining factor for development of PMF is merely the amount of coal dust inhaled. Whatever the cause, the progression of CWP to PMF is an ominous event.

Silicosis

Silicates are inorganic minerals abundant in stone and sand. Consequently, any industrial worker involved in the grinding of stone or sand will be at risk from silicosis. Small particles of silica less than 2 μm in diameter enter the terminal respiratory units where they are ingested by alveolar macrophages. However, in contrast to pure coal dust, silicates are toxic to macrophages, leading to their death with release of proteolytic enzymes and the undigested silica particles. The enzymes cause local tissue destruction and subsequent fibrosis; the silica particles are ingested by other macrophages and the cycle repeats itself.

Nodules tend to form in the lungs after many years of exposure. With progressive fibrosis and increasing numbers of nodules, respiratory impairment increases. Pulmonary function tests show a restrictive defect like any other chronic interstitial lung disease. Some patients develop reactivation of tuberculosis.

The lungs show scattered minute nodules of hard, fibrous tissue with surrounding irregular emphysema. Advanced cases show the typical features of end-stage diffuse pulmonary fibrosis, together with numerous silicotic nodules.

Asbestosis

The name 'asbestos' is derived from a Greek word meaning 'inconsumable', and, indeed, asbestos has been used for its fire-resistant qualities for many centuries. Asbestos is used for insulation and the manufacture of brake linings and other friction materials. There are several types of asbestos: amphiboles are the fibres that cause pulmonary disease in man, and of these crocidolite (Cape blue asbestos) is probably the most dangerous.

Asbestos fibres, although 5–100 μm long, are only 0.25–0.5 μm in diameter, and therefore may collect in the alveoli at lung bases. Many become coated in acid mucopolysaccharide and encrusted with haemosiderin to form 'asbestos bodies', appearing as characteristic beaded structures. However, most fibres are detectable only by electron microscopy.

The first symptoms of asbestosis are dyspnoea and a dry cough; finger-clubbing is common. The typical late inspiratory crackles indicate significant diffuse pulmonary fibrosis. Lower lobes are more severely affected. Asbestos bodies in the sputum help to differentiate asbestosis from fibrosing alveolitis. Histology shows the features of pulmonary fibrosis and honeycomb lung, together with asbestos bodies.

Patients with asbestosis may also develop large areas of fibrosis resembling progressive massive fibrosis in coal-miners, but without the coal-dust pigment. These cases have almost all been exposed to significant amounts of silica as well as asbestos.

Extrinsic allergic alveolitis (hypersensitivity pneumonitis)

In pneumoconiosis caused by organic dusts, the disease results from the individual being already sensitised (hypersensitive) to the inhaled antigen. Many antigens can cause allergic lung disease; these include: cotton fibres, causing byssinosis; sugar cane fibres, causing bagassosis; and bird faeces, causing bird fancier's lung.

The best known and most typical example of extrinsic allergic alveolitis is *farmer's lung*. In this disorder, a fungus present in poorly stored, mouldy hay is inhaled by whoever disturbs the hay. If the individual is already sensitised to the organism, a type III immune complex hypersensitivity reaction follows. One of the earliest features is a bronchiolitis. Later, chronic inflammatory cells are seen in the interstitium, together with non-caseating granulomas in airways. These may either resolve on withdrawal of the antigen, or organise leading to pulmonary fibrosis.

Clinically, there is acute dyspnoea and cough a few hours after inhalation of the antigen. Corticosteroid treatment helps to ameliorate the inflammatory reaction and to prevent the onset of pulmonary fibrosis.

Sarcoidosis

Sarcoidosis of the lung is a common cause of interstitial lung disease. The lung is often involved by this disease; only lymph nodes are involved with greater frequency. The typical, non-caseating granulomas are usually found in, or close to, small lymphatics. They then heal by organisation leading to pulmonary fibrosis. Granulomas also occur in the walls of small airways and blood vessels, especially veins. Clinical symptoms are variable depending on the extent of the disease. The aetiology is unknown. A Kveim test, in which the subcutaneous injection of sterile sarcoid tissue homogenate induces granulomas in affected patients, is a useful diagnostic procedure.

Histiocytosis X

Histiocytosis X is a disease caused by the proliferation of Langerhans' cells; these are a specialised type of histiocyte which contain characteristic racquet-shaped cytoplasmic inclusions (Birbeck granules) visible only on electron microscopy. The cause of the disease is unknown. Infiltrates are seen in the pulmonary interstitium, where they may heal by resolution or organise leading to pulmonary fibrosis. Pulmonary histiocytosis X is confined to the lung in 80% of cases. Overall mortality from pulmonary histiocytosis X is 7%. Systemic spread to bone marrow or lymph nodes carries a poorer prognosis.

Alveolar lipoproteinosis

Alveolar lipoproteinosis (or proteinosis) is a rare condition characterised by the accumulation of eosinophilic material within alveoli. It may complicate other interstitial diseases, notably desquamative interstitial pneumonitis, and occur also following acute exposure to high levels of silica dust. However, in most instances the aetiology is unknown and the pathogenesis is uncertain. Symptoms include dyspnoea and cough, when gelatinous material may be expectorated.

Diffuse malignancies

Diffuse malignancies invading the lung may lead to pulmonary fibrosis if a desmoplastic (fibroblastic) response is prominent. *Lymphangitis carcinomatosa* is the spread of tumour throughout the pulmonary lymphatics; a chest X-ray may show diffuse increase in density. Bronchioloalveolar cell carcinomas may spread widely throughout the lungs, possibly through the airways, and lead to diffuse pulmonary involvement.

Rheumatoid disease

It has been estimated that the lung and/or pleura may be affected in 10–15% of patients with rheumatoid disease (Ch. 25). Usually, such patients have severe rheumatoid disease and are seropositive, with vasculitis and subcutaneous nodules. Pulmonary disease may precede the development of systemic features. The lung may show diffuse pulmonary fibrosis, contain rheumatoid nodules and, if coal-worker's pneumoconiosis is also present, show features of Caplan's syndrome. The pleura may be involved and show fibrosis; pleural effusions are also relatively common. Small airways disease is common, showing either a follicular bronchiolitis with lymphoid aggregates and germinal centres around bronchioles, or bronchiolitis obliterans.

LUNG TUMOURS

Lung tumours may be primary or secondary. Both are common.

Primary carcinoma of the lung

> ► Most common primary malignant tumour in Europe and USA
> ► Directly related to cigarette smoking
> ► Associated with occupational exposure to carcinogens
> ► Overall 5-year survival rate of 4–7%
> ► Squamous cell, small cell, adenocarcinoma, and large cell undifferentiated types

Over 90% of primary lung tumours are carcinomas. Lung cancer is one of the commonest human cancers (it is the commonest in the United Kingdom, for example) and has about the worst overall prognosis, with roughly a 5% 5-year survival. This is due to the aggressive natural history of the disease, only about 15% of cases being operable at diagnosis. Another reason for the dismal prognosis is that the only chance of a cure is by complete surgical resection. However, intensive chemotherapy regimes are beginning to show some benefit for patients with small cell lung cancer.

About one-third of all cancer deaths in males in the United Kingdom are due to lung cancer. The disease is also increasing in incidence among women; it now ranks a close second behind breast cancer and may soon have the grim reputation of being the commonest lethal cancer in females in the United Kingdom. Typically, patients are aged between 40 and 70 years; the disease rarely affects those less than 30 years of age.

Aetiology

Major risk factors for the development of lung cancer are:

- cigarette smoking
- occupational hazards, e.g. inhalation of asbestos and other dusts, radioactive gases
- pulmonary fibrosis.

Cigarette smoking
There is now overwhelming evidence implicating cigarette smoking as the major risk factor for the development of lung cancer (Ch. 11). The rise in the incidence of lung cancer over the last century has closely paralleled the increase in cigarette smoking. For example, in 1941 about 5000 deaths occurred from lung cancer in England and Wales; the figure had risen to 35 000 in 1984, falling to 31 500 in 1992. In 1978 male deaths from lung cancer in England and Wales peaked at 26 771; this figure fell slightly to 26 041 in 1984 and fell further to 21 291 in 1992. At the same time the prevalence of cigarette smoking has fallen, and more people are giving up smoking than ever before, the biggest decrease occurring in professional men. The increase in lung cancer in women since World War II is undoubtedly due to more women smoking cigarettes.

There are progressive changes in the bronchial mucosa associated with smoking. Carcinoma is pre-ceded by squamous metaplasia and, subsequently, dysplasia. Squamous metaplastic and dysplastic cells are seen far more commonly in the sputum of smokers than that of non-smokers. The number of shed abnormal cells is also in proportion to the number of cigarettes smoked daily.

Occupational hazards
There are several occupational hazards associated with an increased incidence of lung cancer. The most important are:

- *Asbestos.* There is a significantly increased risk of lung cancer in those exposed occupationally to asbestos. If an individual also smokes, the risk is greatly increased, possibly 20–100-fold. A latent period of about 20 years is usual between exposure and the development of carcinoma. Adenocarcinoma is the most common tumour.
- *Other inhaled dusts.* There is no evidence that lung cancer is associated with coal-worker's pneumoconiosis. However, a significant proportion of haematite miners die from lung cancer.
- *Radioactive gases.* In the 19th century, the Schneeberg mines in Saxony produced rock rich not only in numerous metals but also in radon; many of the workers died from lung cancer. Survivors of the atomic bombs dropped on Japan in 1945 showed an increased incidence of lung cancer, presumably related to radiation.
- *Other factors.* There is an increased risk of lung cancer in workers in industries involved with nickel, chromates, mustard gas, arsenic, and coal-tar distillates.

Fibrosis
Some peripheral lung cancers (usually adenocarcinomas) apparently arise in areas of fibrous scarring, e.g. wounds, old tuberculous foci or infarcts. The theory is that metaplastic and dysplastic changes occur in pneumocytes within the scar. Such ideas have recently been challenged, the so-called 'scar cancers' being considered carcinomas with a pronounced central desmoplastic (fibroblastic) reaction. Despite this argument, there is undoubtedly a significant increase of lung adenocarcinoma in patients with pulmonary fibrosis and honeycomb lung.

Clinical features

Weight loss, cough and haemoptysis are common presenting features. Weight loss is often severe and may be due to humoral factors from the tumour.

Dyspnoea and chest pain are also common; the latter is often pleuritic and due to obstructive changes. Patients may present with, or ultimately develop, metastases; common sites include lymph nodes, bone, brain, liver and adrenals. Paraneoplastic effects are common and are due to ectopic hormones: ACTH and ADH from small cell lung carcinomas, PTH from squamous cell carcinomas. Finger-clubbing and hypertrophic pulmonary osteoarthropathy are common (Fig. 14.24).

Morphology

Most tumours arise from bronchi close to the hilum (Fig. 14.25); usually an upper lobe or main bronchus is involved. Ulceration is common, so the sputum may be bloodstained and contain malignant cells which can be detected cytologically (Fig. 14.26). Distally, the lung may be consolidated with foamy macrophages, the usual result of proximal bronchial obstruction.

Some adenocarcinomas may arise peripherally. Small peripheral tumours are most amenable to

surgery if detected before the development of metastases.

Histological classification

There are four major types of lung cancer, classified according to their appearance on light microscopy (Fig. 14.27); their approximate incidences are:

- squamous cell carcinoma (SqCC): 52%
- small cell lung carcinoma (SCLC) (including oat cell carcinoma) and bronchial carcinoids: 30%
- adenocarcinoma (AC): 13%
- large cell undifferentiated carcinoma (LCUC): 5%.

The lung cancers are discussed below according to this classification, but it should be noted that LCUC probably represents a group of squamous and adenocarcinomas that are too poorly differentiated to categorise as such by light microscopy. In fact, using electron microscopy it can be seen that many SqCC and AC are mixtures, composed of glandular and squamous cells; sometimes, a few cells

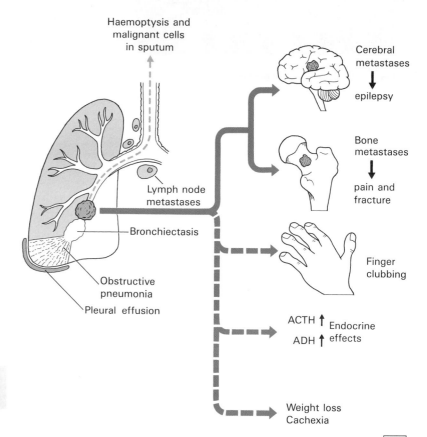

Fig. 14.24 Clinical features and complications of primary lung cancer

See text for details.

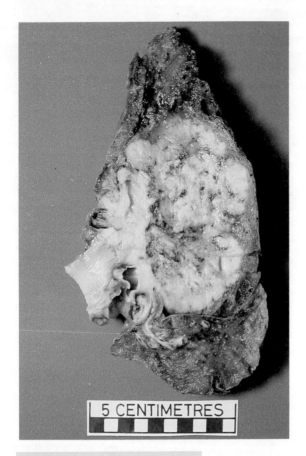

5 CENTIMETRES

Fig. 14.25   Carcinoma of the lung

The tumour is arising at the hilum of the affected lobe and is invading the adjacent lung tissue.

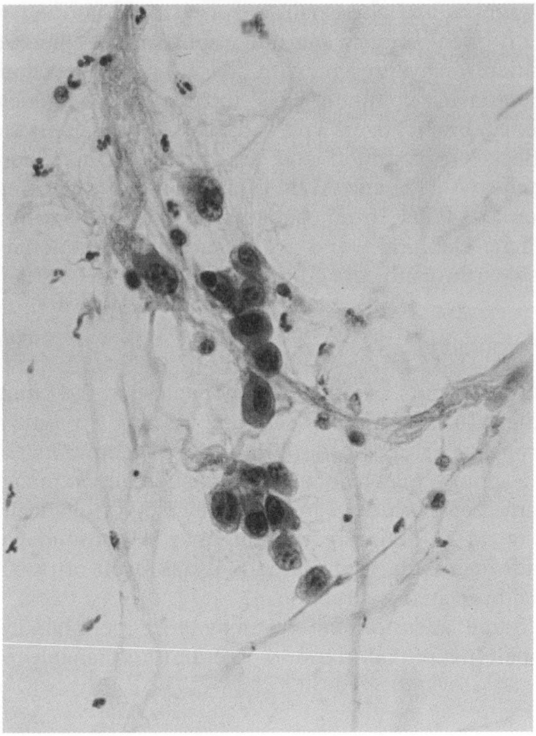

Fig. 14.26   Carcinoma of the lung

Tumour cells found in diagnostic bronchial washings.

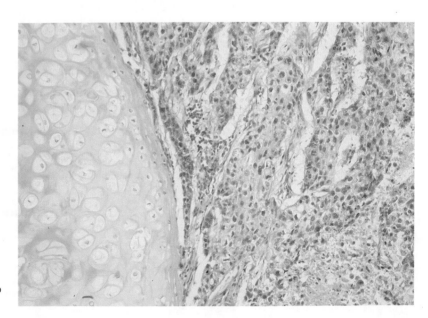

Fig. 14.27   Lung carcinoma

Histology of a poorly differentiated squamous cell carcinoma. Bronchial cartilage (left) is relatively resistant to neoplastic invasion.

with neuro-endocrine granules characteristic of SCLC are also seen. This is not entirely surprising as it is now thought that all lung cancers arise from a primitive stem cell that gives rise to the numerous varied cells seen in the mature respiratory tree.

Squamous cell carcinoma. This is the type of lung cancer most closely associated with cigarette smoking. The tumours are almost always hilar, and are thought to arise from squamous metaplasia through grades of dysplasia. There is often haemorrhage and necrosis with cavitation. Tumours may be well, moderately or poorly differentiated. SqCC tends to metastasise locally to hilar lymph nodes; distant metastases are a later feature.

Small cell lung carcinomas. Also known as 'oat cell' carcinoma because the small nuclei are thought to resemble oat grains, SCLC usually arise in a hilar bronchus. Unlike SqCC, they metastasise very early, producing widespread bulky secondary deposits. Sometimes, the primary tumour can be small and difficult to find. The histology is of a highly cellular tumour composed of small cells with hyperchromatic nuclei and indistinct nucleoli. The cells are very delicate and the chromatin may appear smudged. Electron microscopy shows a few dense core secretory granules in the cytoplasm suggesting that the tumour originates from bronchial endocrine or APUD cells. Similar granules are seen in cells of *bronchial carcinoid* tumours, although in far greater numbers. It is for this reason that SCLC and bronchial carcinoid are thought to represent types of bronchial neuro-endocrine carcinoma; SCLC is aggressive and highly malignant, while bronchial carcinoid is slow-growing and of low-grade malignancy. An intermediate type of bronchial neuro-endocrine carcinoma is also recognised which has some features of SCLC and some of bronchial carcinoid. Bronchial carcinoids are either central or peripheral, and may have a partial capsule. Histologically, they show packets or trabeculae of round cells with bland regular nuclei.

Adenocarcinomas. These are usually peripheral. There is a significant association with diffuse pulmonary fibrosis and honeycomb lung, especially if due to asbestosis. There is a suspicion that AC may arise in discrete areas of scarring such as old infarcts or fibrotic tuberculous foci, but it is also likely that the scar is a product of the adenocarcinoma. Two growth patterns are seen. A discrete nodule in the periphery with pleural tethering is the more common. A few cases, however, show multifocal and bilateral diffuse tumour, so-called *bronchioalveolar cell carcinoma*. In the latter case, the tumour cells creep along alveolar walls. It is not clear whether the multifocal nature of the disease is due to multiple pulmonary tumours or spread by the movement of air or through intrapulmonary lymphatics. Against the latter explanation is the fact that hilar lymph nodes are often uninvolved. Adenocarcinomas arise from glandular cells, such as mucous goblet cells, Clara cells and type II pneumocytes. The histology may, therefore, be of a mucus-secreting AC, forming glands and tubules, or of an AC without significant mucus production.

Large cell undifferentiated carcinomas. Usually central, these are highly aggressive and destructive lesions with necrosis and haemorrhage. Histologically, there is gross nuclear pleomorphism with numerous bizarre mitoses. No squamous or glandular differentiation is seen on light microscopy, although such evidence is often found ultrastructurally.

Staging and treatment

As with all tumours, the stage of the tumour at presentation is of great prognostic significance. The only hope of survival is complete surgical resection, usually only possible with small peripheral tumours without metastases. As previously indicated, SCLC has almost always metastasised at the time of diagnosis and is therefore not amenable to surgery. Combination chemotherapy can induce remission in SCLC, and in a few patients this is sustained.

Other primary tumours

Primary tumours other than carcinomas are rare. They can be classified as:

- benign, e.g. bronchial gland adenomas, benign mesenchymal tumours
- malignant, e.g. sarcomas, adenoid cystic carcinomas, combined tumours, lymphomas.

Benign tumours

Adenomas may arise from bronchial mucous glands. They present as polypoid or sessile lesions in a bronchus. Symptoms are related to obstruction.

Benign mesenchymal tumours may arise anywhere that mesenchyme (connective tissue) occurs. Thus neurofibromas, lipomas, etc., may be found in the lung. More common is the chondroma or adenochondroma; this is probably a hamartoma (Ch. 11). The lesion is hard, white and well circumscribed, and is discovered as an isolated 'coin' lesion on chest X-ray. It is composed of nodules of cartilage with infoldings and clefts lined with bronchial or bronchiolar epithelium.

Malignant tumours

Malignant mesenchymal tumours (sarcomas) are extremely rare.

Primary pulmonary lymphomas are rare tumours presenting as pulmonary disease with or without hilar lymph node involvement, but without clinical evidence of disease elsewhere. They are almost always composed of small B-lymphocytes that may show some plasma cell differentiation (lymphoplasmacytoid cells); monotypic immunoglobulin may be secreted into the blood. These tumours arise from bronchus- and bronchiole-associated lymphoid tissue. Benign reactive lymphoid hyperplasia is the major differential diagnosis; this can be seen with infection, especially in children, or in association with connective tissue disorders, especially rheumatoid disease. Malignant lymphoma of the lung is a slowly progressive disorder leading to respiratory impairment or, eventually, systemic disease.

Lymphomatoid granulomatosis is a rare lymphoma of T-lymphocytes which destroys blood vessels, leading to large cavitating lesions on X-ray. The central nervous system, skin and kidneys are also often involved.

Secondary lung tumours

Secondary lung tumours are more common than primary tumours, although a patient presenting first with a lung tumour is more likely to have a primary. Metastases may arise from blood or lymphatic spread. Usually, discrete nodules are seen scattered throughout both lungs; however, the lymphatics may be diffusely involved, leading to the appearance of *lymphangitis carcinomatosa*. Sarcomas, carcinomas and lymphomas can lead to pulmonary metastases. Carcinomas that commonly give rise to lung secondaries include those from the breast, kidney and gastrointestinal tract.

PLEURA

- ▶ Proteinaceous fluid, blood, lymph or air may form collections
- ▶ Inflammation is common, causing sharp localised chest pain (pleurisy)
- ▶ Pleurisy seen with pneumonia, pulmonary infarction, TB, connective tissue disease, etc.
- ▶ Pleural plaques and mesothelioma are related to asbestos
- ▶ Secondary tumours usually from lung or breast carcinomas

The pleura is composed of connective tissue lined with mesothelial cells forming two apposing surfaces; the *visceral pleura* covers the lungs and the *parietal pleura* covers the thoracic cage wall, diaphragm, heart and mediastinum.

EFFUSIONS AND PNEUMOTHORAX

Various fluids (effusions) and air (pneumothorax) can collect between the two layers of pleura (Table 14.5).

Patients with pleural effusions or pneumothorax suffer shortness of breath and respiratory distress; these symptoms can be relieved by draining the fluid

Table 14.5   Disorders due to collection of fluid and air in the pleural cavities

Disorder	Collection	Causes
Haemothorax	Blood	Chest injury; ruptured aortic aneurysm
Hydrothorax	Low protein fluid (transudate)	Liver failure; Cardiac failure; Renal failure
	High protein fluid (exudate)	Tumours; Infection; Inflammation
Chylothorax	Lymph	Neoplastic obstruction of thoracic lymphatics
Pneumothorax	Air	Spontaneous, following rupture of alveolus or bulla in emphysema or tuberculosis Traumatic, e.g. following penetrating injuries of the chest Spontaneous idiopathic (in young healthy people without pulmonary disease); cause unknown
Pyothorax (empyema)	Pus	Infection

or air from the pleural cavity. Clinically, an effusion is dull to percussion; this is in contrast to a pneumothorax which is hyper-resonant. To investigate the possibility that a pleural effusion might be due to primary or metastatic neoplasia, it is essential to perform a cytological examination of the cells within the fluid.

At autopsy, effusions are usually obvious, but a pneumothorax can be demonstrated only by seeing bubbles of air escaping when the pleural cavity is opened under water.

INFLAMMATORY DISORDERS

Inflammation of the pleura (pleuritis or pleurisy) is common. It can be seen with:

- connective tissue disease: rheumatic fever, rheumatoid disease, systemic lupus erythematosus (SLE)
- infections: any pneumonia, tuberculosis, lung abscess
- pulmonary infarcts
- lung neoplasms.

The inflammation is nearly always accompanied by an effusion. Symptoms are usually of sharp, localised chest pain, worse on breathing. Treatment is of the underlying disorder causing the pleurisy. Depending on the degree of inflammation, pleurisy may resolve or organise to leave an area of fibrosis, sometimes with dystrophic calcification.

Pleural plaques are markers of asbestos exposure. They are asymptomatic patches of thickened fibrotic pleura on the diaphragm and posterior thoracic wall. Histologically, they consist of hyaline acellular connective tissue with a few inflammatory cells at the periphery. *Diffuse pleural fibrosis* and *pleural effusions* may both be related to asbestos exposure in the absence of lung cancer, mesothelioma or asbestosis.

TUMOURS

Benign tumours of the pleura are rare. The *pleural fibroma* consists of fibrous connective tissue and mesothelial cells. It grows as a solitary lump in the pleura, sometimes becoming very large. Hypertrophic pulmonary osteoarthropathy is a frequent association.

Malignant tumours are most often secondary deposits from primary lung adenocarcinomas, breast carcinomas or, less commonly, ovarian carcinomas.

These secondary deposits may grow into the interlobar fissures, thus mimicking a mesothelioma.

Mesothelioma

Primary malignant mesothelioma is strongly associated with occupational exposure to asbestos, especially fibres such as crocidolite ('blue' asbestos) and amosite ('brown' asbestos). These fibres have a diameter of less than $0.25\ \mu$m, even though they may be well over $5.0\ \mu$m long. Other non-asbestos fibres

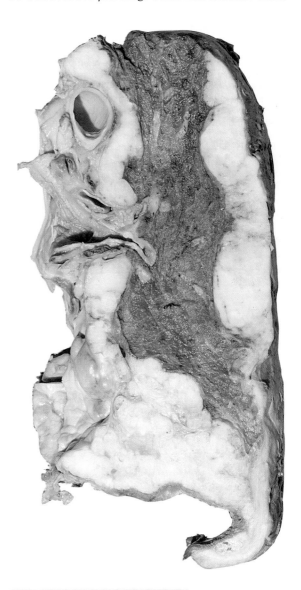

Fig. 14.28 Pleural mesothelioma

The tumour envelops the lung.

of similar diameter, such as volcanic silicate erionite in Turkey, may also cause mesothelioma. The latent interval between exposure and the development of mesothelioma is often about 30 years.

The tumour begins as nodules in the pleura which extend as a confluent sheet to surround the lung and extend into fissures (Fig. 14.28). The chest wall is often invaded, with infiltration of intercostal nerves, giving severe intractable pain. Lymphatics may be invaded, giving hilar node metastases.

Histology is varied; most commonly the appearance is of a mixed epithelial and spindle cell tumour. Rarely, pure epithelial or spindle cell (sarcomatous) mesotheliomas can occur. Special histological techniques are often necessary to distinguish between mesothelioma and adenocarcinoma.

There is no treatment for malignant mesothelioma, and the symptoms of chest pain and dyspnoea become worse until death, usually within two years of diagnosis.

FURTHER READING

Fletcher C M, Pride N B 1984 Definitions of emphysema, chronic bronchitis, asthma and airflow obstruction: 25 years on from the CIBA symposium. Thorax 39: 81–85.

Lamb D 1987 Lung cancer and its classification. In: Anthony P P, MacSween R N M (eds) Recent advances in histopathology 13. Churchill Livingstone, Edinburgh, pp 45–60

Millard P R, Esiri M M 1992 The pathology of AIDS: an update. In: Anthony P P, MacSween R N M (eds) Recent advances in histopathology 15. Churchill Livingstone, Edinburgh, pp 67–92

Seaton A 1983 Coal and the lung. Thorax 38: 241–243

Thurlbeck W M 1988 Pathology of the lung. Thieme-Stratton, New York

Dunnill M S 1987 Pulmonary pathology. Churchill Livingstone, Edinburgh

Alimentary system

The alimentary system is constantly in contact with dietary contaminants, especially infective agents and environmental toxins, so it is not surprising that it is affected by many diseases. This chapter examines these diseases and, in those of major importance, attempts to relate them to the potentially pathogenic factors present in the human diet.

Pathological basis of gastrointestinal signs and symptoms	
Sign or symptom	Pathological basis
Dysphagia (difficulty swallowing)	Impaired neuromuscular function (e.g. multiple sclerosis) Obstruction (intrinsic or extrinsic)
Heartburn (indigestion)	Oesophageal/gastric mucosal irritation, often with inflammation and ulceration
Abdominal pain • visceral • peritoneal	Spasm (colic) of muscular layer in gut wall Irritation or inflammation of peritoneum
Diarrhoea	Excessive secretion or impaired absorption of fluid within lumen of gastrointestinal tract
Steatorrhoea (fatty stools)	Impaired absorption of fat due to reduced lipase secretion or reduced mucosal surface area for absorption
Blood loss • in vomit (haematemesis) • through anus	Ruptured blood vessel in oesophagus (e.g. varices) or stomach (e.g. erosion by ulcer) Ulceration or inflammation of colorectal mucosa, or oozing from surface of a tumour, or ruptured blood vessel (e.g. haemorrhoid, angiodysplasia)
Weight loss	Impaired food intake Malabsorption of food Catabolic state associated with a malignant neoplasm
Anaemia	Blood loss (e.g. tumour, ulcer) or impaired absorption of iron, folate or B_{12} due to mucosal disease

NORMAL STRUCTURE AND FUNCTION

The mouth and teeth masticate the food prior to swallowing and digestion. At the same time digestion is initiated by the addition of salivary amylases and lipases.

The *mouth* is lined by stratified squamous epithelium overlying richly vascular connective tissue. The epithelium is of variable thickness, being thickest over the tongue where there are also papillary projections which account for its rougher texture. The epithelium is mostly non-keratinised, except over the lips, gums and hard palate where slight keratinisation occurs. Elsewhere pathological keratinisation (keratosis) results in the formation of white plaques on the mucosa; this is termed leukoplakia.

The *teeth* consist principally of *dentine* which is similar to bone; it is composed of a collagen matrix mineralised by calcium phosphate (apatite) crystals. It differs from bone, however, in that its cellular constituents (odontoblasts) form a layer over the surface of the dentine, from which long tubular processes ramify through the tissue. The dentine is covered over the exposed part of the tooth (crown) by *enamel*, which is composed almost entirely of inorganic material arranged in stacked crystalline rods. The dentine of the root is covered by a thin layer of *cementum* which, as its name implies, attaches the tooth to the periodontal 'ligament' lining the socket. Centrally, the tooth has a connective tissue core, the *pulp*, which links with the narrow root canal.

The *salivary glands* are usually categorised as either major or minor. The major glands are the parotid, submandibular and sublingual glands; minor glands are scattered throughout the oral cavity. The parotids enclose branches of the facial nerve and a few lymph nodes. The glandular tissue comprises multiple small secretory acini lined by plump cells containing zymogen granules and surrounded by supporting myoepithelial cells. The secretion has a low protein content, hence these glandular units are referred to as *serous* acini. Small ducts lined by cuboidal epithelium drain the glandular lobules and unite to form the main secretory (Stensen's) duct. The submandibular glands contain both serous and mucus-secreting cells in mixed acini; the sublingual and minor salivary glands are predominantly or entirely mucus-secreting. The main ducts of the submandibular glands (Wharton's ducts) are lined by partly ciliated epithelium to facilitate drainage of the more viscid mucous secretion.

CONGENITAL DISORDERS OF THE MOUTH

Hare-lip and cleft palate

Hare-lip may appear as a sporadic defect of development but may also occur as an inherited condition exhibiting male sex linkage. The inherited form occurs both with and without a cleft palate. Where a cleft palate exists alone, a proportion of the cases are due to a dominant gene of low penetrance. Other cases are not genetically determined, as for example in the rubella syndrome (Ch. 5).

Hare-lip may be unilateral or bilateral: it may involve the lip only, or extend upwards and backwards to include the floor of the nose and the alveolar ridge. Cleft palate may vary considerably, from a small defect in the soft palate, which causes little disability, to a complete separation of the hard palate combined with hare-lip. With extensive lesions, there may be considerable difficulty with feeding as the child is unable to suck.

DISEASES OF THE TEETH AND GUMS

While of paramount importance to the dental student, diseases of the mouth, teeth and gums are soon evident to both patient and doctor, and frequently reflect generalised disorders. Their recognition and an understanding of the processes involved is therefore also of wider importance in clinical medicine.

Dental caries

Caries is the result of acid destruction of the calcified components of the teeth (Fig. 15.1). The acid is produced by bacteria, usually specific strains of *Streptococcus mutans*, acting mainly on refined sugar which is trapped in contact with the dentine by 'plaque', a mixture of adhesive sugar residues and bacteria. Penetration of the dentine is followed by bacterial invasion which can infect the pulp, causing *pulpitis*.

Gingivitis

Acute gingivitis (inflammation of the gums) is an

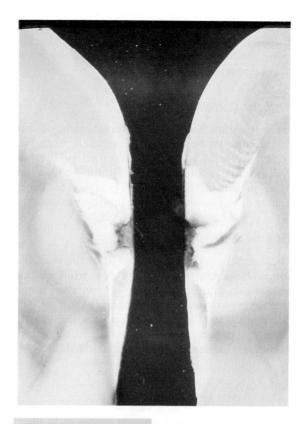

Fig. 15.1 Dental caries

Longitudinal sections of adjacent teeth showing characteristic erosion of enamel and dentine. (Courtesy of Professor C J Smith, Sheffield)

uncommon infection caused by the anaerobic *Borrelia vincentii* and fusiform bacilli. It is a severe ulcerative disease, formerly referred to as Vincent's infection, which can spread widely along the gum margins and deeply to destroy bone.

Chronic gingivitis, by contrast, is a very common condition which represents the response of the gum to adjacent bacterial plaque. Proliferation of anaerobic bacteria, and possibly their production of proteolytic enzymes, leads to chronic periodontitis and gradual destruction of the supporting tissues of the teeth. This results in loosening and eventual loss of teeth.

DISEASES OF THE ORAL MUCOSA

Inflammatory disorders

The oral mucous membrane is affected in a wide variety of mucocutaneous inflammatory disorders such as acute erythema multiforme, lichen planus, Behçet's syndrome and many others. However, some conditions (discussed below) are restricted to the oral mucosa.

Herpetic stomatitis

Herpetic stomatitis is a very common manifestation of infection by herpes simplex virus. It is characterised by vesiculation and ulceration of the oral mucosa and is usually acquired during childhood. Many patients develop recurrences in later life which appear as similar lesions on the lips (herpes labialis).

Oral candidiasis

Oral candidiasis (thrush), is caused by the yeast-like fungus *Candida albicans*. It appears as white plaques on the oral mucosa consisting of enmeshed fungal hyphae, which invade the epithelium, together with polymorphs and fibrin. The infection is seen in neonates, in patients receiving broad-spectrum antibiotics and in immunocompromised individuals.

Aphthous stomatitis

Aphthous stomatitis is a very common disorder in which single or, more usually, multiple small ulcers appear in the oral mucosa. They are shallow, with a grey, necrotic base and a haemorrhagic rim. Many patients suffer from recurrent crops of ulcers which heal spontaneously after several days. The aetiology is unknown but assumed to be immunological; some patients have an associated gastrointestinal disorder, such as coeliac disease or inflammatory bowel disease.

Reparative lesions

The oral mucosa is frequently subjected to minor trauma. In some individuals the reparative processes that follow prove excessive, and the surplus fibrovascular tissue appears as a polyp. Such a reparative lesion in the mouth is termed an *epulis*, of which 'congenital' and giant cell forms are recognised. There is also a similar angiomatous 'tumour' of pregnancy, and many of the so-called haemangiomas and fibromas of the mouth have the same histogenesis.

Leukoplakia

Leukoplakia is a clinical term used to describe patches of keratosis. Its importance is that it can be premalignant. Thus, in leukoplakia there is hyperkeratosis and hyperplasia of the squamous epithelium with, in some cases, dysplastic changes which herald the onset of malignant change.

In the UK and USA leukoplakia is associated with heavy cigarette smoking, excessive alcohol consumption and poor dental hygiene. The high incidence in India and Sri Lanka is attributed to the habit of chewing betel quids made up of tobacco dust, areca nut and lime wrapped up in a betel leaf.

Tumours

Cancer of the lip is more common than intra-oral cancers. It occurs mainly in elderly people and has a definite relationship to sunlight exposure. Thus it is much more common on the lower than the upper lip. Lip cancers are usually well-differentiated squamous carcinomas which spread directly into surrounding tissues, and through lymphatics to the regional nodes.

Intra-oral cancers most frequently affect the tongue and commonly develop in areas of leukoplakia (Fig. 15.2). Like lip cancers, they are squamous carcinomas. Initially they are painless and can remain undetected, especially if situated on the posterior third of the tongue, until fixation and swelling interfere with swallowing and speech. This tendency towards late presentation and towards spread to vital structures underlies the poorer prognosis of cancer of the tongue compared to that of cancer of the lip.

DISEASES OF THE PHARYNX

Pharyngitis

Viral pharyngitis
The commonest cause of pharyngitis is viral infection, but the causative virus is rarely identified. Most cases are thought to be caused by adenoviruses, but other viral infections, notably those directed at the respiratory tract, can be responsible. Patients with these infections either start with a pharyngitis or develop it during the illness. Thus pharyngitis is a common feature of the common cold, influenza, measles and infectious mononucleosis (glandular fever).

Streptococcal pharyngitis
Although less common than viral infections, streptococcal pharyngitis is important for its complications. In non-immune individuals a widespread skin rash (scarlet fever) develops and occasional

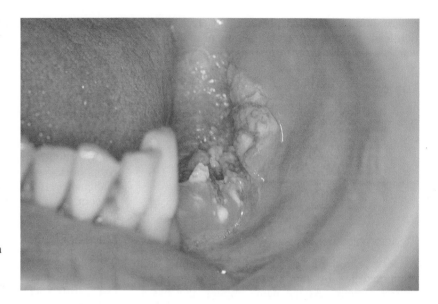

Fig. 15.2 Oral cancer

Ulcerated squamous cell carcinoma arising from buccal mucosa. (Courtesy of Mr P McAndrew, Rotherham)

patients will develop acute proliferative glomerulonephritis, rheumatic fever or Henoch–Schönlein purpura.

Ulcerative pharyngitis

An ulcerative pharyngitis and tonsillitis is a common complication of agranulocytosis (deficiency of polymorphs) due to a leukaemia or marrow failure. Diphtheria was formerly an important cause of an ulcerative pharyngitis, but has now been largely eradicated in many countries by immunisation.

Tonsillitis

The faucial tonsils are collections of lymphoid tissue covered by non-keratinising squamous epithelium thrown into a series of clefts; these can harbour debris and act as a nidus for infection. The tonsils are thus a frequent site for bacterial infection, producing either an acute inflammation or, more frequently, recurring chronic inflammation leading to tonsillar enlargement and general debility.

Tumours

The pharynx can be the site of both squamous carcinoma and intermediate or 'transitional' cell carcinomas that exhibit features of epithelium transitional between squamous and columnar, respiratory-type epithelium. However, most carcinomas in this site are anaplastic (undifferentiated). In addition, the tonsils may be involved by lymphomas.

Nasopharyngeal carcinoma is of interest because of the wide geographical variation in its incidence. It is an uncommon carcinoma in Caucasians (less than 1%), but in some parts of China accounts for over 50% of all malignant disease. A causative agent has not been identified, but patients with nasopharyngeal carcinomas have higher titres of antibody to Epstein–Barr (EB) virus than age-matched controls, and parts of the EB viral genome can be detected in the carcinoma tissue. Genetic factors also appear to be involved; the susceptible Chinese show a higher frequency of the histocompatibility haplotypes HLA-A2 and -BW46 than other populations.

DISEASES OF THE SALIVARY GLANDS

Sialadenitis

Acute bacterial sialadenitis (inflammation of the salivary glands) is uncommon. It arises by ascending infection from the mouth and occurs in patients with abnormal dryness of the mouth (xerostomia) either as part of a generalised dehydration or as a result of an autoimmune induced atrophy of the salivary glands (*Sjögren's syndrome*). Acute enlargement of the salivary glands is usually due to mumps virus infection.

Recurrent sialadenitis is seen in patients who have some degree of duct obstruction, hyposecretion of saliva and ascending infection. Duct obstruction can be due to a stone (calculus) or to fibrosis. Hyposecretion may be a direct consequence of duct obstruction but may also be due to the acinar atrophy resulting from sialadenitis itself. Bacterial infection leads to recurrent acute inflammation and also acts as a nidus for stone formation.

Tumours

> ▶ Pleomorphic adenoma: a benign, mixed tumour
> ▶ Warthin's tumour (adenolymphoma): a benign tumour
> ▶ Muco-epidermoid tumour: both benign and malignant forms exist
> ▶ Adenoid cystic carcinoma: has a tendency for perineural invasion

Pleomorphic adenoma

At least two-thirds of all salivary tumours are accounted for by the pleomorphic adenoma or 'mixed tumour'. As the name implies, this has a varied histological appearance and is composed of a mixture of stromal and epithelial elements (Fig. 15.3). The myxoid stroma, which is rich in proteoglycans, is thought to be produced by myoepithelial cells; thus, despite its biphasic appearance, it is a purely epithelial neoplasm. Occasionally the stroma has a cartilaginous appearance. Pleomorphic adenomas are essentially benign tumours but are prone to local recurrence if surgical removal is incomplete. The facial nerve is vulnerable during attempts at surgical removal. A very small proportion undergo malignant change and are capable of metastasising; these are termed *malignant mixed tumours*. Occasional tumours are composed entirely of ductular epithelial cells arranged in a tubular pattern and are referred to as *monomorphic adenomas*.

Warthin's tumour

Warthin's tumour or adenolymphoma is a relatively common salivary gland tumour (5–10% of total). It has a very characteristic appearance: tall columnar epithelial cells line convoluted cystic spaces separated by a dense lymphoid stroma. The term adenolymphoma, with its connotations of lymphoid malignancy, is a misnomer; this is an entirely benign tumour.

Muco-epidermoid tumour

True adenocarcinomas of the salivary gland do exist, but the malignant epithelial tumours are usually 'special' forms such as the muco-epidermoid tumour which consists of mucus-secreting cells, cells showing squamous differentiation and intermediate cells (small cells that are probable precursors of the mucus-secreting and squamous cells). Malignancy is associated with an increasing proportion of intermediate and squamous cells with fewer mucous cells.

Adenoid cystic carcinoma

Adenoid cystic carcinoma is a distinctive malignancy composed of small epithelial cells arranged in islands showing microcystic change. This tumour has a propensity for perineural spread and is particularly difficult to eradicate surgically.

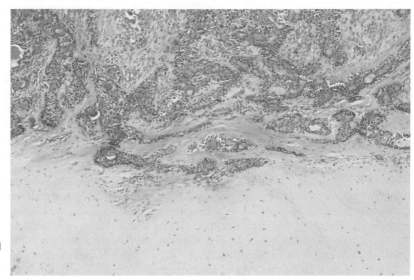

Fig. 15.3 Pleomorphic salivary adenoma

These benign neoplasms consist of a mixture of proliferating epithelium and mucinous connective tissue resembling cartilage.

OESOPHAGUS

NORMAL STRUCTURE AND FUNCTION

The oesophagus is a muscular tube lined mostly by squamous epithelium. It extends from the pharynx to the cardia of the stomach and is about 25 cm long in the adult. At the upper end there is the *cricopharyngeal sphincter*; close to the lower end there is a functional sphincter whose position can be determined only by manometry. The upper sphincter contains striated muscle fibres enabling voluntary control over the initiation of swallowing, whereas the remainder of the muscular tube is composed of smooth muscle which propels the food bolus by peristalsis and is under autonomic control. Entry of food into the stomach is facilitated by relaxation of the distal sphincter. Protection of the lower oesophagus against regurgitation of gastric contents is achieved by the distal sphincter assisted by constricting muscle bands in the diaphragm, and an acute valve-like angle of entry into the stomach. The distal 1.5–2 cm of the oesophagus is situated below the diaphragm and is lined by columnar mucosa of cardiac type. The squamo-columnar junction is clearly visible on endoscopy and is usually found at about 40 cm (measured from the incisor teeth). Proximal extension of this junction is found in hiatus hernia or when there is columnar metaplasia.

The squamous lining of the oesophagus consists of a layer of non-keratinising squamous epithelium overlying connective tissue papillae containing blood vessels and lymphatics. A narrow layer 1–2 cells thick at the base of the epithelium forms the proliferative compartment from where cells migrate upwards, mature and desquamate at the surface (Fig. 15.4). These cells acquire an increasing glycogen content as they mature. Scattered argyrophil cells and melanoblasts can also be found in the basal layer.

CONGENITAL AND MECHANICAL DISORDERS

Heterotopic tissue

Patches of fundic-type gastric mucosa are occasionally found above the distal sphincter and separated from the columnar lining of the distal oesophagus. These are assumed to be congenitally misplaced (heterotopic) gastric tissue rather than an acquired change; they can lead to ulceration and stricturing due to local acid/pepsin secretion.

Atresia

Atresia is a failure of embryological canalisation. It is more frequent than agenesis of the oesophagus, which is extremely rare. Atresia is usually associated with an abnormal connection (fistula) between the patent part of the oesophagus and the trachea. The affected child cannot swallow and develops an aspiration bronchopneumonia.

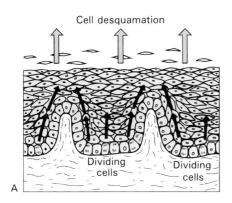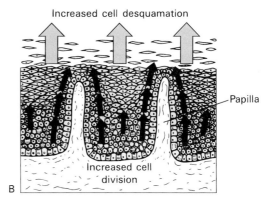

Fig. 15.4   Basal cell hyperplasia in reflux oesophagitis

A. Normal cell proliferation and migration. **B.** In reflux oesophagitis, increased proliferation to compensate for increased cell desquamation results in basal zone hyperplasia and elongation of connective tissue papillae.

Diverticula

Diverticula are outpouchings of the wall of a hollow viscus. Some represent a saccular dilatation of the full thickness of the wall; others are formed by herniation of mucosa through a defect in the muscle coat. Diverticula are more common in the pharynx but can develop in the oesophagus by either *traction* (external forces pulling on the wall) or *pulsion* (forcible distension). These diverticula differ from congenital forms in lacking a muscle coat in their wall. They frequently become permanently distended with retained food and cause difficulties in swallowing (dysphagia).

Hiatus hernia

The commonest mechanical disorder of the oesophagus is hiatus hernia, defined as the presence of part of the stomach above the diaphragmatic orifice. It was formerly believed that this could arise from congenital shortening of the oesophagus, but it is now thought that most, if not all, hiatus hernias are acquired. The herniation of the stomach with subsequent retraction of the oesophagus is largely a consequence of increased intra-abdominal pressure and loss of diaphragmatic muscular tone with ageing. The consequent incompetence of the oesophageal sphincter leads to regurgitation and oesophagitis.

Achalasia

Achalasia is an uncommon condition in which the contractility of the lower oesophagus is lost and there is a failure of relaxation at the sphincter (cardiospasm).

Normal functioning of the oesophagus is dependent upon the integrity of its co-ordinated muscular activity, which in turn relies on normal neuronal transmission of peristaltic signals. Thus dysphagia may arise from fibrosis and atrophy of the smooth muscle, as occurs in progressive systemic sclerosis, or by destruction or degeneration of the intrinsic nerves. The latter can occur in neurotropic infections such as Chagas' disease (South American trypanosomiasis), or by unknown mechanisms as in the condition of achalasia. Achalasia results in slowing or retention of the food bolus with increasing obstruction and dilatation of the oesophagus. The cause of this condition is unknown, but there are reduced numbers of ganglion cells in the myenteric plexus, and both myelinated and unmyelinated axons of the extra-oesophageal vagus nerves show Wallerian degeneration (Ch. 26).

Oesophageal varices

Varices are localised dilatations of veins. The veins of the lower oesophagus are a potential site for porto-systemic shunting of blood when portal venous flow through the liver is impaired. Therefore, in portal hypertension (most commonly resulting from cirrhosis of the liver) the submucosal veins of the oesophagus become congested and dilate (Ch. 16). These enlarged veins elevate the mucosa and protrude into the oesophageal lumen where they are easily traumatised by the passage of food. Haemorrhage is thus a frequent complication and, because of the relatively high pressure within the vascular bed, can be torrential and fatal.

INFLAMMATORY DISORDERS

Oesophagitis

Acute oesophagitis
Acute oesophagitis is clinically of only minor importance. Spread of bacterial infection from the nasopharynx to involve the oesophagus is a rare occurrence. More important are viral and fungal infections in immunocompromised individuals; for example, herpes simplex and cytomegalovirus infections are occasionally encountered in patients with leukaemias, lymphomas or AIDS. *Candidiasis* is a more common infection which may give rise to difficulties in swallowing; it is endoscopically recognisable as white plaques with haemorrhagic margins. Candidiasis is also opportunistic in immunodeficiency states and in diabetes mellitus, but can sometimes be found in otherwise healthy individuals. A further cause of acute inflammation and ulceration is the ingestion of *corrosive substances*; this may be either accidental (as when children swallow chemicals from unlabelled bottles) or taken with suicidal intent.

Chronic oesophagitis
As with chronic inflammation in any site, chronic oesophagitis may be either specific or non-specific. Specific causes are rare, but involvement by tuberculosis and Crohn's disease are recognised. Non-specific oesophagitis is very common and usually results from regurgitation of gastric contents into the lower oesophagus; this is *reflux oesophagitis*.

Reflux oesophagitis

The squamous lining of the oesophagus is easily

damaged by regurgitated gastric contents and soon becomes chronically inflamed. A defective sphincter mechanism at the cardia predisposes to such gastro-oesophageal reflux, which is therefore an invariable accompaniment of hiatus hernia. It may also be a consequence of increased intra-abdominal pressure without herniation, or of gastric surgery. Other patients appear to have an underlying abnormality of upper gastro-intestinal motility which leads to gastro-oesophageal reflux and/or duodeno-gastric reflux. The characteristic symptom is an awareness of acid regurgitation with central chest pain or discomfort ('heartburn').

Morphology
Exposure of the squamous mucosa to refluxed acid (together with bile in patients with entero-gastric reflux) leads to cell injury and accelerated desquamation. The increased cell loss is compensated for by increased proliferation of the germinative cells of the epithelium (basal cell hyperplasia; see Fig. 15.4); this results in less mature cells occupying most of the epithelial thickness and is accompanied by elongation of the connective tissue papillae. Such elongation permits extension of the basal layer and possibly reflects an interaction between the proliferating epithelial cells and underlying mesenchyme. The epithelial injury is accompanied by a low-grade inflammatory cell response so that, in general, relatively small numbers of polymorphs (including eosinophils) and lymphocytes are seen within the epithelium and in the underlying connective tissue. Thus the response to reflux embraces both:

- an epithelial reaction — basal cell hyperplasia and elongation of papillae
- a conventional chronic inflammatory cell reaction.

Unfortunately, there is a poor correlation between the histological findings in biopsy specimens, the endoscopic appearances, symptomatology, and objective tests of reflux. However, the finding of typical histological changes in a patient who has no endoscopic evidence of reflux can be useful in management.

Where reflux is severe, cell proliferation cannot keep pace with cell desquamation and ulceration occurs. These areas of ulceration can be the source of haemorrhage, and may even perforate in the most severe cases. Healing is achieved by fibrosis and epithelial regeneration; subsequent shrinkage of fibrous tissue can produce a segmental narrowing (*stricture*) in the area of healed ulceration.

Restoration of epithelial continuity is usually achieved by proliferation of squamous cells, but in some patients the lost squamous epithelium is replaced by columnar epithelium, giving rise to a condition known as 'Barrett's oesophagus' (see below).

BARRETT'S OESOPHAGUS

As a result of longstanding reflux, the lower oesophagus comes to be lined by columnar mucosa, an appearance referred to as Barrett's oesophagus. Opinions vary as to whether this is due to epithelial 'subsitution' — migration of columnar epithelium from the distal two centimetres or from the ducts of submucosal mucous glands — or to an effect on the differentiation of progeny cells from a common stem cell (metaplasia).

Three kinds of columnar mucosa may be seen in a Barrett's oesophagus:

- a *junctional type* resembling normal gastric cardia
- an *atrophic fundal type* containing scanty specialised gastric secretory cells
- a *'specialised' mucosa* in which the epithelium is undergoing a further metaplastic change towards an intestinal type and has acquired goblet cells.

Barrett's oesophagus has assumed increasing clinical importance in recent years following its recognition as a premalignant condition. Although cancer is not common in absolute terms, the risk of malignancy is about 100 times higher among patients with Barrett's oesophagus than in the general population. Thus, once the condition has been diagnosed, it is advisable to put the patient on regular endoscopic surveillance and take multiple biopsies for the detection of dysplasia.

TUMOURS

Benign tumours

Benign tumours are uncommon and comprise about 5% of all neoplasms of the oesophagus; the type most frequently encountered is a *leiomyoma*. The behaviour of smooth muscle tumours in the alimentary tract is generally difficult to predict (see below) but those arising in the oesophagus are almost invariably benign. Other benign non-epithelial tumours — lipomas, haemangiomas and fibromas — are rare. The only benign epithelial tumour of note is *squamous papilloma*. Compared with squamous carcinoma (see below) these are rare lesions, certainly in terms of clinical presentation, but are of interest because they are likely to share a common pathogenesis with other squamous papillomas in that they result from human papillomavirus (HPV) infection.

Carcinoma

> ▶ Wide geographic variation in incidence
> ▶ Links with environmental factors
> ▶ Two main types: squamous carcinoma and adenocarcinoma
> ▶ Most adenocarcinomas arise from metaplastic columnar epithelium (Barrett's oesophagus)

Carcinoma of the oesophagus accounts for about 2% of all forms of malignant disease in the United Kingdom. However, the incidence shows a remarkable degree of geographic variation and in some countries is much higher than in the UK. For example, the incidence in north-eastern Iran around the Caspian Sea is more than 300 times that found in low-incidence countries such as the UK and USA.

Aetiology and pathogenesis
Epidemiological studies in high-incidence areas have indicated that a high dietary intake of tannic acid, in the form of strong tea or sorghum wheat, or dietary deficiencies of riboflavin, vitamin A and possibly zinc may be important, but other factors such as fungal contamination of foodstuffs, opium usage and thermal injury may also be involved. In Western countries, cigarette smoking and the drinking of alcoholic spirits are associated with a higher incidence.

A factor of current interest is the possible involvement of HPV. Some oesophageal cancers contain HPV in their cells, and viruses of similar subtype can be found in intact and apparently normal oesophageal mucosa. It is therefore possible that virus integrated into the host genome can bring about oncogene activation and carcinogenesis. The involvement of papillomaviruses in the development of bovine oesophageal carcinoma is well established.

Non-specific chronic oesophagitis is common among the general population in high-incidence areas, and biopsies will frequently reveal dysplasia. The squamous epithelium shows cellular pleomorphism: there is disordered maturation with immature cells and mitotic activity appearing close to the surface. The degree of atypia can be categorised as low- or high-grade dysplasia; the latter condition will proceed to invasive carcinoma if surgical resection is not performed. As in the oropharynx, dysplasia is sometimes associated with abnormal keratosis of the squamous mucosa which appears to the endoscopist as an area of leukoplakia.

Histological types
Most carcinomas of the oesophagus are of *squamous* type, although in the lower third of the oesophagus *adenocarcinomas* are the predominant type. These have almost invariably developed on the basis of a Barrett's oesophagus and have risen dramatically in incidence among white, middle-aged men in European countries and the USA in recent years.

Squamous carcinoma (Fig. 15.5) usually commences as an ulcer, but spreads to become annular and constricting so that the patient develops dysphagia. Most patients present with difficulty in swallowing, by which time direct spread to adjacent organs has occurred and the surgical resection rate is only about 40%. Thus a majority of patients can be treated only by radiotherapy, or palliatively by laser therapy. Many receive symptomatic treatment and are simply intubated to facilitate adequate nutrition. The long-term outlook is therefore very poor, with only a 5% survival at five years. Most patients die of local disease and bronchopneumonia exacerbated by malnutrition. Unlike many forms of cancer, metastases are rarely found at autopsy.

Other tumours

Other rare malignant tumours arising in the oesophagus include malignant melanoma (from the melanocytes which are present in very small numbers in normal mucosa), small cell anaplastic (oat cell) carcinoma, mixed adeno-squamous carcinomas and sarcomas.

STOMACH

NORMAL STRUCTURE AND FUNCTION

The stomach acts essentially as a 'mixing' reservoir for food during acid-pepsin digestion. Hydrochloric acid and pepsin are, however, only two of many products of the gastric mucosa.

Histologically, the stomach can be divided into three regions—the *cardia*, *body* and *antrum*. The surface of the gastric mucosa and its pits (*foveolae*), are lined throughout by columnar mucus-secreting epithelium. The mucus secreted by these cells,

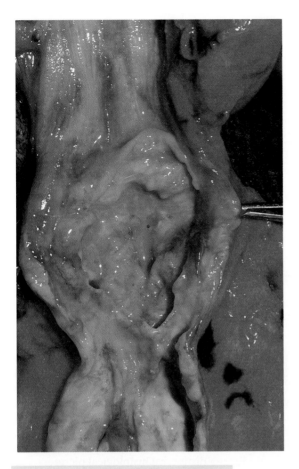

Fig. 15.5   Carcinoma of the oesophagus

The tumour partly obstructs the oesophageal lumen and has an ulcerated surface from which blood loss can lead to anaemia. (Courtesy of Professor L Henry, Sheffield)

together with contributions from the antral mucous glands, forms a viscid gel covering the mucosa — the *gastric mucus barrier* (Fig. 15.6). Bicarbonate and sodium ions, also secreted by surface epithelial cells, diffuse into the unstirred gel and buffer the hydrogen ions entering from the luminal aspect. A pH gradient is thus established, ranging from 1 or 2 at the luminal surface of the barrier, to neutrality at the plasma membrane of the epithelium.

The glandular component varies from region to region.

The *cardiac (or junctional) mucosa* is a narrow zone immediately below the termination of the oesophagus; it comprises simple tubular or cystic glands lined by mucus-secreting cells in which numerous endocrine cells and a few parietal (acid) and chief (pepsinogen) cells are scattered.

Body mucosa lines the proximal two-thirds of the stomach and consists of tightly-packed tubular glands, the upper parts of which are lined by parietal cells and the lower parts by chief cells (Fig. 15.7A). In addition to acid, the parietal cells secrete intrinsic factor, essential for vitamin B_{12} absorption. Other cells present in body mucosa are mucous neck cells and endocrine cells. The neck cells are found at the bases of the gastric pits, i.e. at the junction between foveolar lining cells and glandular cells, and contain the stem cells of the mucosa together with some immature foveolar cells. The majority of the endocrine cells are so-called enterochromaffin-like (ECL) cells (p. 445) which are readily identifiable by silver staining (argyrophil) techniques. These cells mediate parietal cell activity by releasing histamine in response to stimulatory hormones such as gastrin.

Antral (or pyloric) mucosa occupies a roughly triangular region proximal to the pylorus with its base about one-third of the distance along the lesser curvature, and its apex a few centimetres from the pylorus on the greater curve. The antral glands are more branched, tortuous and less tightly packed than those in the body (Fig. 15.7B). The glands are lined by mucus-secreting cells with faintly granular cytoplasm and basal nuclei, together with endocrine cells and scattered parietal cells. The endocrine cells of the antrum produce several hormones: G cells secreting gastrin are the most numerous, but others include D cells (which secrete somatostatin), EC cells (5-hydroxytryptamine, 5-HT), P cells (bombesin) and S cells (secretin).

CONGENITAL DISORDERS

Congenital abnormalities, apart from hypertrophic pyloric stenosis, are rare. They include accessory structures lined by gastric mucosa, which are referred to as 'cysts' when saccular and not communicating with the gastric lumen, 'duplications' if tubular and non-communicating and 'diverticula' if they communicate.

Diaphragmatic hernia

Maldevelopment of the diaphragm can lead to defects though which the stomach, together with parts of the intestine and the spleen, herniate into the left thoracic cavity. Usually only part of the stomach is dislocated into the thorax, but after birth it may become expanded by swallowed air and can rapidly cause death from respiratory failure.

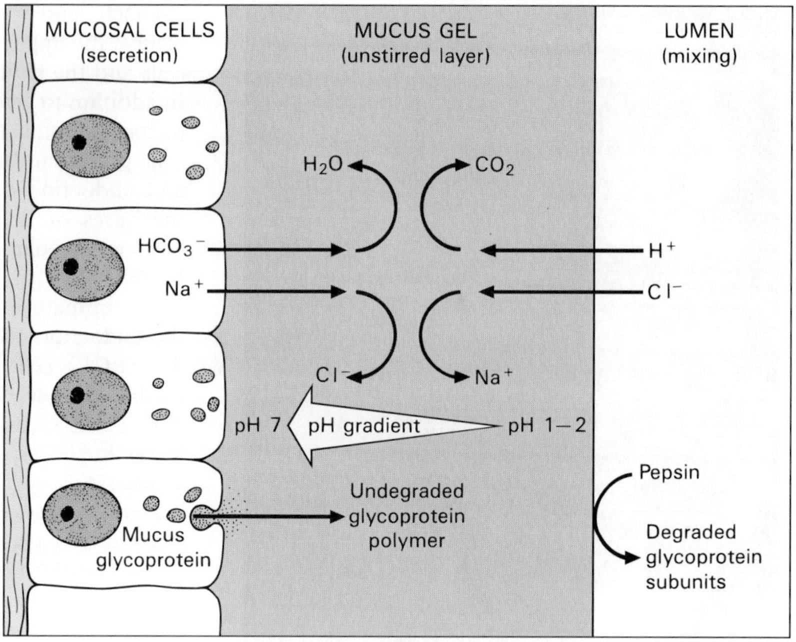

Fig. 15.6 The gastric mucus barrier

The surface epithelial cells (supplemented by foveolar and glandular mucous cells) secrete viscid mucus which forms an unstirred layer between the epithelium and the gastric lumen. The surface cells also secrete sodium and bicarbonate ions into the mucus gel and a pH gradient is established. This constitutes the major defence against acid attack.

Pyloric stenosis

An abnormal hypertrophy of the circular muscle coat at the pylorus can lead to outflow obstruction from the stomach. The condition, found in approximately 4 per 1000 live births, usually presents with projectile vomiting. It is four to five times more common in males than females.

INFLAMMATORY DISORDERS

▶ Acute gastritis is commonly due to chemical injury (e.g. alcohol, drugs)
▶ Commonest form of chronic gastritis results from *Helicobacter pylori* infection
▶ Chronic gastritis can also result from an autoimmune process, often causing vitamin B$_{12}$ deficiency
▶ Chemical (reactive) gastritis is caused by biliary regurgitation or drug-induced damage

Inflammation of the stomach, as with other organs, is usually considered as either acute (often described as 'haemorrhagic' or 'erosive') or chronic gastritis. Until recently chronic gastritis was a rather nebulous condition, ill-defined in pathogenetic terms and poorly correlated with endoscopic findings and symptomatology. One form (type A) has long been recognised as an autoimmune disorder, but this type is uncommon; the generality of chronic gastritis (type B) has been attributed to non-specific irritants, whether exogenous (e.g. hot drinks and spices) or endogenous (e.g. bile reflux). However, it is now recognised that type B gastritis is a response to bacterial infection, and that reflux of bile into the stomach produces a distinctive histological picture.

Acute gastritis

Acute gastritis is almost invariably an acute response to an irritant 'chemical' injury by drugs or alcohol. The principal drugs involved are non-steroidal anti-inflammatory drugs (NSAIDs), notably aspirin, but many others have been implicated. These agents cause a prompt exfoliation of surface epithelial cells and diminished secretion of mucus such that the protective barrier against acid attack (see below) may be compromised. Many of their effects are probably mediated by an inhibition of prostaglandin synthesis.

Depending on the severity of the injury, the mucosal response varies from vasodilatation and oedema of the lamina propria, to erosion and haemorrhage. An erosion is an area of partial loss of the mucosa, as opposed to an ulcer where the full thickness, i.e. below the muscularis mucosae, is lost. The erosions in acute gastritis are frequently multiple and the resultant haemorrhage can be severe and life-threatening. Fortunately the lesions are transient and heal rapidly

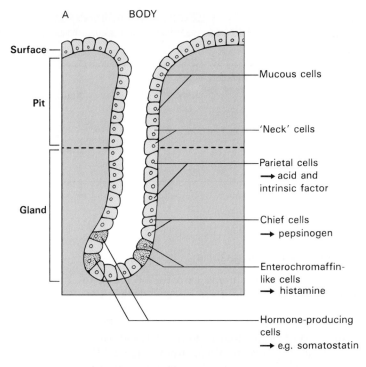

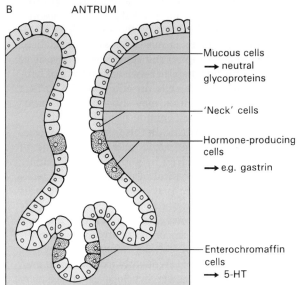

Fig. 15.7 Structure of the gastric mucosa

A. Body (corpus) mucosa where the tubular glands contain specialised secretory cells. The 'neck' cells represent the proliferative compartment of the gastric pit from where the majority of cells migrate upwards to replenish exfoliated surface cells, and a minority move downwards to replace glandular cells.
B. Antral mucosa, predominantly composed of mucus-secreting cells but with scattered endocrine cells.

by regeneration, so that erosions may well have disappeared 24–48 h after the bleeding episode.

An acute neutrophilic gastritis (i.e. one in which polymorph infiltration is a dominant feature) is characteristic of the initial response to *Helicobacter pylori* infection. Acute *Helicobacter* gastritis is a transient phase which in the majority of individuals is subclinical and over the course of 3–4 weeks gives way to chronic gastritis. In a minority of individuals the infection is spontaneously eradicated and the inflammatory response resolves. The pathological features of acute bacterial gastritis are summarised in Table 15.1.

Table 15.1 Pathological features of *Helicobacter*-associated gastritis

Pathological feature	Classification	
Surface epithelial degeneration Regenerative hyperplasia of pit-lining epithelium Vasodilatation/congestion Neutrophil polymorph response	**Acute gastritis**	'Active' chronic gastritis
Lymphocyte and plasma cell response Glandular atrophy Lamina propria fibrosis Intestinal metaplasia	**Chronic gastritis**	

Chronic gastritis

Autoimmune chronic gastritis

A few patients with chronic gastritis are found to have antibodies in their serum directed against gastric parietal cells and intrinsic factor binding sites. These patients exhibit varying degrees of hypochlorhydria (they are often achlorhydric), and have a macrocytic anaemia resulting from vitamin B_{12} deficiency; this association of autoimmune gastritis with macrocytic anaemia is called *pernicious anaemia*.

Histologically, the body of the stomach is maximally affected: there is marked loss of specialised cells (glandular atrophy) and replacement fibrosis of the lamina propria, together with an infiltrate of lymphocytes and plasma cells. In addition, the surface and pit-lining epithelium may show *intestinal metaplasia* (IM), a change common to all forms of long-standing chronic gastritis. In this form of metaplasia, the neutral, mucin-secreting cells characteristic of the stomach are replaced by goblet cells containing acidic glycoproteins typical of the intestine. In well-developed cases there may also be absorptive cells and Paneth cells. Intestinal metaplasia is generally regarded as a premalignant condition, because patients with gastric cancer frequently exhibit intestinal metaplasia elsewhere in the stomach and because the cancers themselves frequently exhibit 'intestinal' features. However, cancer develops in only a very small proportion of patients with IM, and the possession of intestinal features by a cancer does not necessarily imply origin from intestinalised epithelial cells. On the contrary, it is likely that metaplasia is in fact an adaptive response, whereby alteration in a cell's environment inhibits differentiation along the usual pathway in favour of a route which results in the production of 'different', but fully mature, end-cells which are generally better equipped to survive in the adverse environment. Thus, intestinal metaplasia pos-

sibly constitutes a defence response and its association with gastric cancer may represent an epiphenomenon.

Helicobacter-associated chronic gastritis

The cause of the most common form of chronic gastritis is bacterial infection by *Helicobacter pylori*. This is a Gram-negative organism that inhabits a peculiarly protected niche closely applied to the surface epithelium beneath the mucous barrier where the pH approaches neutrality (Fig. 15.8). The organism is not simply a commensal, as it attacks the surface cells, causes accelerated cell desquamation and leads to a polymorph and chronic inflammatory cell response in the gastric mucosa. *H. pylori* is found in over 90% of biopsies showing active chronic (type B) gastritis but is uncommon in type A disease. Interestingly, the organism is found only on gastric epithelium and does not colonise duodenal mucosa or cause intestinal metaplasia.

The acute inflammatory response provoked by *H. pylori* is mediated by complement components which are liberated through activation of the alternative pathway and are chemotactic for polymorphs (Ch. 9) together with low molecular weight chemotactic factors shed by the bacteria and interleukin-8 secreted by epithelial cells, macrophages and endothelial cells. The polymorphs subsequently release proteases and reactive oxygen metabolites which may be responsible for the glandular destruction (resulting in atrophy) which characterises the established disease. In addition, anti-*H. pylori* IgA, IgG and IgM antibodies are produced locally by plasma cells in the lamina propria; these have a role in the prevention of bacterial adhesion and in opsonisation but fail to eliminate the infection.

Histologically, *Helicobacter*-associated gastritis affects the entire stomach but to a variable degree. The majority of patients exhibit diffuse involvement

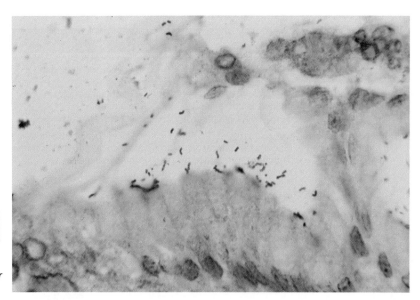

Fig. 15.8 Gastritis associated with *Helicobacter pylori*

High power histology of a gastric biopsy specially stained to reveal numerous minute curved *Helicobacter* adherent to the mucosal surface.

of the antrum and body with the gradual acquisition over time of glandular atrophy, replacement fibrosis and intestinal metaplasia. Patients with this distribution of gastritis are at an increased risk of gastric ulcer and carcinoma than uninfected individuals. A second main pattern is where the antrum is markedly inflamed but with little involvement of body mucosa. These individuals exhibit an increased acid output and are at greater risk of duodenal ulcer. The histological features of acute and chronic gastritis are summarised in Table 15.1.

Chemical (reflux) gastritis

The presence of regurgitated bile and alkaline duodenal juice in the stomach provokes epithelial desquamation, compensatory hyperplasia of the proliferative compartment in the gastric foveolae, and vasodilatation and oedema of the lamina propria; this is reflux gastritis. In 'normal' people there is little or no regurgitation of duodenal contents into the stomach. Reflux gastritis is seen in the post-operative stomach following operations which destroy or bypass the pylorus, as a result of secondary motility disturbances in patients with gallstones and after cholecystectomy, and in some patients who appear to have a disturbance of antro-duodenal motility or co-ordination. Unoperated patients with bile reflux appear to have a failure in pyloric competence resulting from a disturbance in pyloro-antral motor function; this may be either a primary disturbance, or a defective response to hormones, such as cholecystokinin and secretin, which normally increase pyloric

tone during duodenal acidification. The ensuing reflux gastritis stimulates production of gastrin by the antral mucosa; this may also block the effects of cholecystokinin and secretin on the pyloric muscles.

Reflux gastritis may present with bilious vomiting or less severe dyspeptic symptoms; repeated damage to the mucosa may lead to the development of a gastric ulcer.

A similar histological picture to that found with bile reflux can result from long-term usage of non-steroidal anti-inflammatory drugs (NSAIDs); the common denominator is repeated chemical injury. The various types of chronic gastritis are compared in Table 15.2.

Other forms of gastritis

Less common forms of chronic gastritis have been distinguished from the three major types discussed above.

In *lymphocytic gastritis* the main histological feature is the presence of numerous mature lymphocytes within the surface epithelium. This form is occasionally seen in patients who have peculiarly heaped-up erosions running along prominent rugal folds. The aetiology, and its precise relationship to *H. pylori* gastritis, is unknown.

Eosinophilic gastritis is characterised by oedema and a large number of eosinophils in the inflammatory cell infiltrate. It is thought to be an allergic response to a dietary antigen to which the patient has become sensitised.

Granulomatous gastritis is a rare form of gastritis in

Table 15.2 Types of chronic gastritis

Aetiology	Pathogenic mechanisms	Histological findings	Clinical consequences
Autoimmune	Anti-parietal cell and anti-intrinsic factor antibodies Sensitised T-lymphocytes	Glandular atrophy in body mucosa Intestinal metaplasia	Pernicious anaemia
Bacterial infection (*H. pylori*)	Cytotoxins Mucolytic enzymes ?Ammonia production by bacterial urease Tissue damage by immune response	Active chronic inflammation Multifocal atrophy: antrum >body Intestinal metaplasia	Peptic ulceration (DU/GU) ?Gastric cancer
Chemical injury NSAIDs Bile reflux ?Alcohol	Direct injury Disruption of the mucus layer Degranulation of mast cells	Foveolar hyperplasia Oedema Vasodilatation Paucity of inflammatory cells	Gastric erosions Gastric ulcer

DU = duodenal ulcer; GU = gastric ulcer

which epithelioid cell granulomas are found. Such granulomas can be part of Crohn's disease (p. 431) or sarcoidosis, but after exclusion of these causes there remains an isolated granulomatous gastritis of unknown aetiology.

PEPTIC ULCERATION

▶ Major sites: first part of duodenum, junction of antral and body mucosa in stomach, distal oesophagus, and gastro-enterostomy stoma
▶ Main aetiological factors: hyperacidity, *Helicobacter* gastritis, duodenal reflux, NSAIDs, smoking and genetic factors
▶ Ulcers may be acute or chronic
▶ Complications include haemorrhage, penetration of adjacent organs, perforation, anaemia, obstruction due to fibrous strictures, and malignancy

Peptic ulceration is a breach in the mucosa lining the alimentary tract as a result of acid and pepsin attack. Gastric and duodenal ulcers differ in their epidemiology, incidence and pathogenesis (Table 15.3). They arise as either acute or chronic ulcers.

Acute ulcers

Acute peptic ulcers develop:

• as part of an acute *gastritis*
• as a complication of a severe *stress response*
• as a result of extreme *hyperacidity*.

Deeper extension of the erosions in acute gastritis resulting from NSAIDs or acute alcohol overdosage can produce frank ulcers. Acute ulcers occur also in a heterogeneous group of conditions where stress seems to be the common denominator. For example, ulcers may be found following severe burns (Curling's ulcer), major trauma or cerebrovascular accidents. Such ulcers probably arise as a consequence of mucosal ischaemia, which lowers the mucosal resistance to acid. Extreme hyperacidity, as seen for example in patients with gastrin-secreting tumours (Zollinger–Ellison syndrome), can lead to multiple acute ulcers in the antrum, the duodenum and even the jejunum.

Table 15.3 Comparison of the epidemiology, incidence and aetiology of gastric and duodenal ulcers

Feature	Gastric ulcer	Duodenal ulcer
Incidence (relative)	1	3
Age distribution	Increases with age	Increases up to 35 years of age
Social class	Higher in class V	Even distribution
Blood group	A	O
Acid levels	Normal or low	Elevated or normal
***Helicobacter* gastritis**	About 70%	95–100%

Chronic ulcers

Chronic peptic ulcers (Fig. 15.9) seem to occur most frequently at mucosal junctions. Thus gastric ulcers are found in antral mucosa where it meets body-type mucosa; duodenal ulcers are found in the proximal duodenum close to the pylorus; oeso-phageal peptic ulcers are found in the squamous epithelium just above the cardio-oesophageal junction; and stomal ulcers — those occurring following construction of a gastro-enterostomy linking stomach and jejunum — are found in the jejunal mucosa immediately adjacent to the gastric mucosa of the stomal margin. This suggests that ulceration is most likely to occur where acid and pepsin first come into contact with a susceptible mucosa.

Pathogenesis

For many years peptic ulceration has been attributed to excessive acid production. However, there are many problems with this hypothesis. People with gastric ulcers frequently have normal or even sub-normal acid production, and over one-half of duode-nal ulcer patients do not have hyperacidity. Con-versely, many people who are hypersecretors of acid do not get ulcers. Furthermore, while most ulcers respond initially to anti-acid treatment there are fre-quent relapses. It has therefore become increasingly apparent that mucosal defence against acid attack is of considerable importance (Fig. 15.10). Failure of the mucosal defence mechanisms means that ulcers can result from normal or even decreased quantities of acid.

Gastric ulcers
The pH of the gastric juice under fasting conditions is extremely acidic (between 1 and 2) so that any unprotected gastric mucosa would rapidly undergo auto-digestion.

The mucosal defences against acid attack consist of:

- a mucus–bicarbonate barrier
- the surface epithelium.

The *mucus barrier* is the more important of the two lines of defence. The pit-lining and surface epithelial cells of the stomach secrete viscid neutral glycoproteins which form a layer of unstirred mucus on the surface. The mucus itself has acid-resistant properties, but its protective power is greatly enhanced by the establishment of a buffering gradient within the layer brought about by bicarbonate ions.

The *surface epithelium* constitutes a second line of defence; for its proper functioning it requires integrity of both the apical plasma membrane as a barrier to ion transfer, and cellular metabolic functions including the production of bicarbonate. These functions are dependent upon an adequate mucosal blood supply.

Ulceration can follow either destruction or removal of the mucus barrier, or a loss of integrity of the sur-face epithelium. Dissolution of the mucus layer can occur as a primary event as a consequence of duode-no-gastric reflux. The regurgitated bile from the duo-denum strips off the mucus barrier and paves the

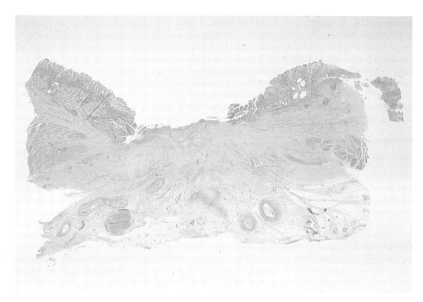

Fig. 15.9 Chronic gastric ulcer

Histological section through the ulcer revealing replacement of the underlying muscularis propria by fibrous tissue.

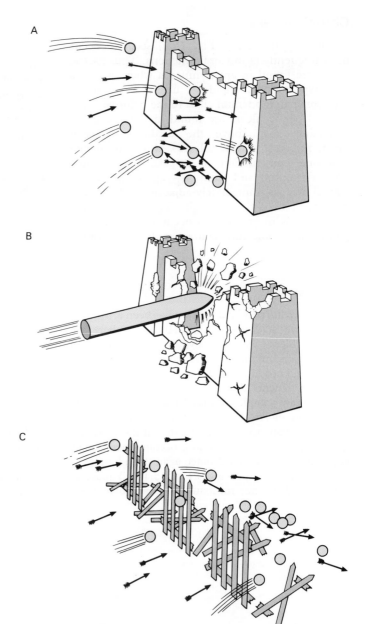

A

B

Fig. 15.10   Peptic ulceration

C

'An ulcer represents the adverse outcome of a conflict between aggressive forces in the stomach or duodenum and the defence mechanisms.' (Sir Francis Avery-Jones) **A. Normal.** Acid/pepsin attack is balanced by the mucus barrier and other defence mechanisms. **B. Increased attack.** Hyperacidity (as in the Zollinger–Ellison syndrome) or NSAIDs may bring about the ulceration of 'normal' mucosa in the stomach and duodenum. **C. Weakened mucosal defence.** This is the major factor in peptic ulceration. Chronic inflammation in the gastric and duodenal mucosa resulting from *Helicobacter pylori* infection can lead to ulceration in the presence of normal or even reduced levels of acid. Duodenal inflammation results from infection of patches of acid-induced gastric metaplasia in the first part of the duodenum.

way for acid attack. Acid and bile in combination damage the surface epithelial cells, increasing the permeability of the mucosa. This causes the congestion and oedema of the lamina propria seen in reflux gastritis.

The epithelial barrier may be damaged by the effect of NSAIDs blocking the synthesis of the prostaglandins which normally protect the epithelium. Epithelial injury is also a consequence of *H. pylori* infection either produced directly by cytotox-

ins and ammonia or indirectly as a result of the inflammatory reaction.

Thus in peptic ulcers in the stomach, breakdown of mucosal defence is much more important than excessive acid production.

Duodenal ulcers
Increased production of acid assumes more importance in the pathogenesis of duodenal ulceration; about one-half of such patients have an elevated max-

imal acid secretion, and even in those with a normal maximal acid output it may be that they have inappropriately sustained acid secretion without the normal sharp fall-off of acid production during sleep. It has been shown that *H. pylori* infected individuals secrete 2–6 times as much acid as non-infected controls when stimulated by gastrin-releasing peptide. Nevertheless, excess acidity is not the entire explanation and mucosal defence is also important.

The factors causing lowered resistance in the stomach do not usually apply in the duodenum: *Helicobacter* does not colonise duodenal epithelium; the duodenal mucosa is tolerant of bile and pancreatic alkaline secretions; and drugs are generally diluted or absorbed before reaching the duodenum. Nevertheless, *Helicobacter* is involved in duodenal ulceration because there is gastric metaplasia in response to excess acid. Gastric metaplasia paves the way for colonisation by *Helicobacter*, which in turn sets up chronic inflammation in the duodenum and predisposes to ulceration.

Morphology

Grossly, chronic peptic ulcers are usually less than 20 mm in diameter but they may be larger and can exceed 100 mm in diameter. The edges are clear-cut and overhang the base. Microscopically, the base consists of necrotic tissue and polymorph exudate overlying inflamed granulation tissue which merges with mature fibrous (scar) tissue. The latter frequently occupies the remainder of the wall, with the muscularis propria completely breached. Arteries within this fibrous base often show extreme narrowing of their lumina by intimal proliferation (*endarteritis obliterans*).

Ulcers heal by epithelial regeneration, which reconstitutes the mucosa, and progressive fibrosis. Later, shrinkage of the fibrous tissue (cicatrisation) may lead to pyloric stenosis or a central narrowing of the stomach, the so-called *hour-glass deformity*.

More immediate complications of peptic ulcers include:

- *perforation*, giving rise to spillage of gastric contents into the peritoneal cavity and peritonitis
- *penetration*, whereby the ulcer erodes into an adjacent organ such as the liver or pancreas
- *haemorrhage*, from eroded vessels in the ulcer base.

Although malignant change is claimed to occur in gastric ulcers, this is a very uncommon event: as far as duodenal ulcers are concerned it can be assumed that they never become malignant.

BENIGN TUMOURS AND POLYPS

A polyp is simply a protuberant mass of tissue; it can either be neoplastic or form as a result of an excessive reparative or regenerative process. The commonest form of polyp involves simple elongation of the gastric pits separated by fibrous tissue or mildly inflamed lamina propria. These are *hyperplastic* or *regenerative* polyps and are generally found against a background of *Helicobacter*-associated gastritis in the gastric antrum. A similar variety is seen in body-type mucosa, but in this instance the main feature is enlargement by cystic dilatation of the specialised fundic glands. These were originally thought to be hamartomatous, but this is questionable and they are best termed *simple fundic polyps*. Much more rarely, true *hamartomas* occur, either as adenomyomas, which, as the term implies, are overgrowths of glandular and smooth muscle elements, or as part of the Peutz–Jeghers syndrome, where the patient has multiple gastrointestinal hamartomatous polyps and circumoral skin pigmentation. A further rare cause of a polypoid mass in the stomach is *heterotopic pancreas*, i.e. the presence of pancreatic tissue separate from the main gland.

A benign epithelial tumour of the stomach (*adenoma*) is uncommon. These polypoid tumours have a strong potential for malignant change and, if subjected to multiple sectioning, around 40% will be found to contain carcinoma on microscopic examination.

The commonest connective tissue neoplasm is the *smooth muscle tumour*. Endoscopically these have a characteristic appearance, with the mucosa heaped up over an intramural tumour projecting into the lumen. There is often a small central ulcer crater which can be a source of haemorrhage. Histologically they consist of interwoven bundles of spindle cells with variable amounts of eosinophilic cytoplasm. However, identical appearances can be seen in some tumours which prove to be of neural origin. Because of this doubt over their histogenesis, these tumours are increasingly referred to as *gastric stromal tumours*. These tumours are of unpredictable behaviour and it is difficult to distinguish between benign and malignant tumours on histological criteria. Those features which indicate a benign course are small size, encapsulation, low mitotic activity and absence of necrosis.

MALIGNANT TUMOURS OF THE STOMACH

Carcinoma of the stomach

▶ Majority are adenocarcinomas
▶ Many arise on a background of chronic gastritis and intestinal metaplasia
▶ Most cases present when clinically advanced
▶ Early cases (carcinoma confined to mucosa or submucosa) have a good prognosis
▶ All gastric ulcers must be regarded as potentially malignant

The incidence of gastric cancer, like that of carcinoma of the oesophagus, varies widely both between and within countries. There is a notably high incidence in Japan, China, Colombia and Finland, but even in these countries, as elsewhere in the world, the incidence of carcinoma of the stomach is declining. Despite this fall, gastric cancer is still the second most common fatal malignancy (after lung cancer) in the world, with an estimated three-quarters of a million new cases diagnosed annually. In many countries gastric cancer remains the most common form of cancer. Migrant studies indicate strong environmental influences; for example, when Japanese move to Hawaii or California the incidence of gastric cancer in that group falls, and after only one generation approximates to that of the local population. While the causative environmental factors remain to be conclusively determined, it appears that *H. pylori* plays a major part.

Aetiology

For many years a sequence of events, starting with chronic gastritis and passing through atrophy and intestinal metaplasia to premalignant dysplasia, has been acknowledged as the precursor to cancer of the stomach. Given that *H. pylori* has now been accepted as the major cause of chronic gastritis, it is logical to implicate this infection in the causation of gastric cancer. The prevalence of *H. pylori* infection frequently runs parallel with the incidence of gastric cancer in the same populations, and epidemiological studies have shown that patients with antibodies to *H. pylori* have a higher risk of gastric cancer. The strength of the epidemiological links is such that the International Agency for Research into Cancer has declared that *H. pylori* is a gastric carcinogen, that is, the infection initiates the events leading to

cancer. Given the high prevalence of infection and the comparative rarity of cancer it is unlikely that the organism or its products are direct-acting mutagens.

There are a number of possible indirect mechanisms linking *H. pylori* infection to gastric cancer. Long-term infection leads to glandular atrophy which leads to a gradual decline in acid secretion. Hypochlorhydria allows other bacteria to proliferate in the gastric juice; these bacteria are capable of reducing nitrate ions to nitrite and can catalyse nitrosation of amines and amides present in the diet to give rise to potentially carcinogenic N-nitroso compounds. *H. pylori* possesses an inducible alcohol dehydrogenase which is capable of producing acetaldehyde from alcohol substrates. Acetaldehyde is a highly reactive product which damages epithelial cells and can cause DNA damage, but its role in vivo is in dispute. A more likely source of genomic DNA damage in *H. pylori* gastritis is reactive oxygen attack by superoxide and hydroxyl radicals, monochloramines and nitric oxide produced by activated polymorphs and macrophages. Interestingly, nitrosation and oxidative damage is minimised by antioxidant vitamins, among which ascorbic acid is the most important, and diets rich in fresh fruit and vegetables have long been recognised as protective against gastric cancer. Ascorbic acid secretion into gastric juice is severely compromised in *H. pylori* gastritis.

Perhaps the most important factor underlying the relationship between *H. pylori* and gastric cancer is a promotional effect through high cell turnover. The production of cytotoxins and ammonia by the organism, and indirect epithelial damage brought about by cytokines and polymorph products, induce increased cell turnover. DNA repair is compromised by increased cell proliferation, and the probability of a mutation escaping repair and being transmitted to daughter cells is increased.

Several molecular genetic changes have been demonstrated in gastric cancer. Mutations and deletions of tumour suppressor genes, notably p53, K-*ras* and the APC gene, and over-expression of oncogenes like c-*myc* and *erb*B-2, have been demonstrated. However, while some of these mutations are consistent with exogenous chemical carcinogens or exposure to endogenous free radical injury, one cannot infer the nature of the mutational agent from the genetic lesions with any certainty.

Nevertheless the overall evidence favours an aetiological link between *H. pylori* infection and gastric cancer. The implications for the prevention of this major cancer are clear. Eradication of this infection, or more practically, vaccination in childhood will have a profound effect on the incidence of gastric cancer.

Premalignant conditions

There are few clearly defined conditions in the stomach where an increased incidence of cancer is observed. In addition to the atrophy and intestinal metaplasia of chronic *H. pylori* gastritis, a higher incidence of gastric cancer is seen in patients with pernicious anaemia and following partial gastrectomy for benign ulcer disease. Patients with pernicious anaemia exhibit a threefold increase in the risk of gastric cancer over the general population, while postgastrectomy patients develop an excess risk about 15–20 years after surgery. A common denominator in all such patients is the presence of hypochlorhydria or achlorhydria as a result of glandular atrophy and/or alkaline reflux; low gastric acidity allows the proliferation of large numbers of bacteria in the gastric juice. It is possible that such individuals have inherited defects in DNA repair genes. Thus it may be that the development of most 'environmental' gastric cancers can be explained in terms of longstanding mucosal injury leading to gastric atrophy and low acid secretion, with a consequent rise in bacterial counts in the gastric juice. These bacteria are capable of nitrate reduction and act as catalysts for the nitrosation of amines to carcinogenic nitrosamines.

There are patients with gastric cancer who have neither a recognised premalignant condition nor chronic gastritis and hypochlorhydria. Genetic factors are likely to be involved, but little is known of these beyond a link with blood group A and the appearance of frequent gastric cancers in certain families often at a young age. It is possible that such individuals have inherited defects in DNA repair genes.

Dysplasia and early gastric cancer

The dysplasia–carcinoma sequence is thought to characterise the development of most if not all gastric cancers, but the finding of dysplasia is relatively uncommon in low-incidence countries such as the UK and USA. Most cancers are advanced at the time of initial diagnosis and potentially curative operations are only possible in about 45% of cases. This accounts for the poor prognosis of gastric cancer, which generally has only a 10–15% survival rate at five years after diagnosis. However, much better results are obtained when patients undergo radical operations with extensive lymph node clearance. Patients who have such 'potentially curative

resections' with removal of all macroscopic cancer have about a 60% chance of survival to 5 years.

Gastric cancers are classified as either 'early' or 'advanced' on the basis of direct spread through the stomach wall. *Early* gastric cancer is confined to either the mucosa (intra-mucosal carcinoma) or submucosa; *advanced* tumours extend into or beyond the main muscle coats. Cancers can thus still be 'early' even if spread has occurred to regional lymph nodes. The importance of this categorisation lies in their differing prognosis, cases of early gastric cancer having a 5-year survival in excess of 90%. The prognosis of advanced cases rests largely on whether or not surgery has been truly 'curative' in removing all the tumour. Thus involvement of the resection margins by carcinoma carries a dire prognosis, as does the presence of covert hepatic or distant lymph node metastases. The best guide to prognosis in curative cases appears to be the number of involved lymph nodes and, to some extent, the histological type of carcinoma.

Morphology

Foci of high-grade dysplasia and intra-mucosal carcinoma may be endoscopically visible as slightly elevated plaques or shallow depressions. If either of these lesions is diagnosed in a gastric biopsy, gastrectomy is essential. Histologically, they may be distinguished according to whether invasion of the lamina propria has occurred, but this can only be excluded in high-grade dysplasia by examination of multiple sections from the entire area of involvement. With increasing size, the elevated lesions develop into *polypoid* and later into *fungating* carcinomas, while the depressed areas present an excavated *ulcerated* appearance mimicking that seen in chronic peptic ulcer. The distinction between carcinoma and chronic peptic ulcer cannot be made with certainty on clinical, endoscopic or radiological grounds, so that all gastric ulcers should be subjected to cytology or multiple biopsy both before and after therapy.

Carcinomas of the stomach are almost exclusively *adenocarcinomas* derived from mucus-secreting epithelial cells. Like other carcinomas, they can be graded according to their degree of differentiation; poorly differentiated carcinomas behave more aggressively than well-differentiated types. However, a better guide to prognosis results from division into either 'intestinal' or 'diffuse' types according to the scheme devised by Lauren.

- *Intestinal carcinomas* show glandular formations lined by mucus-secreting cells with plentiful cytoplasm; they tend to have an expansile growth pattern with a well-demarcated 'pushing' border.

- *Diffuse carcinomas*, on the other hand, consist of chains of single cells infiltrating the wall with a poorly demarcated invasive margin. Mucus secretion is generally less apparent, and usually takes the form of intra-cytoplasmic vacuoles which may compress the nucleus to form so-called 'signet ring' cells.

Intestinal carcinomas carry a better prognosis than the diffuse type. Interestingly, the intestinal form predominates in high-incidence countries and has a strong correlation with pre-existing *H. pylori*-associated chronic gastritis. Diffuse carcinomas form a higher proportion of the total in low-incidence countries; this may reflect the increased contribution of genetic factors to cancer development in these areas.

Carcinomas spread directly to involve the serosa, which can lead to peritoneal dissemination. This can result in the formation of a malignant effusion or involvement of other organs by transcoelomic spread, of which metastases in the ovaries (Krukenberg tumours) are a classical example. Depending upon the site of the tumour, direct spread can also occur into the pancreas, transverse colon (when fistulation can occur), liver and spleen. Lymphatic spread is initially to local nodes along the right and left gastric arteries, extending to coeliac nodes, then to more distant sites like the classical (but rare) involvement of the left supraclavicular nodes (Troisier's sign). Blood stream spread occurs via the portal vein; liver metastases are frequently evident at the time of presentation.

Other malignant tumours

Other malignant tumours include carcinoid tumours (p. 445), malignant stromal tumours and lymphomas.

Stromal tumours

The stomach is the commonest site for gastrointestinal stromal tumours; approximately 45% of these are malignant and can give rise to metastases. They frequently present with symptoms referable to secondary ulceration, namely haemorrhage, anaemia, anorexia and weight loss. Endoscopically they protrude into the lumen and often have a central deep ulcer crater. Malignancy is diagnosed on the basis of mitotic activity, and presence of metastases at the time of surgery.

Lymphomas

The stomach is the commonest site for primary lymphomas to arise in the gastrointestinal tract, accounting for around 40% of all cases, and are steadily increasing in incidence. Lymphomas of the stomach represent about 5% of all gastric malignancies and are most frequently of the non-Hodgkin B-cell type; they are closely related to preceding *H. pylori* infection. The normal gastric mucosa is virtually devoid of lymphocytes. *H. pylori* infection provokes a mucosal immune response characterised by an influx of lymphocytes and plasma cells and an active chronic inflammatory reaction. The appearance of lymphoid follicles with germinal centres in the gastric mucosa together with an increase in intraepithelial lymphocytes in the overlying epithelium recapitulate the features of mucosa-associated lymphoid tissue (MALT) and it is this acquired MALT which provides the tissue of origin for gastric B-cell lymphomas. As with gastric carcinoma, epidemiological studies reveal a much increased risk for the subsequent development of gastric lymphoma when *H. pylori* infected individuals are compared with uninfected controls. The emergence of a monoclonal proliferation of B-lymphocytes associated with aggressive features evidenced by invasion of epithelium (*lympho-epithelial lesions*) and replacement of germinal centres by atypical centrocyte-like B-cells are the characteristic features of a malignant lymphoma. The transition from chronic gastritis to lymphoma is associated with genetic changes but the cause of these DNA changes remains unknown.

Gastric lymphomas have a relatively good prognosis if confined to the stomach (50% survival at 5 years), but the outlook worsens considerably when penetration of the serosa or involvement of regional lymph nodes has occurred. The stomach may also be involved by lymphomas which have arisen elsewhere; the outlook in these systematised cases depends upon the overall extent, histological type and grade.

INTESTINE

NORMAL STRUCTURE AND FUNCTION

Small intestine

The main functions of the small intestine are:

- enzymatic digestion
- absorption of nutrients.

By providing a vast surface area of specialised epithelium, the villous structure of the mucosa optimises absorption; this can be either passive or under active control. The *villi* are covered by tightly packed absorptive cells (*enterocytes*), which themselves have *microvilli* on the luminal surface along their plasma membranes. This microvillous or 'brush' border further increases surface area and, together with the adherent glycoproteins of the glycocalyx, is also the site of hydrolytic enzyme activity, for example, disaccharidases and peptidases.

Endocrine cells
Scattered among the absorptive cells are mucus-secreting goblet cells and endocrine cells; the latter produce a wide variety of 'gut' hormones, such as enteroglucagon, cholecystokinin, gastrin, motilin, secretin and vasoactive intestinal polypeptide (VIP). Endocrine cells are also found among the proliferating cells (*enteroblasts*) of the intestinal crypts. Here, many of the endocrine cells are of the *enterochromaffin* type and produce serotonin (5-HT) which has an important role in the control of gut motility and blood supply. Endocrine cells of the gut are often considered as part of a diffuse system of APUD (amine precursor uptake and decarboxylation) cells, which are found in many organs and from which distinctive neoplasms may originate. They are discussed further on page 445.

Paneth cells
These are distinctive cells also found at the bases of the crypts, which contain prominent lysozyme-rich granules. The role of these cells is unknown, but their close proximity to the stem cells, and their appearance in metaplastic epithelia, suggest that they may produce local factors regulating cell proliferation and differentiation.

Brunner's glands
The duodenal submucosa contains Brunner's glands, collections of mucus-secreting acini most plentiful proximally. They are much less frequent in the jejunum. Besides producing an alkaline mucous secretion essential for mucosal protection against acid attack in the proximal duodenum, Brunner's glands are rich in epidermal growth factor (EGF) and may therefore encourage mucosal regeneration after injury.

Lymphoid tissue
The connective tissue of the mucosa (lamina propria) contains prominent lymphatics (lacteals), blood capillaries, and a cellular infiltrate comprising lymphocytes, plasma cells, eosinophils and mast cells. The lymphoid cells form an important arm of mucosal immunity, known as *mucosa-associated lymphoid tissue* (MALT). Most of those in the lamina propria are T-helper cells, whereas the intraepithelial lymphocytes are predominantly T-suppressor cells which are thought to be important in maintaining tolerance to food antigens. Lymphoid aggregates or follicles with germinal centres are found throughout the intestinal mucosa; they frequently straddle the muscularis mucosae and extend into the superficial submucosa. Dense aggregates are found in the terminal ileum where they form *Peyer's patches*. The flattened epithelium over these aggregates contains *M-cells*, specialised cells capable of antigen binding and processing; they pass antigenic material to adjacent helper T-lymphocytes.

Large intestine

The large intestine has several functions:

- the storage and elimination of food residues
- an important role in maintaining fluid and electrolyte balance
- an important role in permitting bacterial degradation of complex carbohydrates and other nutrients.

The large intestine can be divided into six parts—caecum, ascending colon, transverse colon, descending colon, sigmoid and rectum. These divisions are imprecise, but are useful for describing the sites and extent of disease.

Mucosa
The mucosa of the large bowel is devoid of villi. Instead, it comprises perpendicular crypts extending from the flat surface down to the muscularis mucosae, separated by a little lamina propria. Numerically, the predominant cell is of columnar absorptive type, but in tissue sections such cells often appear less numerous than the intervening goblet cells. As in the small intestine, several types of endocrine (or APUD) cell are present, but in health Paneth cells are confined to the right side of the colon and then only sparsely. Also in contrast to the small intestine, large bowel mucosa has only scanty lymphatics which are concentrated towards the muscularis mucosae. This restricts the metastatic potential of intra-mucosal malignant cells.

Vascular supply
The vascular supply to the colon derives from the superior and inferior mesenteric arteries:

- The caecum, ascending and proximal transverse colon are supplied by branches of the superior mesenteric artery.
- The distal transverse, descending, sigmoid colon and upper rectum are supplied by branches of the inferior mesenteric artery.
- The remainder of the rectum is supplied by the middle and inferior rectal arteries which are branches of the internal iliac and internal pudendal arteries respectively.

These patterns of blood supply are important in determining the sites and consequences of ischaemia (for example, the 'watershed' territory around the splenic flexure is especially vulnerable) and, because lymphatic drainage follows similar patterns, in predicting the likely distribution of lymph node metastases from the site of the tumour.

Nerve supply

The intestine has a complex nerve network comprising autonomic motor and sensory neurones and a separate enteric nervous system. The sympathetic supply originates from ganglia outside the gut in the coeliac and mesenteric plexuses. The parasympathetic ganglia are found within the gut wall, and these, together with the associated neurones, form two nerve networks, the submucosal (Meissner's) plexus and the myenteric (Auerbach's) plexus. The nerve plexuses create and conduct the basic electrical rhythm of the gut. Stimulation of parasympathetic nerves increases muscular contraction (particularly in the inner circular layer), blood supply and secretory activity; stimulation of the sympathetic supply has the opposite effects. The enteric nervous system has sensory receptors in the mucosa and bowel wall which respond to changes in volume and composition of the bowel contents, and through neuronal connections elicits the appropriate response in the effector system. These activities are mediated by a wide variety of neurotransmitters, such as VIP, cholecystokinin and somatostatin, some of which were formerly thought to be gut hormones.

Appendix

The appendix arises from the caecum. It is a blind-ended structure lined internally by colonic-type mucosa, surrounded by submucosa and muscle coats. In children and young adults the mucosa contains numerous prominent lymphoid follicles. In the elderly, the lumen often shows fibrous obliteration.

CONGENITAL DISORDERS

The duodenum derives from the distal end of the primitive foregut; the jejunum, ileum and proximal colon from the midgut; and the distal colon and rectum from the hindgut. Proper development involves canalisation (development of a lumen), temporary herniation into the extra-embryonic coelom, rotation, and eventual retraction back into the abdominal cavity. Defects arising in the course of this complex process are relatively common.

Atresia and stenosis

Atresia represents either a failure of the gut to canalise or a failure of a segment to develop during fetal growth. A congenital stenosis is a constriction of the bowel arising during fetal development. These lesions are most commonly found in the duodenum or small intestine, and are rare in the colon. Duodenal atresia seems to be a failure of organ development, and around 30% of affected children also have Down's syndrome; jejuno-ileal atresia commonly appears to be the result of an intra-uterine accident, such as incarceration of the midgut in the physiological umbilical hernia or some other form of vascular occlusion.

Malrotation

The commonest type of malrotation occurs when the large bowel fails to descend into the right iliac fossa after emerging from the physiological umbilical hernia. This means that the caecum remains high in the abdomen and the bands that should fix it in the right iliac fossa (Ladd's bands) cross the duodenum and compress it, causing extrinsic obstruction.

Duplication and diverticula

Duplication of the bowel may present either as a tubular double-barrelled appearance, or form a cyst in the mesentery. These anomalies can produce an abdominal mass, cause intestinal obstruction, or initiate a volvulus (p. 440). Congenital diverticula are out-pouchings of the full thickness of the bowel wall and are found mainly in the duodenum and jejunum. These rarely have clinical consequences, but some patients develop bacterial overgrowth, steatorrhoea and vitamin B_{12} malabsorption. The diverticula can also undergo perforation and haemorrhage.

Meckel's diverticulum

Meckel's diverticulum arises as a result of incomplete regression of the vitello-intestinal duct, such that a tubular diverticulum is present in the ileum. The diverticulum is usually lined by normal small-intestinal mucosa, but occasionally it may contain heterotopic gastric or pancreatic elements. If gastric elements are present, acid and peptic secretion may lead to ulceration at the mouth of the diverticulum and give rise to haemorrhage and perforation. The diverticulum may also become inflamed and present as an acute abdomen which can mimic appendicitis.

Meconium ileus

The term meconium ileus refers to small-intestinal obstruction resulting from thickening and desiccation (inspissation) of the viscid meconium produced by children with cystic fibrosis (Ch. 7). It is seen in about 15% of affected babies and may be complicated by perforation, secondary atresia or volvulus.

Hirschsprung's disease

Hirschsprung's disease, or aganglionosis of the intestine, results from a failure of migration of neuroblasts from the vagus into the developing gut, such that the intramural parasympathetic nerve plexuses fail to develop. The distal colon and rectum have an additional parasympathetic supply from extramural nerves derived from the sacral plexus. Under normal circumstances the parasympathetic tone, which controls the contraction of the circular muscle coat, is modulated at the ganglia by the sympathetic innervation. However, in the absence of the myenteric ganglia, the intact extramural parasympathetic supply is unchecked by sympathetic modulation and results in spasm of the circular muscle and intestinal obstruction. There is a proliferation of cholinergic nerves derived from this extramural supply throughout the affected segment, and their high content of acetylcholinesterase can be utilised to diagnose Hirschsprung's disease in frozen sections of rectal mucosa.

Hirschsprung's disease affects the distal large intestine extending proximally from the anus for a variable distance. The rectum and distal colon are usually involved, but the extent varies from one or two centimetres to total colonic aganglionosis, or even extension into the small intestine. The effects of the aganglionosis vary from life-threatening total obstruction to mild cases causing chronic constipa-

tion. The main cause of death in Hirschsprung's disease is the development of an acute enterocolitis with endotoxaemia.

Anorectal anomalies

A large variety of malformations have been described which affect the termination of the large bowel. These include:

- a *primitive cloaca*, where the alimentary, urinary and genital tracts open into a single orifice
- *anorectal agenesis* and *rectal atresia*, where there is a failure of development or canalisation from above the level of the levators
- an *ectopic* or *imperforate anus*.

Anorectal anomalies occur in approximately 1:5000 live births. Most are amenable to surgical correction.

MALABSORPTION

Malabsorption can result from pancreatic disease or various biochemical disorders such as lactase and sucrase-isomaltase deficiency, as well as from small-intestinal diseases. Small-intestinal causes include:

- *coeliac disease*, the major small-intestinal cause of malabsorption in Western countries
- *extensive surgical resection*, for example in patients with Crohn's disease
- *lymphatic obstruction*, which gives rise to a protein-losing state
- *'blind loop syndrome'*, where bacterial overgrowth in partly obstructed or bypassed loops robs the patient of vital nutrients.

Coeliac disease

> ► Results from sensitivity to gluten in cereals
> ► Diagnosis by finding villous atrophy and crypt hyperplasia on duodenal or jejunal biopsy
> ► Clinically, results in malabsorption
> ► Complicated by splenic atrophy and, less commonly, lymphoma and small-intestinal ulceration

Coeliac disease is due to an abnormal reaction to a constituent of wheat flour, gluten, which damages the surface enterocytes of the small intestine and severely reduces their absorptive capacity.

Incidence

Coeliac disease affects about 1 in 2000 individuals in the United Kingdom but in the west of Ireland this rises to 1 in 300. However, these incidence rates are set to increase as the range of disturbances resulting from gluten intolerance becomes more widely appreciated. In family studies the incidence of coeliac disease in siblings is between 10 and 20% and there is a raised incidence in their parents.

Aetiology and pathogenesis

It is now fairly certain that the toxic component of gluten is gliadin, but the mechanism by which gliadin induces tissue damage remains unknown. It seems increasingly likely that tissue injury is more a consequence of the immune response than a direct toxic effect. There is an apparent increase in intraepithelial lymphocytes (IELs) in this condition and an increased proportion of a specialised subpopulation of T-lymphocytes among the IELs, but the significance of these findings remains obscure. Genetic factors are also involved and there is a strong association with HLA-B8. Approximately 80% of patients have this phenotype; furthermore, coeliac disease is associated with the skin disease dermatitis herpetiformis which seems to be associated independently with the HLA-B8 antigen. These genetic associations are likely to be linked to mucosal immune responsiveness and thus determine susceptibility to the disease. Sensitivity to gliadin and the development of coeliac disease might be 'triggered' in susceptible individuals by some other factor such as viral infection. This would explain the variable age of onset of the disease and its occasional appearance in middle-aged or even elderly people.

Morphology

Under normal circumstances, enterocytes are constantly shed from the tips of the villi and replenished by migration of cells up the villi from the proliferative compartment in the crypts (Fig. 15.11). The entire cycle from cell birth through functional maturation to extrusion takes about 72 hours. Under conditions of accelerated cell loss, lower rates of loss can be compensated for by increased cell proliferation. With higher rates of cell loss, a stage is soon reached when the increased proliferative compartment cannot maintain a normal number of maturing and functioning 'end cells', the size of this compartment diminishes, and villous atrophy results. Shrinkage of villi and reduction in epithelial surface area are thus inevitable consequences of any injury causing a high rate of cell loss in the small intestine. In coeliac disease the ultimate stage of this process is seen; despite

a marked increase in size of the proliferative compartment, evidenced by elongation, hypercellularity and high mitotic activity of the crypts (crypt hyperplasia), there is a flat surface (total villous atrophy; see Fig. 15.12) and even this is populated by immature cells incapable of proper absorptive activity. The disease is therefore characterised by a total malabsorption, affecting sugars, fatty acids, monoglycerides, amino acids, water and electrolytes; the failure to absorb fat is the dominant abnormality in most cases. The net loss of surface epithelial cells also gives rise to a secondary disaccharidase deficiency, so that patients become intolerant of lactose and other sugars.

The lesion is more severe in the proximal small intestine — the duodenum and proximal jejunum — and may spare the ileum, although the latter is susceptible to injury if exposed to gluten. In addition to malabsorption, intestinal hormone production from

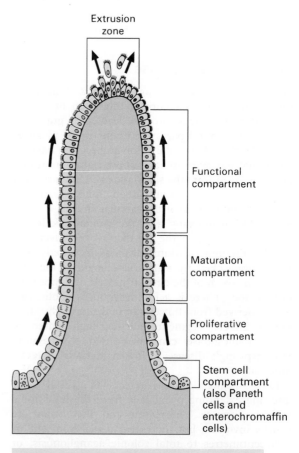

Extrusion zone

Functional compartment

Maturation compartment

Proliferative compartment

Stem cell compartment (also Paneth cells and enterochromaffin cells)

Fig. 15.11 Cell proliferation and maturation in the small intestine

(After Wright, 1984) See text for details.

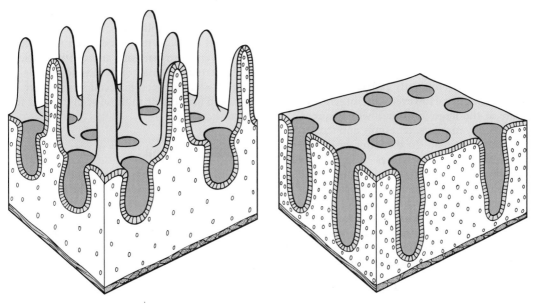

A Normal jejunal mucosa

B Total villous atrophy in coeliac disease. (See text for details.)

Fig. 15.12 Coeliac disease

the proximal small bowel is impaired; there may be secondary reduction in pancreatic secretion and bile flow as a result of reduced production or release of pancreozymin, secretin and cholecystokinin.

Complications
Now that the primary lesion and clinical consequences of coeliac disease can be managed by gluten-free diets, the later effects of the disease are becoming of greater concern. The main long-term problem is the development of malignant lymphomas in the small intestine, but there is also a higher incidence of other gastrointestinal cancers. In general, small bowel lymphomas are of B-cell lineage, but in coeliac disease they are frequently of a large cell type derived from T-cells (enteropathy-associated T-cell lymphoma). The patient presents with either haemorrhage, perforation, small-bowel obstruction or systemic symptoms. A few patients with coeliac disease develop ulceration of the small intestine which is non-lymphomatous; microscopic examination simply reveals non-specific chronic inflammation (chronic ulcerative enteritis).

Tropical sprue

Pathological changes identical to those found in coeliac disease (but usually less severe) are evident in tropical sprue, a form of malabsorption found, as the name indicates, in the tropics and sub-tropics but not apparently in Africa. It is characterised by chronic diarrhoea, weight loss and a macrocytic anaemia due to folate or vitamin B_{12} deficiency. A gluten-free diet has little or no beneficial effect, but the condition may be relieved by broad-spectrum antibiotics. The cause of the disease remains uncertain, but abnormal bacterial colonisation of the upper small bowel is probably involved.

Giardiasis

Mild malabsorption sometimes occurs in giardiasis (see p. 430).

BACTERIAL INFECTIONS

Bacterial infections of the intestinal tract are a major cause of morbidity and mortality throughout the world. Bacterial contamination of water supplies and the consequent diarrhoeal diseases are the major cause of infant mortality in developing countries.

Salmonella

Food poisoning by *Salmonella* organisms is a common and increasing problem in the United Kingdom. Whereas the organisms *S. typhi* and

S. paratyphi cause bacteraemic illnesses, *Salmonella* infection of food poisoning type (salmonellosis) is generally confined to the gastrointestinal tract. In some patients this results in vomiting and profuse watery diarrhoea, usually with colicky, peri-umbilical pain suggesting predominantly gastric and small-intestinal involvement. However, in others the features relate to the large intestine, with frequent, small-volume bloody motions, tenesmus and tenderness over the sigmoid colon. In the latter cases, sigmoidoscopic examination discloses a range of abnormalities varying from mucosal oedema and hyperaemia, to mucosal friability with slough formation and contact or spontaneous haemorrhage. The histological appearances are similarly varied. Some biopsies show oedema, focal interstitial haemorrhage and a mild increase in neutrophil polymorphs; more severe cases show a marked increase in polymorphs, with occasional crypts distended by polymorphs and mucus in the lumen ('mucoid crypt abscesses'). The crypt pattern, however, remains normal.

Bacillary dysentery

Bacillary dysentery is an acute infection of the large intestine characterised by painful diarrhoea, often with blood and mucus in the stools. *Shigella sonnei* is the commonest cause; it produces relatively minor lesions and seldom causes ulceration. However, *Shigella flexneri* and *Shigella dysenteriae* can produce necrosis, sloughing and haemorrhage, giving rise to a picture closely resembling ulcerative colitis.

Cholera

Cholera is a form of enterotoxigenic diarrhoea resulting from infection with *Vibrio cholerae*. The cholera toxin binds to a specific receptor on epithelial cells which leads to increased adenylate cyclase activity; this in turn results in high cyclic-AMP levels in the intestinal mucosa. The affected enterocytes secrete fluid and sodium ions, and the ensuing watery diarrhoea can be extreme, with overwhelming fluid loss and a rapidly fatal outcome. Because the effects are mediated by an exotoxin and there is no bacterial invasion of host tissues, the histological changes are remarkably slight; the mucosa shows mild oedema and goblet cell depletion.

Campylobacter colitis

It has been known since the early 1900s that *Campylobacter* organisms cause dysentery and abortion in cattle and domestic animals, but recognition of their role in human disease is relatively recent. Contamination of milk and water supplies with *C. jejuni* and *C. coli* is now recognised as a frequent cause of severe gastroenteritis and colitis, particularly in debilitated and malnourished individuals. The histological changes seen in rectal biopsies are non-specific, and are similar to those seen in other forms of infective colitis.

Neonatal diarrhoea

In some of the diarrhoeas of neonates and infants, various strains of *Escherichia coli* can be isolated. Such infections are more common in bottle-fed infants, and epidemics may occur in children's wards. Certain defined enteropathogenic serotypes are involved, and these differ from non-pathogenic types in their powers of adhesion to colonocytes and their ability to invade the mucosa. Diarrhoea may be severe and lead to dehydration and death. At autopsy, the small- and large-intestinal mucosa shows mucosal congestion and oedema with focal ulceration.

Staphylococcal enterocolitis

The form of enterocolitis due to staphylococcal infection is rare, but potentially fatal. The injudicious use of broad-spectrum antibiotics can so alter the normal ecology of the intestinal bacterial flora that the way is open for invasion by organisms which are either completely foreign to the bowel or normally present only in small numbers. The most dangerous of these is *Staphylococcus aureus*, which, when present in large numbers, can liberate sufficient endotoxin to produce a severe enterocolitis. Staphylococcal enterocolitis is usually the result of cross-infection, and typically affects the hospital inpatient who has had contact with an antibiotic-resistant staphylococcus.

Patients present with sudden onset of severe diarrhoea, accompanied by shock and dehydration. A smear of the stools stained by Gram's method will reveal numerous staphylococci and often no other organisms. The course can be relatively mild and respond to treatment, but is often severe with a high mortality. There is widespread superficial ulceration predominantly affecting the small intestine. Microscopically there is acute inflammation of the mucosa with intense congestion and widespread necrosis. The surface of the mucosa is covered in an exudate containing numerous staphylococci.

Gonococcal proctitis

Gonococcal proctitis (inflammation of the rectum)

is an acute exudative inflammatory condition which develops by genito-anal spread in females, and results from anal intercourse in males. The histological changes are non-specific, but the demonstration of numerous Gram-negative diplococci in the exudate leads to a presumptive diagnosis. As with other forms of infective colitis, definitive diagnosis depends on culture of the organisms.

Tuberculosis

Tuberculosis is almost entirely confined to the small intestine. In primary infection, an inconspicuous intestinal lesion is accompanied by gross enlargement of mesenteric nodes. This was the form of infection characteristic of bovine tuberculosis, a variety now virtually eliminated from the UK through the introduction of tubercle-free herds of cattle and the pasteurisation of milk.

Secondary tuberculous enteritis is a complication of extensive pulmonary tuberculosis which results from the swallowing of infected sputum. The typical alimentary lesion is ulceration of the ileum, the ulcer having formed by coalescence of caseous foci in the mucosa and submucosa. As the ulcers enlarge they follow the path of the lymphatics around the circumference of the intestine and eventually encircle the bowel. Healing is by fibrosis, and strictures may result from subsequent cicatrisation. The inflammatory exudate on the serosal aspect of the bowel may organise and form fibrous adhesions.

Ileo-caecal tuberculosis is a distinctive form of infection consisting of an ulcerative, granulomatous and fibrotic process occurring around the ileo-caecal valve, with variable extension into both ileum and caecum. The thickening and stenosis present a picture which is frequently indistinguishable from Crohn's disease, although, in tuberculosis, distinct pale tubercles can be seen in the serosa. Patients recognised as having active intra-abdominal tuberculosis are treated by chemotherapy, but surgery may be required for the treatment of complications or for diagnosis. The major complications are intestinal obstruction by adhesions, perforation of ulcers (although this is uncommon because of the marked fibrous reaction), and malabsorption resulting from widespread mucosal involvement or blockage to lymphatic drainage.

Actinomycosis

Actinomycosis usually presents as a localised chronic inflammatory process most commonly related to the appendix or caecal area. The organism, *Actinomyces israelii*, is a normal commensal of the mouth, and when swallowed may resist acid digestion and infect the bowel. The infection is protracted and characterised by chronic suppuration and the formation of sinuses (openings on to the skin) and fistulae (abnormal connections with other hollow viscera). Histology reveals inflamed granulation tissue, and foci of suppuration containing the characteristic colonies of organisms visible to the naked eye as 'sulphur granules' in the watery pus.

Whipple's disease

Whipple's disease is a rare bacterial infection usually involving the small intestine. The causative organism has been recently identified as *Tropheryma whippelii*, and this infection, in combination with alterations in immune responsiveness, produces multisystem involvement with joint pains, weight loss, pigmentation, lymphadenopathy and malabsorption. The mucosa from affected individuals shows infiltration of the lamina propria by numerous granular macrophages containing abundant glycoprotein. On electron microscopy, the Whipple bacillus and granular material derived from the bacterial cell wall can be found in these macrophages. Patients usually respond to prolonged treatment with tetracyclines.

Antibiotic-associated colitis

Many patients taking a broad-spectrum antibiotic develop diarrhoea. In most cases this is not severe and responds to withdrawal of the antibiotic. However, a small proportion develop a fulminant colitis with profuse diarrhoea and dehydration, leading in the more debilitated patients to death. On biopsy, there is superficial loss of epithelial cells and a 'volcano-like' eruption of mucin, polymorphs and fibrin forming a pseudomembrane on the surface; this is *pseudomembranous colitis*. It has been established that this form of colitis results from the suppression of the normal bowel flora and the overgrowth of *Clostridium difficile*, which causes a widespread toxic mucosal injury.

VIRAL INFECTIONS

In many cases of presumed infective gastroenteritis or colitis no bacteria are isolated, and viral infection is probably responsible. Acute viral gastroenteritis is a major public health problem and as a cause of illness is second only to the common cold. However, the positive identification of viruses in contaminated food is difficult. The minute infecting dose required and the insensitivity of the available tests mean that laboratory identification is not always possible.

The principal agents are parvoviruses and 'small round structured' viruses including calicivirus. In the small intestine these viruses produce degenerative changes in absorptive cells, minor shortening of villi and crypt hyperplasia, and inflammatory cell infiltration of the lamina propria.

Rare viral infections of the large bowel include cytomegalovirus and lymphogranuloma venereum. Cytomegalovirus colitis has been described as both a primary infection and as a complication of ulcerative colitis. Infection is readily recognised by the presence of large intranuclear inclusions in cells within the mucosa. Proctitis due to *lymphogranuloma venereum* is principally a disease of females. The infection begins in the genital tract and is thought to spread to the rectum via lymphatics. The deeper tissues are most heavily involved, and rectal stricture is the likely clinical problem. While non-specific chronic inflammation is usually pronounced, granulomas are a characteristic histological finding and these may show central necrosis when the disease is active.

FUNGAL INFECTIONS

Fungal infections of the alimentary tract are rare. Histoplasmosis may produce a striking picture of multiple inflammatory polyps in the small and large intestines, and on microscopy the intracellular *Histoplasma capsulatum* can be identified.

Mucor and *Rhizopus* are phycomycetes with non-septate hyphae which are widely distributed in nature. Though these organisms are usually non-pathogenic, gastrointestinal involvement in debilitated or immunosuppressed patients is becoming increasingly common. The oesophagus, stomach and colon are most frequently involved, and in addition to ulceration there is thrombosis of submucosal vessels with intravascular growth of the fungi. Despite this propensity for vascular infection, distant spread is surprisingly rare.

PARASITIC DISEASES

Giardiasis

Infection with the protozoan parasite *Giardia lamblia*

produces a generally mild malabsorption state. It is a cause of 'traveller's diarrhoea', and of diarrhoea in childhood, in people with IgA deficiency, and following gastric surgery. It has been suggested that the malabsorption state is due to heavy infestation blocking access of nutrients to the surface epithelium; however, this is unlikely, as the numbers of organisms are rarely sufficient.

Amoebiasis

Amoebiasis is a disease of the large intestine resulting from infection with the protozoan *Entamoeba histolytica*. It is worldwide in its distribution, though more prevalent in the tropics than in temperate climates. Vegetative forms are present in the large bowel in infected individuals; these are passed in the stools, encyst into a more resistant form, and may survive in food and fluid and be reingested later. The cysts pass unharmed through the stomach and on reaching the intestine the cyst wall is dissolved, liberating the active amoebae. These secrete a cytolytic enzyme which enables them to pass through the intestinal epithelium and, in disrupting the mucosa, release red blood cells which they then ingest. Contamination of food and water is brought about by human carriers, infected rats, or flies. Carriers may either be individuals known to have suffered an attack in the past, or be apparently healthy people, some of whom may have symptomless lesions in the bowel.

The disease can lead to discrete oval ulcers, which are characteristically 'flask-shaped' in section, or to a diffuse colitis.

Balantidiasis

Balantidiasis is a rare form of colitis caused by the ciliated protozoan *Balantidium coli*. It may be acute or chronic. Most cases are found in tropical or subtropical countries among debilitated, malnourished individuals. Gross and microscopic findings in the tissues are much like those in amoebiasis. The organism is readily detected by microscopy in both the lumen and the mucosa: it is so large as to dwarf the surrounding host cells.

Schistosomiasis

Infestation of the large intestine by *Schistosoma* occurs most commonly with *Schistosoma mansoni* and *S. japonicum* but can also be found with *S. haematobium*. Humans may become infected while wading or bathing in water contaminated with the second larval stage (cercaria) of the fluke. The cercariae penetrate the skin, enter venules, and are carried through the circulation to the portal veins in the liver where they mature to form the adult flukes (Fig. 15.13). The adults migrate to either the submucosal veins of the gut, or the venous plexus in the bladder, where they lay their eggs. The ova pass through the intestinal wall into the faeces or through the bladder wall into the urine. The cycle is completed in water contaminated with egg-containing urine or faeces. The eggs hatch out, liberating miracidia (first larval stage) which infect a snail, the intermediate host within which the second larval stage of cercariae develop, later to emerge in their free-swimming form.

The pathological changes in schistosomiasis are essentially the result of an inflammatory reaction to the eggs in the tissues of the intestinal wall. Lesions are commonest in the rectum and left colon and are then nearly always due to *S. mansoni*; if the lesions are in the right side of the colon and the appendix then *S. haematobium* may be responsible.

Cryptosporidiosis

Cryptosporidiosis is caused by a coccidial organism of the genus *Cryptosporidium*. These are common parasites in a variety of reptiles, birds and mammals, but were not believed until recently to infect or cause diarrhoea in humans. It is now appreciated that they are a frequent cause of diarrhoea in children, and they are increasingly encountered in AIDS sufferers. A severe acute colitis with surface exudation and ulceration may be produced. Cryptosporidia cannot be recognised in stool specimens, so that a biopsy or mucosal scraping is needed to make the diagnosis.

INFLAMMATORY DISORDERS

Crohn's disease

▶ Chronic inflammatory disorder of unknown aetiology
▶ Small bowel most commonly affected, but any part of the gut may be involved
▶ Characterised by transmural inflammation with granulomas
▶ Thickened and fissured bowel leads to intestinal obstruction and fistulation

It was not until 1932 that Burrill Bernard Crohn and

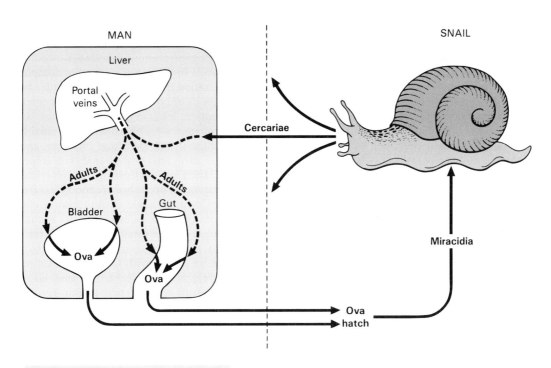

Fig. 15.13 Life-cycle of *Schistosoma*

See text for details.

his colleagues established regional enteritis as a distinct entity. Previously, the condition had been confused with intestinal tuberculosis, then a common disease in Western countries. The chronic inflammation and ulceration in Crohn's disease predominantly affect the terminal ileum, but all parts of the alimentary tract from the mouth to the anus may be involved and more than one site may be affected. 'Satellite' lesions can also occur in skin remote from the peri-anal area. However, involvement outside the small and large intestine is uncommon. About two-thirds of patients have only small-intestinal involvement, about one-sixth only large-intestinal involvement, and in one-sixth of patients both small and large bowel are affected.

Crohn's disease usually presents with either small-intestinal obstruction or abdominal pain which may mimic acute appendicitis; other presentations can relate to its complications (see below). The course of the disease is chronic, with exacerbations and remissions not always linked to therapy. Onset is usually in early adult life, with about half of all cases beginning between the ages of 20 and 30 years and 90% between 10 and 40 years. Slightly more males than females are affected.

Morphology

Involvement by Crohn's disease is frequently segmental, that is lengths of diseased bowel are separated by apparently normal tissue. Such separated segments of disease are referred to as 'skip lesions'.

The earliest evidence of involvement visible with the naked eye is presence of small discrete shallow ulcers with a haemorrhagic rim. These ulcers have been likened to the common aphthous ulcers of the mouth and are thus often described as 'aphthoid'; however there is no aetiological link between the two conditions. Later, the more characteristic longitudinal ulcers develop which progress into deep fissures (Fig. 15.14). The process comes to involve the full thickness of the wall and subsequent fibrosis leads to considerable narrowing in the diseased segments (Fig. 15.15). This produces a characteristic radiological sign where only a trickle of contrast medium passes through the affected segment (the 'string sign'). Where longitudinal fissures cross oedematous transverse mucosal folds, a 'cobblestone' appearance results. The mesenteric lymph nodes are enlarged by reactive hyperplasia and may also contain granulomas.

Microscopy reflects the gross appearances. Inflammatory involvement is discontinuous: it is focal or patchy. Collections of lymphocytes and plasma cells are found, mainly in the mucosa and submucosa but usually affecting all layers (transmural inflammation). The classical microscopic feature of Crohn's disease is the presence of granulomas. These consist of epithelioid macrophages and giant cells surrounded by a cuff of lymphocytes. The giant cells are usually of the Langhans' type, but may resemble foreign body giant cells. The granulomas are distinguished from those of tuberculosis by the absence of central caseous necrosis. While they are virtually diagnostic of the condition, granulomas are found in only 60% of cases of Crohn's disease; in their absence the diagnosis must be based on a summation of the less specific histological changes. In addition to the aggregated transmural pattern of inflammation, these changes include the finding of vertical fissure ulcers and marked submucosal oedema, lymphangiectasia, fibrosis and neuromatoid hyperplasia (enlargement and proliferation of submucosal nerves).

Complications

The complications of Crohn's disease are summarised in Table 15.4. Widespread involvement of the small intestine can lead to a malabsorption syndrome, but the commonest cause of malabsorption in Crohn's disease is iatrogenic. Repeated resections of small intestine can lead to a 'short bowel syndrome' in which adequate nutrition can be maintained only by intravenous or intraperitoneal alimentation. Fistula formation is a frequent complication; deep penetration by ulcers produces fistulae between adherent loops of bowel and, particularly after surgical intervention, leads to entero-cutaneous fistulae.

Approximately 60% of patients have anal lesions. These include simple skin 'tags', fissures, and fistulae into the anal canal or peri-anal skin. Acute complications such as perforation, haemorrhage and toxic dilatation do occur but are much less frequently seen in Crohn's disease than ulcerative colitis. In the long term, there is an increased risk of malignancy, particularly in the small intestine, but the overall risk is less than in patients with ulcerative colitis because more people with Crohn's disease have the affected areas resected. Systemic amyloidosis is a rare, long-term complication which results from excessive production of serum amyloid A protein (Ch. 7).

Aetiology and pathogenesis

The incidence of idiopathic inflammatory bowel disease (Crohn's disease and ulcerative colitis) shows

A　　　　　　CROHN'S DISEASE

B　　　　　　ULCERATIVE COLITIS

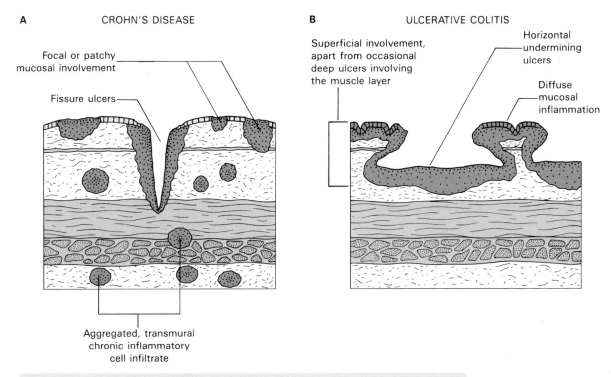

Focal or patchy
mucosal involvement

Fissure ulcers

Aggregated, transmural
chronic inflammatory
cell infiltrate

Superficial involvement,
apart from occasional
deep ulcers involving
the muscle layer

Horizontal
undermining
ulcers

Diffuse
mucosal
inflammation

Fig. 15.14　Comparison of the lesions of Crohn's disease and those of ulcerative colitis

considerable geographic variation. These diseases have a much higher incidence in northern Europe and the United States than in countries of southern Europe, Africa, South America and Asia, although increasing urbanisation and prosperity is leading to a higher incidence in parts of southern Europe and Japan. Even within Europe and the USA the incidence of Crohn's disease varies widely from around 4 to 65 affected persons per 100 000 population. There are, however, interesting ethnic differences: Jewish populations in Israel have a much higher incidence than Bedouin Arabs in the same locality. On

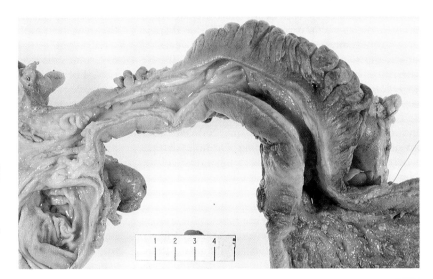

Fig. 15.15　Crohn's disease

The terminal ileum is severely narrowed due to thickening of the bowel wall by the chronic inflammatory process. On the right, the lumen is passively dilated in response to the presence of the obstructive lesion.

Table 15.4   Complications of Crohn's disease

Complication	Comment/Example
Malabsorption syndrome	Often iatrogenic ('short bowel syndrome')
Fistula formation	Causes malabsorption when loops of bowel are bypassed
Anal lesions	Skin tags, fissures, fistulae
Acute complications	Perforation (haemorrhage, toxic dilatation — rare)
Malignancy	Increased risk — adenocarcinoma
Systemic amyloidosis	Rare

the other hand, Ashkenazi Jews living in Israel have a lower incidence than those living in the United States. Such data indicate a stronger role for environmental than genetic factors. On epidemiological grounds, both Crohn's disease and ulcerative colitis are thought to be diseases brought about by genetic susceptibility to as yet undetermined environmental agents.

In Crohn's disease it has been proposed that a genetic defect, possibly in a major recessive gene, prevents the patient from mounting a controlled and effective immune response to the causative agent. Support for a genetic role comes from a twin study in Sweden where 44% of monozygous twins had Crohn's disease compared with 4% of dizygous twins. Other studies have sought a linkage to HLA types, and a higher prevalence of HLA-DR1 and DQw5 has been found in Crohn's disease. However, genetic links may be obscured by the heterogeneity within Crohn's disease; clinically there are two main groups, the first comprising patients whose disease goes into lasting remission within three years of onset, the second comprising patients with disease persisting beyond three years. Clearer links may emerge if these clinical subgroups were considered separately.

The most clearly determined environmental influence is that of cigarette smoking. Smokers have an increased risk of developing Crohn's disease whereas the opposite applies with ulcerative colitis. Nevertheless smoking is not incriminated as an *aetiological* agent in Crohn's disease. It has been suggested that, in genetically predisposed individuals, smoking habit will determine the type of inflammatory bowel disease that will develop. The most likely candidates as aetiological factors are infective agents.

Ever since a Scottish surgeon and farmer, Dalziel,

recognised the similarity between a mycobacterial infection, Johne's disease, affecting his pedigree cattle and Crohn's disease affecting some of his patients, there has been varying interest in the role of *Mycobacterium paratuberculosis* in Crohn's disease. Indeed, slow-growing mycobacteria biochemically and genetically identical to *M. paratuberculosis* have been isolated on rare occasions from Crohn's disease patients. However, similar organisms have also been isolated from patients with ulcerative colitis and other colonic disorders, and no specific serological response to *M. paratuberculosis* antigens can be found in Crohn's disease. Likewise, the results of tests for mycobacterial DNA by the polymerase chain reaction have also produced conflicting results, and trials of anti-mycobacterial treatment in Crohn's disease do not show any convincing improvement separate from the anti-inflammatory effects of some of the regimes. The case against *M. paratuberculosis* as an aetiological agent in Crohn's disease remains unproven.

Another line of investigation has pursued the role of microvascular infarction in the aetiology of Crohn's disease. Occlusion of the microcirculation is demonstrable in affected segments of intestine and there may even be granulomatous involvement of intramural and mesenteric arteries. Allied to this, there are the promoting effects of smoking and use of the contraceptive pill, which together with the finding of other pro-coagulant changes in Crohn's disease patients, lend circumstantial support to microthrombosis as a cause. It has been proposed that the triggering event is measles virus infection, which in certain genetically predisposed individuals leads to chronic endothelial injury, intravascular accumulation of monocytes and platelet aggregation, followed by occlusion of the microcirculation. This theory is even more controversial than the mycobacterial hypothesis. Public discussion of the aetiology of Crohn's disease invariably leads to inflamed opinions. The cause of inflammation, however, remains a mystery.

Whatever the aetiology, there is evidence of persistent and inappropriate T-cell and macrophage activation in Crohn's disease with increased production of pro-inflammatory cytokines, in particular interleukins 1, 2, 6 and 8, and interferon γ and TNFα. Crohn's disease is characterised by sustained (chronic) inflammation accompanied by fibrosis. The process of fibroblastic proliferation and collagen deposition may be mediated by transforming growth factor β which has certain anti-inflammatory actions, namely fibroblast recruitment, matrix synthesis and down-regulation of inflammatory cells, but it is likely that many other mediators will be implicated.

Ulcerative colitis

> ▶ Chronic relapsing inflammatory disorder, but may have an acute fulminating presentation
> ▶ Aetiology is unknown
> ▶ Affects only colon and rectum, sometimes confined to the latter
> ▶ Diffuse superficial inflammation
> ▶ Acute complications include toxic dilatation, perforation, haemorrhage and dehydration; the chronic complications are anaemia, liver disease and malignant change

In temperate climates ulcerative colitis is the commonest cause of diarrhoea associated with the passage of blood, mucus and pus. It is a non-specific inflammatory disorder of the large intestine, usually commencing in the rectum and extending proximally to a varying extent. Unlike Crohn's disease, ulcerative colitis is confined to the large intestine. Involvement of the terminal ileum in a so-called 'backwash ileitis' is occasionally seen, but this is thought to represent chronic inflammation provoked by incompetence of the ileo-caecal valve, rather than an actual part of the disease.

Aetiology

The geographic variation in the incidence of inflammatory bowel diseases has already been remarked upon (see p. 433). In northern Europe and the USA the incidence of ulcerative colitis varies between 12 and 140 per 100 000 population, but lower rates occur in underdeveloped countries with warmer climates. Part of the wide variation found in the northern, developed countries is attributable to a lack of uniformity in the inclusion of proctitis, some believing this to be ulcerative colitis confined to the rectum while others argue that it is a different disease entity. In low-incidence countries there may be diagnostic confusion with chronic infective colitis.

The consensus of opinion is in favour of a strong genetic predisposition towards ulcerative colitis; these genetic factors may operate at both the level of the host response and in the colonic mucosa. Differences in host response will be reflected in links to particular HLA types, cytokine genes and immunoglobulin marker genes. In ulcerative colitis there is an association with HLA-DR2 and with certain alleles of cytokine genes, and preferential pro-

duction of IgG1 compared with IgG2, the latter being increased in Crohn's disease. At the mucosal level, changes in permeability and in mucin glycoprotein composition have been found in ulcerative colitis but increased permeability may well be a consequence rather than a cause of the disease. Other evidence of a role for genetic factors comes from increased aggregations in families, a higher concordance rate in monozygotic twins, an increased prevalence in certain ethnic groups and association with diseases which have a known genetic predisposition such as ankylosing spondylitis, psoriasis and primary sclerosing cholangitis.

There is growing evidence to indicate that ulcerative colitis is a consequence of altered autoimmune reactivity but mucosal injury could also result from inappropriate T-cell activation and indirect damage brought about by cytokines, proteases and reactive oxygen metabolites from macrophages and neutrophils. This latter mechanism of damage to the colonic epithelium has been termed 'innocent bystander' injury. Evidence in favour of autoimmunity is the presence of self-reactive T-lymphocytes and auto-antibodies directed against colonic epithelial cells and endothelial cells, and anti-neutrophil cytoplasmic auto-antibodies (ANCA). However, these antibodies and self-reactive lymphocytes are not considered to be responsible for the tissue damage, and ulcerative colitis should not be thought of as an *autoimmune disease* in which mucosal injury is a *direct* consequence of an immunological reaction to self-antigens. Thus some of these autoimmune aspects are considered to be epiphenomena.

Inappropriate and persistent T-cell activation may lie at the centre of both ulcerative colitis and Crohn's disease. Under normal circumstances the mucosal immune system is tolerant of luminal foreign antigens, and this tolerance is dependent upon the relationship between colonic epithelium and suppressor T-cells. Changes in epithelial cell antigen presentation consequent upon the acquired expression of class II (HLA-DR) major histocompatibility molecules activate helper T-lymphocytes and initiate a cascade of cytokine-mediated effects which induce and sustain a mucosal immune reaction. The nature of the antigen or putative triggering factors is not known, but microbial antigens from the gut flora are likely candidates. This could account for the well-known triggering of ulcerative colitis by enteric infections. Interactions between the immune system and smoking, and the effects of stress and neuropeptide release on immune reactivity and mucosal inflammation, are capable of modulating the response to such triggering factors.

Whatever the initiating events it seems clear that the mucosal injury in ulcerative colitis is largely a consequence of polymorph accumulation in the mucosa and release of destructive proteases, nitric oxide and superoxide radicals. Polymorph emigration from mucosal vessels follows up-regulation of endothelial adhesion receptors, including E-selectin, ICAM-1 and VCAM (Ch. 10), by pro-inflammatory cytokines. Subsequent neutrophil production of leukotriene B4 and interleukin-8 attracts more polymorphs into the inflamed mucosa and amplifies their accumulation. Increased permeability and absorption of bacterial antigens may give rise to immune complex phenomena and some of the extra-intestinal complications.

Morphology

Ulcerative colitis is continuous in its distribution. Thus the disease, which is typically maximal in the rectum, extends proximally and continuously to involve the colon. Some cases are confined to the rectum (proctitis), others to the recto-sigmoid (distal colitis) while others may exhibit a total colitis extending into the caecum. The disease does not involve the mucosa of the anal transitional zone or the anal canal, but a small proportion of patients do have anal tags and fissures.

The ulcers are irregular in outline and orientation and become confluent (Fig. 15.16); they extend horizontally to undermine adjacent, less involved, mucosa which remains as discrete islands. Usually the ulceration remains superficial (Fig. 15.14), in-

volving mucosa and submucosa, but in severe cases there is extension into the main muscle coats and perforation is likely. There is intense hyperaemia of the intact mucosa and haemorrhage from the ulcers.

Microscopically, there is diffuse infiltration of the mucosa by mixed acute and chronic inflammatory cells. Polymorphs are seen in the interstitium, but are particularly evident as aggregates within distended crypts (crypt abscesses). There are widespread degenerative changes in surface and crypt lining epithelium, with marked depletion of their mucin content. Crypts undergo destruction during the acute phase, and when regeneration occurs they are frequently distorted by branching or dilatation. This disturbance of the crypt pattern is a useful diagnostic pointer in quiescent cases, when the inflammatory features may have totally subsided. Thus, in long-standing disease, rectal biopsy will reveal crypt atrophy and distortion, and there may be metaplastic features such as the acquisition of Paneth cells. Ulcerative colitis is a recognised premalignant condition, and a few cases will reveal epithelial dysplasia.

Complications

The complications of ulcerative colitis are summarised in Table 15.5.

Malignancy
The overall incidence of colorectal cancer in ulcerative colitis is low, around 2%, but this rises to about 10% in patients who have had the disease for

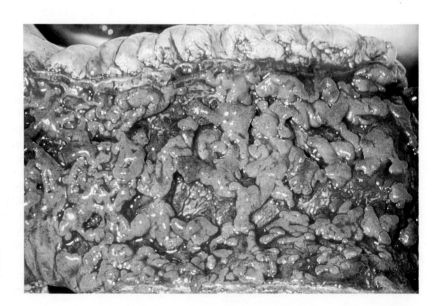

Fig. 15.16 Ulcerative colitis

The colonic mucosa is extensively ulcerated and haemorrhagic.

Table 15.5 Complications of ulcerative colitis

Complication	Comment/Example
Blood loss	May be: acute (haemorrhage)
	chronic, leading to anaemia
Electrolyte disturbances	Due to severe diarrhoea in acute phase
Toxic dilatation	May develop insidiously
Colorectal cancer	Overall incidence 2%
Skin involvement	Pigmentation, erythema nodosum, pyoderma gangrenosum
Liver involvement	Fatty change, chronic pericholangitis, sclerosing cholangitis, cirrhosis, hepatitis
Eye involvement	Iritis, uveitis, episcleritis
Joint involvement	Ankylosing spondylitis, arthritis

25 years. The increased risk over that for the general population warrants colonoscopic surveillance of longstanding cases. The clinical factors apparently associated with a higher cancer risk are:

- onset of the disease in childhood
- clinically severe first attack
- total involvement of the colon
- continuous rather than intermittent symptoms.

In practice, patients with extensive colitis of longer than 8–10 years' duration are usually admitted into surveillance programmes and undergo regular (usually annual) colonoscopy and multiple biopsy. If high-grade (severe) dysplasia is seen, then probably the patient already has a focus of cancer somewhere in the bowel and total resection is warranted.

Local complications
Haemorrhage is occasionally massive and life-threatening, but more often occurs as chronic blood loss leading to iron-deficiency anaemia. In the acute phase, severe diarrhoea with a markedly increased loss of water and mucus can lead to serious electrolyte disturbances. A further hazard of the acute phase is toxic dilatation. When ulceration affects large areas of muscle the viability and contractile strength is impaired. The resultant adynamic segment — commonly the transverse colon — becomes progressively distended, and the consequent thinning of the wall predisposes to perforation. Since there are few adhesions to localise its spread, perforation into the peritoneal cavity results in generalised faecal peritonitis and a fatal outcome is likely. Frequent radiographs should be taken in the seriously ill patient, since toxic dilatation may develop insidiously.

Systemic complications
Patients with ulcerative colitis are at risk of developing systemic problems (Table 15.5). These include:

- skin — *erythema nodosum* (subcutaneous

inflammation) and *pyoderma gangrenosum* (sterile dermal abscesses)
- liver — *pericholangitis* (inflammation around bile ducts), *sclerosing cholangitis* (fibrous constriction and obliteration of bile ducts), *cholangiocarcinoma*, and *chronic active hepatitis*
- eyes — *iritis, uveitis* and *episcleritis*
- joints — increased incidence of *ankylosing spondylitis*.

VASCULAR DISORDERS

Ischaemic injury to the intestine occurs either as a consequence of obstruction to the mesenteric arterial supply (*occlusive ischaemia*) or in circumstances where, despite patency of the vessels, the blood supply falls to a level at which the nutrition of mucosa cannot be maintained (*non-occlusive ischaemia*). Thus occlusive ischaemia results from arterial thrombosis (usually on the basis of atherosclerosis) or thrombo-embolism originating from atrial or ventricular mural thrombosis; non-occlusive ischaemia is a consequence of systemic hypotension, vasoconstriction, viscosity disturbances, arterial narrowing, and of certain drugs, such as digitalis and cocaine.

Pathogenesis

Total vascular occlusion results in segmental anoxic or hypoxic injury, the extent of which depends on the adequacy of the collateral supply; cell death appears to ensue from a lethal ingress of calcium ions through the damaged plasma membrane. However, much of the mucosal injury in non-occlusive ischaemia develops after the period of hypoperfusion, i.e. when normal perfusion and oxygenation have been restored. This is an example of a 'reperfusion injury' of the kind seen after myocardial and cerebral ischaemia and following iatrogenic ischaemia in organ transplantation. Reperfusion injuries are thought to be mediated by free radical formation (Ch. 6). These oxygen-derived free radicals are responsible for the membrane injuries which bring about mucosal disintegration in the reperfusion phase.

Acute ischaemia

Acute ischaemia results in varying degrees of infarction of the bowel wall. Such infarcts can be classified, according to the depth of involvement, as either mucosal, mural or transmural (Fig. 15.17).

Mucosal infarction
Mucosal infarction is usually considered transient or reversible because the lesion can be followed by complete regeneration. However, mucosal damage leads to release of proteolytic enzymes and increased permeability to toxic substances; this can bring about further cardiovascular deterioration and gradual progression of the intestinal lesion to transmural infarction.

Mural infarction
Mural infarction reaches into the submucosa or into, but not through, the muscularis propria. The mucosa is variably ulcerated and, where intact, is haemorrhagic and elevated by marked submucosal oedema. The deeper extent of necrosis with involvement of connective tissues necessitates healing by granulation tissue formation and a more prolonged process of repair. If the patient recovers, this is likely to lead to fibrous stricture formation.

Transmural infarction
Transmural infarction of the intestine extends through the muscularis propria and is synonymous with gangrene. The bowel becomes flaccid and dilates, and the serosal aspect is deeply congested and coated in a thin layer of fibrin. The wall becomes friable and liable to perforation. Segmental infarction results either from occlusion of distal mesenteric vessels which is sufficiently widespread to impair the collateral supply, or by mechanical obstruction of the supply to a loop of intestine. This type of involvement is amenable to surgical treatment, but many patients already have peritonitis, endotoxaemia and severe circulatory problems at the time of diagnosis so that operative results remain poor. Massive infarction, most commonly seen in the small intestine following complete occlusion of the superior mesenteric artery, has a hopeless prognosis.

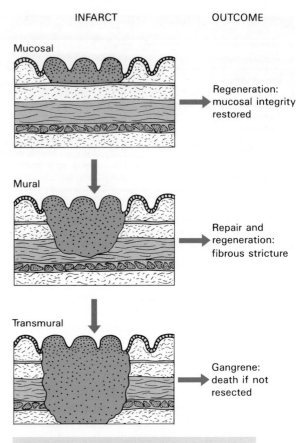

INFARCT OUTCOME

Mucosal

Regeneration: mucosal integrity restored

Mural

Repair and regeneration: fibrous stricture

Transmural

Gangrene: death if not resected

Fig. 15.17 Acute intestinal infarction and its outcome

Chronic ischaemia

Chronic ischaemia leads to two main problems:

- fibrous stricture formation following segmental mural infarction
- chronic mesenteric insufficiency.

Strictures are encountered most often in the large intestine, particularly in the 'watershed' area around the splenic flexure of the colon. The patients generally present with the consequences of large bowel obstruction. Chronic mesenteric insufficiency is used to describe a condition in which there is insufficient blood flow to the small intestine to satisfy the demands of increased motility, secretion and absorption that develop after meals. The insufficiency is usually manifest as pain (so-called *mesenteric angina*), but patients may also have diarrhoea and malabsorption.

Necrotising enterocolitis

Necrotising enterocolitis is an uncommon condition which arises through a combination of ischaemia and infection. The disease is manifested as severe abdominal pain, distension and diarrhoea. Paralytic ileus develops and progresses to intestinal infarction, sepsis and shock. The appearances are typically those of gas gangrene, with either segmental or total involvement of the small and large intestines by coagulative necrosis and intramural gas bubble formation.

Most cases of necrotising enterocolitis are seen in neonates, where the interplay of intestinal ischaemia, bacterial colonisation and excess protein substrate in the intestinal lumen in bottle-fed babies is the main cause. In adults the disease is related to *Clostridium perfringens* infection.

Vascular anomalies

Vascular anomalies in the gut are uncommon but enter into the differential diagnosis of gastrointestinal haemorrhage. Their classification is confused; some are congenital malformations which form part of recognised syndromes, while other, possibly identical, lesions are claimed to be acquired. Congenital types include arteriovenous malformations and telangiectasias; acquired forms are usually termed angiodysplasias. *Angiodysplasia* of the colon is an occasional cause of blood loss from the large bowel. This condition is more common in the elderly and can be diagnosed by mesenteric angiography.

DISORDERS RESULTING FROM ABNORMAL GUT MOTILITY

Diverticular disease

Diverticula are herniations of mucosa into the intestinal wall. The herniations are of the pulsion type and form at sites of potential weakness, notably where lymphoid aggregates breach the muscularis mucosae. They extend through the muscularis propria at the point of entry or exit of blood vessels and bulge into the subserosa.

Diverticula can be found anywhere in the intestinal tract, but the colon, and particularly the sigmoid, is by far the commonest site (Fig. 15.18). Most diverticula occur between the mesenteric and anti-mesenteric longitudinal muscle bands — the taenia coli. The affected segment of colon shows thickening of the muscularis propria, and prominence of the mucosal folds so that they almost occlude the lumen. The disease is generally acknowledged to result from a deficiency of fibre in the diet. Sigmoid motility is peculiarly sensitive to the bulk of the colonic contents and when this is low, due to a low-fibre diet, abnormally high intra-luminal pressures are generated which push the diverticula into the wall.

Complications

Diverticular disease presents as abdominal pain and altered bowel habit, but it is also prone to develop some serious complications, ˙the most common

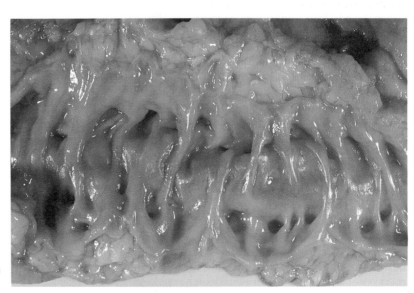

Fig. 15.18 Diverticulosis of the sigmoid colon

The mucosal surface is ridged due to hypertrophy of the underlying muscle. The openings of the diverticula can be seen between the mucosal ridges.

being *diverticulitis*. The faecal contents can lead to abrasion of the herniated mucosa, or a microscopic perforation in the apex of a diverticulum can occur, which allows infection by faecal organisms and the development of a suppurative diverticulitis. This in turn can cause a peri-colic abscess and a *fistula* may form into the bladder, vagina or small intestine; more seriously, a peri-diverticular abscess may perforate and produce a generalised faecal peritonitis.

Diverticula can be the source of *haemorrhage* from the colon. This usually arises from areas of granulation tissue in an inflamed diverticulum, but the precise source is sometimes difficult to identify.

Intussusception

An intussusception is an invagination of one segment of bowel into another thus causing intestinal obstruction. A lesion in the wall of the bowel disturbs normal peristaltic contractions, forcing the lesion and a segment of proximal bowel into a distal segment. Several lesions can act as the apex of an intussusception, including polyps, ingested foreign bodies, a Meckel's diverticulum, an area of intramural haemorrhage, and lymphoid hyperplasia. Such hyperplasia close to the ileo-caecal valve is the cause of the ileo-colic intussusception, the most common form of this disorder.

Volvulus and strangulation

Intestinal obstruction can result from a twist in the bowel which occludes its lumen (*volvulus*) or when a segment of bowel becomes trapped in a defect in either the posterior peritoneum or mesentery (internal herniation), or herniates into an inguinal or para-umbilical peritoneal sac. The neck of the sac may then constrict the bowel and compromise its blood supply (*strangulation*). Volvulus occurs around a 'fulcrum' such as a Meckel's diverticulum or a congenital band of fibrous tissue, or around an abnormally long mesentery. About two-thirds of cases affect the small intestine; most of the remaining one-third affect the sigmoid colon.

TUMOURS

Paradoxically, the small intestine, with its vast surface area and a higher cell turnover rate than any other tissue in the body, is an uncommon site for primary neoplasms. For example, benign epithelial neoplasms (adenomas) and adenocarcinomas are distinctly rare in the small intestine, yet in the large bowel represent a very common form of neoplasia. The low incidence of carcinoma means that other neoplasms, such as endocrine cell tumours and lymphomas, assume more importance in the small intestine where they are relatively more common than in the large bowel.

Polyps

A polyp is simply a protuberant growth and there is thus a wide variety of histological types. These can be broadly divided into *epithelial* and *mesenchymal* polyps (of which the latter are distinctly uncommon), and into *benign* and *malignant* categories (Table 15.6). Even epithelial polyps are rare in the small intestine and some, such as metaplastic polyps, are confined to the large bowel. Thus, the following account is confined to large-intestinal polyps.

Benign epithelial polyps

Benign epithelial polyps fall into four categories: adenomas, and inflammatory, hamartomatous and metaplastic polyps.

Adenomas
The most important of the epithelial polyps are the neoplastic polyps; these, being derived from a secretory epithelium, are termed adenomas. Adenomas are very common; there is an increase in incidence with age so that at 60 years they are found in about

Table 15.6	Polyps of the large intestine	
Type of polyp	Benign	Malignant
Epithelial	Neoplastic Adenoma Inflammatory (e.g. in inflammatory bowel disease) Hamartomatous Juvenile polyp Peutz–Jeghers syndrome Metaplastic (or hyperplastic)	Polypoid adenocarcinomas Carcinoid polyps
Mesenchymal	Lipoma Lymphangioma Haemangiomas Fibromas Leiomyoma	Sarcomas Lymphomatous polyps

20% of the population. There are two main histological types — *tubular* (75%) and *villous* (10%); the remaining 15% are intermediate in pattern and are designated *tubulo-villous*.

Tubular adenomas are generally small (usually less than 10 mm in diameter), and macroscopically resemble a raspberry. Most have a stalk (pedunculated) and a minority have a broad base (sessile). Microscopically, they consist of numerous cross-sectioned crypt profiles lined by mucus-secreting epithelium showing varying degrees of dysplasia.

Villous adenomas are usually sessile; they are often over 20 mm in diameter and some extend over a wide area as a thick, carpet-like growth. Microscopically, they consist of elongated villi in a papillary growth pattern; the villi are again lined by columnar epithelium showing dysplasia. Large adenomas may secrete copious electrolyte-rich mucus resulting in hypokalaemia and acute renal failure, but their real importance lies in their propensity for malignant change.

Inflammatory polyps
These usually arise in the context of inflammatory bowel disease, and represent excessive reparative and regenerative tissue formed in the aftermath of mucosal ulceration. In most cases there is a preponderance of granulation or mature fibrovascular tissue, so their categorisation as epithelial is somewhat debatable.

Hamartomatous polyps
These rare polyps may be solitary, like the majority of so-called 'juvenile' polyps, or be multiple and occur throughout the gastrointestinal tract, as in *Peutz–Jeghers syndrome*.

Metaplastic (or hyperplastic) polyps
These polyps are of unknown histogenesis, but the surface cells are hypermature compared to normal epithelium. They are common lesions, being found with increasing age, and are most frequently situated in the rectum. Microscopically they are sessile with elongated crypts, but the majority show no dysplasia. Their characteristic feature is the 'serrated' appearance of the cells lining the upper crypt and at the surface. Unlike adenomas, these polyps have no malignant potential.

Malignant epithelial polyps

Examples of malignant epithelial polyps are polypoid carcinomas and carcinoid (EEC — from entero-endocrine cells) polyps. Some adenocarcinomas develop as protuberant growths and appear endoscopically as polyps, hence the term 'polypoid carcinoma'. The vast majority of adenocarcinomas, however, arise within pre-existing adenomas and these constitute the bulk of 'malignant polyps'. A very small minority of polyps are neoplasms derived from entero-endocrine cells; such carcinoid polyps have a low malignant potential and only give rise to metastases late in their course. Thus, complete local removal is usually curative.

Benign mesenchymal polyps

Mesenchymal polyps are uncommon. The benign forms are lipomas, haemangiomas, lymphangiomas and fibromas. Smooth muscle tumours are less likely to present as polyps, and are of uncertain malignant potential.

Malignant mesenchymal polyps

Malignant varieties include the sarcomas equivalent to the benign tumours, and lymphomatous polyps.

The adenoma–carcinoma sequence

Adenomas are probably the precursors of most, if not all, colorectal cancers. Evidence in favour of a link comes from a number of sources, but one of the strongest associations is illustrated by the condition of *familial adenomatous polyposis* (FAP). FAP is a rare autosomal disease carried by either parent and transmitted as a Mendelian dominant. Both sexes are equally affected. Adenomas, mainly in the large intestine (Fig. 15.19) but also in the small, develop during the second and third decades and subsequently undergo malignant change with an almost inevitable progression to cancer by the age of 35. The gene responsible for FAP is on the long arm of chromosome 5; interestingly, a somatic mutation has been identified on chromosome 5 in cases of sporadic (non-inherited) colorectal cancer (see below).

Epidemiological support comes from the marked geographic variation in the prevalence of adenomas, and a strong correlation with the incidence of colorectal carcinoma in the same countries.

Adenomas and carcinomas are frequently found together in a resected segment of bowel. Such patients have an increased risk of developing a second cancer, compared with patients having carcinoma alone. Histologically, the finding of residual adenomatous tissue in many cancers, and the observation of early invasive malignancy developing in

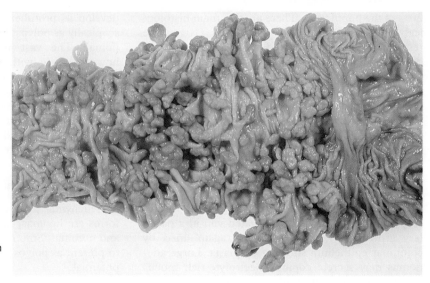

Fig. 15.19 Familial adenomatous polyposis

The colonic mucosa is studded with numerous adenomatous polyps. These are premalignant.

adenomas, is further supportive evidence of a link. Examination of adenomas showing early malignancy has demonstrated in association with increasing size, villous growth pattern and more severe degrees of dysplasia.

Molecular pathology of the adenoma–carcinoma sequence

In no other tumour system are the genetic events underlying the development of carcinoma as clearly understood as they are in colorectal cancer. In general, these genetic defects are:

- activation of oncogenes
- loss or mutations of tumour suppressor genes
- defective genes of the DNA repair pathway leading to genomic instability.

The oncogenes most frequently altered in colorectal cancer are c-Ki-*ras* and c-*myc*. Point mutations in Ki-*ras* mean that the protein can no longer hydrolyse bound GTP to GDP. Persistence of GTP-*ras*, the active form of the protein, results in continual signalling of cell division. Over-expression of c-*myc* is a feature of most colorectal cancers; c-*myc* encodes a nuclear phosphoprotein which is required for DNA synthesis and increased expression may well be followed by increased cellular proliferation.

Tumour suppressor genes appear to be very important in colorectal carcinoma. FAP results from point mutations in a tumour suppressor gene, APC, localised on chromosome 5q, and subsequent deletion of the accompanying normal allele results in loss of tumour suppressor function which leads to colo-

rectal cancer. Mutations and deletions of the APC gene, and in other tumour suppressor genes, have also been identified in sporadic (i.e. non-hereditary) colorectal cancer. Other genes implicated are MCC (mutated in colorectal cancer), DCC (deleted in colorectal cancer), c-*yes*, *bcl*-2 and p53 genes. *bcl*-2 is a key inhibitor of apoptosis; over-expression renders the cell more resistant to degrees of damage which would normally result in apoptosis and elimination of the cell. As a consequence 'faulty' cells may remain in the stem cell pool. The p53 gene product is a nuclear protein which can apply a checkpoint in the G_1 phase of the cell cycle and allow time for successful DNA repair or divert the cell towards apoptosis and elimination.

Mutation or loss of the p53 gene is not the only way in which DNA repair can be compromised. Highly conserved genes have been discovered which recognise mismatched nucleotides in complementary DNA strands and orchestrate the enzymes that effect repairs. Alterations in two mismatch repair genes, hMLH1 and hMSH2, have been identified in kindreds with hereditary non-polyposis colorectal cancer and it seems likely that similar alterations in these and other 'housekeeper' genes will be found in sporadic cancers. Finally, deletion of the nm23 gene may be related to an increased metastatic potential.

The sequence of these genetic events in causing colorectal cancer is not as critical as the accumulation of changes, but the different prevalences of mutations and deletions between premalignant lesions and invasive carcinoma does suggest that there is a preferred order (Fig. 15.20).

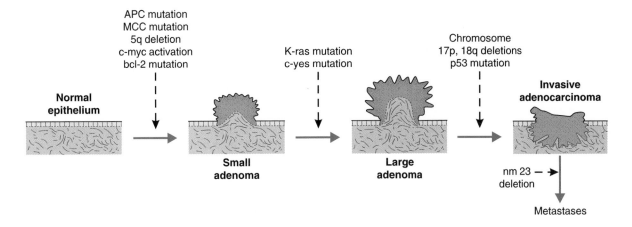

Fig. 15.20   Molecular genetics of adenoma–carcinoma sequence
Analysis of adenomas, small and large, and of invasive carcinomas and their metastases reveals a cascade of gene mutations, deletions and activations corresponding to the altered behaviour of the tumour cells.

Colorectal cancer

▶ Common malignancy in developed countries
▶ All are adenocarcinomas
▶ Increased risk in patients with adenomatous polyps and longstanding ulcerative colitis
▶ Dukes' staging, based on local extent and metastatic status, is the best guide to prognosis

Cancer of the colon and rectum is one of the commonest forms of malignancy in developed countries. It accounts for about 10% of all cancer registrations in the United Kingdom, where the death rate is second only to that of lung cancer, with gastric cancer a close third. The incidence appears to be rising.

Aetiology
Apart from the role played by inherited genetic factors, and a few cases developing in the unstable mucosa of ulcerative colitis, the most important factor in the aetiology of colorectal cancer appears to be environmental. Epidemiological evidence indicates that this is dietary. Diet affects the bacterial flora of the large bowel, the bowel transit time, and the amount of cellulose, amino acids and bile acids in the bowel contents. It is known that certain kinds of bacteria, the nuclear dehydrogenating clostridia (NDC), can act on bile acids to produce carcinogens. Similarly, bacterial transformation of amino acids may result in carcinogen (or co-carcinogen) production. On the other hand, a high content of fermentable cellulose leads to high levels of volatile fatty acids which appear to be 'protective' in that they provide nutrition and aid maturation of the epithelial cells. Thus, the type of diet which is linked to colorectal cancer is a high-fat, high-protein, low-fibre diet. High fat leads to an increase in bile salt production and higher load of faecal bile acids to react with NDC; high protein favours the transformation of amino acids by bacteria; low fibre reduces volatile fatty acids and prolongs intestinal transit so that there is more time for bacterial action on the contents and more prolonged contact between any carcinogen generated and the mucosa. These factors, more than anything else, account for the high incidence of colorectal cancer in developed countries.

Clinicopathological features
Approximately 50% of cancers occur in the rectum, where they are equally divided between the upper, middle and lower thirds; about 30% occur in the sigmoid colon and the rest are equally distributed in the ascending, transverse and descending colon. This anatomical distribution is of practical importance, since about 50% of large bowel cancers can be reached with the examining finger and 80% with the sigmoidoscope.

In the rectum, the majority of cancers are of the ulcerating type (Fig. 15.21) which usually present with rectal bleeding. The stenosing type is more common in the descending colon and sigmoid, where it usually produces obstruction relatively early

443

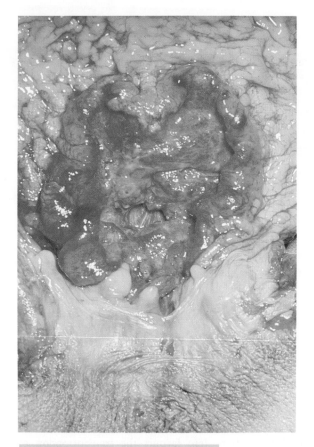

Fig. 15.21 Carcinoma of the rectum

Ulcerated carcinoma arising in the lower rectum close to and invading the anal canal.

because of the narrowing of the lumen and the solid consistency of the faeces at this site. Polypoid and larger fungating cancers are more common in the right colon, where they tend to give rise to recurrent occult bleeding; the patient may present late with iron-deficiency anaemia or change in bowel habit.

Microscopically the cancers are adenocarcinomas, showing varying degrees of mucin production and differentiation. To a limited extent, the degree of differentiation (grade) determines the outlook for the patient after surgery, but a much more valuable guide to prognosis is the completeness of excision and the extent of spread. If microscopic examination of the resection margins (especially the circumferential margin) establishes that the operation has been potentially curative, then the extent of spread through the bowel wall and the presence of lymph node metastases are the major prognostic determi-

nants. The extent of spread is given by the Dukes' stage (Fig. 15.22). Unfortunately, only about 70% of patients with colorectal cancer undergo a potentially curative operation; in about 15–25% of patients only a palliative operation is possible because they have widespread peritoneal deposits or liver secondaries, and the remainder are totally inoperable. However, with technical advances, patients formerly considered inoperable are undergoing resection of liver metastases, so that the number of operations for 'cure' will increase.

APUD cell tumours

The endocrine cells of the gut are part of a diffuse system present thoughout many tissues which utilises amino acids, or derivatives of amino acids, as chemical messengers mediating paracrine and neurocrine effects. They are known by the acronym APUD (amine precursor uptake and decarboxylation) cells and may be divided into two broad categories (Fig. 15.23).

- *Enterochromaffin cells.* These are cells found in small groups at the bases of the intestinal crypts which are named for their staining after chromate fixation. They secrete 5-hydroxytryptamine (5-HT) and kallikrein, and give rise to carcinoid tumours.
- *Entero-endocrine cells.* More dispersed single cells are found scattered in the crypt and villous epithelium, and in the bowel wall. They are nonchromaffin, and secrete a multiplicity of gut regulatory peptides. These are generally referred to as entero-endocrine cells. Although the cells are capable of producing more than one peptide, when neoplasms develop they are identified by their major product and are therefore designated as gastrinoma, somatostatinoma, etc. Most of these neoplasms, which are rare, arise in the pancreas rather than in the intestine.

The great majority of APUD cell tumours of the gastrointestinal tract are carcinoid tumours ('argentaffinomas') of mid-gut origin and are found in the appendix and ileum. Those in the appendix are generally small (less than 20 mm diameter), situated at or near the tip, and are discovered incidentally in specimens removed for abdominal pain. Such tumours can be considered benign, and no further treatment is necessary. However, larger tumours in the appendix and carcinoids of the ileum exhibit a tendency to spread to regional lymph nodes and the liver, and must be considered as tumours of low-grade malignancy. Mid-gut carcinoids produce vary-

DUKES' STAGE   FIVE-YEAR SURVIVAL

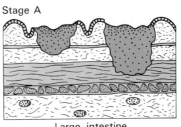

Stage A

Large intestine

90+%

Stage B

70%

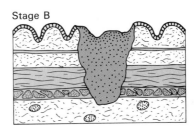

Stage C

35%

Fig. 15.22   Dukes' staging

A. The tumour is confined to the submucosa or muscle layer. **B.** The tumour has spread through the muscle layer, but does not yet involve the lymph nodes. **C.** Any tumour involving lymph nodes.

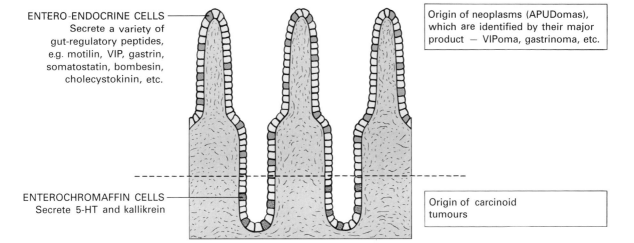

ENTERO-ENDOCRINE CELLS
Secrete a variety of gut-regulatory peptides, e.g. motilin, VIP, gastrin, somatostatin, bombesin, cholecystokinin, etc.

Origin of neoplasms (APUDomas), which are identified by their major product — VIPoma, gastrinoma, etc.

ENTEROCHROMAFFIN CELLS
Secrete 5-HT and kallikrein

Origin of carcinoid tumours

Fig. 15.23   APUD cell tumours of the gastrointestinal tract

ing amounts of 5-HT which exerts local effects but is inactivated in the liver by monoamine oxidases to form 5-hydroxyindole acetic acid (5-HIAA), and this is excreted in the urine. The local effects comprise diarrhoea and borborygmi (excessive bowel sounds) because 5-HT stimulates intestinal contractility. Once metastases have formed in the liver the products (5-HT and kinins) are released into the hepatic veins and can affect the right side of the heart and the lungs before oxidation takes place in the pulmonary vasculature; this results in the *carcinoid syndrome*. The patient develops flushing of the face, cyanosis, and stenosis or incompetence of the pulmonary and tricuspid valves. The heart shows smooth muscle proliferation within the endocardium; this is thought to result from bradykinin stimulation of mesenchymal cells which undergo differentiation to muscle cells. The development of carcinoid tumours and their effects are summarised in Figure 15.24.

Lymphomas

Lymphomas are the commonest form of malignancy in the small intestine but are rare in the large bowel. Mention has already been made of the development of malignant lymphoma in coeliac disease, but this accounts for only a small proportion of the total; the majority of cases in developed countries have no predisposing cause. In the Middle East and South Africa, however, lymphoma of the small intestine frequently follows alpha heavy chain disease, a condition in which there is an initially benign proliferation of plasma cells secreting incomplete immunoglobulins.

The non-coeliac-associated lymphomas are most commonly of B-cell lineage and of centrocytic or centroblastic types. They appear as plaques or polypoid masses and may be multiple, and give rise to abdominal pain, obstruction (either directly or by intussusception), and anaemia through intestinal blood loss.

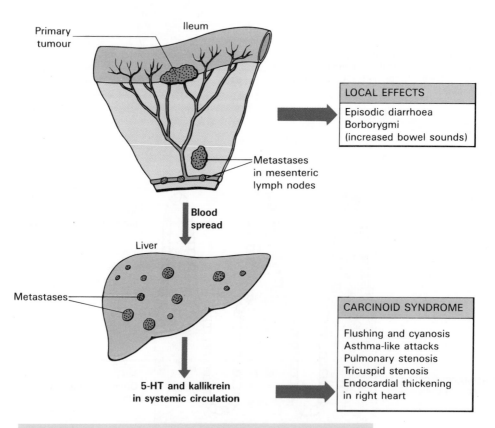

Fig. 15.24 Carcinoid tumours of the small intestine and their effects

See text for details.

The appendix can be the site for carcinoid tumours, adenocarcinomas and lymphomas, but these are rare compared with the frequency of non-specific suppurative inflammation.

APPENDICITIS

> ▶ Commmon cause of the 'acute abdomen'
> ▶ Inflammation often precipitated by obstruction due to faecolith, lymphoid hyperplasia or tumour
> ▶ Complications include peritonitis, portal pyaemia and hepatic abscesses

Aetiology

Several factors are claimed to predispose to acute inflammation of the appendix, including faecoliths (hard pellets of faeces arising from dehydration and compaction) and food residues, lymphoid hyperplasia (as occurs in childhood and with some viral infections), diverticulosis of the appendix, and the presence of a carcinoid tumour.

Specific inflammations can also affect the appendix, and very occasional cases are due to *Yersinia pseudotuberculosis*, typhoid, tuberculosis and actinomycosis. The appendix is also involved by ulcerative colitis and Crohn's disease.

Pathogenesis

Acute inflammation commences in the mucosa following a breach in the epithelium which permits infection by bowel flora. Infection leads to mucosal ulceration and a polymorph response, with exudation of cells and fibrin into the lumen. Further spread involves all the layers of the appendix and eventually causes a peritonitis over the serosal aspect. The build-up of fluid exudate within the wall increases tissue pressure and this, together with toxic damage to blood vessels and thrombosis, can lead to superimposed ischaemia. In this way the distal part of the appendix can become gangrenous and perforate.

Complications

Complications of acute appendicitis include those arising as a result of perforation, such as generalised peritonitis, abscess and fistula formation, and the consequences of blood spread, suppurative pyelophlebitis (inflammation and thrombosis of the portal vein), liver abscess and septicaemia. The inflammation may become chronic, or obstruction to the neck of the appendix may lead to mucus retention causing a *mucocele*. This does not often give rise to clinical problems but, on rare occasions, may rupture and disseminate mucus-secreting epithelial cells into the peritoneal cavity.

NORMAL STRUCTURE AND FUNCTION

The anal canal begins at the upper border of the internal sphincter at the level of the insertion of the puborectalis portion of levator ani (the so-called anorectal ring), and extends down to the groove between the terminal ends of the internal and external sphincters. It is 30–40 mm long.

The upper part of the canal is lined by rectal-type glandular mucosa, the lower part by non-keratinising squamous epithelium. The upper end of the squamous portion is clearly delineated by the pectinate (or dentate) line. Proximal to this is a narrow zone of 'transitional' mucosa, consisting of columnar epithelium with multilayered small basal cells, which merges with the rectal-type mucosa of the upper segment.

The sensory nerves of the anal canal and the muscle sphincters are of vital importance in the control of defecation.

DISEASES OF THE ANUS AND ANAL CANAL

Fissures, fistulae and abscesses are common anal conditions which arise either in isolation or as part of Crohn's disease. Anorectal tuberculosis is very rare in the United Kingdom, but is common in countries with a high incidence of pulmonary tuberculosis. Lesions of syphilis and other sexually transmitted diseases may occur at the anus.

Haemorrhoids

Haemorrhoids are varicosities resulting from dilatation of the internal haemorrhoidal venous plexus.

The mechanisms involved in their formation are not clearly understood, although chronic constipation with straining at stool is most commonly invoked.

Tumours

Warts

Warts (condyloma acuminata) are the commonest benign neoplasm of the anus. They are often multiple and are almost always attributable to human papillomavirus (HPV) infection. Their high incidence in homosexual males suggests venereal transmission through anal intercourse. There is also an increased risk of anal carcinoma.

Carcinoma

There are three main categories of carcinoma corresponding to the three kinds of epithelium found in the anal canal:

- adenocarcinoma in the upper part
- squamous carcinoma in the lower part
- 'basaloid' carcinoma arising from the transitional zone.

Squamous carcinomas are the predominant tumours at the anal verge and arising in peri-anal skin. They appear as ulcerated lesions with rolled margins, and cause pain or bleeding. They spread upwards into the lower rectum, outwards to involve the sphincters, and via lymphatics to involve the lateral pelvic and inguinal nodes. Squamous carcinomas have a higher incidence in homosexual males. Some are known to have developed in pre-existing viral warts (condyloma acuminata), and a relationship between HPV infection and the development of squamous carcinoma, akin to that seen in the uterine cervix, therefore seems likely.

Melanoma

The anus and anal canal are also rare sites for a malignant melanoma.

FURTHER READING

Fenoglio-Preiser C M, Lantz P E, Listrom M B, Davis M, Rilke F O 1989 Gastrointestinal pathology: an atlas and text. Raven Press, New York
Morson B C, Dawson I M P 1990 Gastrointestinal pathology, 3rd edn. Blackwell Scientific Publications, Oxford
Quirke P (ed) 1994 Molecular biology of digestive disease. BMJ Publishing Group, London

Shearman D J C, Finlayson N D C (eds) 1994 Diseases of the gastrointestinal tract and liver, 3rd edn. Churchill Livingstone, Edinburgh
Whitehead R (ed) 1995 Gastrointestinal and oesophageal pathology, 2nd edn. Churchill Livingstone, Edinburgh

Liver, biliary system and exocrine pancreas

LIVER

NORMAL STRUCTURE AND FUNCTION

The liver is a wedge-shaped organ weighing approximately 1.5 kg in the adult. It is situated in the right hypochondrial region of the abdominal cavity and is divisible into four lobes; the right is larger than the left; the smaller caudate lobe is situated posteriorly and the quadrate lobe is anterior. The liver receives blood from two sources:

- *arterial blood* from the right and left hepatic arteries, which are branches of the coeliac axis
- *venous blood* from the hepatic portal vein, which drains much of the alimentary tract, from the stomach to the rectum, and the spleen.

Blood leaves the liver through the hepatic veins, which drain into the inferior vena cava.

Bile is formed in the liver and drains from it into the right and left hepatic ducts; these fuse to form the common bile duct to be joined by the cystic duct, which communicates with the gallbladder where the bile is stored and concentrated.

Most of the liver volume is occupied by the liver cells (*hepatocytes*). These are arranged in plates one cell thick, bordering the vascular sinusoids through which flows hepatic arterial and portal venous blood. The blood flowing through the vascular sinusoids is separated from the liver cells by a thin fenestrated (porous) barrier of cells (*endothelial cells* and *phagocytic Kupffer cells*) and the *space of Disse*. Within the space of Disse the liver cells do not have a continuous basement membrane, thus allowing free interchange of molecules at the liver cell membrane. Blood flowing through the vascular sinusoids drains into hepatic vein branches (central veins or terminal hepatic venules). Bile formed by the liver cells is secreted from them into minute canaliculi which run along the centre of the liver cell plates to drain into the bile duct branches in the portal tracts. Close to the vascular sinusoids in the vicinity of the terminal hepatic venules are the *perisinusoidal cells of Ito*; these are thought to participate in certain forms of hepatic fibrosis by synthesising collagen.

The portal tracts each contain three structures, which are branches of:

- the bile duct
- the hepatic artery
- the portal vein.

These constitute the *portal triad* and are supported by collagen-rich connective tissue. The hepatic artery and portal vein branches give origin to the axial vessels on which the so-called 'acinar concept' is centred.

The microanatomy of the liver can be regarded conceptually to consist of either acini or lobules (Fig. 16.1):

- *Acini* are centred on the axial vessels, emanating from the hepatic artery and portal venous channels in the adjacent portal tract. Their periphery is demarcated by the surrounding hepatic veins.
- *Lobules* are centred on terminal hepatic venules ('central veins'). Their periphery is demarcated by imaginary lines joining each of the surrounding portal tracts.

Of the two microanatomical concepts—acinar or lobular—the 'acinar concept' is now considered to be more useful because it explains better many of the pathophysiological disturbances in liver disease. The zone of liver cells most remote from the axial vessels in the centre of the acinus (acinar zone 3) is the most susceptible to injury resulting from vascular insufficiency, as in circulatory shock or cardiac failure. As adjacent zones 3 are contiguous, liver cell necrosis affecting this zone is often confluent.

The portal tracts are circumscribed by a boundary of liver cells, known as the 'limiting plate', which is breached in certain forms of chronic liver injury; breaching of the limiting plate, when seen in biopsies, denotes that progression to cirrhosis is likely. The liver cells at the portal tract boundary can, in response to bile duct injury or obstruction, undergo a metaplastic change and proliferate to form new bile ductules.

Liver cells have ultrastructural features that are characteristic of cells involved in a wide variety of metabolic functions. They are rich in organelles, including numerous mitochondria, lysosomes, peroxisomes (microbodies), and rough and smooth endoplasmic reticulum (Fig. 16.2). The cytoplasm is also laden with finely granular glycogen; this glycogen can be excessive in diabetes and in congenital deficiencies of glycogen debranching enzymes (the glycogenoses).

Liver cells synthesise albumin, clotting factors including fibrinogen, some complement components, α_1-antitrypsin, etc., and remove from the body many waste products and potentially toxic substances. Liver cells are also involved in the metabolism of many drugs. Extensive disease of the liver therefore affects many vital functions and has profound effects on the body.

The liver cells contain many enzymes, some of which are diagnostically important because their

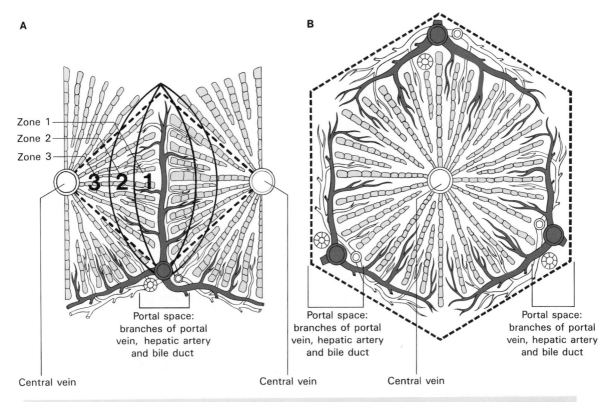

A

Zone 1
Zone 2
Zone 3

3 2 1

Portal space:
branches of portal
vein, hepatic artery
and bile duct

Central vein

B

Portal space:
branches of portal
vein, hepatic artery
and bile duct

Central vein

Portal space:
branches of portal
vein, hepatic artery
and bile duct

Central vein

Fig. 16.1 Diagrammatic comparison of acinar and lobular concepts of the microanatomical units of the liver

A. The acinar concept explains better the pathophysiology of the liver, in that injury to liver cells in zone 3 results in the observed necrosis bridging between portal tracts and central veins in severe liver injury. Cells in zone 3, being the most remote from the vascular supply in the hilum of the acinus, are consequently the most vulnerable to injury. **B.** Lobular units are, however, often easier to perceive in histological sections.

release into the blood, where their activity can be measured, indicates the presence and severity of liver disease (Table 16.1). These enzymes include:

- aspartate aminotransferase (AST)
- alanine aminotransferase (ALT)
- γ-glutamyltransferase (γ-GT).

All cells in the liver are capable of regeneration. The liver cells are considered to be stable — that is, they are not normally replicating but can be induced to do so if the liver is injured. This regenerative capacity is vital in the recovery of patients with liver damage due to viruses, drugs or trauma, but if the damage is persistent or occurs repeatedly, it can result in loss of the normal acinar or lobular structure and its replacement by regenerative liver cell nodules which are functionally inefficient. This is the condition called *cirrhosis*.

Some changes occur naturally in the liver with age. In the fetus, the liver is a relatively larger organ compared to the rest of the body. It is a major site of

haemopoiesis and the adult liver can revert to this activity in some haematological disorders. The fetal liver synthesises α-fetoprotein, a fetal serum protein, and this is replaced by albumin towards the end of gestation. α-Fetoprotein synthesis by the adult liver usually denotes the presence of a primary liver cell carcinoma. With advancing age, the liver shrinks and often assumes a dark brown colour due to an increased concentration of lipofuscin in the liver cells ('brown atrophy').

INVESTIGATION OF LIVER DISEASE

Techniques commonly used in the investigation of a patient with liver disease include:

- analysis of serum concentrations of bilirubin, hepatic enzymes, albumin, clotting factors, etc.
- immunological testing for auto-antibodies

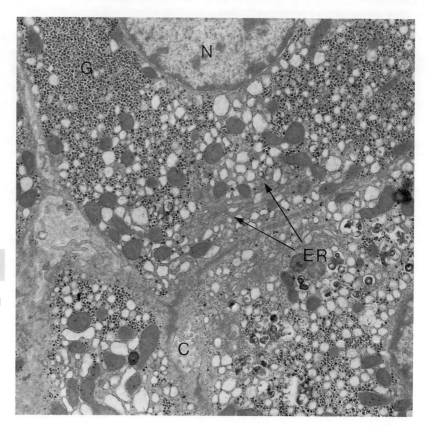

Fig. 16.2 Ultrastructure of the human liver

The liver cell nucleus (N) is unremarkable. The cytoplasm is filled with organelles including mitochondria, peroxisomes (microbodies) and lysosomes. The electron-dense granular material is glycogen (G). There are profiles of rough and smooth endoplasmic reticulum (ER). The bile canaliculus (C) between adjacent liver cells is bordered by microvilli.

- liver biopsy
- imaging techniques.

These procedures complement careful history-taking and a thorough clinical examination.

Biochemistry

Bilirubin

Bilirubin pigment is a breakdown product of the haem moiety of haemoglobin (Fig. 16.3). It is produced at sites of red cell destruction (e.g. spleen) and circulates in the blood in an unconjugated water-insoluble form bound to albumin. In the liver it is conjugated to glucuronic acid by the enzyme glucuronyl transferase. Conjugated bilirubin is water-soluble and can therefore appear in the urine if the outflow of bile from the liver is interrupted; the patient's urine then becomes stained with conjugated bilirubin. Bilirubin is converted by bacteria in the intestine to faecal urobilinogen (stercobilinogen), some of which is absorbed and then excreted, mostly in the bile to complete its enterohepatic circulation

or, in only trace amounts normally, by the kidneys to appear in the urine as urobilinogen. Stercobilinogen is oxidised to stercobilin (faecal urobilin), the principal faecal pigment.

In early or recovering viral hepatitis, impaired biliary excretion results in pre-formed stercobilinogen appearing in the urine in excess as urobilinogen; this is one sensitive marker of early liver injury. In well-established biliary obstruction, the urinary urobilinogen concentration falls, because the cessation of biliary excretion into the gut results in sustained absence of synthesis of faecal urobilinogen.

Enzymes

In liver cell injury, damage to the membranes of cells and organelles allows intracellular enzymes to leak into the blood, where their now-elevated concentrations can be measured. Examples include ALT, AST and γ-GT. Their diagnostic usefulness is summarised in Table 16.1.

The enzyme alkaline phosphatase is normally present in bile. Obstruction to the flow of bile, by gallstones for example, causes regurgitation of alka-

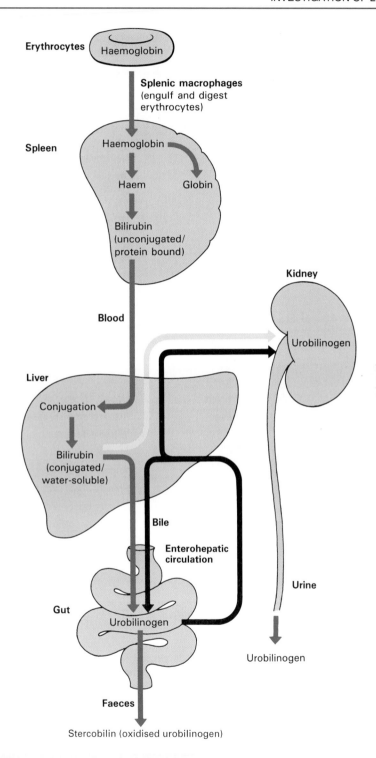

Fig. 16.3   Simplified pathways of bilirubin metabolism

Excessive breakdown of haemoglobin, as in haemolytic anaemias, will lead to increased biliary excretion of bilirubin. Biliary obstruction will cause regurgitation of conjugated, water-soluble bilirubin into the blood which is then excreted in the urine. Liver cell damage in hepatitis will cause impaired biliary excretion of urobilinogen and conjugated bilirubin; these are excreted in the urine, causing it to darken. The enterohepatic circulation returns *cholic* and *chenodeoxycholic acid* to the liver; this enhances bile secretion.

Table 16.1   Diagnostic usefulness of serum analyses in liver disease

Test	Deviation from normal	Interpretation
Albumin Normal 35–50 g/l	↓	Liver failure
Prothrombin time Normal <15s	↑	Liver failure
Alanine aminotransferase (ALT) Normal <40 IU/l	↑	Hepatocellular injury
Aspartate aminotransferase (AST) Normal <40 IU/l	↑	Hepatocellular injury
γ-Glutamyltransferase (γ-GT) Normal <50 IU/l	↑	Hepatocellular injury (centrilobular)
Alkaline phosphatase Normal <100 IU/l	↑	Biliary obstruction Hepatic metastases
Bilirubin Normal 5–12 μmol/l	↑	Hepatocellular injury Biliary obstruction Liver failure Congenital hyperbilirubinaemia Haemolysis
IgM anti-HAV antibody	Present	Hepatitis A
HBsAg	Present	Hepatitis B or carrier
HBeAg	Present	Active hepatitis B infection
Anti-HCV antibody	Present	Hepatitis C virus exposure
HCV RNA	Present	Active hepatitis C infection
Caeruloplasmin	↓	Wilson's disease
IgA	↑	Alcoholic cirrhosis
IgG	↑	'Lupoid' hepatitis
IgM	↑	Primary biliary cirrhosis
Anti-mitochondrial antibody	Present	Primary biliary cirrhosis
Anti-smooth muscle antibody	Present	'Lupoid' hepatitis
Ferritin	↑	Haemochromatosis
α_1-Antitrypsin	↓	α_1-Antitrypsin deficiency
α-Fetoprotein (AFP) (normally undetectable)	↑	Liver cell carcinoma

HAV=hepatitis A virus; HBsAg=hepatitis B surface antigen; HCV=hepatitis C virus.

line phosphatase into the blood, resulting in increased serum concentrations.

Many of these enzymes are not exclusively specific to the liver, therefore the result of diagnostic serum assays need careful interpretation.

Albumin

Albumin is a major serum protein synthesised by the liver cells. It has a relatively long half-life, compared to that of clotting factors (see below), so liver damage has to be sustained for some time before decreased serum levels are found. In chronic liver disease, such as cirrhosis, a low serum albumin concentration is an important manifestation of liver failure, which results in peripheral oedema and contributes to the presence of ascites, due to a reduction in plasma oncotic pressure.

Clotting factors

Liver cells synthesise the vitamin K-dependent clotting factors, deficiency of which results in a bleeding tendency. This can be detected in the laboratory by

Pathological basis of hepatic signs and symptoms

Sign or symptom	Pathological basis
Jaundice	Haemolysis (increased formation of bilirubin), liver disease (impaired conjugation and/or excretion) or biliary obstruction
Dark urine	Conjugated hyperbilirubinaemia (water soluble)
Pale faeces	Biliary obstruction causing lack of bile pigments
Spider naevi Gynaecomastia	Secondary to hyperoestrogenism
Oedema	Reduced plasma oncotic pressure due to hypoalbuminaemia
Xanthelasma	Cutaneous lipid deposits due to hypercholesterolaemia in chronic biliary obstruction
Steatorrhoea	Malabsorption of fat due to lack of bile (e.g. biliary obstruction)
Pruritus	Biliary obstruction resulting in bile salt accumulation
Ascites	Combination of hypoalbuminaemia, portal hypertension, and secondary hyperaldosteronism
Bruising or bleeding	Impaired hepatic synthesis of clotting factors
Hepatomegaly	Increased size of liver due to inflammation (e.g. hepatitis), infiltration (e.g. amyloid, fat), or tumour (primary or secondary)
Haematemesis	Ruptured oesophageal varices due to portal hypertension
Encephalopathy	Failure of liver to remove exogenous or endogenous mimicking or altering balance of neurotransmitters

measuring the prothrombin time. A prolonged bleeding and prothrombin time is a further manifestation of liver failure and, because these clotting factors have a relatively short half-life, deficiency may be found quite early in the course of the illness. It is mandatory to measure the prothrombin time before performing a liver biopsy or undertaking surgery on a patient with liver disease, to avoid the risk of unexpected haemor-

rhage. These clotting factor deficiencies can be corrected by administration of high doses of vitamin K or of the clotting factors themselves.

Immunology

Although insignificant amounts of immunoglobulins are synthesised in the liver, immunological abnormalities often accompany liver disease and are useful diagnostic markers. These abnormalities include the appearance in the patient's serum of auto-antibodies to normal tissue antigens. The antibodies are *not* thought to participate in the liver diseases with which they are associated. Examples include:

- anti-mitochondrial antibodies found in primary biliary cirrhosis
- anti-nuclear antibodies and anti-smooth muscle antibodies found in the 'lupoid' (autoimmune) type of chronic hepatitis.

Polyclonal immunologloglobulin elevations also occur:

- raised IgG in autoimmune (lupoid) hepatitis
- raised IgM in primary biliary cirrhosis
- raised IgA in alcoholic cirrhosis.

Biopsy

Current knowledge of the pathology of the liver owes much to advances in liver biopsy techniques. The two common types of liver biopsy are:

- wedge biopsies, taken during the course of an abdominal operation
- needle biopsies, which are done percutaneously under local anaesthesia.

Both procedures carry a small but significant risk of haemorrhage and biliary leakage from the biopsy site. Bile duct obstruction is a contraindication to liver biopsy because of the increased risk of biliary peritonitis from bile leakage from the biopsy site. The risk must be outweighed by the likely therapeutic benefit to the patient resulting from an accurate diagnosis.

Most liver diseases produce diffuse abnormalities in the organ and a biopsy from any part of it will therefore be representative. Focal lesions such as tumours may be missed, particularly by percutaneous needle sampling, but the biopsy needle can be guided to focal lesions by using ultrasound or computed axial tomography (CAT) imaging.

Liver biopsies are examined by light microscopy after sectioning and staining. Unlike renal biopsies, little additional clinically useful information is obtained by examining liver biopsies with the electron microscope.

Imaging

Techniques used to visualise the liver and detect lesions within it include:

- scintigraphy after the injection of ^{99m}Tc-labelled colloids, which are taken up by the phagocytic Kupffer cells
- ultrasound
- computed axial tomography (CAT)
- magnetic resonance imaging (MRI).

JAUNDICE

Jaundice (or icterus) is the name given to yellowing of the skin and mucosal surfaces due to the presence of bilirubin. Usually jaundice is observable when the serum bilirubin concentration exceeds 40 μmol/l. It is important to emphasise that:

1. Many patients with significant liver disease, often severe, are not jaundiced.
2. Liver disease is not the only cause of jaundice.

The accumulation of bilirubin in the skin may cause some embarrassment to the patient and, often if due to biliary obstruction, discomfort due to pruritus from bile salt accumulation.

Jaundice in infants

Physiological neonatal jaundice is relatively common, particularly in premature infants. Although it causes understandable parental anxiety, the jaundice is rarely severe and it fades as liver function matures. However, high bilirubin levels in infancy can be directly harmful: because the neonatal blood–brain barrier is relatively permeable, unconjugated bilirubin can accumulate in the lipid-rich brain tissue causing *bilirubin encephalopathy* or *kernicterus*; this can be avoided by phototherapy or, in severe cases, exchange transfusion.

Worsening jaundice may be one of the clinical features alerting to the presence of a congenital abnormality within the hepato-biliary system. Such abnormalities may be:

- structural
- functional.

Structural congenital abnormalities include biliary atresia, a condition in which the bile ducts have failed to develop normally, resulting in obstruction to the biliary outflow from the liver. Functional abnormalities include congenital metabolic defects involving the liver and congenital hyperbilirubinaemias.

Classification of jaundice

Jaundice may be classified into *pre-hepatic*, *intra-hepatic* or *post-hepatic* causes, depending on the site of the lesion, or into *conjugated* and *unconjugated* forms, based on chemical analysis of the bilirubin in the blood or by deduction from the colour of the patient's urine. Only conjugated bilirubin is sufficiently water-soluble to be excreted in the urine.

Pre-hepatic causes

The main cause of 'pre-hepatic jaundice' is *haemolysis*, due for example to hereditary spherocytosis or autoimmune red cell destruction (Ch. 23). In these conditions there is excessive production of bilirubin from the haemoglobin released from lysed red cells. Because the excess bilirubin is unconjugated, it is not excretable in the urine; the urine colour is normal (hence the synonym 'acholuric jaundice'). The bile, however, may contain so much bilirubin that there is a risk of pigment gallstone formation (see p. 477).

Intra-hepatic causes

Hepatic disorders in which jaundice may be a feature include:

- acute viral hepatitis
- drug-induced liver injury
- alcoholic hepatitis
- decompensated cirrhosis
- intra-hepatic bile duct loss (e.g. primary biliary cirrhosis, sclerosing cholangitis, biliary hypoplasia)
- in pregnancy, intra-hepatic cholestasis and acute fatty liver.

In these conditions there is accumulation of bilirubin within the liver (intra-hepatic cholestasis), often histologically evident in biopsies as plugs of bile pigment distending canaliculi or bile ducts. The excess bilirubin is predominantly conjugated, is therefore water soluble and is excreted in the urine causing darkening; this is a simple but diagnostically useful observation.

Congenital hyperbilirubinaemia
Congenital metabolic defects in the intra-hepatic conjugation, transport or excretion of bilirubin are relatively rare causes of jaundice. These include:

- Gilbert's syndrome (predominantly unconjugated)
- Crigler–Najjar syndrome (predominantly unconjugated)
- Dubin–Johnson syndrome (predominantly conjugated)
- Rotor syndrome (predominantly conjugated).

Post-hepatic causes

Obstruction of the extra-hepatic bile ducts is an important cause of jaundice necessitating urgent investigation and alleviation in order to prevent serious damage to the liver. Important causes are:

- congenital biliary atresia — often accompanied by a reduction in the number of intra-hepatic ducts
- gallstones — usually associated with biliary colic and a non-distendable chronically inflamed gallbladder
- strictures — often following previous biliary surgery
- tumours — notably carcinoma of the head of the pancreas compressing the common bile duct.

As with intra-hepatic causes, some of which also directly interfere with biliary drainage (e.g. primary biliary cirrhosis, sclerosing cholangitis), the excess bilirubin is conjugated and darkens the urine. Conversely, the patient's faeces are pale.

ACUTE LIVER INJURY

> ▶ May present with acute onset of jaundice
> ▶ Causes include viruses, alcohol, drugs, bile duct obstruction
> ▶ Possible outcomes include complete recovery, chronic liver disease, or death from liver failure

Liver injury is conveniently divided into acute and chronic for the purposes of description and clinical management. However, in practice, the same agent may produce either an acute or a chronic illness, in the latter event not necessarily with any preceding clinically evident acute phase. For example, viral hepatitis is considered here under the heading of acute liver injury, but it can lead to chronic liver damage.

Aetiology

The major causes of acute liver injury are:

- viral infections
- high alcohol consumption
- adverse drug reactions
- biliary obstruction, commonly due to gallstones.

Direct physical injury to the liver, such as laceration in a road traffic accident, is another important form of acute liver injury, but the focal nature of the injury contrasts with the diffuse injury produced by the agents listed above. Recovery from acute liver injury, focal or diffuse, is attributable to the capacity of the organ for cellular regeneration.

Clinicopathological features

The clinical and laboratory manifestations of acute liver injury are:

- malaise
- jaundice
- raised serum bilirubin and transaminases
- in severe cases, evidence of liver failure.

Most of the signs and symptoms of acute liver damage are predictable from the known functions of the liver. The best-known is jaundice (or icterus) due to failure of the liver to secrete bile at the rate at which it is formed in the body from the destruction of red cells. The accumulation of bile salts causes itching (pruritus). Severe acute liver damage can lead to bruising and haemorrhage, due to clotting factor deficiency, and coma due to the accumulation of toxic metabolites which mimic neurotransmitters ('false neurotransmitters').

Laboratory investigations

Laboratory investigations will reveal evidence of liver cell damage in that there will be elevated levels of serum enzymes, particularly the transaminases, and bilirubin. Liver cell damage results in some impairment of bilirubin conjugation, but also failure to excrete conjugated bilirubin and any stercobilinogen absorbed from the gut. Consequently, the urine is darkened by the presence of excess conjugated bilirubin and urobilin (derived by oxidation from urobilinogen) that cannot be excreted by the liver (Fig. 16.3). Eventually, as the liver damage persists, urobilinogen disappears from the urine because little or no bilirubin is being excreted by the liver. Jaundice due to bile duct obstruction — commonly by gallstones — also results in dark urine due to excess conjugated bilirubin that cannot be excreted by the liver; urobilinogen is usually absent, unless the obstruction is of very recent onset or intermittent, because no bilirubin reaches the intestine. Examination of urine and faeces (for colour) can therefore assist in the differential diagnosis of jaundice (Table 16.2).

Histology

In almost all cases of acute liver injury there will be histological evidence of liver cell degeneration or death and an inflammatory reaction. Superimposed

Table 16.2 Differential diagnosis of jaundice from bile abnormalities in urine and faeces, and from serum biochemistry

Colour		Serum biochemistry*	Interpretation
Faeces	Urine		
Dark	Normal	Unconjugated hyperbilirubinaemia	Haemolysis
Pale	Dark	Conjugated hyperbilirubinaemia and raised alkaline phosphatase	Cholestasis Biliary obstruction
Pale	Dark	Mixed hyperbilirubinaemia and raised transaminases	Acute hepatitis
Variable	Variable	Unconjugated or conjugated hyperbilirubinaemia; other tests normal; no evidence of haemolysis	Congenital hyperbilirubinaemia (e.g. Gilbert's syndrome)

*Dominant abnormalities are listed; cholestasis and hepatitis are usually associated with other minor abnormalities of serum biochemistry.

on this uniform reaction to acute injury are, in many cases, diagnostic changes specific to the causative agent.

Also evident will be the pattern of liver cell damage, from which the clinical implications can be deduced (Fig. 16.4):

- Death of individual liver cells (*apoptosis*) is the most frequent pattern of cell loss in viral hepatitis and usually denotes certain recovery with no long-term sequelae.
- Death of periportal hepatocytes (*piecemeal necrosis*) or entire acinar zones, usually zone 3 (*bridging necrosis*), disturbs the hepatic architecture and leads to a risk of cirrhosis developing.
- Necrosis substantially affecting the entire acinus (*panacinar necrosis*) leads to liver failure and a significant risk of immediate death.

Viral hepatitis

▶ Common cause of acute liver injury
▶ Hepatitis viruses A, B, C and delta agent
▶ Other viruses causing liver damage include Epstein–Barr virus, yellow fever virus, herpes simplex virus and cytomegalovirus

The main hepatitis viruses (Table 16.3) are:

- hepatitis A virus (HAV)
- hepatitis B virus (HBV)
- hepatitis C virus (HCV)
- hepatitis E virus (HEV)
- delta agent, a defective virus requiring HBV for pathogenicity.

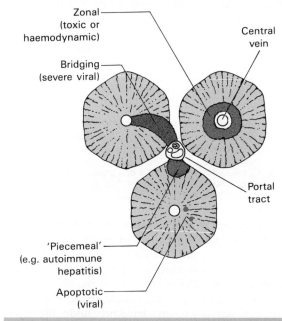

Fig. 16.4 Patterns of hepatic apoptosis and necrosis and their clinicopathological significance

Necrosis of the liver cells immediately surrounding central veins denotes cardiac failure, some other impediment to venous drainage, or some toxic cause (e.g. paracetamol overdose). Bridging necrosis (in acinar zone 3) is a feature of severe hepatitis. 'Piecemeal' necrosis refers to apoptosis of liver cells at the margin of the portal tracts; this apoptosis is a feature of chronic active hepatitis due to variety of causes. Apoptotic necrosis is typical of acute viral hepatitis.

These hepatitis viruses are immunologically distinct and infection usually confers life-long immunity to the infecting virus but not to the others.

The clinical features range from a trivial illness

Table 16.3 Hepatitis viruses: their characteristics and associated diseases (Delta agent, a defective virus, is not included)

Virus	Type of virus	Incubation period (days)	Illness	Carriers	Serological markers	Patient susceptibility	Transmission
HAV	ssRNA enterovirus	15–40	Mild; very low mortality	No	IgM anti-HAV antibody	Young	'Faecal–oral'
HBV	dsRNA hepadnavirus	50–180	Significant risk of chronicity and mortality	Yes	HBsAg, HBeAg	Any age	Blood and blood products; needles; venereal
HCV	ss+RNA flavivirus	40–55	Fluctuating; risk of chronicity and mortality	Yes	Anti-HCV antibody, HCV RNA	Any age	Blood and blood products; needles; possibly venereal
HEV	ssRNA virus	30–50	No risk of chronicity; high mortality in pregnancy	No	Anti-HEV antibody	Any age	'Faecal–oral'

HAV=hepatitis A virus; HBV=hepatitis B virus; HCV=hepatitis C virus; HBsAg=hepatitis B surface antigen; HEV=hepatitis E virus.

without jaundice (*anicteric hepatitis*) which may escape detection (this is a common result of HAV infection) to a more significant illness with jaundice and other clinical evidence of disturbed liver function. Sometimes the illness is dominated by jaundice, with little elevation of serum transaminases (*cholestatic hepatitis*). Severe infection leads to overt liver failure.

Yellow fever, caused by a group B arbovirus, shares many clinical and histological features with the illness usually designated viral hepatitis, but it is not normally included within this group for the purposes of description, mainly because its geographical distribution is very restricted.

The liver may also become infected by many other viruses, but these are not necessarily considered to be 'hepatitis viruses' because the infection is not just confined to the liver. Examples include:

- infectious mononucleosis due to Epstein–Barr virus
- herpes simplex virus 1
- cytomegalovirus.

Hepatitis A virus

The main characteristics of hepatitis A are:

- 'faecal–oral' spread
- relatively short incubation period

- sporadic or epidemic
- directly cytopathic
- no carrier state
- mild illness, full recovery usual.

Infection by HAV used to be called 'infectious hepatitis' because of its common occurrence in epidemics, though it also occurs sporadically. In most countries, infection by the virus is common, usually in youth; the resulting illness is often very mild and jaundice absent or so slight that it escapes notice. Overt jaundice and clinical recognition of the infection is less common. Hepatitis sufficiently severe to warrant hospital admission is rare, and long-term sequelae or death are exceptional rarities. It is therefore a relatively benign infection.

HAV passes from one individual to another by 'faecal–oral' transmission — usually indirectly, such as by the contamination of food and drinking water with sewage. Because the virus is excreted in the faeces before jaundice appears, thus leading to the recognition of the illness and isolation of the patient, many other individuals can be rapidly exposed to the risk of infection. The incubation period is relatively short. HAV produces liver cell damage by a direct cytopathic effect.

Specific diagnosis is made by seeking an IgM-class antibody to HAV in the patient's serum; this indicates recent infection. A carrier state does not exist.

Hepatitis B virus

The main characteristics of hepatitis B are:

- spread by blood, blood-contaminated instruments, blood products and venereally
- relatively long incubation period
- liver damage by antiviral immune reaction
- carrier state exists
- relatively serious infection.

Infection by HBV used to be called 'serum hepatitis' because it was known to be transmitted by blood and blood products. This is because infected, but apparently healthy, individuals can carry the virus in their blood and pass it on to others by the transfusion of blood or its products. This mode of transmission is much less common now that blood donors are screened by testing for the presence of the virus. However, the term 'serum hepatitis' should be abandoned because it misleadingly excludes transmission of the virus by other methods, notably venereally; the disease is not uncommon in homosexual males. HBV can also be transmitted by contaminated needles, such as may be used for tattooing or by drug addicts. There is a relatively high incidence of the carrier state in underdeveloped countries and the virus can be transmitted vertically from mother to child—in utero, during delivery or through intimate post-natal contact.

Specific diagnosis is made by seeking the hepatitis B surface antigen (HBsAg, formerly known as 'Australia antigen' because it was first detected in the serum of an Australian aborigine). The presence of the 'e' antigen of HBV in the patient's serum is considered to indicate the presence of active liver disease.

Virus B produces liver cell damage not by a direct cytopathic effect but by causing viral antigens to appear on the cell surface (HBsAg); these are then recognised by the body's immune system and the infected liver cells that bear them are destroyed (Fig. 16.5). Thus, if immunity is impaired or there is tolerance to the antigen, the virus can survive in the liver cells without causing damage; the patient becomes an asymptomatic carrier of the virus and his or her body fluids are a risk to other individuals. Liver biopsies of HBV-infected carriers show that the liver cells have a ground-glass texture to their cytoplasm due to the abundance of virus particles.

Virus B infection is much more serious than virus A. Infection is more likely to produce a clinical illness and jaundice, and it is more likely to result in long-term sequelae such as chronic hepatitis and cirrhosis, or even death due to fulminating acute infec-

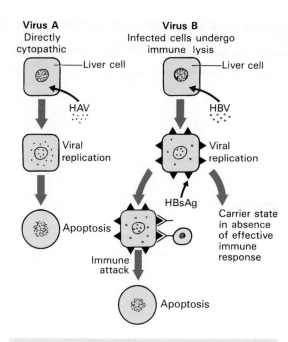

Fig. 16.5 Comparison of the pathogenesis of HAV and HBV hepatitis

The A virus, in contrast to the B virus, appears to be directly cytopathic. The B virus evokes liver cell injury by causing viral antigens to be expressed on the liver cell surface (HBsAg=hepatitis B surface antigen). The infected cells are eliminated immunologically, but an asymptomatic carrier state can ensue in the absence of specific immunity. The pathogenesis of other hepatitis viral infections is uncertain.

tion causing extensive hepatic necrosis. Hepatitis B virus is also implicated in the pathogenesis of liver cell carcinoma.

Hepatitis C virus

Hepatitis C virus has been characterised more recently. Its main features are:

- spread by blood, blood-contaminated instruments, blood products and possibly venereally
- relatively short incubation period
- often asymptomatic
- fluctuating liver biochemistry
- tendency to chronicity.

HCV is an important cause of hepatitis following blood transfusion and the administration of clotting factor concentrates. Indeed, its existence was first suspected after HBV had been excluded as a possible cause by antibody testing; it used to be known as 'non-A/non-B' hepatitis.

The initial illness is often asymptomatic and the abnormalities of liver biochemistry (e.g. raised serum transaminases) are usually fluctuant. However, despite these misleadingly benign signals, the infection is prone to chronicity and cirrhosis is a frequent consequence eventually.

The risk of post-transfusion HCV infection is being reduced by routine screening of blood donors.

Hepatitis E virus and other non-A, non-B viruses

There are possibly up to three other authentic hepatitis viruses. The best characterised is a waterborne agent, distinct from HAV, that has been responsible for outbreaks of hepatitis in India; it has been designated hepatitis E virus (HEV). Fortunately, the disease rarely progresses to chronicity and, as with HAV, full recovery is usual except in pregnancy, when it is associated with a high mortality rate.

Experimental studies involving transmission of hepatitis by blood transfusion to apes have produced evidence of other viruses distinct from HBV and HCV as the cause of a small number of cases of post-transfusion hepatitis.

Delta agent

Delta agent is a defective RNA virus which requires the presence of HBV, which supplies the outer layers of the viral coat, for its replication and assumed role as a pathogen. Its main effect is to aggravate the consequences of HBV infection.

Histology

Histological features of viral hepatitis are:

- apoptosis (Councilman or acidophil bodies)
- portal tract inflammation
- cholestasis.

Although the pathogenesis of the liver cell damage resulting from HAV and HBV infection is different, the morphology of the liver in a typical case is very similar (Fig. 16.6). The principal features are:

- cytoplasmic swelling of liver cells
- apoptosis of individual liver cells recognisable by the formation of eosinophilic Councilman bodies (first described in yellow fever)
- infiltration of portal tracts by mixed inflammatory cells and expansion by oedema
- hyperplasia of Kupffer cells; in the later stages of the disease, during recovery, cellular debris (ceroid) accumulates in their cytoplasm
- accumulation of bile in liver cells, which are often swollen, and within the intercellular canaliculi where it is sometimes misleadingly referred to as 'bile thrombi'; this pooling of bile within the liver cells and the canaliculi is called *cholestasis*.

The swelling of liver cells, portal oedema and the infiltration by inflammatory cells are responsible for hepatomegaly in viral hepatitis.

In severe viral hepatitis there may be confluent liver cell necrosis, resulting in a risk of death

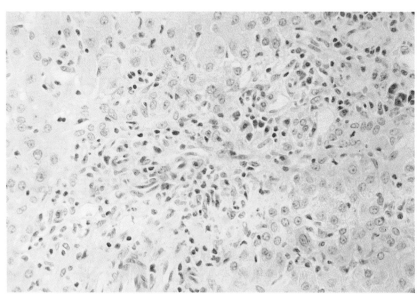

Fig. 16.6 Liver histology in acute viral hepatitis

The portal tract bears an inflammatory infiltrate. Hepatocytes are undergoing apoptotic necrosis.

from liver failure. In such a case at autopsy the liver will be small, have a wrinkled instead of smooth capsule, and show extensive necrosis on the cut surfaces.

HCV hepatitis is often characterised by the presence of lymphocytes within the vascular sinusoids and fatty change in the hepatocytes, often with relatively little evidence of active liver cell necrosis. This combination of features is unusual in HAV or HBV infection.

Alcoholic liver injury

▶ Common cause of acute and chronic liver disease
▶ Liver may show fatty change, hepatitis, fibrosis or cirrhosis, or a combination of these features
▶ Mechanisms include diversion of metabolic resources, direct hepatotoxicity, and stimulation of collagen synthesis

Alcohol (ethyl alcohol) is a common cause of acute and chronic liver injury. The spectrum of alcoholic liver injury observed in biopsies includes:

- fatty change in liver cells, a relatively benign abnormality
- acute hepatitis with Mallory's hyalin
- architectural damage ranging from portal fibrosis to cirrhosis.

Histology

The fatty change (*steatosis*) is evident as fat globules within the cytoplasm of the liver cells; those in the centrilobular or acinar zone 3 areas are usually most severely affected. Fatty change by itself is a relatively non-specific event because it is seen in many disorders. More specific, but not exclusive, to alcoholic liver injury is *Mallory's hyalin*; this is an intracytoplasmic aggregate of intermediate filaments in the liver cells (Fig. 16.7). This is usually associated with acute inflammation and, in contrast to pure fatty change, carries an appreciable risk of progression to irreversible architectural disturbance and possibly cirrhosis.

Pathogenesis

Alcohol produces liver injury by a variety of mechanisms (Fig. 16.8):

- Cellular energy is diverted from essential metabolic pathways, such as fat metabolism, to the metabolism of alcohol so fat accumulates in the liver cells.
- Alcohol appears to be directly cytotoxic at high concentrations, resulting in injured hepatocytes and an inflammatory reaction.
- Alcohol stimulates collagen synthesis in the liver, leading to fibrosis and eventually cirrhosis.

Sustained alcoholic liver injury results in irreversible architectural disturbance, initially the linking of portal tracts and/or terminal hepatic venules by fibrous tissue, and ultimately nodular regeneration of the liver cells; this is alcoholic cirrhosis. It is estimated that a male consuming 120 g alcohol (for example, two bottles of wine or two-thirds of a bottle of spirits or eight pints of beer) per day for 5 years has a

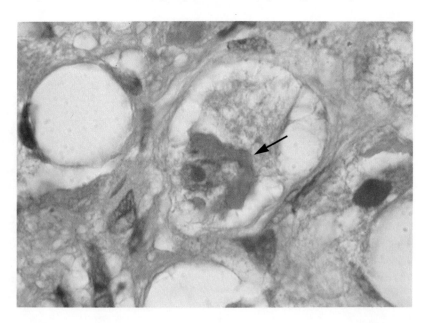

Fig. 16.7 Histology of alcoholic liver disease

Fatty change is conspicuous, and there is Mallory's hyalin (arrowed) in the cytoplasm of an injured hepatocyte.

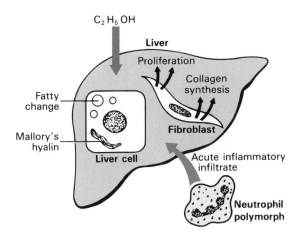

C_2H_5OH

Liver

Proliferation

Collagen synthesis

Fatty change

Fibroblast

Mallory's hyalin

Liver cell

Acute inflammatory infiltrate

Neutrophil polymorph

Fig. 16.8 Pathogenesis of alcoholic liver disease

There is increased peripheral release of fatty acids, and increased synthesis of fatty acids and triglycerides within the liver cells. Acetaldehyde, a product of alcohol metabolism, is probably responsible for liver cell injury, manifested by the formation of Mallory's hyalin. There is increased collagen synthesis by fibroblasts and by the perisinusoidal cells of Ito.

significant risk of developing cirrhosis. The equivalent risk for females is approximately 90 g daily.

Drug-induced liver injury

▸ At least 10% of drug reactions involve the liver
▸ May be cholestatic or hepatocellular
▸ Pathogenesis may be dose-related (predictable) or idiosyncratic (unpredictable)

Approximately 10% of all adverse reactions to drugs involve the liver. This is not surprising in view of the central role played by the liver in metabolism and in the conjugation and elimination of toxic substances from the body. A full drug history should therefore be taken from any patient presenting with liver disease, and any suspected or proven association reported to the appropriate body (in the UK, the Committee on the Safety of Medicines).

Adverse drug reactions may be predictable or unpredictable (Ch. 2). They may be caused through injury to the liver cells (hepatocellular), which is pathologically indistinguishable from viral hepatitis, or to bile production or excretion (cholestatic). Predictable reactions will occur in any individual if a sufficient dose is administered; examples include coagulative centrilobular necrosis due to paracetamol overdose and cholestatic jaundice due to methyl testosterone. Unpredictable reactions include an

idiosyncratic response to a drug and are not necessarily dose-related; examples include cholestatic jaundice due to chlorpromazine.

Acute biliary obstruction

▸ Usually due to gallstones
▸ Clinically characterised by colicky pain and jaundice
▸ May be complicated by infection (cholangitis)
▸ Liver shows portal tract oedema and inflammation, and cholestasis.

Acute obstruction of the main bile ducts is most commonly due to gallstones. Clinically, it usually results in colicky pain and jaundice. If there is superimposed infection of the biliary tract, the ducts become inflamed (*cholangitis*) and the patient develops a fever. Cholangitis can lead to the formation of liver abscesses.

Bile accumulates within the liver, initially in the canaliculi (Fig. 16.9) and later within the intrahepatic bile ducts. Rupture of these may result in extravasation of bile into the adjacent liver tissue where the resulting necrosis is often referred to as a *'bile infarct'*. The portal tracts are oedematous and infiltrated with neutrophil polymorphs. The hepatocytes at the edge of the portal tract undergo ductular metaplasia. Cholangitis is recognised histologically by the presence of neutrophil polymorphs in the bile ducts.

Repeated episodes of biliary obstruction lead to portal tract fibrosis and nodular regeneration of the liver cells — *secondary biliary cirrhosis*.

CHRONIC LIVER DISEASES

Chronic liver diseases, of which there are many, are a common clinical problem. Some follow a clinically evident episode of acute liver injury; others present insidiously and may be asymptomatic until the later stages. Many forms of chronic liver disease culminate in hepatic cirrhosis, which is dealt with separately.

Chronic hepatitis

▸ Defined as clinical or biopsy evidence of hepatitis lasting more than 6 months
▸ Causes include hepatitis viruses, drugs, alcohol, autoimmune ('lupoid') hepatitis
▸ Biopsy appearances categorised as either mild (termed chronic persistent) or severe (termed chronic active) hepatitis

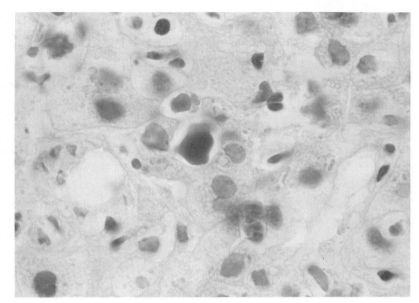

Fig. 16.9 Intrahepatic cholestasis in biliary obstruction

The bile canaliculi are stuffed with stagnant bile unable to be discharged from the liver because the common bile duct is blocked by a gallstone. Similar appearances result from viral hepatitis and some adverse drug reactions.

Chronic hepatitis is generally defined as inflammation of the liver lasting at least 6 months without evidence of resolution. The inflammation and consequent liver cell injury cause a sustained elevation of the serum transaminases, but confirmation of the diagnosis and precise classification of the disease in an individual patient usually requires a liver biopsy.

Aetiology

Chronic hepatitis is due to a variety of causes. Important causes include:

- hepatitis viruses, principally HBV and HCV
- alcohol
- drugs
- autoimmune processes, as in 'lupoid' chronic hepatitis.

Histological classification

The severity of the chronic hepatitis and its likely course is deduced from interpretation of the histology of the liver biopsy. This can be classified as showing either:

- chronic persistent hepatitis (CPH)
- chronic active hepatitis (CAH).

These are merely *histological descriptions* of the extent

and activity of the inflammatory process and are not specific disease labels. There is also considerable prognostic and morphological overlap between CPH and CAH, such that some experts suggest that this classification should be abandoned in favour of a uniform numerical scoring of the inflammatory activity and architectural disturbance. The scheme devised by *Knodell* and colleagues is most widely used.

Clues to the aetiology, enabling a specific diagnosis to be made, may be evident from the immunological, biochemical, or detailed biopsy features (Table 16.4).

Chronic persistent hepatitis
Chronic persistent hepatitis is characterised by:

- lymphocytic infiltration confined to portal tracts
- normal hepatic architecture
- little or no liver cell death
- good prognosis.

Biopsies showing the appearance described above (Fig. 16.10) usually denote a favourable prognosis and probable resolution without specific treatment. An exception seems to be chronic persistent hepatitis due to HCV infection, where progression to chronic active hepatitis and cirrhosis has been observed.

Table 16.4   Principal diagnostic features of chronic disease

Disease	Feature		
	Serological	Biochemical	Biopsy
Lupoid hepatitis	Anti-smooth muscle antibody and anti-nuclear factor	Raised IgG and transaminases	Liver cell rosettes and plasma cells
Chronic virus B hepatitis	HBsAg, HBeAg	Raised transaminases	Piecemeal necrosis
Chronic virus C hepatitis	Anti-HCV HCV RNA	Raised transaminases	Fatty change and sinusoidal infiltration
Primary biliary cirrhosis	Anti-mitochondrial antibody	Raised IgM and alkaline phosphatase	Depleted interlobular ducts and granulomas
Alcoholic cirrhosis		Raised IgA and γ-GT	Mallory's hyalin and fat
Wilson's disease		Low caeruloplasmin	Excess copper
α_1-Antitrypsin deficiency		Low α_1-antitrypsin	Hyaline globules
Haemochromatosis		Raised ferritin	Haemosiderin

HBsAg=hepatitis B surface antigen; γ-GT=gamma-glutamyltransferase.

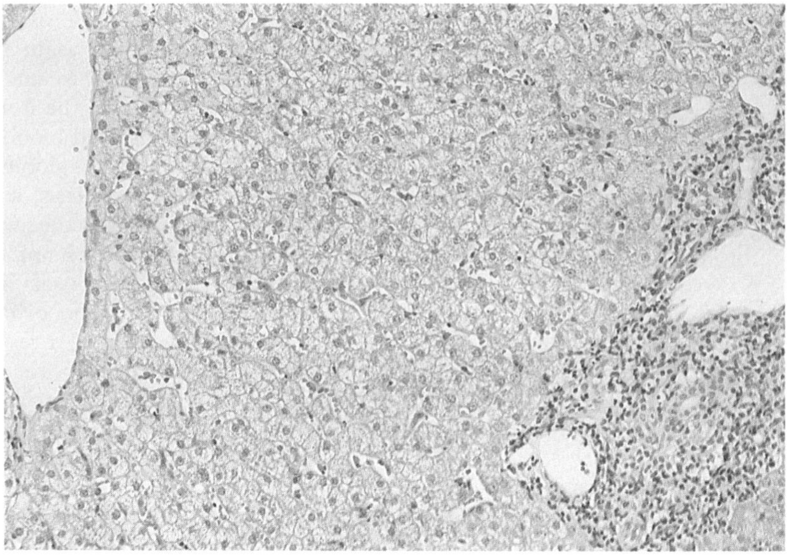

Fig. 16.10   Liver biopsy appearances denoting mild chronic hepatitis (chronic persistent hepatitis)

The dense lymphocytic infiltrate is confined to portal tracts and there is no erosion of hepatic architecture. This abnormality progresses only rarely to cirrhosis.

Chronic active hepatitis

Chronic active hepatitis is characterised by:

- piecemeal necrosis and bridging
- inflammation extending from portal tracts into adjacent parenchyma
- risk of progression to cirrhosis.

The histological hallmark of chronic active hepatitis is the presence of *piecemeal necrosis* (interface hepatitis), which is inflammatory destruction of groups of liver cells immediately adjacent to the portal tracts (Fig. 16.11). This results in disruption of the limiting plate of liver cells surrounding each portal tract and eventual erosion of hepatic architecture. Biopsies showing this appearance usually convey a significant risk of progression to cirrhosis.

Sometimes the biopsy additionally shows evidence of a specific aetiology. Examples include Mallory's hyalin in alcoholic injury, and large numbers of plasma cells and rosette-like arrangements of swollen

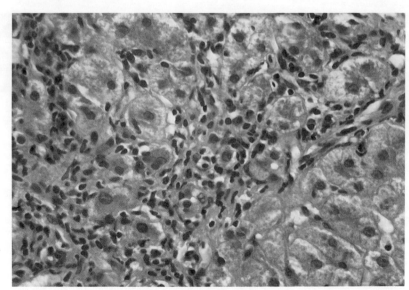

Fig. 16.11   Piecemeal necrosis

This pattern of liver cell death characterises chronic active hepatitis. Degenerate liver cells adjacent to the edge of a portal tract are associated with dense inflammatory cell infiltration. It leads to progressive erosion of liver architecture, frequently culminating in cirrhosis.

liver cells in autoimmune or 'lupoid' hepatitis (Table 16.4).

Iron overload and the liver

▶ Excessive accumulation of iron, as haemosiderin, in the liver causes it to appear dark brown
▶ Haemosiderosis: excess iron with normal architecture
▶ Haemochromatosis: excess iron with consequent cirrhosis
▶ Primary haemochromatosis (congenital): excess iron absorption, deposited in liver (cirrhosis) and endocrine glands (e.g. 'bronze diabetes')
▶ Secondary haemochromatosis (acquired): excess dietary iron or parenteral administration (e.g. multiple blood transfusions)

In haemosiderosis and haemochromatosis the liver is dark brown due to the deposition of excess iron in the form of haemosiderin (an iron-rich protein). The haemosiderin is visible in histological sections as light brown granules; its identity can be confirmed by Perls' stain.

The distinction between these two entities is as follows:

- *Haemosiderosis* is the name given to the mere presence of excess iron, in the form of haemosiderin, in the liver. The liver architecture is usually normal.
- *Haemochromatosis* is a more serious disorder in which the presence of excess iron, as haemosiderin, is associated with a risk of progression to cirrhosis.

Haemosiderosis

Haemosiderosis usually results from parenteral iron overload as in the case of a patient with aplastic anaemia treated with blood transfusions. In this instance, the iron liberated from degradation of the transfused blood cannot be reutilised in the patient for haemoglobin synthesis, because of absence of haemopoiesis, so it accumulates in various organs, notably in the liver where it is stored as haemosiderin, mainly in Kupffer cells. Haemosiderosis is not commonly associated with significant liver damage or progression to cirrhosis; however, if cirrhosis does develop as a result of massive iron overload by this mechanism, the condition is referred to as *secondary haemochromatosis*.

Haemosiderosis can also occur in alcoholic liver disease because alcohol enhances iron absorption from the gut. Any hepatic architectural disturbance is more likely to be due to the alcohol than the iron in these cases.

Primary haemochromatosis

Primary haemochromatosis is the most common form of iron overload. It is a congenital disorder due to a gene defect on chromosome 6 near the HLA-A locus. Heterozygotes show increased absorption of iron, but only in homozygotes does this reach dangerous levels. The defect causes excessive absorption of iron in the small intestine even when transferrin, the iron-binding protein in the blood, is fully saturated. By adult life the total body iron stores may reach as high as 40–60 g (normal about 4 g). The disease is clinically manifested more commonly in men than women; women compensate for the excessive iron absorption through natural iron loss due to menstrual bleeding.

For many years the iron is deposited, as haemosiderin, in the hepatocytes without any clinical effects. Eventually, however, the iron deposition becomes more extensive, involving Kupffer cells, bile duct epithelium and portal tract connective tissue (Fig. 16.12). Hepatic fibrosis ensues, followed by cirrhosis. In advanced cases the haemosiderin is deposited in other tissues, notably in endocrine organs; the clinical syndrome of 'bronze diabetes' is due to concomitant iron-induced damage to the pancreatic islets (resulting in diabetes) and the effect of raised melanotrophin levels on the skin (resulting in bronze coloration). Cardiac failure and impotence may also result.

If the condition is diagnosed in the pre-cirrhotic phase, the process may be arrested by depleting the body's iron stores by regular venesection or by the administration of desferrioxamine, a chelating agent. The genetic aetiology of primary haemochromatosis means that it is important to screen first-degree relatives by measuring the serum ferritin concentration, which is typically elevated in affected individuals.

Secondary haemochromatosis

Unlike primary haemochromatosis, secondary haemochromatosis is not a single discrete disease entity.

It may be due to increased iron in the diet (e.g. excessive medicinal iron tablets) or to parenteral iron loading. For example, secondary haemochromatosis may be seen in patients with aplastic anaemia and haemoglobinopathies who have received multiple transfusions. It is possible, however, that the liver damage in some cases is due to co-existent post-transfusion viral hepatitis rather than iron overload.

Wilson's disease (hepatolenticular degeneration)

▶ Inherited disorder of copper metabolism
▶ Copper accumulates in liver and brain
▶ Kayser–Fleischer rings at corneal limbus
▶ Low serum caeruloplasmin

Wilson's disease is a rare but treatable inherited autosomal recessive disorder in which copper accumulates in the liver and in the basal ganglia of the brain. The underlying defect is failure of the liver to excrete copper in the bile. Copper accumulation in the liver causes chronic hepatitis and, ultimately, cirrhosis. Copper deposition in the brain causes severe progressive neurological disability. Surplus copper released into the blood may cause episodes of haemolysis.

Clinically Wilson's disease is recognised by the combination of hepatic and neurological abnormalities and from the presence of characteristic brown Kayser–Fleischer rings at the corneal limbus. Diagnosis is confirmed by finding a low concentration of

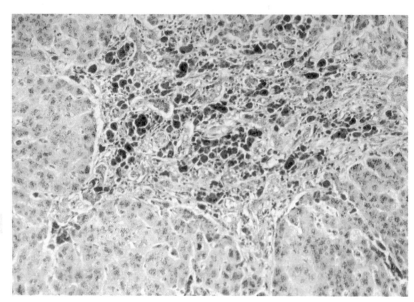

Fig. 16.12 Haemochromatosis
The portal tract and the liver cells contain brown granules of haemosiderin. This has caused portal fibrosis and, if untreated, will eventually lead to cirrhosis.

caeruloplasmin (a copper-containing protein) in the serum and an excess of copper in the liver biopsy. It is treated with penicillamine, a chelating agent that binds the copper and eliminates it in the urine.

α_1-Antitrypsin deficiency

> ▶ Congenital defect of synthesis
> ▶ Hyaline globular inclusions in liver
> ▶ Risk of emphysema and cirrhosis

α_1-Antitrypsin is a serum protein with alpha mobility on electrophoresis. It is normally synthesised in the liver and is immediately secreted into the blood, where it has antiproteolytic properties. Several phenotypes occur in the population. The normal phenotype is referred to as MM.

Phenotypes of α_1-antitrypsin which can be associated with a serum deficiency are not uncommon. They are recognised in the laboratory by their unusually fast or slow electrophoretic mobility. Heterozygous states, such as MZ or MS, are not considered to have any significance, but homozygous states, such as ZZ, are associated with a predisposition to pulmonary emphysema and hepatic cirrhosis. These unusual phenotypes of α_1-antitrypsin are not readily released from the liver cell after synthesis; low serum levels are therefore found and the unreleased protein accumulates in the cytoplasm of periportal hepatocytes as hyaline intracytoplasmic globules.

Autoimmune liver disease

There are two chronic liver diseases that are considered to have an autoimmune basis:

- autoimmune ('lupoid') hepatitis
- primary biliary cirrhosis.

In most cases these autoimmune diseases are distinguishable on investigation, including liver biopsy. However, in a small proportion, there appears to be some overlap and a clear-cut distinction may not be possible. Like almost all other autoimmune diseases, they are more common in females.

Autoimmune ('lupoid') hepatitis

> ▶ Females>males
> ▶ Liver biopsy shows chronic active hepatitis with plasma cells and liver cell rosettes
> ▶ Anti-smooth muscle antibody, raised IgG and transaminases

'Lupoid' hepatitis is most commonly seen in females and is histologically characterised by the appearance of chronic active hepatitis dominated by numerous plasma cells and rosette-like arrangements of swollen liver cells. It is not related to systemic lupus erythematosus, although it shares the presence of antinuclear antibodies in the serum with that condition. Auto-antibodies to smooth muscle antigens are often present also. Associated biochemical factors include raised serum IgG and transaminases. Patients sometimes benefit from treatment with steroids.

Primary biliary cirrhosis

> ▶ Females>males
> ▶ Liver biopsy shows bile duct destruction, granulomas, ductular proliferation, fibrosis, and eventual cirrhosis
> ▶ Raised IgM and alkaline phosphatase, antimitochondrial antibody, pruritus, jaundice, xanthelasmas

Primary biliary cirrhosis is misleadingly named because cirrhosis is a late manifestation of the disease and many patients have the condition diagnosed before this stage is reached.

The stages in the development of the disease are:

- autoimmune destruction of bile duct epithelium, particularly that of the smaller intrahepatic ducts; histologically, the damaged ducts are seen to be surrounded by a dense lymphocytic infiltrate and granulomas are often present (Fig. 16.13)
- later proliferation of small bile ductules, perhaps in a vain attempt to replace those that have been deleted by the autoimmune process
- architectural disturbance due to portal and bridging fibrosis
- cirrhosis.

Copper accumulates in the liver because it can no longer be adequately excreted in the bile.

In addition to the biopsy appearances, which may not be absolutely diagnostic in the later stages, other important features of primary biliary cirrhosis include:

- elevated serum alkaline phosphatase and IgM levels
- an anti-mitochondrial auto-antibody in the serum
- pruritus, jaundice and xanthelasmas (yellow deposits of lipid-laden macrophages in the skin around the eyes).

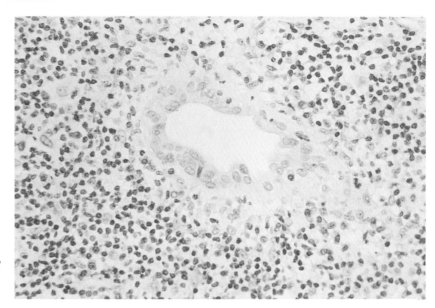

Fig. 16.13   Primary biliary cirrhosis

Lymphocytes surround a bile duct, the epithelium of which is damaged as a result of the autoimmune process.

Sclerosing cholangitis

Primary sclerosing cholangitis is a chronic inflammatory process affecting intrahepatic, and sometimes extrahepatic, bile ducts. Initially, the ducts are surrounded by a mantle of chronic inflammatory cells, but this is eventually replaced by fibrosis and obliteration of the ducts.

There is an association with chronic inflammatory bowel disease, particularly ulcerative colitis.

CIRRHOSIS

▶ Diffuse and irreversible process
▶ Characterised by fibrosis and nodular regeneration
▶ Classified morphologically and aetiologically
▶ Causes include HBV, HCV, alcohol and haemochromatosis
▶ Complications are liver failure, portal hypertension and liver cell carcinoma

The liver has considerable powers of regeneration such that quite severe loss of liver cells can be restored and normal architecture retained. However, if the loss of liver cells is recurrent or takes place against a background of severe architectural disturbance (e.g. bridging necrosis) then cirrhosis can result.

Cirrhosis is not specific disease; it is the end result of a variety of diseases causing chronic liver injury. It is an irreversible disturbance of hepatic architecture, affecting the entire liver, and is characterised by:

• fibrosis
• nodular regeneration.

The amount of fibrous tissue greatly exceeds that in the normal liver and the liver cells are no longer arranged in acini or lobules, but regenerate after various forms of injury in a nodular pattern (Fig. 16.14).

The regeneration nodules lack the well-organised zonal structure of the normal liver lobules or acini. The blood perfuses them in a haphazard fashion, resulting in a relatively inefficient organ that is prone to failure.

Classification

Cirrhosis is classified in two ways:

• morphologically
• aetiologically.

The two classification systems are complementary and not mutually exclusive. Greater emphasis should be placed on the aetiological classification.

Morphological classification

Cirrhosis can be classified according to the average size of the regeneration nodules:

• *micronodular* — nodules up to 3 mm diameter

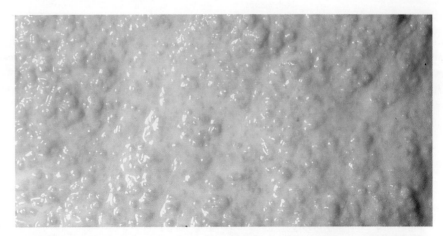

Fig. 16.14 Cirrhotic (micronodular) liver

A. External surface of a cirrhotic liver studded with regeneration nodules about 2 mm in diameter.

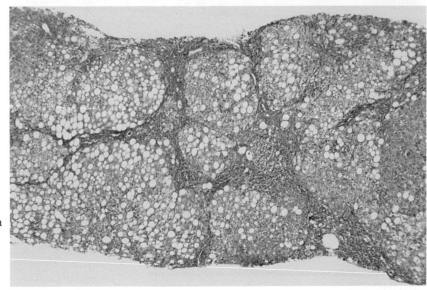

B. Histology of a needle biopsy of a cirrhotic liver revealing regeneration nodules surrounded by dense connective tissue. (Masson trichrome stain in which connective tissue is green.)

- *macronodular*—nodules greater than 3 mm diameter.

A cirrhotic liver intermediate between these two categories is described as 'mixed'.

One of the commonest causes of micronodular cirrhosis is alcoholic liver disease. The significance of macronodular cirrhosis, irrespective of cause, is that it is believed to carry a greater risk of complication by liver cell carcinoma. Macronodular cirrhosis may also be difficult to diagnose with certainty in needle biopsies because the abnormal architecture is not often seen clearly in such small tissue samples.

Aetiological classification

The aetiological classification of a cirrhotic liver can often be deduced from clinical, biochemical, immunological or biopsy features (Fig. 16.15). Important causes include:

- viral hepatitis (HBV and HCV)
- alcohol
- haemochromatosis
- autoimmune liver disease ('lupoid' hepatitis and primary biliary cirrhosis)
- recurrent biliary obstruction (e.g. gallstones)
- Wilson's disease.

In countries such as the UK, alcohol is one of the commonest causes. If the cause is unknown, then the cirrhosis is labelled 'cryptogenic' (hidden cause), although with modern investigations the proportion of cases thus designated is falling.

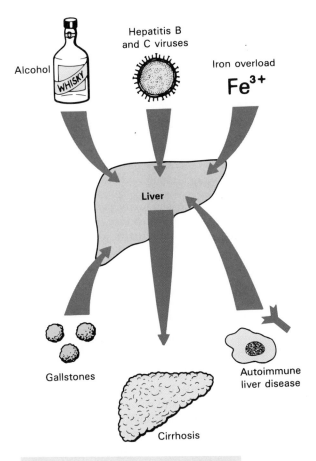

Fig. 16.15 Common causes of cirrhosis

Complications

The major complications of cirrhosis are:

- liver failure
- portal hypertension
- liver cell carcinoma.

Liver failure

Liver failure results in:

- inadequate synthesis of albumin, clotting factors, etc.
- failure to eliminate endogenous products such as hormones, nitrogenous waste, etc.

Cirrhosis may be functionally compensated or decompensated. Indeed, if the disease process which led to the cirrhosis is now inactive, then there may be no detectable abnormalities of liver function. Liver failure is a manifestation of decompensation

(Table 16.5) and is characterised clinically by:

- hypoalbuminaemia, causing oedema due to reduced plasma oncotic pressure
- clotting factor deficiencies, causing bruising, etc.
- ascites
- encephalopathy, sometimes leading to coma.

Hepatic encephalopathy is due to the failure of the liver to eliminate toxic nitrogenous products of gut bacteria; some of these mimic the effect of neurotransmitters (i.e. they are 'false neurotransmitters'). Renal failure may also occur with hepatic failure (hepato-renal syndrome). The patient's breath has a characteristic odour (foetor hepaticus).

Failure to eliminate endogenous steroid hormones results in secondary hyperaldosteronism, causing sodium and water retention and, in the male, loss of secondary sexual characteristics and gynaecomastia due to hyperoestrogenism. 'Spider naevi' are small vascular lesions on the skin, commonly seen in pregnancy, associated with hyperoestrogenism in cirrhosis.

Defective Kupffer cell function may be responsible for the increased incidence of bacteraemia in patients with cirrhosis in the absence of other manifestations of liver failure.

Portal hypertension

Cirrhosis is the commonest cause of portal hyperten-

Table 16.5 Pathophysiological basis of clinical features of chronic liver disease	
Clinical feature	Explanation
Oedema	Reduced albumin synthesis resulting in hypoalbuminaemia
Ascites	Hypoalbuminaemia, secondary hyperaldosteronism, portal hypertension
Haematemesis	Ruptured oesophageal varices due to portal hypertension
Spider naevi Gynaecomastia	Hyperoestrogenism
Purpura and bleeding	Reduced clotting factor synthesis
Coma	Failure to eliminate toxic gut bacterial metabolites ('false neurotransmitters')
Infection	Reduced Kupffer cell number and function

sion (Fig. 16.16). In cirrhosis the increased blood pressure(>7 mmHg) in the hepatic portal vein is probably due to a combination of:

- increased portal blood flow
- increased hepatic vascular resistance
- intrahepatic arterio-venous shunting.

Portal hypertension leads to oesophageal varices (Fig. 16.17) and haemorrhoids (because normal anastomoses between the portal and systemic venous systems at these sites are enlarged) and also contributes to the development of ascites. Oesophageal varices are a particularly serious complication because these thin-walled dilated veins are prone to rupture, causing massive haematemesis which can be fatal. Other manifestations of portal hypertension include the less common 'caput medusae' around the umbilicus. Portal hypertension may be further complicated by portal vein thrombosis; this complication can lead to sudden clinical deterioration.

Liver cell carcinoma

Cirrhosis is a premalignant condition; it is associated with an increased risk of liver cell carcinoma. The tumour often appears to be multifocal, arising at multiple sites within the liver. The risk is greatest in macronodular cirrhosis and applies to all aetiological types. Liver cell carcinoma is considered in more detail below.

TUMOURS OF THE LIVER

> ▶ Benign tumours are rarely of clinical significance
> ▶ Metastatic carcinoma is the most common hepatic tumour
> ▶ Primary malignant tumours include liver cell carcinoma, cholangiocarcinoma, angiosarcoma and hepatoblastoma

Benign tumours

Benign tumours of the liver rarely give rise to serious clinical problems, except when they cause confusion with their malignant counterparts. Benign tumours of the liver include:

- liver cell adenoma
- angioma
- bile duct hamartoma
- focal nodular hyperplasia.

Liver cell adenoma

Liver cell adenoma is a benign, well-differentiated neoplasm of liver cells. It forms a well-circumscribed nodule, with a texture and colour resembling that of the normal liver. Adenomas may arise spontaneously, but an increased incidence occurs in patients taking anabolic, androgenic or oestrogenic steroids. They

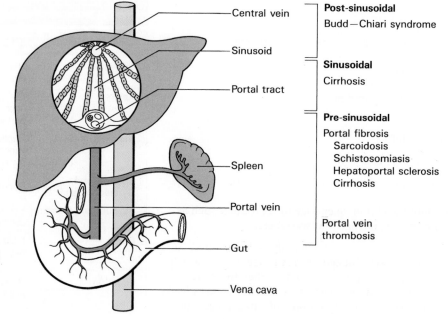

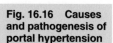

Fig. 16.16 Causes and pathogenesis of portal hypertension

Portal hypertension may be due to haemodynamic abnormalities proximal or distal to the sinusoids or at the sinusoidal level. Increased portal vascular resistance and intrahepatic shunting between high-pressure hepatic arterial and low-pressure portal venous channels are postulated explanations for portal hypertension in cirrhosis.

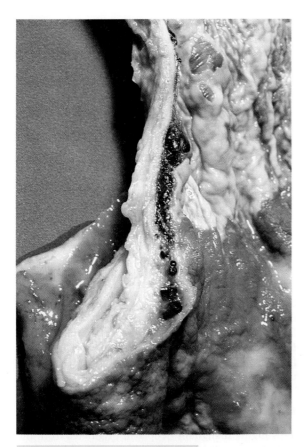

Fig. 16.17 Oesophageal varices

The cardio-oesophageal junction has been opened to reveal numerous dilated, thin-walled veins in a cirrhotic patient who died from a massive haematemesis.

may be clinically silent or cause hepatomegaly. Occasionally haemoperitoneum due to spontaneous rupture may be the first manifestation.

Angioma

Angioma, a benign vascular neoplasm, is sometimes multiple, rarely exceeding a few centimetres in diameter. Angiomas are rarely of clinical significance, but they may be mistaken for something more sinister when found unexpectedly during a laparotomy.

Bile duct hamartoma

Bile duct hamartomas are not strictly tumours but are tumour-like congenital malformations. They are usually small and often multiple, sometimes referred to as *von Meyenberg complexes*. They are often seen in association with congenital hepatic fibrosis.

Focal nodular hyperplasia

Focal nodular hyperplasia is neither a true neoplasm nor, despite its name, a hyperplastic disorder; it is thought to be another hamartomatous entity. It is usually solitary and up to 50 mm in diameter. At its centre is a stellate mass of fibrous connective tissue in which there are numerous small bile ducts. The rest of the lesion comprises liver cells and vascular sinusoids. These lesions are usually clinically occult, but they can become abnormally vascular, enlarge and rupture in patients receiving oestrogenic steroids such as oral contraceptives.

Malignant tumours

Malignant tumours in the liver often present with jaundice and weight loss. Most often they are metastases from other organs.

Primary malignant tumours of the liver include:

- liver cell carcinoma (hepatocellular carcinoma)
- cholangiocarcinoma (adenocarcinoma of bile ducts)
- angiosarcoma (malignant neoplasm of vascular endothelium)
- hepatoblastoma (primary liver tumour in childhood).

Metastases

The commonest malignant neoplasm to be found in the liver is metastatic carcinoma from a primary malignant tumour in another organ. These metastases usually form multiple deposits with central necrosis, causing an umbilicated appearance when they are visible on the liver surface. They are usually white unless they are derived from a malignant melanoma, in which case they may be dark brown or black. Common primary origins for hepatic metastases include the entire gastrointestinal tract including pancreas and bowel, the lung and the breast.

Metastases receive their vascular supply from the hepatic arterial system and this is sometimes selectively perfused with cytotoxic drugs or artificially embolised to occlude the vascular supply.

Liver cell carcinoma

Liver cell carcinoma (hepatocellular carcinoma) is one of the commonest tumours in certain parts of the world (Fig. 16.18). Known or suspected aetiological factors include:

- aflatoxins, carcinogenic mycotoxins produced by

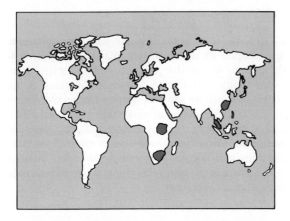

Fig. 16.18   Geographic areas of high incidence of liver cell carcinoma

The tumour occurs in all countries, particularly in patients with cirrhosis. Regions with a well-documented, very high incidence are shaded.

the fungus *Aspergillus flavus*, which contaminates food stored in humid conditions
• hepatitis B virus
• hepatic cirrhosis, irrespective of its cause (Fig. 16.19).

Various growth patterns are recognised, resembling to a variable extent the normal trabecular arrangement of liver cells. If the tumour is sufficiently well differentiated it retains the capacity to secrete bile, so that the tumour and any metastases from it

appear bile-stained. In cirrhotic livers, liver cell carcinomas often appear multifocal.

A type of liver cell carcinoma with specific features is the *fibrolamellar variant* in which the neoplastic liver cells are arranged in broad bands or lamellae separated by dense fibrous tissue. This variant occurs most often in young women, without cirrhosis as a predisposing cause.

Liver cell carcinomas often produce α-fetoprotein. This is a normal serum protein of the fetus, synthesis of which declines towards the end of gestation, when it is replaced by albumin. α-Fetoprotein is secreted by the tumour cells into the patient's blood, where it is a useful diagnostic marker.

Cholangiocarcinoma

Cholangiocarcinoma is an adenocarcinoma of bile duct epithelium. In liver biopsies it can be extremely difficult to distinguish from metastatic adenocarcinoma from some other organ. Known aetiological factors include infestation with the Chinese liver fluke, *Clonorchis sinensis*. There is also an increased incidence of cholangiocarcinoma in patients with ulcerative colitis.

Angiosarcoma

This highly malignant neoplasm originates from the endothelium of the vascular sinusoids and infiltrates the liver by spreading along the vascular sinusoids. Known aetiological factors include vinyl chloride,

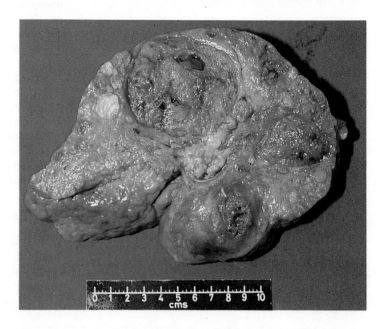

Fig. 16.19   Liver cell carcinoma arising in a cirrhotic liver

Cirrhosis is a pre-neoplastic condition. Several tumour nodules are present, perhaps reflecting the multifocal origin in cirrhotic livers.

used in the manufacture of polyvinyl chloride (PVC), and administration of the now-obsolete radiological contrast medium Thorotrast (Ch. 11). Thorotrast was a colloidal suspension of thorium dioxide, a naturally radioactive emitter of α-radiation with an extremely long half-life.

Hepatoblastoma

Hepatoblastoma is a rare malignant neoplasm of the liver occurring almost exclusively in children below the age of 5 years. In a significant proportion of cases it is associated with various developmental abnormalities. Histologically, its growth pattern resembles some features of the embryonic liver, but it is not uncommon to find unexpected tissues such as muscle. The prognosis is poor.

LIVER CYSTS

Liver cysts can often be distinguished from solid tumours by modern imaging techniques, although some malignant tumours may be so necrotic in the centre that they mimic cysts.

The main varieties are:

- simple cysts
- hydatid cysts
- choledochal cysts.

Simple cysts

Simple cysts are common, relatively small (10–20 mm diameter), and often multiple. Sometimes they are associated with lesions elsewhere, as in the rare von Hippel–Lindau syndrome. They have little or no intrinsic clinical importance.

Hydatid cysts

Hydatid cysts are due to the parasite *Echinococcus granulosus*. They are usually many centimetres in diameter, have a fibrous laminated wall and contain numerous daughter cysts (Fig. 16.20). Great care must be taken during surgical removal, because spillage of the cyst fluid into the peritoneum may precipitate anaphylactic shock due to the presence of hydatid antigens in a patient already sensitised to them.

Choledochal cysts

Choledochal cysts are uncommon congenital cysts of the bile ducts which may be intra- or extra-hepatic. Their presence predisposes to cholangitis.

LIVER INVOLVEMENT BY SYSTEMIC DISEASE

The liver is commonly affected by disease primarily arising in other organs or systems; this often causes hepatomegaly. Examples include:

- centrilobular congestion and liver cell necrosis in right ventricular heart failure
- granulomas in sarcoidosis
- infiltration by amyloid
- metastatic solid tumours
- infiltration by leukaemic cells in leukaemias
- extramedullary haemopoiesis in myelofibrosis
- fatty change as a non-specific feature in patients ill from a variety of causes.

Liver biopsy is often indicated in the diagnosis and investigation of systemic diseases such as suspected sarcoidosis or carcinomatosis. The biopsy may be diagnostic of the systemic problem.

The commonest liver involvement by systemic disease is seen in cardiac failure. At autopsy in such cases, the liver appears to have a finely mottled surface due to an acinar pattern of central congestion surrounded by fatty change. This is the so-called 'nutmeg liver'.

TRANSPLANTATION AND THE LIVER

The pathology of transplantation and the liver is important for two reasons. First, although liver transplants are relatively well tolerated, immunological rejection of the grafted organ can occur. Second, the liver is frequently affected by graft-versus-host disease following bone marrow transplantation.

Liver transplants

Liver transplants have been performed successfully since the 1960s. The most frequent indication in the UK is primary biliary cirrhosis. The 5-year survival in experienced centres exceeds 60%.

Experimental studies showed that the immunogenicity of the liver was relatively low, for example compared with the kidney, but in clinical practice there is a significant risk of rejection. The most vulnerable cells are biliary epithelium and vascular endothelium; these express MHC class II antigens. Rejection may be:

- *acute* — occurring within 2 weeks of transplantation in most cases and characterised by a mixed inflammatory cell infiltrate in portal tracts and in the endothelial layer of portal and hepatic vein branches (endotheliitis)
- *chronic* — characterised by cell-mediated destruction of intrahepatic bile ducts (vanishing bile duct syndrome) and occlusion of hepatic arteries by macrophages with lipid-laden cytoplasm accumulating in the intima.

Fortunately, close monitoring of liver transplants and improvements in immunosuppressive therapy are gradually reducing the probability of graft loss by rejection.

Graft-versus-host disease

Patients with leukaemia or lymphoma may be treated by bone marrow transplantation after whole-body irradiation to eliminate the neoplastic cells. Although every effort is made to find a closely matched donor by histocompatibility testing, there is a risk that the lymphocytes in the marrow allograft will recognise and react to the normal antigens on the host's tissues; the result is graft-versus-host disease. Skin, gut epithelium and the liver are especially vulnerable. In the liver, the principal target for the immune reaction is biliary epithelium. If the condition is untreated, many bile ducts will be destroyed resulting in jaundice.

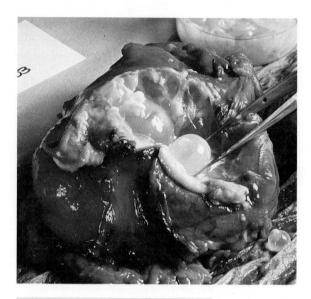

Fig. 16.20   Hydatid cyst of the liver
The surgically resected cyst has been opened to reveal the enclosed daughter cysts.

through the ampulla of Vater as the sphincter of Oddi relaxes.

CONGENITAL ABNORMALITIES

Malformations of the biliary system include:

- *biliary atresia*, in which there is failure of the biliary tree to develop and normally anastomose with intrahepatic structures
- *choledochal cysts* (see above), sometimes associated with *congenital hepatic fibrosis*.

Intrahepatic malformations of the biliary system are inaccessible to surgical correction and, if life-threatening, may be an indication for liver transplantation.

In addition to these malformations, the liver is often affected by the production of abnormally viscous bile in patients with cystic fibrosis (mucoviscidosis) (Ch. 7).

BILIARY SYSTEM

NORMAL STRUCTURE AND FUNCTION

The biliary system comprises the intrahepatic and extrahepatic bile ducts and the gallbladder. The system is lined by a glandular mucus-secreting epithelial cell layer. Bile is secreted by the liver along the right and left hepatic ducts which fuse to form the common bile duct. The bile consists of micelles of cholesterol, phospholipid and bile salts, and of course bilirubin.

Bile enters the gallbladder through the cystic duct; it is then stored and concentrated in the gallbladder. In response to the ingestion of food, particularly with a high fat content, the gallbladder contracts by stimulation with cholecystokinin and expels the concentrated bile into the second part of the duodenum,

DISEASES OF THE GALLBLADDER

Gallbladder disease is extremely common and in almost every case it is associated with or due to the presence of gallstones.

Cholelithiasis (gallstones)

> ► Risk factors include female gender, obesity, diabetes mellitus
> ► Gallstones consist of pure cholesterol, bile pigment or a mixture
> ► Complications include cholecystitis, obstructive jaundice, carcinoma of the gallbladder

Cholelithiasis is the name given to the common condition in which *gallstones* form within the biliary system. Risk factors for cholesterol-rich stones include female gender and obesity (hence 'fat, fair, forty, fertile, female', an alliterative description of the typical patient) and diabetes mellitus. Stones are prone to occur if there is a relative excess of cholesterol in the bile. Gallstones are usually composed of a mixture of cholesterol and bile pigment (Fig. 16.21), although almost pure cholesterol or pigment stones are occasionally found. Pure pigment gallstones occur notably in patients with haemolytic anaemia where there is consequent excessive excretion of bilirubin. Calcium carbonate stones are also found rarely.

The stones often have a laminated internal structure and, if multiple (as they commonly are), have faceted surfaces.

Pathogenesis

Cholesterol stones may form if there is an imbalance between the ratio of cholesterol and bile salts; the latter form micelles which have a hydrophilic exterior enclosing the hydrophobic cholesterol. Thus, gallstones can result from:

- an excess of cholesterol
- a deficit of bile salts.

Pathological effects

The pathological effects of gallstones include (Fig. 16.22):

- inflammation of the gallbladder (cholecystitis)
- mucocele
- predisposition to carcinoma of the gallbladder
- obstruction of the biliary system resulting in biliary colic and jaundice
- infection of static bile, causing cholangitis and liver abscesses
- gallstone ileus due to intestinal obstruction by a gallstone which has entered the gut through a fistulous connection with the gallbladder
- pancreatitis.

Cholesterosis

Cholesterosis is the name given to the clinically unimportant occurrence of cholesterol-laden macrophages in the lamina propria of the gallbladder mucosa. This occurrence gives the mucosa a yellow-speckled appearance known as 'strawberry gallbladder'.

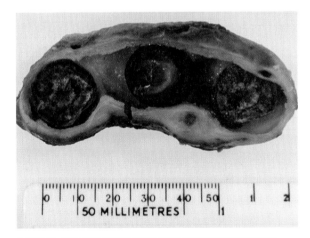

Fig. 16.21 Gallstones and chronic cholecystitis

The thickened gallbladder has been opened to reveal several large cholesterol-rich stones.

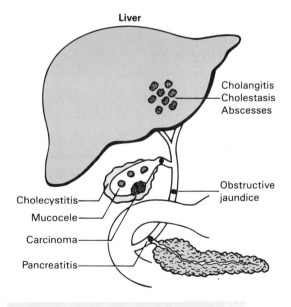

Fig. 16.22 Pathological effects of gallstones

Cholecystitis

Cholecystitis is an inflammatory condition of the gallbladder. It is almost always associated with gallstones and occurs as an acute or chronic condition. It is a common cause of abdominal pain in the right hypochondrium.

Acute cholecystitis

> ▶ Usually associated with gallstones
> ▶ Initially sterile, then infected
> ▶ Complications include empyema and/or rupture

Acute cholecystitis is usually due to obstruction of the outflow from the gallbladder by a gallstone. The initial inflammatory reaction is due to the irritant effects of bile and is therefore usually sterile at this stage. However, stasis of bile predisposes to infection which then stimulates a more vigorous and often pyogenic acute inflammatory response. The gallbladder wall becomes oedematous, due to increased vascular permeability, and infiltrated with acute inflammatory cells. The lumen distends with pus, and stretching of the wall already weakened by inflammation leads to a risk of perforation and peritonitis. Alternatively a fistula may form with the second part of the duodenum and allow stones to be passed into the bowel lumen. Large stones may occasionally lodge at the ileocaecal valve and cause intestinal obstruction (gallstone ileus).

An inflamed gallbladder grossly distended with pus is called an *empyema*.

Chronic cholecystitis

> ▶ Invariably associated with gallstones
> ▶ Fibrosis and Aschoff–Rokitansky sinuses

Chronic cholecystitis may develop insidiously or after repeated episodes of acute cholecystitis.

The gallbladder wall is thickened by fibrosis and is relatively rigid. Thus obstructive jaundice due to gallstones is not usually associated with a palpable gallbladder because the stones will be associated with chronic cholecystitis and therefore a rigid gallbladder. Conversely, obstructive jaundice due to carcinoma of the head of the pancreas often results in a palpable distended gallbladder; this is the pathological basis of *Courvoisier's law*.

The thick gallbladder wall has within it Aschoff–Rokitansky sinuses, mucosal herniations

(diverticula) often containing inspissated bile or even small stones. The wall bears an infiltrate of chronic inflammatory cells and the blood vessels often show endarteritis obliterans (Fig. 16.23). A stone is often found in Hartmann's pouch, a pathological dilatation in the neck of the gallbladder formed by increased intraluminal pressure or impaction of the stone.

A rare variant is *xanthogranulomatous cholecystitis* in which lipid-laden macrophages and giant cells accumulate in large numbers; they mimic a neoplasm grossly and, specifically, a clear-cell carcinoma histologically. The lesion, like its more common renal counterpart, xanthogranulomatous pyelonephritis, is prone to give rise to fistulae.

Mucocele

A mucocele of the gallbladder is the result of sterile obstruction of the neck by a gallstone. The lack of inflammation permits the gallbladder to distend

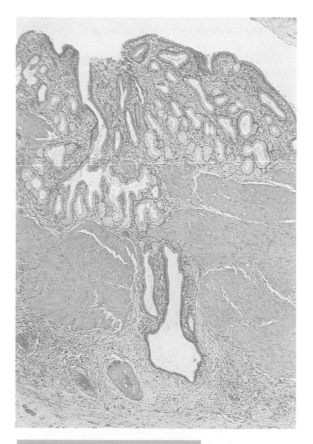

Fig. 16.23   Chronic cholecystitis

Histology showing a thickened gallbladder wall, diffuse chronic inflammatory infiltration, and Aschoff–Rokitansky sinuses.

with mucus without rupturing. The mucocele has a thin wall and demands careful handling during surgical removal to avoid the risk of spillage of mucus into the peritoneal cavity and thus the risk of pseudomyxoma peritonei, a rare complication in which the peritoneum becomes seeded with mucus-producing epithelial cells and the cavity fills with mucus.

Carcinoma of the gallbladder

> ▶ Usually an adenocarcinoma
> ▶ Invariably associated with gallstones

Carcinoma of the gallbladder is almost always associated with the presence of gallstones; this relationship may be causal. The tumour is most often an adenocarcinoma, although squamous cell carcinoma is also seen. As the gallbladder is not a vital organ, the tumour is often advanced at the time of clinical presentation, and invasion of the liver and other adjacent structures defeats attempts at operative removal. It therefore has a poor prognosis.

Carcinoma of the bile duct

> ▶ Adenocarcinoma
> ▶ Increased incidence in ulcerative colitis
> ▶ Presents with jaundice

Carcinoma of the bile duct is most commonly an adenocarcinoma. There is an increased incidence in patients with chronic ulcerative colitis. It tends to present at a relatively early stage with obstructive jaundice.

Biliary obstruction

Bile duct obstruction is a fairly common event and may be due to:

- gallstones
- carcinoma of the common bile duct
- carcinoma of the head of the pancreas
- inflammatory stricture of the common bile duct
- accidental surgical ligation of the common bile duct.

The patient becomes jaundiced, deeply so if the obstruction is not relieved, with a raised conjugated serum bilirubin, pale stools and dark urine. A raised serum alkaline phosphatase with only modest elevation of transaminases is usual.

If the biliary obstruction persists, there is a risk that the static bile becomes infected, causing cholangitis and liver abscesses. Lack of bile in the small intestine interferes with the absorption of fat and fat-soluble substances (e.g. some vitamins).

Diseases of intrahepatic bile ducts

A clinical picture similar to that of biliary obstruction can result from diseases of intrahepatic bile ducts such as:

- biliary atresia
- primary biliary cirrhosis
- sclerosing cholangitis
- cholestatic drug reactions.

These conditions can usually be distinguished by careful clinical assessment, liver biopsy and imaging techniques.

EXOCRINE PANCREAS

NORMAL STRUCTURE AND FUNCTION

The pancreas is a retroperitoneal organ, the head and uncinate process lying within the duodenal loop, the body crossing the aorta and inferior vena cava, and the tail abutting onto the splenic hilum.

The pancreas is a mixed exocrine and endocrine organ. Scattered through the gland are the islets of Langerhans consisting of endocrine cells producing peptide hormones, the most important of which are insulin and glucagon (Ch. 17); their secretion drains directly into the blood and ultimately into the liver through the hepatic portal vein.

The exocrine pancreas comprises the bulk of the organ and is composed of glands and ducts, with a lobular arrangement, the latter fusing to form the pancreatic and accessory ducts which convey the exocrine secretions into the duodenum. The exocrine glands contain numerous zymogen granules and produce trypsin, lipase, phospholipase, amylase and elastase; these enzymes require activation, normally in the duodenum. The pancreas also secretes a bicarbonate-rich alkaline medium.

Some of the exocrine glands are perfused with blood that has already perfused islets in the vicinity (i.e. they have a portal blood supply); this almost certainly provides some physiological advantages, but it does mean that these glands are specially vulnerable if the circulation is impaired.

INVESTIGATION OF PANCREATIC DISEASE

Disorders of the exocrine pancreas can be investigated radiologically by the technique of ERCP (endoscopic retrograde cholangiopancreatography). The pancreatic duct is cannulated under endoscopic visualisation, and contrast medium is injected to permit radiological delineation of the duct and thus reveal any deformities due to inflammatory fibrosis or tumours. Pancreatic juice can be collected through the cannula and examined biochemically for enzymes, or cytologically for abnormal cells such as may be shed from a carcinoma.

Operative biopsies of the pancreas are hazardous because there is a significant risk of precipitating acute pancreatitis (inflammation of the pancreas) due to extravasation of exocrine secretions. Nevertheless, an intra-operative frozen section diagnosis may be required in cases of suspected pancreatic carcinoma before attempting to remove the lesion, a procedure with a relatively high post-operative complication rate. Fine-needle aspiration cytology is possible through the unopened abdomen under ultrasound or computed axial tomography (CAT) guidance.

Serum amylase is an important marker of pancreatic inflammation. The concentration is greatly elevated in acute pancreatitis; lesser elevations may occur following a perforated peptic ulcer.

CONGENITAL ABNORMALITIES

Congenital abnormalities of the pancreas include:

- *annular pancreas* encircling, and sometimes obstructing, the duodenum
- *pancreas divisum* due to failure of fusion of the two embryological anlagen
- *ectopic pancreatic tissue* (in the stomach or in a Meckel's diverticulum)
- *cysts.*

In addition, the pancreas is severely affected in cystic fibrosis (mucoviscidosis), a congenital disorder of exocrine secretions in which they are abnormally vis-cous (Ch. 7). The mucus plugs the pancreatic ducts resulting in retention of secretions and damage to the exocrine glands.

DISEASES OF THE PANCREAS

Pancreatitis

Pancreatitis (inflammation of the pancreas) can be classified into acute and chronic forms. There is, however, overlap in that patients with chronic pancreatitis may have acute exacerbations.

Acute pancreatitis

> ▶ Aetiological factors include duct obstruction, shock, alcohol, etc.
> ▶ Amylase is released into blood (diagnostically useful)
> ▶ Often haemorrhagic
> ▶ Fat necrosis in surrounding tissue binds calcium

Aetiology
Acute pancreatitis (Fig. 16.24) may be due to:

- obstruction of the pancreatic duct
- bile reflux
- alcohol, particularly acute intoxication
- vascular insufficiency (e.g. shock)
- mumps virus infection
- hyperparathyroidism
- hypothermia
- trauma
- iatrogenic factors (e.g. after ERCP).

Although many cases are mild, acute pancreatitis is often a serious disorder with a high mortality. It is more common in adults than in children. The condition is serious because the gland, once injured, releases its lytic enzymes into the blood, contributing to the severe shock, and into the surrounding tissue, causing tissue digestion.

Clinical features
Patients present with a sudden onset of severe abdominal pain, often radiating into the back, and nausea and vomiting. The upper abdomen is tender. The clinical deterioration may be rapid, the patient becoming severely shocked. Diagnosis is made by finding a greatly elevated serum amylase concentration.

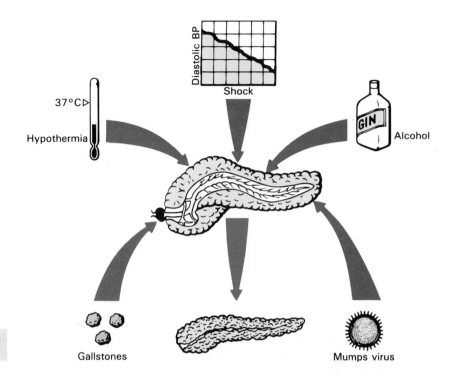

Fig. 16.24 Common causes of pancreatitis

Pathogenesis

The pathogenesis of the early stages varies according to the aetiology. For example, when the pancreatic duct is obstructed by a gallstone at the ampulla of Vater, or where there is biliary reflux into the pancreatic duct for any other reason, the duct epithelium is damaged, particularly if the bile is infected or admixed with trypsin. The damage extends into the gland and results in the leakage and activation of pancreatic enzymes. In contrast, when pancreatitis is attributable to vascular insufficiency, the hypoxic injury due to reduced blood flow occurs first in the acini at the periphery of the lobules; they are precariously remote from the vascular supply and some are fed by portal vessels from islets in the vicinity. Irrespective of the initiating event, the liberation of lytic enzymes causes further damage and diffuse pancreatitis develops rapidly.

The gland becomes swollen and often haemorrhagic if the inflammation is severe. Proteases digest the walls of blood vessels, causing extravasation of blood. Amylase is released into the blood, where measurement of its concentration is an important diagnostic marker of the condition.

Lipolytic action causes fat necrosis, which can be quite extensive within the abdomen and subcutaneous tissue. Sometimes the necrosis extends anteriorly around the abdominal wall to produce discoloration of the skin (Grey Turner's sign). The released fatty acids bind calcium ions, and the resulting white precipitates are readily visible; severe fat necrosis can bind so much calcium that hypocalcaemia results, sometimes causing tetany.

Concomitant destruction of the adjacent islets can result in hyperglycaemia.

Other complications include the formation of abscesses and cysts within the pancreas or adjacent tissues. These often necessitate surgical drainage.

Chronic pancreatitis

▶ Commonest cause is alcohol (long-term excess)
▶ Pancreas shows fibrosis and exocrine atrophy
▶ May result in intestinal malabsorption due to loss of pancreatic secretions

Aetiology

Chronic pancreatitis is a relapsing disorder that may either be the result of repeated episodes of clinically evident acute pancreatitis or may develop insidiously without previous symptoms of pancreatic disease. The commonest cause is chronic excessive alcohol consumption. Chronic pancreatitis is also a feature of cystic fibrosis (mucoviscidosis). There is

481

also a rare familial pancreatitis inherited as an auto-somal dominant trait, in some cases associated with aminoaciduria or hyperparathyroidism.

Clinicopathological features
Chronic pancreatitis is more common in adults than in children, and presents with intermittent upper abdominal and back pain and weight loss. A plain X-ray of the upper abdomen often reveals flecks of calcification due to previous fat necrosis. An ERCP often shows that the pancreatic ducts are distorted by scar tissue resulting from the chronic inflammatory process.

The exocrine tissue is eventually replaced by fibrosis (Fig. 16.25) and, if localised, its hard texture mimics that of a carcinoma when the gland is palpated during laparotomy. The endocrine component of the gland is relatively unaffected except at an advanced stage.

Pancreatic malabsorption
Chronic pancreatitis, with loss of exocrine secretions, results in malabsorption of fat because of the relative lack of lipases. The patient's faeces contain abnormally high quantities of fat (steatorrhoea), and absorption of fat-soluble substances such as vitamins A, D, E and K is impaired.

Carcinoma of the pancreas

▶ Usually adenocarcinoma
▶ May present with obstructive jaundice
▶ Very poor prognosis

Aetiology
Pancreatic carcinoma is increasing in incidence in many countries. Just under 6000 cases occur annually in England and Wales. There is an association with cigarette smoking and with diabetes mellitus. There appears to be an increased risk in the rare entity of familial pancreatitis. The prognosis is dismal even in operable cases.

Weight loss is a common presenting feature; other symptoms are attributable to the precise location of the tumour. Some cases develop flitting venous thromboses (thrombophlebitis migrans): this is *Trousseau's sign.*

Clinicopathological features
Most pancreatic carcinomas are adenocarcinomas with a marked desmoplastic stromal reaction (Fig. 16.26), making them very firm on palpation during surgery. They arise most commonly in the head of the organ, where they tend to compress the common bile duct and cause obstructive jaundice. Elsewhere in the gland, they can present at a relatively late stage because they cause few signs or symptoms. Extensive replacement of the gland by carcinoma can lead to diabetes mellitus due to destruction of the islets of Langerhans.

Pancreatic adenocarcinomas spread by the blood stream to the liver and via lymphatics to regional lymph nodes. Prognosis is relatively poor because metastases are often present at the time of surgery. If surgical removal is attempted, it involves excision of at least part of the pancreas, the duodenum and

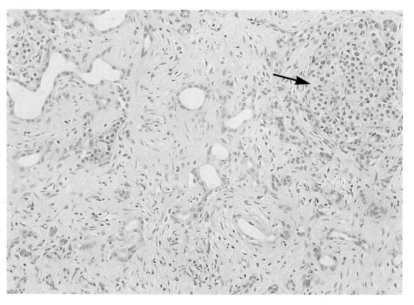

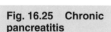
Fig. 16.25 Chronic pancreatitis

Histology showing considerable loss of acini and replacement by fibrosis. Inflammatory cells are relatively inconspicuous at this late stage. Islets of Langerhans (one is arrowed) sometimes escape destruction, but their loss can result in diabetes mellitus.

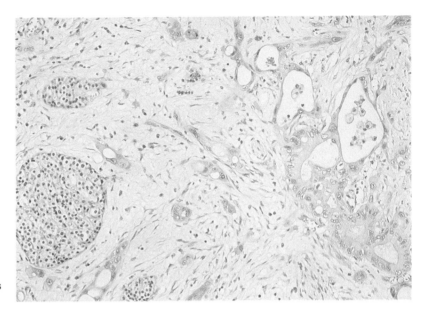

Fig. 16.26 Pancreatic adenocarcinoma

The neoplastic glands with pleomorphic atypical nuclei are invested by dense fibrous connective tissue, thus mimicking the texture of chronic pancreatitis when the gland is palpated during surgery.

regional nodes with anastomotic restoration of intestinal, biliary, and residual pancreatic flow; this procedure is associated with a high risk of operative mortality.

Cysts and cystic tumours

Pancreatic cysts are of two types:

- *true cysts*, which are lined by epithelium and may be congenital
- *pseudocysts*, which lack an epithelial lining and are often the result of acute pancreatitis; they can be drained surgically.

True cystic tumours also occur; the benign *cystadenoma* and its malignant variant, *cystadenocarcinoma*.

FURTHER READING

MacSween RNM, Antony PP, Scheuer PJ, Burt AD, Portman BC 1995 Pathology of the liver, 3rd edn. Churchill Livingstone, Edinburgh
Rosai J 1989 Ackerman's surgical pathology, 7th edn. Mosby, St Louis, pp 737–788

Scheuer PJ, Lefkowitch JH 1994 Liver biopsy interpretation, 5th edn. Harcourt Brace, London

Endocrine system

NORMAL STRUCTURE AND FUNCTION

An *endocrine gland* secretes hormones directly into the blood stream to reach distant 'target organs' where the secretory products exert their effects. Endocrine glands are thus distinguished from *exocrine glands*, whose secretions pass into the gut or respiratory tract, or on to the exterior of the body; examples of exocrine glands include the exocrine pancreas and the bronchial mucous glands. Closely related to the endocrine system is the *paracrine (diffuse endocrine) system*, consisting of regional distributions of specialised cells producing locally acting hormones, such as those regulating gut motility, and forming part of the APUD system (Ch. 15); *autocrine effects* are those acting on the cell producing the hormone (Fig. 17.1).

Hormones exert their effects on the target organs by binding to receptors, protein molecules with high and specific affinity for the hormone. These hormone receptors may be either on the cell surface (for example, thyroid-stimulating hormone receptors on the thyroid epithelium) or intracellular (for example, nuclear receptors for steroid hormones). The binding of a hormone to its cell surface receptor sets off a series of intracellular signals via secondary 'messenger' molecules (cyclic nucleotides), which results in changes in metabolic activity, differentiation or mitosis of the stimulated cell.

ENDOCRINE PATHOLOGY

The major disorders of an endocrine gland are:

* hyperfunction
* hypofunction
* benign and malignant tumours, which themselves may cause disordered function.

There are several important general considerations in endocrine pathology. First, disease of one endocrine gland cannot usually be considered in isolation, because it almost always has implications for other endocrine glands:

* Many glands are interdependent, for example hypersecretion of a hormone by one gland may stimulate a target endocrine gland into overactivity.
* Tumours or hyperfunction of one endocrine gland may be associated with similar disease in other glands in the multiple endocrine neoplasia (MEN) syndromes.
* Organ-specific autoimmune disease may affect more than one endocrine gland.

Second, one hormone may have many diverse clinical effects, so that malfunction of one endocrine gland may produce numerous clinical features.

Third, the same hormone may be produced in more than one site; thus, ectopic hormone production by tumours of non-endocrine tissues may simulate primary endocrine disease.

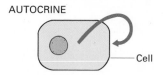

AUTOCRINE

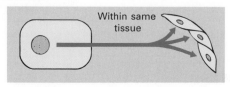

Cell

PARACRINE

Within same tissue

ENDOCRINE

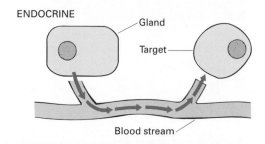

Gland

Target

Blood stream

Fig. 17.1 Comparison of the autocrine, paracrine and endocrine systems (see text for details)

THE PITUITARY

The pituitary is a small gland, weighing only 500–1000 mg. It is situated in the sella turcica of the skull beneath the hypothalamus. Despite its small size, it exerts many essential control functions over the rest of the endocrine system, earning it the title 'conductor of the endocrine orchestra'. It consists of two parts (Fig. 17.2), each with separate functions. The anterior pituitary, the *adenohypophysis*, is developed from Rathke's pouch, an outpouching of the roof of the embryonic oral cavity; it comprises about 75% of the bulk of the gland. The posterior pituitary, the *neurohypophysis*, is derived from a downgrowth of the hypothalamus.

Pathological basis of endocrine signs and symptoms	
Sign or symptom	Pathological basis
Signs or symptoms of hormone excess (hyperfunction)	Endocrine gland hyperplasia caused by increased trophic stimulus to secretion Functioning neoplasm of endocrine gland
Signs or symptoms of hormone deficiency (hypofunction)	Endocrine gland atrophy due to loss of trophic stimulus to secretion Destruction of endocrine gland by inflammation, ischaemia or non-functioning tumour
Diffuse enlargement of gland	Inflammatory cell infiltration Hyperplasia
Nodular enlargement of gland	Tumour (benign or malignant)
Some organ-specific features	
• headache, bitemporal hemianopia	Pituitary tumour
• anxiety, sweating, tremor	Increased thyroid hormone secretion due to hyperplasia or neoplasia of gland
• exophthalmos	Autoimmune involvement of retrobulbar connective tissue in Graves' disease
• hypertension	Adrenocortical hyperplasia or neoplasia Adrenal medullary neoplasm (phaeochromocytoma)
• excessive growth (features vary according to whether prepubertal or postpubertal)	Growth-hormone secreting pituitary tumour
• glycosuria	Absolute or relative deficiency of insulin (diabetes mellitus)

ADENOHYPOPHYSIS

Classification of cell types

Modern histological classification of the types of hormone-secreting cell is based on immunohisto-chemistry, a technique in which antibodies raised

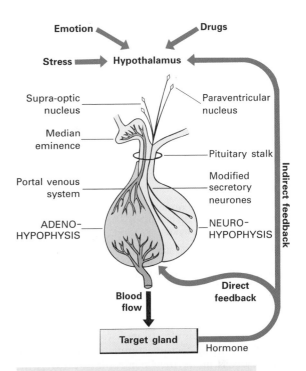

Fig. 17.2 The pituitary and its physiological relationships

The pituitary is controlled both by hormones from its target glands, and via the hypothalamus.

to a hormone bind to the cells containing that hormone in tissue sections, leading to a coloured stain (Fig. 17.3). This has enabled the true hormone content of the cells to be determined, and has rendered obsolete the traditional classification of the cells into eosinophil, basophil and chromophobe types according to their staining by haematoxylin and eosin (H&E). By electron microscopy, the cells of the adenohypophysis are seen to contain electron-dense granules ranging from 50 to 500 nm in diameter (Fig. 17.4); these contain stored secretory products. The six types of hormone-secreting cells are shown in Table 17.1.

Control of hormone secretion

Hormonal control factors

The adenohypophysis lacks any direct arterial supply. Blood from the hypothalamus passes down venous portal channels in the pituitary stalk (Fig. 17.2) into sinusoids which ramify within the gland. In this way hormonal control factors produced by neurosecretory cells in the hypothalamus are carried directly to the hormone-producing cells

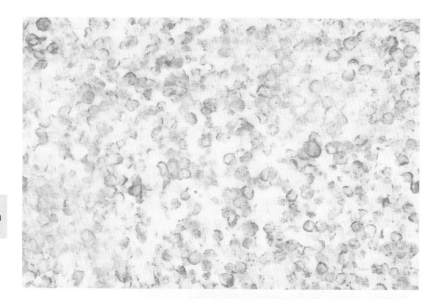

Fig. 17.3 Growth hormone-containing cells in an adenoma of the adenohypophysis

Immunoperoxidase localisation of growth hormone. Cells containing growth hormone are stained brown by this technique.

of the adenohypophysis. The known hormonal control factors and their effects are listed in Table 17.2. In general, these factors stimulate the particular secretory cells under their control into activity; the exception is prolactin-inhibiting factor, whose effect on the lactotrophs is inhibitory.

Secretion of these hormonal control factors by the hypothalamus is under two types of control:

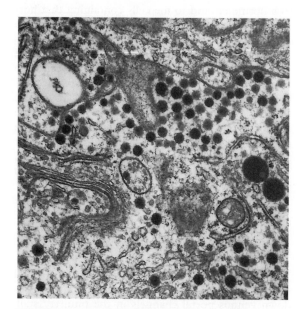

Fig. 17.4 Electron micrograph of a secretory cell of the adenohypophysis

The hormonal products are stored as electron-dense membrane-bound granules (×300 000).

Table 17.1 Hormone-secreting cells of the adenohypophysis

Cell type	Staining reaction with H&E	Hormonal product
Corticotroph	Basophilic	Adrenocorticotrophic hormone (ACTH)
Thyrotroph	Basophilic	Thyroid-stimulating hormone (TSH)
Gonadotroph	Basophilic	Follicle-stimulating hormone (FSH)
		Luteinising hormone (LH)
Somatotroph	Eosinophilic	Growth hormone (GH)
Lactotroph	Eosinophilic	Prolactin (PL)
Chromophobe	Pale	Unknown

Table 17.2 Hormonal control factors and their effects on the adenohypophysis

Hormonal control factor	Effect
Corticotrophin-releasing factor (CRF)	Corticotrophs release ACTH
Thyrotrophin-releasing factor (TRF)	Thyrotrophs release TSH
Gonadotrophin-releasing factor (FSH/LH-RF)	Gonadotrophs release FSH/LH
Growth hormone-releasing factor (GHRF)	Somatotrophs release GH
Prolactin-inhibiting factor (PIF)	Lactotrophs inhibited from releasing PL

neural and hormonal. *Neural control* is via nerves from other parts of the central nervous system, and is important in reactions to stress and in changes during sleep. *Hormonal control* is a negative feedback mechanism in which the hypothalamus monitors the level of adenohypophysial hormones in the blood and adjusts its output of hormonal control factors accordingly, so as to stabilise the level of each adenohypophysial hormone at the optimum level. This is called the *hypothalamic–hypophysial feedback control*.

Feedback control

In addition to control via the hypothalamus, a more direct method of control of the adenohypophysis also exists, whereby its cells respond directly to the levels of hormones and metabolites in the blood. Most adenohypophysial hormones stimulate another endocrine gland, termed the 'target' gland; for example, ACTH stimulates the adrenal cortex to produce steroid hormones, and TSH stimulates the thyroid to produce thyroxine.

In these examples, the level of hormone from the target gland is monitored for feedback control. However, in the case of growth hormone (GH), which has no single target gland, it is the level of metabolites such as glucose which is monitored. A general scheme of the feedback control mechanisms operating in the regulation of a hypophysial hormone is shown in Figure 17.2.

Adenohypophysial hormones

Adrenocorticotrophic hormone

Adrenocorticotrophic hormone (ACTH), a peptide consisting of 39 amino acids, causes increased cell numbers (hyperplasia) and increased secretory activity in the adrenal cortex. Glucocorticoid output is elevated, but there is no effect on the output of mineralocorticoids, such as aldosterone, which are not under anterior pituitary control. ACTH levels may be measured by radio-immunoassay and show a marked circadian variation, being highest early in the morning.

Thyroid-stimulating hormone

Thyroid-stimulating hormone (TSH) is a glycoprotein which induces proliferation of the follicular cells of the thyroid, synthesis of thyroxine (T_4) and tri-iodothyronine (T_3), and secretion of these into the blood. Radio-immunoassay of TSH provides information on the state of the control system of the thy-

roid and is valuable in the diagnosis of thyroid malfunction.

Gonadotrophic hormones

In the female, follicle-stimulating hormone (FSH) induces growth of Graafian follicles in the ovaries; these secrete oestrogens, which in turn cause endometrial proliferation. After rupture of the follicle at ovulation, luteinising hormone (LH) causes a change in the follicle cells known as luteinisation, whereby their secretory product changes from oestrogens to progesterone which induces secretory changes in the endometrium. Both gonadotrophic hormones are glycoproteins.

The hypothalamus monitors circulating levels of the sex steroids including oestrogens and progesterone, and releases probably a single hormonal control factor, FSH/LH-releasing factor (FSH/LH-RF), to control the adenohypophysial gonadotrophs. Their response to this factor depends on the prevailing levels of sex steroids. Cyclical changes in this feedback loop form the hormonal basis for the menstrual cycle.

In the male, FSH and LH both exist but, in the absence of ovaries as the target organ, their names are inappropriate to their actions. LH stimulates testosterone production by the interstitial cells of Leydig in the testes, while FSH stimulates spermatogenesis.

The circulating levels of FSH and LH vary markedly with age: they increase at puberty and are very high in females after the menopause.

Growth hormone

Growth hormone (GH) is a protein containing 191 amino acids; it binds to receptors on the surface of various cells and thus causes increased protein synthesis, accelerates breakdown of fatty tissue to produce energy, and tends to raise the blood glucose. It is vital for normal growth and deficiency causes dwarfism. Part of its action at tissue level is mediated by a group of peptide growth factors known as somatomedins. The hypothalamic control of GH release from the hypothalamus is complex, there being both a growth hormone-releasing factor (GH-RF) and an inhibitory factor, somatostatin.

Prolactin

Prolactin (PL) is a protein hormone with a structure very similar to that of GH. Although it is present in individuals of both sexes, its function in males remains uncertain. In females, it can produce lactation, provided that the breast has already been prepared during pregnancy by appropriate levels of sex steroids. Prolactin release is a good example of the neural form of hypothalamic control: the sensation of suckling causes reduction in hypothalamic pro-lactin-inhibiting factor (PIF) release and a consequent rise in PL levels.

Hypofunction

> ▸ Most cases due to destruction by tumour or extrinsic compression
> ▸ Causes include adenomas, craniopharyngiomas and ischaemic necrosis
> ▸ Leads to secondary hypofunction of adenohypophysial-dependent endocrine glands

Like other endocrine organs, the adenohypophysis has considerable reserve capacity, and deficiency of its hormones becomes manifest only after extensive destruction; hypofunction is therefore uncommon. Since the pituitary is tightly encased within the sella turcica, any expansile lesion, such as an adenoma, produces compression damage to the adjacent pituitary tissue in addition to any effect from its own hormonal production. Damage to the hypothalamus or pituitary stalk may also produce adenohypophysial hypofunction through failure of control. Table 17.3 sets out the main causes of hypofunction. These conditions lead to a deficiency of all adenohypophysial hormones, a state known as *panhypopituitarism*. This is a life-threatening condition, since deficiency of ACTH leads to atrophy of the adrenal cortex and failure of production of vital adrenocorticoids. Diagnosis of hypopituitarism is by radioimmunoassay of the individual hormones. The commonest causes of pituitary hypofunction are compression by metastatic carcinoma or by an ade-

Table 17.3   Causes of adenohypophysial hypofunction

Site	Lesions
Pituitary	Adenoma
	Metastatic carcinoma
	Trauma
	Post-partum ischaemic necrosis (Sheehan's syndrome)
	Craniopharyngioma
	Infections
	Granulomatous diseases
	Autoimmunity
	Iatrogenic
Hypothalamus	Craniopharyngioma
	Gliomas

noma, but two specific rarer syndromes will be mentioned because they illustrate how congenital and acquired disease may affect the pituitary.

Pituitary dwarfism

Pituitary dwarfism is due to deficiency of GH, sometimes associated with deficiency of other adenohypophysial hormones. The child fails to grow, although remaining well-proportioned. There are a variety of known causes including adenomas, craniopharyngiomas (rare tumours derived from remnants of Rathke's pouch) and familial forms.

Post-partum ischaemic necrosis

During pregnancy, the pituitary enlarges and becomes highly vascular. Hypotensive shock due to haemorrhage at the time of birth, compounded by the lack of direct arterial supply to the adenohypophysis, may cause ischaemic necrosis. This specific cause of necrosis is known as *Sheehan's syndrome* and the effects of the resulting adenohypophysial hypofunction are termed *Simmond's disease*. The neurohypophysis is usually spared. The first symptom following delivery is failure of lactation due to PL deficiency; the effects of lack of FSH/LH, TSH and ACTH then follow—loss of sexual function, hypothyroidism, and the diverse effects of glucocorticoid deficiency. Improvements in obstetric management mean that Sheehan's syndrome is now rare, although hypotensive shock due to trauma may produce similar effects.

Tumours: adenomas

> ▸ Primary pituitary tumours are almost always benign
> ▸ May be derived from any hormone-producing cell
> ▸ If functional, the clinical effects of the tumour are secondary to the hormone being produced (e.g. acromegaly, Cushing's disease)
> ▸ Local effects are due to pressure on optic chiasma or adjacent pituitary cells

Pituitary tumours account for approximately 10% of primary intracranial neoplasms. They may be derived from any of the hormone-secreting cells and thus may be clinically manifest by virtue of single hormone overproduction, destruction of surrounding normal pituitary and consequent hypofunction, and mechanical effects due to intracranial pressure rise and specific location.

Adenomas are the commonest adenohypophysial tumours; carcinomas are rare. Small adenomas may be subclinical and found only at postmortem. Histologically, adenomas consist of nodules containing cells similar to those of the normal adenohypophysis, with many small blood vessels between them (Fig. 17.5). They may produce clinical disease in two ways: excess hormone production and pressure effects.

Excess hormone production. Adenomas may produce any adenohypophysial hormone depending on their cell of origin (Table 17.4); hence presentation may be via excess production of one of the hormones, for example acromegaly due to excess growth hormone production in an adult (Fig. 17.6), or gigantism if this occurs during childhood.

Pressure effects. These may be either on the surrounding pituitary to produce hypofunction, or on the overlying optic chiasma (Fig. 17.7) producing a characteristic visual field defect called bitemporal hemianopia. Further growth may compress the hypothalamus.

Table 17.4 Types of adenohypophysial adenoma	
Type	Remarks
Prolactinoma (chromophobe)	Commonest type Produces galactorrhoea and menstrual disturbances
GH-secreting (eosinophil)	Produces gigantism in children and acromegaly in adults (Fig. 17.6)
ACTH-secreting (basophil)	Produces Cushing's disease (p. 498)
Other	Exceptionally rare

Types of adenoma

All the following adenomas comprise, histologically, nests and cords of a monotonous single cell type, the islands of cells being supported on a richly vascular sinusoidal framework. Amyloid deposition is not infrequent and calcification may occur.

Chromophobe adenoma. The commonest tumour is one derived from apparently inactive cells; thus hormonal manifestations may be absent but more sensitive biochemical assessments suggest that prolactin may be produced by many of these adenomas. The clinical effects may thus be limited to infertility and be discovered only because of failed conception in the female.

Eosinophil adenoma. Approximately one-third of lesions are derived from the growth hormone-producing cells and are thus manifest by gigantism in the pre-pubertal patient and acromegaly in the adult.

Basophil adenoma. The rarer ACTH-producing adenoma has its effects by stimulating bilateral adrenocortical hyperplasia and hyperfunction, resulting in Cushing's syndrome. Though rare, this remains the commonest cause of Cushing's syndrome in the adult.

Microadenoma. The microadenoma is a small neoplasm measuring less than 10 mm with no mechanical effects, usually discovered only during intensive investigation of infertility; the lesion often produces prolactin in excess.

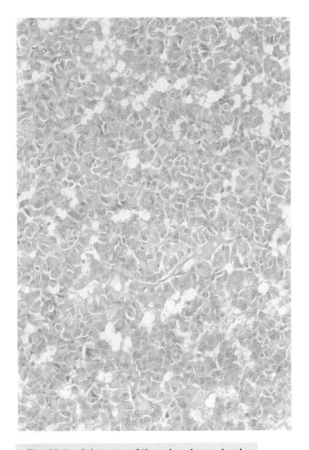

Fig. 17.5 Adenoma of the adenohypophysis

The packeted arrangement of cells resembles that of the anterior pituitary, together with a prominent vascular network.

NEUROHYPOPHYSIS

Neurosecretory cells in the supra-optic and paraventricular nuclei of the hypothalamus give rise to modified nerve fibres which carry the two neurohy-

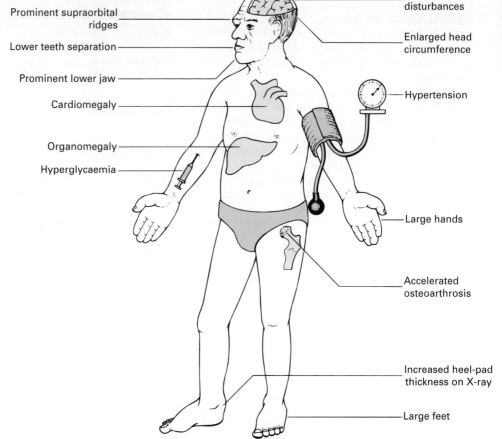

Prominent supraorbital ridges

Lower teeth separation

Prominent lower jaw

Cardiomegaly

Organomegaly

Hyperglycaemia

Mental disturbances

Enlarged head circumference

Hypertension

Large hands

Accelerated osteoarthrosis

Increased heel-pad thickness on X-ray

Large feet

Fig. 17.6   The systemic features of acromegaly

Acromegaly is the clinical syndrome resulting from growth hormone excess in adult life. The chief presenting features are enlargement of the hands, feet and head, but it may also present with secondary diabetes. The cardiovascular effects may be life-threatening.

pophysial hormones—antidiuretic hormone and oxytocin—into the posterior lobe of the pituitary (Fig. 17.2); both hormones are octapeptides, and are stored until released on response to hypothalamic stimuli.

Antidiuretic hormone

Antidiuretic hormone (ADH) controls plasma osmolarity and body water content by increasing the permeability of the renal collecting ducts; this means that more water is reabsorbed and the urine becomes more concentrated. ADH release is stimulated by increased plasma osmolarity and by hypovolaemia.

Damage to the hypothalamus, for example through trauma or tumours, causes deficiency of ADH leading to production of large volumes of dilute urine accompanied by compensatory polydipsia (excess drinking). This is called *diabetes insipidus*, from the

days when tasting of the patient's urine was part of the diagnostic armamentarium: the urine is tasteless in this condition, whereas in diabetes mellitus it is sweet due to its glucose content.

Excess ADH is occasionally produced by the neurohypophysis in response to head injury or meningitis, but most clinical cases of ADH excess are due to its ectopic production by tumours, including bronchial carcinomas. The tumours are almost certainly of APUD origin and thus equipped for the synthesis of peptide hormones.

The rarity of any neurohypophysial tumour secreting ADH (or oxytocin) is perhaps due to the incapacity of the neurones producing these hormones to undergo mitotic division.

Oxytocin

Oxytocin is an aptly named hormone (it is the Greek word for quick birth) as it stimulates the uterine

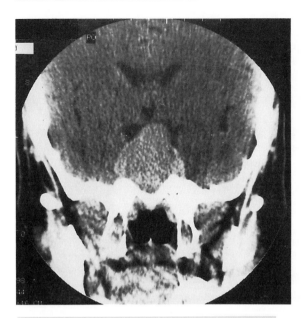

Fig. 17.7 Coronal plane CT scan of the pituitary fossa showing a pituitary adenoma

The sella turcica is widened by a pituitary adenoma which is compressing the optic chiasma and hypothalamus.

smooth muscle to contract. Interestingly, it is oxytocin from the fetal pituitary which plays the greater role in initiating parturition, suggesting that the fetus orders its own birth. Oxytocin also causes ejection of milk during lactation. The hormone is present in males although its function, if any, is unknown.

PINEAL GLAND

The pineal gland is a tiny organ lying above the third ventricle of the brain. Little is known of its function, although its secretory product, melatonin, is thought to be involved in circadian rhythm control and gonadal maturation. The most important tumours of the pineal gland are *malignant germ cell tumours* (teratomas and seminomas), and *pinealoblastomas*, resembling neuroblastomas.

ADRENALS

The adrenals consist essentially of two separate endocrine glands within a single anatomical organ. The *medulla*, of neural crest embryological origin, is

part of the sympathetic nervous system; it secretes catecholamines, which are essential in the physiological responses to stress, e.g. infection, shock or injury. The *cortex*, derived from mesoderm, synthesises a range of steroid hormones with generalised effects on metabolism, the immune system, and water and electrolyte balance.

ADRENAL MEDULLA

Histologically, the adrenal medulla consists of chromaffin cells (so called because they produce brown pigments when fixed in solutions of chrome salts) and sympathetic nerve endings. The adrenal medulla is the main source of adrenaline (epinephrine), since it is produced there from noradrenaline (norepinephrine) by the enzyme phenylethanolamine-N-methyl transferase. Elsewhere in the body, sympathetic nerve endings lack this enxyme and their secretory product is thus noradrenaline. Electron microscopy reveals electron-dense granules in the chromaffin cells (Fig. 17.8), similar to those found in other tissues of the so-called amine precursor uptake and decarboxylation (APUD) system. Islands of similar tissue, known as the organs of Zuckerkandl, are sometimes found in other retroperitoneal sites; these have similar functions and a similar pattern of diseases to that seen in the adrenal medulla. Catecholamines are secreted in states of stress and of hypovolaemic shock, when they are vital in the maintenance of blood pressure by causing vasoconstriction in the skin, gut and skeletal muscles. At tissue level, these hormones bind to cell surface receptors, altering cellular levels of a second messenger, cyclic-AMP, which brings about rapid functional changes in the cell.

Tumours

Phaeochromocytoma

- ▶ Derived from adrenal medullary chromaffin cells
- ▶ Symptoms due to excess catecholamine secretion (e.g. hypertension, sweating)
- ▶ May be familial and associated with other endocrine tumours
- ▶ Occasionally malignant
- ▶ A curable cause of secondary hypertension

A phaeochromocytoma is derived from the adrenal medullary chromaffin cells (or from those lying in other sites); it is classified as a paraganglioma. The

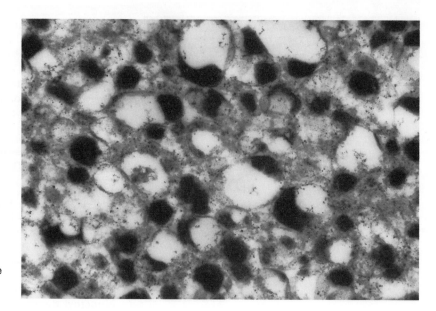

Fig. 17.8 Electron micrograph of noradrenaline granules in a chromaffin cell

The granules characteristically have eccentric electron-dense cores ($\times$ 75 000).

tumour presents through the effects of its catecholamine secretions: hypertension (which is sometimes intermittent), pallor, headaches, sweating and nervousness. Its presence should be suspected especially in younger hypertensive patients. Although it is a rare cause of hypertension, phaeochromocytoma must not be overlooked since it is one of the few curable causes of elevated blood pressure; other causes include adrenal cortical adenoma, renal artery stenosis, and aortic coarctation.

The diagnosis of phaeochromocytoma is usually based on estimating the urinary excretion of vanillylmandelic acid (VMA), a catecholamine metabolite, which is generally at least doubled in the presence of the tumour. Localisation of the tumour is assisted by computerised tomography of the abdomen and by radio-isotope scanning with ^{131}I-mIBG, a catecholamine precursor which accumulates in the tumour.

Phaeochromocytoma may be familial, associated with medullary carcinoma of the thyroid or with hyperparathyroidism as part of a multiple endocrine neoplasia (MEN) syndrome. The familial cases are frequently bilateral. Other associations are with neurofibromatosis and the rare von Hippel–Lindau syndrome.

Phaeochromocytomas are brown, solid nodules, usually under 50 mm in diameter, often with areas of haemorrhagic necrosis (Fig. 17.9). Histologically, they consist of groups of polyhedral cells which give the chromaffin reaction, and are highly vascular (Fig. 17.10).

Although most are benign, a few phaeochromocytomas pursue a malignant course. It is not generally possible to predict this behaviour from the histological appearance.

Neuroblastoma

Neuroblastoma is a rare and highly malignant tumour found in infants and children. Derived from sympathetic nerve cells it may, like phaeochromocytoma, secrete catecholamines, and there may be elevated levels of their metabolites in the urine. It may also originate from parts of the sympathetic chain outside the adrenal medulla. Secondary spread to liver, skin and bones (especially those of the skull) is common. Surprisingly, neuroblastoma may occasionally mature spontaneously to *ganglioneuroma*, a benign tumour.

ADRENAL CORTEX

Histologically, the adrenal cortex can be divided into three zones. Beneath the capsule lies the *zona glomerulosa*, so called because the cells are grouped into spherical clusters superficially resembling glomeruli. This zone produces mineralocorticoid steroids such as aldosterone. Most of the adrenal cortex comprises the middle and inner zones — *zona fasciculata* and *zona reticularis* respectively. The middle zone is rich in lipid. The inner zone is

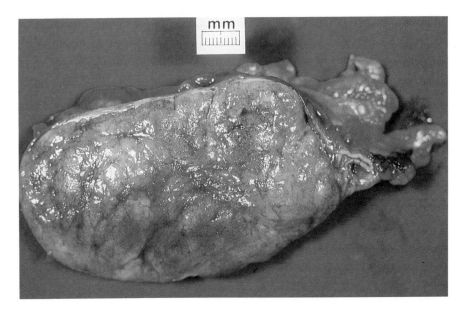

**Fig. 17.9
Phaeochromocytoma**

The adrenal medulla is expanded by a dark-coloured tumour with areas of degeneration and haemorrhage.

engaged in the conversion of lipid into corticosteroids, principally glucocorticoids and sex steroids, for secretion.

The cells of the adrenal cortex appear clear on histology (Fig. 17.11) because their secretory contents are lipids and are dissolved out in tissue processing. Depletion of the adrenal steroid content, which occurs as a response to the stress of prolonged illness, causes the cells to appear smaller and more eosinophilic in autopsy material.

Steroid hormones

Glucocorticoids

The glucocorticoids have important effects on a wide range of tissues and organs. At physiological levels they:

- inhibit protein synthesis
- increase protein breakdown
- increase gluconeogenesis.

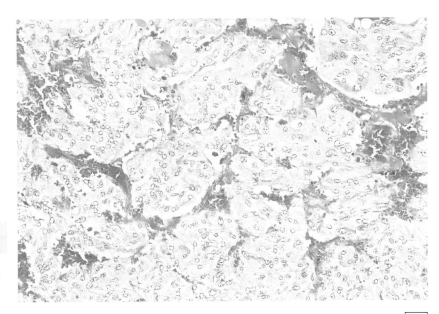

Fig. 17.10   Chromaffin cells in a phaeochromocytoma

There are groups of cells with granular cytoplasm, amidst which there are numerous branching capillaries.

In excess, as a result of therapeutic administration or high levels of endogenous secretion, they:

- cause adiposity of face and trunk
- cause hypertension
- suppress wound healing
- are anti-inflammatory
- are immunosuppressive
- inhibit growth
- cause osteoporosis
- cause peptic ulceration
- cause a diabetic state.

The most important of the hormones is cortisol (hydrocortisone), but other steroid metabolites have similar effects. The synthesis and secretion of glucocorticoids are controlled by ACTH from the pituitary (p. 489).

Mineralocorticoids

The most important of the mineralocorticoids, aldosterone, acts on the renal tubules to increase reabsorption of sodium and chloride, reducing their loss in urine at the expense of potassium exchange. Unlike the production of glucocorticoids, the synthesis and release of aldosterone is not under pituitary control, but is regulated instead by the *renin–angiotensin* system (Fig. 17.12). Low perfusion pressure in the kidney stimulates release of renin, an

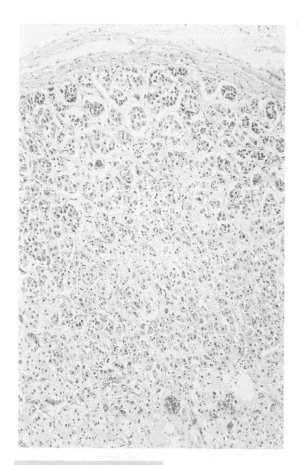

Fig. 17.11 Adrenal cortex

The normal zones are: zona glomerulosa (top), zona fasciculata (middle) and zona reticularis (bottom).

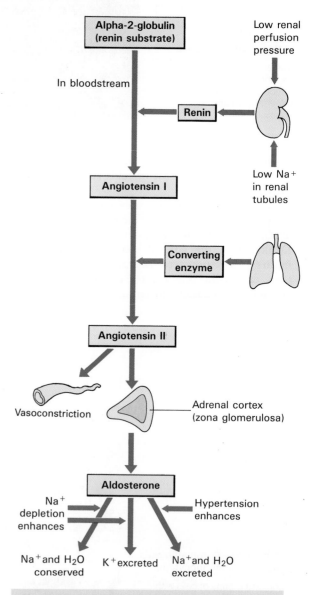

Fig. 17.12 Schematic diagram of the renin–angiotensin–aldosterone system (see text for details)

enzyme, from the juxtaglomerular apparatus of the kidney. This cleaves off a decapeptide, angiotensin I, from a carrier molecule, α_2-globulin. Angiotensin I is then converted to angiotensin II (an octapeptide) by a converting enzyme, mainly in the lung. Angiotensin II stimulates secretion of aldosterone from the adrenal cortex. Thus, aldosterone is released to combat fluid depletion.

Sex steroids

The production of sex steroids in the adrenal cortex is low compared with that in the gonads and may not be physiologically important. However, virilising androgens may be produced in conditions such as certain congenital enzyme defects and adrenal cortical tumours, especially if these are malignant.

Hyperfunction

Hyperfunction of the adrenal cortex produces generalised effects, the nature of which depends on whether glucocorticoids, mineralocorticoids or sex steroids are produced in excess.

Cushing's syndrome

> ▶ Due to excess glucocorticoids
> ▶ Main features include central obesity, hirsutism, hypertension, diabetes and osteoporosis
> ▶ Main causes are excess ACTH secretion from the pituitary, adrenal cortical neoplasms, or the iatrogenic effects of ACTH or steroid administration

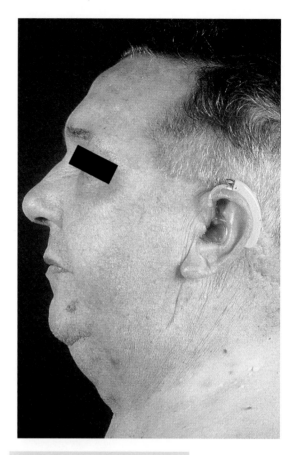

Fig. 17.13 Cushing's syndrome
There is rounding of the face, acne and central obesity causing double chin.

Cushing's syndrome refers to the constellation of bodily responses to excess glucocorticoids, whatever the underlying cause. Exogenous administration of glucocorticoids or ACTH is a common iatrogenic cause of Cushing's syndrome. The syndrome occurs most commonly in adult women, and sometimes there is also excess androgen production causing virilisation. The main physical features of the syndrome in an adult are shown in Figures 17.13 and 17.14. In children, there is also growth retardation.

Diagnosis
Diagnosis is by demonstration of glucocorticoid excess, either as elevated plasma levels of cortisol or as elevated urinary excretion of 17-hydroxysteroids, degradation products of glucocorticoids. Further tests, such as estimation of plasma ACTH by radioimmunoassay, are essential to determine the cause of the Cushing's syndrome (see below).

Pathogenesis
Iatrogenic disease. The therapeutic administration of glucocorticoids to the patient is by far the commonest cause of the features of Cushing's syndrome.

In addition, three different types of *natural disease* can cause the syndrome:

- excess ACTH secretion by the adenohypophysis
- adrenal cortical neoplasms
- ectopic ACTH secretion.

Excess ACTH secretion by the adenohypophysis. This was the cause of the syndrome originally described

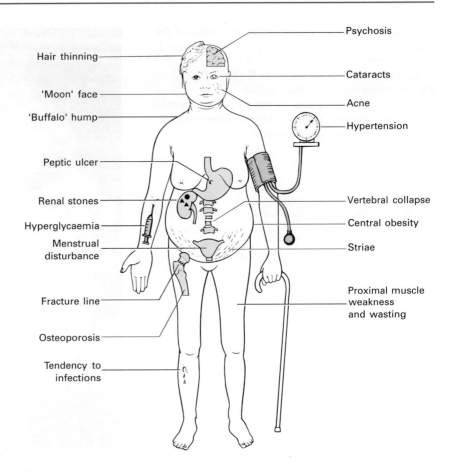

Psychosis

Hair thinning

Cataracts

'Moon' face

Acne

'Buffalo' hump

Hypertension

Peptic ulcer

Renal stones

Vertebral collapse

Hyperglycaemia

Central obesity

Menstrual
disturbance

Striae

Proximal muscle
weakness
and wasting

Fracture line

Osteoporosis

Tendency to
infections

Fig. 17.14 The systemic features of Cushing's syndrome

by Harvey Williams Cushing, a Boston neurosurgeon with an interest in the pituitary. Hypersecretion of ACTH by an adenoma of the corticotrophs leads to bilateral adrenal cortical hyperplasia; this combination is termed *Cushing's disease*. Histologically, the cells of the adrenal cortex may appear depleted of lipid, indicating that they have discharged their secretions into the blood. Plasma ACTH is raised, and if the dexamethasone suppression test is performed — administration of the synthetic potent steroid, dexamethasone — a fall in cortisol levels will result due to the suppression of pituitary ACTH secretion.

The ideal treatment of this common cause of Cushing's syndrome is surgical removal of the pituitary adenoma; this not only abolishes the excess ACTH secretion, but also avoids the serious pressure effects which may be produced by a pituitary space-occupying lesion (p. 491). Removal of the adrenals (once the main form of treatment) is unsatisfactory, because the adenohypophysial tumour is left to grow and, in addition to secreting ACTH, may produce a peptide (melanocyte-stimulating hormone) with an amino acid sequence similar to that of the ACTH molecule. In 20% of cases this leads to marked enlargement of the pituitary adenoma (Nelson's syndrome). Skin pigmentation will occur in most cases.

Adrenal cortical neoplasms. These may secrete cortisol autonomously, independently of ACTH control; low ACTH levels are then found in the presence of elevated cortisol. This is the commonest cause of Cushing's syndrome in children. The neoplasm is usually an adenoma, but 5–10% of cases it is a carcinoma, in which case virilising steroid production may be prominent. Treatment is by excision of the neoplasm.

Ectopic ACTH secretion. Certain tumours unrelated to the adenohypophysis may secrete ACTH. Oat cell (small cell) carcinoma of the bronchus (Ch. 14) is the commonest example, although carcinoids, pancreatic islet cell tumours and renal adenocarcinoma (hypernephroma) may occasionally be responsible. Plasma ACTH levels are very high and are not suppressed in the dexamethasone suppression test.

Hyperaldosteronism

Primary hyperaldosteronism (Conn's syndrome). This is the autonomous secretion of excess aldosterone. The usual cause is an adenoma of the zona glomerulosa, but generalised hyperplasia of the zona is sometimes responsible. The resulting renal retention of sodium and water leads to hypertension, while potassium loss leads to muscular weakness and cardiac arrhythmias. The hypokalaemia is associated with metabolic alkalosis, causing tetany and paraesthesiae.

Secondary hyperaldosteronism. When renal glomerular perfusion is reduced, for example through a fall in blood volume, the *renin–angiotensin* system (Fig. 17.12) stimulates aldosterone secretion from the zona glomerulosa in an attempt to correct this. This physiological response is known as secondary hyperaldosteronism, which is by far the commonest type of hyperaldosteronism.

Diagnosis

The diagnosis of primary hyperaldosteronism rests on two criteria: plasma aldosterone must be *raised* while renin is *low*. This is to distinguish it from secondary hyperaldosteronism, in which aldosterone levels are raised but are an appropriate response to high renin levels.

Hypersecretion of sex steroids

Some adrenal cortical adenomas secrete sex steroids, most commonly androgens. In Cushing's syndrome, quantities of androgens are occasionally secreted along with the glucocorticoids, causing virilisation of females, especially those with adrenocortical carcinomas.

Rarely, congenital enzyme defects of the pathways of steroid synthesis may result in excess production of sex steroids. The least rare example is '*congenital adrenal hyperplasia*' due to deficiency of the enzyme 21-hydroxylase, needed for the synthesis of both cortisol and aldosterone (Fig. 17.15). Failure of cortisol production leads to increased ACTH secretion, resulting in hyperplasia of the adrenal cortex. The production of androgens occurs before the metabolic block caused by the enzyme deficiency, and their excessive secretion results in masculinisation of females and precocious puberty in males. 21-hydroxylase deficiency is serious, because deficiency of mineralocorticoids causes life-threatening salt loss unless replacement therapy is given.

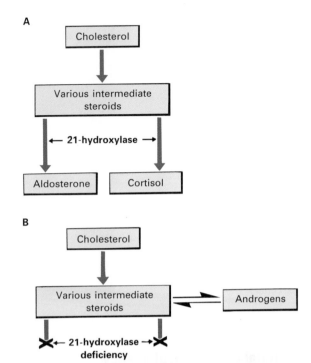

Fig. 17.15   21-hydroxylase deficiency: the commonest cause of congenital adrenal hyperplasia

A. Normal metabolism. B. 21-hydroxylase deficiency.
Failure of aldosterone production leads to salt-wasting, while cortisol lack causes the anterior pituitary to release ACTH, resulting in adrenal cortical hyperplasia. The resulting excess intermediate steroids are converted to androgens, leading to virilisation.

Tumours

Adenoma. In addition to those 'functioning' adrenal cortical adenomas which present by causing Cushing's or Conn's syndromes, a clinically unsuspected 'non-functioning' adenoma may be found in about 2% of adult autopsies. The adenoma is a pale yellow circumscribed nodule, perhaps 20–30 mm in diameter (Fig. 17.16). The cells have clear cytoplasm owing to their high lipid content (Fig. 17.17).

Carcinoma. Adrenal cortical carcinoma is rare; these tumours are usually hormone-secreting, with a tendency to produce androgens. They are commonly large (over 100 g) and exhibit invasive growth. Examination of the adjacent adrenal cortex and that of the opposite gland may give a clue as to the function of the neoplasm; glucocorticoid-secreting tumours will suppress ACTH, resulting in atrophy of the non-neoplastic adrenal cortex.

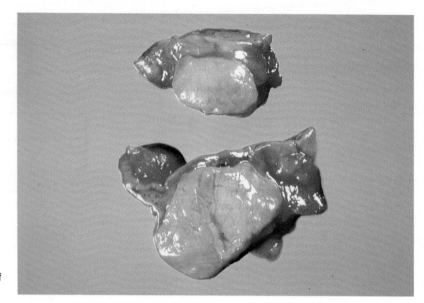

Fig. 17.16 Adrenal cortical adenoma

A pale-coloured fleshy nodule in the adrenal cortex is displacing the medulla and stretching out the rest of the cortex.

Adrenal cortical insufficiency

► Clinical effects are due to lack of mineralocorticoids and glucocorticoids
► Main features include weight loss, lethargy, hypotension, pigmentation and hyponatraemia
► Causes include tuberculosis and Waterhouse–Friderichsen syndrome

Adrenocortical hypofunction can be *primary*, due to lesions within the adrenal gland, or *secondary*, due to failure of ACTH secretion by the adenohypophysis. Acute primary insufficiency is called *Waterhouse–Friderichsen syndrome*. Causes of chronic primary insufficiency include:

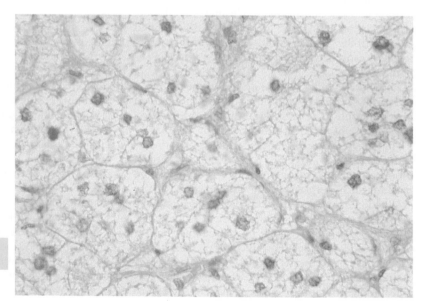

Fig. 17.17 Cells comprising an adrenal cortical adenoma

The cells are large with clear cytoplasm and compact nuclei.

- tuberculosis
- autoimmune adrenalitis
- amyloidosis
- haemochromatosis
- metastatic tumours
- atrophy due to prolonged steroid therapy.

Autoimmune adrenalitis selectively damages and destroys the adrenal cortex, sparing the medulla; tuberculosis destroys the cortex and medulla.

Acute insufficiency

Acute insufficiency ('adrenal apoplexy') was first noted in children by Waterhouse and Friderichsen who, in 1911 and 1918 respectively, independently described acute haemorrhagic necrosis of the adrenals in the course of meningococcal septicaemia. Other acute septicaemias, especially those due to Gram-negative bacteria, may cause a similar effect. The adrenal cortices are necrotic and the medullae contain acute haemorrhage (Fig. 17.18). The adrenal necrosis is probably due to disseminated intravascular coagulation (DIC). The symptoms are attributable to lack of mineralocorticoids (salt and water loss with hypovolaemic shock) and of glucocorticoids (failure of gluconeogenesis resulting in hypoglycaemia).

Chronic insufficiency

Thomas Addison first described an association between destruction of the adrenal cortex and the constellation of symptoms caused by the resulting chronic insufficiency of adrenal cortical hormones (*Addison's disease*). The effects are due to a combined lack of mineralocorticoids and glucocorticoids:

- anorexia, weight loss, vomiting
- weakness
- lethargy
- hypotension
- skin pigmentation
- hyponatraemia with hyperkalaemia
- chronic dehydration
- sexual dysfunction.

Patients with chronic adrenocortical insufficiency may develop an *acute Addisonian crisis*, in which even minor illnesses such as infections may cause vomiting, fluid loss, electrolyte disturbances and circulatory collapse.

The commonest cause of Addison's disease was once caseous necrosis of the adrenal cortices due to tuberculosis. Autoimmune destruction of the cortex is now a commoner cause; this is associated with other 'organ-specific' autoimmune diseases, such as pernicious anaemia (also described by Addison), thyroiditis, insulin-dependent diabetes mellitus and parathyroid failure.

In all cases of Addison's disease, plasma cortisol levels are low. Estimation of ACTH levels enables a distinction to be made between primary adrenocorti-

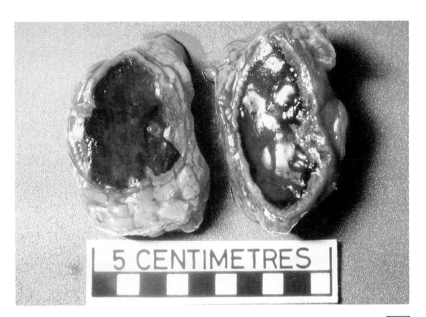

Fig. 17.18 Appearance of the adrenals in Waterhouse–Friderichsen syndrome

The adrenals from a child dying of meningococcal septicaemia are destroyed by haemorrhage.

cal insufficiency (ACTH raised) and secondary insufficiency (ACTH low).

THYROID

The thyroid gland (normal weight 20–30 g) is composed of follicles which are lined by cuboidal epithelial cells (Fig. 17.19) and contain a proteinaceous stored secretion ('colloid'). The main function of the thyroid epithelial cells is the synthesis of the iodinated amino acids, thyroxine (T_4) and tri-iodothyronine (T_3).

The secretion of T_3 and T_4 is under negative feedback control by TSH from the anterior pituitary. For example, a fall in the plasma level of these thyroid hormones causes increased TSH secretion by both direct effects on the adenohypophysis and effects on the hypothalamus (p. 489).

The thyroid also contains a population of cells known as C-cells; these are sparsely scattered throughout the gland and secrete calcitonin, a peptide hormone involved in calcium metabolism. Medullary carcinoma, a tumour of these cells, is discussed on page 512.

There are three main types of clinical thyroid disease:

- *secretory malfunction*: hyper- or hypothyroidism
- *swelling of the entire gland*: goitre

- *solitary masses*: one large nodule in a nodular goitre, adenoma or carcinoma.

SECRETORY MALFUNCTION

Hyperthyroidism

> ▶ Syndrome due to excess T_3 and T_4
> ▶ Very rarely due to excess TSH
> ▶ Commonest cause is Graves' disease, in which there is a long-acting thyroid-stimulating immunoglobulin (LATS)
> ▶ Also may be due to functioning adenoma

Hyperthyroidism (thyrotoxicosis) is the clinical syndrome resulting from the effect on the tissues of excess circulating T_3 and T_4; the overall result is an increased metabolic rate. The features are summarised in Figure 17.20. Hyperthyroidism may result from three main pathological lesions:

- Graves' thyroiditis
- functioning adenoma
- toxic nodular goitre.

Graves' thyroiditis

Graves' thyroiditis is the commonest cause of thyrotoxicosis, usually associated with a diffuse goitre. The thyroid is moderately enlarged, firm and beefy-

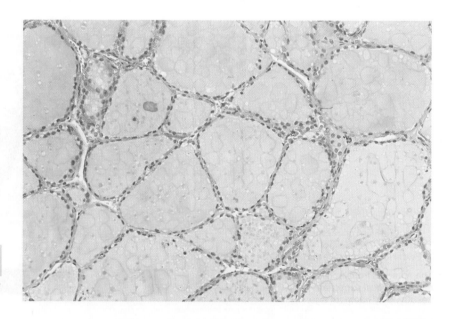

Fig. 17.19 Normal thyroid histology

Colloid-filled follicles are lined by regular cuboidal epithelium.

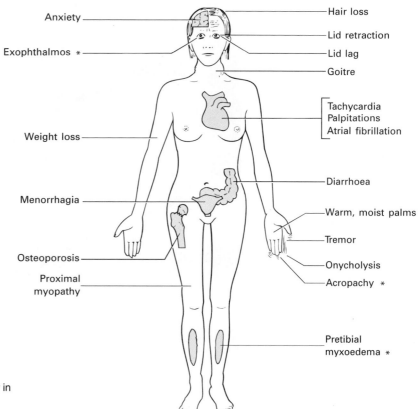

Anxiety

Exophthalmos *

Weight loss

Menorrhagia

Osteoporosis

Proximal
myopathy

Hair loss

Lid retraction

Lid lag

Goitre

Tachycardia
Palpitations
Atrial fibrillation

Diarrhoea

Warm, moist palms

Tremor

Onycholysis

Acropachy *

Pretibial
myxoedema *

Fig. 17.20 The systemic features of thyrotoxicosis

The features marked* are seen only in thyrotoxicosis due to Graves' thyroiditis.

red due to increased vascularity (Fig. 17.21). Histologically, the gland shows hyperplasia of the acinar epithelium, reduction of stored colloid, and local accumulations of lymphocytes with lymphoid follicle formation (Fig. 17.22). This full spectrum of features is now rarely seen in subtotal thyroidectomy specimens of the condition, because antithyroid drugs are given before surgery.

Graves' thyroiditis is one of the so-called 'organ-specific' autoimmune diseases. The pathogenesis is the production of an auto-antibody of the IgG class which binds to the thyroid epithelial cells and mimics the stimulatory action of TSH. The auto-antibody is known as long-acting thyroid stimulator (LATS) and its effect on the thyroid can be classed as a form of hypersensitivity reaction, 'stimulatory hypersensitivity'. LATS stimulates the function and growth of thyroid follicular epithelium. In addition to showing the usual features of thyrotoxicosis, patients with Graves' thyroiditis may also show exophthalmos, pretibial myxoedema (accumulation of mucopolysaccharides in the deep dermis of the skin) and finger-clubbing. The latter

two signs are rare effects, but exophthalmos is common. It results from infiltration of the orbital tissues by fat (interestingly, adipocytes have been shown to have cell surface TSH receptors), mucopolysaccharides and lymphocytes, and may be due to an additional auto-antibody reacting with these tissues.

Functioning adenoma

Functioning adenomas of the thyroid may cause thyrotoxicosis, but less than 1% of adenomas show enough secretory activity to do so. Histologically, the tumour is composed of thyroid follicles and is sometimes so small that it is visualised only on a ^{131}I radio-isotope scan. Occasionally it may present as a solitary thyroid mass.

Toxic nodular goitre

Rarely one or two nodules in a nodular goitre (p. 507) may develop hypersecretory activity, a condition termed *toxic nodular goitre*.

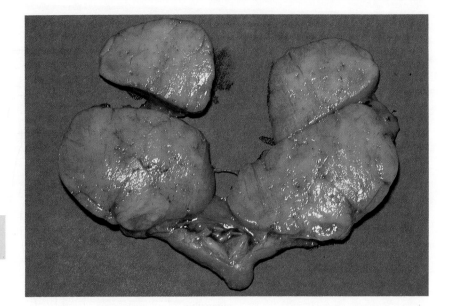

Fig. 17.21 Subtotal thyroidectomy for treatment of Graves' thyroiditis

The gland is diffusely enlarged, fleshy and dark-coloured due to increased vascularity.

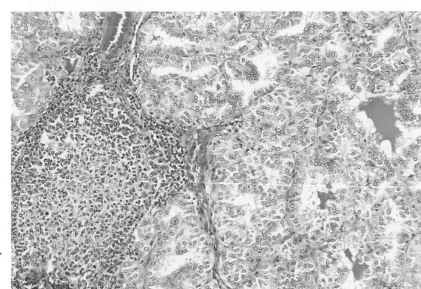

Fig. 17.22 Graves' thyroiditis

There is hyperplasia of the follicular epithelium with nuclear irregularity, depletion of colloid and focal lymphoid aggregates.

Hypothyroidism

▶ Syndrome due to insufficient circulating T_3 and T_4
▶ If congenital, causes cretinism
▶ Commonest cause is Hashimoto's thyroiditis, an autoimmune disorder

Hypothyroidism (myxoedema) is the clinical syndrome resulting from inadequate levels of circulating T_3 and T_4. The metabolic rate is lowered and mucopolysaccharides accumulate in the dermal connective tissues to produce the typical myxoedema face (Fig. 17.23). The general features of hypothyroidism are summarised in Figure 17.24. If hypothyroidism is present in the newborn, physical growth and mental development are impaired, sometimes irreversibly; this condition is known as *cretinism*. Cretinism may be endemic in geographical areas where the diet contains insufficient iodine for thyroid hormone synthesis. Sporadic cases are usually due to a congenital absence of thyroid tissue, or to enzyme defects blocking hormone synthesis.

The commonest cause of acquired hypothyroidism in adults is *Hashimoto's thyroiditis* (see below), but

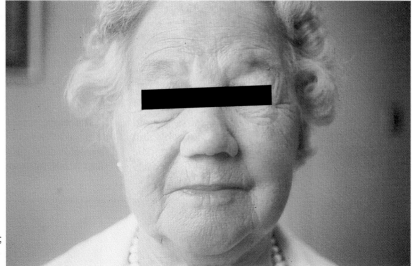

Fig. 17.23 Myxoedemic face

The skin is coarse and puffy due to accumulation of mucopolysaccharides; the outer third of the eyebrows is lost.

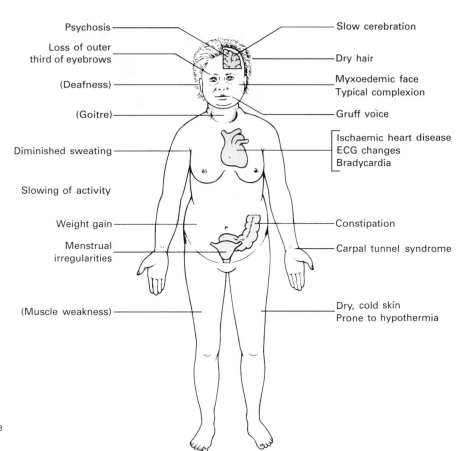

Psychosis
Loss of outer third of eyebrows
(Deafness)
(Goitre)
Diminished sweating
Slowing of activity
Weight gain
Menstrual irregularities
(Muscle weakness)

Slow cerebration
Dry hair
Myxoedemic face
Typical complexion
Gruff voice
Ischaemic heart disease
ECG changes
Bradycardia
Constipation
Carpal tunnel syndrome
Dry, cold skin
Prone to hypothermia

Fig. 17.24 The systemic features of hypothyroidism (myxoedema)

The features in brackets are neither common nor essential.

occasional cases are iatrogenic; for example due to surgical removal of thyroid tissue or to certain drugs which cause unwanted hypothyroidism, such as sulphonylureas, resorcinol, lithium and amiodarone.

Hashimoto's thyroiditis

Hashimoto's thyroiditis may initially cause thyroid enlargement, but later there may be atrophy and fibrosis. The gland appears firm, fleshy and pale (Fig. 17.25). Histologically, the gland is densely infiltrated by lymphocytes and plasma cells, with lymphoid follicle formation. Colloid content is reduced, and the thyroid epithelial cells show a characteristic change in which they enlarge and develop eosinophilic granular cytoplasm due to proliferation of mitochondria; they are then termed Askanazy cells, Hürthle cells or oncocytes (Fig. 17.26). In advanced cases there may be fibrosis. Paradoxically, in the early stages of Hashimoto's thyroiditis, the damage to the thyroid follicles may lead to release of thyroglobulin into the circulation, causing a transient phase of thyrotoxicosis.

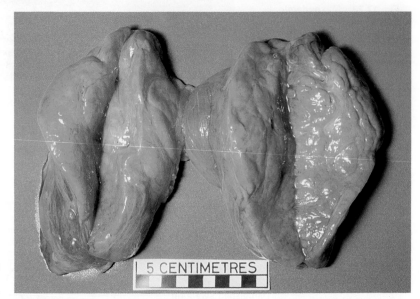

Fig. 17.25 Thyroid removed at autopsy from a patient with Hashimoto's thyroiditis

The gland is slightly enlarged and the lobes have been sliced to show the uniformly pale and fleshy cut surface.

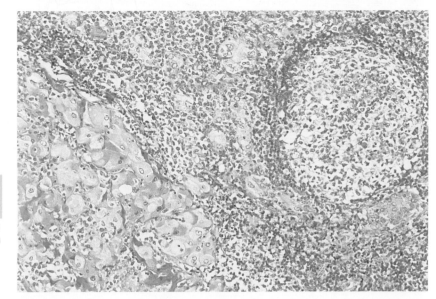

Fig. 17.26 The histological features of Hashimoto's thyroiditis

There is destruction of follicles by a dense lymphocytic infiltrate with germinal centre formation (right). Some of the surviving epithelial cells show Hürthle cell change (left).

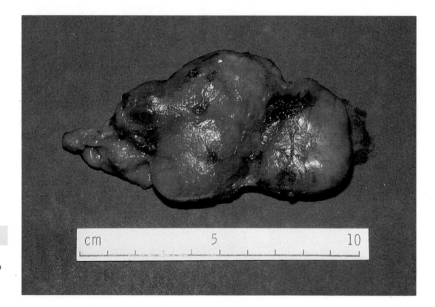

Fig. 17.27   Multinodular goitre

Thyroid lobectomy tissue showing irregular nodular enlargement due to hyperplasia, fibrosis and focally excessive colloid.

Like Graves' thyroiditis, Hashimoto's thyroiditis is one of the 'organ-specific' autoimmune diseases (Ch. 9). Two auto-antibodies can be detected in the serum of most patients with Hashimoto's thyroiditis, one reacting with the endoplasmic reticulum of thyroid epithelial cells, and the other with thyroglobulin. These auto-antibodies are probably formed locally by the plasma cells infiltrating the thyroid, and are possibly the result of a loss of specific suppressor T-lymphocytes. In common with other organ-specific autoimmune diseases, there is a female preponderance, and certain HLA antigens (Ch. 3) are commonly found in affected individuals — especially HLA-B8 and -DR5.

GOITRE (ENLARGEMENT OF THE WHOLE GLAND)

The term goitre denotes an enlargement of the thyroid without hyperthyroidism.

Simple goitre

A spectrum of pathological changes may occur, ranging from parenchymatous goitre to colloid goitre.

In *parenchymatous goitre* there is at first hyperplasia of the thyroid epithelium with loss of stored colloid, but eventually less active areas appear and are compressed by the hyperplastic areas. Tracts of fibrosis may separate these areas, resulting in *multinodular goitre* (Fig. 17.27). The multiple nodules of this type

of goitre can usually be palpated clinically, but occasionally one large nodule may be noted and give rise to suspicion of neoplasia.

In *colloid goitre* there is no epithelial hyperplasia, but follicles accumulate large volumes of colloid (Fig. 17.28), and coalesce to form colloid-filled cysts. There may be areas of haemorrhage, fibrosis and dystrophic calcification. The thyroid may be diffusely enlarged or multinodular. A complication of this condition is haemorrhage into a cyst, giving rise to rapid enlargement of the cyst which may cause tracheal compression and stridor.

Aetiology

The aetiology of simple goitre is thought to involve a phase of relative lack of T_3 and T_4 so that TSH rises and causes hyperplasia of the thyroid epithelium. This lack of T_3 and T_4 can be brought about in three main ways:

- iodine deficiency, due to endemic goitre or food faddism
- rare inherited enzyme defects in T_3 and T_4 synthesis
- drugs which induce hypothyroidism (p. 506).

Endemic goitre was formerly common in areas remote from the sea, where the soil contains little iodine, for example in the Derbyshire hills, parts of Switzerland and mountainous regions. The addition of iodine to the diet by iodination of table salt has reduced the incidence of goitre in some areas.

507

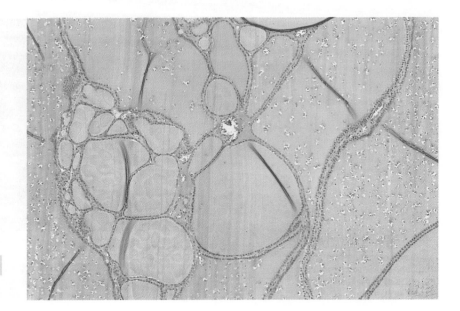

Fig. 17.28   Colloid goitre
The follicles are distended by accumulated colloid.

Rare causes of goitre

Giant cell thyroiditis

Giant cell thyroiditis (de Quervain's thyroiditis) is a distinctive form of slight thyroid swelling with tenderness on palpation, and fever, usually with fairly abrupt onset. Histologically, the gland is infiltrated by a mixture of neutrophil polymorphs and lymphocytes, with a focal giant cell reaction possibly due to epithelial cell fusion. The disease is thought to be induced by viral infections such as mumps, but the reason why only a few individuals develop this rare disease is not known.

Riedel's thyroiditis

Riedel's thyroiditis is an exceptionally rare cause of thyroid enlargement with dense fibrosis which may involve adjacent muscles; this renders the thyroid firm and immobile on palpation, thus mimicking carcinoma. Histologically, there is dense fibrous replacement of the gland and, characteristically, occlusion of thyroid veins by fibrosis. The condition is of unknown aetiology, but may be associated with retroperitoneal fibrosis.

SOLITARY MASSES

The patient with a solitary mass in the thyroid pre-

sents a common clinical problem. The investigation of such a patient, following clinical examination, first involves checking the thyroid secretory status (serum T_3, T_4 and TSH).

Diagnostic imaging of the thyroid gland may be performed with ^{99m}Technetium which localises to the gland in a similar distribution to iodine (Fig. 17.29). 'Cold' lesions (which do not take up the radio-isotope) may be cysts or solid tumours; these can be distinguished by ultrasound (Fig. 17.30) or by fine-needle aspiration cytology. Cytology enables a preoperative diagnosis of thyroid neoplasia to be made and has revolutionised the management of thyroid nodules.

Many apparently solitary nodules turn out to be merely one large nodule in an otherwise multi-nodular goitre. Others, however, are neoplastic.

Tumours

> ▶ Usually benign (follicular adenoma)
> ▶ Malignant forms include carcinomas and lymphoma:
>   – Papillary adenocarcinoma (often multifocal, lymphatic spread)
>   – Follicular adenocarcinoma (usually solitary, haematogenous spread)
>   – Medullary carcinoma (derived from calcitonin-producing C-cells, sometimes associated with multiple endocrine neoplasia syndromes)
>   – Lymphoma (usually non-Hodgkin's lymphoma of B-cell type)

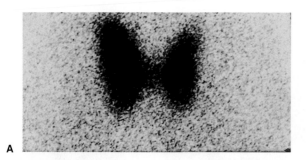

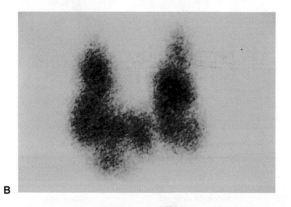

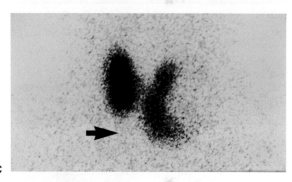

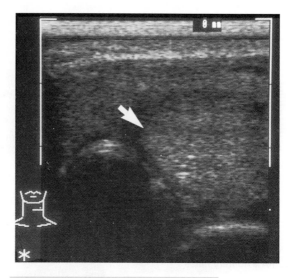

Fig. 17.30   Ultrasound scan of thyroid

There is a solid solitary nodule (arrowed) which may be neoplastic.

Fig. 17.29 ^{99m}Technetium thyroid scans

A. Normal thyroid showing symmetrical uptake of the isotope by both lobes.
B. Multiple 'hot' nodules taking up the isotope, consistent with a multinodular goitre.
C. Solitary 'cold' nodule (arrowed); this may be a cyst or a solid tumour.

Benign tumours

Follicular adenoma is a common cause of a solitary thyroid nodule. It usually consists of a solid mass within a fibrous capsule, compressing the adjacent gland (Fig. 17.31), but the centre may show areas of haemorrhage and cystic changes. Microscopically, a range of appearances may be seen, but the commonest type consists of very compact follicles, lined by epithelial cells with slight nuclear hyperchromaticism, containing little colloid. There is a surrounding fibrous capsule which is not breached by the tumour. Rarely, follicular adenomas may synthesise excess T_3 and T_4, appearing 'hot' on a radio-isotope scan, and sometimes causing thyrotoxicosis.

Malignant tumours

Carcinoma of the thyroid is not a common tumour and, because the majority of these tumours are well-differentiated types with a good prognosis, it accounts for less than 1% of cancer deaths. It is one of the malignancies known to be associated with radiation exposure, whether as X-rays to the neck or as nuclear fall-out, which contains radio-isotopes of iodine which are selectively trapped by the gland. The main features of the four types of thyroid carcinoma are summarised in Table 17.5. In addition, some of the thyroid tumours once classified as anaplastic carcinoma are now known to be lymphomas.

Tumours of the thyroid are generally benign. Carcinomas are rare at this site, and lymphomas rarer still. Those tumours which are malignant have a variable behaviour that dictates the clinical management. Histological classification is, therefore, of vital importance.

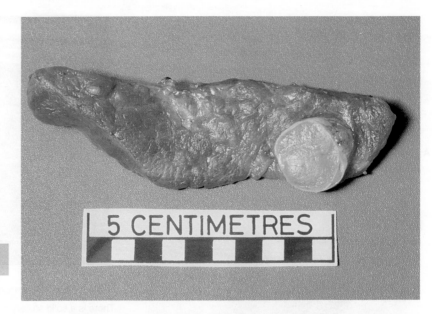

Fig. 17.31 Thyroid lobectomy for a solitary mass

There is an encapsulated follicular adenoma.

Table 17.5	Carcinoma of the thyroid			
Type	Proportion of all cases (%)	Typical age range	Mode of spread	Prognosis
Papillary	60–70	Children–young adults	Lymphatic, to local nodes	Excellent
Follicular	20–25	Young–middle age	Blood stream, especially to bone	Good
Anaplastic	10–15	Elderly	Aggressive local extension	Very poor
Medullary	5–10	Usually elderly, but familial cases occur	Local, lymphatic, blood stream	Variable. More aggressive in familial cases

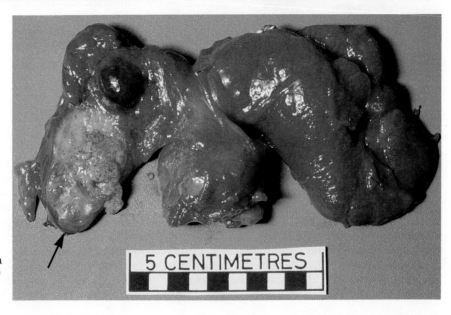

Fig. 17.32 Thyroidectomy showing papillary adenocarcinoma and multinodular goitre

At the lower pole of the right lobe there is an infiltrating white mass (arrowed) which histologically was found to be a papillary adenocarcinoma. The gland also shows multinodular goitre.

Papillary adenocarcinoma

Papillary adenocarcinoma is a well-differentiated form of adenocarcinoma most commonly found in younger (less than 45 years old) patients. It presents as a non-encapsulated infiltrative mass (Fig. 17.32) which may be firm and white due to fibrosis. Histologically, it consists of epithelial papillary projections (Fig. 17.33) between which calcified spherules (psammoma bodies) may be present. The epithelial cell nuclei are characteristically large with central clear areas; for this reason, they are sometimes termed 'Orphan Annie' nuclei (Fig. 17.34).

Papillary adenocarcinoma metastasises via the lymphatics within the thyroid gland, which may give a multifocal appearance, and to the cervical lymph nodes. However, it is a slow-growing tumour which may even regress; thus the prognosis is excellent.

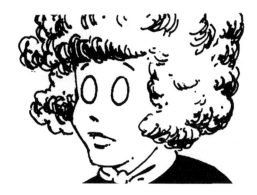

Fig. 17.34   Orphan Annie

This cartoon-strip character first appeared in the New York News in 1926. Her forlorn-looking eyes inspired the name 'Orphan Annie' for the nuclei seen in papillary adenocarcinoma.

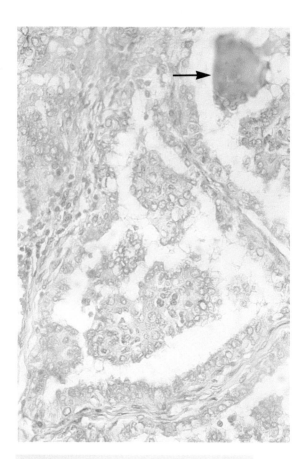

Fig. 17.33   Papillary adenocarcinoma of the thyroid

High-power photomicrograph showing atypical epithelial cells with large vesicular ('Orphan Annie') nuclei forming papillae. The dark laminated sphere (arrowed) is a psammoma body.

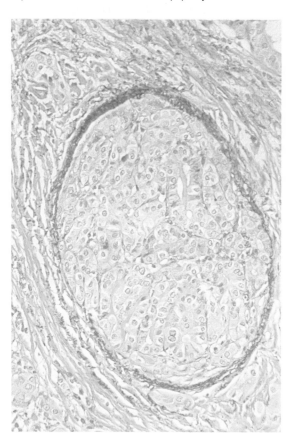

Fig. 17.35   Vascular invasion by follicular carcinoma of the thyroid

Medium-power photomicrograph of a section stained for elastin which appears dark brown in the wall of the large vein (centre). The vein is plugged by infiltrating follicular carcinoma.

Follicular adenocarcinoma

Follicular adenocarcinomas usually present in a similar way to follicular adenomas and on naked-eye inspection are often round encapsulated nodules. However, histology reveals invasion of the capsule, blood vessels (Fig. 17.35) or the surrounding gland.

Metastasis characteristically occurs via the blood stream, with the bones and lungs the commonest sites of secondary spread. However, many of the tumours retain the ability to take up ^{131}I, which may be used as a highly effective targeted form of radiotherapy. The prognosis is therefore good.

Anaplastic carcinoma

Anaplastic carcinomas (undifferentiated) usually present in the elderly as diffusely infiltrative masses. There are various histological appearances, but spindle cell and giant cell types are common (Fig. 17.36). There is evidence that anaplastic carcinomas are poorly-differentiated adenocarcinomas derived from thyroid epithelium. The prognosis is very poor, due to rapid local invasion of structures such as the trachea, producing respiratory obstruction.

Medullary carcinoma

Medullary carcinoma is derived from the thyroid C-cells and commonly both synthesises and secretes calcitonin. Histologically, the tumour is composed of sheets of neoplastic cells with, between them, a hyaline stroma with the staining reactions of amyloid; this is due to polymerisation of calcitonin into a β-pleated sheet (Fig. 17.37).

Although the patient often has very high circulatory levels of calcitonin, this produces no clinical effects. Being a tumour of APUD cells (Ch. 15) medullary carcinoma may produce other secretory products, such as 5-HT, and may lead to symptoms of the carcinoid syndrome (Ch. 15).

Some cases, especially those presenting in young patients, are familial and may be part of one of the so-called multiple endocrine neoplasia (MEN) syndromes (Table 17.6). These syndromes are rare, but it is important to recognise them in order to suspect, and diagnose early, associated endocrine neoplasms.

The tumour usually pursues a rather indolent course, but some familial cases are aggressive.

Table 17.6 The multiple endocrine neoplasia (MEN) syndromes	
Syndrome	**Features**
MEN type 1	Hyperparathyroidism (parathyroid adenoma or hyperplasia) Pancreatic islet cell tumours Pituitary adenomas
MEN type II	Medullary carcinoma of thyroid Phaeochromocytoma (may be bilateral) Hyperparathyroidism Sometimes neuromas/ganglioneuromas

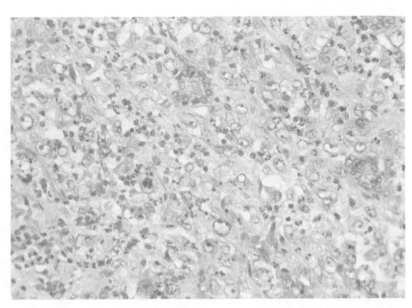

Fig. 17.36 Anaplastic carcinoma of the thyroid

High-power photomicrograph showing pleomorphic hyperchromatic nuclei, some lying in tumour giant cells. Aberrant mitotic figures are present.

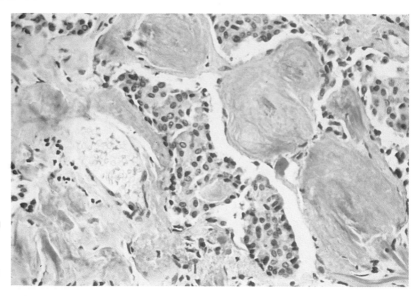

Fig. 17.37   Medullary carcinoma of the thyroid

High-power photomicrograph showing small spherical tumour cells adjacent to masses of amorphous hyaline material; the latter can be demonstrated, using special stains, to be amyloid.

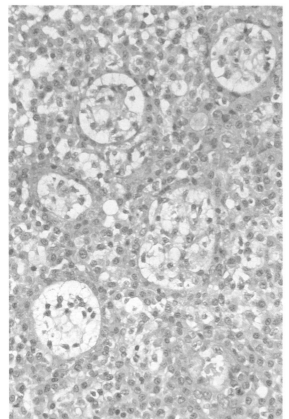

Fig. 17.38   Non-Hodgkin's lymphoma of the thyroid

High-power photomicrograph showing a uniform population of lymphocytes with nuclear morphology similar to centrocytes over-running the thyroid tissue and invading through follicular epithelium.

Lymphoma

Some thyroid tumours which in the past would have been classified as anaplastic carcinoma are now known on the basis of electron microscopy and immunohistochemistry to be mostly non-Hodgkin's lymphomas of follicular centre cell type (Fig. 17.38). There is an increased incidence of these types of lymphoma originating in the thyroid in Hashimoto's thyroiditis.

PARATHYROIDS

NORMAL STRUCTURE AND FUNCTION

About 90% of individuals have four parathyroid glands, the remainder having three or five. The upper pair are derived from the endoderm of the fourth pharyngeal pouch and lie close to the upper posterior surface of the thyroid. The lower pair, derived from endoderm of the third pharyngeal pouch, are variable in position lying anywhere from the lower pole of the thyroid to the upper mediastinum. Three types of cell can be recognised — chief cells, water-clear cells and oxyphil cells — but these may represent different functional states of the same cell lineage (Fig. 17.39). Despite having a combined weight of only 120 mg, these tiny glands play a major role in the control of calcium homeosta-

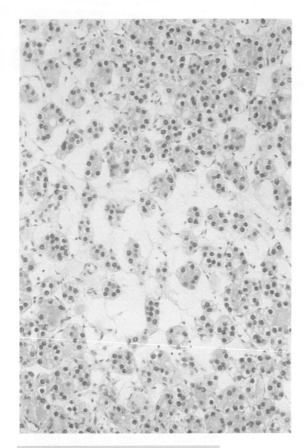

Fig. 17.39   Normal parathyroid gland

Low-power photomicrograph showing groups and small acini of the different types of parathyroid cells, between which there are islands of adipose tissue.

sis through their secretion of parathyroid hormone (PTH).

Calcium homeostasis

Parathyroid hormone, a polypeptide of 84 amino acids, plays a major part in the regulation of bone metabolism and plasma calcium levels. Plasma calcium levels are normally stabilised to within a very narrow range because differences in calcium concentrations across cell membranes are essential in excitable tissues such as muscle. The chief actions of PTH are shown in Table 17.7. The net effect of an increase in PTH secretion is to raise plasma calcium and reduce plasma phosphate levels. The actions of PTH cannot be considered in isolation because of its close relationship with vitamin D and calcitonin in the control of plasma calcium levels.

Table 17.7	The chief actions of PTH
Site	**Action**
Bone	Stimulates osteoclastic resorption Inhibits osteoblasts from forming bone matrix Releases calcium from bone
Kidney	Acts on renal tubular epithelium to cause reabsorption of calcium while inhibiting phosphate reabsorption Increases 1-hydroxylation in the epithelium of the proximal convoluted tubule of 25-hydroxyvitamin D to yield 1,25-dihydroxyvitamin D, the most active form

Vitamin D is acquired in two ways: either by synthesis from 7-dihydrocholesterol in the skin in the presence of sunlight, or from dietary sources such as eggs, butter and fortified margarine. The chief circulating form is 25-hydroxyvitamin D produced in the liver. Under the influence of PTH, the kidney hydroxylates this further to 1,25-dihydroxyvitamin D, the most active form. The actions of vitamin D are shown in Table 17.8.

Calcitonin is secreted by the C-cells of the thyroid (p. 502) in response to a rise in plasma calcium. It inhibits resorption of bone by osteoclasts and increases renal phosphate excretion. This tends to lower plasma calcium; however, hypersecretion of the hormone does not cause significant hypocalcaemia in otherwise normal individuals.

Table 17.8	The actions of vitamin D
Site	**Action**
Intestine	Increases calcium absorption
Bone	In conjunction with PTH, releases calcium into the circulation Is essential for normal mineralisation of osteoid

DISEASES OF THE PARATHYROIDS

The most important diseases of the parathyroids are hyperparathyroidism, hypoparathyroidism and tumours.

Hyperparathyroidism

> ▶ Primary: usually due to parathyroid adenoma
> ▶ Secondary: a physiological response to hypocalcaemia (e.g. malabsorption, renal failure)
> ▶ Tertiary: adenoma rarely arising in patients with secondary hyperparathyroidism
> ▶ Manifestations include bone resorption and, if primary or tertiary, the consequences of hypercalcaemia

Hyperparathyroidism is classified into primary, secondary and tertiary types according to the circumstances in which it occurs (Table 17.9). Primary and tertiary hyperparathyroidism are pathological states with inappropriate excess PTH secretion for the prevailing plasma calcium levels. Secondary hyperparathyroidism, however, is an appropriate physiological response to hypocalcaemia, for example in renal failure.

Primary hyperparathyroidism

Primary hyperparathyroidism is a fairly common condition, occurring in almost 0.1% of the population, most frequently in post-menopausal females. It presents through the symptoms of hypercalcaemia:

- renal stones, due to hypercalciuria
- muscle weakness
- tiredness
- thirst and polyuria
- anorexia and constipation
- rarely, peptic ulceration (gastrin secretion is enhanced).

In rare cases the effects of hyperparathyroidism

Table 17.9 Classification of hyperparathyroidism	
Hyperparathyroidism	Cause
Primary	Hypersecretion of PTH by an adenoma or hyperplasia of the gland
Secondary	The physiological increase in PTH secretions in response to hypocalcaemia of any cause
Tertiary	The supervention of an autonomous hypersecreting adenoma in longstanding secondary hyperparathyroidism

on bone — osteitis fibrosa and brown tumour (Ch. 25) — are also apparent clinically.

Hyperparathyroidism is only one of several important possible causes of hypercalcaemia. The commonest causes of hypercalcaemia are:

- disseminated malignancy in the bones
- hyperparathyroidism
- vitamin D intoxication
- milk–alkali syndrome
- sarcoidosis
- multiple myeloma
- rarely, PTH production by malignant tumours.

In the investigation of a patient with hypercalcaemia, the results which point to hyperparathyroidism as the cause are:

- a raised plasma calcium with a lowered plasma phosphate (due to the phosphaturic effect of PTH)
- mild metabolic acidosis
- importantly, raised PTH levels measured by radio-immunoassay.

In about 80% of cases, primary hyperparathyroidism is due to a secretory *adenoma* of one of the parathyroid glands; this consists of a neoplastic mass of functioning parathyroid cells surrounded by a compressed rim of inactive parathyroid tissue (Fig. 17.40). The remainder of cases are usually due to *hyperplasia* of all the parathyroid glands, especially when hyperparathyroidism forms part of one of the MEN syndromes (Ch. 11).

The management of hyperparathyroidism usually consists of operative inspection of all four parathyroid glands wherever possible, followed by removal of any suspected adenoma which is then submitted for intra-operative frozen section diagnosis.

Hypoparathyroidism

Hypoparathyroidism results in a fall in plasma calcium levels accompanied by elevated plasma phosphate levels. The patient presents with the clinical features of hypocalcaemia:

- tetany (spasm of the skeletal muscles)
- convulsions
- paraesthesiae
- psychiatric disturbances
- rarely, cataracts and brittle nails.

Diagnosis is confirmed by low or absent plasma PTH levels in the presence of hypocalcaemia.

In addition to hypoparathyroidism, other important causes of hypocalcaemia include:

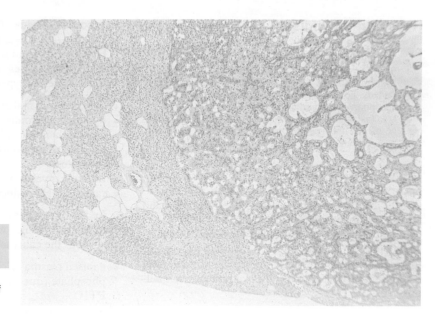

Fig. 17.40 Parathyroid adenoma from a patient with primary hyperparathyroidism

The adenomatous nodule is surrounded by a compressed rim of parathyroid tissue.

- hyperphosphataemia occurring in chronic renal failure
- rickets due to vitamin D deficiency (Ch. 25)
- excessive loss during lactation.

Even when the total plasma calcium levels are normal, symptoms of hypocalcaemia, such as tetany, may be produced by alkalosis; this lowers the proportion of plasma calcium in the ionised state, an important factor in the control of muscle excitability.

The leading causes of hypoparathyroidism are:

- removal of or damage to the parathyroid glands during thyroidectomy
- idiopathic hypoparathyroidism
- congenital deficiency (di George syndrome; Ch. 9).

Iatrogenic disease, such as accidental removal of the parathyroid glands during thyroidectomy, remains a common cause. Idiopathic hypoparathyroidism is now known to be due to destruction of the parathyroid cells by an auto-antibody. It is associated with other 'organ-specific' autoimmune diseases (Ch. 9).

Tumours

The commonest tumours, adenomas, are benign neoplasms of one of the three types of parathyroid cell. They are usually small (less than 50 mm in diameter) and only become clinically apparent through hypersecretion of PTH. Very rarely, they may occur in more than one parathyroid gland. Adenocarcinoma of the parathyroid glands is exceptionally rare.

ENDOCRINE PANCREAS

The pancreas consists of two functionally distinct components:

- the *exocrine* pancreas which secretes digestive enzymes into the duodenum (Ch. 16)
- the islets of Langerhans, scattered within the tissues of the exocrine pancreas, which together act as an *endocrine* gland.

Numbering about a million, the islets of Langerhans are derived from endoderm bordering the pancreatic ductal system. Although they comprise only 1–1.5 g of the pancreatic tissue (about 1% of its mass), their endocrine secretions have profound metabolic effects and are essential for life.

The islets consist of clusters of compact cells interspersed with small blood vessels (Fig. 17.41); they contain at least four distinct cell types, classified according to their hormone content as demonstrated by immunohistochemistry (Fig. 17.42). There are regional differences in hormone content of the islet cells in different parts of the pancreas, but the

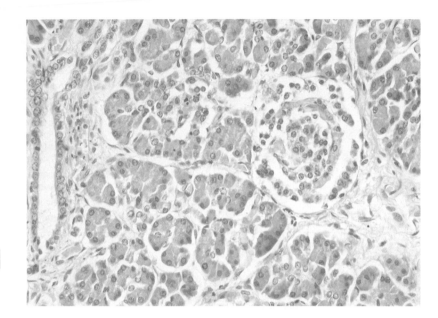

Fig. 17.41 Normal pancreas

An islet of Langerhans (right) is surrounded by exocrine pancreatic acini and a duct (left).

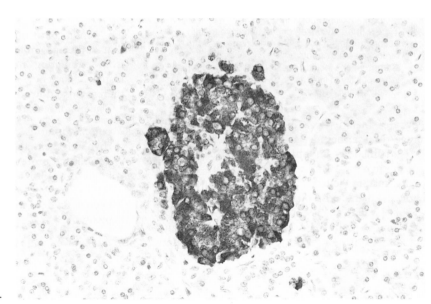

Fig. 17.42 β-Cells in an islet of Langerhans

This normal pancreas has been stained by the immunoperoxidase technique for insulin. The insulin-containing cells are darkly stained.

average hormonal composition is as shown in Table 17.10.

On electron microscopy, these endocrine cells contain membrane-bound electron-dense granules, some of which have characteristic shapes revealing their hormone content, and they have the histochemical features of APUD cells (Ch. 15).

The effects of two of the islet hormones, insulin and glucagon, are virtually antagonistic (Table 17.10). It seems that the secretion of pancreatic hormones is controlled locally; for example, a rising blood glucose level appears to stimulate the β-cells to secrete insulin directly.

The principal diseases of the endocrine pancreas are hypofunction, especially of the β-cells (diabetes mellitus), and tumours of the islet or other APUD cells which may produce widespread effects due to hypersecretion of their hormones.

Table 17.10 Cell types in the islets of Langerhans

Cell type	Average prevalence (%) in islets	Hormone produced	
		Identity	Actions
β	70	Insulin	Promotes glucose entry into cells, glycogen synthesis (and inhibits breakdown), lipogenesis (and inhibits lipolysis), and protein synthesis (together with growth hormone)
α	20	Glucagon	Promotes breakdown of glycogen (only in liver) and gluconeogenesis (from proteins)
δ	8	Somatostatin	Inhibits insulin and glucagon secretion
PP	2	Pancreatic polypeptide	Function in man unknown

Diabetes mellitus

▶ Abnormal metabolic state characterised by glucose intolerance due to inadequate insulin action
▶ Type I (juvenile onset) due to destruction of β-cells (probably a result of virus infection and genetic factors); insulin-dependent
▶ Type II (maturity onset) due to defective insulin action; treatment by weight reduction and oral hypoglycaemic agents
▶ Complications include accelerated atherosclerosis, susceptibility to infections, and microangiopathy affecting many organs

Diabetes mellitus is a disease state rather than a single disease, because it may have several causes. It is defined as an abnormal metabolic state in which there is glucose intolerance due to inadequate insulin action. Diagnosis is based on the clinical demonstration of glucose intolerance (Table 17.11).

Insulin is unique, in that it is the only hormone with a hypoglycaemic effect; there are five hormones which tend to exert a hyperglycaemic effect — glucagon, glucocorticoids, growth hormone, adrenaline and noradrenaline. Thus, the hyperglycaemic effects of these hormones cannot be counterbalanced if there is inadequate insulin action.

Pathogenesis

The actions of insulin (Table 17.10) are all *anabolic*, that is, they promote the laying down of tissue stores from circulating nutrients. The consequences of insulin deficiency are therefore *catabolic*, that is, there is breakdown of tissue energy stores.

The major features of diabetes mellitus are:

• inability to utilise, and overproduction of, glucose (hyperglycaemia)
• diminished protein synthesis
• lipolysis resulting in hyperlipidaemia, hence there is rapid wasting and weight loss. This state has been aptly described as 'starvation in the midst of plenty'.

In hyperglycaemia the renal threshold for glucose conservation is exceeded, so that there is osmotic diuresis resulting in polyuria, dehydration and

---

Table 17.11 Diagnosis of diabetes

Test	Diagnosis		
	Normal	Impaired GT	Diabetes
Random glucose	2.2–11.1	>10.0 on more than one occasion implies impaired GT or diabetes mellitus	
Fasting glucose	2.2–6.7	6.7–10.0	>10.0
2 hours after 75 g glucose	6.7	6.7–10.0	>10.0

Samples taken from venous blood; measurements in mmol/l; all figures apply to non-pregnant adults. GT=glucose tolerance

thirst. Lipolysis may also have serious consequences. Free fatty acids are converted in the liver to ketone bodies, such as acetoacetate, acetone and 3-hydroxybutyrate. These dissociate to release hydrogen ions, and a profound metabolic acidosis may ensue.

The combined result of severe ketosis, acidosis, hyperglycaemia, hyperosmolarity and electrolyte disturbance is to impair cerebral function, producing *diabetic ketoacidotic coma*. This is quite distinct from the *hypoglycaemic coma* which may also be found in diabetic patients; this is due to insulin overdosage, and has entirely different clinical features.

Classification

The two major types of diabetes mellitus are defined according to the clinical setting in which they occur. Research into pathogenesis of the disease has reinforced this classification, as the two types appear to have distinct pathogeneses. In addition, diabetes sometimes appears as a secondary consequence of other diseases.

Type I (juvenile-onset, insulin-dependent diabetes)
Type I diabetes mellitus (also called juvenile-onset, or insulin-dependent diabetes) typically presents in childhood. The patient usually shows the catabolic effects described above and is prone to develop ketoacidosis. The central defect is inadequate insulin secretion by the β-cells of the pancreas, and this can only be corrected by the life-long administration of exogenous insulin.

Post-mortem examination of the pancreas in patients who had recently developed type I diabetes but died from other causes (e.g. road traffic accident) shows lymphocytic infiltration of the islets with specific destruction of the β-cells. There are three major theories concerning the aetiology of these changes: autoimmune destruction, genetic factors and viral infection.

Autoimmune destruction. The majority of patients who have recently developed type I diabetes have circulatory antibodies to several different types of islet cells. Patients with this type of diabetes are also prone to develop other 'organ-specific' autoimmune diseases (Ch. 9).

Genetic factors. As with other 'organ-specific' autoimmune diseases, there is an association with certain HLA types (Ch. 3), notably HLA-DR4, especially if HLA-B8 or -DR3 is also present. It seems that environmental factors also play a role, since identical twins show only 40% concordance in development of the disease.

Viral infection. Titres of antibodies to viruses such as Coxsackie B types and mumps are elevated in some patients developing this type of diabetes; these viruses may act as a trigger for direct or autoimmune destruction of the islets.

Type II (maturity-onset, non-insulin-dependent diabetes)
Type II diabetes mellitus (also called maturity-onset, or non-insulin-dependent diabetes) is more common than type I and usually presents in middle age, being commonest in the obese. Patients are not prone to ketoacidosis, but occasionally develop a non-ketotic coma in which there is extreme hyperosmolarity of the plasma. Insulin secretion is normal or increased and the central defect may therefore be a reduction in the number of cell surface receptors for insulin.

Genetic factors clearly play an important part in the aetiology of type II diabetes, since identical twins show nearly a 100% concordance in development of the disease. No clear Mendelian pattern of inheritance can be recognised. The evidence is against this being an autoimmune disease.

Treatment is usually by weight reduction coupled with orally administered drugs which potentiate the action of insulin.

Secondary diabetes
Hypersecretion of any of the hormones which tend to exert a hyperglycaemic effect (p. 518) may cause glucose intolerance. Thus Cushing's syndrome, phaeochromocytoma, acromegaly and glucagonomas (p. 521) may cause secondary diabetes. Generalised destruction of the pancreas (see Ch. 16) by acute and chronic pancreatitis, haemochromatosis and, occasionally, carcinoma may cause insulin deficiency.

Complications

The major complications of diabetes mellitus are shown in Table 17.12. The commonest complications are seen in blood vessels. Atheroma, often ultimately severe and extensive, develops at an earlier age than in the non-diabetic population. Small blood vessels show basal lamina thickening and endothelial cell proliferation (diabetic microangiopathy), frequently causing retinal and renal damage. About 80% of adult diabetics die from cardiovascular disease, while patients with longstanding diabetes, especially type I, frequently develop serious renal and retinal disease. Improved metabolic control through modern insulin regimes has only partial-

Table 17.12 Complications of diabetes	
Situation	Complication
Large blood vessels	Accelerated atheroma, leading to: myocardial infarction cerebrovascular disease ischaemic limbs 80% of adult diabetic deaths
Small blood vessels	Endothelial cells and basal lamina damage Retinopathy (a major cause of blindness) Nephropathy, including Kimmelstiel–Wilson lesion (Ch. 21)
Peripheral nerves	Neuropathy, possibly due to disease of small vessels supplying the nerves
Neutrophils	Susceptibility to infection
Pregnancy	Pre-eclamptic toxaemia Large babies Neonatal hypoglycaemia
Skin	Necrobiosis lipoidica diabeticorum Granuloma annulare Gangrene of extremities

ly reduced the incidence of such serious complications.

Tumours

- ▶ Less common than pancreatic adenocarcinoma
- ▶ Present with endocrine effects and may be malignant
- ▶ Insulinoma: causes hypoglycaemia
- ▶ Glucagonoma: causes secondary diabetes and skin rash

Adenomas and carcinomas derived from the islet cells are quite rare. They usually present clinically through hypersecretion of their normal hormonal product, producing widespread symptoms; consequently these tumours may be small at the time of presentation. Most consist of cellular nodules within the pancreatic tissue. Histologically, they are composed of cells resembling normal islet cells (Fig. 17.43) and immunohistochemistry may be used to identify the hormonal content of the cells. Like other tumours of APUD tissues (Ch. 11), they contain dense-core secretory granules on electron microscopy. It is usually not possible to predict whether an islet cell tumour will pursue a benign or malignant course on the basis of histological appearance.

Insulinoma
Insulinoma is the commonest islet cell tumour, and produces hypoglycaemia through hypersecre-

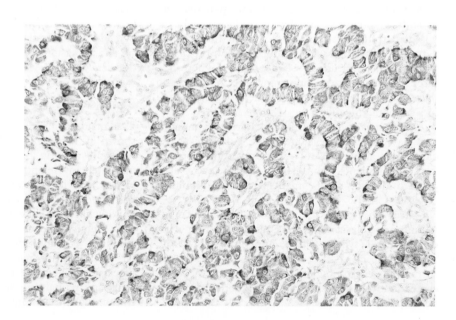

Fig. 17.43 Insulinoma
Ribbons of brown-stained cells resembling those of the normal islet of Langerhans.

tion of insulin. During hypoglycaemic attacks, the patient develops confusion, psychiatric disturbances and possibly coma. Diagnosis is urgent since hypoglycaemia may produce permanent cerebral damage.

Glucagonoma

Glucagonoma is much less common; it leads to hypersecretion of glucagon producing secondary diabetes and a distinctive skin rash known as necrolytic migratory erythema.

Other islet cell tumours

Other islet cell tumours are very rare, but include somatostatinomas, and tumours secreting vasoactive intestinal peptide (VIP) which leads to watery diarrhoea.

Gastrinomas

Although gastrin is usually produced in the G-cells of the stomach, tumours of the G-cells called gastrinomas most commonly originate in the pancreas. These APUD tumours lead to intractable hypersecretion of gastric acid due to the action of gastrin, resulting in widespread severe peptic ulceration (Zollinger–Ellison syndrome). Most gastrinomas are malignant.

Islet cell tumours and gastrinomas may occur as part of one of the MEN syndromes (Ch. 11), most commonly MEN type I.

FURTHER READING

Bloodworth J M B 1982 Endocrine pathology, general and surgical, 2nd edn. Williams and Wilkins, Baltimore

Brown C L 1981 The solitary thyroid nodule. In: Anthony P P, Woolf N (eds) Recent advances in histopathology 11. Churchill Livingstone, Edinburgh

Edwards C R W 1986 Endocrinology. Heinemann, London

Gould R P 1978 The APUD cell system. In: Anthony P P, Woolf N (eds) Recent advances in histopathology 10. Churchill Livingstone, Edinburgh

Klöppel G, Heitz P U 1984 Pancreatic pathology. Churchill Livingstone, Edinburgh

Lack E E 1990 Pathology of the adrenal glands. Churchill Livingstone, Edinburgh

LiVolsi V A 1990 Surgical pathology of the thyroid. W B Saunders, Philadelphia

Ney R L 1985 Investigation of endocrine disorder. Clinics in endocrinology and metabolism 14.1. W B Saunders, London

Scheithauer B W 1984 Surgical pathology of the pituitary: the adenomas, part II. In: Sommers S C, Rosen P P (eds) Pathology Annual, part 2. Appleton-Century-Crofts, Norwalk

Williams R N 1981 Textbook of endocrinology, 6th edn. W B Saunders, Philadelphia

18

Breast

NORMAL STRUCTURE AND FUNCTION

The physiological and pathological changes in a woman's breasts vary during different phases of her life. This is due to the variations in hormone levels that occur before, during and after the period of reproductive life; hormones are important in the regulation of growth, development and function of the breast.

Development

Before puberty, the breast consists of a few ducts which are connected to the nipple and open to the surface, but there are no glandular structures. Shortly before menarche, lengthening and branching of the ducts occurs and the terminal buds appear. There is increased volume of fat and connective tissue. With the onset of menses, further growth takes place and continues until at least the age of 25, unless accelerated by the intervention of pregnancy.

Developmental abnormalities

Failure of breast development in the female is very rare; in some cases it is due to ovarian agenesis (Turner's syndrome). *Accessory nipples* are the commonest abnormality; these can occur anywhere along the 'milk line', from axilla to groin. *Juvenile hypertrophy* is characterised by rapid and disproportionate breast growth during puberty; it can cause psychological distress and may warrant surgical reduction.

Hormonal regulation

Development of the breast requires the co-ordinated action of many hormones. The precise role of each hormone is difficult to determine since they may have both growth and secretory effects, and may regulate the activity of each other (Fig. 18.1).

Structure

The main function of the breast is the production and expression of milk (Fig. 18.2).

Lobules

The lobules are the secretory units of the breast. Each lobule consists of a variable number of *acini*, or glands, embedded within loose connective tissue and connecting to the intralobular duct (Fig. 18.3). Each acinus is composed of two types of cells, *epithelial*

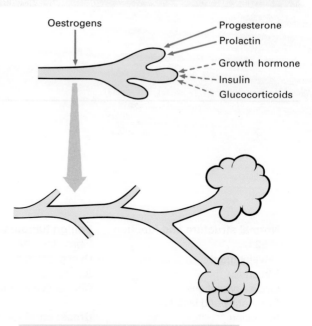

Fig. 18.1   The action of hormones in the development of the breast

Some hormones have a definite effect (→), whereas the role of others is less certain (– →).

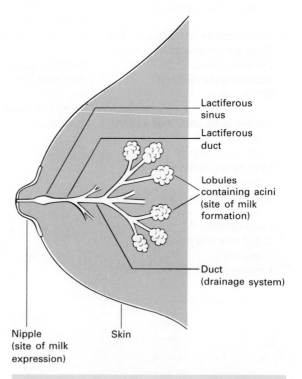

Fig. 18.2   Structure of the adult female breast, showing the major components and their functions

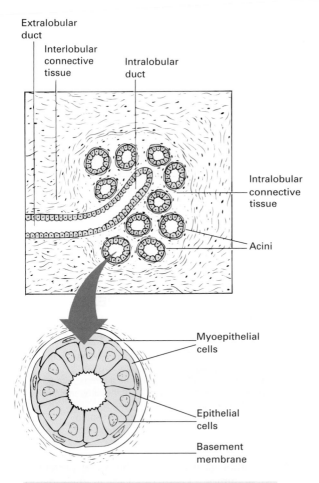

Fig. 18.3 A breast lobule showing the different components

The acinus is lined by epithelial cells surrounded by myoepithelial cells and the basement membrane.

and *myoepithelial*. The epithelial cells are secretory. Although synthesising milk only during the later stages of pregnancy and post-partum, they continuously secrete a variety of glycoproteins into the glandular lumens. They are surrounded by myoepithelial cells which contain contractile proteins and whose function is mechanical. The intralobular duct connects with the extralobular duct and this, together with the lobule, is called the *terminal ductal lobular unit*.

Ducts

The extralobular ducts within the same area link together to form subsegmental ducts, which link in turn to form segmental ducts. These drain into the lactiferous ducts and sinuses (Fig. 18.2) which empty

on to the surface of the nipple through separate orifices. There are 15–20 lactiferous ducts, each draining a segment of breast. The ducts are lined by epithelial cells surrounded by myoepithelial cells. The connective tissue in which they lie is denser than that of the lobules, and they are surrounded by elastic tissue which helps in the drainage function of the ducts.

Cyclical variations

The breast undergoes minor changes during each menstrual cycle but these will vary if there is a failure of ovulation or if pregnancy intervenes. The breast is sensitive to changes in the levels of sex steroids during the different phases (Fig. 18.4). The lobular stroma becomes quite oedematous during the secretory phase, due to the effects of oestrogens, and this accounts for the breast fullness often felt in the premenstrual phase. An increase in the number of cells in

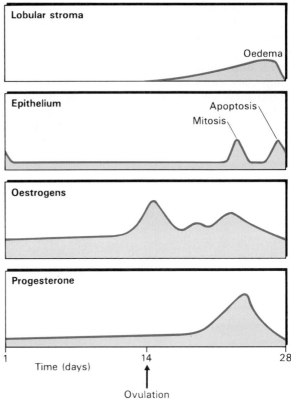

Fig. 18.4 Changes in breast epithelium and stroma in relation to the levels of oestrogen and progesterone during the menstrual cycle

Mitotic activity peaks at 22–24 days and apoptosis at 26 days.

mitosis occurs at days 22–24 of the cycle, coincident with the high peaks of oestrogen and progesterone; however, the numbers are never very high. A loss of cells occurs by apoptosis (Ch. 5) at the end of the cycle, due to a fall in hormone levels, so that an overall balance is maintained. In view of the changes that can occur in the breast in the second half of the menstrual cycle, it is better to examine clinically the breasts of a pre-menopausal woman in the first half of the cycle.

Pregnancy and lactation

During pregnancy, the lobules undergo controlled proliferation and enlargement in preparation for the synthetic and secretory activity of lactation. By the third trimester the number of acini in each lobule and the overall size of the lobules have markedly increased. The epithelial cells have become differentiated and they synthesise and secrete milk (Fig. 18.5). The various components of milk (casein, α-lactalbumin and milk fat globule membranes derived from the luminal surface of breast cells) are useful markers of the state of differentiation of breast cells, and because of this they have been extensively studied in breast disease.

Oestrogens, progesterone and prolactin, together with other hormones shown in Figure 18.1, are important in the development of the breast during pregnancy; however, once delivery occurs the levels of sex steroids fall and it is prolactin which is necessary for the initiation of lactation. When breast feeding ceases there is a rapid involution of the differentiated lobular structure, and the breast returns to the pre-pregnancy structure.

Involution

Changes occur in the breast with increasing age; these involutional changes relate to the altered sex steroid levels that accompany decreasing ovarian function. The connective tissue of the lobules changes from a loose to a dense structure, the basement membranes around acini become thicker, and the lining cells of the acini are lost. These changes start in the premenopausal period and continue past the menopause; they often occur at an uneven rate, producing clinically palpable lumps. In elderly women, the major component of the breast is adipose tissue.

CLINICAL FEATURES OF BREAST LESIONS

▶ Physiological changes must be distinguished from pathological lesions
▶ Many breast conditions present as a lump or lumps
▶ Always note the characteristics of the lump and the age of the patient
▶ Discharge from the nipple occurs with some conditions

Most pathological lesions of the breast present as a lump or lumps. These can vary in their nature

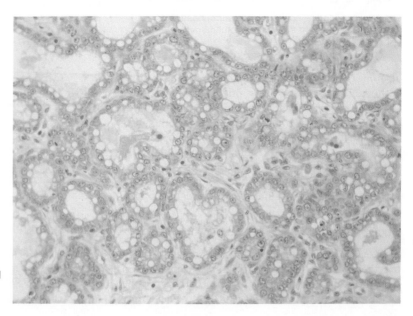

Fig. 18.5 Lactation

Breast histology from a woman 30 weeks pregnant, showing the acini lined by cells containing secretory vacuoles, and with secretions in their lumens.

depending on their cause: well-circumscribed or ill-defined; single or multiple small nodules; soft or firm; mobile or attached to skin or underlying muscle. These features assist in the clinical distinction between benign breast lesions and breast carcinomas, but they are relatively weak discriminators on their own. Below the age of about 35, benign breast lumps are much more common than carcinomas. Most women with breast cancer are peri- or post-menopausal. The most likely type of lesion will vary with the age of the patient, although overlaps occur (Table 18.1). However, there can be exceptions and histological examination is mandatory for a definite diagnosis.

Physiological conditions can be confused with, or mimic, pathological conditions. A degree of tenderness and swelling of the breast in the premenstrual phase is common. Some women have naturally 'lumpy' breasts and this may become exaggerated in this phase of the menstrual cycle. Uneven proliferation of the glandular substance during pregnancy, and irregular involution after pregnancy and during and after the menopause can result in lumps that are the outcome of physiological and not pathological events. Other manifestations of a pathological lesion within the breast are discharge from the nipple, eczema and ulceration of the skin of the nipple.

DIAGNOSTIC METHODS

Several methods are currently used to investigate breast lesions. These include:

- fine-needle aspiration cytology
- Tru-Cut biopsy
- examination of frozen section
- mammography and ultrasound.

Fine-needle aspiration cytology

This technique is increasingly employed. When a woman presents at a clinic with a breast lump, a needle can be inserted into the area (guided, if necessary, by radiological imaging or by ultrasound) and cells aspirated without the need for even a local anaesthetic. After smearing and staining, the cells are examined by a pathologist, and if the specimen is adequate a diagnosis can be made. The advantages of this approach are that it is relatively painless and that management can be planned so that the patient is fully aware of the extent of any surgery that may be required.

Tru-Cut biopsy

Another approach which can be used in the clinic is Tru-Cut biopsy, in which a core of tissue is removed using a biopsy needle. This technique has the disadvantage that the tissue has to be processed overnight for histological examination, whereas it is often possible to prepare and interpret fine-needle aspiration cytology in the clinic. In addition, the procedure requires a local anaesthetic and can be more painful.

Examination of frozen section

Breast lesions can be diagnosed very rapidly by frozen section at the time of surgery. A small sample is frozen, and sections are cut, stained and interpreted by a pathologist within a few minutes. However,

Table 18.1 The probable pathological causes of presenting clinical lesions at different ages in women

Clinical presentation	Probable pathological cause			
	<25 years	25–35 years	35–55 years	>55 years
Mobile lump	Fibroadenoma	Fibroadenoma	Fibroadenoma Phyllodes tumour	Phyllodes tumour
Ill-defined lump or lumpy areas	Uncommon	Fibrocystic change Sclerosing adenosis	Fibrocystic change	Uncommon
Firm lump ± tethering	Uncommon	Carcinoma*	Carcinoma	Carcinoma Fat necrosis
Nipple discharge Clear Bloody	Uncommon Uncommon	Uncommon Uncommon	Duct ectasia Duct papilloma	Duct ectasia Duct papilloma
Nipple ulceration, eczema	Nipple adenoma	Nipple adenoma	Paget's disease Nipple adenoma	Paget's disease Nipple adenoma

*Carcinoma is unusual in this age group, but can occur.

Pathological basis of breast signs and symptoms	
Sign or symptom	Pathological basis
Lump	
• diffuse	Fibrosis, epithelial hyperplasia and cysts in fibrocystic change
• discrete	Neoplasm or solitary cyst
• mobile	Benign neoplasm (usually fibroadenoma)
• tethered	Invasive neoplasm (carcinoma)
Skin features	
• oedema (peau d'orange)	Impaired lymphatic drainage due to carcinoma
• puckering and tethering	Invasion of skin by carcinoma
• erythema	Increased blood flow due to inflammation or tumour
Nipple	
• discharge	Milky—pregnancy or prolactinoma Bloody—duct papilloma or carcinoma
• retraction	Tethering by invasive carcinoma
• erythema and scaling	Paget's disease of nipple or eczema
Breast pain	
• cyclical	Benign breast disease
• on palpation	Inflammatory lesion (e.g. mastitis)
Microcalcification (on mammography)	Dystrophic calcification often, but not always, associated with in-situ or invasive carcinoma
Axillary node enlargement	Often due to metastatic breast carcinoma
Bone pain or fracture	Possibly due to metastatic breast carcinoma or associated with hypercalcaemia

since the patient does not know definitely before her operation the extent of surgery she may receive, the use of this technique is declining in comparison to fine-needle aspiration cytology or Tru-Cut biopsy. It may be used when unsatisfactory results are obtained by the other procedures and the surgeon considers the lesion to be clinically worrying.

Mammography and ultrasound
X-raying of the breasts (mammography) is used to help in the diagnosis of both palpable and impalpable lesions. This technique is the basis of screening programmes, which try to detect impalpable small breast cancers, i.e. 'early' tumours. Lesions detected in this way require an X-ray-directed guidewire to be inserted into them before surgery to help the surgeon find the right area. It is important that the pathologist care-

fully examines the tissue to ensure that the lesion has been removed. Ultrasound imaging can also be used.

Screening for breast cancer

In several developed countries with a high incidence of breast cancer, such as the UK, screening programmes for the detection of early breast cancer have been or are being introduced. Trials in Sweden and the USA strongly suggest that women whose cancers have been detected by regular mammographic screening have an increased survival rate. This is because the tumours are detected when they are either pre-invasive (in-situ carcinoma) or invasive but small, with less risk of metastasis. Unscreened women present when the tumour has grown to a size sufficient to be felt, at which stage there is a higher probability of metastases.

In the UK, women between the ages of 50 and 64 are invited to attend for breast screening by mammography every 3 years. Suspicious features on the X-ray image, such as microcalcification and localised densities, are further investigated by ultrasound and clinical examination, with cytology of aspirated cells and histology of biopsy samples providing the definitive diagnosis.

Besides being smaller, the invasive tumours have a higher frequency of being of a special, more favourable type. This, along with the lower incidence of lymph node metastasis, will contribute to the improved prognosis. The surgery for these early lesions is more likely to be conservative.

The greater density of the pre-menopausal breast means that mammography is less reliable for screening women under 50 years.

INFLAMMATORY CONDITIONS

▶ Infections of the breast are uncommon, usually complications of lactation
▶ Duct ectasia can cause nipple discharge, commoner in older women
▶ Fat necrosis is due to trauma, more frequent in the obese

Acute pyogenic mastitis

Acute pyogenic mastitis is a painful acute inflammatory condition which usually occurs in the first few weeks after delivery, and *Staphylococcus aureus* is the commonest organism. The usual portal of entry is a crack in the nipple, although persistence of the keratotic plug at the orifice of a duct may be a factor.

The organisms spread via the lymphatics, and the infection tends to be confined to one segment of the breast resulting in localised swelling and erythema. The infection can spread to other segments and, if *Streptococcus pyogenes* is the causative organism, a more widespread inflammation occurs with systemic symptoms. If antibiotics are given but there is inadequate drainage, a localised breast abscess will result.

Other infections

Tuberculosis of the breast
This is rare and usually results from haematogenous spread. The infection results in a fibrocaseous mass with the formation of sinuses, although a marked fibrous reaction can occur giving a firm mass that will mimic a carcinoma.

Actinomycosis
Also rare, actinomycosis is none the less the commonest fungal infection of the breast in the United Kingdom. It can be due to extension of infection from the lung through the thoracic cage, or occur as a primary infection. The usual presentation is as a hard lump beneath the nipple, which may be painful, but with no temperature change, so mimicking a tumour. It results in abscess formation, within which are the fungal colonies.

Mammary duct ectasia

Mammary duct ectasia involves the larger ducts within the breast but, in severe cases, can also extend to the smaller interlobular ducts. It occurs predominantly in women in the second half of reproductive life and after the menopause, and mild degrees of the condition are often an incidental finding in breast tissue excised for other conditions. Severe forms, in which it is the primary presenting condition, are less frequent. Severe cases can be mistaken clinically for a carcinoma since there may be a discharge from the nipple which may be blood-stained. Fibrosis around the ducts may result in nipple retraction, and there may be a firm palpable mass. However, mammary duct ectasia is a purely inflammatory condition with no relationship to malignancy.

The aetiology is unknown but the affected women are usually parous. The ducts are dilated and filled with white–green viscid matter; this material may be discharged from the nipple. The matter can usually be seen with the naked eye in excised tissue. The tissue around the ducts contains lymphocytes, plasma cells, and macrophages, with a significant degree of fibrosis. Due to the inflammatory reaction, the condition is sometimes known as *periductal mastitis*.

Fat necrosis

Trauma is thought to be the cause of fat necrosis, although a history is not always obtained. It is more frequent in obese women and after the menopause, when the breast has a proportionally greater amount of adipose tissue. It usually presents as a discrete lump and can therefore mimic a carcinoma clinically.

Macroscopically, the tissue is yellow and haemorrhagic, with flecks of calcification. Fibrous tissue is also present, the amount depending on the duration of the condition.

Histologically, the appearances are the same as those of any adipose tissue that undergoes necrosis (Ch. 6): collections of macrophages and giant cells containing lipid material may be seen, and there is an associated reaction with lymphocytes, fibroblasts and small vascular channels. The necrotic fat acts as a persistent irritant, resulting in a chronic inflammatory process and hence fibrous tissue formation.

Similar foreign body reactions can occur in the breast around prosthetic implants, in which silicone fluid is frequently used; a very dense fibrous tissue reaction can result, causing considerable distortion.

PROLIFERATIVE CONDITIONS OF THE BREAST

> ▶ Increase in frequency towards menopause, then rapid decrease
> ▶ Present as diffuse granularity, ill-defined lump or discrete swelling
> ▶ Variety of histological changes
> ▶ Adenosis commoner in younger age group, cysts commoner nearer the menopause
> ▶ Women with atypical hyperplasia are at increased risk of developing breast cancer
> ▶ Gynaecomastia is enlargement of breasts in men

Proliferative conditions of the breast include a wide variety of morphological changes with consequently varied clinical features; because of this there has been much confusion about the terminology and significance of these conditions.

Fibrocystic change

The commonest proliferative condition of the breast is fibrocystic change. Although benign and non-neoplastic, it is important because:

- in many women, it causes severe periodic discomfort

- one component, epithelial hyperplasia, is associated with an increased breast cancer risk
- it causes palpable lumps mimicking breast cancer.

Terminology

The old term for proliferative conditions of the breast was 'chronic mastitis'; this is incorrect, as these are not inflammatory conditions, but the name may have arisen because of the tenderness that can occur in some cases. Other names include fibroadenosis, epithelial hyperplasia, fibrocystic disease, cystic hyperplasia and mammary dysplasia. Since some of the features are similar to physiological changes the term 'fibrocystic change', rather than 'disease', is now used.

The terms *fibroadenosis* and *epithelial hyperplasia* describe the proliferative changes that occur in the condition (see below), and are appropriate terms for the changes that occur in the 30–45-year age group. *Fibrocystic change* and *cystic hyperplasia* are descriptive of the changes that occur from 40–45 years to the menopause, when cysts are more prominent. The term 'mammary dysplasia' is not really correct, since true dysplasia occurs only in a few cases.

Incidence

Estimates indicate that at least 10% of women develop clinically apparent benign proliferative breast disease, although breast tissue from women at postmortem shows such changes to be present in 50% or more, suggesting that lesser degrees of change are much more common.

Aetiology and pathogenesis

Although benign proliferative breast disease is not uncommon, the aetiology is poorly understood. There is no doubt that ovarian hormones participate in its causation but the means by which the changes are produced are still obscure.

The fact that the incidence of benign proliferative changes increases as the menopause gets nearer, and that failure of ovulation also increases in this time period, suggests that the relative imbalance between oestrogen and progesterone in each menstrual cycle could be an important aetiological factor. The disturbance may involve interaction of the pituitary and the ovaries. Alternatively, the fault may lie in the responsiveness of the breast tissue to the hormonal influences. Not all parts of the breast are equally affected by the hormonal changes occurring in each menstrual cycle, and this may account for the focal nature of the changes.

Cystic change is considered to be due to an imbalance between epithelial hyperplasia, together with ductal and lobular dilatation, that occurs with each menstrual cycle, and subsequent regressive changes. The cystic dilatation thus occurs because of a distortion of cyclical changes rather than as a consequence of obstruction, which is the usual cause in other organs.

Clinical and gross features

Proliferative lesions and their associated tissue responses generally occur between the ages of 30 and 55, with a marked decrease in incidence after the menopause. The incidence reaches a maximum in the years just before the menopause (Fig. 18.6).

The clinical features tend to vary with the age of the patient and the underlying pathological changes. In younger women, there is usually a diffuse granularity in one or more segments of the breast, with nodules up to 5 mm in diameter. The area may be tender, particularly in the premenstrual period. In women nearer the menopause, there is usually an ill-defined rubbery mass. The finding of discrete swelling indicates the presence of cysts. If fibrosis is a component of the proliferative lesion, the lump will be firm and therefore more difficult to differentiate clinically from carcinoma.

The gross appearance of the breast tissue shows variation from case to case. In younger women, it is

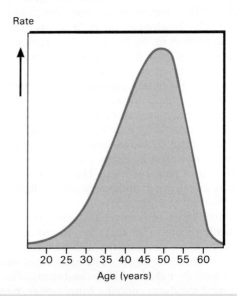

Rate

Age (years)

Fig. 18.6   Incidence rates of benign proliferative breast changes, occurring in women at different ages

more common to find nodules of soft pink or grey tissue, up to 3 mm in diameter, which represent areas of epithelial proliferation, whereas in women nearer the menopause cysts are frequently seen. These cysts can vary in size from 2 to 20 mm (Fig. 18.7) and, rarely, a solitary large cyst can be seen. The small cysts are often multiple. They frequently have a dark blue surface and, on opening, contain clear, yellowish or blood-stained fluid. The intervening tissue is usually firm due to the increase in fibrous tissue but the softer foci of epithelial proliferation can be seen and felt.

Histological features

A variety of histological changes can occur (Fig. 18.8). These are:

- adenosis
- sclerosing adenosis
- epithelial hyperplasia
- papillomatosis
- cysts
- apocrine metaplasia
- fibrosis.

An individual woman may show one, some or all of these changes. However, the types of changes do tend to vary with the age of the patient.

Adenosis

Adenosis is enlargement of the lobules which contain many, up to hundreds, of acini. In other respects they are structurally normal. The term is often used to refer to *blunt duct adenosis* in which the acini of the lobules are larger than normal and are lined by cells

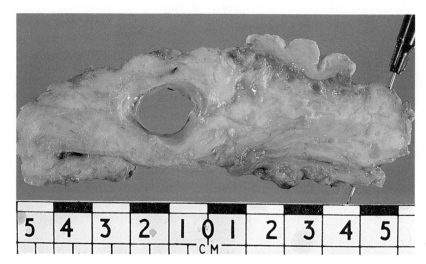

Fig. 18.7 Fibrocystic change: cysts

Breast tissue from a 48-year-old woman showing one large cyst and multiple smaller ones, with areas of fibrosis.

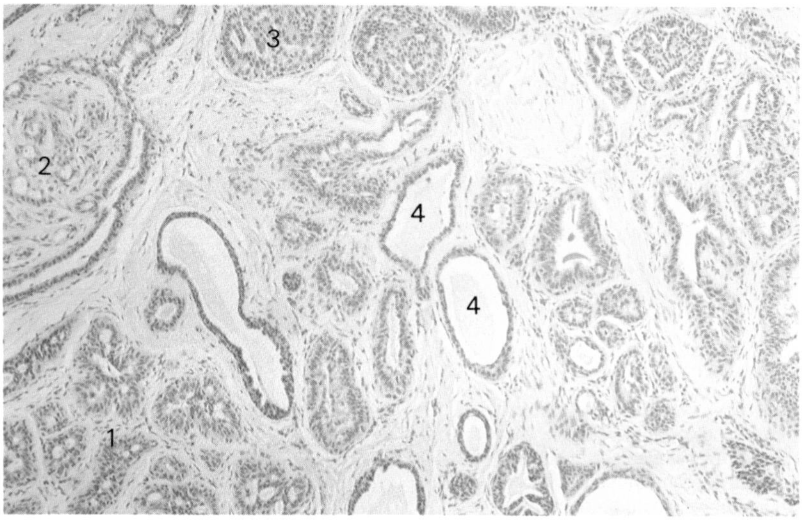

Fig. 18.8 Fibrocystic change

There is adenosis (1), papilloma formation (2), epithelial hyperplasia (3) and small cysts (4).

which are increased in size and may also be more numerous, although the acinar lumen is always clearly seen. The lobular stroma may also increase. The changes are not confined to the epithelium and can involve the surrounding myoepithelium. Such areas correspond to the grey–pink nodules seen macroscopically and the fine nodules felt clinically.

Sclerosing adenosis

In sclerosing adenosis there is lobular proliferation but the acini become distorted. The proliferation involves both epithelium and myoepithelium, but the latter tends to predominate. Large amounts of collagen can intervene between the glandular components, although the extent of this varies both within the same breast and between patients (Fig. 18.9). Due to the collagen component these lesions can mimic carcinomas clinically, and their bizarre architecture can cause difficulties in the interpretation of frozen sections.

Epithelial hyperplasia

Epithelial hyperplasia, previously called epitheliosis, is the proliferation of epithelial cells which occurs in the small interlobular ducts, the intralobular ducts and the acini, resulting in a solid or almost solid mass obliterating the lumens (Fig. 18.10).

Papillomatosis

Papillomatosis comprises simple papillary processes projecting into the lumens of dilated ducts or small cysts. The papillae have a fine connective tissue core and are covered by one or two layers of epithelium; they may undergo branching.

Cysts

Cysts develop through dilatation of the acini of the lobules and the terminal ducts. These cysts may remain small, or enlarge to sizes up to 20–30 mm. They may be fairly evenly distributed, with little variation in size, or show quite marked variation in size, shape or number. They may be lined by simple cuboidal or flattened epithelium, or focal proliferative change may occur. Occasionally cysts can rupture, causing an inflammatory reaction.

Apocrine metaplasia

Frequently the cysts, both large and small, are lined entirely or partly by cells which resemble the epithelium of the apocrine sweat glands. This condition is called apocrine metaplasia. The lining cells are large columnar cells with pink-staining (eosinophilic) cytoplasm, hence the alternative name 'pink cell metaplasia'. It has no special clinical or prognostic significance.

Fibrosis

Fibrosis can occur in association with the various proliferative conditions, or as an isolated lesion. When associated with proliferative conditions it is probably due to the hormonal imbalances causing changes in the typical loose connective tissue of the lobules, making it denser with fewer glycosaminoglycans. The solitary form of fibrosis produces a poorly-defined area of rubbery consistency consisting of dense connective tissue with few atrophic epithelial areas. This condition is found mainly in women with a clear history of hormone imbalance.

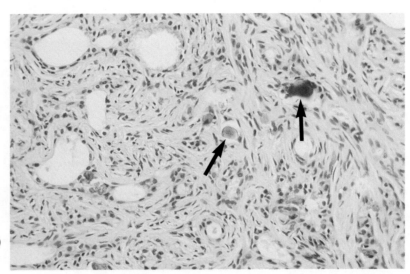

Fig. 18.9 Sclerosing adenosis

There are glandular structures with intervening cords of cells in a fibrous stroma. Areas of calcification (arrowed) are also present; these would render the lesion visible on mammography.

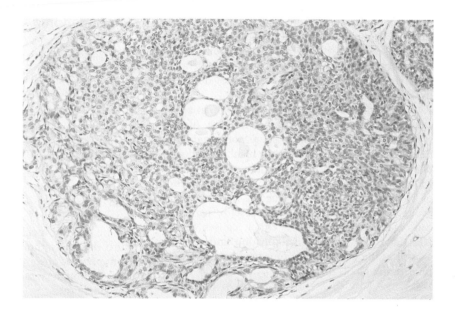

Fig. 18.10 Epithelial hyperplasia

The duct lumen is filled by hyperplastic epithelium.

Atypical hyperplasia

The epithelial hyperplasia that can result in total or partial occlusion of the acini and small ducts may sometimes show abnormalities of cellular growth, with disordered orientation of cells, nuclear pleomorphism and occasional mitotic figures. This is termed either atypical ductal or atypical lobular hyperplasia, depending on its situation. It is important for the pathologist to identify these cellular changes (see below).

Lesions in women aged 30–45 years

In the 30–45-year age group, lesions are more likely to consist of areas of adenosis, possibly with epithelial hyperplasia, and a mild degree of fibrosis. Sclerosing adenosis may also be present. Microcysts with apocrine metaplasia start to develop in the late thirties, but are generally not a major feature. Between 40 and 45 years the changes may be predominantly proliferative, with adenosis and epithelial hyperplasia, or may be more cystic.

Lesions in women aged 45–55 years

Cysts are the more prominent feature in this age group and can be quite large. The terms 'blue domed cyst' and 'Bloodgood's cyst' used to be applied. Apocrine metaplasia is often present. Proliferative features, such as adenosis, epithelial hyperplasia and papillomatosis, can be seen, and fibrosis is quite common.

Radial scars

Radial scars are benign focal lesions commonly detected by mammography in post-menopausal women. They are stellate fibrous structures with foci of ductal epithelial proliferation. Their structure mimics radiologically the appearance of invasive carcinoma. When larger than 10 mm, they are named *complex sclerosing lesions*.

Significance of proliferative lesions

Clinically, the presence of a lump can cause anxiety in the patient, who may believe it is a cancer when it is benign; excision and histological confirmation can reassure her.

Up to 70% of women who undergo breast biopsy for benign fibrocystic change are not at an increased risk of developing cancer. However, if the biopsy contains areas of atypical hyperplasia, the woman has a risk of developing cancer 5 times higher than that of a woman with non-proliferative lesions, and the risk increases if there is a family history of breast cancer. Cysts alone do not appear to increase the risk.

Lesions in men: gynaecomastia

The breast tissue in men contains only ductular structures with no evidence of acini; it is similar in appearance to the pre-pubertal female breast.

Gynaecomastia is benign enlargement of the male breast tissue. The breast may resemble that of a young adolescent female in appearance and consistency, or there may be a firm, mobile disc beneath the nipple. The condition is unilateral in 75% of cases. The ducts are dilated and there is a variable degree of epithelial proliferation. The stroma around the ducts is often oedematous and myxoid, but in longstanding cases the stroma becomes dense and hyalinised (Fig. 18.11).

Gynaecomastia occurs most commonly in adolescence and in older age groups. In both of these groups it is probably due to some hormonal effects relating to oestrogens, possibly a result of endocrine disturbances such as hyperthyroidism, pituitary disorders and tumours of the adrenals and testis. Both of the latter can secrete oestrogens. In the older age group, stilboestrol therapy of prostatic carcinoma can cause gynaecomastia. Other causes include Klinefelter's syndrome, malnutrition and cirrhosis, as well as the drugs chlorpromazine and spironolactone, and digitalis therapy.

BENIGN TUMOURS

Unlike the situation in other glandular tissues, the commonest type of benign tumour of the breast is a combined product of both connective tissue and epithelial cells; purely epithelial tumours are less frequent.

The benign breast tumours comprise:

- fibroadenomas
- duct papillomas
- adenomas
- connective tissue tumours.

Fibroadenoma

> ▶ Commonest type of benign tumour, mainly in young women
> ▶ Arises from connective tissue and epithelium
> ▶ Clinically, mobile on palpation

Fibroadenomas are the commonest type of benign tumour of the breast, and are the commonest primary tumour in younger age groups. In a study in New York, fibroadenomas were seen with a quarter of the frequency of carcinomas, but six times more frequently than duct papillomas. However, not all fibroadenomas are excised, so their actual frequency may be higher.

The greatest incidence of fibroadenomas is in the third decade, although they can occur at any time from puberty onwards. The tumours are usually solitary, although some women do develop multiple fibroadenomas.

Fibroadenomas arise from the breast lobule, from both the loose connective tissue stroma and the glands. As they are mixed tumours, fibroadenomas will undergo some of the same hormonally induced changes as the surrounding breast. Thus, during pregnancy the glands will show lactational changes, and in older women the stroma will become more dense and fibrous. During pregnancy, fibroadenomas may grow rapidly in size, but this is due to hormonal affects and is not a sign of malignancy.

Gross appearance

Fibroadenomas are well circumscribed with a lobulated appearance (Fig. 18.12), and range in size

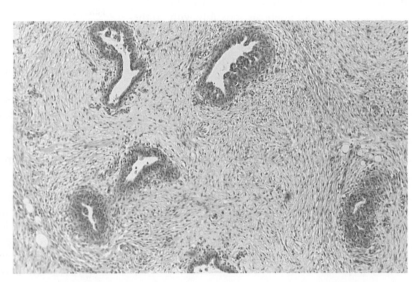

Fig. 18.11 Gynaecomastia

Male breast in which the ducts are lined by an increased number of cells, and are surrounded by loose connective tissue.

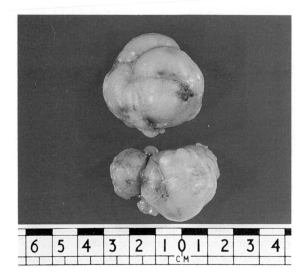

Fig. 18.12 Fibroadenoma

The outer surface is smooth, well circumscribed, and has a lobulated appearance.

from 10–40 mm in diameter although larger tumours can occur in juvenile fibroadenoma (see below). The surrounding breast tissue can become compressed, but the tumour is not tethered; this lack of fixation accounts for its mobility on clinical examination, and the nickname of 'breast mouse'. In young women, the tumours are soft and have a slightly gelatinous cut surface due to the loose connective tissue component; however, in older women they tend to be firmer since the connective tissue becomes more fibrous and sometimes calcified.

Histology

Fibroadenomas show duct-like structures or elongated and thinned ductular structures associated with overgrown connective tissue masses (Fig. 18.13). Fibroadenoma does not progress to malignancy, although very occasionally a tumour, such as lobular carcinoma, will involve a fibroadenoma.

Juvenile fibroadenoma

Large (50–100 mm diameter) fibroadenomas can occur in the breast of girls, the tumours growing quite rapidly. They are more frequent in Africans and West Indians than in Caucasians. The tumours are benign and should not be confused with phyllodes tumour (p. 550).

Duct papilloma

- ► Less common, occurring in middle-aged women
- ► Presents as blood-stained nipple discharge
- ► Usually solitary lesion, occurring in large ducts
- ► Papillary structures, with fibrovascular core covered by benign epithelium

Duct papillomas are considerably less frequent than fibroadenomas. They also differ in several other respects. Although they can occur in the young and the elderly, they more frequently arise in middle-aged women. Duct papillomas are the commonest cause of nipple discharge. About 80% of patients present with a discharge, which is often blood-stained, and a mass can often be felt. The tumours arise from ductal epithelium.

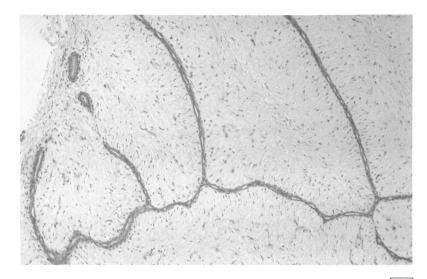

Fig. 18.13 Fibroadenoma

Elongated duct-like structures are surrounded by loose connective tissue.

Duct papillomas arise as a solitary lesion within a large duct, up to 40 mm from the nipple. They appear either as an elongated structure extending along a duct, or as a spheroid which causes distension of the duct, making it cyst-like. The tumours have soft, pink or white outgrowths except when haemorrhage has occurred, in which case the surface will be brown from altered blood. Duct papillomas consist of branching fibrovascular cores covered by epithelium, which is cytologically benign (Fig. 18.14). Solitary duct papillomas are not premalignant; there is no increased risk of carcinoma. There is a rare condition in which multiple ductal papillomas occur, but these arise in the smaller ducts, away from the nipple, and so present as a mass rather than as nipple discharge. These tend to occur in a younger age group than do solitary papillomas and there is an increased risk of carcinoma developing.

Adenomas

> ▸ Rare, arise only from epithelium
> ▸ Tubular and lactating adenomas occur in young women
> ▸ Nipple adenomas occur at all ages; there is a mass beneath the nipple which can ulcerate the skin

Adenomas are much rarer than fibroadenomas and duct papillomas. *Tubular adenomas* are well-circumscribed tumours between 10 and 40 mm in diameter, occurring mainly in women in their early twenties. They are composed of closely packed, uniform tubular structures with little connective tissue in between; hence the only tumorous component is the glands.

Lactating adenomas are tubular adenomas which undergo secretory changes during pregnancy.

Nipple adenomas occur as a nodule under the nipple, usually less than 15 mm in diameter, in women of any age. The overlying skin is often ulcerated, and there may be a blood-stained discharge, so that clinically nipple adenomas may be mistaken for Paget's disease. They are well circumscribed, and contain small and larger ducts filled with masses of cells and surrounded by a dense stroma.

Connective tissue tumours

Lipomas and haemangiomas can occur in the breast, but are often hamartomas. Leiomyomas may occur deep in the breast or in the nipple, arising from the smooth muscle which is abundant there.

BREAST CARCINOMA

> ▸ 20% of all cancers in women
> ▸ Commonest cause of death in women in 35–55 age group
> ▸ In the UK, any woman has a 1 in 10–12 chance of developing breast cancer

In North America, North-west Europe and Australia, breast cancer is the commonest type of malignancy in women. In the United Kingdom it accounts for 20% of all cancers, and is the commonest cause of death amongst women in the 35–55 age

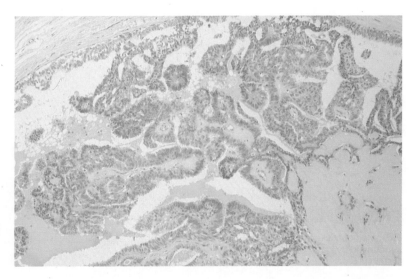

Fig. 18.14 Duct papilloma

A duct containing finger-like projections covered by a layer of epithelial and underlying myoepithelial cells, with a fibrous core.

group. There are 24 000 new cases each year. It is estimated, in the high-risk areas, that any individual woman has a 1 in 10–12 chance of developing the disease in her lifetime.

Many risk factors have been identified, and these, together with advances in the analysis of genetic and hormonal factors, have resulted in several aetiological hypotheses (Fig. 18.15). An understanding of these can help in the development of programmes directed towards the prevention of breast cancer. At present, schemes aimed at the early detection of breast cancer are being introduced.

Risk factors

The risk factors identified to date are:

- female sex; risk increases with age
- long interval between menarche and menopause
- older age at first full-term pregnancy
- obesity and high-fat diet
- family history of breast cancer
- geographic factors
- atypical hyperplasia in previous breast biopsy.

Female sex and age

Less than 1% of all breast cancers occur in men, so being female is an important risk factor. As with all carcinomas, increasing age is another significant factor. Up to the age of 40–45 years, the rate of increase is steep; it then slows down, although the incidence of breast cancer continues to increase into old age (Fig. 18.16).

Age at menarche and menopause

There is a significantly higher risk of developing breast cancer amongst women with an early age at menarche. At the other end of the reproductive life, women whose natural menopause occurs before 45 years have only half the breast cancer risk of those whose menopause occurs after 55 years. Therefore women with 40 or more years of active menstruation have twice the breast cancer risk of those with fewer than 30 years of menstrual activity.

Age at first full-term pregnancy

Nulliparous women have an increased risk of develop-

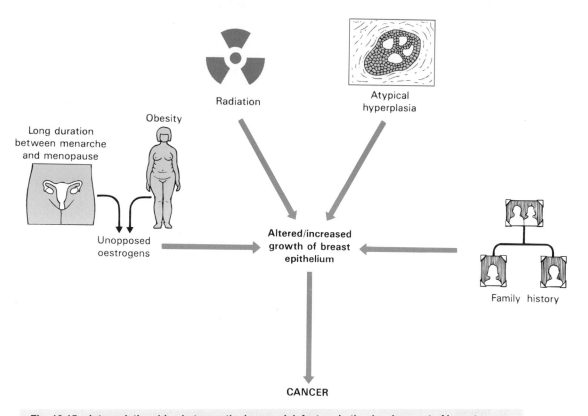

Fig. 18.15   Inter-relationships between the known risk factors in the development of breast cancer

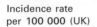

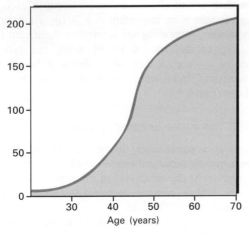

Incidence rate
per 100 000 (UK)

Age (years)

Fig. 18.16   The incidence of breast cancer in the UK related to age

There is a marked increase between the ages of 40 and 50, but the highest incidence is in those aged 60–70 years.

ing breast cancer. However, among parous women protection is related to early age for the first full-term pregnancy. If the first birth is delayed to the mid or late thirties, the woman is at a greater risk of developing breast cancer than is a nulliparous woman.

Weight and diet

For women of above average weight but below 50 years of age there is little or no increased risk of developing breast cancer. However, women aged 60 or over whose weight is increased have a higher cancer risk. Diet, obviously, can be a determinant for weight. In rodents, a high-fat diet increases the incidence of breast tumours, and international breast cancer incidence rates correlate with the consumption of fat. Although these observations suggest that a high-fat diet may be a risk factor, the evidence is not as clear as it is for weight.

Family history and genetic factors

Breast cancer is common, thus a history of a relative having breast cancer can be found in at least 10% of new cases. However, a proportion of these will be sporadic cancers and not due to familial (inherited genetic) factors. The risk of developing breast cancer is increased in first-degree relatives (e.g. sister, daughter) of breast cancer cases, particularly if that

person is pre-menopausal. For example, the risk increases to nine-fold for first-degree relatives of pre-menopausal women with bilateral breast cancer. Up to five-fold increases in risk have been found for women with multiple first-degree relatives with breast cancer.

There are rare familial syndromes such as Li–Fraumeni, in which there is an association between sarcomas, brain tumours and breast cancer at a young age. This is linked in some families to abnormalities of the p53 gene. Approximately 4% of breast cancers are associated with a very strong family history and in certain families there is breast and ovarian cancer. A gene on the long arm of chromosome 17 (BRCA1) is responsible for almost all families with susceptibility to female breast and ovarian cancer. It is a tumour suppressor gene. Another susceptibility gene, BRCA2, located on chromosome 13q12–13, is linked to families with early onset breast cancer and there are likely to be yet more genes that confer susceptibility. It must be remembered that this explains only a small proportion of breast cancers.

Geographic variation

There is a marked variation in breast cancer rates between different countries. The highest rates are in North America, North-west Europe, Australia and New Zealand, with the lowest in South-East Asia and Africa. Several factors probably contribute to this difference: age at menarche, age at first full-term pregnancy, age at menopause and post-menopausal weight. The length of time between age at menarche and first pregnancy may be quite short in some of these low-incidence countries.

Atypical hyperplasia

Women with benign breast disease whose breast biopsies show atypical epithelial hyperplasia have a definite increased risk of developing breast cancer. Ordinary epithelial hyperplasia is associated with a slightly increased risk. The risk is augmented by a family history of breast cancer.

Aetiological mechanisms

- ▶ Overexposure to oestrogens and underexposure to progesterone important
- ▶ No definite relationship to oral contraceptives
- ▶ Some tumours contain receptors for oestrogen and progesterone and respond to hormone manipulation
- ▶ No good evidence for viral involvement

Hormones

The association of breast cancer risk with menarche, menopause and first full-term pregnancy indicates that hormones must have some role in the development of carcinomas, but they are much more likely to be promoters than initiators.

Oestrogen activity appears to be important, with overexposure to oestrogens and underexposure to progesterone being significant. Early menarche and late menopause will result in a higher number of menstrual cycles, with repeated surges of oestrogen having a stimulatory effect on breast epithelium. The beneficial effect of early full-term pregnancy could be due to the high concentrations of progesterone and/or prolactin protecting the breast cells against oestrogens in the long term. The risks associated with obesity may be partly due to the ability of fat cells to synthesise oestrogens, or to altered levels of sex hormone-binding protein levels.

Oral contraceptives

Contraceptive preparations consisting of a low oestrogen-to-progesterone ratio are currently considered safe and may even be protective. One report has suggested a higher incidence in young women taking oral contraceptives since just after the menarche. High-oestrogen pills have been linked with an increased risk of endometrial cancer and, possibly, breast cancer.

Hormone receptors

Hormones have an effect on cells only after interacting with specific receptors present on or in their target cells. The sex steroid, oestrogen, interacts with a nuclear receptor. Subsequent interaction with DNA results in the formation of differentiation- and proliferation-associated factors. Prolactin and other polypeptides interact with receptors on the cell surface (Fig. 18.17).

Oestrogen receptors can be detected in varying amounts in about 70% of breast cancers. The progesterone receptor, which can normally only be formed when the oestrogen receptor is present and active, is present in about 35% of tumours, and women whose tumours contain both types of receptors are more likely to respond to some form of hormone manipulation therapy. This suggests that hormones are important in the growth and maintenance of these carcinomas.

Viruses

In mice there is evidence of a tumorigenic virus transmitted via milk (the Bittner factor). However,

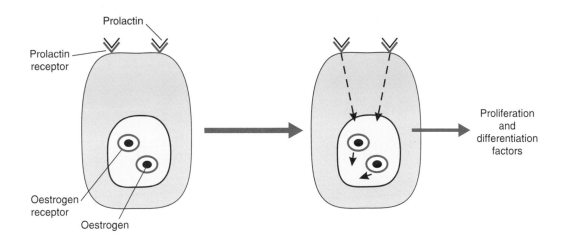

A. Hormones pass from the bloodstream and interact either with membrane receptors (prolactin) or nuclear receptors (oestrogen)

B. The hormone-receptor interactions result in activation of DNA response elements with the resulting production of differentiation and proliferation factors

Fig. 18.17   Hormone-responsive breast epithelium

no such clear-cut association has been found for human breast cancer.

Non-invasive carcinomas

> ▶ Tumour is confined to ducts (ductal carcinoma in situ) or acini (lobular carcinoma in situ)
> ▶ Ductal carcinoma in situ carcinoma is unilateral, in pre- and post-menopausal women, and has several forms
> ▶ Lobular carcinoma in situ carcinoma occurs in pre-menopausal women, has no clinical features, is often bilateral, and can be multifocal

Virtually all breast carcinomas are *adenocarcinomas* derived from the epithelial cells of the ducts or glands.

The term 'non-invasive' means that the malignant cells are confined to either the ducts or the acini of the lobules, with no evidence of penetration of the tumour cells through the basement membranes around these two types of structures into the surrounding fibrous tissue. There are two forms of non-invasive carcinoma:

- ductal carcinoma in situ
- lobular carcinoma in situ.

Ductal carcinoma in situ

Ductal carcinoma in situ can occur in both pre- and post-menopausal women, usually in the 40–60-year age group. It can present as a palpable mass, especially if extensive and associated with fibrosis. If the larger ducts are involved, presentation can be as a nipple discharge, or as Paget's disease of the nipple. The disease can be found incidentally in surgical biopsies or detected by mammography screening. Pure ductal carcinoma in situ accounts for about 5% of breast carcinomas which present clinically.

The size of the area involved in the breast can range from 10–80 mm in length. It is usually unifocal, being confined within one quadrant of the breast, although multicentricity can occur with larger lesions. Bilateral disease is uncommon. The macroscopic appearances depend on the type of ductal carcinoma in situ. If it is *comedo carcinoma*, creamy necrotic material exudes from the cut surface of the breast, rather similar in appearance to comedones. Other types have less characteristic appearances.

Histologically, the changes are to be found in the small and medium-sized ducts, although, in older women, the larger ducts tend to be involved. Several different patterns can be seen, but all the ducts involved contain cells which show cytoplasmic and nuclear pleomorphism to varying degrees. Mitotic figures may be frequent and can be abnormal. The ducts may be completely filled with cells (solid type), or have central necrosis (comedo type; Fig. 18.18) which may calcify, rendering the lesion mammographically detectable. The cribriform pattern of ductal carcinoma in situ has numerous gland-like structures within the sheets of cells. Ductal carcinoma in situ can spread along the duct system or into the lobules.

Most cases of ductal carcinoma in situ have been treated by mastectomy, so it is difficult to know the fate of these lesions if left. Estimates of residual car-

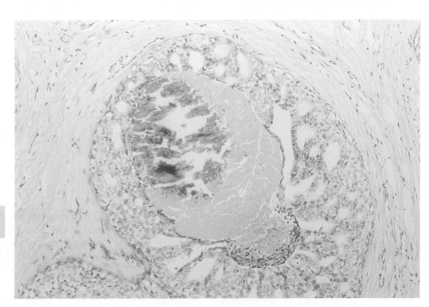

Fig. 18.18 Ductal carcinoma in situ

The duct is filled with cells. There is a central necrotic area which has calcified and would show on a mammogram. The basement membrane is intact.

cinoma changing from non-invasive to invasive range from one-third to one-half, based on studies where only local excision has been performed.

Lobular carcinoma in situ

Lobular carcinoma in situ (intralobular carcinoma) occurs predominantly in pre-menopausal women. If it is found after the menopause it is usually associated with an infiltrating tumour. Lobular carcinoma in situ accounts for about 6% of all breast carcinomas. A major problem is that it does not present as a palpable lump and is usually found in biopsies removed because of cysts or other palpable benign lesions. A further important clinical feature is that it is often multifocal within the one breast and is frequently bilateral. Not surprisingly, there are no specific macroscopic features.

Histologically, the changes are found in the acini — hence the term, 'lobular' — although they may extend into extralobular ducts and replace ductal epithelium (Fig. 18.19). Within the acini, the normal cells are replaced by relatively uniform cells with clear cytoplasm that appear loose and non-cohesive. The overall size of the acini increases, but the lobular shape is retained. Unlike the situation in ductal carcinoma in situ, necrosis is unusual.

About one-quarter to one-third of all patients with lobular carcinoma in situ who are treated by biopsy alone will go on to develop an invasive carcinoma. This may occur in either or both breasts and there may be a long time interval.

Invasive carcinomas

> ▶ Occur in pre- and post-menopausal women
> ▶ Most are invasive duct type
> ▶ Infiltrating lobular carcinomas can be multifocal
> ▶ Less common types include mucinous, medullary, papillary and tubular carcinomas

An 'invasive' tumour is one whose cells have broken through the basement membrane around the breast structure in which they have arisen, and spread into the surrounding tissue. Invasive carcinomas are categorised into different histological types, but the name given to them does not always mean that the tumour arises only from that site; for example, invasive duct or ductal carcinomas and invasive lobular carcinomas may both arise from the cells at the junction of the extralobular and intralobular duct. If an invasive tumour develops in a patient with previous intralobular carcinomas it can be ductal in morphology.

The histological types of invasive carcinoma and their relative incidence for palpable tumours are:

- invasive ductal (85%)
- invasive lobular (10%)
- mucinous (2%)
- tubular (2%)
- medullary (<1%)
- papillary (<1%)
- others (<1%)

There is a higher frequency of tubular carcinoma in mammographically detected tumours.

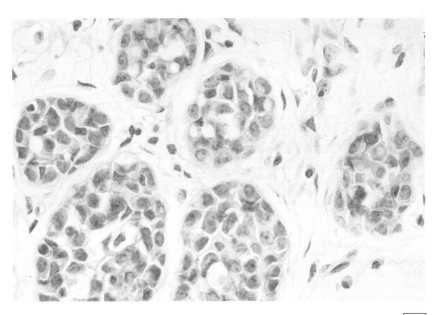

Fig. 18.19   Lobular carcinoma in situ

A breast lobule in which the acini are expanded. There is complete loss of the lumen and of the two-cell layer.

Carcinomas vary in size from less than 10 mm in diameter to over 80 mm, but are often 20–30 mm at presentation. Clinically, they are firm on palpation and may show evidence of tethering to the overlying skin or underlying muscle. The skin also shows *peau d'orange*, dimpling due to lymphatic permeation. The nipple may be retracted due to tethering and contraction of the intramammary ligaments.

Gross features

The macroscopic appearance of the tumours tends to depend on the amount or type of stroma within the carcinoma. It is this which gave rise to the terms previously applied to tumours: scirrhous, medullary (or encephaloid) and mucinous (or colloid).

The term *scirrhous* implies that there is a prominent fibrous tissue reaction, usually in the central part of the tumour. This results in the carcinoma having a dense white appearance, which grates when cut. Yellow streaks may be seen; these are due to the presence of elastic tissue within the tumour. Carcinomas with a prominent stromal reaction usually have irregular edges, extending into the adjacent fat or breast parenchyma (Fig. 18.20).

Medullary (brain-like) tumours are very cellular with little stroma. The edges of the carcinoma are often more rounded and discrete than those of the scirrhous tumours (Fig. 18.21). Necrosis is common. When palpated the tumours feel much softer.

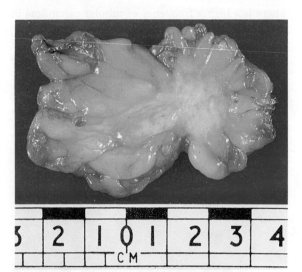

Fig. 18.20 Invasive carcinoma of breast

Excised breast tissue, consisting mainly of fat, contains an irregular white area which has caused contraction of the surrounding fat. The white tissue represents the fibrous (scirrhous) reaction within this carcinoma.

Mucinous carcinomas have a predominance of mucin, or jelly-like, material within them. They usually have a well-defined edge.

Some of the changes that occur within carcinomas explain their clinical features, for example skin and nipple retraction due to the fibrous reaction.

Invasive ductal carcinomas

Invasive duct or ductal carcinomas comprise the majority (up to 85%) of infiltrating breast carcinomas. Macroscopically, they can usually have a scirrhous consistency. The size of the tumours varies between patients. They can occur in both pre- and post-menopausal women.

Histologically, the tumour cells are arranged in groups, cords and gland-like structures. Quite marked variations can be seen between different carcinomas even though they are of the same type (Fig. 18.22). For example, the size of the solid groups of cells can be variable, and ductal carcinoma in situ is often present. The amount of stroma between the tumour cells can also vary, but in those carcinomas in which it is prominent it is most marked at the centre, with the periphery being more cellullar. Collections of elastic tissue (elastosis) around ducts or within the stroma are common in tumours with a scirrhous reaction.

The degree of differentiation of the tumour is based on the extent to which it resembles non-tumorous breast: whether the cells are in a gland-like pattern or as solid sheets; the degree of nuclear pleomorphism; and the number of mitotic figures present. A well-differentiated infiltrating duct carcinoma tends to behave less aggressively than a poorly-differentiated tumour, which is composed of sheets of pleomorphic cells with large numbers of mitotic figures.

Invasive lobular carcinomas

While lobular carcinoma in situ usually occurs in pre-menopausal women, the infiltrating lesion can also occur in post-menopausal women. In the United Kingdom, invasive lobular carcinomas constitute about 10% of invasive breast carcinomas, but the incidence may vary in other parts of the world.

Invasive lobular carcinomas have abundant fibrous stroma, so that macroscopically they are always scirrhous. While invasive ductal carcinomas usually form at one focus in the breast, invasive lobular carcinomas can be multifocal throughout the breast.

Histologically the cells are small and uniform and are dispersed singly, or in columns one cell wide ('Indian files'; Fig. 18.23), in a dense stroma. Elastosis

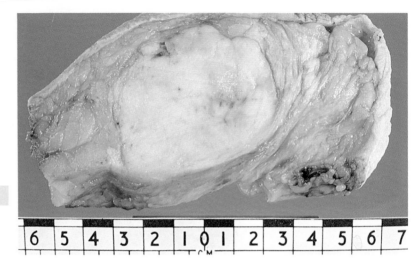

Fig. 18.21   Medullary carcinoma

Breast tissue containing a 60 mm diameter carcinoma with a rounded edge, and no evidence of a fibrous reaction.

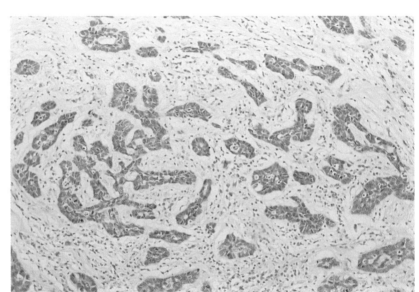

Fig. 18.22   Invasive ductal carcinoma

The lesion is composed of irregular solid groups of cells in a dense fibrous stroma, with an associated lymphocytic infiltrate.

can be present. The cells infiltrate around pre-existing breast ducts and acini, rather than destroying them as occurs with invasive duct carcinomas. This method of infiltration may account for the occasional multifocal nature of the tumours, although this could also be due to pre-existing multifocal lobular carcinoma in situ. The cells in some carcinomas may appear signet-ring in shape due to the accumulation of mucin within an intracytoplasmic acinus, displacing the nucleus to one side. Residual lobular carcinoma in situ can usually be found in the invasive tumours.

Mucinous carcinomas

Mucinous carcinomas (also known as colloid, mucoid and gelatinous carcinomas) usually arise in post-menopausal women and comprise 2–3% of invasive carcinomas.

Macroscopically, the tumours are well circumscribed and have a soft, grey, gelatinous cut surface. They vary in size from 10–50 mm in diameter. Since there is no dense stroma and the edges are rounded, these tumours do not cause retraction of the nipple or tethering of the skin.

These carcinomas comprise small nests and cords of tumour cells, which show little pleomorphism, embedded in large amounts of mucin (Fig. 18.24). The latter is composed of neutral or weakly acidic glycoproteins, which are secreted by the tumour cells and are different from the proteoglycans of the stroma.

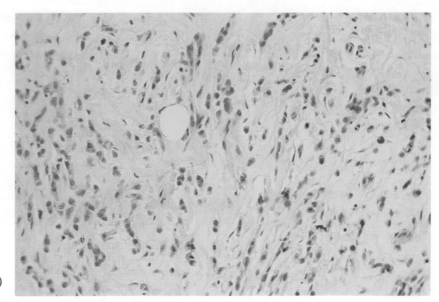

Fig. 18.23 Infiltrating lobular carcinoma

Strands of single cells (Indian file) invade fibrous stroma.

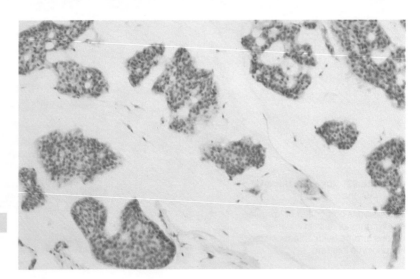

Fig. 18.24 Mucinous carcinoma

Small solid and tubular groups of cells lie in pools of mucin, or jelly-like material.

The survival of women with mucinous carcinomas is better than that of those having invasive duct or lobular carcinomas.

Tubular carcinomas

As the name implies, tubular carcinomas are well-differentiated carcinomas composed of cells arranged as tubules. They are usually small lesions, less than 10 mm in diameter, and are firm, gritty tumours with irregular outlines. Tubular carcinomas form 1–2% of invasive carcinomas but constitute a higher proportion of screen-detected tumours.

Histologically, they are composed of well-formed tubular structures, the cells of which show little pleomorphism or mitotic activity. The stroma is dense, often with elastosis (Fig. 18.25).

Patients with tubular carcinomas do extremely well—better than those with well-differentiated invasive duct carcinomas.

Medullary carcinoma

The incidence of medullary carcinomas is difficult to assess since not all the criteria for diagnosis have been strictly adhered to in some studies; hence figures have ranged from very rare to 5%. These tumours probably

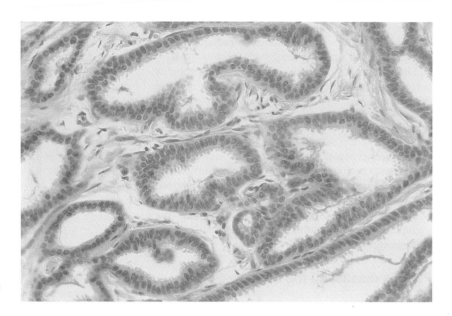

Fig. 18.25 Tubular carcinoma

Tubular structures lie in a fibrous stroma.

form less than 1% of invasive carcinomas, and usually occur in post-menopausal women.

Medullary carcinomas are circumscribed and often large with areas of necrosis. Histologically, they are composed of large tracts of confluent cells with little stroma in between them. The cells show quite marked nuclear pleomorphism, and mitotic figures are frequent. There is never evidence of gland formation. These cytological appearances put them into the 'poorly-differentiated' category. Around the islands of tumour cells there is a prominent lymphocytic infiltrate, predominantly T-lymphocytes, with macrophages (Fig. 18.26).

Despite the aggressive cytological features of these tumours, the patients have a significantly better 10-year survival than women with invasive duct carcinomas. It may be that the lymphocytic and macrophage infiltrate has a beneficial effect, and this has stimulated much research into the immunological responses to tumours generally.

Papillary carcinoma

Papillary carcinomas are rare tumours which occur in post-menopausal women. They are usually circumscribed and can be focally necrotic, with little

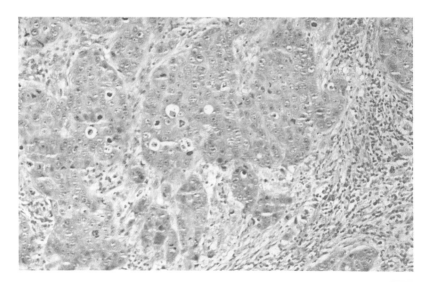

Fig. 18.26 Medullary carcinoma

Large groups of irregularly shaped tumour cells are surrounded by an infiltrate of lymphocytes.

stromal reaction. The tumours are in the form of papillary structures, and areas of intraductal papillary growths are usually found.

The prognosis of these carcinomas is probably better than that of the much more common invasive duct carcinoma.

Other types

Much rarer types of breast carcinoma include: adenoid cystic carcinomas; secretory carcinomas, which occur predominantly in juveniles; apocrine carcinomas, which are composed of cells with abundant eosinophilic cytoplasm; and carcinomas showing metaplasia, e.g. squamous, spindle cell, cartilaginous and osseous features.

Paget's disease of the nipple

> ▶ Erosion of the nipple clinically resembling eczema
> ▶ Associated with underlying ductal carcinoma in situ or invasive carcinoma

Paget's disease of the nipple was first described by Sir James Paget in 1874. Clinically, there is roughening, reddening and slight ulceration of the nipple, similar to the skin changes of eczema. Recognition is important, since it is associated with an underlying carcinoma, mainly in the subareolar region. Paget's disease of the nipple occurs with about 2% of all breast carcinomas, and is associated with a higher frequency of multicentric breast carcinomas.

Within the epidermis of the nipple, large, pale-staining malignant cells can be seen histologically and these cause the changes seen clinically. The malignant cells are derived from the adjacent breast carcinomas. A direct connection may not be seen. The relationship between Paget's disease of the nipple and an underlying carcinoma is shown in Figure 18.27.

Spread of breast carcinomas

> ▶ Directly into skin and muscle
> ▶ Via lymphatics to axillary and other local lymph nodes
> ▶ Via blood stream to lungs, bone, liver and brain
> ▶ May be considerable delay before metastasis occurs

Breast carcinomas can infiltrate locally (direct spread) or metastasise to more distant sites via lymphatics and the blood stream and to pleura (Fig. 18.28).

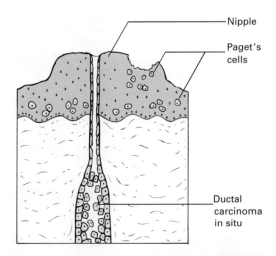

Nipple

Paget's cells

Ductal carcinoma in situ

Fig. 18.27 Relationship between Paget's disease of the nipple and underlying ductal carcinoma in situ

Note the epidermis infiltrated by individual tumour (Paget's) cells.

Direct spread. Local infiltration (direct spread) into the underlying muscles and the overlying skin can be detected clinically, the latter because of ulceration or tethering.

Via lymphatics. Permeation of the lymphatic channels of the skin results in the clinical sign of *peau d'orange.* The axillary lymph nodes are the commonest initial site of metastasis via lymphatics, and between 40 and 50% of women with breast carcinoma will have axillary lymph node metastases at the time of presentation. It is important that the lymph nodes are examined histologically, since clinical palpation is not always reliable. Metastasis to intramammary, supraclavicular and tracheobronchial lymph nodes also occurs.

Via blood stream. Blood-borne metastasis most frequently involves the lungs and bones, but the liver, adrenals and brain are also common sites. The pleura on the same side as the breast carcinoma can be a site of metastasis, causing an effusion.

Invasive lobular carcinomas can metastasise to more unusual sites, and this may be due to their single-cell method of spread as seen within the breast.

Extensive infiltration of bone marrow can cause leukoerythroblastic anaemia. Destruction of bone can result in hypercalcaemia, with renal complications.

Breast carcinomas exhibit quite marked variation in the length of time between presentation of the primary carcinoma and the appearance of recurrent/ metastatic

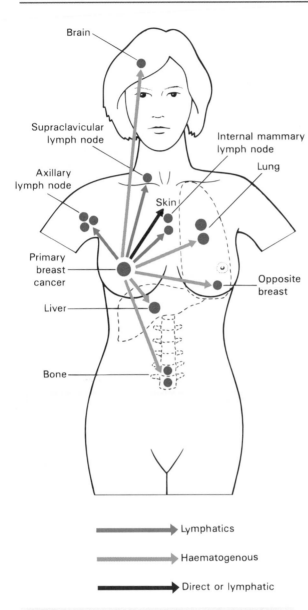

Brain

Supraclavicular
lymph node

Axillary
lymph node

Internal mammary
lymph node

Lung

Skin

Primary
breast
cancer

Opposite
breast

Liver

Bone

→ Lymphatics

→ Haematogenous

→ Direct or lymphatic

Fig. 18.28   The common sites of metastasis from breast carcinoma via the lymphatic system or blood stream

site, causing them to alter their behaviour, and/or to changes in the host response to the tumour.

Prognostic factors

> ▶ These can be gross and histological features — type, grade, size
> ▶ Spread, local to lymph nodes or distant
> ▶ Behavioural characteristics of carcinomas, such as growth rates and hormone receptor status

Some women have carcinomas for several years before seeking medical help; in this time the tumour may ulcerate into the skin and become large. However, despite the horrifying features the tumour may present, such patients may survive for many years after treatment. Other women seek medical help promptly after palpating a lump but die of the disease within a short time. There are thus obviously quite marked differences between individual breast carcinomas and in the host response of patients to them.

Several factors have been identified which may help to predict how an individual carcinoma will behave, and may help in planning therapy. However, despite the great effort expended in this area, the only major changes made clinically have been in lengthening the disease-free interval (time before development of recurrence/metastasis) rather than in improving patient survival.

Type of carcinoma

Medullary, mucinous, tubular and, possibly, invasive lobular carcinomas generally behave less aggressively than other types, but these constitute the minority of types so that this knowledge is of value to only a few patients.

Histological differentiation

As described above, tumours can be graded for their degree of differentiation. Patients whose tumours are well differentiated (grade 1), showing greater resemblance to non-malignant breast, do better, while those whose tumours are poorly differentiated (grade 3) do worse; however, prediction of how the group with moderately-differentiated carcinomas will do is more difficult.

Stage

When a woman presents with a breast carcinoma,

disease. Some breast carcinomas never recur; in some patients reappearance of the disease may not be until as much as 20 years after the original excision, while for others it can be within 2–5 years. Tumour can recur at the site of the original excision and/or as distant metastases. The mechanisms by which a metastasis becomes clinically apparent after a long time interval are not known. They may relate to changes in tumour cells which have been lying dormant at that

staging is undertaken so as to assess the absence or presence and extent of spread both locally and distantly. The management of the patient will depend on the stage of the disease. The two main systems used are the International Classification of Staging and the TNM (Tumour, Node, Metastasis) system (Table 18.2 and Fig. 18.21).

If there is evidence of metastatic spread to axillary lymph nodes when the patient presents with the primary carcinoma, both the 5- and 10-year survival figures are worse than in those with no evidence of metastasis. The outlook for the patient is also worse if there is evidence of more distant spread.

Oestrogen receptors

The presence of oestrogen receptors within a carcinoma indicates that the tumour cells have a higher degree of functional differentiation. It is thus not surprising that women whose tumours are oestrogen-receptor-positive have better 5- and 10-year sur-

vival figures than those whose carcinomas are oestrogen-receptor-negative and they are more likely to benefit from tamoxifen, an oestrogen receptor antagonist.

Growth kinetics

The growth activity of carcinomas can be measured by several methods; that of breast carcinomas may be low, medium or high. Tumours with lower cell growth rates tend to behave better clinically. It must

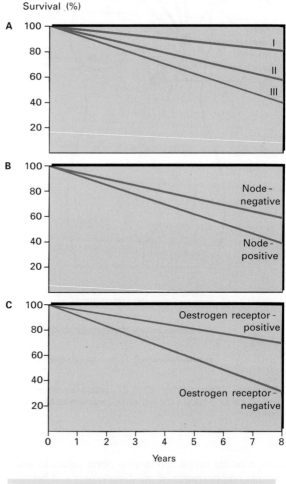

Fig. 18.29 Relationship of various prognostic factors with survival of patients up to 8 years after initial surgery

A. Degree of tumour differentiation (I = well differentiated; II = moderately differentiated; III = poorly differentiated).
B. Presence or absence of lymph node metastasis.
C. Presence or absence of oestrogen receptors within the tumour.

Table 18.2 The main staging systems used to assess the extent of spread of breast carcinomas	
Stage	Extent of spread
International classification	
I	Lump with slight tethering to skin, but node-negative
II	Lump with lymph node metastasis or skin tethering
III	Tumour which is extensively adherent to skin and/or underlying muscles, or ulcerating or lymph nodes are fixed
IV	Distant metastases
TNM	
T_1	Tumour 20 mm or less; no fixation or nipple retraction. Includes Paget's disease
T_2	Tumour 20–50 mm, or less than 20 mm but with tethering
T_3	Tumour greater than 50 mm but less than 100 mm; or less than 50 mm but with infiltration, ulceration or fixation
T_4	Any tumour with ulceration or infiltration wide of it, or chest wall fixation, or greater than 100 mm in diameter
N_0	Node-negative
N_1	Axillary nodes mobile
N_2	Axillary nodes fixed
N_3	Supraclavicular nodes or oedema of arm
M_0	No distant metastases
M_1	Distant metastases

be remembered that tumours with a high rate of division may also have a high cell death rate by apoptosis, and that not all cell divisions result in doubling of the population since the division may be abnormal.

Examples of the effects some of these prognostic factors may have on survival are shown in Figure 18.29.

Breast carcinomas in men

About 1% of breast carcinomas occur in males, but the incidence varies throughout the world. The tumour is rare in young men. There is an increased risk in patients with Klinefelter's syndrome, but no other risk factors have been identified.

The tumour usually presents as a lump, but there can be nipple discharge or retraction. Paget's disease is relatively commoner in men, probably because of the small size of the male breast.

Ductal carcinoma in situ and all types of invasive carcinoma can occur, although lobular carcinoma in situ has not been reported. The prognosis in males is similar to that in females, and is affected by such fac-

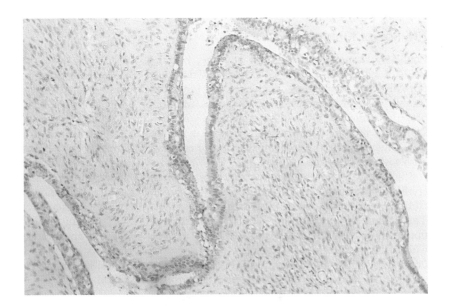

Fig. 18.30 Phyllodes tumour

The stroma is cellular and it is forming club-like fingers covered with epithelium.

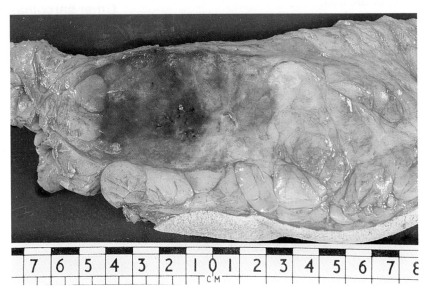

Fig. 18.31 Angiosarcoma of the breast

There is a large haemorrhagic tumour in the breast.

tors as lymph node status and size. Oestrogen receptors can be detected in male breast carcinomas.

OTHER TUMOURS

> ▶ Phyllodes tumours used to be called 'giant fibroadenoma' and 'cystosarcoma phyllodes'
> ▶ The stroma of phyllodes tumours is the part which becomes aggressive if the tumours recur
> ▶ Cutaneous angiosarcomas can occur after radical mastectomy, but can arise spontaneously in younger women.

Phyllodes tumours

Phyllodes tumours can occur at any age, but the median age is 45 years. This is older than for fibroadenoma and the incidence of phyllodes tumours is considerably lower. Phyllodes tumours present clinically as a discrete lump. Macroscopically, they are circumscribed and vary in size up to as much as 450 mm in diameter. They may have both soft and firm areas.

Phyllodes tumours have two characteristic parts, epithelium and stroma. The epithelium covers large, club-like projections which push into cystic spaces. The stroma is much more cellular than that of fibroadenomas (Fig. 18.30) and can vary in type within the same tumour. The cells may resemble fibroblasts, or they may show marked pleomorphism with mitotic figures. In some tumours, the stromal changes are so marked that they have the appearances of sarcomas.

Recurrence is a major problem with phyllodes tumours. The risk of recurrence is less if the tumours are small, with a low mitotic rate and minimal cellular atypia, and have a rounded rather than an infiltrative edge. With each recurrence, the stroma of the tumour tends to become more atypical with a higher mitotic rate. The chance of metastasis then increases, and this is usually via the blood stream to

lung and bones; lymph node involvement is rare. In one series of cases, recurrence occurred in 30% of cases and 16% died of metastatic disease; however, these patients were a pre-selected group whose original tumours had a more aggressive-looking stroma.

Angiosarcomas

Angiosarcomas are rare tumours which can occur at any time from adolescence to old age but are commoner in young women. Although most cases occur spontaneously, angiosarcomas can arise in irradiated mastectomy scars and in lymphoedematous arms after radical mastectomy for breast cancer (Stewart–Treves syndrome).

Angiosarcomas can present as a lump, or cause a diffuse enlargement of the breast. Discoloration of the overlying skin can be seen in some cases. Macroscopically, they can be haemorrhagic or appear as ill-defined areas of induration (Fig. 18.31).

Histologically, the tumours consist of numerous vascular channels which infiltrate into fat and around normal breast structures. The channels are lined by endothelial cells which have hyperchromatic nuclei. Papillary areas can be present and, in the more undifferentiated tumours, there can be sheets of large, pleomorphic endothelial cells with little evidence of vascular channels.

The clinical outcome tends to parallel the histological appearances. Those tumours with well-formed vascular spaces and little atypia of the endothelium are less aggressive. Metastasis is by the blood stream to lungs, bone, liver and brain.

Other sarcomas

Fibrosarcoma, liposarcoma and leiomyosarcoma can all occur in the breast but are rare.

Lymphomas

Lymphomas may be primary, but are more usually secondary to disease elsewhere in the body.

FURTHER READING

Breast Cancer Screening Report to Health Ministers of England, Wales, Scotland and Northern Ireland 1986 HMSO, London
Harris J R, Hellman S, Henderson I C, Kinne D W, 1991 Breast diseases, 2nd edn. J B Lippincott, Philadelphia

Page D L, Anderson T J, 1987 Diagnostic histopathology of the breast. Churchill Livingstone, Edinburgh
Sloane J P 1985 Biopsy pathology of the breast. Chapman and Hall Medical, London

19

Female genital tract

Diseases of the female genital tract include inflammation, neoplasia, hormonal disturbances and complications of pregnancy. The commonest disorders are discussed here on a topographical basis.

NORMAL DEVELOPMENT

Female sexual development

Female development does not require the presence of a gonad, and the ovary plays no part in primary sexual development. This means that a neuter embryo will always develop along female lines. The testis-determining factor is the SRY gene carried in the sex-determining region of the Y chromosome. The indifferent gonad develops into an ovary when no Y chromosome is present. Disorders of female sexual development are listed in Table 19.1.

Embryological development

Germ cells arise in the wall of the yolk sac, and migrate to the region of the coelomic germinal epithelium. In the sixth week cords of cells appear within the indifferent gonad, but it is not until after the seventh week that ovarian differentiation is apparent and by 14 weeks these cell cords surround the primordial follicles.

The paired paramesonephric Müllerian ducts arise as an invagination of the coelomic epithelium of the mesonephric ridge lateral to the mesonephric duct. The paramesonephric duct follows the mesonephric duct. Near the cloaca, the paramesonephric ducts cross from the lateral to the medial side of the mesonephric ducts (Fig. 19.1A); together they carry with them some mesoderm from the side walls of the pelvis to create the transverse bar which helps to form the septum dividing the rectum from the urogenital sinus.

At the 30 mm stage (eight weeks), fusion of the paramesonephric ducts creates the utero-vaginal canal which ultimately forms the uterus and proximal part of the vagina (Fig. 19.1B); the unfused parts form the uterine tubes. The trans-pelvic bar, which is a continuation of the mesonephric mesentery, forms the broad ligament; the ovary, projecting medially from the mesonephric ridge in the early stage, comes to lie posterior to the broad ligament. The inferior free end of the fused paramesonephric ducts (utero-vaginal canal) is still solid, and the sino-vaginal bulbs grow out from the posterior wall of the urogenital sinus to fuse with it and, later, give rise to the lower part of the vagina. The hymen occupies the position where the sino-vaginal bulb and urogenital sinus meet. The gonads are at first elongated and lie in the long axis of the embryo. Later, each gonad assumes a transverse lie. The gubernaculum is formed in the inguinal fold as a fibromuscular band which burrows from the gonad to gain attachment to the genital swelling; thus the caudal pole of the gonad becomes relatively fixed. The gubernaculum persists as the round ligament of the uterus. The ovaries retain attachment to the posterior aspect of the broad ligament. The genital swellings form the labia majora, the genital folds form the labia minora, and the genital tubercle forms the clitoris.

Table 19.1 Abnormalities of female sexual development		
Sex chromosomes	Gonads	Possible abnormalities
Normal XX	Bilateral normal ovaries	Congenital adrenal hyperplasia Maternal androgen or progestagen administration in pregnancy Maternal virilising tumour in pregnancy
Normal XX or XY	Abnormal (streak gonads)* Ovaries (XY) or testes (XX)*	Gonadal dysgenesis Inappropriate gonads for chromosomes
Abnormal		Turner's syndrome Mixed gonadal dysgenesis True hermaphroditism
*Diagnosis of a specific type of intersex requires histological confirmation of gonadal status; ovotestis can look macroscopically exactly like a normal ovary, or the patient could have one macroscopically normal testis on one side and an ovary on the other.		

VULVA

A variety of skin disorders, including inflammatory lesions, may manifest themselves in the vulva. Candidal infection may occur, particularly in diabetics. These disorders are discussed in Chapter 24. Vulval condylomata (viral warts) are discussed below.

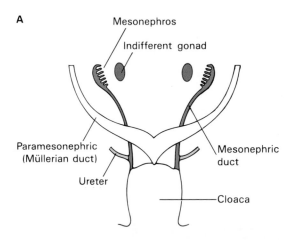

A

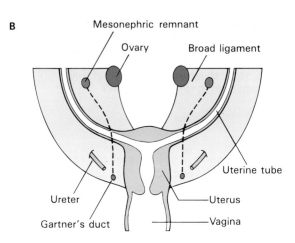

B

Fig. 19.1   Development of the female genital tract

A. Frontal view of the posterior wall of seven-week embryo showing the mesonephric and paramesonephric ducts during the indifferent stage of development. **B.** Female genital tract in a newborn infant.

Pathological basis of signs and symptoms in the female genital tract

Sign or symptom	Pathological basis
Vaginal bleeding	
• in pregnancy	Haemorrhage from placenta (e.g. placenta praevia), placental bed (e.g. miscarriage) or decidua (e.g. ectopic pregnancy)
• post-coital	Haemorrhage from lesion on cervix (e.g. carcinoma)
• post-menopausal	Haemorrhage from uterine lesion (e.g. polyp, carcinoma)
Abnormal menstruation (timing or volume of loss)	Psychological disturbance Hormonal dysfunction Defects in local haemostasis Fibroids
Pain	Pathological distension or rupture (e.g. tubal ectopic pregnancy) Muscular spasm (e.g. uterine contractions) Ischaemia or inflammation (e.g. ovarian torsion) Menstrual pain due to adenomyosis
Abdominal distension	Ascites (e.g. peritoneal involvement by ovarian carcinoma) Uterine enlargement (e.g. pregnancy) Ovarian cyst

Herpes virus infection

Sexually transmitted herpes virus infection is usually due to Herpes simplex type 2, and produces painful ulceration of the vulval skin. Histologically, intra-epithelial blisters are seen, accompanied by specific cytopathic effects characterised by intranuclear viral inclusions and eosinophilic cytoplasmic swelling.

Cysts and tumours

Benign cysts and tumours of the skin may be seen in the vulva. Two benign tumours are worthy of comment because of their distinct histological appearance: papillary hidradenoma and granular cell tumour.

Papillary hidradenoma

Papillary hidradenoma is a benign skin adnexal tumour. It presents as a localised lump, and is composed of interlacing papillae lined with epithelium.

Granular cell tumour

Granular cell tumour is uncommon and presents as a well-circumscribed vulval lump. It is composed of uniform large cells with pink granular cytoplasm. The histogenesis of this tumour remains controversial.

Bartholin's glands

Bartholin's glands are common sites of cysts and of abscesses secondary to infection of a cyst. Bartholin's gland adenoma is uncommon, and adenocarcinoma arising at this site is rare.

NON-NEOPLASTIC EPITHELIAL DISORDERS

The term 'non-neoplastic epithelial disorders' (Fig. 19.2), encompasses a group of vulval disorders of uncertain aetiology which affect all age groups, although predominantly peri- and postmenopausal women. In the past, these disorders have been given a confusing variety of clinical labels. They often appear clinically as 'leukoplakia', a term which refers to the white appearance of the skin and which should never be used in a pathological context. The clinical appearance of 'leukoplakia' is due to hyperkeratosis. In about 5% of cases there is a risk of superimposed neoplastic change developing, so that the presence or absence of cytological atypia (vulval intraepithelial neoplasia) in biopsies should always be reported. There are two basic types of non-neoplastic epithelial disorders of the vulva: squamous hyperplasia and lichen sclerosus; these may sometimes co-exist.

Squamous hyperplasia

Vulval squamous hyperplasia is characterised by hyperkeratosis, irregular thickening of the epidermal rete ridges, and chronic inflammation of the superficial dermis.

Lichen sclerosus

Lichen sclerosus, like hyperplasia, shows hyperker-

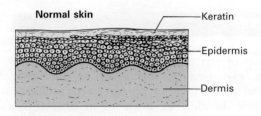

Normal skin

Keratin

Epidermis

Dermis

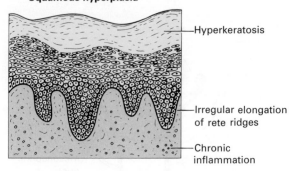

Squamous hyperplasia

Hyperkeratosis

Irregular elongation of rete ridges

Chronic inflammation

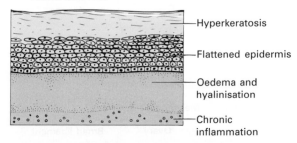

Lichen sclerosus

Hyperkeratosis

Flattened epidermis

Oedema and hyalinisation

Chronic inflammation

Fig. 19.2 Morphological features of vulval non-neoplastic epithelial disorders

atosis, but there is thinning of the epidermis with flattening of the rete ridges. The most characteristic feature is a broad band of oedema and hyalinised connective tissue in the superficial dermis. Beneath this, there may be mild chronic inflammation. Lichen sclerosus has a lower neoplastic potential than squamous hyperplasia.

NEOPLASTIC EPITHELIAL DISORDERS

Intraepithelial neoplasia

The term *intraepithelial neoplasia* refers to the spectrum of pre-invasive neoplastic change affecting the vulva. Its classification is the same as that of similar lesions in the cervix, although it may be incorrect to draw too close an analogy with the cervix as far as natural history is concerned. It is a condition that predominantly affects young women, and may be associated with human papillomavirus infection (see below). In severe cases, there may be extensive involvement of the perineum, including the peri-anal area. The incidence of malignant change occurring in these lesions is surprisingly low as compared to the cervix. There is a tendency for intraepithelial neoplasia to occur multifocally with synchronous or metachronous involvement of vulva, vagina and cervix.

Squamous carcinoma

Squamous carcinoma (Fig. 19.3) is a tumour predominantly affecting elderly women. It is often difficult to find evidence of associated intraepithelial neoplasia, suggesting that its aetiology and natural history differ from that of vulval neoplasia in young women. The appearances are those of squamous carcinoma in any site; thus the tumour may be well, moderately or poorly differentiated. The prognosis is determined by the size, depth of invasion and degree of histological differentiation of the tumour and the presence and extent of lymph node metastases, which predominantly affect the inguinal lymph nodes. The pathological criteria for describing early invasive disease are not clearly established

in the vulva. In contrast to squamous carcinoma of the cervix, even minimally invasive disease in the vulva is associated with a definite risk of local lymph node metastasis, though this risk seems to be negligible for carcinoma invading to a depth of less than 1 mm. Tumour thickness of greater than 5 mm and positive lymph nodes are associated with a poor prognosis.

Paget's disease

The rare occurrence of mucin-containing adenocarcinoma cells within the squamous epithelium of the vulva is analogous to Paget's disease of the breast (Ch.18). Paget's disease of the vulva tends to be chronic, with multiple recurrences. It may be indicative of an underlying invasive adenocarcinoma (in about 25% of cases), usually of skin adnexal origin although, unlike the equivalent breast lesion, this is not usual. Adenocarcinomatous differentiation within the squamous epithelium has been proposed as a possible explanation.

Other malignant tumours

Other malignant tumours of the vulva are rare. The most important of these are *basal cell carcinoma*, for which local excision is usually curative, and *malignant melanoma* which, as in other sites, generally has a poor prognosis.

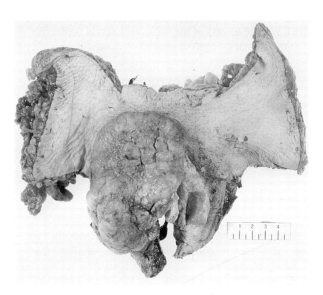

Fig. 19.3   Vulval squamous carcinoma

This large, fungating and invasive tumour is on the vulva of an elderly patient.

VAGINA AND CERVIX

The commonest diseases affecting the vagina and cervix are infections, many of which are transmitted venereally. Tumours and pre-neoplastic lesions of the cervix, of which squamous cell carcinoma is the most important, are associated with viral infection.

Infections

Vaginal infections are common and often transmitted venereally. The organisms of most importance are: *Gardnerella vaginalis*, *Neisseria gonorrhoeae*, *Candida albicans* and *Trichomonas vaginalis*.

Vaginal adenosis

The occurrence of glands within the subepithelial connective tissue of the vagina is uncommon, and is believed to be due to a defect in embryological development. The lining of these glands is usually a mucinous cuboidal epithelium which may undergo squamous metaplasia. Vaginal adenosis is particularly likely to occur in young females who have been exposed to diethylstilbestrol in utero. This synthetic oestrogenic agent was used in the 1950s in the treatment of threatened abortion (miscarriage) in the USA and, to a lesser extent, in the UK. Clear cell adenocarcinoma of the vagina may rarely complicate adenosis.

Vaginal intraepithelial neoplasia

Vaginal intraepithelial neoplasia is much less common than cervical intraepithelial neoplasia but the same diagnostic criteria are applied. The lesion may co-exist with similar lesions of the vulva and cervix (reflecting the multicentric origin of squamous neoplasia).

Vaginal squamous carcinoma

Vaginal squamous carcinoma is an uncommon tumour predominantly occurring in older women. Pathologically, the tumour resembles squamous carcinoma of the cervix but it has a propensity to local invasion and radical surgery may be necessary.

Cervicitis

Non-specific acute and/or chronic inflammation is common in the cervix, particularly in the presence of an intra-uterine contraceptive device, ectopy (see below) or prolapse.

Chlamydiae are obligate intracellular organisms containing DNA and RNA, and are larger than viruses. *Chlamydia trachomatis* is a common venereal infection which is often recognised by its persistence following treatment for gonorrhoea in males (post-gonococcal urethritis). Chlamydiae can be isolated from the cervices of about 50% of asymptomatic female partners of these infected males and from women with chronic cervicitis. Chlamydial infection may produce subepithelial reactive lymphoid follicles, a condition sometimes given the label of 'follicular cervicitis'.

Cervical polyps

Benign polyps of the cervix are common. They are composed of columnar mucus-secreting epithelium and oedematous stroma. Vessels may be prominent and there may be acute or chronic inflammation of varying severity. These polyps have no malignant potential.

Cervical microglandular hyperplasia

Cervical microglandular hyperplasia is a commonly seen complex glandular proliferation that may be confused with carcinoma. Small, tightly packed glands, lined by low columnar or cuboidal epithelium, may form polypoid projections into the endocervical canal. Accompanying acute inflammation and reserve cell hyperplasia (see below) are often seen. These changes are usually seen in pregnancy and in users of the oral contraceptive pill, where they are the result of high levels of progesterone. Microglandular hyperplasia may also rarely be seen in post-menopausal women. It appears to have no malignant potential.

CERVICAL SQUAMOUS NEOPLASIA

- ▶ Incidence associated with sexual intercourse (especially number of male partners)
- ▶ Human papillomavirus postulated as main causative factor
- ▶ Pre-invasive phase of intraepithelial neoplasia can be detected by cervical cytology

Aetiology

Squamous neoplasia of the cervix is associated with sexual activity; early age at first intercourse, frequency of intercourse and number of sexual partners are all risk factors. The sexual behaviour of the male partner is probably also of importance. There is probably no one single cause of cervical cancer or pre-cancer, but epidemiological evidence points to a sexually transmitted agent or agents. There is now compelling evidence that human papillomaviruses are implicated in the aetiology of cervical squamous neoplasia. Cigarette smoking is an independent risk factor: some contents of cigarette smoke, which can be detected in cervical mucus, may act as co-carcinogenic agents. The polycyclic aromatic hydrocarbons in cigarette smoke form damaging adducts with DNA; these have been demonstrated in cervical tissue at higher levels in current smokers.

Human papillomaviruses and neoplasia of the lower female genital tract

Genital warts or condylomata have been recognised for centuries. Only comparatively recently, however, has their viral aetiology been established. Electron microscopy has shown the presence of viral particles, and immunohistochemistry (using antibodies to viral capsid antigen) and in situ hybridisation (using DNA probes) have also confirmed their viral nature. Warts may affect the vulva but may also involve the cervix (Fig. 19.4). Moreover, it is now appreciated that human papillomaviruses (HPV) may infect the vulva, vagina and cervix in a non-condylomatous manner. Such infections show characteristic morphological features: most important of these is a specific cytoplasmic vacuolation called *koilocytosis* (Fig. 19.5). The features associated with human papillomavirus infection are:

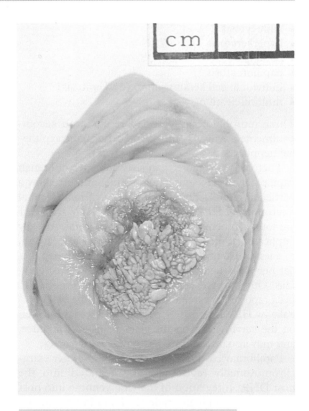

Fig. 19.4   Florid condyloma of the cervix

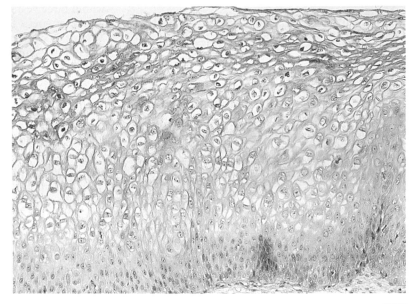

· Fig. 19.5   Koilocytosis

Cytoplasmic vacuolation and pyknotic nuclei indicative of human papillomavirus infection of the cervix.

- koilocytosis
- hyperkeratosis
- parakeratosis
- papillomatosis
- individual cell keratinisation (dyskeratosis)
- multinucleation.

These morphological features are common accompaniments of vulval, vaginal and cervical intraepithelial neoplasia.

There are now more than sixty subtypes of human papillomavirus recognised and certain of these show a particular predilection for the lower female genital tract, notably HPV 6, 11, 16 and 18. HPV 6 and 11 are found in benign condylomata and are not usually implicated in malignant transformation. HPV 16 and, to a lesser extent, 18 are found in cervical intraepithelial neoplasia and in about 90% of cervical carcinomas. Other types, such as HPV 31 and 33, have also been reported in carcinoma. Infection of the male genitalia by HPV is also seen; similar lesions to those seen on the cervix occur on the glans penis and prepuce, and may also be associated with neoplastic change.

Papillomavirus DNA may be present either extrachromosomally (episomal) or integrated into the host DNA. Integration of the viral genome into host DNA is usual in high-grade CIN and invasive cervical squamous carcinoma. The protein coding sequences of the viral early (E) or late (L) open reading frames appear to have a major role in oncogenesis. Most interestingly, the E6 protein of HPV type 16 is capable of binding to the cellular p53 protein to form a complex which neutralises the normal response of cervical epithelial cells to DNA damage (apoptosis mediated by p53), which may thereby allow the accumulation of genetic abnormalities. E6 protein of low risk HPV types (e.g. 6 and 11) does not appear to form a complex with p53.

These events may explain why, unlike many other solid tumours, mutation of the p53 gene is an uncommon event in cervical carcinogenesis, since there is an alternative mechanism for its inactivation.

Formerly, Herpes simplex virus 2 was thought to be implicated in the aetiology of cervical neoplasia, but the virus has never been isolated from a cervical tumour, and interest in this virus as the cause of neoplasia of the lower female genital tract has waned. It has been suggested, however, that papillomaviruses and Herpes simplex may act synergistically.

Physiological and neoplastic changes in the cervical transformation zone

Before puberty, the squamo-columnar junction lies within the endocervical canal (Fig. 19.6). With the onset of puberty and in pregnancy, there is eversion of the columnar epithelium of the endocervix so that the squamo-columnar junction comes to lie beyond and on the vaginal aspect of the external os. This produces the clinical appearance of a cervical 'erosion', an unfortunate term, since the change is physiological. The term *ectopy* is more appropriate. The columnar epithelium is then exposed to the low pH of the vaginal mucus and undergoes squamous metaplasia. This is a physiological phenomenon, and takes place through the stages of reserve cell hyperplasia and immature squamous metaplasia. Reserve cells, which may be derived from the cervical stroma, undermine the columnar mucus-secreting cells and multiply. This labile epithelium is called the transformation zone and is the predominant site for the development of cervical neoplasia.

Cervical intraepithelial neoplasia (CIN) refers to the spectrum of epithelial changes that take place in squamous epithelium as the precursors of invasive squamous carcinoma. The severity of the lesion is assessed subjectively as grade (CIN) 1, 2 or 3, according to the level in the epithelium at which cytoplasmic maturation is taking place (Fig. 19.7). Abnormal nuclei are present throughout the thickness of the epithelium, and mitotic figures are not confined to the basal cell layer (Fig. 19.8). Any grade of cervical intraepithelial neoplasia is potentially invasive, although the risk of invasion becomes greater as the severity of the lesion increases. The rate at which these intraepithelial lesions progress and the proportion of cases that would progress if left untreated is uncertain, but probably about 11% of CIN 1 cases will progress to CIN 3 within three years. More than 12% of cases of CIN 3 would progress to invasion if left untreated; about 30% of cases would regress. The presence of abnormal mitotic figures is associated with progression. It is also the case that, in some young women, the lesions progress to invasive carcinoma more quickly (3 years or less). Due to inconsistencies in reporting these lesions there is a growing tendency to consider cervical neoplasia in terms of low (CIN 1) and high (CIN 2 and 3) grade intraepithelial neoplasia.

Cytology screening programmes

Cytology screening programmes are sometimes referred to erroneously as cervical cancer screening. This is incorrect because the aim is to detect atypical cells in a cervical smear in the pre-invasive stage of the disease. The abnormal epithelium can then be eradicated by local measures, such as diathermy large loop excision of the transformation zone

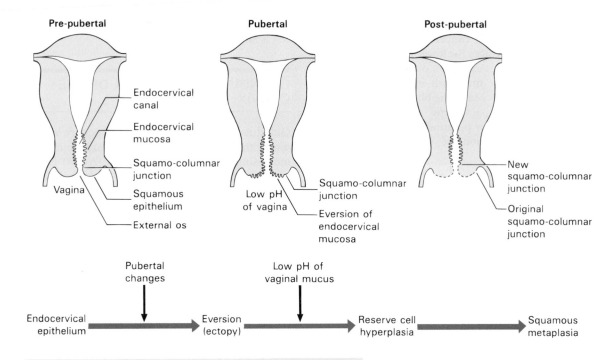

Pre-pubertal

Pubertal

Post-pubertal

Endocervical canal

Endocervical mucosa

Squamo-columnar junction

Squamous epithelium

External os

Vagina

Low pH of vagina

Squamo-columnar junction

Eversion of endocervical mucosa

New squamo-columnar junction

Original squamo-columnar junction

| Endocervical epithelium | Pubertal changes | Eversion (ectopy) | Low pH of vaginal mucus | Reserve cell hyperplasia | Squamous metaplasia |

Fig. 19.6   Epithelial changes in the cervical transformation zone

(LLETZ). Cervical cytology is a simple, safe, non-invasive method of detecting precancerous changes in the cervix. The majority of smears submitted to the pathology laboratory are taken from asymptomatic women as part of a national screening programme. The incidence of and mortality from invasive cervical cancer has fallen in communities where intensive screening has been carried out. In the United Kingdom the annual mortality from cervical cancer has remained static for many years at about 2000 women per year, but is now falling. The increasing incidence of cervical cancer in women under the age of 35 years is a worrying trend. The examination of a cervical smear relies on the identification of abnormal (dyskaryotic) nuclei. The degree of abnormality may be mild, moderate or severe, but does not always correlate with subsequent histological findings in a biopsy specimen. Therefore, even patients with mildly dyskaryotic smears should be referred for colposcopy. Cytology may not always be a reliable means of detecting an invasive tumour; the diagnosis of invasive carcinoma of the cervix is largely clinical and is confirmed by biopsy of suspicious areas of the cervix. The morphological abnormalities of the nucleus (dyskaryosis) in cervical smears are:

- disproportionate nuclear enlargement
- irregularity in form and outline

- hyperchromasia
- irregular chromatin condensation
- abnormalities of the number, size, and form of nucleoli
- multinucleation.

Invasive squamous carcinoma

The earliest sign of malignancy is early stromal invasion when small foci (less than 1 mm) are seen to arise from the basal epithelium and to breach the integrity of the basement membrane (Fig. 19.7). The concept of a microinvasive carcinoma is one in which there is a negligible risk of lymph node metastasis so that conservative management is appropriate. The tumour spreads by local and lymphatic invasion. The two principal factors that determine the prognosis of cervical carcinoma are:

- the size and depth of invasion of the primary tumour
- the presence and (more importantly) the extent of lymph node metastases.

The staging of cervical cancer is based on clinical and pathological assessment. Stage I cervical cancer is strictly confined to the cervix, stage II cancer extends beyond the cervix but has not extended onto the pelvic wall. It involves the vagina but not the lower third. Stage III cancer may extend onto the pelvic wall and involves the lower third of the vagina, and stage IV implies extension outside the reproductive tract. Tumour may then involve the adjacent organs, e.g. the mucosa of the bladder or rectum.

Involvement of para-aortic nodes is associated with a uniformly poor prognosis. The degree of histological differentiation of squamous carcinoma (whether it is well, moderately or poorly differentiated) is also an important factor.

GLANDULAR NEOPLASIA OF THE CERVIX

Glandular neoplasia of the cervix occurs less commonly than squamous neoplasia, but its incidence is increasing. *Adenocarcinoma in situ* (ACIS) is recognised as the precursor of invasive adenocarcinoma, and precursor lesions of a lesser severity than ACIS are also being recognised more frequently. These occur at a younger age than malignant glandular neoplasia. The widespread use of oral hormonal contraceptive preparations may be implicated in the aetiology of glandular neoplasia.

The mode of spread of the malignant tumour is the same as that of squamous carcinoma, although there is some evidence that adenocarcinoma may have a poorer prognosis. It is increasingly recognised that a significant proportion of cervical cancers (perhaps as high as 25%) are mixed adenosquamous carcinomas. This is understandable if one considers that 'atypical' reserve cells may differentiate along squamous or glandular lines to give pure or mixed tumours.

OTHER MALIGNANT TUMOURS

Other malignant tumours of the cervix are rare; they include sarcoma, malignant melanoma and lymphoma. Small cell carcinoma of the cervix is an uncommon, but highly malignant, tumour at this site analogous to the oat or small cell carcinoma of the lung (Ch. 14).

A. Cervical intra-epithelial neoplasia

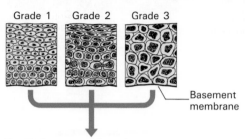

Grade 1   Grade 2   Grade 3

Basement membrane

B. Early stromal invasion
Stage 1A

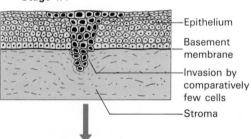

Epithelium

Basement membrane

Invasion by comparatively few cells

Stroma

C. Microinvasive carcinoma
Stage 1A

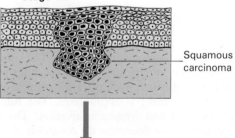

Squamous carcinoma

D. Occult invasive carcinoma
Stage 1B

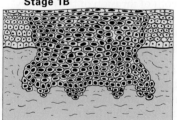

Fig. 19.7 Cervical intraepithelial neoplasia (CIN) and invasive squamous carcinoma

A. Cervical intraepithelial neoplasia. The concept of CIN refers to the level in the epithelium at which cytoplasmic maturation occurs. Grade 1 represents mild dysplasia; nuclear abnormalities throughout the epithelium, and cytoplasmic differentiation in the upper two-thirds are present. Grade 2 represents moderate dysplasia, with differentiation in the upper third of the epithelium. Grade 3 represents severe dysplasia and carcinoma in situ. **B. Early stromal invasion.** Invasion is <1 mm and there is a negligible risk of lymph node spread. **C. Microinvasive carcinoma.** Invasion is ≤ 3 mm depth and the maximum horizontal dimension of the tumour is ≤7 mm. There is still < 1% risk of lymph node spread. The presence of tumour within local lymphatic or vascular channels does not affect this definition. **D. Occult invasive carcinoma.** Invasion is >500 mm^3 and there is some risk of lymph node spread, but the tumour is still clinically undetectable.

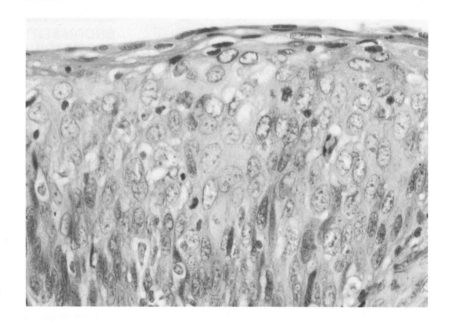

Fig. 19.8 Cervical intraepithelial neoplasia (CIN) grade 3

Note that there is minimal surface differentiation.

UTERINE CORPUS

Diseases affecting the uterine corpus (body of the uterus) may arise primarily within the endometrial lining (e.g. adenocarcinoma) or the myometrial wall (e.g. 'fibroids'). Pathological complications of pregnancy may also affect the uterus, but these conditions are dealt with in a separate section.

CONGENITAL ABNORMALITIES

Atresias and aplasias of the female genital tract are rare, with the exception of imperforate hymen. The majority of congenital abnormalities result from a partial or complete failure of the paramesonephric (Müllerian) ducts to fuse (Fig. 19.9). The major problems associated with these anomalies relate to pregnancy, with abortion and obstetric complications being the most common.

THE NORMAL ENDOMETRIUM AND MENSTRUAL CYCLE

At the onset of puberty, the first signs of oestrogenic stimulation of the endometrium appear and are soon followed by the first menstrual cycles, most of which are anovulatory.

The following discussion relates to a normal menstrual cycle of 28 days. The normal endometrium responds to the cyclical production of hormones by the ovary. During the follicular or proliferative phase of the cycle, rising levels of pituitary follicle stimulating hormone (FSH) stimulate the ovary to produce oestrogens, which in turn stimulate the endometrium to proliferate. There is growth of endometrial glands and stroma, both of which show mitotic activity, and vessels become increasingly coiled. Following ovulation at about day 14 of the cycle (mediated by pituitary luteinising hormone and a further output of FSH) the follicle is transformed into a corpus luteum, which continues to secrete oestrogens and also large quantities of progesterone. This post-ovulatory or luteal phase is associated with secretory changes in the endometrium which can be recognised in three stages:

- *early secretory* (post-ovulatory days 2–5), characterised by prominent sub-nuclear vacuolation
- *mid-secretory* (post-ovulatory days 5–9), characterised by stromal oedema and luminal secretion
- *late secretory* (post-ovulatory days 10–14), characterised by stromal changes referred to as pre-decidualisation in which there is increased prominence of periarterial stroma, increased tortuosity of stromal vessels (now referred to as spiral arteries) and prominent stromal granulocytes.

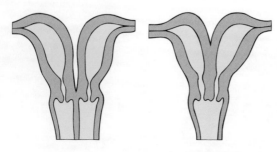

A. Uterus didelphys   B. Uterus bicornis bicollis

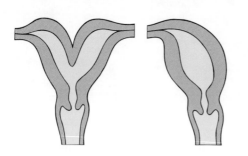

C. Uterus bicornis   D. Uterus unicornis
   unicollis

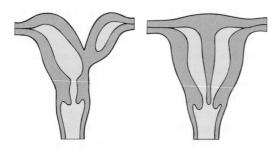

E. Uterus unicornis with   F. Uterus septus
   rudimentary horn

Fig. 19.9   Congenital abnormalities of the uterus

These changes prepare the endometrium for implantation of the blastocyst following fertilisation. If this does not occur there is functional decline as the corpus luteum atrophies, with falling levels of oestrogens and progesterone. This leads to the stromal haemorrhage and crumbling of the menstrual phase endometrium, which is quite variable in duration. Further proliferative activity is initiated with the development of a new follicle.

ABNORMALITIES OF THE ENDOMETRIUM

Disorders of the menstrual cycle leading to abnormal appearances of the endometrium will be discussed, followed by iatrogenic changes, polyps, endometrial hyperplasia and neoplasia. It must be remembered that many cases of abnormal uterine bleeding show a morphologically normal uterus. Defects in local haemostasis and hormonal dysfunction are important causes of bleeding in this context.

Luteal phase insufficiency

In some cases of primary or secondary infertility, endometrium examined in the secretory or luteal phase of the cycle shows inadequate secretory maturation for the appropriate estimated post-ovulatory day. Glandular and stromal maturation may also appear to be out of phase (so-called 'irregular ripening'). These changes are due to diminished production of progesterone by the corpus luteum.

Irregular shedding

Irregular shedding presents with abnormal uterine bleeding, and a confusing combination of secretory, menstrual and proliferative changes are seen in endometrial curettings. The changes are the result of a persistent corpus luteum.

Arias-Stella phenomenon

The Arias-Stella phenomenon is a hypersecretory response of the endometrium to high levels of circulating progesterone. It is characterised by cytoplasmic vacuolation and cytological atypia (Fig. 19.10). The presence of the Arias-Stella phenomenon in the absence of other evidence of intra-uterine pregnancy suggests the possibility of extra-uterine pregnancy, but it must be emphasised that this change is not pathognomonic of pregnancy. It may also occur in the absence of pregnancy and, rarely, in other sites, such as the mucosa of the endocervix or fallopian tube.

Endometritis

It is unusual for the endometrium to be the site of inflammation. The commonest situation in which this occurs is after intra-uterine pregnancy, when the appearances are of non-specific acute or chronic inflammation. This may follow instrumentation or the retention of products of conception. Inflamma-

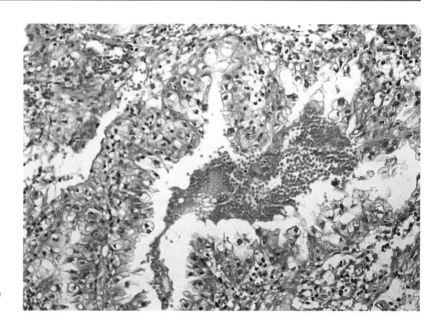

Fig. 19.10 Arias-Stella phenomenon

Note the intraluminal tufting and the hyperchromatic nuclei.

tion may also result from the presence of an intra-uterine contraceptive device (see below).

Two important specific infections of the endometrium are chlamydial infection and tuberculosis.

Chlamydial infection

Chlamydial infection produces a severe acute inflammation or chronic endometritis, with an extensive lymphocytic infiltrate and lymphoid follicle formation.

Tuberculosis

Secondary tuberculous infection of the endometrium may occur. Typical caseating or non-caseating granulomas are best seen in the secretory phase of the menstrual cycle. Definitive diagnosis rests on the demonstration of acid-alcohol-fast bacilli by the Ziehl–Neelsen technique. Endometrial infection may be associated with other evidence of pelvic or peritoneal tuberculosis.

Iatrogenic changes in the endometrium

Changes may be induced in the endometrium as a result of:

- exogenous hormones, including oral contraceptive preparations and hormone replacement therapy
- the use of a mechanical intra-uterine contraceptive device

- tamoxifen administration for patients with breast cancer.

Oral contraceptive preparations

There are two main types of oral contraceptive 'pill':

- *combined* — both oestrogen and progestogen are taken throughout the cycle; the dose may vary through the cycle and these are then called multiphasic preparations
- *progestogen* only.

The commoner pill now in use is the combined preparation and much smaller doses of oestrogen and progestogen are currently used. The commonest appearance in the endometrium is that of small, tubular, relatively inactive glands in a poorly developed stroma. Long-term use of the contraceptive pill in women over the age of 35 (particularly smokers) may be associated with hypertension, subarachnoid haemorrhage, thrombo-embolic phenomena and gallstones.

For the purpose of contraception, progestogens alone may be administered as a long-term intramuscular injection or as a daily oral preparation. Glandular atrophy and stromal pseudo-decidualisation are the usual changes produced. Oral progesterone given for the treatment of uterine bleeding secondary to ovarian dysfunction or endometrial hyperplasia produces similar effects.

Hormone replacement therapy

Exogenous oestrogen is used in the treatment of

peri- and post-menopausal symptoms. It is of great potential benefit in the prevention of post-menopausal osteoporosis. There is, however, a risk of endometrial hyperplasia and adenocarcinoma with unopposed exogenous oestrogen so that post-menopausal hormone replacement therapy in the presence of a uterus should involve a combination of oestrogen and progesterone. The progesterone opposes the potentially deleterious effects of oestrogen on the endometrium.

Intra-uterine devices

The precise mode of action of intra-uterine contraceptive devices is uncertain (Fig. 19.11). They may act by preventing fertilisation or blastocyst implantation, or by inducing very early abortion of an implanted pregnancy. The following pathological changes related to the presence of an intra-uterine device may be seen in the endometrium:

- chronic inflammation
- focal acute inflammation
- ulceration
- focal irregular ripening
- papillary metaplasia
- vascular thrombosis
- pseudo-decidual change.

Not all of these changes produce symptoms. Pelvic infection with *Actinomyces*-like organisms may occur with any of these devices.

Some intra-uterine devices contain a progestogen preparation, in which case the endometrial changes associated with exogenous progestogen administration (see above) are also seen.

Tamoxifen

Tamoxifen is an anti-oestrogenic agent used in the treatment of breast cancer. Paradoxically it also has oestrogenic effects and in recent years endometrial abnormalities have been reported following its long-term use; these include endometrial polyps and adenocarcinomas. The risk of developing endometrial cancer in patients treated with tamoxifen is still low (1.2 per 1000 person-years).

Endometrial polyps

Endometrial polyps are common in peri-menopausal and post-menopausal endometrium, and may be single or multiple. They are the result of the inappropriate reaction of foci of endometrium to oestrogenic stimulation. They are composed of variably sized glands, which are often cystic and are set in a cellular stroma which characteristically contains thick-walled blood vessels. The epithelium lining the glands may show variable metaplasia and secondary inflammatory changes may occur. Malignant change is rare.

Endometrial hyperplasia

The endometrium undergoes hyperplasia in response to unopposed oestrogenic stimulation. The source of oestrogenic stimulation may be endogenous, such as an ovarian tumour, the polycystic ovary syndrome (see below) or exogenous. Obesity is an important cause of a hyperoestrogenic state, since there is peripheral conversion of androstenedione to oestrone by the enzyme, aromatase, in fat cells. The various

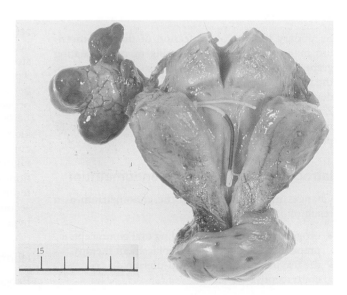

Fig. 19.11 An intra-uterine contraceptive device (Copper-7)

types of endometrial hyperplasia discussed below are associated with a variable risk of malignant change. The precise factors which determine which type will develop in a particular patient are unknown.

Simple hyperplasia

Simple hyperplasia is a diffuse abnormality affecting the whole of the endometrium. Many of the glands are dilated, and the epithelium shows increased nuclear stratification. The stroma also shows increased mitotic activity but there is no nuclear atypia (Fig. 19.12). This form of hyperplasia is associated with no increased risk of malignancy.

Complex hyperplasia

Complex hyperplasia is usually a focal architectural change in the endometrium. Characteristically, the glands are crowded and irregularly branched (Fig. 19.13). There is a low risk of malignant change.

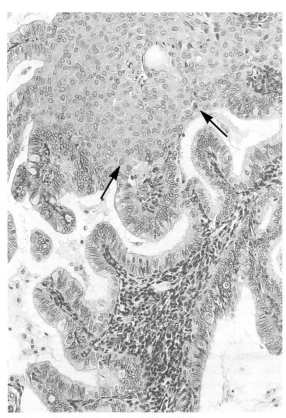

Fig. 19.13 Complex hyperplasia of the endometrium

There is architectural, but no cytological, abnormality. Note the associated squamous metaplasia (arrowed).

Atypical hyperplasia

In atypical hyperplasia (intraendometrial neoplasia) architectural and cytological changes are combined. The nuclei of the epithelial cells may show a variable degree of cytological atypia (Fig. 19.14). There is a close correlation between the risk of malignant change and the severity of the atypia. Thus, for atypical hyperplasia showing a severe degree of cytological atypia, the risk is probably about 25% after three years.

Endometrial adenocarcinoma

▶ May result from unopposed oestrogenic action or in atrophic post-menopausal endometrium
▶ Spreads via lymphatic and haematogenous routes

There are two clinicopathological types of endometrial adenocarcinoma.

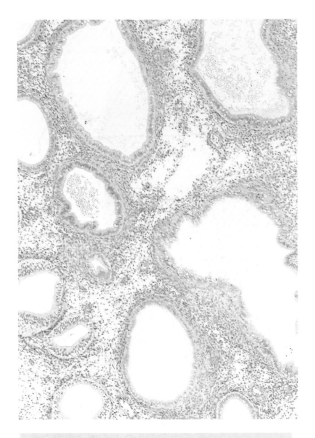

Fig. 19.12 Simple hyperplasia of the endometrium

There is prominent cystic dilatation of glands.

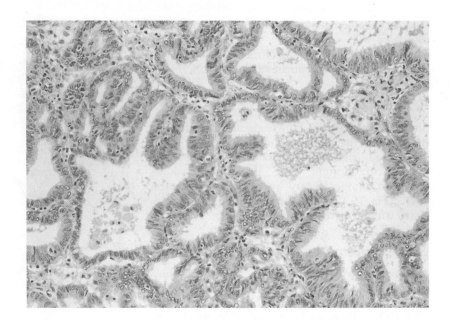

Fig. 19.14 Atypical hyperplasia of the endometrium

There is a combination of architectural abnormality and cytological abnormality (nuclear pleomorphism).

The first type is due to unopposed oestrogenic stimulation and arises from atypical hyperplasia. This type of tumour characteristically occurs in young women with the polycystic ovary syndrome or in association with obesity. It also affects peri-menopausal women, and may complicate post-menopausal oestrogen replacement therapy. It is generally associated with a good prognosis.

The second type of endometrial adenocarcinoma affects elderly post-menopausal women and probably arises on the basis of a pre-existing inactive or atrophic endometrium. Unusual histological types are sometimes encountered which are associated with a poor prognosis:

- adenosquamous
- papillary serous
- clear cell.

Endometrial adenocarcinoma may be confined to the endometrium. Since the endometrium is composed of glands and stroma, it is possible for a carcinoma to invade its own stroma and still be intra-endometrial. Alternatively, there may be invasion of the myometrium (Fig. 19.15). The extent of myometrial invasion at the time of diagnosis is the single most important prognostic factor. Involvement of the endocervix also has

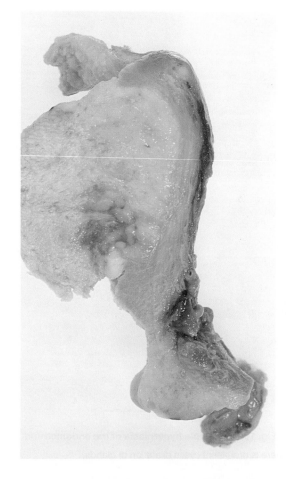

Fig. 19.15 Endometrial adenocarcinoma

There is extensive myometrial invasion by this poorly differentiated endometrial adenocarcinoma.

an adverse effect on prognosis. Thereafter, spread of the tumour occurs via the lymphatic and venous routes to the vagina and pelvic and para-aortic lymph nodes.

Endometrial stromal sarcoma

Neoplastic change can occur in the endometrial stroma as well as the endometrial glands, but stromal neoplasms are much less common. Low-grade stromal sarcoma occurs in the uterus of peri- and post-menopausal women and may be diagnosed as an incidental finding in a hysterectomy specimen or following a clinical diagnosis of fibroids. Nodules of bland-looking stroma infiltrate the myometrium, with little or no mitotic activity. The natural history of these tumours is one of local recurrence, sometimes after many years. Histologically, these recurrences resemble the original tumour. High-grade stromal sarcoma is a highly malignant tumour which may show extensive invasion of the myometrium at the time of diagnosis, with high mitotic activity and focal necrosis.

Mixed Müllerian neoplasia

Not only do both glandular and stromal components of the endometrium have the propensity to undergo neoplastic change, but they may do so concurrently. This gives rise to the spectrum of mixed Müllerian (mesodermal) neoplasia. Either component may be benign or malignant. Several variants are recognised, but carcinosarcoma or malignant mixed Müllerian tumour is the most important type and is discussed in more detail below.

Malignant mixed Müllerian tumour

Malignant mixed Müllerian tumour is a highly malignant tumour with a poor prognosis that occurs in elderly women. Clinically, it presents in the same way as endometrial adenocarcinoma, but the tumour is usually advanced with extensive myometrial invasion at the time of diagnosis. Diagnosis can usually be made on a curettage specimen, where obviously malignant glands and stroma are characterised by cellular pleomorphism, increased mitotic activity and abnormal mitoses. The tumours are usually polypoid and fill the endometrial cavity (Fig. 19.16). If the tumour shows only those components derived from endometrium or myometrium, it is of *homologous type*. Often, other components foreign to the uterus are seen, including cartilage and bone; it is then of *heterologous type*.

ABNORMALITIES OF THE MYOMETRIUM

Adenomyosis

Adenomyosis is a common finding in hysterectomy specimens and refers to the presence of endometrial glands and stroma deep within the myometrium. It characteristically occurs in peri-menopausal multiparous women and is of uncertain aetiology, although it may be regarded as a form of 'diverticulosis' since there is continuity between adenomyotic foci and the lining endometrium of the uterine cavity. Neoplastic change may occur within these foci but should not be regarded as evidence of myometrial invasion.

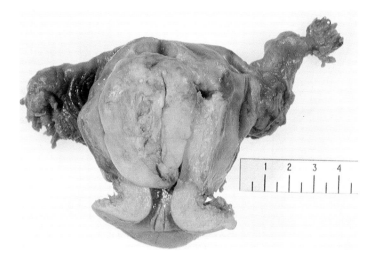

Fig. 19.16 Malignant mixed Müllerian tumour

This polypoid tumour fills the uterine cavity of an elderly patient.

Smooth muscle tumours

> ► Uterine leiomyomas (fibroids) are the commonest benign tumours
> ► Associated with infertility
> ► Leiomyosarcomas have varying malignant potential correlated with their mitotic activity

The commonest tumour of the female genital tract is the benign fibroid or *leiomyoma*. These commonly present in later reproductive life and around the time of the menopause. They are associated with low parity, although it is uncertain whether this is a common cause or an effect. The precise aetiology of leiomyomas is unknown. They may present clinically with:

- abdominal mass
- urinary problems due to pressure on the bladder
- abnormal uterine bleeding.

Characteristically, they are multiple, round, well-circumscribed tumours varying in diameter from 5 mm to, in some cases, 200 mm or more (Fig. 19.17). They may show cystic change or focal necrosis. On section, they have a white, whorled appearance. Histologically, they are composed of complex interlacing bundles of smooth muscle fibres showing little or no mitotic activity. Sometimes, nodules of tumour may be seen within veins (intravenous leiomyomatosis); this is not a sinister feature. Smooth muscle tumours contain steroid hormone receptors, and at least a proportion are oestrogen-dependent.

The crucial factor in the assessment of potential malignancy in smooth muscle tumours is their mitotic activity. There is a very good correlation between clinical behaviour and the mitotic count. The latter is usually expressed in terms of numbers of mitoses per 10 high power fields (hpf) of the microscope (the field area should always be stated). Leiomyomas contain 0–3 mitoses/10 hpf. If there are 10 or more in association with atypia, then a tumour must be regarded as a leomyosarcoma and will behave as a malignant tumour with all the risks of recurrence and metastases. If there are between 3 and 10 mitoses/10 hpf the behaviour of smooth muscle tumours is unpredictable. They are referred to as 'smooth muscle tumours of uncertain malignant potential', and the patients must be placed under periodical surveillance. Although these criteria may appear arbitrary, their application has proved useful in practice.

Adenomatoid tumour

The adenomatoid tumour is a small (20 mm in diameter) myometrial tumour that may resemble a fibroid on gross examination. Microscopically, it is composed of complex channels lined by flattened cells of mesothelial origin.

OVARY

Ovarian lesions present either with pain due to inflammation or swelling of the organ, or with the remote effects of an endocrine secretion.

OVARIAN CYSTS

Ovarian cysts may be non-neoplastic or neoplastic; many ovarian tumours are partially cystic. The various types of non-neoplastic cysts are:

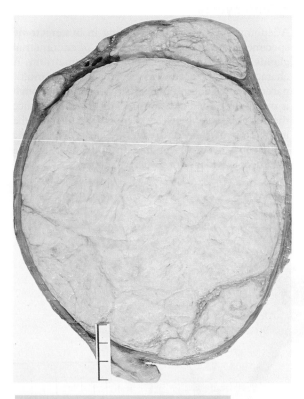

Fig. 19.17 Benign fibroid or leiomyoma
Note the classical white whorled appearance of its cut surface. This is an enormous example; the remaining uterus, adjacent to the scale, is small by comparison.

- mesothelial-lined
- epithelial inclusion
- follicular
- luteinised follicular
- corpus luteum
- corpus albicans
- corpus luteum cyst of pregnancy
- endometriotic.

Inclusion cysts occur in the ovarian cortex probably as a result of surface trauma at the time of ovulation; they may be lined by original peritoneal mesothelium or metaplastic epithelium. This is discussed in more detail below. The nature and origin of many of the non-neoplastic cysts that occur in the ovary can only be appreciated with knowledge of the normal histology of the ovary, as well as of the development of the follicle (Fig. 19.18) and corpus luteum.

Polycystic ovary syndrome

The polycystic ovary syndrome is the association of amenorrhoea, hyperoestrogenism and multiple follicular cysts of the ovary. There is usually stromal hyperplasia and little evidence that ovulation has occurred. The syndrome is an important cause of infertility, endometrial hyperplasia and, rarely, endometrial adenocarcinoma in young women.

Ovarian hyperstimulation syndrome

This may be induced by gonadotrophins or clomiphene used in the treatment of infertility. It is characterised by bilateral ovarian enlargement due to multiple luteinised follicular cysts. The condition may be complicated by ascites and pericardial effusion, hypovolaemic shock and renal failure.

OVARIAN STROMAL HYPERPLASIA AND STROMAL LUTEINISATION

The stroma of the ovary is unlike stromal tissue at other sites because, in addition to a general metabolic and supportive function, the cells may also be directly involved in the endocrine activity of the organ. Ovarian stromal hyperplasia is a proliferative change seen to some extent in the ovaries of most peri- and post-menopausal women. It is characterised by the non-neoplastic proliferation of stromal cells resulting in varying degrees of bilateral ovarian enlargement. It begins as localised nodules in the

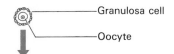

A. **Primordial follicle**

- Granulosa cell
- Oocyte

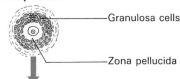

B. **Primary follicle**

- Granulosa cells
- Zona pellucida

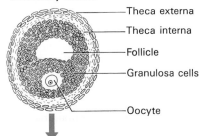

C. **Secondary follicle**

- Theca externa
- Theca interna
- Follicle
- Granulosa cells
- Oocyte

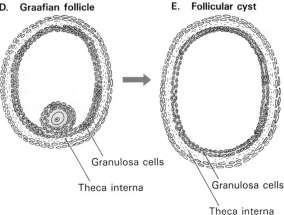

D. **Graafian follicle**   E. **Follicular cyst**

- Granulosa cells
- Theca interna
- Granulosa cells
- Theca interna

Fig. 19.18   Follicle development in the ovary and the origin of a follicular cyst

A. Primordial follicle. B. Primary follicle. The primordial follicle responds to follicle stimulating hormone (FSH) to form a primary follicle comprising the oocyte, a mucopolysaccharide layer (zona pellucida) and proliferating granulosa cells. **C and D. Secondary and Graafian follicles.** With continuing FSH stimulation a secondary or Graafian follicle is produced, comprising an eccentrically placed oocyte, a cavity containing clear liquid (the antrum), surrounding granulosa cells and condensed ovarian stromal cells, the theca interna and theca externa. The maximum diameter should be 25–30 mm. **E. Follicular cysts**, which are probably due to disordered hormonal function, are larger than 30 mm.

cortex or medulla of ovaries of women in the latter part of reproductive life. It later becomes more diffuse and, in extreme cases, the entire ovary may be replaced by cellular stromal tissue. The proliferation reaches a peak in the sixth and seventh decades. Thereafter there is a tendency towards atrophy. Atrophic ovaries tend to be small, wrinkled, hard and pearly-white. The proliferating cells resemble normal stromal cells but are typically plumper. Large, polyhedral, often lipid-laden cells of the theca interna may be present in isolation or in groups.

Hyperplastic stroma is associated with increased levels of androgens and oestrogens. Thus there is an association between stromal hyperplasia and endometrial hyperplasia, carcinoma, and polyps. Other steroidogenic cells may be scattered throughout the stroma; such 'luteinised' cells may secrete androgens and, if hyperplastic or neoplastic, may cause virilism. Stromal hyperplasia and luteinisation may also be observed in ovaries containing primary or secondary neoplasms.

ENDOMETRIOSIS

Endometriosis is the presence of endometrial glands and stroma in sites other than the uterine corpus. It is a very important cause of morbidity in women and may be responsible for pelvic inflammation, infertility and pain. The common sites include the pouch of Douglas, the pelvic peritoneum and the ovary. Endometriosis may also involve the serosal surface of the uterus, cervix, vulva and vagina, and extragenital sites such as the bladder and the small and large intestines. The occurrence of endometriosis in extra-abdominal sites is very rare.

The aetiology of endometriosis is unknown, but retrograde menstruation into the peritoneal cavity along the fallopian tube, or metaplasia of mesothelium to Müllerian-type epithelium are possible explanations. The glands and stroma are usually subject to the same hormone-induced changes that occur in the endometrium. Thus, haemorrhage in endometriotic foci may cause pain. In the ovary especially, recurrent haemorrhage may produce cysts containing altered blood; these are the so-called 'chocolate cysts'. Uncommonly, hyperplastic or atypical changes may be seen in the epithelial component, with appearances similar to those that affect the endometrium. At least a proportion of endometrioid tumours of the ovary arise from pre-existing foci of endometriosis.

OVARIAN NEOPLASMS

> ▶ May be solid or cystic, benign or malignant
> ▶ Borderline lesions have unpredictable behaviour
> ▶ Nomenclature based on cellular origin
> ▶ Some produce oestrogens
> ▶ Commonest fatal gynaecological malignancy in many countries

Ovarian tumours may be divided into five broad categories:

- epithelial
- germ cell
- sex-cord stromal
- metastatic
- miscellaneous.

The further subdivisions of these categories are shown in Table 19.2.

Epithelial tumours

Epithelial tumours are believed to arise from the mesothelial cell layer covering the peritoneal surface of the ovary. This mesothelium has the propensity to undergo metaplasia to Müllerian differentiation as, indeed, does the entire mesothelial lining of the peritoneal cavity. Thus, differentiation may take place to resemble tubal mucosa (serous tumours), endocervical mucosa (mucinous tumours) or endometrium (endometrioid tumours). Brenner tumours do not fit neatly into this histogenetic theory since they resemble the transitional epithelium of the bladder. Each of these tumours may be benign or malignant (Fig. 19.19), but there is a third category of *borderline malignancy* or tumours of low malignant potential. These tumours show some of the features associated with malignancy, such as irregular architecture, nuclear stratification and pleomorphism and mitotic activity, but lack the most important criterion of invasion. Their biological behaviour is intermediate between that of clearly benign and overtly malignant tumours (Figs 19.20 and 19.21). The application of flow cytometry to borderline tumours has shown that aneuploid tumours are more likely to behave in a malignant manner. A significant proportion of mucinous tumours, particularly in the borderline category, contain intestinal-type rather than endocervical-type epithelium. These tumours may be complicated by peritoneal implants producing copious amounts of mucus (*pseudomyxoma peritonei*). This condition has a poor prognosis and is often complicated by intestinal obstruction.

Table 19.2 Classification of ovarian neoplasms

Origin	Tumour	
	Types	Subtypes
Epithelium	Serous Mucinous Endometrioid* Brenner	Benign, borderline or malignant
Germ cells	Dysgerminoma Teratoma Extraembryonic Malignant mixed germ cell tumours	Mature cystic, immature solid or monodermal (e.g. carcinoid, struma ovarii) Yolk sac (endodermal sinus tumour) Choriocarcinoma
Sex-cord stroma	Thecoma Granulosa cell tumour Sertoli–Leydig cell tumour Mixed germ cell stromal tumour (gonadoblastoma) Steroid cell tumour	
Metastatic	Various	
Miscellaneous	Haemangioma, lipoma, etc.	

*Clear cell carcinoma is a variant of endometrioid tumour

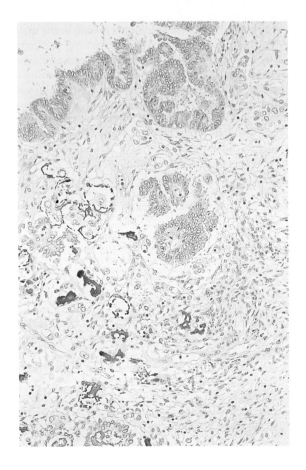

The diagnosis of borderline tumour is made on the primary tumour but associated peritoneal implants may be borderline or invasive. The latter are associated with an adverse prognosis.

Benign mucinous and serous tumours are commonly smooth-walled and cystic (Fig. 19.22), while Brenner tumours are solid but may show cystic areas. Endometrioid tumours of the ovary may show the full range of mixed Müllerian neoplasia already referred to in the context of uterine tumours, such as endometrioid adenofibroma and malignant mixed Müllerian tumours.

The aetiology of these epithelial tumours remains uncertain but certain facts are known. First, ovarian cancer is a disorder of developed societies and shows a higher incidence among women of higher social classes. Second, the oral contraceptive pill and pregnancy offer a protective effect; these probably act by reducing ovulation, although the reduced risk conferred by one pregnancy is much greater than would be expected. Exposure of the ovary to talc from powder applied to the vulva has been suggested as an aetiological factor, although there is little experimental evidence to support this. A common factor may be repeated trauma to the surface epithelium.

Fig. 19.19 Papillary serous adenocarcinoma

Note the presence of microcalcification (psammoma body formation).

A. Benign mucinous cystadenoma

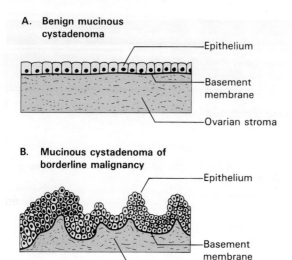

Epithelium

Basement membrane

Ovarian stroma

B. Mucinous cystadenoma of borderline malignancy

Epithelium

Basement membrane

Ovarian stroma

C. Mucinous cystadenocarcinoma

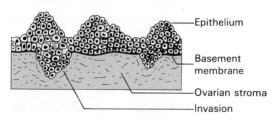

Epithelium

Basement membrane

Ovarian stroma

Invasion

Fig. 19.20 Epithelial morphology of ovarian mucinous neoplasms

A. Benign mucinous cystadenoma. Note the monolayer of cuboidal mucinous cells and basally located nuclei.
B. Mucinous cystadenoma of borderline malignancy. There is irregular architecture, multilayering of cells and mitotic activity, but the basement membrane is intact.
C. Mucinous cystadenocarcinoma. There is invasion through the original basement membrane.

Studies of ovarian cancer in families have shown that sisters and mothers of affected individuals have an approximately 5-fold increased risk of ovarian cancer. Among all of the common cancers this is the largest excess risk to relatives and implies genetic susceptibility. Family studies also show that first-degree relatives are at an increased risk of breast cancer. A rare dominant gene, termed BRCA-1, which increases the risk of cancer at both sites, has recently been identified on chromosome 17q. It must be emphasised, however, that only about 5% of cases of ovarian cancer are hereditary; 95% are sporadic.

Ovarian cancers show complex genetic abnormalities with a high incidence of p53 point mutations. Loss of heterozygosity has been demonstrated at a number of other chromosomal sites close to known tumour suppressor genes. Amplification of the *erb*B-2 (HER-2/neu) oncogene is associated with a poor prognosis.

Ovarian cancer is responsible for more deaths than any other gynaecological malignancy (Table 19.3). This is largely because it often presents at an advanced stage, due to its anatomically obscure site. Malignant tumours may be solid and/or cystic and there may be areas of haemorrhage and necrosis, with the tumour projecting into the lumen of a cyst or projecting exophytically into the peritoneal cavity. Tumour spread occurs predominantly intra-abdominally. The ovarian cancer related protein CA125 is now used routinely as a serum tumour marker, particularly to aid in the recognition of early relapse.

Germ cell tumours

A potentially confusing range of tumours may arise from primitive germ cells in the ovary. These may be benign or malignant.

Dysgerminoma

The fundamental or undifferentiated female ovarian germ cell tumour is the dysgerminoma, which is the exact counterpart of the seminoma arising in the male testis. It is a rare malignant tumour arising predominantly in young females; it is usually confined to one ovary and has a fleshy cut surface. Histologically, it shows a uniform appearance of germ cells admixed with lymphocytes. Occasional giant cells containing human chorionic gonadotrophin may be present, but these do not imply a poorer prognosis. These tumours are highly radiosensitive.

Teratomas

Germ cells may differentiate along embryonic lines when they give rise to teratomas, that is, a tumour that contains elements of all three germ cell layers — ectoderm, endoderm and mesoderm.

Mature cystic teratoma
The commonest germ cell tumour and, indeed, the commonest ovarian tumour is the benign or mature cystic teratoma (dermoid cyst). The majority of ovarian mature cystic teratomas arise from an oocyte that has completed the first meiotic division, in a manner analogous to parthenogenesis. It may present at any age, although usually in younger patients, as a smooth-walled, unilateral ovarian cyst. These tumours characteristically contain hair, sebaceous material and teeth (Fig. 19.23). Histologically, they show a wide range of tissues which, though haphaz-

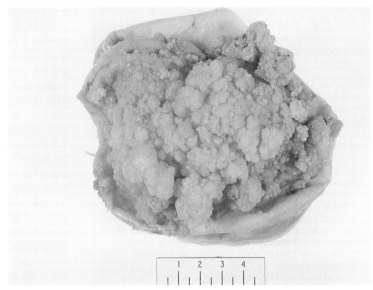

Fig. 19.21 Serous cystadenoma of borderline malignancy

An ovarian cyst containing abundant papillary tumour that was found on subsequent histological examination to be a serous cystadenoma of borderline malignancy.

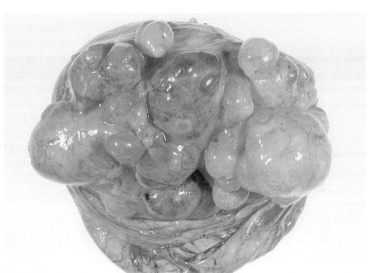

Fig. 19.22 Mucinous cystadenoma of the ovary

ardly arranged, are indistinguishable from those seen in the normal adult. Squamous epithelium, bronchial epithelium, cartilage and intestinal epithelium may all be seen. These tumours are benign, although in elderly women malignancy (usually squamous carcinoma) may develop very rarely.

Immature teratoma
In contrast to the mature cystic type, teratomas may also be predominantly solid and composed of immature tissues similar to those in the early embryo. These tumours are potentially malignant, and the predominant components are immature neural tissue and immature mesenchyme. These tumours occur in young patients, and the prognosis is related to the amount of immature neural tissue present. Such tumours may metastasise to the peritoneum, where the assessment of tissue maturity is crucial. Immature neural tissue within the peritoneum may mature, or mature glial tissue may be present from the outset (gliomatosis peritonei).

Monodermal teratoma
Germ cell tumours may be composed entirely, or almost entirely, of one tissue type; these are monodermal teratomas. The best examples are *struma ovarii*, composed of thyroid tissue which may be benign or malignant and rarely cause thyrotoxicosis, and *carci-*

Table 19.3 Number of cases of, and deaths from, various forms of gynaecological cancer in England and Wales in 1989

	Incidence*	Deaths†
Ovary	5032	3911
Cervix uteri	4147	1820
Body of uterus	3693	929
Vulva	776	384
Uterus, part unspecified	380	515
Vagina	210	106
Fallopian tube	44	20
Placenta	9	7

There are more deaths than incident cases of 'unspecified uterus' because many death certificates are less clearly defined than the pathology reports and other sources of registration.
*Taken from: Cancer statistics, registrations 1989. Series MB1 no 22
†Taken from: Mortality statistics, cause 1989. Series DH 2 no 16

noid tumours, which are similar to carcinoid tumours arising in the gut. The carcinoid syndrome may occur even with benign tumours, since metabolic products are released directly into the systemic circulation and are therefore not denatured by hepatic enzymes.

Extraembryonic germ cell tumours

Differentiation of germ cells may take place along extraembryonic (as opposed to embryonic) lines to form the neoplastic counterpart of the non-fetal parts of the conceptus (the primitive yolk sac and the trophoblast of the placenta). These elements may give rise to yolk sac tumours (also known as endodermal sinus tumours because of their resemblance to the endodermal sinuses of Duval in the developing rat placenta) and choriocarcinoma. These are highly malignant tumours which may be associated with other germ cell elements.

Yolk sac tumours

Yolk sac tumours usually affect young females below the age of 30 years. The tumours are cystic and solid and often haemorrhagic. Histologically, characteristic structures (Duval–Schiller bodies), composed of central vessels with a rosette of tumour cells, may be seen. Alpha-fetoprotein may be demonstrated immunohistologically and is used as a serum marker. Intra-abdominal metastasis occurs, and the prognosis for untreated patients is poor. Modern combination chemotherapy, however, has considerably improved the outlook for patients with this tumour.

Choriocarcinoma

Pure choriocarcinoma of the ovary is extremely rare and is associated with beta human chorionic gonadotrophin (βhCG) production. Theoretically, it could occur either as a germ cell tumour or as a primary or secondary gestational neoplasm (see below), in which case the tumour would contain the paternal haplotype on chromosomal analysis. When choriocarcinoma is seen, it is more usually one component of a malignant mixed germ cell tumour.

Sex-cord stromal tumours

During the fourth month of fetal life and onwards

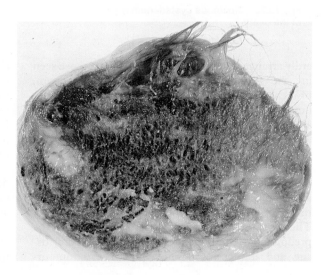

Fig. 19.23 Ovarian dermoid cyst
This benign cystic teratoma is filled with matted hair.

cell cords grow down from the surface epithelium of the ovary to surround the primordial follicles. Sex-cord stromal tumours comprise a range of ovarian neoplasms which frequently produce steroid hormones and are considered to arise from the cells which are the adult derivatives of these primitive sex cords in the fetal ovary. The detailed classification of these tumours is complex, but there are five broad groups (see Table 19.2).

Thecoma

Thecoma is the commonest sex-cord stromal tumour. It presents in the reproductive years as an abdominal mass, and is a benign tumour of the ovarian stroma. It is usually a unilateral, well-circumscribed tumour with a pale, fleshy cut surface. Histologically, it is a cellular, spindle-celled tumour containing abundant lipid. Its particular importance clinically is that it may be associated with the production of oestrogens, and may therefore give rise to abnormal uterine bleeding, endometrial hyperplasia or endometrial adenocarcinoma.

Granulosa cell tumour

Granulosa cell tumours can occur at any age and all cases are potentially malignant, although there is a close correlation between large size at presentation and malignant behaviour. It is particularly associated with oestrogenic manifestations. (It should, however, be remembered that granulosa cells do not synthesise oestrogens, but merely convert hormonal precursors to oestrogens.) They present as unilateral multicystic tumours that may be focally haemorrhagic or necrotic. Histologically, they are composed of nests and cords of granulosa cells with characteristically grooved nuclei. Often, cells surround a central space containing eosinophilic hyaline material; this structure is called the Call–Exner body. Patients often have concomitant endometrial pathology, either hyperplasia or adenocarcinoma. Granulosa cell tumours are characterised by their propensity for late recurrence, in some cases many years after removal of the original tumour. Granulosa cells produce *inhibin* and this may now be used as a serum marker for the tumour.

Sertoli–Leydig cell tumours

Sertoli–Leydig cell tumours are rare tumours composed of a variable mixture of cell types normally seen in the testis. Pure Sertoli and Leydig cell tumours may also occur. The tumours may be well, moderately or poorly differentiated and may present with androgenic signs and symptoms. Leydig cells may be identified by the presence of Reinke's crystals within their cytoplasm.

Gonadoblastoma

Gonadoblastoma is a rare lesion, which may not be a true neoplasm, in which primitive germ cells and sex-cord stromal derivatives are present. The latter usually resemble immature Sertoli cells and granulosa cells. These lesions typically develop in the dysgenetic streak gonads of phenotypic females carrying a Y chromosome. The germ cell component may undergo malignant change, usually to form a dysgerminoma.

Steroid cell tumours

Steroid cell tumours are uncommon and are usually benign and unilateral. In most cases the patient presents with virilisation due to androgen production (Fig. 19.24). Microscopically, the tumour is well circumscribed and composed of cells that resemble adrenal cortical cells and contain abundant intracellular lipid. The precise origin of these tumours is still debated. Although other sex-cord stromal tumours may secrete steroids, the term 'steroid cell tumour' is conventionally reserved for this particular variant.

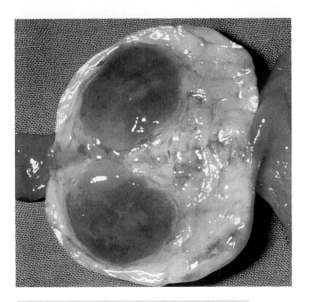

Fig. 19.24   Steroid cell tumour of the ovary

A well-circumscribed benign ovarian stromal tumour that caused virilisation in the patient.

Metastatic tumours

Tumour metastatic to the ovary may be genital or extra-genital. Endometrial adenocarcinoma may spread to the ovary, but it should be remembered that primary endometrial adenocarcinoma may co-exist with primary endometrioid adenocarcinoma of the ovary and be associated with a favourable prognosis. Large intestine, stomach and breast adenocarcinomas are the most important extra-genital tumours. Metastatic colonic adenocarcinoma may be confused with primary mucinous cystadenocarcinoma. The term 'Krukenberg tumour' refers to bilateral ovarian neoplasms composed of malignant, mucin-containing, signet ring cells, usually of gastric origin. Breast carcinoma frequently metastasises to the ovary, but usually these metastases do not manifest themselves clinically.

FALLOPIAN TUBES

The fallopian tubes may be the site of inflammation, pregnancy (pp. 582–583), cysts or neoplasia. Inflammatory lesions and tubal ectopic pregnancies commonly present clinically with acute lower abdominal pain, mimicking, for example, acute appendicitis. Whenever possible it is important to preserve the patency of the fallopian tubes; blockage is an important cause of female infertility.

Inflammation (salpingitis)

Inflammation of the fallopian tube (salpingitis) is usually secondary to endometrial infection or the presence of an intra-uterine device; it may be acute or chronic. Chlamydial infection is now an important cause of chronic inflammation and subsequent secondary infertility due to loss of tubal patency. Anaerobic organisms, such as *Bacteroides*, are also important as causes of salpingitis, whereas gonococcal infection is uncommon. Infection may be complicated by the accumulation of pus within the lumen of the tube *(pyosalpinx)*. Longstanding chronic inflammation may lead to distension of the tube, loss of mucosa and the accumulation of serous fluid within the lumen *(hydrosalpinx)*.

Cysts and tumours

Benign fimbrial cysts and *paratubal cysts* are common. They are usually lined by tubal-type epithelium. Rarely, *benign papillary serous neoplasms* may arise in paratubal or paraovarian cysts.

Tumours of the fallopian tube are rare. Of most clinical importance is *primary adenocarcinoma of the fallopian tube epithelium*. This tumour has a similar appearance to that of papillary serous adenocarcinoma of the ovary, for which it may be mistaken. The mode of spread is via lymphatics and the peritoneum. The tumour usually has a poor prognosis.

PATHOLOGY OF PREGNANCY

There is a high rate of fetal loss in early pregnancy, and many early abortions are subclinical. Clinical spontaneous abortion is usually the result of chromosomal abnormalities (see Ch. 3). The chorionic villi of the immature placenta may be oedematous *(hydropic abortion)*, or the stroma may be fibrotic, which is an involutional change following fetal death.

HYDATIDIFORM MOLE

> ► Characterised by swollen chorionic villi and trophoblastic hyperplasia
> ► Associated with high hCG levels
> ► Complete mole: 46,XX karyotype; no fetus
> ► Partial mole: triploid karyotype; fetus may be present
> ► May be complicated by choriocarcinoma

The hydatidiform mole is a disorder of pregnancy affecting approximately 1 in 1000 pregnancies in the Western world. It is characterised by swollen, oedematous chorionic villi and trophoblastic hyperplasia. Macroscopically, the placenta appears to be composed of multiple cystic, 'grape-like' structures (Fig. 19.25). A hydatidiform mole usually grows faster than a normal pregnancy, and the patient may present with either a 'large for dates' pregnant uterus, or with bleeding in early pregnancy. If an ultrasound scan is performed, the abnormal cysts can be clearly seen and uterine evacuation is indicated. There are two types of hydatidiform mole — complete mole and partial mole (Fig. 19.26) — which are genetically quite different.

Complete mole

The chromosomal constitution of the complete mole

is androgenetic (i.e. of paternal origin), characteristically 46XX, and is probably due to the fertilisation of an 'empty' ovum by a spermatozoon carrying an X chromosome which is then reduplicated. Grossly, the placenta is obviously abnormal with swollen villi. Histologically, the oedema is confirmed; there is an absence of stromal vessels and circumferential trophoblastic hyperplasia affecting all villi. The constituent trophoblast may show varying degrees of cytological atypia.

Partial mole

The partial mole is triploid, and may not be diagnosed clinically but only identified histologically in abortion material. Most contain one maternal and two paternal haploid sets of chromosomes, with all three sex chromosome patterns possible (XXY, XXX and XYY). It must be remembered, however, that not all triploids are partial moles. A fetus may be present and only a proportion of the villi abnormal; the rest may be fibrotic or may simply be hydropic without trophoblastic hyperplasia. Stromal vessels are present.

Complications

The importance of correctly diagnosing hydatidiform mole is that, in a small number of cases, the disorder may be complicated by *persistent trophoblastic disease*. This term encompasses two main pathological entities with similar clinical manifestations, diagnosed by persistently elevated or rising urinary hCG levels following evacuation of molar tissue.

- *Invasive mole*; chorionic villi are present within the myometrium and myometrial vessels. The main complication is uterine perforation.
- *Choriocarcinoma*; this is a very rare, malignant neoplasm of trophoblast with a propensity to systemic metastasis. Although there is usually a preceding history of hydatidiform mole, choriocarcinoma may follow a spontaneous abortion or very rarely an apparently normal pregnancy. It is more common in the Far East and, without treatment, has a high mortality. A biphasic pattern of invading cyto- and syncytiotrophoblast is the characteristic appearance of this tumour.

Cases of hydatidiform mole are monitored by estimation of the serum and urinary hCG. If the level rises, or does not fall, then the patient will receive

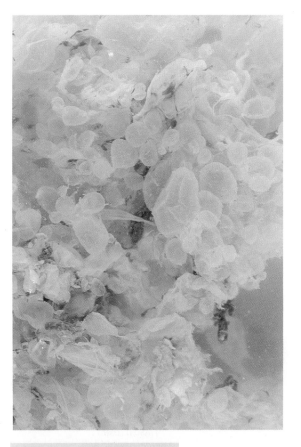

Fig. 19.25　Hydatidiform mole
Note the characteristic 'grape-like' clusters.

chemotherapy irrespective of the precise pathological diagnosis. The role of the pathologist in the management of persistent trophoblastic disease is thus limited. The neoplastic potential of complete mole is greater than that of partial mole. Therefore, all cases of molar disease are followed up although this may prove to be unnecessary in many cases.

PATHOLOGY OF THE FULL-TERM PLACENTA

The pathology of the full-term placenta is a large complex topic, the details of which are beyond the scope of this book. Only the commoner and/or clinically significant lesions are mentioned here. These may be considered under the following headings:

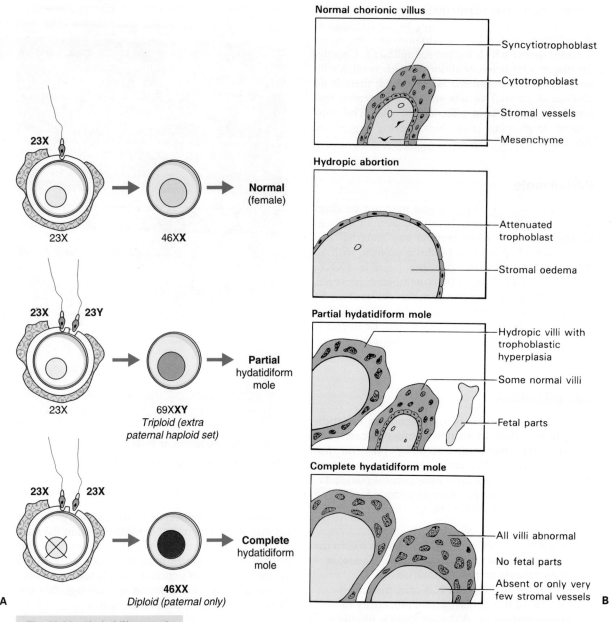

Fig. 19.26 Hydatidiform mole

A. Genetic analysis. Partial moles are triploid and result from fertilisation of one ovum by two spermatozoa. Complete moles are diploid, but comprise only paternal chromosomes. **B. Morphology.** See text for details.

- abnormalities of placentation
  - extrachorial (may be circumvallate or circum-marginate)
  - accessory lobe
  - placenta accreta
- inflammation (villitis)
- vascular lesions
  - perivillous fibrin deposition
  - fetal artery thrombosis
  - placental infarct
  - haemangioma
- immaturity of villous development.

Fascinatingly, long-term follow-up of individuals whose placental weights were accurately recorded earlier this century has shown a strong correlation between low placental weight and adult (e.g. cardio-vascular) disease.

Abnormalities of placentation

Abnormalities of placental shape are usually of no clinical significance. Placenta accreta is an abnormality of implantation.

Extrachorial placentation

Extrachorial placentation is a developmental abnormality in which the fetal surface of the placenta from which the chorionic villi arise (the chorionic plate) is smaller than the maternal surface attached to the uterine decidua (the basal plate). Thus, the border between the extravillous chorionic membrane and chorionic villi is not at the placental margin but is present circumferentially on the fetal surface of the placenta (Fig. 19.27). This border may be flat ('circum-marginate') or raised ('circumvallate'). Circum-marginate placentation is of no clinical significance, but circumvallate placentation is associated with a higher incidence of low birthweight babies, although the causal relationship between the two is still obscure.

Accessory lobe

An accessory lobe to the placenta is usually of no clinical importance, but occasionally the lobe may be retained in utero after delivery of the main placenta.

Placenta accreta

Placenta accreta is a rare disorder in which the chorionic villi are immediately adjacent to, or penetrate, the myometrium to a varying degree. This is associated with a deficiency of decidua, and may be the result of previous operative intervention, such as curettage or Caesarian section, infection or uterine malformation. The main clinical significance is the risk of ante-partum bleeding. Post-partum bleeding may also occur due to a failure of placental separation resulting from the abnormally adherent chorionic villi.

Inflammation

Inflammation of the placental tissues may involve either the chorionic villi (villitis) or the extraplacen-tal membranes (chorioamnionitis). Inflammation of chorionic villi is usually due to infection through the maternal blood stream. Specific infections, such as listeriosis, toxoplasmosis or cytomegalovirus, are responsible for only a small proportion of cases (Fig. 19.28). Most examples are of unknown aetiology, and are seen in approximately 5% of all pregnancies as a focal infiltrate of lymphocytes and histiocytes. Villitis is associated with a high incidence of fetal intra-uterine growth retardation but, again, the pathogenesis is unclear.

Chorioamnionitis occurs by infection into the amniotic sac from the vagina and cervix. It may be associated with prolonged rupture of membranes before delivery.

A. **Normal placenta**

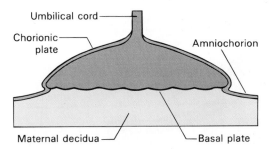

B. **Circum-marginate placenta**

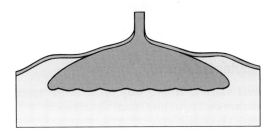

C. **Circumvallate placenta**

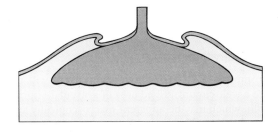

Fig. 19.27 Extrachorial placentation

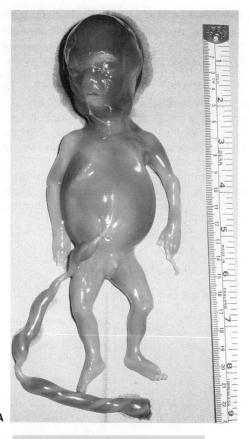

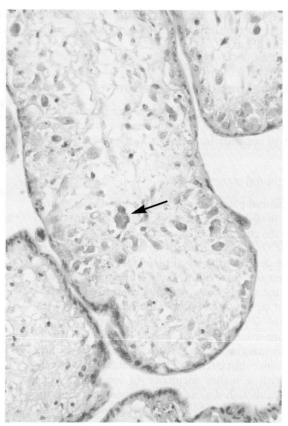

A

B

Fig. 19.28   Chorionic inflammation

A. Intra-uterine fetal death at 17 weeks' gestation due to cytomegalovirus infection. **B.** Chorionic villi from the placenta showing the characteristic inclusion bodies (arrowed) of cytomegalovirus infection.

Vascular lesions

Several vascular lesions may occur in the placenta which are usually of no clinical significance.

Perivillous fibrin deposition

Perivillous fibrin deposition occurs to some extent in all placentae and quite commonly is macroscopically apparent as a firm white plaque. The lesion is of no clinical significance.

Fetal artery thrombosis

Thrombosis of a fetal villous stem artery will produce a well-circumscribed area of avascular chorionic villi, which may be apparent macroscopically as an area of pallor. The inter-villous space appears normal. The aetiology is unknown, although there is an association with maternal diabetes mellitus.

Although usually of no clinical significance, extensive thrombosis of fetal villous stem vessels can, rarely, be responsible for fetal death.

Placental infarct

A placental infarct is a localised area of ischaemic villous necrosis due to thrombotic occlusion of a maternal uteroplacental (spiral) artery. (It must be remembered that chorionic villi have a dual blood supply). Macroscopically, fresh infarcts are red but progressively undergo fibrosis. When extensive, placental infarction is a manifestation of maternal vascular disease and is thus particularly associated with hypertensive disorders of pregnancy.

Haemangioma

Haemangiomas are uncommon tumours that occur

as well-circumscribed, dark nodules. They are of no clinical significance except when large or multiple. They may then be associated with polyhydramnios, premature labour and intra-uterine growth retardation due to diversion of blood through the tumour rather than through normal placental tissue.

Immaturity of villous development

Maturation of the placenta during pregnancy is associated with increased branching of chorionic villi with the production of small terminal villi to maximise the surface area available for materno-fetal transfer. Syncytiotrophoblast at the tips of villi thins to form vasculosyncytial membranes closely apposed to fetal stromal vessels. These are important sites of oxygen transfer between mother and fetus. Immaturity of chorionic villi and inadequate formation of vasculosyncytial membranes may be associated with intra-uterine fetal hypoxia, low birthweight and perinatal death.

PATHOLOGY OF THE UMBILICAL CORD AND MEMBRANES

Umbilical cord

Mechanical lesions of the umbilical cord include knots, rupture, torsion and stricture, all of which may lead to fetal complications. Abnormal (velamentous) insertion of the cord into the membranes, rather than the chorionic plate, may lead to serious haemorrhage during pregnancy or labour, since unprotected vessels run from the membranes to the surface of the placenta. A single umbilical artery is often accompanied by congenital fetal malformation. Visible oedema of the cord is associated with a relatively high incidence of fetal respiratory distress, although the reason for this is unclear.

Membranes

Amnion nodosum is the occurrence of nodules on the fetal surface of the amnion, particularly around the site of the insertion of the cord. Histologically, these are composed of amorphous material in which cell fragments, and sometimes fetal hair, are embedded. The lesion is usually associated with oligohydramnios.

Chorioamnionitis, or acute inflammation of the membranes, is usually the result of ascending bacter-

ial infection and is often associated with prolonged rupture of membranes. Some experts believe that chorioamnionitis itself is a cause of premature labour.

PATHOLOGY OF THE PLACENTAL BED

Within the placental bed there is an intimate admixture of maternal and fetal cells. The former comprise the decidua, residual endometrial glands and a population of macrophages and stromal granulocytes. The cells of fetal origin are composed of the various populations of non-villous trophoblast. These cells develop from the proliferating cytotrophoblast columns of the implanted blastocyst in the early weeks of pregnancy, and invade maternal decidua in a manner reminiscent of a malignant neoplasm. However, this biologically unique and physiologically controlled invasion is essential for the establishment of normal placentation. The most important types of non-villous trophoblast are the interstitial trophoblast cells, some of which fuse to form giant cells (Fig. 19.29), and the endovascular trophoblast, which invades maternal spiral arteries destroying the muscular media and replacing it with a fibrinoid matrix. In this way, these vessels lose their elasticity and become of wide calibre to meet the growing nutritional demands of the developing feto-placental unit. The invasion of non-villous trophoblast occurs in two waves, the first wave occurring in the first weeks of pregnancy and the second between 14 and 16 weeks.

Pre-eclampsia and fetal intra-uterine growth retardation

Pre-eclampsia is a common syndrome of pregnancy characterised by maternal hypertension and proteinuria. It is potentially dangerous for both mother and fetus.

It is now established that in pre-eclampsia, especially when associated with intra-uterine fetal growth retardation, there is a failure of the second wave of endovascular trophoblast migration into the myometrial segments of the spiral arteries. This may also occur in intra-uterine growth retardation uncomplicated by hypertension. Examination of the placental bed shows that the physiological changes mediated by endovascular trophoblast are confined to the intradecidual segments of the spiral arteries. The pathogenesis of this lesion is still uncertain.

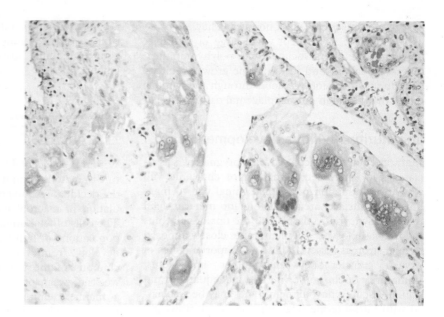

Fig. 19.29 Placental bed
Typical appearance showing interstitial trophoblast giant cells.

Acute atherosis

Acute atherosis is a necrotising lesion of the uterine spiral arteries characterised by infiltrates of foam cells. It occurs in the hypertensive disorders of pregnancy — pre-eclampsia and eclampsia — either alone or superimposed on other hypertensive disorders, such as renal disease. Pathological changes in the placental bed or implantation site may be difficult to distinguish from the physiological changes of pregnancy. The decidua away from the implantation site (decidua vera or parietalis) are thus the optimum sites to see this lesion.

Post-partum haemorrhage

There are three main causes of post-partum haemorrhage:

- retained chorionic villi
- infection
- inadequate involution of placental bed vessels.

Retained chorionic villi are unusual after normal pregnancy, but are more common following abortion. Normally, after parturition, the myometrial segments of the uteroplacental spiral arteries are left behind, and rapidly undergo thrombosis to prevent torrential haemorrhage. Other involutory changes then take place, and over the course of a few weeks the vessels resume their non-pregnant appearance. However, in a substantial number of cases of post-partum haemorrhage, the vessels are seen to be still distended and only partially thrombosed, so-called *inadequate involution* (Fig. 19.30).

The control mechanisms of normal involution and the causes of its failure are unknown.

ECTOPIC PREGNANCY

► Pregnancy outside uterine cavity
► Fallopian tube is commonest site
► Leads to pain and haemorrhage when it ruptures
► Pregnancy-associated changes in endometrium

An ectopic pregnancy is the occurrence of pregnancy outside the uterine cavity; its incidence is increasing. The incidence of ectopic pregnancy in the United Kingdom is 10–12 per 1000 pregnancies. 65% of cases occur in the 25–34-year age range. After one ectopic pregnancy the risk of recurrence is 10–20%. By far the commonest site of ectopic pregnancy is the fallopian tube (Fig. 19.31); the ovary is a much rarer site. In some cases, there is evidence of a fallopian tube abnormality such as chronic inflammation. The apparently increasing incidence of ectopic pregnancy may be related to increasing tubal infection. In most cases, however, there is no obvious cause, and a functional defect in tubal transport is assumed. Whether the presence of an intra-uterine device leads to a real increased risk of ectopic pregnancy is controversial.

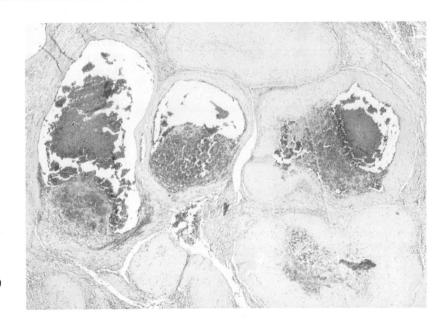

Fig. 19.30 Inadequate involution of placental bed vessels

Widely patent, only partially thrombosed uteroplacental (spiral) arteries in a case of post-partum haemorrhage.

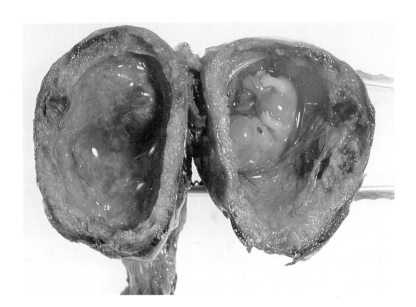

Fig. 19.31 A tubal ectopic pregnancy

The presenting symptoms are due to the physical expansion of the developing pregnancy within the limited space of the tube. Thus pain, with or without rupture, and haemoperitoneum are the commonest presenting features. In most cases, the pregnancy and fetus per se are not abnormal, and the same physiological changes associated with implantation can be seen in the fallopian tube as are seen in the uterus. The finding of pregnancy-associated changes in the endometrium in the absence of trophoblast or a fetus should always alert the pathologist to the possibility of an ectopic pregnancy (Arias-Stella phenomenon, p. 562).

MATERNAL DEATH

The maternal mortality rate is 10 per 100 000 maternities. The main causes of direct maternal death are:

- thrombosis and thrombo-embolism (including amniotic fluid embolism)
- hypertensive disorders of pregnancy
- haemorrhage.

Early pregnancy deaths are usually due to ectopic pregnancy and abortion, which includes rare cases of legal termination of pregnancy and spontaneous abortion. Rare causes of maternal mortality include anaesthetic-related deaths, uterine rupture and genital tract sepsis.

FURTHER READING

Fox H, Wells M (eds) 1995 Haines and Taylor: Obstetrical and Gynaecological Pathology, 4th edn. Churchill Livingstone, Edinburgh

20

Male genital tract

PROSTATE GLAND

NORMAL STRUCTURE AND FUNCTION

The prostate gland surrounds the bladder neck and proximal urethra (Fig. 20.1). It consists of five lobes, separated by the urethra and ejaculatory ducts. Two lateral lobes and an anterior lobe enclose the urethra. The two lateral lobes are marked by a posterior midline groove, palpable on rectal examination. The middle lobe lies between the urethra and ejaculatory ducts and the posterior lobe lies behind the ejaculatory ducts. The normal gland weighs about 20 g and is enclosed in a fibrous capsule.

Within the prostate there are three main groups of glands arranged concentrically around the urethra: an inner peri-urethral group, submucosal glands and the external group or main prostatic glands. From all three groups, ducts converge and open into the prostatic urethra.

Individual glandular acini have a convoluted outline, the epithelium varying from cuboidal to a pseudostratified columnar cell type depending upon the degree of activity of the prostate and androgenic stimulation. The epithelial cells produce acid phosphatase and the prostatic secretion that forms a large proportion of the seminal fluid for the transport of

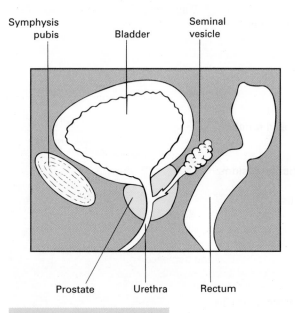

Fig. 20.1   Male pelvic organs

Sagittal section showing that the prostate can be palpated easily by inserting a finger into the rectum.

Pathological basis of clinical signs and symptoms in the male genital tract	
Sign or symptom	Pathological basis
Abnormal micturition	
• dysuria (pain)	Inflammation of the urethra, often accompanying a urinary tract infection
• hesitation and dribbling	Obstructed urinary outflow, usually due to prostate gland enlargement
• frequency	Incomplete bladder emptying due to obstructed urinary outflow
• urinary retention	Severe obstruction to bladder outflow, usually due to prostate gland enlargement
Urethral discharge	Urethritis, possibly due to venereal infections
Scrotal swelling	
• painful	Inflammation or ischaemia of the testis
• painless	Enlargement of scrotal contents due to hernia, fluid (e.g. hydrocele), varicocele, or tumour
Genital ulceration	Often venereal infection (e.g. syphilis)
Bone pain	If associated with male genital tract disease, possibly due to metastases from prostatic adenocarcinoma
Raised serum acid phosphatase	Secreted by prostatic carcinoma
Raised serum alphafetoprotein and/ or human chorionic gonadotrophin	Testicular germ cell neoplasia, particularly teratoma
Gynaecomastia	Possible manifestation of interstitial cell tumour of testis
Infertility	Impaired spermatogenesis due to endocrine disorders or to testicular lesions, or impaired ejaculation due to obstruction or to neurological disorders

sperm. The normal gland acini often contain rounded concretions of inspissated secretions (corpora amylacea). The acini are surrounded by a stroma of fibrous tissue and smooth muscle.

Table 20.1 Differences between the three most common types of prostatic pathology

Condition	Incidence	Location in gland	Pathology	Serum acid phosphatase	Metastases
Benign nodular hyperplasia	75% of men over 70 years	Peri-urethral zone	Nodular hyperplasia of glands and stroma	Normal	None
Clinical carcinoma of prostate	Common tumour — peak 60–85 years	Posterior subcapsular zone	Infiltrating adenocarcinoma	Raised in 2 out of 3 cases	Bone Lymph node Lung Liver
Latent carcinoma	Commoner than clinical carcinoma; 80% of glands over 75 years	Any site	Microscopic focus of adenocarcinoma	Normal	Rare

The blood supply to the prostate gland is from the internal iliac artery by the inferior vesical and middle rectal branches. The prostatic veins drain to the prostatic plexus around the gland and then to the internal iliac veins.

INCIDENCE OF PROSTATIC DISEASE

Diseases of the prostate are common causes of urinary problems in men, the incidence of which increases with age, particularly beyond 60 years. Most prostatic diseases cause enlargement of the organ resulting in compression of the intraprostatic portion of the urethra; this leads to impaired urine flow, an increased risk of urinary infections, and, in some cases, acute retention of urine requiring urgent relief by catheterisation. The most important and common causes of these signs and symptoms are *prostatic hyperplasia* and *prostatic carcinoma*. Inflammation of the prostate gland — *prostatitis* — is also common, but it less often gives rise to serious clinical problems; indeed, small foci of prostatic inflammation are not uncommon coincidental findings in prostatic tissue removed because of hyperplasia or carcinoma.

The principal clinicopathological features of the common types of prostatic pathology are compared in Table 20.1.

PROSTATITIS

A variable inflammatory infiltrate is commonly seen in the prostatic stroma in glands enlarged by benign nodular hyperplasia. Its significance is sometimes uncertain; it may simply be associated with leakage of material from distended ducts into the stroma. A marked degree of stromal oedema and periductal inflammation may, however, contribute to urethral obstruction.

Prostatitis implies a more prominent inflammatory lesion of the gland, often associated with a specific infective cause. Prostatitis may be:

- *acute suppurative prostatitis* — caused by coliforms, *Staphylococcus*, or *Neisseria gonorrhoeae* (gonococcus)
- *chronic non-specific prostatitis*
- *granulomatous prostatitis* — idiopathic, tuberculous, following transurethral resection, or allergic.

Acute suppurative prostatitis

Acute prostatitis usually results from spread of infection along the prostatic ducts secondary to urethritis or cystitis. Common causative micro-organisms include coliforms, staphylococci and gonococci. Acute prostatitis may occasionally follow urethral catheterisation or endoscopy; more rarely, the infection is blood-borne. The lesion is characterised by difficulty in micturition with perineal or rectal pain. There is general malaise and pyrexia and the prostate is palpably enlarged, soft and tender. Histology reveals acute inflammation with acini distended by polymorphs, macrophages and damaged epithelial cells. There may be necrosis with formation of an abscess which may eventually discharge into the urethra.

Chronic non-specific prostatitis

Chronic non-specific prostatitis may develop from

recurrent episodes of acute infective prostatitis. The prostate gland shows increased stromal fibrosis with an infiltrate of lymphocytes and plasma cells, associated with acinar atrophy.

Granulomatous prostatitis

Granulomatous prostatitis is a heterogeneous group of lesions, all of which may cause enlargement of the gland and urethral obstruction. The inflammatory component and associated fibrosis produce a firm, indurated gland on rectal examination which may mimic a neoplasm clinically; thus the importance of correctly diagnosing this uncommon group of conditions.

Idiopathic prostatitis may result from leakage of material from distended ducts in a gland enlarged by nodular hyperplasia. There is a periductal inflammatory infiltrate which includes macrophages, multinucleated giant cells, lymphocytes and plasma cells, with associated fibrosis.

The prostate is often involved in cases of genito-urinary *tuberculosis*. This condition is usually secondary to tuberculous cystitis or epididymitis, the infection spreading along the prostatic ducts or vas deferens. The histological features are of caseating granulomas distributed among the prostatic glands and through the stroma.

Some patients may require a second transurethral resection for benign nodular hyperplasia or carcinoma if the first operation fails to relieve the obstructive symptoms. The second biopsy often contains granulomas with necrosis; this lesion may be *ischaemic*, related to damaged blood vessels.

Allergic (eosinophilic) prostatitis is a rare lesion, occurring usually in men with bronchial asthma. There may be a sudden onset of prostatic symptoms. The gland contains granulomas with areas of fibrinoid necrosis and a surrounding zone of histiocytes, giant cells and numerous eosinophils.

BENIGN NODULAR HYPERPLASIA

▶ A common non-neoplastic lesion
▶ Involves peri-urethral zone
▶ Nodular hyperplasia of glands and stroma

Benign nodular hyperplasia is a non-neoplastic enlargement of the prostate gland which occurs commonly after the age of 50 years. About 75% of men aged 70–80 years are affected and develop vari-

able symptoms of urinary tract obstruction. If severe and untreated, benign nodular hyperplasia may lead to recurrent urinary infections and, ultimately, impaired renal function.

Aetiology

Benign nodular hyperplasia is thought to be related to a hormonal imbalance, although the exact mechanism is uncertain. With increasing age, the androgen levels fall, with a relative rise in oestrogens. Oestrogens also increase the prostatic tissue sensitivity to androgens. The central or peri-urethral group of prostatic glands, which are oestrogen-responsive, undergo consequent hyperplasia.

Morphology

The hyperplastic process usually involves both lateral lobes of the gland. In addition, there may be a localised hyperplasia of peri-urethral glands posterior to the urethra and projecting into the bladder adjacent to the internal urethral meatus (Fig. 20.2). This hyperplasia is described as 'median' lobe enlargement but does not correspond to the anatomical middle lobe.

The cut surface of the enlarged prostate shows multiple circumscribed solid nodules and cysts (Fig. 20.3). Histological examination reveals two components: hyperplasia of both glands and of stro-

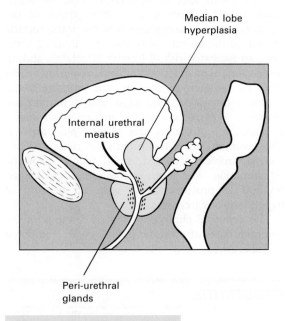

Fig. 20.2 Prostatic hyperplasia

Sagittal section showing the hyperplastic median lobe protruding into the bladder.

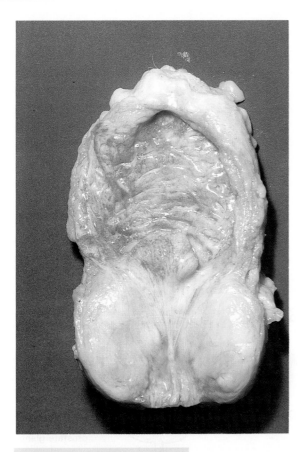

Fig. 20.3 Prostatic hyperplasia

The prostatic lobes are symmetrically enlarged and nodular. The bladder mucosa has a trabecular pattern due to hypertrophy of the underlying muscle bundles.

ma. The acini are larger than normal (some may be cystic) and are lined by columnar epithelium covering papillary infoldings (Fig. 20.4). The acini may contain numerous corpora amylacea. Phosphates and oxalates may be deposited around these to form prostatic calculi.

The stromal hyperplasia includes both smooth muscle and fibrous tissue. Some of the nodules are solid, being composed predominantly of stroma, and others also contain hyperplastic acini. Stromal oedema and periductal inflammation are common and may contribute to the urinary obstruction. Areas of infarction commonly occur, evident as yellowish necrotic areas with a haemorrhagic margin; these may result from a mechanical disturbance to the blood supply by the hyperplastic nodules. There is often squamous metaplasia of prostatic ducts and acini at the edges of the infarct. Benign nodular hyperplasia is not a premalignant lesion.

Clinical features

There are two main factors in the development of obstructive symptoms:

- The hyperplastic nodules compress and elongate the prostatic urethra, distorting its course.
- Involvement of the peri-urethral zone at the internal urethral meatus interferes with the sphincter mechanism.

As a result of these two factors, the severity of obstructive symptoms is not necessarily related to the size of the gland.

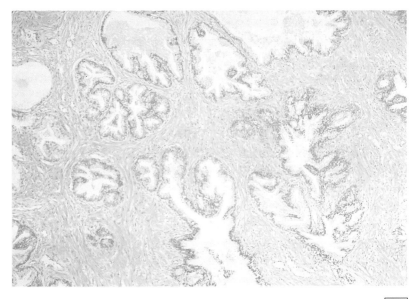

Fig. 20.4 Prostatic hyperplasia

The acini are lined by columnar epithelium with numerous infoldings. The muscular stroma is abnormally abundant.

The resulting obstruction to the bladder outflow produces difficulty in micturition. There is a delay in starting to pass urine with a poor or intermittent stream and dribbling at the end of micturition ('prostatism'). Haematuria may occur but is not common.

Digital examination of the gland per rectum reveals enlargement of the lateral lobes, often asymmetrical. The gland has a firm, rubbery consistency, and the median groove is still palpable.

Acute urinary retention may develop in a man with previous symptoms of prostatism; the bladder is palpably enlarged and tender, requiring catheterisation. This condition may be precipitated by voluntarily withholding micturition for some time, or by recent infarction causing sudden enlargement of a hyperplastic nodule.

Chronic retention of urine is relatively painless. There may be increasing frequency and overflow incontinence, usually at night. The bladder is distended, often palpable up to the umbilicus, but is not tender since the distension is more gradual.

Complications

Continued obstruction of the bladder outflow results in gradual *hypertrophy* of the bladder musculature. *Trabeculation* of the bladder wall develops due to prominent bands of thickened smooth muscle between which *diverticula* may protrude. This compensatory mechanism eventually fails, with resulting dilatation of the bladder. The ureters gradually dilate (*hydroureter*), allowing reflux of urine; if untreated, bilateral *hydronephrosis* may develop, with dilatation of renal pelvis and calyces (Fig. 20.5).

As the bladder fails to empty completely after micturition a small volume of urine remains in the bladder. This *residual urine* is liable to *infection*, usually by coliform organisms. The resulting cystitis is characterised by painful micturition with increased frequency and haematuria. An ascending infection in the presence of an obstructed urinary tract may result in *pyelonephritis* and *impaired renal function*. Repeated infections predispose to the development of *calculi*, often containing phosphates, within the bladder. *Septicaemia* may complicate pyelonephritis.

Clinical diagnosis and management

Further investigation of a man with suspected benign prostatic enlargement includes:

- microbiological examination of the urine to detect any infection requiring treatment

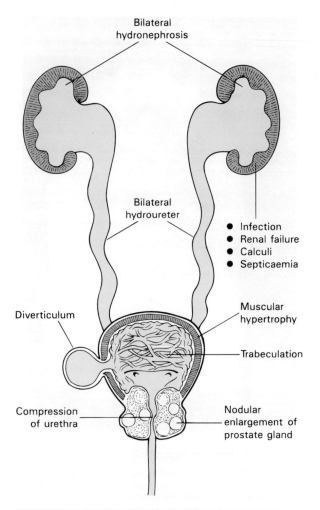

Fig. 20.5 Complications of prostatic hyperplasia

- a blood urea or creatinine measurement to monitor renal function; the serum prostatic acid phosphatase activity is not usually raised, although a slight, transient rise may occur following rectal examination or urethral catheterisation
- urinary tract ultrasound to provide an assessment of the upper urinary tract, indicating the severity of obstruction; it may demonstrate an enlarged prostate as a filling defect in the bladder. Ultrasound also provides an assessment of the quantity of residual urine after micturition
- cystoscopy to reveal median lobe enlargement not palpable on rectal examination
- histological examination of a prostatectomy specimen.

Surgical treatment of the condition may be by endoscopic transurethral resection of the hyperplastic peri-urethral zone, yielding numerous tissue fragments for histology. An alternative retropubic prostatectomy allows enucleation of the hyperplastic nodules from the compressed false capsule of the prostate. Both types of surgical specimen require histological examination to confirm the diagnosis and exclude a co-existent carcinoma.

If the symptoms are less severe, α-blocker drugs or anti-androgens may be of value, or a surgical bladder neck incision.

IDIOPATHIC BLADDER NECK OBSTRUCTION

Idiopathic bladder neck obstruction, an uncommon obstructive lesion at the bladder outlet, usually occurs in young men. Its cause is unknown. A prominent transverse ridge develops at the internal urethral meatus, resulting from a localised hypertrophy of smooth muscle.

The clinical symptoms are similar to those of benign nodular hyperplasia. As the pathological lesion is very localised, the gland is not palpably enlarged on rectal examination. Treatment is by bladder neck incision.

PROSTATIC CARCINOMA

> ► Adenocarcinoma occurring in males usually > 50 years
> ► Metastasises mainly to bone (osteosclerotic metastases)
> ► Obstructs bladder outflow
> ► Many are hormone (androgen)-dependent

Carcinoma of the prostate is one of the commonest forms of malignant disease; it caused approximately 8000 deaths in 1990 in England and Wales (11% of male cancer deaths). The tumour is rare below 50 years of age; peak incidence is between 60 and 85 years. The incidence is increasing.

Aetiology

The aetiology of prostatic carcinoma is unknown, although it is probable that the hormonal changes which occur with increasing age are involved. With advancing age there is a decrease in circulating androgen levels. This decrease is associated with involution of the outer zone of the prostate, the area in which most tumours arise. Benign nodular hyperplasia is not considered a pre-neoplastic lesion although it is often found in the same gland as a carcinoma, since both lesions are common.

Clinicopathological types

Two clinicopathological types of prostatic carcinoma are recognised, differing in their behaviour:

- clinical (active) carcinoma
- latent (incidental) carcinoma

Clinical (active) carcinoma

> ► Origin in posterior subcapsular area of gland
> ► Adenocarcinoma
> ► Architectural disturbance — invasion of stroma and perineural spaces
> ► Metastasises, especially to bone

Clinical carcinoma is the important form of the disease, producing metastases and urinary tract obstruction. Sometimes, the primary tumour in the prostate remains small — an *occult carcinoma* — yet produces widespread symptomatic metastases before the primary is clinically manifest. About two-thirds of patients will have locally advanced disease or metastases at the time of initial presentation.

Most active tumours arise in the posterior lobe of the gland, in the subcapsular area. Figure 20.6 compares location of lesions in benign hyperplasia and prostatic carcinoma. A retropubic prostatectomy for benign hyperplasia does not remove the posterior zone; this explains why carcinoma may develop following such a 'prostatectomy'. The tumour appears as an ill-defined, grey or yellow, firm or gritty area. Fragments of tissue from a transurethral resection may show these suspicious yellow areas.

In the majority of cases the tumour is an *adenocarcinoma*, usually well differentiated, forming acini, tubules or a cribriform pattern (Fig. 20.7). The convoluted outline of the glands is lost and neoplastic acini are formed from a single layer of cells, unlike the glands in benign hyperplasia which have a double-layered epithelium. There is a variable degree of cellular and nuclear pleomorphism, but often the epithelial cells are so well differentiated that it may be difficult to identify the lesion as a neoplasm. There is a variable amount of *fibrous stroma*.

Various histological grading systems have been devised for assessing the prognosis of prostatic carci-

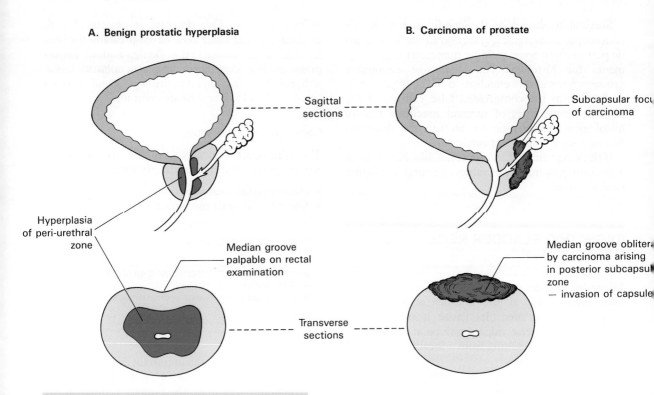

A. Benign prostatic hyperplasia

B. Carcinoma of prostate

Sagittal sections

Subcapsular focus of carcinoma

Hyperplasia of peri-urethral zone

Median groove palpable on rectal examination

Median groove obliterated by carcinoma arising in posterior subcapsular zone — invasion of capsule

Transverse sections

Fig. 20.6   Prostatic hyperplasia versus carcinoma

A. Hyperplasia commonly affects the peri-urethral zone. **B.** In contrast, most carcinomas are peripheral.

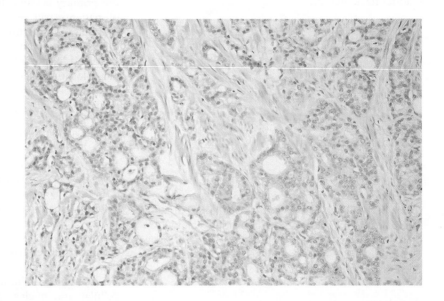

Fig. 20.7   Histology of prostatic carcinoma

The tumour is an adenocarcinoma consisting of neoplastic glands infiltrating a fibrous stroma.

noma. The most widely used is that devised by Gleason which grades tumours on a scale of 1–5.

The neoplastic acini invade the stroma of the gland, lymphatics, and perineural spaces. The tumour cells contain cytoplasmic lipid which gives the lesion a yellow appearance grossly. There may also be slight mucin secretion within the cells and acini. Immunohistological techniques are helpful to identify metastases as prostatic in origin and thus indicate specific hormonal treatment of an occult primary.

Latent (incidental) carcinoma

> ▶ Microscopic focus of tumour found incidentally
> ▶ Common; incidence high in old age
> ▶ Dormant lesions; metastases in 30% after 10 years

Latent carcinomas are microscopic foci of carcinoma found incidentally on histological examination of prostatectomy specimens removed for benign hyperplasia or at autopsy. These minute tumours were formerly thought not to produce clinical manifestations. Such foci are found in about 30% of prostates over the age of 50 years, the incidence rising to about 80% of glands over the age of 75 years. It is, therefore, much commoner than the clinically active form of the disease.

The natural history of these microscopic tumours is uncertain. Recently, the concept of latent carcinoma has been questioned with the recognition that some of them eventually progress and metastasise. Disease progression is related to the length of follow-up and probably occurs in about 30% of these patients after ten years; it may also be related to the histological grade of tumour. The majority, however, probably remain as latent or dormant lesions and, in practical terms, the finding of such minute foci of tumour in a prostatectomy specimen is not an indication for immediate hormonal therapy. Latent tumours have the same histological features as the clinically active type of the disease — a well-differentiated adenocarcinoma. Currently, there are no laboratory techniques available to identify which of these microscopic tumours will progress, and most surgeons will follow up the patient without any initial therapy if such tumours are identified in a prostatectomy specimen for benign hyperplasia.

Diagnosis may be attempted at an early stage when the disease is potentially curable; this can be done by screening procedures using rectal examination, serum prostatic antigen and transrectal ultrasound. There are also advocates for radical prostatectomy for the treatment of these small tumours.

Mode of spread

Spread of prostatic carcinoma may be:

- *direct* — stromal invasion, prostatic capsule, urethra, bladder base, seminal vesicle
- *via lymphatics* to sacral, iliac and para-aortic nodes

- *via blood* to bone (pelvis, lumbo-sacral spine, femur), lungs and liver.

Direct spread

Direct spread of the prostatic tumour occurs both within the gland and to extracapsular adjacent structures. There is invasion of the prostatic stroma towards the peri-urethral tissues and the base of the bladder is also commonly involved. Extension through the prostatic capsule is common, involving the seminal vesicles. The rectal wall is rarely invaded, being protected by the recto-vesical fascia. This extracapsular invasion results in the prostate becoming fixed to adjacent tissues.

Spread via lymphatics

Lymphatics provide an important route of dissemination of prostatic carcinoma, producing metastases in the sacral, iliac and para-aortic nodes. These may result in lymphatic obstruction and oedema of the legs. Less often, the inguinal nodes are involved.

Spread via blood

Vascular invasion by the tumour results in blood-borne metastases, most commonly to bone, lungs and liver. The most frequent sites of bone metastases are the pelvis, lumbo-sacral spine and proximal femur, less frequently the ribs and skull. Tumour emboli may reach the vertebrae by venous spread to the lung, then by passing through the pulmonary capillaries to enter the arterial circulation. An alternative mechanism is by retrograde venous spread through the vertebral venous plexus, because the blood flow in these veins may reverse due to physiological variation in the intra-abdominal pressure.

Bone metastases are usually *osteosclerotic*, with proliferation of osteoblasts and areas of new bone formation occurring in association with the neoplastic cells (Fig. 20.8). The osteoblast proliferation results in a raised serum alkaline phosphatase level.

Clinical features

The clinical presentation and features of prostatic carcinoma include:

- urinary symptoms — difficulty or increased frequency of micturition, urinary retention
- rectal examination revealing hard craggy prostate
- bone metastases — presenting with pain, pathological fracture, anaemia
- lymph node metastases.

Urinary outflow obstructive symptoms caused by

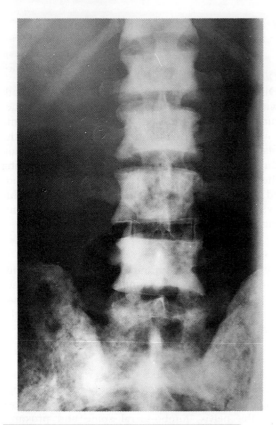

Fig. 20.8   Metastases from carcinoma of the prostate

X-ray of lumbar spine, including part of iliac bones, showing numerous sclerotic (white) metastases.

prostatic carcinoma usually progress more rapidly than those due to benign hyperplasia.

Digital rectal examination is a very important clinical procedure, revealing a hard nodule of tumour in the posterior lobe; the induration is due to the fibrous stroma of the tumour. The gland may be enlarged. If capsular invasion has occurred, the capsule is irregular and the median groove is obliterated. Less often, the rectal mucosa is fixed to the prostate. Induration may, however, be due to a non-neoplastic lesion such as prostatic calculi or granulomatous prostatitis.

Bone metastases often present as *localised bone pain*, back pain from vertebral metastases being a common initial manifestation of the tumour. *Pathological fracture* is another clinical presentation. *Anaemia* may result from extensive neoplastic infiltration of several bones with replacement of haemopoietic tissue.

Finally, peripheral *lymphadenopathy* due to

metastatic carcinoma is occasionally the initial presentation.

Diagnosis

Useful diagnostic investigations include:

- *diagnostic imaging* — ultrasound, skeletal X-rays, isotope bone scan
- *cystoscopy* — including transurethral resection
- *chemical pathology* — serum acid and alkaline phosphatase
- *haematology* — leukoerythroblastic anaemia
- *biopsy* — transurethral resection, needle biopsy, fine-needle aspiration cytology.

Ultrasound examination is important to assess upper urinary tract dilatation caused by the tumour. Transrectal ultrasound identifies suspicious areas within the prostate and aids selection of sites for needle biopsy. *Skeletal X-rays* are also vital to detect bone metastases. However, Paget's disease of bone (Ch. 25) is also a common lesion in the lumbo-sacral spine in elderly men and may produce similar radiological appearances to osteosclerotic metastases. An isotopic bone scan is also helpful in the detection of small metastases in the bones.

About 60% of patients with a localised carcinoma of the prostate and about 80% of patients with associated bone metastases have a raised level of *serum acid phosphatase*; this enzyme is produced by the neoplastic cells. Most of the increase is due to the prostatic iso-enzyme of acid phosphatase. The *serum alkaline phosphatase* is increased by the presence of osteosclerotic bone metastases as a result of osteoblast proliferation.

With widespread carcinomatous infiltration of the bone marrow a *leukoerythroblastic anaemia* develops, evinced by the presence of primitive red and white cell precursors in the peripheral blood (Ch. 23). In about 10% of patients with prostatic carcinoma the tumour stimulates *increased fibrinolytic activity* in the serum, which may cause excessive haemorrhage after prostatectomy.

Clinical management

About 75% of patients with clinical prostatic carcinoma benefit from treatment which reduces androgen levels. This reduces the rate of growth of both the primary tumour and its metastases, and relieves the pain from bone metastases.

Oestrogens suppress the production of pituitary gonadotrophic hormones, thereby inhibiting Leydig cells and reducing androgen production in the testis; this was the first clinical application of the hormonal treatment of malignancy, instituted by Huggins in Chicago in 1941. A successful therapeutic effect is indicated by histological changes in the tumour, which include cytoplasmic vacuolation and nuclear pyknosis in tumour cells or actual necrosis of the tumour. Oestrogens also cause squamous metaplasia of normal prostatic duct epithelium and the bladder neck mucosa, often seen in a post-treatment transurethral resection. The side effects of oestrogen therapy include gynaecomastia (Ch. 18) and retention of sodium and water. The latter factor may produce oedema and precipitate cardiac failure in elderly men with pre-existing ischaemic heart disease. There is also an increased incidence of both arterial and venous thromboses.

Gonadorelin (gonadotrophin-releasing hormone) analogues are also effective. They act by stimulating luteinising hormone (LH) release from the pituitary which then stimulates testicular testosterone secretion; the high testosterone levels achieved then suppress LH release.

Orchidectomy is also used to reduce androgen levels. More recently, a progestagenic anti-androgen, *cyproterone*, has been used therapeutically. Cyproterone competes with testosterone at prostatic androgen receptors, thereby blocking the effects of testicular androgens.

Radiotherapy is an alternative effective means of palliation for bone metastases.

PENIS AND SCROTUM

Diseases affecting the penis, ranked in order of frequency, are:

- venereal infections
- congenital malformations
- tumours.

It is common practice to examine carefully the external genital region of male neonates to detect major malformations; minor abnormalities may remain undetected until the prepuce can be fully retracted. In adolescents and adults, venereal infections (e.g. gonorrhoea) constitute a major public health problem in many countries; the penis is also one route of transmission of other serious infections, notably HIV — the cause of AIDS. The commonest tumours are benign warts, occurring usually in young adults; carcinomas are relatively uncommon.

CONGENITAL LESIONS

Congenital lesions of the penis and scrotum include:

- hypospadias
- epispadias.

Hypospadias

Hypospadias is the commonest congenital abnormality of the male urethra, resulting from a failure of fusion of the urethral folds over the urogenital sinus. Normal fusion of these folds starts at the posterior end and extends forward along the penile shaft to the tip. If fusion is incomplete, the urethra does not reach the tip of the penis, but opens on to its inferior aspect. The commonest site is a meatus on the inferior aspect of the glans. Less often, the meatus is on the penile shaft, and is associated with a downward curvature of the penis (congenital chordee). Rarely, there is a complete hypospadias with the urethral opening on the perineum behind the scrotum.

Epispadias

The congenital abnormality epispadias is much less common than hypospadias. The urethra opens on to the dorsum of the penis, the commonest site being at the base of the shaft near the pubis. This lesion results in urinary incontinence and infections. Epispadias is sometimes associated with exstrophy of the bladder.

INFLAMMATION AND INFECTIONS

Balanoposthitis

Inflammation of the inner surface of the prepuce (posthitis) is usually accompanied by inflammation of the adjacent surface of the glans penis (balanitis). Such a balanoposthitis is often associated with a tight prepuce (*phimosis*). Sebaceous material and keratin may accumulate beneath the prepuce, which may become infected by pyogenic bacteria. These bacteria include staphylococci, coliforms or gonococci. In diabetic patients, *Candida* infection is a further risk.

There is redness and swelling of the prepuce and glans with an associated purulent exudate. If treatment is delayed or there are recurrent episodes of infection, fibrous scarring can occur with the formation of preputial adhesions or severe phimosis.

Phimosis

Phimosis, and the closely related condition of para-phimosis, are the commonest medical indications for male circumcision.

In phimosis, the prepuce cannot be retracted over the glans penis. In most cases this is an acquired lesion, being the late sequel of an ammoniacal preputial dermatitis in the infant. Ammonia is formed by the action of some bacteria on the urine, producing blisters over the glans and inner aspect of the prepuce. This blistering results in the formation of numerous minute skin ulcers with associated acute inflammation and eventual fibrosis, reducing the opening in the prepuce.

Paraphimosis

If a tight prepuce is retracted behind the glans it may obstruct the venous return from the glans and pre-puce. The resulting oedematous swelling of the glans and prepuce produces a paraphimosis in which the prepuce cannot be returned easily to its normal position.

Balanitis xerotica obliterans

Balanitis xerotica obliterans is an uncommon penile lesion characterised by the appearance of thickened white plaques and fissures on the glans and pre-puce. The symptoms are of a non-retractile prepuce or preputial discharge, often necessitating circumcision. Similar lesions may develop around the urethral meatus with resulting scarring. The condition most commonly affects men of 30–50 years of age.

The histological features are of hyperkeratosis and atrophy of the epidermis with basal layer degeneration. The papillary dermis shows hyalinisation of the collagen with an underlying infiltrate of lymphoid cells. Similar changes are seen in lichen sclerosus of the vulval skin.

Genital herpes

Aetiology

Herpes is an acute infectious disease caused by herpes simplex virus (HSV). There are two antigenic types of the virus: HSV types 1 and 2. The majority of genital tract lesions are caused by type 2 as a sexually transmitted disease. HSV type 2 produces a recurrent, acute vesicular eruption on the skin, usu-ally around the mouth or on the genitalia. The incidence of genital herpes is increasing.

The majority of *primary herpes infections* are sub-clinical, but following this initial infection the virus may remain *latent* for many years. It is thought that the virus remains either locally in the skin or in the nerve ganglion supplying that skin segment, by migrating along the axons to the ganglia. *Recurrent herpes infections* are caused by reactivation of the virus and may be precipitated by a febrile illness, immune suppression, emotional stress or by ultraviolet light.

Clinicopathological features

The primary lesion of herpes genitalis in the male is preceded by itching followed by the appearance of several closely grouped *vesicles* surrounded by ery-thema on the glans penis or the coronal sulcus. The acute skin lesion is an intra-epidermal vesicle with evidence of cellular damage associated with the virus. There may be vacuolation of the epidermal cells, some of which are multinucleated and contain viral inclusions. The vesicles soon burst to produce shallow painful *ulcers*. Less often, there is a more diffuse bal-anitis which may heal with a resulting phimosis, and occasionally vesicles develop on the shaft of the penis or on the scrotum. Herpetic lesions are less common in circumcised men. In some patients, the infection is asymptomatic with no visible lesions, although these patients may still transmit the disease.

The clinical features may be sufficient to enable a diagnosis but laboratory confirmation can be obtained by isolation of the virus from vesicular fluid. A swab or scrape from this source, collected in a suitable viral transport medium, can be used to demonstrate a cytopathic effect in tissue culture. Viral particles may also be identified by examining vesicle fluid by electron microscopy.

Genital warts

Genital warts are increasing in prevalence and are now probably the commonest type of lesion seen in patients attending departments of genito-urinary medicine.

Aetiology

Genital warts are caused by the human papillo-mavirus (HPV), a DNA virus of the papovavirus group. The HPV type causing genital warts (HPV6) differs from those causing the common skin wart (HPV1, 2 and 4). Other HPV types are incriminated in the aetiology of cervical cancer (Ch. 19).

Clinicopathological features

In the male, the characteristic lesion is a hyperplastic, fleshy wart or *condyloma acuminatum*. This wart occurs most commonly on the glans penis and inner lining of the prepuce or in the terminal urethra. Less often, lesions develop on the shaft of the penis, the peri-anal region or the scrotum.

Histologically, the epidermis shows papillomatous hyperplasia. Many of the epidermal cells show cytoplasmic vacuolation, a feature indicating a viral aetiology. There is no epidermal dysplasia and these lesions are not premalignant.

The clinical diagnosis is usually obvious and laboratory diagnosis is rarely required. The clinical management is complicated by a high infectivity and a tendency to multiple recurrences.

Syphilis

> ▶ Causative organism is a spirochaete: *Treponema pallidum*
> ▶ Primary chancre on penis: ulcerated nodule and endarteritis with lymphocytes and plasma cells; associated inguinal lymphadenitis
> ▶ Secondary stage: condylomata lata, generalised lymphadenitis
> ▶ Tertiary stage: gumma, often in the testis

Aetiology

Syphilis is now a less prevalent sexually transmitted infection. It is caused by a spirochaete, *Treponema pallidum*. In the male, the primary lesion develops between one and 12 weeks after infection, usually on the penis at the site of inoculation. The organism probably enters the tissues through a mucosal abrasion and, by the time the primary lesion develops, the organism has already disseminated via lymphatics.

Clinicopathological features

The *primary chancre* usually develops on the inner aspect of the prepuce, the glans penis or corona. It forms a painless indurated nodule which soon becomes an ulcer with rounded margins. Examination by dark-ground microscopy of the serous exudate in the base of the ulcer reveals numerous spirochaetes. Initially, the tissue response consists of oedema with necrosis and an associated exudate of fibrin and polymorphs. At a later stage there is an endarteritis with a perivascular infiltrate of lymphocytes and plasma

cells. Thrombotic occlusion of these vessels produces necrosis and ulceration of the epidermis. There is usually an associated unilateral or bilateral inguinal lymphadenitis. Without treatment the primary chancre heals in a few weeks, leaving an atrophic scar.

The secondary and tertiary stages of syphilis develop later as a result of dissemination of the infection and are accompanied by an immunological reaction. Secondary syphilis develops within two years of the primary lesion and may include several different cutaneous manifestations. One of these is the development of *condylomata lata* on the prepuce and scrotum — proliferative epithelial lesions containing numerous spirochaetes. There is a generalised lymphadenitis in many cases.

The tertiary stage of syphilis may involve the formation of a *gumma* in the testis, but is also associated with thoracic aortic aneurysms and central nervous system changes.

Clinical diagnosis and management

Syphilis is diagnosed in the primary stage by microscopy of the exudate in the chancre or ulcer; the characteristic spirochaetes can be seen by dark-ground illumination. In the later stages, the diagnosis is confirmed serologically by seeking specific antibodies in the patient's blood; the fluorescent treponemal antibody absorption (FTA-Abs) test and the *Treponema pallidum* haemagglutination assay (TPHA) are the most specific.

Treatment is usually with penicillin, but it is essential to trace and possibly treat the patient's sexual partners.

Lymphogranuloma venereum

> ▶ Caused by *Chlamydia trachomatis*, serotypes L1–L3
> ▶ Primary genital lesion
> ▶ Inguinal lymphadenitis: acute suppurative inflammation with necrosis; chlamydial inclusions

Lymphogranuloma venereum is a sexually transmitted disease seen more commonly in the tropics. Infections seen in the UK, for example, have usually been acquired abroad.

Aetiology

The disease is caused by the bacterium *Chlamydia trachomatis*, serotypes L1–L3 (different from those associated with non-specific urethritis).

Clinicopathological features

Following a short incubation period of two to five days, about 50% of infected males give a history of a *primary genital lesion*. This lesion is a painless papule on the penis which may ulcerate but usually heals within a few days.

Between one and four weeks later the patient develops an *inguinal lymphadenitis* and this is the usual manifestation of the disease in the male. There is usually unilateral enlargement of the inguinal lymph nodes. The nodes are tender and initially discrete, becoming matted together as a result of pericapsular inflammation. The nodes may also become fluctuant. This lymphadenitis is often accompanied by constitutional symptoms with pyrexia and malaise. If untreated, the lymphadenitis may resolve but with some residual local lymphoedema.

The histological features are of an acute inflammation of the node with foci of necrosis surrounded by a margin of polymorphs, histiocytes and plasma cells. This inflammatory infiltrate extends through the capsule of the lymph node into the perinodal adipose tissue and may result in the development of sinuses to the overlying skin.

Clinical diagnosis

Surgical biopsy of the lymph node may be performed if the diagnosis is unsuspected; the histological features are almost pathognomonic. The diagnosis may also be made by aspirating pus from the lymph node and examining smears by specific immunofluorescence or stained by the Giemsa technique for the presence of chlamydial inclusions. A serum complement fixation test is also available.

Elephantiasis

In elephantiasis, the skin of the penis, scrotum and legs is greatly thickened by chronic oedema resulting from lymphatic obstruction. Two main groups can be distinguished:

* non-tropical elephantiasis
* tropical elephantiasis.

The tropical form is relatively common in parts of Africa and other countries with a similar climate in which the causative parasite is prevalent.

Non-tropical elephantiasis

In non-tropical elephantiasis, an earlier inflammatory process such as a recurrent cellulitis results in obliteration of the lymphatics in the skin. Another cause is trauma to lymphatics following surgical dissection of the inguinal lymph nodes as treatment for metastatic carcinoma of the penis or scrotum.

Tropical elephantiasis

Tropical elephantiasis is a late sequel of infection by the nematode parasite *Wuchereria bancrofti*. The adult worm lives in the lymphatic spaces, where the female produces microfilariae which re-enter the blood. These are ingested by blood-sucking mosquitoes, developing further in the insects' salivary glands. They re-infect man at the time of a further bite, passing back to the lymphatics. In this site the parasite induces a granulomatous inflammation with associated fibrosis, leading to lymphatic obstruction. Mechanical blockage of the lymphatic lumen by numerous parasites contributes to the oedema.

Peyronie's disease

Peyronie's disease is a rare penile lesion presenting usually in the fifth and sixth decades with painful curvature of the penis on erection and, sometimes, difficulty in micturition. The lesions may gradually progress for a few years, and some later resolve spontaneously.

One or more ill-defined plaques of fibrous tissue develop along the dorsal aspect of the shaft of the penis, initially involving the corpora cavernosa. Histological examination shows fibroblast proliferation, with increasing amounts of collagen as the lesion progresses. In the early stages of Peyronie's disease, there is also an inflammatory component with an infiltrate composed predominantly of lymphocytes and plasma cells.

The nature of the lesion is uncertain. Some cases are associated with palmar fibromatosis (Dupuytren's contracture) although the inflammatory component is unlike most fibromatoses. Peyronie's disease may be related to idiopathic retroperitoneal fibrosis.

Idiopathic gangrene of the scrotum (Fournier's syndrome)

Idiopathic gangrene of the scrotum (Fournier's syndrome) is a rare necrotising subcutaneous infection which involves the scrotum and sometimes extends to involve the penis, perineum and abdominal wall. It usually affects middle-aged to elderly men.

Aetiology

Several predisposing factors may be associated with Fournier's syndrome: local trauma, anal fistula or ischiorectal abscess. There is an increased risk in patients with diabetes mellitus. The common aetiological factor of local tissue trauma allows bacteria to enter the subcutaneous tissue. The causative organisms are of the faecal flora, including coliforms and anaerobes such as *Bacteroides*, some of which are gas-forming organisms. A mixed infection is common.

Clinicopathological features

The scrotum is red and swollen with crepitus on palpation due to the presence of subcutaneous gas. This initial stage is soon followed by necrosis of the skin and subcutaneous tissue, eventually exposing the testes. Later, the tissue slough separates, sharply demarcated from the adjacent viable skin. Finally, if the patient survives, there is regeneration of the skin.

Thrombosis of blood vessels in the scrotal skin results in necrosis of the subcutaneous tissue and dermal gangrene.

TUMOURS OF THE PENIS

Tumours of the penis are of two types:

- intra-epidermal carcinoma (Bowen's disease)
- invasive squamous carcinoma.

Intra-epidermal carcinoma

A localised area of intra-epidermal carcinoma (Bowen's disease; see Ch. 24) may develop on the penis as on other sites on the body surface, presenting as a sharply delineated erythematous patch with a moist keratotic surface. On the glans penis this lesion is sometimes termed *erythroplasia of Queyrat*, with the appearance of a well-defined slightly raised red plaque.

The histological features are of a pre-invasive squamous cell carcinoma. The epidermis is thickened with loss of cellular polarity and stratification. There is cellular and nuclear pleomorphism with hyperchromatic nuclei and an increased number of mitoses. Many of these abnormal cells keratinise at deeper levels within the epidermis (dyskeratosis). The basal layer of the epidermis remains sharply demarcated from the dermis at this stage, although this lesion carries a significant risk of progression to invasive squamous carcinoma.

Invasive squamous carcinoma

Carcinoma of the penis is a rare form of malignancy in the UK although common in parts of Africa and the Far East. It occurs only in uncircumcised men and does not occur in Jews, circumcised at birth. Human papillomavirus infection may be an aetiological factor.

The usual site at which the tumours develop is on the glans penis or inner aspect of the prepuce, forming an indurated nodule or plaque which later ulcerates. It rarely develops on the outer surface of the prepuce or on the shaft of the penis.

The tumour is usually a well-differentiated squamous carcinoma and invades the corpora cavernosa. Infiltration down to the urethra occurs late in the course of the disease. Metastases may develop in the inguinal lymph nodes.

CARCINOMA OF THE SCROTUM

Carcinoma of the scrotum was the first recognised example of a tumour caused by occupational exposure to carcinogens. In 1775, Percival Pott recognised this association in chimney sweeps. During the sweeps' work, soot containing carcinogens became retained in the rugose skin of the scrotum, later inducing a tumour. Since that time, other occupational factors have been identified in the development of this type of tumour, such as Lancashire cotton mill workers being exposed to mineral oils used to lubricate the machinery. Workers handling arsenic or tar are also at risk.

Nevertheless, this tumour is now rare in the UK. It develops in elderly men, often many years after possible exposure to industrial carcinogens. It presents as a nodular, often ulcerated mass which may involve an extensive area of the scrotal skin. The tumour is a squamous carcinoma, usually well-differentiated with keratinisation. The inguinal lymph nodes may be enlarged by metastatic carcinoma or as a result of reactive changes resulting from ulceration of the primary tumour.

URETHRA

URETHRAL OBSTRUCTION

The commonest cause of urethral obstruction is extrinsic compression due to prostate gland enlargement. Intrinsic lesions include:

- congenital valves
- rupture
- stricture.

Congenital urethral valves

Congenital urethral valves are a rare cause of urinary tract obstruction in the male neonate. In most cases this presents acutely with urinary obstruction and resulting bladder distension and muscle hypertrophy. The causative lesion is single or paired mucosal folds in the prostatic part of the urethra. Less often, a milder degree of this abnormality is first diagnosed in early adult life.

Traumatic rupture of the urethra

Traumatic rupture of the urethra is a rare event confined to males, and results from trauma such as a fall astride a hard object or complicating a fractured pelvis. The resulting damage to the wall of the urethra may involve its whole circumference or only part of it and may involve both the mucosa and muscle layers. Any part of the urethra may be involved.

The rupture leads to *extravasation of urine* into the peri-urethral tissues, which may later become the site of a *secondary infection*. There is *difficulty in passing urine* with *bleeding* from the urethral orifice and *localised pain*. A late complication of this lesion is the development of a *urethral stricture*.

Urethral stricture

A urethral stricture is usually an acquired lesion developing secondary to some other pathological condition of the urethra. The commonest cause is a *post-inflammatory stricture* following a *gonococcal urethritis*. This infection usually involves the peri-urethral glands and, if treatment is delayed, this condition may be associated with fibrosis around the glands and a fibrous stricture which encircles the urethra. Proximal to the stricture, the urethra becomes dilated, with hypertrophy of bladder muscle and urinary obstruction. The patient complains of difficulty in micturition with a poor stream and dribbling of urine. The retention of urine may be complicated further by the development of cystitis.

Urethral strictures may also be *post-traumatic*, complicating a rupture of the urethra, or develop after transurethral instrumentation or resection. A congenital stricture of the urethra occurs more rarely.

URETHRITIS

Urethritis (inflammation of the urethra) may occur in association with a more proximal infection in the urinary tract or adjacent to a local urethral lesion such as a calculus or an indwelling urinary catheter. The commonest causes, however, are the following specific primary infections of the urethra occurring as a sexually transmitted disease:

- gonococcal urethritis (gonorrhoea)
- non-gonococcal (non-specific) urethritis.

Gonococcal urethritis (gonorrhoea)

In gonococcal urethritis, the bacterial organism *Neisseria gonorrhoeae* (syn. gonococcus) produces an acute inflammation of the urethra. Following a short incubation period of two to five days after intercourse, a purulent urethral discharge develops, with pain on passing urine. If the infection spreads to the proximal urethra there may also be increased frequency of micturition. About 90% of males develop such symptoms as a result of infection, in contrast to females in whom about 70% of gonococcal infections are asymptomatic.

The gonococcus can penetrate an intact urethral mucosa, producing an infection in the submucosa which extends to the corpus spongiosum. This is an acute suppurative inflammation with increased vascularity, oedema and an infiltrate of polymorph leukocytes.

The inflammation commonly involves the *peri-urethral glands* and may also extend to the *prostate* and *epididymis* (Fig. 20.9). In all these sites *abscesses* may develop containing numerous polymorphs and bacteria with localised tissue destruction. A *urethral stricture* may develop many years after the initial infection as a result of fibrosis in relation to damaged peri-urethral glands. Gonorrhoea is a common infection, mainly occurring in young adults, and has a high infectivity.

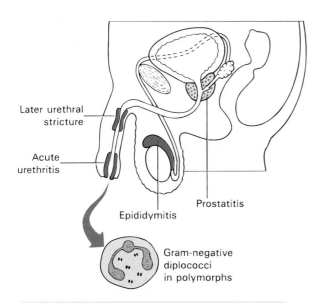

Later urethral stricture

Acute urethritis

Epididymitis

Prostatitis

Gram-negative diplococci in polymorphs

Fig. 20.9   Complications of gonococcal urethritis

Diagnosis

The gonococcus is a delicate organism and careful collection and transport of specimens is required for a laboratory diagnosis. A swab from the urethral mucosa may give a rapid diagnosis of gonococcal urethritis in the clinic, enabling immediate antibiotic treatment of the infection to be started. *Microscopy* demonstrates Gram-negative gonococci within polymorphs (Fig. 20.10).

Microbiological culture of the organism requires urethral swabs to be transferred promptly to the laboratory. Such a culture will provide confirmation of the diagnosis. Laboratory *antibiotic sensitivity tests* may also be required because of the recent emergence of strains of gonococci resistant to penicillin due to penicillinase (β-lactamase) production.

Non-gonococcal (non-specific) urethritis

Non-gonococcal urethritis (synonymous with non-specific urethritis) is the commonest sexually transmitted disease. In males, a mucopurulent urethral discharge and dysuria develop within a few days to a few weeks of the infecting intercourse. The discharge contains pus cells but gonococci cannot be detected by microscopy or culture.

Aetiology

Evidence from both microbiological culture and serological studies suggests that at least two micro-organisms are a significant cause of non-specific urethritis, although their exact importance as aetiological factors is still uncertain. These organisms are *Chlamydia trachomatis* and *Ureaplasma urealyticum*.

Chlamydia trachomatis is an obligate intracellular organism which structurally resembles a bacterium. Serotypes D–K are associated with genital tract infections. The infectious form of the agent, the elementary body, enters the urethral mucosal cell, enlarging to produce an initial body which is meta-

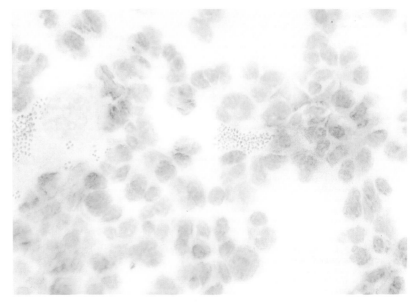

Fig. 20.10   Gonococcal urethritis

Gram-stained pus showing numerous neutrophil polymorphs and clusters of gonococci.

bolically active. This body multiplies to form more organisms within a vacuole, seen on microscopy as a basophilic cytoplasmic inclusion. These organisms are released by cell rupture to infect adjacent cells.

Ureaplasma urealyticum is a mycoplasma, a related type of micro-organism.

TUMOURS

Tumours of the urethra include:

- viral condyloma
- transitional cell carcinoma.

Viral condyloma

Recent studies have shown that minute viral 'warts' may occur in the penile urethra. These 'warts' may be associated with the better-known condyloma of the female ectocervical epithelium, caused by a human papillomavirus. The relationship of this type of lesion to neoplasia and its possible premalignant potential are still uncertain.

Transitional cell carcinoma

A papillary transitional cell carcinoma may rarely develop in the urethra, in association with a similar tumour in the bladder. This condition may be a separate, multifocal tumour of the urothelium, or may develop occasionally as a result of tumour implantation in the urethra following instrumentation of the bladder.

TESTIS

NORMAL STRUCTURE AND FUNCTION

During its development, each testis descends from the posterior abdominal wall to the scrotum, carrying with it a covering layer of peritoneum which forms the *tunica vaginalis*, a closed serous cavity around the testis (Fig. 20.11). Blood vessels and lymphatics enter and leave the testis on its posterior surface at the hilum which is not covered by tunica vaginalis.

Blood is supplied by the *spermatic artery*, a branch of the aorta, which passes along the spermatic cord. The venous return surrounds the spermatic artery as a network of intercommunicating veins, the *pampiniform plexus*. This plexus becomes the main testicular vein which, on the right side, drains to the inferior vena cava and, on the left, joins the left renal vein.

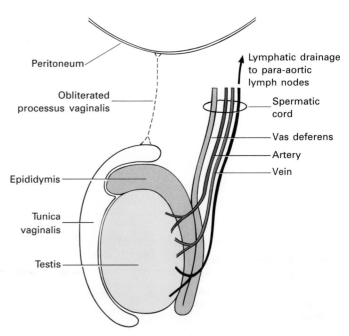

Peritoneum

Obliterated processus vaginalis

Epididymis

Tunica vaginalis

Testis

Lymphatic drainage to para-aortic lymph nodes

Spermatic cord

Vas deferens

Artery

Vein

Fig. 20.11 Anatomy of testis and vascular connections

Note that the lymphatic drainage of the testis is to the para-aortic lymph nodes.

Lymphatic drainage of the testis is to the *iliac* and *para-aortic lymph nodes*.

The testis has a fibrous capsule, the *tunica albuginea*. From this capsule, fibrous septa divide the testis into about 250 lobules, each containing up to four convoluted *seminiferous tubules*. These tubules converge on to a network of spaces, the rete testis, at the hilum, from where 10–12 *efferent ductules* lead to the *epididymis*. The rete testis and the efferent ductules are both lined by a ciliated epithelium.

The epididymis lies along the posterior aspect of the testis and is the main storage site for freshly formed sperm. The epididymis is a convoluted tubular structure lined by columnar epithelium.

The seminiferous tubules are each lined by a layer of *germinal epithelium* four or five cells thick; the more immature spermatogonia are situated close to the basement membrane. During spermatogenesis, meiotic division occurs at the spermatocyte stage; maturation of spermatids into sperm occurs near the tubular lumen. *Sertoli cells* lie in contact with the tubular basement membrane and insinuate between the germinal epithelial cells, providing local support and phagocytic function. In the interstitium between the seminiferous tubules, *Leydig cells* occur in small groups. These cells produce the hormone testosterone, which promotes spermatogenesis and the development of secondary sex characteristics, in response to stimulation by the pituitary gonadotrophic hormone, luteinising hormone.

From birth until puberty, the seminiferous tubules are small, being lined by Sertoli cells and primitive germ cells only. Spermatogenic activity starts at puberty.

INCIDENCE OF TESTICULAR LESIONS

Most testicular lesions are non-neoplastic disorders (e.g. mumps orchitis, torsion), but the possibility of a tumour must be considered fully in each case of testicular swelling or pain. Many testicular lesions present with a hydrocele, an accumulation of fluid around the testis; when this has been drained the testis must be examined carefully by palpation and, if necessary, by ultrasound imaging to exclude the possibility of an underlying testicular tumour.

The incidence of testicular tumours is rising slowly in many countries, but improvements in therapy are having a beneficial impact on patient survival.

Undescended testis (cryptorchidism)

During fetal development, the testis descends from the posterior abdominal wall to the scrotum and in most cases is intrascrotal at birth. In about 5% of boys, one or both testes are undescended at birth, although many descend by the first birthday.

An undescended testis cannot be palpated in the scrotum because the testis is situated in the inguinal canal or in the abdominal cavity. This condition must be distinguished clinically from a retractile testis, in which a normally situated testis is drawn up into the inguinal canal by contraction of the cremaster muscle.

If an undescended testis is not surgically drawn down to the scrotum before puberty, adequate spermatogenic activity does not develop. The seminiferous tubules remain small and are lined by Sertoli cells only. There is associated peritubular fibrosis. A longer-term risk of undescended testis is neoplasia; an undescended testis carries a higher risk of tumour development than a normally situated testis.

Hydrocele

The commonest intrascrotal swelling is a *hydrocele*, an accumulation of serous fluid within the tunica vaginalis of the testis. The smooth, pear-shaped swelling may be tense but is usually fluctuant and can be transilluminated. The contained testis is not palpable as it is surrounded by a layer of fluid (Fig. 20.12).

A *congenital hydrocele*, appearing in the first few weeks of life, results from persistence of the processus vaginalis, the channel between the peritoneal cavity and the tunica.

A *secondary hydrocele* may be associated with an underlying lesion of the testis or epididymis. This may be either *inflammatory*, such as mumps orchitis or gonococcal epididymitis, or *neoplastic*. The accompanying inflammation of the mesothelial lining of the tunica vaginalis results in the overproduction of fluid which cannot be drained adequately by the lymphatics in the tunica outer layer.

An *acute inflammatory hydrocele* accumulates rapidly and may produce pain. The straw-coloured fluid contains protein, fibrin, erythrocytes and polymorphs. A *chronic hydrocele*, however, causes only gradual stretching of the tunica and although it may become large and produce a dragging sensation, it rarely produces pain. In this instance the fluid may also contain cholesterol crystals. A rough exudate of fibrin lines the hydrocele sac with an associated proliferation of mesothelial cells and the

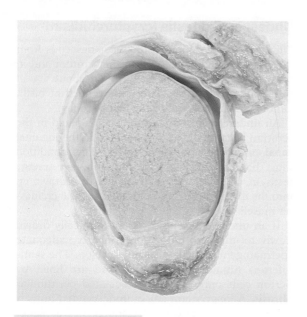

Fig. 20.12   Hydrocele

The tunica vaginalis is dilated. In this case, the testis was normal.

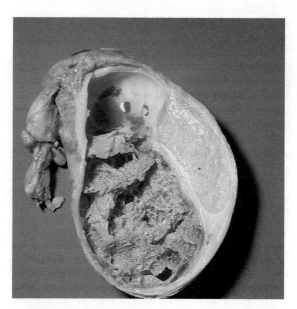

Fig. 20.13   Haematocele

The tunica vaginalis is distended with blood clot compressing the testis.

wall of the sac gradually becomes thickened by fibrosis.

Haematocele

A haematocele is haemorrhage into the tunica vaginalis. The usual cause is local trauma to the scrotal contents; this includes trauma to a blood vessel in a hydrocele sac as a result of a therapeutic tap. Another cause is an underlying testicular neoplasm.

In this condition, the tunica is lined by a shaggy layer of organising blood clot (Fig. 20.13). Microscopy of the tunica reveals fibrosis, haemosiderin-containing macrophages and an associated reactive proliferation of mesothelial cells.

ORCHITIS

Orchitis is the name given to any inflammatory condition of the testes.

Mumps orchitis

Mumps is an acute infectious febrile illness with parotitis, usually occurring in children. In adults,

about 25% of cases are complicated by an orchitis, which develops as the parotitis begins to subside. The condition is usually unilateral. The testis is enlarged and very tender due to stretching of the tunica albuginea.

There is vascular dilatation and oedema of the interstitium of the testis, with an infiltrate of lymphocytes. Increasing pressure within the swollen testis produces ischaemia from blood vessel compression and necrosis of seminiferous tubules.

If the inflammation is mild, resolution may be complete. In many cases, however, the testis becomes atrophic with increased fibrosis in the interstitium. Spermatogenesis is then reduced; the tubules are lined by Sertoli cells only. If the involvement is bilateral, this scarring may result in subfertility.

Idiopathic granulomatous orchitis

Granulomatous orchitis is an uncommon chronic inflammatory lesion of the testis of unknown aetiology. The peak age incidence is 45–60 years. Granulomatous orchitis produces a firm, unilateral testicular enlargement which may mimic a neoplasm clinically.

The testis is enlarged with a firm or rubbery consistency and a lobulated appearance on its cut surface; there may also be a secondary hydrocele. Histology reveals loss of the germinal epithelium in the seminiferous tubules. The tubular architecture remains recognisable, but there is a dense granulomatous inflammatory infiltrate centred on the tubules and extending into the interstitium. This infiltrate comprises lymphocytes, plasma cells, macrophages and giant cells.

Although the aetiology is unknown, there is often a history of a *urinary tract infection*, suggesting that reflux of urine along the vas may be an aetiological factor. A reaction to *extravasated sperm* in the interstitium is another possible explanation.

Syphilitic orchitis

Although the lesion is now rarely seen, the testis was a common site for the development of a *gumma* in the tertiary stage of syphilis (p. 597). There is unilateral painless enlargement of the testis which may mimic a neoplasm clinically. There is an irregular area of necrosis on the cut surface of the body of the testis and there may be a hydrocele. Histology shows tissue necrosis, although the architectural outline of the seminiferous tubules remains. At the edge of the necrotic area, there is an infiltrate of lymphocytes and plasma cells with an endarteritis.

TESTICULAR TUMOURS

Tumours of the testis are relatively uncommon although their incidence has increased in recent years. They account for less than 1% of all cancer deaths in the UK. Testicular tumours are important, however, since many occur in young men and are the commonest form of malignancy in this age group. Many are highly malignant, although recent advances in chemotherapy have greatly improved the prognosis.

Aetiology

Maldescent of the testis is the only known risk factor for tumour development. An undescended testis is 10 times more likely to develop a tumour than an intrascrotal testis. About 10% of all testicular tumours develop in testes that are, or have been, cryptorchid.

Local trauma is not considered a causative factor, but trauma to a testis containing a tumour may first draw attention to its presence.

Finally, there is current interest in in situ neoplastic changes within seminiferous tubules adjacent to an established tumour. Patients exhibiting this fea-

ture have a significantly increased risk of developing a contralateral tumour.

Clinical features

Testicular tumours (Fig. 20.14) may present with:

- painless unilateral enlargement of testis
- secondary hydrocele
- symptoms from metastases
- retroperitoneal mass
- gynaecomastia.

The majority of testicular tumours present as slow, painless enlargement of one testis. On examination, there is a smooth or irregular firm enlargement of the testis. There may be a loss of testicular sensation on palpation. Less often, the patient notices a more

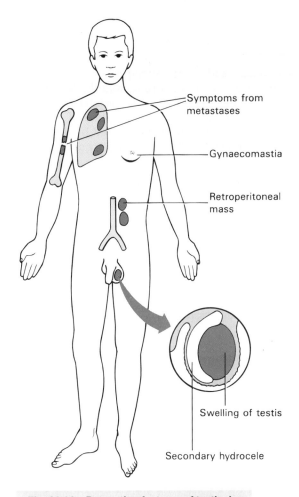

Fig. 20.14 Presenting features of testicular tumours.

rapidly enlarging scrotal swelling due to a secondary hydrocele around the tumour.

Some of the more malignant tumours may produce symptoms from metastases initially, for example haemoptysis from lung deposits, or hepatomegaly.

A retroperitoneal mass may be the presenting feature. This mass may be a para-aortic lymph node metastasis from either a small viable primary tumour in the testis or a regressed testicular primary. Regressed testicular tumours are rare, but are almost always seminomas as evinced by the histology of their metastases; all that remains in the testis is a small hyaline scar.

Gynaecomastia is occasionally the initial feature of sex hormone-secreting interstitial cell tumours, before a testicular swelling is noted.

Classification

Testicular tumours may be derived from germ cells or non-germ cells; 85–90% are of germ cell origin (Fig. 20.15). Germ cell tumours include seminomas, teratomas and their subtypes. Non-germ cell tumours include those arising from the Sertoli cells of the seminiferous tubules and the interstitial cells.

The most widely used classification of testicular neoplasms in the UK is that devised by the British Testicular Tumour Panel and Registry as follows:

- seminoma
- teratoma
- combined (mixed) germ cell tumour — seminoma and teratoma
- malignant lymphoma
- yolk sac tumour
- interstitial (Leydig) cell tumour
- Sertoli cell tumour
- metastatic tumours
- adenomatoid tumour
- paratesticular sarcoma.

Germ cell tumours

Seminoma

> ► Commonest type of testicular tumour
> ► Germ cell origin
> ► Peak incidence 30–50 years
> ► Histological subtypes: classical — lymphocytic stromal infiltrate; spermatocytic; anaplastic; with syncytiotrophoblast giant cells — contain human chorionic gonadotrophin (hCG); combined with other types of tumour

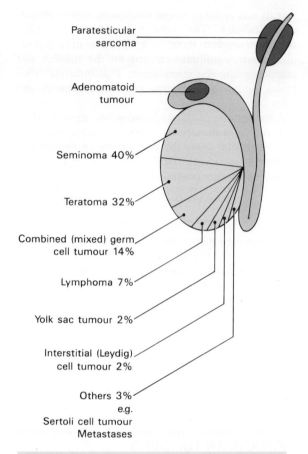

Paratesticular sarcoma

Adenomatoid tumour

Seminoma 40%

Teratoma 32%

Combined (mixed) germ cell tumour 14%

Lymphoma 7%

Yolk sac tumour 2%

Interstitial (Leydig) cell tumour 2%

Others 3% e.g. Sertoli cell tumour Metastases

Fig. 20.15 Relative incidence of different types of testicular tumour

Seminoma has a germ cell origin, arising in the seminiferous epithelium.

Incidence
Seminoma is the commonest type of testicular tumour, comprising 40% of the total incidence. The peak age incidence is between 30 and 50 years (Fig. 20.16). It is the commonest type of tumour to develop in a maldescended testis.

Morphology and classification
The testis is enlarged by a homogeneous firm white solid tumour (Fig. 20.17). This tumour replaces all or part of the body of the testis. A rim of residual testis may be compressed at one edge of the tumour.

Five histological subtypes of seminoma are recognised:

- classical
- spermatocytic

% of
tumours

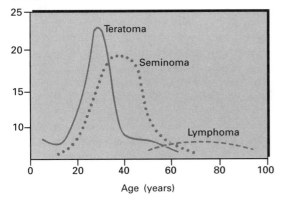

Fig. 20.16   **Age incidence of testicular tumours**

- anaplastic
- with syncytiotrophoblast giant cells
- combined with other types of germ cell tumour
  (p. 610.).

Classical seminoma. This is the commonest sub-type. It is composed of uniform cells with well-defined cell borders. The cytoplasm is vacuolated and contains glycogen. In most of these tumours the stroma contains a variable lymphocytic infiltrate, a favourable prognostic feature (Fig. 20.18). Some tumours may have a histiocytic granulomatous response in the stroma with fibrosis, which correlates with a better prognosis.

Spermatocytic seminoma. About 3–5% of semino-mas are of the spermatocytic type, which occurs in an older age group. The tumour cells resemble spermatocytes and show a marked degree of nuclear pleomorphism with a high mitotic rate. The tumour cells do not contain cytoplasmic glycogen. There is no lymphocytic or granulomatous response in the stroma. Although the histological features suggest an aggressive tumour, the prognosis of this subtype is excellent.

Anaplastic seminoma. This is a histological subtype with marked cellular pleomorphism and a high mitotic rate. The prognosis is slightly worse than for the classical seminoma.

Seminoma with syncytiotrophoblast giant cells. About 5–10% of seminomas contain multi-nucleated syncytiotrophoblast giant cells, distributed through the tumour. Immunocytochemistry demonstrates the presence of human chorionic gonadotrophin (hCG) within these cells (Fig. 20.19). The prognostic implication of this finding is uncertain.

Teratoma

► Germ cell origin
► Peak incidence 20–30 years
► More aggressive than seminomas
► Histological subtypes: differentiated; intermediate; undifferentiated; trophoblastic
► βhCG and alpha-fetoprotein are useful tumour markers

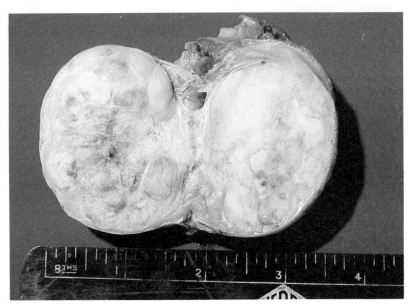

Fig. 20.17   Seminoma

The testis is replaced by a solid and relatively homogeneous neoplasm. Contrast this with the more variegated appearance of a teratoma (Fig. 20.20).

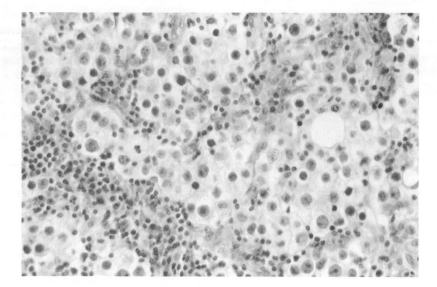

Fig. 20.18   Seminoma

Histology showing the characteristic combination of the large neoplastic cells with clear cytoplasm and the lymphocyte-rich stroma.

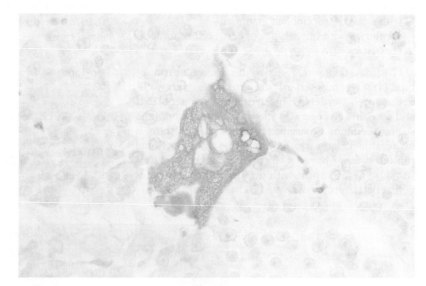

Fig. 20.19   Seminoma

Immunohistology showing a trophoblastic giant cell containing human chorionic gonadotrophin (brown).

Teratomas are composed of several types of tissue representing endoderm, ectoderm and mesoderm (Fig. 20.20). They are now thought to be of germ cell origin, and not from totipotent cells which have escaped the influence of organisers in the embryo. Teratomas have a peak incidence between 20 and 30 years of age and are more aggressive tumours than seminomas.

Classification
In the classification used in the UK and elsewhere, there are four histological subgroups of teratoma:

- differentiated

- malignant intermediate
- malignant undifferentiated
- malignant trophoblastic.

A similar classification, based on the World Health Organization system, is used in the USA. The main differences between the UK and USA classifications are with regard to teratoma undifferentiated and teratoma trophoblastic, which approximate respectively to *embryonal carcinoma* and *choriocarcinoma* in the USA (WHO) classification.

Differentiated teratoma. In this type of teratoma all the component tissues are fully differentiated; there are no histological features of malignancy. Such tumours are rare, usually occurring in infancy. The differentiated tumour (TD) is cystic; the cysts are lined by different types of epithelia. The stroma contains mature cartilage, muscle and bone.

Malignant teratoma intermediate. The malignant teratoma intermediate (MTI) group of tumours are partly solid and partly cystic. There are areas of organoid differentiation, with muscle and stromal cells arranged in a circumferential pattern around spaces lined by bronchial or alimentary type epithelium (Fig. 20.21). There are also histologically malignant areas with cellular pleomorphism and necrosis.

Malignant teratoma undifferentiated. Malignant teratoma undifferentiated (MTU) tumours are composed entirely of sheets and trabeculae of undifferentiated cells with marked nuclear pleomorphism and a high mitotic rate. There is usually extensive tumour necrosis. There are no areas of organoid differentiation (Fig. 20.22).

Malignant teratoma trophoblastic. The malignant teratoma trophoblastic (MTT) contains areas of syncytiotrophoblast and cytotrophoblast arranged in a villous pattern. A teratoma should be included in this category even if only a small area of the tumour is composed of trophoblastic tissue. Trophoblastic teratomas are often haemorrhagic. Vascular invasion by the tumour is a characteristic feature and blood-borne metastases are common. HCG and alpha-fetoprotein (AFP) are valuable markers for this type of teratoma and may be measured in the serum and also demonstrated in the syncytiotrophoblast cells by immunocytochemistry (Fig. 20.23).

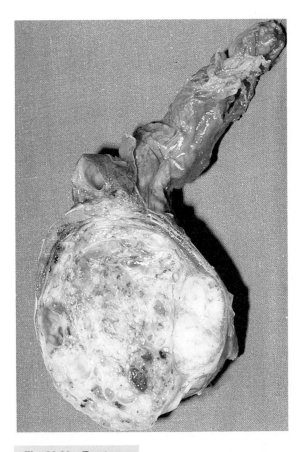

Fig. 20.20   Teratoma

A cystic and haemorrhagic tumour replaces the testis. Contrast this with the more uniform appearance of a seminoma (Fig. 20.17).

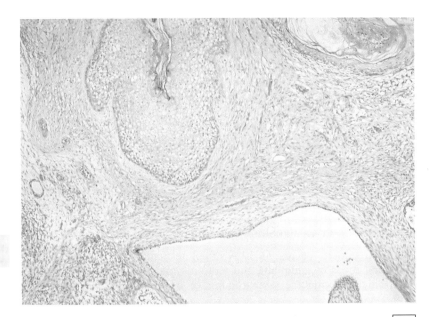

Fig. 20.21   Malignant teratoma intermediate

Histology showing neoplastic epithelium and stroma forming organoid structures.

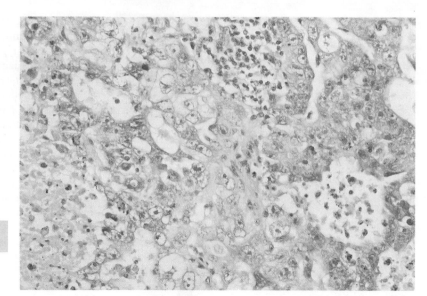

Fig. 20.22 Malignant teratoma undifferentiated

This lesion lacks recognisable organoid structures and shows extensive tumour necrosis (at left).

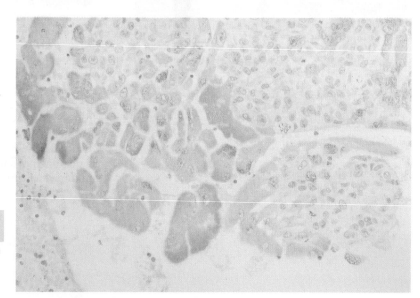

Fig. 20.23 Malignant teratoma trophoblastic

Immunohistology for human chorionic gonadotrophin (brown) revealing evidence of trophoblastic differentiation.

The above classification has prognostic value, with differentiated teratomas having an excellent prognosis and trophoblastic teratomas a poor prognosis.

Combined germ cell tumours

A mixed pattern occurs in 14% of all testicular tumours. Areas of seminoma and teratoma may be intermingled within the same tumour or occur as separate nodules.

In these combined tumours, immunocytochemistry is of value in identifying small foci of more aggressive tissue components such as trophoblast. The prognosis in mixed tumours is determined by the subtype of teratoma.

Non-germ cell tumours

Malignant lymphoma

Malignant lymphoma comprises about 7% of testicular tumours with a peak incidence between 60 and 80 years. The tumours are often bilateral and, in some cases, may be the first manifestation of a diffuse disease involving lymph nodes, liver and spleen.

The testis is enlarged and replaced by a homogeneous fleshy white tumour. This is a *non-Hodgkin's lymphoma*, usually a poorly differentiated B-cell lymphoma with a diffuse pattern (Ch. 22). Typically, the neoplastic cells infiltrate between the seminiferous tubules without destroying the tubular architecture. There is also neoplastic infiltration of the walls of veins within the tumour.

Yolk sac tumour

Yolk sac tumour usually occurs before the age of three years and is the commonest type of testicular tumour in the child; its other name is *orchioblastoma*. It may also occur in adults, usually as one component of a mixed germ cell tumour and less often in pure form.

Histology shows an adenopapillary pattern with columnar or flattened cells containing intracytoplasmic eosinophilic globules. There are also characteristic structures termed Schiller–Duval bodies formed by a perivascular layer of tumour cells (Fig. 20.24). AFP is a valuable marker for this type of tumour and may be detected in the serum and by immunocytochemistry within the neoplastic cells. Occasionally foci of yolk sac differentiation are seen in malignant teratomas.

Interstitial (Leydig) cell tumour

Tumours arising from the interstitial or Leydig cells of the testis are uncommon, comprising only 2% of testicular tumours. The peak age incidence is between 30 and 45 years. This type of tumour may produce androgens and cause precocious sexual development in boys. Paradoxically, gynaecomastia may be the initial manifestation.

An interstitial cell tumour forms a solid yellow–brown nodule within the body of the testis, composed of uniform eosinophilic cells arranged in sheets or columns. The majority of interstitial cell tumours are benign.

Sertoli cell tumour

The Sertoli cell tumour is a type of benign testicular tumour which is rare in man. It more commonly develops in dogs, producing feminising features.

Metastatic tumours

Various tumours may occasionally metastasise to the testis but such metastases are usually found only incidentally at autopsy and very rarely present clinically as testicular enlargement. Carcinoma of the bronchus or prostate and malignant melanoma are among the more frequent primary tumours involved.

Testicular infiltrates of acute lymphoblastic leukaemia cells resist chemotherapy; the testes and central nervous system are 'privileged sites' in this

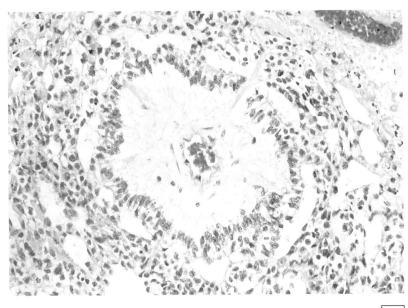

Fig. 20.24   Yolk sac tumour

Histology showing the characteristic arrangement of tumour cells around a blood vessel (Schiller–Duval body).

respect. Consequently, irradiation of the testes has been advocated, even though this causes hypogonadism and infertility.

Dissemination

Testicular tumours initially invade the body of the testis and spread locally to the rete testis and epididymis. Invasion of the fibrous tunica albuginea occurs at a late stage. Invasion of lymphatic spaces leads to spread along the spermatic cord to the internal iliac and para-aortic lymph nodes and then to the mediastinal nodes. Vascular invasion results in visceral metastases, most frequently in the lungs and liver, as well as skeletal deposits. Seminomas tend to spread by lymphatics to para-aortic nodes; teratomas tend to spread haematogenously and, occasionally, to lymph nodes.

The microscopic structure of the metastases usually reflects the histology of the primary tumour but sometimes it may consist of one or more other histological types. This discrepancy may be explained by further differentiation of the tumour in the metastasis, either spontaneously or as a result of chemotherapy. Alternatively, a small focus of some other tumour type may have been missed in the initial histological examination of a mixed germ cell tumour.

Clinical diagnosis and management

If a testicular neoplasm is suspected clinically, a surgical exploration of the testis is required. If the testis is enlarged or nodular, orchidectomy is performed. There is no place for open biopsy, frozen section diagnosis or needle biopsy in the diagnosis of these tumours. Such techniques carry the risk of tumour implantation and may lead to a sampling error in the diagnosis of a heterogeneous tumour. An inguinal orchidectomy is the treatment of choice; a scrotal incision carries the risk of scrotal recurrence if the tunica albuginea is incised. Histology of the orchidectomy specimen is essential to confirm the clinical diagnosis of a neoplasm and determine its type. This examination must include adequate sampling of the tumour to detect more aggressive components such as yolk sac tumour or choriocarcinoma. Immunocytochemical staining of the tumour may aid the detection of areas of yolk sac tumour or trophoblastic tissue.

The degree of local spread is assessed by examination of the rete testis and the resection margin of the spermatic cord.

A variety of imaging techiques are available for the detection of metastases. These include conventional radiography using chest X-ray to identify mediastinal lymph node or pulmonary metastases. Intravenous urography will indicate ureteric distortion by para-aortic lymph node metastases. A more accurate assessment of possible iliac and para-aortic lymph node metastases is available by non-invasive imaging techniques including abdominal ultrasound and computer assisted tomography (CAT scan) for the detection of small visceral and nodal metastases.

In the investigation of a patient with a testicular neoplasm, these techniques are used after the orchidectomy to assess the presence and extent of metastatic disease before planning therapy. They enable an accurate *staging* of the disease to be made, as follows:

Stage I — tumour confined to the testis and its coverings
Stage II — tumour involving the testis and para-aortic lymph nodes
IIA — radiological evidence of node metastases
IIB — bulky, palpable retroperitoneal disease
Stage III — involvement of lymph nodes in the mediastinum and/or supraclavicular region
Stage IV — visceral metastases.

Tumour markers

Certain tumour products appear in the serum with some testicular tumours and are of value in monitoring the response to therapy (Fig. 20.25). These tumour products also provide an early indication of tumour recurrence. This allows a lead time for further courses of treatment, enabling early detection of relapse when the tumour load is minimal and therefore chemotherapy is more effective.

The most useful markers are alpha-fetoprotein (AFP), produced by elements of yolk sac tumour, and the β subunit of human chorionic gonadotrophin (βhCG) produced by trophoblastic components. More recently, the placental-like iso-enzyme of alkaline phosphatase (PLAP) is proving a useful marker for seminoma.

An ideal protocol for the measurement of serum markers includes a pre-operative sample followed by frequent post-orchidectomy samples. Levels should be measured twice each week during the first two months post-operatively, or until basal levels return, then weekly for six months. If tumour recurrence is detected, more frequent measurements will be required. Tumour markers have biological half-life

Alpha-fetoprotein level

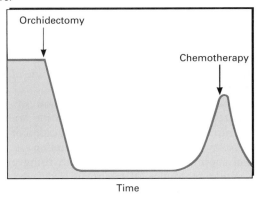

The blood level of the tumour marker (alpha-fetoprotein in this instance) is high at presentation but falls when the tumour is removed. Regular monitoring, however, shows a rise in blood levels of alpha-fetoprotein corresponding to a tumour recurrence. The levels again fall with chemotherapy.

decay times of four days for AFP and one day in the case of βhCG.

Prognosis

There has been a marked improvement in the prognosis for patients with testicular tumours during the last few years. Seminoma is a very radiosensitive tumour which has an excellent prognosis. The main improvements, however, have occurred in patients with non-seminomatous germ cell tumours and are due to three main factors: the development of more precise imaging techniques to improve staging; the development of assays fot tumour markers; and the use of improved chemotherapeutic agents. As a result, the cure rate is now similar to that of seminoma.

Until recently, the management usually involved orchidectomy followed by prophylactic irradiation of the para-aortic lymph nodes. This regime resulted in a 90–95% cure rate for seminoma. A more recent and now accepted management of both seminoma and teratoma is orchidectomy followed by surveillance with imaging techniques and serum markers; recurrences of tumour are then treated with chemotherapy. If the patient survives for two years after completion of chemotherapy with no evidence of recurrence then cure is likely.

MALE INFERTILITY

Male infertility may be due to:

- endocrine disorders — e.g. gonadotrophin deficiency; oestrogen excess — hepatic cirrhosis
- testicular lesions — cryptorchidism; Klinefelter's syndrome; maturation arrest of spermatogenesis — idiopathic, varicocele, pyrexial illness; irradiation; defective spermatozoa (e.g. immotile cilia)
- post-testicular lesions — blockage of efferent ducts, congenital or secondary to an inflammatory process; impotence — neurological disorders.

The clinical assessment of infertile men includes thorough investigation to determine the precise nature of the problem. This may include a testicular biopsy to assess the integrity of the seminiferous tubules and the degree of spermatogenesis.

EPIDIDYMIS AND CORD

Congenital anomalies

In about 10% of men, the epididymis is situated anterior to a normal intrascrotal testis, instead of in its usual posterior position. This abnormality may cause diagnostic problems in palpation of other lesions. *Maldescent* of the testis may be accompanied by an abnormality in the position of the epididymis, which then lies along the course of the spermatic cord.

Rarely, an *extra vas deferens* is present on one side, or one may be *absent*. This latter condition may be associated with absence or hypoplasia of the corresponding epididymis. These abnormalities are of practical importance to the surgeon at vasectomy.

Several vestigial structures adjacent to the epididymis or mesorchium may become enlarged and cystic. These include aberrant ductules and the appendix of the epididymis. They usually remain small but may undergo torsion, with resulting infarction, presenting as an acute painful swelling.

Epididymal cysts

Acquired cysts of the epididymis are more common than the congenital types. An obstruction to the passage of sperm along the narrow lumen of the vas or obstruction of an epididymal tubule results in cystic dilatation of the duct system in the epididymis and efferent ductules of the testis. The resulting spermatocele forms a swelling in the epididymis, above and behind the testis on palpation (Fig. 20.26). It is usually a multilocular cyst with opalescent fluid containing sperms.

Varicocele

A varicocele is varicosity of the pampiniform plexus of veins around the spermatic cord (Fig. 20.26). This may be a *primary varicocele* with no obvious underlying cause, more common on the left side. It may be related to maldevelopment of valves in the pampiniform veins or the testicular vein; on the left side the testicular vein drains into the left renal vein almost at 90°.

A *secondary varicocele* is the result of venous obstruction and occurs with equal frequency on both sides. One cause is a carcinoma of the kidney invading the renal vein and obstructing the testicular vein.

A varicocele may raise the intrascrotal temperature as a result of increased blood flow, reducing spermatogenesis and causing *subfertility*.

Torsion of the spermatic cord

Torsion of the spermatic cord involves twisting of the testis and epididymis together on their axis. It is an acute surgical emergency, presenting as a swollen, hard, painful testis. The patient is usually aged 13–16 years. An earlier peak incidence occurs under the age of one year. Torsion of the spermatic cord is often precipitated by exertion, which causes contraction of the cremaster muscle. There is sometimes a history of preceding minor, less painful episodes of testicular pain.

Several anatomical abnormalities, often bilateral, predispose to this lesion. They include maldescent of the testis, an abnormally long spermatic cord, or an abnormally long mesorchium. The torsion usually occurs within the tunica vaginalis, involving only the testis and epididymis. If it occurs above the level of the tunica it involves all structures in that side of the scrotum.

Torsion produces an initial occlusion of the venous return from the testis, although the arterial flow continues for a time. There is congestion of the testis followed by haemorrhagic infarction as the arterial supply becomes impaired with rising pressure within the tunica. If treatment is delayed the infarction progresses, finally resulting in a shrunken, fibrotic testis and epididymis.

Inflammatory lesions

Acute epididymo-orchitis

An acute inflammation of the body of the testis (*orchitis*) most frequently develops in association with an initial *epididymitis* which later spreads to the testis. The commonest underlying cause is a *urinary tract infection* with coliform organisms; it may also develop after a *prostatectomy* if the vasa deferentia are not ligated. A *urethritis*, either gonococcal or nonspecific, may be complicated by an epididymo-orchitis. In all these instances, the infection spreads along the vas deferens or the lymphatics of the spermatic cord to the epididymis.

The process may be unilateral or bilateral. The epididymis and testis are enlarged, warm and painful. These signs are accompanied by fever and malaise. Histology shows an acute inflammatory process. There may be a secondary hydrocele. The

A

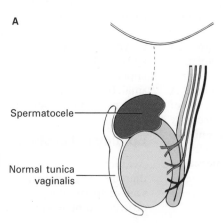

B

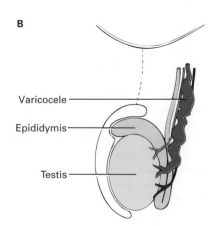

**Fig. 20.26
Spermatocele
and varicocele**

A. Spermatoceles are derived from the epididymis.
B. Varicoceles are lesions of the pampiniform venous plexus in which there is excessive tortuosity and dilatation.

Spermatocele

Normal tunica vaginalis

Varicocele

Epididymis

Testis

inflammation is usually mild and resolves either spontaneously or with antibiotic therapy; in severe cases it may, however, progress to suppuration.

Less often, an epididymo-orchitis may complicate a septicaemia (e.g. meningococcal).

Tuberculous epididymo-orchitis

Tuberculous infection of the male genital tract is now rare but the epididymis used to be the commonest site of involvement in the male. Infection of the epididymis is secondary to a tuberculous lesion elsewhere in the urinary tract, such as the kidney or bladder, with extension of the infection along the vas deferens.

In about one-third of cases the infection is bilateral, resulting in nodular enlargement of the epididymis. There may be a secondary hydrocele and, in an advanced infection, the inflamed epididymis becomes adherent to the scrotal skin with the formation of sinuses. The infection may spread directly to the *testis* with the formation of areas of caseation necrosis and the characteristic granulomatous inflammation. There may also be extension to the prostate or seminal vesicles. Microscopy of the urine shows a 'sterile' pyuria with acid-alcohol-fast bacilli.

Sperm granuloma

Sperm granuloma is an uncommon chronic inflammatory lesion involving the epididymis and resulting from extravasation of sperm from the tubules into the interstitium. There is an associated inflammatory reaction composed mainly of histiocytes and polymorphs, with secondary fibrosis. The process results in the formation of a firm swelling in the epididymis. The cause is uncertain, although there may be a preceding history of an epididymitis.

A similar cellular response to extravasated sperm may sometimes be seen in the spermatic cord at the site of recent vasectomy, forming a localised nodule at the operation site.

Tumours

Tumours of the epididymis and spermatic cord are relatively rare, together forming only 1–2% of the total group of testicular tumours. They include:

- adenomatoid tumour
- paratesticular sarcoma.

Adenomatoid tumour

Adenomatoid tumour is an uncommon, benign neoplasm of the epididymis, which may develop over a wide age range, and presents as a slowly enlarging painless firm nodule in the epididymis. Examination reveals a circumscribed solid nodule 10–20 mm in diameter, composed of irregular clefts and spaces lined by flattened or cuboidal cells. These cells merge with an intervening stroma of fibrous tissue and smooth muscle. The histogenesis of this lesion is debatable, but current opinion favours a mesothelial origin. A similar neoplasm may occur in the female over the uterine serosa or in the fallopian tube. This localisation to the genital tract has led to the alternative view that these tumours arise from Müllerian remnants.

Paratesticular sarcoma

Paratesticular sarcomas of the spermatic cord are rare neoplasms which present as an inguinal or scrotal swelling, the tumour forming a mass separate from the body of the testis and epididymis. The types of tumour which occur vary with age: in children and adolescents the majority are rhabdomyosarcomas; in adults, the lesion may be a leiomyosarcoma, liposarcoma or fibrosarcoma. These tumours have a poor prognosis and metastasise by lymphatics and veins.

FURTHER READING

Ansell I D 1985 Atlas of male reproductive pathology. MTP Press, Lancaster

Ansell I D 1994 Carcinoma of prostate. In: Current diagnostic pathology, vol 1, no 3. Churchill Livingstone, Edinburgh, pp 167–173

Dearnley D P 1994 Cancer of the prostate. British Medical Journal 308: 780–784

Hill G S (ed) 1989 Uropathology, vol 2. Churchill Livingstone, New York, pp 1165–1380

Jacobsen G K, Talerman A 1989 Atlas of germ cell tumours. Munksgaard, Copenhagen

Kidneys and urinary tract

NORMAL STRUCTURE AND FUNCTION OF THE KIDNEYS

The kidneys contribute to the body's biochemical homeostasis by:

- eliminating metabolic waste products
- regulating fluid and electrolyte balance
- influencing acid–base balance.

These vital functions are effected by the filtration of blood plasma in the glomeruli and subsequent processing of the filtrate by the tubules to eventually produce urine.

The kidneys also produce the following hormones:

- *prostaglandins*, which are thought to affect salt and water regulation and influence vascular tone
- *erythropoietin*, which stimulates red cell production
- *1,25-dihydroxycholecalciferol*, which enhances calcium absorption from the gut and phosphate reabsorption by the renal tubules
- *renin*, which acts on the angiotensin pathway to increase vascular tone and aldosterone production.

The kidneys have a large functional reserve; the loss of one kidney produces no ill-effects. However, in renal disease waste products can accumulate, causing a condition known as *uraemia*. If the glomerular filters become excessively leaky, large protein molecules are lost in the urine — *proteinuria*. If the glomeruli are severely damaged, erythrocytes pass through causing *haematuria*.

The basic unit of the kidney is the *nephron*; each comprises a glomerulus connected to a tubule. Each kidney contains approximately 1 million nephrons. These form in the embryonic metanephros, after the physiological involution of the pronephros and mesonephros. The ureter, calyceal system and collecting ducts form from the ureteric bud arising from the original duct of the pronephros — the Wolffian duct. These two separately derived structures must fuse; failure results in developmental abnormalities.

The kidneys are in the retroperitoneum; the upper poles lie beneath the 12th rib. There is considerable movement with respiration which must be controlled to avoid tearing when the kidneys are biopsied. Each adult kidney weighs approximately 150 g and has a smooth encapsulated surface. Deep clefts occasionally divide the surface into several lobes, a developmental abnormality of no pathological significance. The medial aspect of each kidney is indented to form the hilum, where the renal artery

and vein and the ureter join with the organ. The cut surface reveals a clearly defined outer cortex and an inner medulla. The medulla comprises the pyramids, which show striations converging into the 8–11 papillae projecting into the calyceal system. Columns of cortical tissue extend between the pyramids towards the hilum. The cortex and cortical columns contain glomeruli and the proximal and distal convoluted tubules. The medulla contains very thin tubules, the loops of Henle, and the collecting ducts.

Glomerular structure and function

The formation of urine begins in the glomeruli, where the filtration of approximately 800 litres of plasma each day results in 180 litres of filtrate, most of which is reabsorbed in the tubules. Each glomerulus consists of a complex tuft of capillaries projecting into Bowman's space (Fig. 21.1). The glomerular capillary comprises:

- endothelial cells
- basement membrane
- epithelial cells.

The capillary tuft is supported by relatively inconspicuous *mesangial cells*, which proliferate and become more prominent in some diseases. Glomeruli have a lobulated architecture which is very difficult to appreciate normally, but becomes pronounced in some renal diseases. Glomerular endothelial cells are fenestrated; they have small 'windows', allowing the plasma direct contact with the underlying basement membrane (Fig. 21.2). The endothelial cells thereby act as a crude sieve, retaining only the cellular elements of the blood.

The *basement membrane* is the most important filtration component of the capillary wall. The basement membrane proteoglycans (particularly heparan sulphate) are anionic and thus carry a negative charge. These account for the charge-dependent filtration that normally retains proteins in the plasma. The basement membrane also contains type IV collagen, which limits the effective pore size to 3.5 nm, just below the diameter of albumin molecules, which are normally retained. Smaller molecules traverse the membrane with relative ease.

The external aspect of the basement membrane is covered by the epithelial cells. These have long cellular processes (foot processes) which envelop the capillary loops. The glycocalyx covering the endothelial and epithelial cells contains anionic sialoglycoproteins, also contributing to the charge-dependent filtration barrier.

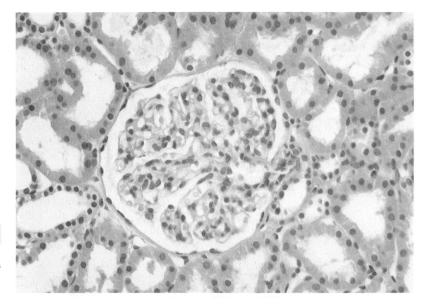

Fig. 21.1 Normal glomerulus

Each glomerulus consists of capillaries invested by epithelial cells and is surrounded by Bowman's space.

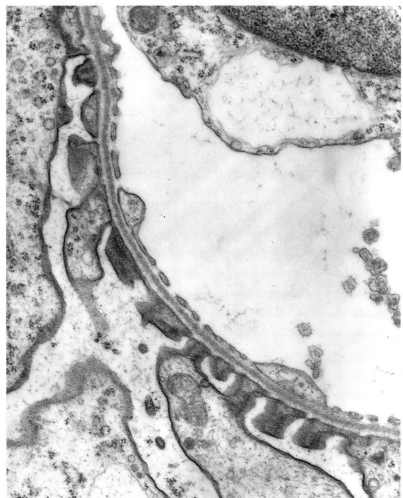

Fig. 21.2 Ultrastructure of the glomerular capillary

The wall of each glomerular capillary comprises an inner thin layer of fenestrated vascular endothelium, the basement membrane and an outer epithelial layer characterised by cytoplasmic ('foot') processes. (Transmission electron micrograph)

Blood enters and leaves the glomerular capillaries by arterioles. Thus, in contrast to all other systemic capillaries in which there is a fall in pressure towards the venous end, the pressure remains high in the glomerular capillary throughout its length—a feature which is essential to efficient filtration.

Juxtaglomerular apparatus

At the vascular pole of the glomerulus is the juxtaglomerular apparatus. This cluster of specialised cells secretes renin, one of the hormones produced by the kidney. Renin is released in response to:

- reduced blood volume
- low sodium concentration in distal tubular fluid

- sympathetic nervous stimulation
- renal ischaemia.

Renin acts on precursor molecules to form, ultimately, angiotensin II (Ch. 17) which, among other effects, stimulates the zona glomerulosa of the adrenal cortex to produce aldosterone. In turn, aldosterone acts on the distal renal tubular epithelium to increase the reabsorption of sodium.

The glomerular filtrate, which is isotonic with the plasma, has to be substantially modified osmotically so that water and electrolytes are conserved and the waste metabolites are concentrated for elimination as urine. This process occurs as the filtrate flows through the tubules, each segment having specific roles (Fig. 21.3).

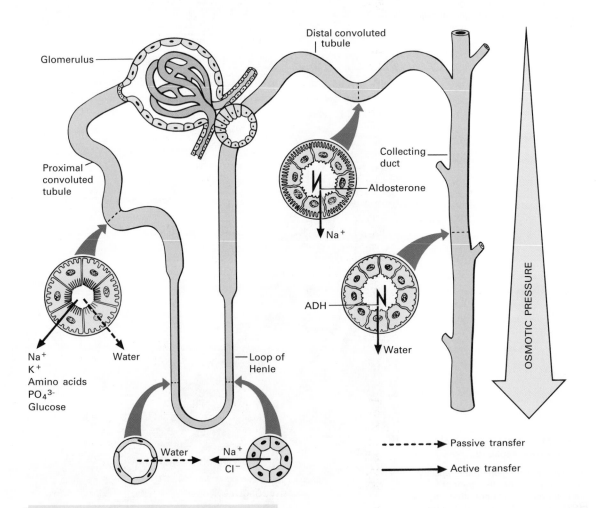

Fig. 21.3   Renal tubular structure and function

Schematic representation of a single nephron showing the function of each part of the tubule. The composition of the glomerular filtrate is modified as it flows along the tubule to form urine.

Tubular structure and function

In the *proximal convoluted tubule*, 60–80% of the sodium in the filtrate is selectively reabsorbed. Amino acids, potassium and phosphate, together with all of the glucose, are also actively reabsorbed. All of these substances are osmotically active, and as a consequence 60–80% of the water in the filtrate moves passively from the lumen of the proximal convoluted tubule into the blood in the peritubular capillaries. The high level of metabolic activity of the proximal convoluted tubule cells renders them vulnerable to ischaemia and toxins.

The *loop of Henle* is the next part of the nephron through which the now reduced volume of filtrate must pass. The loop of Henle is responsible for the development of a high osmotic pressure within the medulla by a process known as the countercurrent system. The active transfer of sodium from the tubular fluid into the interstitium by the cells of the ascending limb is the essential factor in the countercurrent mechanism. This transfer creates a hypertonic environment in the interstitium of the medulla, with the highest osmotic pressures in the depths of the medulla.

The *distal tubule* is continuous with the ascending limb of the loop of Henle. Where it comes close to the vascular pole of the glomerulus, there is a specialised arrangement of closely packed cells known as the *macula densa*. The convoluted part of the distal tubule is fairly short and soon empties into the collecting duct. The final adjustment to the sodium concentration in the tubular fluid is made in the distal convoluted tubule, where sodium is exchanged for potassium and hydrogen ions under the influence of aldosterone. The cells of the distal convoluted tubule also de-aminate amino acids to produce ammonia, which passes into the lumen and combines with hydrogen ions to produce ammonium salts. Thus, the distal tubule plays an important role in acid–base balance.

The *collecting ducts* receive modified filtrate from the distal convoluted tubules and pass through the medulla. The epithelial cells of the collecting ducts are selectively permeable to water under the influence of antidiuretic hormone (ADH). Thus, as the tubular fluid passes through the hypertonic renal medulla, ADH released from the posterior pituitary allows water to be osmotically reabsorbed, producing a hypertonic urine.

Renal papillae and urinary reflux

The collecting ducts open onto the surface of the renal papillae projecting into the calyces. The shape of the duct orifice is relevant to the development of pyelonephritis (p. 646). Two patterns have been described:

- In the *mid-zone papillae*, the ducts open obliquely onto the surface of the papilla. In the event of urinary reflux from the bladder, these duct orifices will close under the increased pressure in the pelvicalyceal system.
- In contrast, those in the *polar papillae* have no valve effect and remain widely patent, thus allowing the refluxed urine and any bacteria within it to be transmitted into the parenchyma of the kidney.

Physiological changes

During pregnancy

During pregnancy the size and weight of the kidneys increases and the glomeruli are enlarged. These changes are reflected in the raised glomerular filtration rate and renal plasma flow which reach a peak by 16 weeks and persist until the end of pregnancy.

Ageing

The weight of the kidneys begins to fall abruptly after the age of 60 years. Gradual shrinkage of the tubules commences at about 40 years. Arteries display intimal thickening, with progressive reduplication of elastic laminae. Small arteries develop medial hypertrophy and hyalinosis. The number of sclerosed or scarred glomeruli increases with age, thus reducing renal reserve. Drugs that are usually excreted by the kidneys must, therefore, be used with caution in the elderly to avoid toxic accumulation.

URINARY TRACT DISEASE

Clinicopathological features

Diseases of the urinary tract can present with a variety of features, alone or in combination. As the kidneys are so often affected by a primary disease elsewhere in the body, a simple urine examination (e.g. colour, glucose, protein, haemoglobin) is routine practice in patients being investigated for a variety of disorders.

Investigation

The investigation of patients with known or suspected urinary tract disease is multidisciplinary (Table 21.1). Urine and blood analyses are essential;

imaging, biopsies and cystoscopy are optional depending on the nature of the clinical problem. Tests with the greatest general clinical utility are urine testing for glucose (to exclude uncontrolled diabetes mellitus), protein (to determine the permeability characteristics of the glomerular basement membrane), and determination of the blood concentrations of urea and/or creatinine, the latter being a more reliable indicator of renal function.

Renal biopsy is performed only when justified by the clinical circumstances, because of the attendant risk of haemorrhage. The biopsy is examined by light microscopy with additional information revealed by immunofluorescence and electron microscopy.

Accurate information about the incidence of diseases of the urinary tract is available from transplant and dialysis registries. However, two important factors conspire to make the true incidence of renal disease almost impossible to ascertain. First, not all countries have registries for the accurate recording of cases. Second, transplantation and dialysis registries record severe and end-stage disease only, making no allowance for mild and subliminal disease. Clinical experience suggests that the prevalence of post-infectious glomerulonephritis is much higher in Africa and India than in Europe and North America.

Table 21.1 Investigation of patients with urinary tract disease

Investigation	Diagnostic utility
Urine analysis Volume Specific gravity Culture Protein content Glucose Haemoglobin Microscopy (casts, etc.)	Determination of urine production rate and concentrating power of the kidneys; investigation of urinary tract infections; urinary protein indicates integrity of glomerular filter; exclusion of diabetes mellitus; investigation of glomerular or tubular lesions
Blood analysis Urea Creatinine Electrolytes	Determination of integrity of renal function; glomerular filtration rate can be calculated from urinary and plasma creatinine concentration and urine flow rate
Imaging Plain X-ray Ultrasound Contrast urography Angiography	Determination of kidney size and symmetry; investigation of suspected tumours, cysts, etc.; detection of calculi; position and integrity of ureters
Renal biopsy Histology Electron microscopy Immunofluorescence	Diagnosis of glomerular, tubular and interstitial renal diseases
Cystoscopy	Investigation of haematuria and other symptoms; biopsy of bladder lesions

Pathological basis for urinary tract symptoms and signs

Symptom or sign	Pathological basis
Proteinuria	Increased permeability of the glomerular basement membrane
Uraemia	Renal failure
Haematuria	Severe glomerular injury (red cell casts on urine microscopy) Renal tumours or trauma Bladder tumours or trauma
Urinary casts • Hyaline casts	Formed in tubules as a result of protein loss from glomeruli
• Granular casts	Formed in tubules from aggregates of inflammatory cells
• Red cell casts	Formed in tubules from red cells in filtrate from severely damaged glomeruli
Hypertension	Renal ischaemia releasing renin
Oliguria or anuria	Severe renal failure (acute or chronic), obstruction or dehydration
Polyuria	Excessive fluid intake (e.g. beer) Osmotic diuresis (e.g. diabetes mellitus) Impaired tubular concentration (e.g. diabetes insipidus)
Renal (ureteric) colic	Calculus, blood clot or tumour in ureter
Oedema	Hypoalbuminaemia due to albumin loss in urine (nephrotic syndrome)
Dysuria	Stimulation of pain receptors in urethra due to inflammation

CONGENITAL DISEASES

Approximately 10% of individuals have a congenital abnormality of the urinary tract. Some are hereditary.

Congenital renal diseases may be:

- malformations related to the volume of renal tissue formed or its differentiation
- anatomical abnormalities of position of vascular or ureteric connections
- metabolic lesions such as enzyme defects which affect tubular transport (e.g. cystinuria and renal tubular acidosis).

Conditions affecting the volume of renal tissue

Bilateral agenesis of the kidneys (Potter's syndrome) is not compatible with independent life. It occurs in 0.04% of all pregnancies. Children with this condition have a characteristic appearance — low-set ears, a receding chin, wide-set eyes and a 'parrot beak' nose. There is always a reduced volume of amniotic fluid (oligohydramnios) due to the absence of fetal urine. The majority of such cases are stillborn. The most likely cause is a failure of the ureteric bud to develop; there are developmental abnormalities also of other tissues derived from the mesonephros, e.g. bladder and genitalia. However, the commonly associated spinal cord abnormalities and pulmonary hypoplasia suggest that the defect is more generalised.

Unilateral agenesis of a kidney is infrequent. The opposite kidney undergoes marked hypertrophy and is subsequently prone to infections and trauma. Children with this condition often do not survive long because of associated multiple developmental abnormalities, including congenital heart disease, spina bifida and meningomyelocele.

In *renal hypoplasia*, the kidney is abnormally small but not otherwise malformed. Hypoplastic kidneys are prone to infection or stone formation.

Disorders of differentiation

Renal dysplasia is a cause of a cystic kidney, which may present in childhood as an abdominal mass requiring surgical excision if only to exclude a malignant tumour (e.g. nephroblastoma). The lesion is characterised by islands of undifferentiated mesenchyme or cartilage within the parenchyma. If the lesion is unilateral, the prognosis is good.

Anatomical abnormalities

Ectopic kidneys form in an abnormal site, usually the pelvis, and may be associated with intestinal malrotation. The principal clinical importance lies in their presenting as a suspicious pelvic mass, and in the risk of infection due to the ureteric kinking that often accompanies this condition.

Horseshoe kidney results from fusion of the two nephrogenic blastemas during fetal life. The majority are fused at the lower pole. The condition is not rare and renal function is usually normal. There may be a susceptibility to infection and stone formation.

Reduplication of vessels or ureters is not uncommon, achieving clinical significance either when an anomalous polar artery passing anterior to the ureter causes ureteric obstruction, or during renal transplantation.

Metabolic abnormalities

Cystinuria (Ch. 7) results from defective tubular reabsorption of several amino acids including cystine, lysine, ornithine and arginine. The precise enzyme defect is unknown, but some patients also have impaired intestinal transport. Cystine crystals are found in the urine and calculi may develop. The disease is inherited as an autosomal recessive. Cystinuria is quite distinct from cystinosis.

Renal tubular acidosis type 1 is probably due to a defect in the enzyme system which enables hydrogen ions to be exchanged for bicarbonate in the proximal tubule. There is loss of bicarbonate and failure to acidify and concentrate the urine. Renal function is otherwise good, but there is a tendency to form stones and develop infections. This condition is inherited as an autosomal dominant gene, although an identical deficiency may be acquired as a result of tubular damage.

Congenital nephrotic syndrome

This rare condition has an autosomal recessive pattern of inheritance. It was originally described in Finland, but has subsequently been shown to occur in other countries. The microcystic appearance of the kidneys arises from dilatation of the proximal tubules and Bowman's capsule. A defect in glycosaminoglycan synthesis has been suggested, which would correlate with the abnormal ultrastructural appearance of the glomerular basement membrane and the development of nephrotic syndrome due to excessive proteinuria. These patients are particularly vulnerable to pneumococcal infection. Congenital nephrotic syndrome can be predicted in utero by the detection of high levels of alpha-fetoprotein in the amniotic fluid and maternal blood. There is no treatment for this condition, but the lesion does not recur in a transplanted kidney.

Alport's disease

Alport's disease is recognised clinically by the triad of:

- nephritis
- deafness
- ocular lesions.

The condition is inherited as a dominant trait which is variably expressed. Males are affected more severely and more frequently than females. Renal involvement is heralded by haematuria commencing usually in the first decade, but may be delayed until the twenties, especially in females. Renal failure by the second decade is the eventual outcome in the majority of males. In contrast, in females renal function may be preserved until the fifth decade. The deafness, which is for high-pitched sounds, is often difficult to demonstrate. Ocular disease occurs only in severely affected patients and involves dislocation of the lens, cataracts and corneal dystrophy. The pathogenesis of this condition has been clarified by the finding that some patients with Alport's disease lack the Goodpasture antigen (p. 628). Mutations in one of the collagen genes for the synthesis of basement membrane material could provide the common factor for the glomerular and ocular pathology.

CYSTIC DISEASE

> - Cysts may be solitary or multiple, congenital or acquired
> - A solitary cyst may simulate a tumour
> - Congenital polycystic disease may not present until adult life
> - Acquired cysts may be due to renal scarring

Cystic disease of the kidney comprises a heterogeneous group of conditions which are congenital or acquired (Fig. 21.4). Some are an important cause of renal failure. Accurate diagnosis is essential so that, where the disease is genetically transmitted, the appropriate counselling can be given to patients and their relatives.

Cysts in the kidney are classified as:

- simple renal cysts

- adult polycystic disease
- childhood polycystic disease
- congenital nephrotic syndrome (see above)
- renal dialysis-associated.

In two further conditions the cysts are localised to the cortico-medullary junction and the papillae respectively:

- uraemic medullary cystic disease
- medullary sponge kidney.

Simple renal cysts

Simple renal cysts are a common finding both at autopsy and, increasingly, with ultrasound imaging. The incidence increases with age. They may be single or multiple, and vary in size from a few millimetres to several centimetres. They have a smooth lining, usually contain clear fluid, and do not affect renal function. Occasionally, haemorrhage occurs into a cyst, causing pain. Their principal significance lies in circumstances where the distinction between cyst and tumour has to be made.

Adult polycystic disease

Adult polycystic disease is the primary renal disease in 8% of adult patients in the European Dialysis and Transplantation Registry. The condition is always bilateral; the kidneys are grossly enlarged, each commonly weighing 1000 g or more (Fig. 21.5). The kidneys are distorted by numerous cysts, from a few millimetres up to almost 100 mm in diameter, with thin bands of renal parenchyma stretched and compressed between them. Most of the cysts contain clear fluid, but previous haemorrhage can result in the contents being brown due to haemosiderin. Microdissection studies have shown that the cysts are formed at all levels of the nephron.

Adult polycystic disease is inherited as an autosomal dominant trait with a high degree of penetrance; this is relevant to genetic counselling and screening. Patients present with this condition at any age from childhood to late adult life. They maintain their renal function until the enlarging cysts press on the adjacent parenchyma, causing ischaemic changes leading to hypertension or renal failure. There is an association with berry aneurysms of the circle of Willis, a frequent source of an often fatal subarachnoid haemorrhage (Ch. 26). Cysts also occur within the liver, pancreas and lungs, but have no functional significance in these organs.

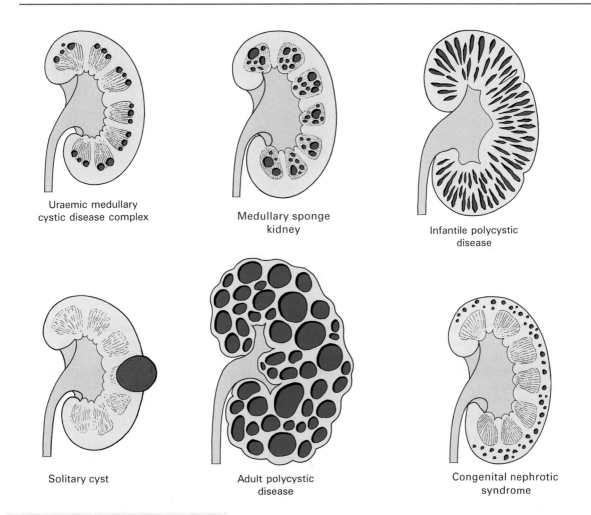

Uraemic medullary
cystic disease complex

Medullary sponge
kidney

Infantile polycystic
disease

Solitary cyst

Adult polycystic
disease

Congenital nephrotic
syndrome

Fig. 21.4   Cystic diseases of the kidneys

Each disease is distinguished by the characteristic distribution of cysts.

Childhood polycystic disease

Childhood polycystic disease is a rare condition which has an autosomal recessive pattern of inheritance. There are several subgroups related to the degree of renal involvement, and more than one gene may be involved.

In the *perinatal subgroup*, which accounts for about 10% of patients with childhood polycystic disease, some 90% of nephrons are involved. There are severe abnormalities at birth, and the baby is either stillborn or dies of renal failure and respiratory distress soon after birth. The kidneys are usually enlarged and show a characteristic radial pattern of rather fusiform cysts which replace both the medulla and cortex and extend nearly to the capsular surface. The cysts are dilated collecting ducts. The enlarged kidneys are usually palpable and may impair delivery.

Neonatal, infantile and juvenile subgroups reflect progressively less severe involvement of the kidney and a longer survival.

All patients with childhood polycystic disease have some abnormality of the liver, ranging from bile duct proliferation and cysts, to substantial hepatic fibrosis which will eventually interfere with hepatic function and produce portal hypertension (Ch. 16).

Dialysis-associated cysts

Dialysis-associated cysts occur in the kidneys of patients in chronic renal failure who have received dialysis treatment for some years. The kidneys,

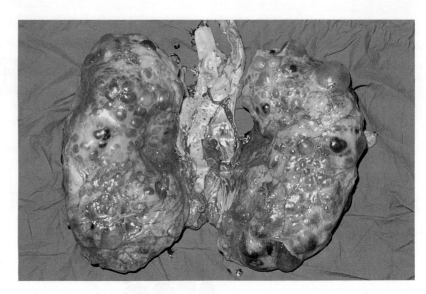

Fig. 21.5   Adult polycystic disease

Both kidneys are greatly enlarged by numerous cysts.

which are severely scarred by the original disease prompting dialysis treatment, contain multiple small cysts throughout the cortex and medulla. The cysts are often associated with oxalate crystals and are thought to arise as a result of obstruction of the tubules by interstitial fibrosis or by the crystals.

Uraemic medullary cystic disease

Uraemic medullary cystic disease (UMCD) complex, or nephronophthisis, is a recently recognised group of conditions accounting for 20–25% of chronic renal failure in children and adolescents. In many cases there is a family history; there is one sub-group showing recessive inheritance and another in which the inheritance is dominant. There is also an association with retinitis pigmentosa. The affected kidneys show numerous cysts at the cortico-medullary junction with interstitial fibrosis and thickened tubular basement membranes.

Medullary sponge kidney

Medullary sponge kidney results from dilated collecting ducts in the medulla, causing cysts mainly in the papillae. It is usually bilateral, but may be unilateral. Renal function is usually normal but calculi may form in the cysts, causing pain and infection.

GLOMERULAR DISEASE

The introduction of percutaneous renal biopsy in the mid-1950s greatly improved knowledge about renal disease by allowing the abnormalities to be studied as they evolved. Before this, kidneys were studied mostly at postmortem, but the changes were so advanced that they essentially represented end-stage disease. Immunofluorescence confirmed that many glomerular diseases are due to immunological reactions (e.g. immune complex deposition). Similarly, electron microscopy enabled visualisation of abnormalities that were undetectable with the light microscope. All of these techniques are used in the assessment of renal biopsies.

Classification

- ► Glomerular disease may be classified by aetiology, immunological reaction or histological pattern
- ► Aetiological classification includes immunological and non-immunological injury
- ► Immunological injury may be due to anti-glomerular basement antibody (anti-GBM) or to immune complex deposition
- ► In immune complex glomerular injury, antigens may be derived from bacteria, parasites, drugs, etc.
- ► Histological classification is based on the reaction of the glomerulus to injury (e.g. proliferative, membranous thickening)
- ► Histological features assist in the identification of aetiology and in therapeutic decisions

Classification of glomerular disease usually presents major difficulties for students of renal disease. As with many aspects of human disease, it is impossible to provide a satisfactory classification of glomerular disease on the basis of one set of features. There are three parallel and complementary classifications:

- aetiological
- immunological
- morphological.

Clinicopathologically, diseases affecting the glomeruli are best grouped initially into the following broad categories:

- *immunological reactions* involving either
  - glomerular antigens (e.g. anti-glomerular basement membrane glomerulonephritis),
  - non-glomerular antigens (e.g. immune complex glomerulonephritis)
- *non-immunological disorders* (e.g. diabetes mellitus); in most cases, the glomerular injury is secondary to events elsewhere in the body.

Nomenclature of glomerular injury

Glomeruli show a limited range of reactions to injury. The following nomenclature is used to describe the pattern of injury:

- *diffuse*: a lesion affecting all glomeruli
- *focal*: a lesion involving some glomeruli, but leaving others unaffected
- *global*: affecting the whole glomerulus
- *segmental*: affecting only part of the glomerulus.

Additional terms are used to describe the character of the light microscopic changes within the glomeruli:

- *proliferative*: increased numbers of cells within the glomerulus; due to proliferation of indigenous cells and to recruitment of polymorphs and macrophages from the circulation as a consequence of activation of the complement cascade
- *membranous change*: the peripheral loops are thickened due to basement membrane expansion
- *membrano-proliferative*: a combination of the two preceding features, often with accentuation of the lobular architecture
- *crescentic*: florid proliferation of cells including macrophages lining Bowman's capsule, often compressing the glomerulus.

Recognition of these changes and the use of this nomenclature have important clinical implications; for example, when crescents are present in >80% of glomeruli, this condition is said to be *crescentic nephritis*, associated with the clinical condition of *rapidly progressive glomerulonephritis*, and heralds a poor prognosis for renal function unless it is treated quickly and vigorously.

Morphology alone gives little indication of the precise nature of the underlying or primary abnormality. Similar morphological features occur in entirely different conditions. To establish as accurate a diagnosis as possible, both immunological and ultrastructural features need to be taken into account. Even so, we remain dismally ignorant of the initiating agent in the majority of cases of glomerular injury.

Clinical presentations

Patients with glomerular disease usually present with one of five possible conditions:

1. *Recurrent painless haematuria* which varies considerably in degree, ranging from macroscopic haematuria to that which may be detected only at a medical examination due to:

- exercise haematuria
- mesangial IgA nephropathy (Berger's disease)
- Henoch–Schönlein purpura
- bacterial endocarditis
- systemic lupus erythematosus (SLE)
- vasculitis–polyarteritis.

2. *Asymptomatic proteinuria*, varying in severity, and detected at a routine or insurance medical examination due to:

- Henoch–Schönlein purpura
- SLE
- polyarteritis
- bacterial endocarditis
- shunt nephritis
- focal segmental glomerulosclerosis
- mesangiocapillary glomerulonephritis (MCGN).

3. *Acute nephritis*, characterised by haematuria, oliguria and hypertension. Loin pain and headache may be present and the patient will often feel unwell. In post-infective cases the relation to the preceding infection can usually be ascertained. This may be due to:

- post-streptococcal glomerulonephritis
- idiopathic rapidly progressive glomerulonephritis (RPGN)
- post-infectious RPGN
- Goodpasture's syndrome (anti-glomerular basement membrane disease)
- SLE
- polyarteritis
- Wegener's granulomatosis
- Henoch–Schönlein purpura
- essential cryoglobulinaemia.

4. *Nephrotic syndrome*, characterised by heavy proteinuria and, as a consequence, hypoalbuminaemia which leads to severe oedema: there is also hypercholesterolaemia. This may be due to:

a. Primary glomerular diseases
   - minimal change disease
   - membranous glomerulonephritis
   - membrano-proliferative GN (mesangiocapillary GN)
   - focal glomerulosclerosis
   - mesangial IgA nephropathy
   - bacterial endocarditis
   - shunt nephritis

b. Secondary glomerular disease
   - SLE
   - Henoch–Schönlein purpura
   - immune complex disease related to tumours, e.g. carcinoma of bronchus, lymphomas
   - diabetes mellitus
   - amyloid
   - drugs — e.g. penicillamine, gold, 'street heroin', phenytoin, captopril
   - infections — malaria, syphilis, leprosy, hepatitis B
   - cardiovascular — constrictive pericarditis
   - bee sting allergy

c. Inherited disease
   - congenital nephrotic syndrome (Finnish type).

5. *Chronic renal failure*, characterised by elevated blood urea (uraemia) and vague features including anaemia, nausea, vomiting, gastrointestinal bleeding and itching; there is often polyuria and nocturia. The gradual loss of nephrons leads initially to a reduction in renal reserve, so that a relatively minor insult, such as an episode of diarrhoea and vomiting, will reveal renal impairment in an otherwise healthy patient. Patients with established chronic renal failure fall into two groups: those with known renal disease which has caused gradual parenchymal destruction, and those who present de novo, the initial disease having been undetected in its active stage.

Some clinical features of chronic renal failure (CRF) reflect the important functions of the kidney. Clearly waste products accumulate as a result of the failure of the kidney to filter the blood. Anaemia results from failure to produce erythropoietin by the damaged kidney in addition to chronic blood loss and haemolysis. Genetically engineered erythropoietin is now available to patients, ameliorating this aspect of CRF. Chronic bone disease (renal osteodystrophy) is present in patients with CRF. This is very similar to rickets because the conversion of the vita-

min D molecule is impaired in the damaged kidney and this in turn reduces intestinal absorption of calcium, resulting in stimulation of parathyroid secretion. This in turn is exacerbated by the phosphate retention which accompanies CRF. Renal osteodystrophy can be treated with the active metabolite of vitamin D, 1-alpha-hydroxycholecalciferol. Renin production is increased whenever renal scarring occurs, and contributes to the hypertension found in CRF.

It is important to remember that there is considerable overlap of the conditions within these clinical states. Several diseases, therefore, may give rise to the same clinical picture; conversely, many diseases fall into more than one of the presenting clinical conditions.

All patients presenting with these features must be investigated thoroughly. In most cases this will include a renal biopsy so that the pathological basis of the disease can be established. This is vital because some conditions require prompt and specific treatment. In contrast, there are other conditions for which there is no effective treatment. It is just as important to establish the correct diagnosis in these patients, thereby avoiding a course of useless and potentially harmful therapy, since the drugs used to treat renal disease cause serious side-effects.

Mechanisms of glomerular damage

Glomeruli can be damaged by immunological or non-immunological mechanisms.

Immune glomerular injury

Immunological damage accounts for most human glomerular disease. There are two mechanisms:

- nephrotoxic antibody, as in anti-glomerular basement membrane (anti-GBM) disease
- immune complex deposition.

The resulting disease is usually referred to as *glomerulonephritis*, but this term is inappropriate in those cases with little inflammation. Glomerulopathy might be a better term, but it does not have wide acceptance.

Nephrotoxic antibody
Anti-GBM disease occurs when the individual forms an IgG antibody against an antigenic glycoprotein within the glomerular basement membrane (Figs 21.6 and 21.7). The antibody binds to the antigen in the collagenase-resistant component of collagen IV located in the lamina rara interna; this

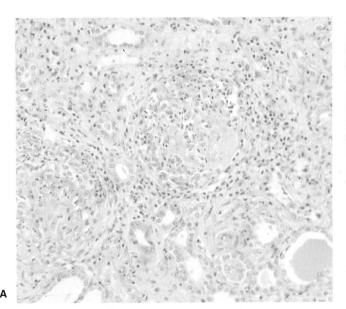
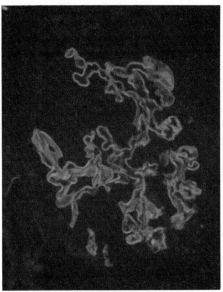

A   B

Fig. 21.6 Anti-glomerular basement membrane disease

The glomerular injury in this case is due to anti-glomerular basement membrane antibody. **A.** The resulting damage causes obliteration of Bowman's space by a crescentic mass of epithelial cells. **B.** Immunofluorescence reveals linear deposition of immunoglobulin on the glomerular basement membrane.

binding is revealed by the linear pattern seen after immunofluorescent staining for IgG. The binding of IgG to the basement membrane antigen activates the complement cascade; polymorphs are attracted and a florid proliferative glomerulonephritis results.

Anti-GBM disease is an uncommon cause of glomerulonephritis. It occurs in *Goodpasture's syndrome*, in which the glomerulonephritis is associated with pulmonary haemorrhages, because the antigen is also present in alveolar basement membrane. Clinical and histological features of anti-GBM disease are discussed below.

Immune complex deposition
The kidney is probably one of the routes by which immune complexes are normally cleared from the body. Experimentally, immune complex glomerulonephritis occurs in a proportion of animals given intravenous protein from another species, as part of the so-called serum sickness reaction.

The glomeruli are vulnerable to the deposition of immune complexes because they filter large volumes of blood (Fig. 21.7). However, the size and charge of the complexes influence glomerular entrapment. Positively-charged molecules gain access readily to the subepithelial location by virtue of the polyanionic nature of the basement membrane. Large-latticed complexes formed with antibodies of high avidity localise predominantly in the mesangium. In contrast, when antibodies have a moderate or low avidity, small complexes result which locate along the peripheral loops in the subepithelial position.

In situ formation of glomerular immune deposits can result from either the interaction between antibodies and a native component of the glomerulus, or between non-glomerular antigens which have been previously 'planted'. The concept of in situ formation has been developed by studies of an animal model known as Heymann nephritis or autologous immune complex (AIC) nephritis. These animals develop antibodies to a glycoprotein occurring on the microvilli of tubular epithelial cells. The histological picture is very similar to that of membranous glomerulonephritis in humans. A membrane-bound glycoprotein associated with coated pits on the epithelial cells is the site of interaction of the antibody. Having formed at the cell surface, the complexes are shed into the underlying basement membrane and undergo a dynamic process of remodelling and modification leading either to enlargement or elimination.

The *planted antigen* involves an extrinsic antigen bound to the basement membrane (Fig. 21.7). For example, in systemic lupus erythematosus (SLE) the antigen is DNA, which has a strong affinity for collagen molecules, and will therefore bind to the basement membrane. Circulating antibody subsequently forms complexes in situ with the now fixed planted antigen within the basement membrane.

The deposition of immune complexes can be visualised ultrastructurally and immunohistochemically as granular deposits within the peripheral glomerular loops or in the mesangium.

The two aspects of in situ formation are not mutually exclusive and both mechanisms may work together.

The role of complement in the elimination of complexes, both within the glomerulus and systemically, should be emphasised. Immune complexes are known to be attached to circulating erythrocytes and other cells by a receptor for C3b known as complement receptor 1 (CR1). In this way the complexes can be further modified and subsequently eliminated by the monocyte-macrophage system. This protective role is highlighted by the tendency of patients with complement deficiencies to develop glomerulonephritis.

Mediators of glomerular damage

When immune reactants become localised within the glomerular basement membrane, there is activation of the complement cascade and release of vasoactive substances. These are the mediators of acute inflammation, and they are responsible for the

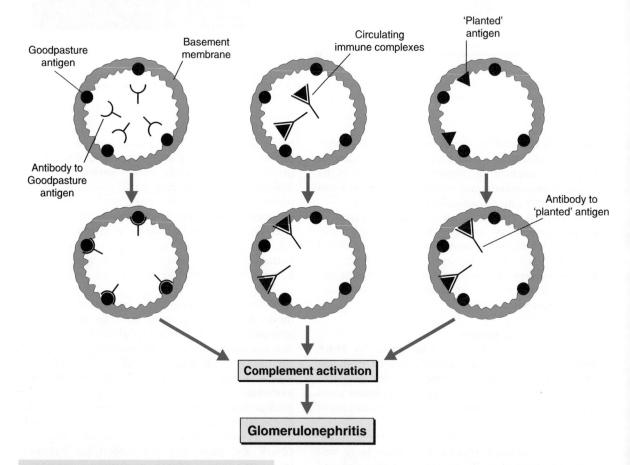

Fig. 21.7 Pathogenesis of glomerulonephritis

Glomerulonephritis is due either to an antibody reaction to glomerular antigen (Goodpasture's antigen), to circulating immune complexes that become deposited in the glomeruli, or to antibody reacting to a foreign antigen that has become 'planted' in the basement membrane. The final common pathway of glomerular injury is complement activation resulting in varying degrees of cell damage and inflammatory cell recruitment.

damage to the basement membrane, altering its properties to result in some of the urinary abnormalities observed clinically. These substances are as follows:

- *Complement* (Ch. 9) has a major role in the inflammatory process in glomerulonephritis. The classical pathway is activated by immune complexes fixed within the glomeruli. This process attracts neutrophil polymorphs, increases vascular permeability, and causes membrane damage.
- *Nephritic factors* (NeF-AP and NeF-CP) are immunoglobulins which bind to and inactivate inhibitors of the converting enzymes of the complement cascade. Consequently, the breakdown of C3 continues unchecked, resulting in the depletion of C3 from the plasma, a situation termed hypocomplementaemia.
- *Polymorphonuclear leukocytes* are attracted by the chemotactic influence of C5a. The polymorphs bind to the complexes by their C3 and Fc receptors. However, they are unable to phagocytose the complexes, which are fixed, and as a result release their lysosomal enzymes in the vicinity of the complexes, augmenting the damage to the glomerular basement membrane.
- *Clotting factors* also mediate glomerular damage. Fibrin is commonly found in glomerulonephritis. Fibrin entraps platelets which, because of their C3 and Fc receptors, form microthrombi, degranulate and release their vasoactive peptides, thus increasing vascular permeability.

Not every mediator is involved in every case. Permutations of mediators are common and account for the range of histological patterns in glomerulonephritis.

PRIMARY GLOMERULAR DISEASES

Anti-glomerular basement membrane disease

Anti-glomerular basement membrane (anti-GBM) disease occurs predominantly in young men. The mechanism of this disease is discussed above. The usual presenting feature is rapidly progressive renal failure, but occasional patients have haematuria and proteinuria, or nephrotic syndrome. Haemoptysis may be present. The prognosis is poor without treatment, but the introduction of plasma exchange (plasmapheresis) has substantially improved the outlook, particularly in patients treated early.

Histologically the characteristic lesion is a focal and segmental glomerulonephritis. With increasing severity, segmental necrosis with fibrin deposition, and a florid crescentic glomerulonephritis occur (Fig. 21.6).

Immune-complex-mediated lesions

Immune-complex-mediated glomerular injury (for mechanism, see above) results in a variety of glomerular reactions depending on the nature of the complexes.

Diffuse proliferative glomerulonephritis

Acute diffuse proliferative glomerulonephritis is one of the patterns of glomerular damage associated with a post-infective aetiology. It is usually an acute lesion following a transient infection. For many years it has been associated with a preceding β-haemolytic streptococcal infection (post-streptococcal glomerulonephritis). However, acute proliferative glomerulonephritis is associated with a variety of other causative organisms and conditions including:

- staphylococci
- meningococci
- pneumococci
- viruses
- malaria
- toxoplasmosis
- schistosomiasis.

Only for convenience, therefore, is post-streptococcal glomerulonephritis discussed as an example below, keeping in mind that this type of lesion is not unique to a streptococcal aetiology.

Post-streptococcal glomerulonephritis
β-haemolytic streptococci of Lancefield group A cause the post-streptococcal glomerulonephritis reaction; within that group, Griffith's subtypes 12, 4 and 1 are nephritogenic. The primary infection usually causes pharyngitis, but may also involve the middle ear or skin. There are considerable geographic differences in the incidence and severity of post-streptococcal glomerulonephritis throughout the world. For example, it is the commonest renal disease in India, contrasting with a falling incidence in the UK.

Clinical features. Post-streptococcal glomerulonephritis affects all ages, but children are more commonly affected, with the onset of malaise, fever and nausea 7–14 days after a sore throat. There is oliguria (a significant reduction in urine volume), and the urine is dark or 'smokey' due to the presence of microscopic haematuria. Facial oedema, often periorbital, and a mild degree of hypertension are apparent on examination. A raised anti-streptolysin O (ASO) titre and a significant reduction in complement (C3) levels are present. A raised blood urea indicates mild renal impairment. Urine analysis confirms the presence of haematuria, together with white cells and casts, and reveals a variable degree of proteinuria.

The kidneys are swollen by oedema, with scattered petechiae beneath the capsule and internally.

Histological features. The glomeruli are distended and hypercellular (Fig. 21.8). All of the glomeruli are involved, hence the use of the term 'diffuse'. The increase in cellularity is due to the proliferation and swelling of mesangial, endothelial and epithelial cells, together with a variable infiltration of polymorphonuclear leukocytes. Some glomeruli may show proliferation of cells lining Bowman's capsule to form a crescent; the presence of crescents in 80% or more of the glomeruli indicates a rapidly progressive disease and heralds a poor prognosis. There is usually interstitial oedema and a variable inflammatory cell infiltrate. The tubules contain red cell casts and the tubular epithelial cells may show degenerative changes.

Using immunofluorescence techniques, granular deposits of IgG and C3 are identified on the peripheral basement membranes and within the mesangium. The precise streptococcal antigen is not yet known; several antigens, some of which are cationic, have been demonstrated in the glomeruli in this condition. Ultrastructurally, electron-dense deposits situated beneath the epithelial cells on the outer aspect of the basement membrane are the principal feature (Fig. 21.9). These are termed subepithelial deposits, and are often referred to as 'humps' or 'lumpy deposits'; they correspond to the granular IgG and C3 demonstrated by the immunological studies. There is usually a mild degree of foot process effacement or fusion.

Prognosis. This is good in children, but only 60% of adults recover fully. Patients with acute post-streptococcal glomerulonephritis are usually treated conservatively, and renal biopsy does not feature in the management unless the anticipated improvement fails to occur. In most cases the characteristic morphological changes will have resolved by 6–8 weeks after the onset of the illness. All that remains is mild mesangial hypercellularity which may persist for many months or even years. The relationship between post-streptococcal glomerulonephritis and subsequent chronic glomerulonephritis remains controversial.

Focal proliferative glomerulonephritis

'Focal' implies uneven involvement of the glomeruli with some affected and others normal. In addition, involvement of only parts of individual glomeruli is common, and the term 'segmental' is also appropriate. Thus, focal and segmental lesions are often found together. A focal glomerulonephritis is a fairly

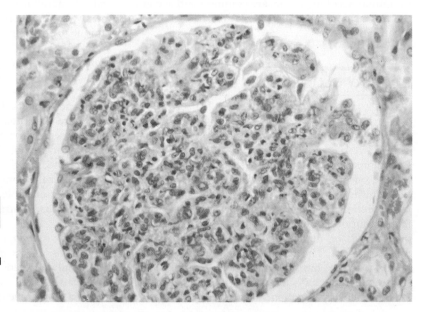

Fig. 21.8 Diffuse proliferative glomerulonephritis

The glomerular injury in this case is due to immune complex deposition. The glomerular injury is characterised by hypercellularity owing to cellular proliferation and acute inflammatory cell infiltration.

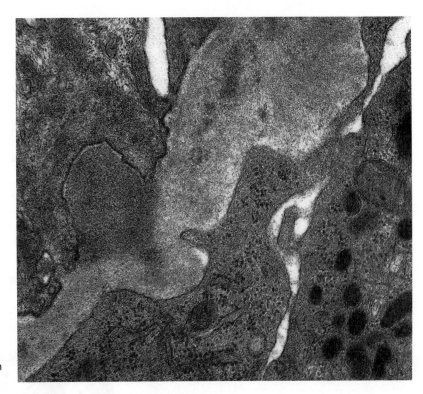

Fig. 21.9 Ultrastructure of diffuse proliferative glomerulonephritis

The principal abnormality is the presence of electron-dense immune complexes deposited between the epithelium and the basement membrane. The granule-containing cytoplasm of a neutrophil polymorph can be seen in the capillary. (Electron micrograph)

common pattern of reaction which is found in a variety of systemic diseases including:

- systemic lupus erythematosus
- Henoch–Schönlein purpura
- infective endocarditis
- microscopic polyarteritis
- Goodpasture's syndrome
- Wegener's granulomatosis.

Some of these conditions are immunologically mediated, and a possible explanation for the focal involvement is that it reflects an overloading of the mesangium's capacity to clear immune complexes. Complexes, unable to be removed from some of the glomerular tufts, accumulate and activate the complement cascade, causing localised inflammation within that part of the glomerulus.

Use of the unqualified term 'focal glomerulonephritis' is not helpful clinically. The immunological and ultrastructural profile of the glomerular lesion in the renal biopsy must be ascertained so that a more precise diagnosis can be made in each case.

There is one significant condition having a focal pattern that affects the kidney primarily: IgA disease. IgA deposition also occurs systemically, giving rise to Henoch–Schönlein purpura, a systemic vasculitis with involvement of the kidney.

IgA disease
IgA disease is now recognised as the major cause of chronic renal failure and insufficiency throughout the world. The features include:

- affects children and young adults
- episodic haematuria coinciding with upper respiratory tract infections
- mild proteinuria, very occasionally nephrotic syndrome
- hypertension
- raised serum IgA levels.

Aetiology. Little is known of the aetiological factors but reports indicate a geographic localisation, with a high incidence in France, Australia and Singapore. There is a weak association with HLA-DR4, but most attention has been directed to finding factors which will cause an excess of IgA; viruses and food proteins have been incriminated. The prognosis in patients with IgA disease is not as good as was first thought. As a consequence of the recurrent nature of the disease, repeated damage to the glomeruli eventually causes their sclerosis.

Histological features. A wide spectrum of changes is seen histologically. A mild focal mesangial proliferation, with IgA and C3 located in the mesangium in all of the glomeruli with corresponding electron-

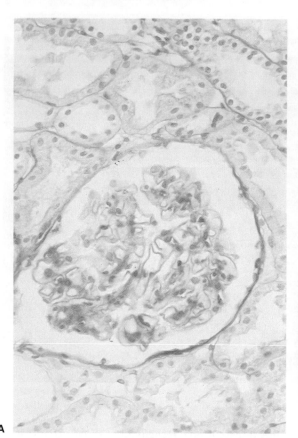

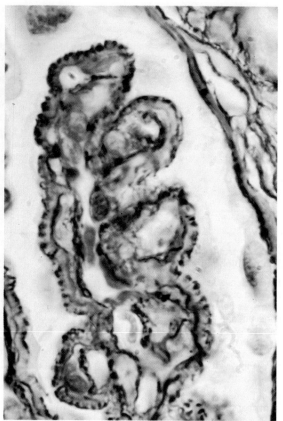

A

B

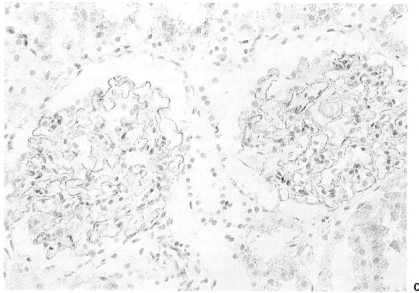

Fig. 21.10   Membranous glomerulonephritis

A. The glomerular capillary walls are thickened due to expansion of their basement membrane.
B. Histological staining by a silver-impregnation method reveals minute 'spikes' of basement membrane material.
C. Immunohistology (by the immunoperoxidase method) reveals granular deposition of IgG in the glomerular basement membranes.

C

dense paramesangial deposits, is associated with a good prognosis. In contrast the other end of the spectrum, represented by a mesangiocapillary pattern, sometimes with segmental necrosis, is associated with a more rapid deterioration of renal function.

Membranous glomerulonephritis

Membranous glomerulonephritis (MGN), a chronic immune-complex-mediated disorder, has distinctive histology but many causes. The morphological change is thought to reflect the size and rate of formation of the complexes.

Aetiology. A small proportion of cases have identifiable causes as follows and are best termed secondary membranous glomerulopathies:

- infective — syphilis, malaria, hepatitis B
- drugs — penicillamine, gold, mercury, heroin
- tumours — lymphomas, melanomas, carcinoma of the bronchus.

These patients are important to identify because the renal lesions may subside when the causative factor is treated or removed. Patients with systemic lupus erythematosus (SLE) form another important group; approximately 10% have MGN. However, approximately 85% of patients with MGN have no identifiable cause and their disease is said to be idiopathic.

Clinical features and prognosis. MGN affects all age groups, but adults are affected more commonly, with the highest incidence in the fifth to seventh decades. Males are affected more frequently than females. The presenting feature is usually proteinuria or nephrotic syndrome. Hypertension features at some time in the clinical course in about half of the patients. The majority of cases are unresponsive to steroids; they progress, over a variable and unpredictable period of between 2 and 20 years, to renal failure due to glomerulosclerosis. The prognosis in children is much better, however, particularly when there is proteinuria alone. In these cases, only 10% develop renal failure, and 50% remit. The prognosis in cases secondary to treatable antecedent causes is excellent.

Histological features. Capillary wall thickening without proliferation or inflammation is present in all glomeruli (Fig. 21.10). Immunopathological studies show granular deposits of IgG and C3 in the thickened capillary walls. Electron microscopy reveals the immune complexes deposited on the outer aspect of the basement membrane beneath the epithelial cells. As the disease progresses the walls become thicker due to the incorporation of the deposits, which eventually undergo degradation and

lysis. Eventually the affected glomeruli become sclerosed.

Thrombosis of the renal vein may complicate MGN, reflecting the increased coagulability of the blood in this condition.

Membrano-proliferative glomerulonephritis

Membrano-proliferative glomerulonephritis (MPGN) includes both proliferation and membrane thickening. The lobular architecture of the glomerulus is also accentuated (Fig. 21.11).

MPGN is not a diagnostic label for one disease; it is only a description of a pattern of reaction to a variety of causes. Since the first description in 1965, two main types have been recognised, with the addition of a rare third variant some 10 years ago.

Type I MPGN
Type I MPGN is an immune-complex-mediated lesion, alternatively named *mesangiocapillary glomerulonephritis* (MCGN), with sub-endothelial deposits. This lesion occurs in a wide range of conditions including infections, tumours, systemic connective tissue disorders, complement deficiencies, drug reactions and genetic disorders. However, the cause in most patients is not apparent. The majority of patients present with nephrotic syndrome, but some have haematuria. A persistently low serum complement C3 (hypocomplementaemia) is present in two-thirds of patients. The clinical course is one of progressive deterioration over 10 or more years.

Type II MPGN
The pathogenesis of type II MPGN, although not yet fully clarified, appears to be related to activation of the alternative complement pathway, and does not seem to involve immune complex deposition. The alternative name — *dense deposit disease* (DDD) — is preferable. DDD may follow an infection, but the absence of immunoglobulins in the glomerular deposits excludes the involvement of immune complexes.

Type III MPGN
Type III MPGN is very rare and is related to immune complex deposition. The capillary walls are markedly eosinophilic. Clinically, there are no distinguishing features.

Crescentic glomerulonephritis

Crescentic glomerulonephritis — rapidly progressive glomerulonephritis (RPGN) — is a manifestation of

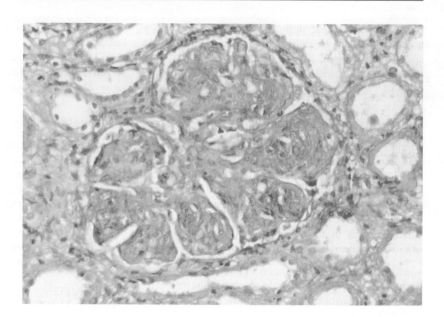

Fig. 21.11 Membrano-proliferative glomerulonephritis

The combination of mesangial cell proliferation and basement membrane thickening exaggerates the lobular architecture of the glomerulus. (PAS stain)

severe glomerular injury characterised by the presence of cellular crescents that eventually compress the glomeruli. It occurs as an uncommon primary renal condition in the small proportion of patients with post-streptococcal glomerulonephritis who have a stormy clinical course and a poor prognosis, but it can be associated with many other forms of glomerular damage.

Clinical features. The salient clinical feature is rapid deterioration, with loss of useful renal function within a matter of weeks. If treated vigorously, with immunosuppression and plasma exchange (plasmapheresis), some patients improve. Nevertheless, there is a high risk of permanent scarring of the kidney with the likelihood of subsequent hypertension.

Histological features. The crescents lining Bowman's capsule are composed of a mixture of epithelial cells and macrophages proliferating in response to the leakage of fibrin from the damaged glomerulus.

Minimal change disease

Minimal change disease is also known as *lipoid nephrosis*, a name which reflects the presence of fat in the renal tubular epithelial cells and is the most noticeable feature microscopically. Glomerular changes are absent or minimal using light microscopy; the diagnostic loss of epithelial foot processes is evident only by electron microscopy.

Pathogenesis. This is still not clear, though ulti-mately there is a loss of polyanion from the glomerular basement membrane. In a few patients it follows an upper respiratory infection or prophylactic immunisation.

Clinical features and prognosis. Minimal change disease affects all ages, but is much more common in children, with a peak incidence between the ages of 2 and 4 years and with a male preponderance. Nephrotic syndrome responsive to steroid therapy is the classical presentation. The prognosis in children is good with no permanent renal damage, but in adults the outlook is variable.

Focal glomerulosclerosis

Focal glomerulosclerosis is an important disease; it is the cause of nephrotic syndrome in some 10% of children and 15% of adults. The pathogenesis is unknown: many experts regard it as part of a spectrum including minimal change disease, implying progression from one to the other.

Segmental sclerosis is seen in a variety of other diseases (e.g. IgA nephropathy, diabetes and reflux nephropathy), but these cases lack the distinctive immunopathological and ultrastructural features of focal glomerulosclerosis.

Clinical features. Focal glomerulosclerosis presents with nephrotic syndrome or alternatively heavy proteinuria. Renal failure ensues within 10 years in most cases. Focal glomerulosclerosis tends to recur in transplanted kidneys.

SECONDARY GLOMERULAR DISEASES

> ► Many systemic disorders can result in glomerular damage
> ► Immune complexes in autoimmune disease (e.g. SLE) can damage basement membranes
> ► Diabetes mellitus may be complicated by glomerulopathy and renal papillary necrosis
> ► Glomerular vascular lesions can result from systemic vasculitis and hypertension

Secondary glomerular disease implies renal damage occurring as part of a systemic condition. These systemic conditions may be:

- immune-complex-mediated
- metabolic
- vascular.

Immune-complex-mediated conditions

Immune-complex-mediated systemic conditions which may involve renal damage include:

- systemic lupus erythematosus
- Henoch–Schönlein purpura
- infective endocarditis.

Systemic lupus erythematosus

Systemic lupus erythematosus (SLE) is a systemic condition affecting multiple organs including the skin, joints, serosal membranes, heart and lungs (Ch. 25). The kidneys are involved in about 70% of cases. The glomerular lesions, found in descending order of frequency, are:

- diffuse proliferative glomerulonephritis
- focal proliferative glomerulonephritis
- membranous glomerulonephritis.

Patients with membranous changes have heavy proteinuria or the nephrotic syndrome.

Henoch–Schönlein purpura

Henoch–Schönlein purpura is a systemic vasculitis affecting the skin, joints, intestine and kidneys, and occurs most commonly in childhood. A purpuric rash typically affects the extensor aspects of the arms and legs and the buttocks. Joint pains, and abdominal pain with or without intestinal haemorrhage, are also present. The proportion of patients with renal involvement is difficult to assess, but it may be the majority. Significant renal damage occurs in over one-third of cases, ranging from proteinuria, possibly with nephrotic syndrome, to rapidly progressive glomerulonephritis.

There is good evidence to suggest an immune complex aetiology. A preceding respiratory infection is noted in about one-third of cases, but there is no association with any specific organism.

Infective endocarditis

Renal complications of infective endocarditis (Ch. 13) are:

- infarcts due to embolic vegetations from the heart valves
- focal and segmental glomerulonephritis ('focal embolic nephritis')
- diffuse proliferative glomerulonephritis.

The last two complications are almost certainly due to immune complex deposition.

In cases with a focal and segmental glomerulonephritis the kidney shows multiple haemorrhagic foci throughout the cortex and beneath the capsule; it is one of the causes of a 'flea-bitten' kidney. The renal lesions subside when the bacterial source of the antigen is removed by intensive antibiotic therapy.

Metabolic conditions

Metabolic conditions which may involve renal damage include:

- diabetes mellitus
- renal amyloidosis
- multiple myeloma.

Diabetes mellitus

Diabetes mellitus is associated with damage involving both large and small vessels throughout the body. The presence of severe atheroma involving the renal artery may cause renal ischaemic lesions and hypertension. Involvement of the microcirculation, in addition to causing lesions in the retina, nerves and skin, significantly affects the kidneys, leading to glomerulopathy, arteriolar hyalinosis, and tubulo-interstitial lesions. The combination of changes that occur in individual cases is varied and often referred to collectively as diabetic nephropathy.

Diabetic glomerulopathy
Glomerular disease in diabetics causes proteinuria, which becomes heavier as the disease progresses, leading to nephrotic syndrome and chronic renal fail-

ure. Approximately 10% of all diabetics die in renal failure. However, when patients developing diabetes in childhood (usually insulin-dependent) are considered separately, death from renal failure occurs in approximately 50% of cases. This correlates with the fact that renal disease occurs more often, and is more severe, when the onset of diabetes is early in life; glomerulosclerosis eventually occurs in these cases.

Pathogenesis. The pathogenesis of the basement membrane changes is not known. All the features point to a basement membrane which is more leaky than normal. The increased permeability may be due to:

- an excess of type IV collagen in the membrane
- a deficiency of proteoglycans, such as heparan sulphate, which are responsible for the polyanionic nature of the membrane
- non-enzymic glycosylation of proteins; this occurs in hyperglycaemia, and may alter the polyanionic state of the basement membrane and also alter the physicochemical properties of the circulating proteins
- hyperfiltration due to increased glomerular blood flow in diabetes.

Histologically, three types of glomerular lesion occur representing a continuous spectrum of increasing severity:

- *Capillary wall thickening* is the initial change.
- The addition of *mesangial matrix expansion* to the capillary thickening eventually encroaches on

the capillaries, and is termed diffuse glomerulosclerosis.
- The nodular expansion of the mesangium at the tips of the glomerular lobules is very characteristic of diabetes, and is known as *nodular glomerulosclerosis* or *Kimmelstiel–Wilson lesion* (Fig. 21.12).

The glomerular changes are accompanied by arteriolar hyalinosis affecting both the afferent and efferent arterioles.

Renal papillary necrosis

Renal papillary necrosis is frequently seen in diabetics with acute pyelonephritis. The blood supply to the renal papillae via the vasa recta is tenuous, and the vasculopathy together with the effects of the inflammation result in ischaemia of the papillae, which become infarcted. The necrotic papillae may then become detached (Fig. 21.13) and either cause an obstruction or are passed in the urine.

Renal amyloidosis

Renal involvement is present in 80–90% of cases of secondary amyloidosis (Ch. 7). The affected patients have heavy proteinuria or the nephrotic syndrome. Renal involvement is the presenting feature in over 50% of patients, and leads inevitably to chronic renal failure, with extensive glomerulosclerosis within 1–2 years.

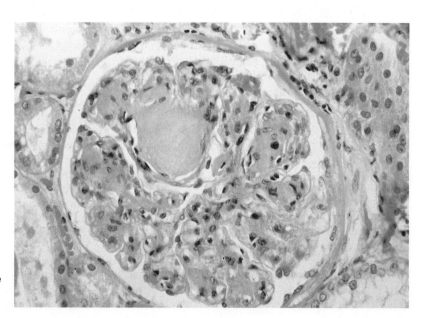

Fig. 21.12 Diabetic glomerulopathy (nodular glomerulosclerosis)

This lesion is characterised by hyaline sclerotic nodules at the glomerular periphery.

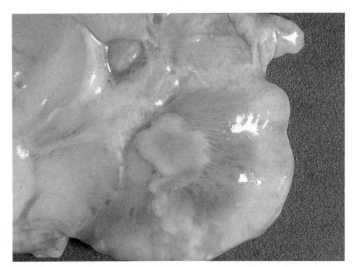

Fig. 21.13 Renal papillary necrosis

The renal papillae in this diabetic appear yellow and structureless due to necrosis. Necrotic papillae may detach and cause ureteric colic or obstruction.

Multiple myeloma

Renal damage occurs frequently in patients with multiple myeloma. Renal failure may be the presenting feature. The most significant lesions are tubulo-interstitial, characterised by proteinaceous casts to which there is a giant cell reaction. Glomerular involvement is uncommon in myeloma, but includes amyloid infiltration in about 10% of cases and the deposition of monoclonal cryoglobulin in a smaller proportion.

Vascular damage

Glomerular diseases due to vascular damage include:

- polyarteritis nodosa
- Wegener's granulomatosis
- haemolytic–uraemic syndrome
- idiopathic thrombocytopenic purpura
- disseminated intravascular coagulation.

Thus, the group includes glomerular damage in systemic vasculitis (polyarteritis and Wegener's granulomatosis) and in thrombotic microangiopathies (haemolytic–uraemic syndrome, idiopathic thrombocytopenic purpura and disseminated intravascular coagulation). The glomerular lesions in systemic vasculitis are usually characterised by segmental necrosis, sometimes with crescents. Circulating auto-antibodies against neutrophil cytoplasmic antigens (ANCA) have been described in these patients. Two patterns are found:

- cytoplasmic (C–) ANCA reacts with proteinase 3
- perinuclear (P–) ANCA reacts with myeloperoxidase.

The majority of patients with Wegener's granulomatosis react with C–ANCA. Patients with microscopic polyarteritis react with P–ANCA but the reaction is less specific. In thrombotic microangiopathies the glomerular capillaries contain fibrin or platelets or both.

Polyarteritis nodosa

Polyarteritis nodosa (Chs 13 and 25) involves medium to small arteries throughout the body. Involvement of renal vessels results in haematuria and loin pain due to renal infarcts, often with hypertension developing later.

Microscopic polyarteritis (also referred to as hypersensitivity angiitis) contrasts with the classical (nodosa) form in that smaller arteries, arterioles, capillaries and venules are damaged. Renal involvement presents not infrequently as rapidly progressive renal failure. Untreated patients die within a few months to years, but there is a good response to immunosuppressive therapy.

Wegener's granulomatosis

Wegener's granulomatosis is a rare necrotising vasculitis affecting the nose and upper respiratory tract (Ch. 14) in addition to the kidneys. It occurs more commonly in males in their fourth and fifth decades, although it can occur at any age. The clinical indicators of renal involvement vary from microscopic haematuria to rapidly progressive renal failure. If the condition remains untreated, progressive renal impairment is inevitable, but cyclophosphamide induces a remission in the majority of patients, with complete resolution of the glomerular lesions if treated early enough.

Haemolytic–uraemic syndrome

Haemolytic–uraemic syndrome (HUS) is a complex condition in which there is:

- acute nephropathy
- haemolysis
- thrombocytopenia.

Fibrin strands are deposited in small vessels, including the glomerular capillaries. The resultant mesh, through which the blood has to pass, deforms the erythrocytes ('helmet' and 'burr' cells) and platelets with subsequent destruction. This process is microangiopathic haemolysis. There are three subgroups of HUS:

- childhood
- adult
- secondary.

Childhood HUS
Childhood HUS carries a much better prognosis than that occurring in adults. There is often a prodromal episode of diarrhoea or a flu-like illness which lasts 5–15 days. There is a sudden onset of oliguria, with haematuria and occasionally melaena. There is increasing anaemia. Approximately half the patients develop hypertension. The pathogenesis is uncertain, but geographic variations point to a specific infective agent; verotoxin-producing *E. coli* are thought to be responsible in some cases.

Adult HUS
Adult HUS is more frequently fatal and is seen in a variety of situations:

- pregnancy — sometimes occurring post-partum even several months after delivery
- oestrogen therapy — occurring in women taking contraceptive pills and, rarely, in men treated with oestrogens for prostatic carcinoma
- infections, e.g. typhoid, viruses and shigellosis.

Secondary HUS
Secondary HUS occurs as a complication of:

- malignant hypertension
- progressive systemic sclerosis
- systemic lupus erythematosus
- transplant rejection.

Clinically and morphologically, secondary HUS is identical with the other types.

Histological features of HUS
The glomeruli contain thrombi within the capillary lumen, and there is segmental endothelial and mesangial swelling. The capillary walls are thickened. Arterioles and small arteries show fibrin and erythrocytes in the walls, often with thrombosis. Cortical necrosis can result when there is extensive arterial thrombosis.

Idiopathic thrombocytopenic purpura

Idiopathic thrombocytopenic purpura (ITP) (Ch. 23) occurs predominantly in women, mostly under 40 years. There are neurological symptoms together with haemolytic anaemia and thrombocytopenia. Renal involvement is seen in approximately half the patients and is manifested by proteinuria, microscopic haematuria and renal impairment.

Histological features. Eosinophilic granular platelet thrombi are identified in glomerular capillaries, afferent arterioles and interlobular arteries.

Disseminated intravascular coagulation

Disseminated intravascular coagulation (Ch. 23) is a systemic problem involving generalised endothelial damage. The most common cause is a Gram-negative septicaemia, analogous to the experimental generalised Shwartzman reaction. Fibrin thrombi fill the lumina of glomerular capillaries, afferent arterioles and small arteries, causing severe renal impairment.

RENAL TRANSPLANTATION

Patients in chronic renal failure, who in the past would have died, are now effectively maintained on either peritoneal dialysis or haemodialysis, both of which place restrictions on the patient's lifestyle. For young and otherwise fit patients with domestic and occupational responsibilities, renal transplantation offers freedom from the restrictions of regular dialysis and has transformed the quality of their lives.

The transplanted kidney may be rejected. Rejection may be rapid or slow in onset, and is designated hyperacute, acute or chronic.

Hyperacute rejection

Hyperacute rejection is due to preformed complement-fixing antibodies in the blood of the recipient. The immune damage is directed at the endothelial cells of the graft, and the speed of onset is related to the antibody concentration, so that when high, damage occurs within minutes or hours, compared with 1–2 days when levels are low. In some cases the reaction is immediate, and is apparent to the surgeon on establishing a flow of blood through the graft: the kidney becomes flaccid, cyanosed and mottled, suggesting intrarenal vasoconstriction. Thrombi form in arterioles and glomeruli, and cortical infarcts occur as a result of vascular thrombosis.

Acute rejection

Acute rejection may occur at any time from a few days to months or years after transplantation, and involves both cellular and humoral immunity (Ch. 9). Acute vascular rejection is evinced by a necrotising vasculitis with immunoglobulin, complement and fibrin in the vessel wall. Superimposed thrombosis may lead to infarction. Cellular rejection is characterised by a mononuclear cell infiltrate, interstitial oedema and haemorrhage together with a tubulitis.

Chronic rejection

Chronic rejection is an important cause of failure of grafts months or years after transplantation. Vascular changes dominate, resulting in ischaemic changes in the renal parenchyma. There is progressive interstitial fibrosis and tubular atrophy.

DISEASES AFFECTING BLOOD VESSELS

In addition to the conditions mentioned above, the renal vasculature may be damaged in:

- progressive systemic sclerosis (scleroderma; Ch. 25)
- systemic hypertension (Ch. 13).

Renal infarction

Two mechanisms of infarction are recognised:

- embolic infarction
- diffuse cortical necrosis.

Embolic infarction

Most renal infarcts result from embolisation of:

- *atheromatous material*, responsible for the small subcapsular pits in benign-phase hypertension
- *thrombotic material* arising from the left side of the heart
- *bacterial vegetations* from infective endocarditis.

Many renal infarcts are clinically silent, but some result in haematuria and loin pain.

Renal infarcts are pale or white, and have a characteristic wedge shape with the apex directed towards the hilum.

Diffuse cortical necrosis

Diffuse cortical necrosis is a rare condition complicating pregnancy or trauma associated with severe haemorrhage or severe sepsis. Profound hypotension occurs in these situations, but there is considerable controversy relating to the pathogenesis of this condition. Vasoconstriction is important since infarction can be avoided by the use of angiotensin antagonists.

Diffuse cortical necrosis is a cause of acute anuric renal failure. The prognosis is poor when the infarction is generalised, but is less ominous when the infarction is focal.

Macroscopically, the appearance is striking: the external surface bears irregular yellowish areas with intervening congestion and haemorrhage. The cut surface shows the infarction to be confined to the cortex.

RENAL DISEASE IN PREGNANCY

The kidneys undergo morphological and functional changes during pregnancy. Some of these changes have a bearing on the renal response to disease and are relevant in the context of interpreting function tests. Renal impairment, whatever the cause, which is present at the beginning of pregnancy, has important implications because the risks to both the mother and fetus are significant. The risk of deteriorating renal function and hypertension is increased, and there is a rise in fetal morbidity and mortality.

Infection

Infection is the most frequent urinary tract abnormality in pregnant women and is usually detected on routine testing of the urine during antenatal care. Asymptomatic bacteriuria occurs in up to 10% of pregnant women, and there is good evidence to suggest that such patients run a high risk of developing acute pyelonephritis. Prompt diagnosis and early treatment are therefore essential. Renal abnormalities such as the coarse polar scarring of vesico-ureteric reflux (p. 646) are detected radiologically in a high proportion of these patients. In addition, physiological changes occur in the smooth muscle cells of the lower urinary tract in pregnancy, with slower ureteric peristaltic activity and pelvi-ureteric dilatation. This leads to stasis which, combined with infection particularly with urea-splitting organisms, predisposes to stone formation; existing stones may enlarge considerably during pregnancy.

Hypertension

Hypertension is an important development in the pregnant patient. The patient may have latent essential hypertension or may have intercurrent renal disease. Alternatively, a condition peculiar to pregnancy called pre-eclampsia or eclampsia may be present. *Pre-eclampsia* is a condition characterised by hypertension, proteinuria and oedema; *eclampsia* supervenes when fits occur. In severe cases the glomeruli are large and relatively bloodless due to marked swelling of the endothelial and mesangial cells. Arteries and arterioles display endothelial swelling and myo-intimal proliferation. The tubules and interstitium are relatively normal. The vascular and glomerular lesions are reversible when the hypertension has been corrected. However, disseminated intravascular coagulation is frequently superimposed during the course of pre-eclampsia, and when fibrinoid necrosis of the arterioles has occurred then persistent hypertension may ensue.

TUBULO-INTERSTITIAL DISORDERS

In tubulo-interstitial conditions there is damage to the tubular epithelial cells and the interstitium. These disorders account for a significant proportion of patients presenting with impaired renal function.

Infections of the kidney affect the tubules and the interstitium, and may present as acute renal failure if there are complications such as tubular or papillary necrosis. These are discussed in a later section because of their clinical importance as a separate entity.

Acute tubular epithelial cell damage causes the condition known as acute tubular necrosis.

Acute tubular necrosis

- ► Important cause of acute renal failure
- ► May be due to toxic or haemodynamic causes (e.g. shock)
- ► Regeneration of renal tubular epithelium often permits clinical recovery

Acute tubular necrosis (ATN) is a very important cause of acute renal failure; patients often present with extreme oliguria (less than 100 ml of urine each 24 h). The importance of ATN is that it is fully recoverable if the patient is given adequate supportive fluid and electrolyte therapy. Following the initial oliguria due to tubular obstruction by swollen and necrotic epithelial cells, there is a later diuretic phase due to the loss of urinary concentration. In the oliguric phase, hyperkalaemia with the risk of cardiac arrhythmias presents a serious threat to life. This situation contrasts with hypokalaemia which can occur in the early diuretic phase.

The histological features range from sublethal cell injury to necrosis of the epithelial cells.

The principal causes of acute tubular necrosis are:

- ischaemia
- toxins.

Ischaemic ATN
Ischaemic ATN follows a variety of clinical situations, such as trauma, burns, and infections in which the patient becomes shocked. Profound hypotension is usually responsible for the hypoperfusion of the peritubular circulation. The kidneys are pale and swollen. Histology reveals epithelial cell injury along the entire length of the tubules; the cells are flattened and vacuolated. Inflammatory cells pack the vasa recta in response to the necrotic cells; the interstitium is oedematous. Casts occur frequently in the distal tubules and collecting ducts; they are composed of cellular debris and protein including Tamm–Horsfall protein. In the case of ATN resulting from a crush injury, myoglobin is present in the casts. Following a mismatched blood transfusion haemoglobin would be present.

Toxic ATN
Toxic ATN results from a wide variety of substances:

- *heavy metals* (lead, mercury, arsenic, gold, chromium, bismuth and uranium)
- *organic solvents* (carbon tetrachloride, chloroform)
- *glycols* (ethylene glycol, propylene glycol, dioxane and diethylene glycol)

- *therapeutic substances* (antibiotics — methicillin, sulphonamides, polymyxin, cephalosporins; non-steroidal anti-inflammatory drugs; mercurial diuretics; anaesthetics — methoxyflurane)
- *iodinated radiographic contrast medium*
- *phenol*
- *pesticides*
- *paraquat.*

The kidneys are swollen and red. Histologically, there is often marked vacuolation of the tubular epithelial cytoplasm. The damage is characteristically restricted to the proximal tubular cells, those of the distal tubule being spared. This situation contrasts with the picture in ischaemic ATN in which the tubular cells along the entire length of the tubule are affected. Recovery is indicated in biopsies by the presence of mitotic figures within the flattened cells.

Interstitial nephritis

Interstitial nephritis is a term used for a heterogeneous group of conditions which have morphological and clinical features in common, but have a wide range of causes. The common morphology is an inflammatory reaction composed mainly of T-cells in the intertubular (interstitial) connective tissue. The pathogenesis in many instances is not understood. Classification is therefore based mainly on aetiological factors:

- *toxins* — heavy metals (e.g. lead, gold, mercury), or drugs (e.g. gentamicin, cephaloridine, cyclosporin A)
- *immunological*
- *metabolic* — urate, etc.
- *physical* — obstruction
- *neoplastic* — myeloma.

Acute interstitial nephritis

With acute interstitial nephritis there is acute onset of renal failure; a careful history should be taken to exclude exposure to one of the known substances which can damage the kidney. There is considerable overlap between the many substances which cause acute toxic tubular necrosis and acute interstitial nephritis.

Histologically, there is interstitial oedema, together with a mononuclear cell infiltrate, and evidence of tubular degeneration.

Chronic interstitial nephritis

Patients with chronic interstitial nephritis present in chronic renal failure, and establishing a cause is often very difficult. Histologically, there is marked interstitial fibrosis and tubular atrophy with a variable cellular infiltrate.

Analgesic nephropathy

Analgesic nephropathy is a well-known adverse reaction to analgesics. It occurs worldwide but shows areas of high incidence, first described in 1953 in Switzerland. Epidemiological and experimental research has shown that the chronic ingestion of large quantities of aspirin combined with phenacetin is particularly harmful. The phenacetin produces a metabolite which binds to the cellular proteins, depleting cellular glutathione, and is thus toxic. The aspirin is thought to induce papillary ischaemia by inhibiting the synthesis of vasodilatory prostaglandins. The toxic and ischaemic effects, therefore, are thought to be synergistic to produce, initially, selective damage and, subsequently, necrosis of the papillae.

Transitional cell carcinomas of the renal pelvis and ureter occur more frequently in patients with analgesic nephropathy.

Lesions associated with metabolic disorders

A variety of metabolic diseases and disturbances affect the tubules and interstitium. These include:

- hypokalaemia
- urate nephropathy
- hypercalcaemia
- oxalosis.

Hypokalaemic nephropathy

Persistently low plasma levels of potassium occur in:

- chronic diarrhoea
- hyperaldosteronism, either primary or secondary
- chronic abuse of laxatives or diuretics.

Hypokalaemia causes coarse vacuolation of the tubular epithelial cells principally in the proximal tubules, but in severe states those of the distal tubules are also involved; the medullary tubules are spared.

Urate (gouty) nephropathy

Renal damage due to elevated levels of uric acid in the blood occurs in gout (Ch. 7). Additionally, patients with chronic renal damage due to pyelonephritis or glomerulonephritis have impaired filtration and reduced tubular secretion of uric acid; this leads to retention of uric acid and its subsequent deposition in the kidney. Uric acid crystallises in an acid environment such as that found in the distal tubules, collecting ducts, and interstitium of the papillae.

Acute urate nephropathy

Acute urate nephropathy presents as acute renal failure and is seen principally in patients with myeloproliferative diseases. It is often precipitated by chemotherapy, when extensive breakdown of cells releases vast quantities of nucleic acids. The cut surface of affected kidneys displays yellow streaks within the medulla due to precipitation of urate crystals filling the tubular lumina; this precipitation causes obstruction and tubular dilatation.

Chronic urate nephropathy

Chronic urate nephropathy is more insidious and occurs in patients with persistently elevated uric acid levels, as in gout. The crystals in the tubular lumina cause chronic obstruction and tubulo-interstitial nephritis in the cortex, which becomes atrophic and thinned.

Urate stones may occur in both acute and chronic nephropathy, and there is an increased incidence of pyelonephritis.

Hypercalcaemic nephropathy (nephrocalcinosis)

Calcium deposition in the kidneys occurs when there is hypercalcaemia: this is 'metastatic' calcification (Ch. 7). The onset of renal symptoms is insidious; the tubular disturbance results in an inability to concentrate urine, with consequent polyuria often causing the patient to complain of nocturia. The kidney is often scarred and focally calcified. The cut surface of the kidneys reveals stones within the pelvicalyceal system, and linear white streaks and flecks. There is interstitial fibrosis, a non-specific inflammatory infiltrate and tubular atrophy in relation to the calcification.

Oxalate nephropathy

Calcium oxalate deposition occurs systemically in the tissues when blood levels are high. Increased urinary excretion of oxalate also occurs and the kidneys may be damaged. Hyperoxalaemia and the resulting hyperoxaluria are either primary or secondary. The primary form is due to deficiencies of hepatic enzymes, which are concerned with the decarboxylation of glyoxylate, which accumulates and is oxidised by an alternative pathway to oxalate. Secondary hyperoxaluria is seen in poisoning with ethylene glycol (anti-freeze), or the anaesthetic agent methoxyflurane, and in pyridoxine (vitamin B_6) deficiency. Oxalate deposition is also seen in the kidneys in a variety of chronic renal disorders.

In advanced cases, the kidneys are small, granular and scarred, the thinned cortex reflecting the fibrosis and tubular disruption that occurs with the deposition of oxalate. Stones are often present in the pelvis and calyceal system.

Lesions due to physical agents

Radiation nephritis

The renal tubular cells are sensitive to radiation, and care must be taken to avoid injury to the kidneys during therapeutic irradiation to the upper abdomen. Affected patients present with hypertension and renal insufficiency.

Histologically, there is glomerulosclerosis, marked vascular changes, and interstitial fibrosis. The tubules are lined by atypical epithelial cells and display characteristic thick multilayered basement membranes.

Obstructive uropathy

Obstructive uropathy is an important cause of interstitial nephritis. The causes of urinary tract obstruction include:

- *congenital anomalies* (uretero-pelvic stenosis, vesico-ureteric reflux)
- *tumours* (carcinoma of the bladder and prostate)
- *hyperplastic lesions* (benign prostatic hyperplasia)
- *calculi*.

Clinical features. The signs, symptoms and prognosis depend on the level of the obstruction. Thus, a renal calculus or a fragment of sloughed papilla will cause renal colic, whereas obstruction due to carcinoma of the bladder or benign prostatic hyperplasia will be accompanied by bladder symptoms. Acute obstruction in the lower urinary tract will result in anuria and pain, and if not relieved is incompatible with survival.

Partial, and particularly unilateral, obstruction is much more insidious. There are few symptoms, the condition remaining unnoticed for many years in some patients. There is usually polyuria and nocturia. Poor urinary concentration, tubular acidosis and salt wasting can sometimes be demonstrated in the early stages, all of which are expressions of the tubular epithelial cell damage that occurs. Systemic hypertension is common in these patients.

Pathogenesis. The pelvis and calyceal system become dilated due to back pressure; the dilatation is mild in cases of acute obstruction. The peristaltic activity of the ureters is increased in obstruction, which raises the intrapelvic pressure, which in turn is transmitted into the renal parenchyma. Initially, the filtrate formed is reabsorbed through lymphatic and vascular channels. The continued rapid rise in pressure, however, reduces glomerular and medullary blood flow and eventually impairs glomerular filtration.

Gross dilatation occurs as a result of prolonged back pressure. The kidney becomes a dilated sac-like structure: this is *hydronephrosis* (Fig. 21.14).

Pyelonephritis

> ► A common and important cause of renal disease
> ► Causative bacteria may reach the kidneys either through the blood (as in septicaemia) or by reflux of contaminated urine from the bladder
> ► Acute pyelonephritis is characterised by pus in the tubules and by abscess formation
> ► Chronic pyelonephritis is characterised by coarse scarring and contraction of the kidneys

Pyelonephritis is an infection in the kidney which may arise by haematogenous or retrograde ureteric routes. Due to their rich blood supply, the kidneys are often involved in severe systemic infections by direct spread of organisms through septicaemia. The commonest infecting organisms are bacteria. Urinary tract infections are common within the community, second only to upper respiratory infections. However, not all urinary tract infections are associated with pyelonephritis; organisms can gain access to the kidney only if there is vesico-ureteric reflux.

The incidence of pyelonephritis parallels that of obstructive uropathy. In infancy, boys are mainly affected because of anatomical abnormalities. From puberty to middle age females show the highest incidence, related to urethral trauma and pregnancy. After 40 years, prostatic disease provides an obstructive aetiology in ageing men. Other factors include instrumentation (e.g. catheterisation, cystoscopy) and diabetes mellitus.

The clinical distinction between acute and chronic pyelonephritis is quite clear.

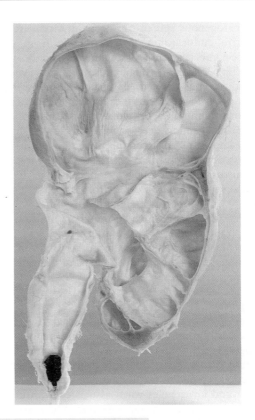

Fig. 21.14   Hydronephrosis

The renal pelvis and calyces are grossly dilated, causing compression atrophy of the renal tissue. In this case, hydronephrosis is due to blockage of the ureter by a stone.

Acute pyelonephritis

Acute pyelonephritis is due to infection of the kidney by pyogenic organisms. It presents with malaise and fever, and pain and tenderness in the loins is not uncommon. Dysuria and urgency of micturition indicate an associated infection in the lower urinary tract. The finding of pus cells in the urine (pyuria) is helpful, but the finding of white cell casts provides unequivocal evidence of pyelonephritis. Urine culture in suspected cases is imperative, but bacteriuria is regarded as significant only when in excess of 10^5 culture-forming units/ml; this result eliminates cases of extraneous bacterial contamination.

Pathogenesis
The pathogenesis of acute pyelonephritis is either:

- haematogenous spread
- retrograde ureteric spread.

Haematogenous spread can occur in a patient with infective endocarditis or bacteraemia from other sources; the spectrum of organisms can be wide, including bacteria, fungi, rickettsia and viruses. Previous renal damage or structural abnormality predisposes to organisms localising in the kidney.

More commonly, pyelonephritis results from organisms gaining access from the lower urinary tract, known as an ascending infection, in association with reflux of urine. In these cases the infecting organisms are Gram-negative bacilli (e.g. *E. coli, Proteus* spp. and *Enterobacter*) from the patient's faecal flora. This occurs frequently in young women; predisposing factors include the short urethra, urethral trauma during sexual intercourse, and pregnancy. Instrumentation of the urinary tract in both sexes increases both the incidence and the variety of infecting organisms.

Morphology
Acute pyelonephritis is characterised by either abscesses throughout the cortex and medulla, or wedge-shaped confluent areas of suppuration. The minute abscesses are randomly distributed when the infection is blood-borne, but tend to be located at the upper and lower poles when associated with urinary reflux. A lower urinary tract infection may be associated with inflammation of the pelvic and calyceal mucosa, and pus may be present in the pelvis.

Histology reveals intratubular polymorphs together with interstitial oedema and inflammation (Fig. 21.15). With healing, fibrosis occurs in the interstitium and the inflammatory infiltrate becomes dominated by lymphocytes and plasma cells.

Complications
Three important complications may develop in acute pyelonephritis:

- *Renal papillary necrosis.* As a result of the inflammation, the medullary blood supply is compromised and renal papillary necrosis may ensue, particularly in diabetics or where there is obstruction.
- *Pyonephrosis.* Ths arises when there is complete obstruction high in the urinary tract near the kidney. The stagnant fluid in the pelvis and calyceal system suppurates. Eventually, the kidney becomes grossly distended with pus.
- *Perinephric abscess.* When the infection breaches the renal capsule and extends into the perirenal tissues, it gives rise to a perinephric abscess.

Chronic pyelonephritis

Chronic pyelonephritis occurs in association with *vesico-ureteric reflux* (VUR), which commences either early in life due to congenital lesions (Fig. 21.16) or with obstruction developing during adulthood.

Vesico-ureteric reflux enables organisms to gain access to the kidney from the bladder. The primary abnormality is the angle at which the terminal ureteric segment traverses the bladder wall. Normally the course taken is oblique, at an acute

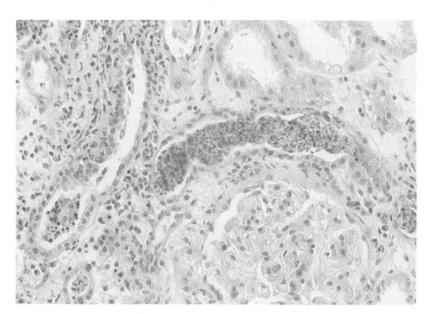

Fig. 21.15 Acute pyelonephritis

The tubules contain casts consisting of neutrophil polymorphs and the intertubular connective tissue is oedematous.

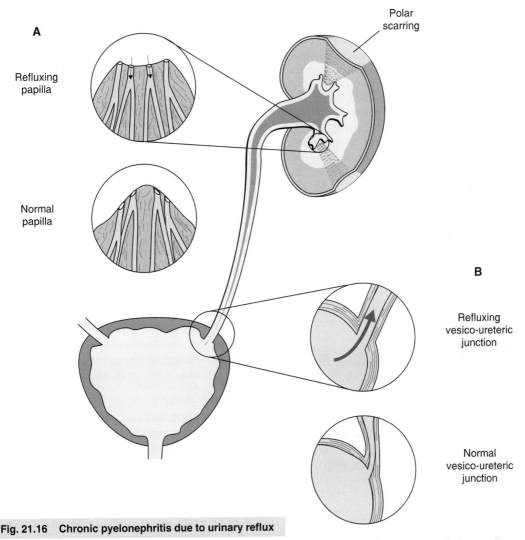

Fig. 21.16   Chronic pyelonephritis due to urinary reflux

Urinary reflux can occur either due to obstruction of urinary flow or, as shown in this diagram, congenital anomalies.
A. Refluxing papilla. Contrasting with the normal convex papilla, refluxing papillae have concave surfaces without valve-like openings of the collecting ducts. **B. Refluxing vesico-ureteric junction.** Normally, the terminal ureter runs through the bladder wall beneath the surface and enters the lumen at an angle forming a valve; refluxing junctions result from the absence of the valve-like structure.

angle to the mucosal surface, so that contraction of the bladder wall during micturition closes the ureteric orifice. In patients with VUR, the terminal portion is short and orientated at approximately 90° to the mucosal surface; contraction of the bladder tends to hold the ureteric orifice open and facilitates reflux of urine.

Pathogenesis

Reflux of urine into the kidney during micturition raises the intrapelvic and intracalyceal pressure, but intra-parenchymal reflux remains the crucial factor for development of pyelonephritis. In cases prone to intra-parenchymal reflux, the renal papillae are flattened rather than conical, and the terminal ducts open on to the surface at right angles. This situation facilitates reflux into the collecting ducts when the intrapelvic pressure is high, in contrast to the oblique angle of opening of the ducts in non-refluxing papillae. Refluxing papillae tend to be situated at the poles of the kidney, and it is in these areas that the pyelonephritic damage is predominantly seen. The presence of infection accelerates scarring due to reflux.

Morphology

The macroscopic appearance of chronic reflux-associated pyelonephritis is so characteristic as to be diagnostic. Deep irregular scars are seen towards the poles of the kidney. Involvement may be unilateral, or if bilateral is characteristically asymmetrical. There is a distinctive relationship between the scarred areas and the underlying deformed and dilated calyces.

Microscopically there is interstitial fibrosis with atrophic and dilated tubules containing eosinophilic casts, giving the appearance of 'thyroidisation' of the kidney, so-called because of the resemblance to thyroid histology.

Xanthogranulomatous pyelonephritis

Xanthogranulomatous pyelonephritis is an uncommon condition, which develops in patients with chronic pyelonephritis, and is associated with *Proteus* and *E. coli* infection and intrapelvic stones.

Clinicopathological features

A renal mass is present in the majority of cases; it may distort the external surface of the kidney and resemble a neoplasm. The cut surface shows a yellowish mass surrounding distorted calyces, and small abscesses are often seen in the adjacent areas. Histologically, foamy macrophages dominate the lesion and are admixed with a varied population of inflammatory cells. The clinical significance of this lesion relates to the potential confusion with renal cell carcinoma, and the risk of fistulae.

Renal tuberculosis

The kidneys can be affected by tuberculosis as part of generalised miliary spread from an active tuberculous lesion elsewhere (usually in the lungs); the kidneys become dotted with numerous minute white granulomas.

Solitary tuberculous lesions occur in the kidneys of adults. These may or may not be associated with other active tuberculous lesions elsewhere; they may represent reactivation of a dormant lesion. The kidney contains an irregular white mass filled with caseous material. This arises within the renal parenchyma but may eventually rupture into the calyceal system leaving an open, ragged cavity and enabling tubercle bacilli to seed along the ureter and into the bladder. Severe and longstanding tuberculosis may produce a tuberculous pyonephrosis with complete destruction of the kidney. 'Sterile' pyuria is an important feature in renal tuberculosis and should stimulate an active search for the acid-alcohol-fast bacilli in the urine.

Viral infections

Virus infection of the kidney is probably a common occurrence. Tubular and glomerular involvement has been demonstrated in cases of measles, mumps, herpes zoster, influenza and other viral infections. Nevertheless, viruses do not appear to be involved in pyelonephritis. Cytomegalovirus, which gives characteristic cytoplasmic and intranuclear acidophilic inclusions in the tubular cells, is very common but appears to cause little damage under normal circumstances.

URINARY CALCULI

Urinary calculi (stones) occur in 1–5% of the population in the UK, mainly those over 30 years, and with a male preponderance. They may form anywhere in the urinary tract, but the commonest site is within the renal pelvis. They present as renal colic, an exquisitely painful symptom due to the passage of a small stone along the ureter, or only as a dull ache in the loins, or as a recurrent and intractable urinary tract infection.

Calculi form in the urine either because substances are in such an excess that they precipitate, or because other factors affecting solubility are upset. Factors influencing stone formation include the pH of the urine, which can be influenced by both bacterial activity and metabolic factors. Substances in the urine normally inhibit precipitation of crystals, notably pyrophosphates and citrates. The mucoproteins in the urine are thought to provide the organic nidus on which the crystals focus.

Classification

Calculi are classified according to their composition. The categories are:

- calcium oxalate, often mixed with calcium phosphate and uric acid (75–80% of all calculi)
- triple (stuivite) stones composed of magnesium ammonium phosphate (15%); these form the large 'staghorn' calculi (Fig. 21.17)
- uric acid stones (6%)
- calculi in cystinuria and oxalosis (1%).

Only 10% of patients with *calcium-containing stones* have hyperparathyroidism or some other cause of hypercalcaemia. However, most have increased levels of calcium in the urine, which is attributable to a defect in the tubular reabsorption. In the remaining patients, with idiopathic hypercalciuria, no known cause has been identified. The association of uric acid with calcium stones is probably because urates can initiate precipitation of oxalate from solution.

Magnesium ammonium phosphate stones are particularly associated with urinary tract infections with bacteria, such as *Proteus*, which are able to break down urea to form ammonia. The alkaline conditions thus produced, together with sluggish flow, cause precipitation of these salts and large staghorn calculi form a cast of the pelvicalyceal system. Staghorn calculi remain in the pelvis for many years and may cause irritation, with subsequent squamous metaplasia or in some cases squamous carcinoma.

Uric acid stones occur in patients with gout (Ch. 7). Uric acid precipitates in acid urine. The stones are radiolucent.

TUMOURS OF THE KIDNEY

> ▶ Benign tumours (e.g. fibroma, adenoma) infrequently cause clinical problems
> ▶ Malignant tumours are renal cell carcinoma (hypernephroma), Wilms' tumour (nephroblastoma) and transitional cell carcinoma
> ▶ Renal cell carcinoma often presents with metastases (occult primary)
> ▶ Malignant tumours present with pain and/or haematuria

Primary tumours and metastases occur in the kidneys, but metastases are less frequent than would be expected in view of the generous blood supply of the kidneys.

Benign renal tumours

Renal fibroma

The commonest benign renal tumour is the renal fibroma or *reno-medullary interstitial cell tumour*. This tumour is usually an incidental finding at autopsy with no clinical significance. Renal fibromas are firm white nodules, usually less than 10 mm in diameter, situated in the medulla or in the papillae and composed of spindle cells tending to surround the adjacent tubules.

Benign cortical adenoma

Benign cortical adenomas are discrete yellowish-grey nodules, usually less than 20 mm in diameter, situated in the cortex of the kidney. They are not uncom-

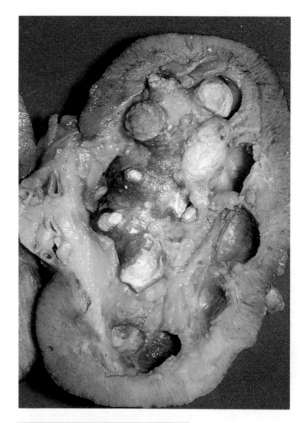

Fig. 21.17 'Staghorn' calculus

The shape of the stone is moulded to that of the pelvis and calyceal system in which it has formed.

mon, being discovered in up to 20% of autopsies. Histologically, there is nothing to distinguish the adenoma from a renal tubular carcinoma; both are composed of large clear cells with small nuclei. The distinction is often made only by size: those below 30 mm in diameter are regarded as benign. This distinction is entirely arbitrary and unreliable, since an early carcinoma may not have achieved the 30 mm threshold. Malignancy may develop in cortical adenomas.

Oncocytoma
Oncocytoma is a subtype of adenoma in which the granular cytoplasm, attributable to abundant large and distorted mitochondria, is the most prominent feature. Oncocytomas occasionally attain a considerable size and thus are easily confused with renal cell carcinomas.

Other benign tumours

Benign tumours can arise from any cell type within

the kidney. Few cause clinical problems, other than *haemangiomas* which may bleed, thus causing pain or predisposing to severe blood loss in the event of trauma.

A rare *tumour of the juxtaglomerular cells* produces renin and is a cause of hypertension in young patients.

Angiomyolipoma is an intra-renal mass composed of a mixture of blood vessels, muscle and mature fat. The lesion is not a true tumour, but is best regarded as a hamartoma. The clinical importance of this lesion lies in the association with tuberous sclerosis, an inherited disorder involving the central nervous system, skin and other viscera.

Malignant renal tumours

The clinically important malignant tumours of the kidney are:

- renal cell carcinoma (hypernephroma)
- Wilms' tumour (nephroblastoma)
- transitional cell carcinoma of the renal pelvis.

Renal cell carcinoma

Renal cell carcinoma (*hypernephroma, Grawitz tumour*) is the commonest primary kidney tumour in adults, but it accounts for only 1–3% of all visceral tumours. It occurs most frequently over the age of 50 years; there is a male preponderance. The common presenting clinical features of haematuria, loin pain and a mass, are late manifestations and account for the relatively poor prognosis. In patients with no evidence of metastasis at presentation, the 5-year survival may be as high as 70%, but it falls to 15–20% when the renal vein is involved or there is extension into the perinephric fat.

Aetiology. There is an increased incidence of renal carcinoma in those who smoke tobacco. There is no evidence to suggest any other known aetiological agents to be relevant in man. A genetic predisposition is indicated by the strong association with von Hippel–Lindau disease (Ch. 11), a rare hereditary condition.

The behaviour of these tumours is very difficult to predict. Hypernephromas are not uncommonly associated with paraneoplastic manifestations including:

- hypercalcaemia
- hypertension
- polycythaemia.

Additionally, some cases develop an eosinophilia or leukaemoid reaction in the blood, and a small proportion of patients develop amyloidosis.

Morphology. Macroscopically, the kidney is distorted by a large bossellated tumour which most often occurs in the upper pole (Fig. 21.18). The cut surface reveals a solid yellowish-grey tumour with areas of haemorrhage and necrosis. Hypernephromas are sometimes cystic; this can present diagnostic problems. The margins of the tumour are usually well demarcated, but some breach the renal capsule and invade the perinephric fat. Extension into the renal vein is sometimes seen grossly; occasionally, a solid mass of tumour extends into the inferior vena cava and, rarely, into the right atrium.

Histologically, renal cell carcinomas are composed

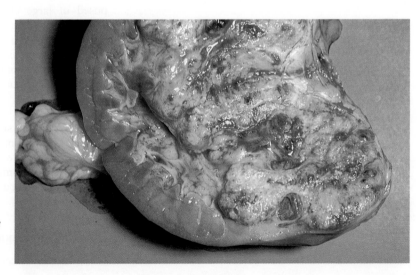

Fig. 21.18 Renal cell carcinoma (hypernephroma)

These tumours occur most commonly at the upper pole of a kidney. The cut surface is typically variegated due to areas of haemorrhage and necrosis.

of either clear or granular cells. The small nuclei belie the malignant nature of this tumour. The clear cytoplasm is due to glycogen and fat; the similarity to adrenal cortical cells is responsible for the name 'hypernephroma', since these tumours were originally thought to arise from embryonic adrenal rests!

Wilms' tumour

Wilms' tumour is the commonest intra-abdominal tumour in children under the age of 10 years; the peak incidence is between the ages of 1 and 4 years, and the sexes are equally involved. The most common presentation is with an abdominal mass. Haematuria, hypertension, abdominal pain and intestinal obstruction may also be the initial clinical features. The tumour is aggressive and rapidly growing; spread to the lungs is identified in a high proportion of cases at the time of diagnosis. Aggressive therapy involving radiotherapy, chemotherapy and surgery has greatly improved the prognosis in these cases.

Morphology. Macroscopically the tumour is often large, and frequently extends beyond the capsule into the perinephric fat and even into the root of the mesentery. The cut surface is variegated and reflects the component tissues seen histologically. Areas of haemorrhagic necrosis are common, merging with solid tumour composed of firm white tissue, together with cartilaginous and mucinous areas.

Histologically, both epithelial and mesenchymal tissues are seen, the tumour being derived from the mesonephric mesoderm. There are poorly developed glomeruli and tubules in a spindle cell stroma. Striated muscle is frequently present in these tumours together with myxoid fibrous tissue, cartilage, bone and fat, thus creating a rather bizarre mixture.

Carcinoma of the renal pelvis

While the majority of renal tumours in adults are renal cell carcinomas, the greater proportion of those remaining (5–10%) are transitional cell carcinomas arising from the urothelium of the renal pelvis. As they project into the pelvicalyceal cavity, they present early with haematuria or obstruction (Fig. 21.19). They frequently infiltrate the wall of the pelvis and may involve the renal vein. The prognosis is not good, especially for those patients with poorly differentiated tumours, and multiple tumours are not uncommon in the ureters and bladder.

Aetiology. There is an association with analgesic abuse, and exposure to aniline dyes used in the dye, rubber, plastics and gas industries (Ch. 11). A few

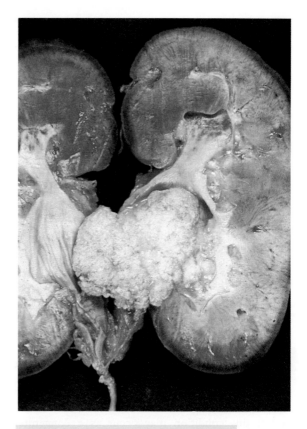

Fig. 21.19   Carcinoma of the renal pelvis

These malignant tumours arise from the transitional cell epithelium (urothelium) lining the renal pelvis. These patients commonly develop synchronous or metachronous urothelial tumours elsewhere in the ureters or bladder.

patients have been reported with transitional cell carcinoma many years following the use of Thorotrast, an α-emitter, in retrograde pyelography.

Clinicopathological features. These are fronded transitional cell neoplasms, identical to their counterparts in the ureter and urinary bladder. It is not uncommon to find multiple transitional cell tumours throughout the urinary tract, suggesting a urothelial field change. The papillary form of the tumours results in fragments breaking off from the tips of the fronds; atypical tumour cells can be detected in the urine, making these lesions particularly amenable to cytological diagnosis and screening.

In the presence of pelvic stones the urothelium may undergo squamous metaplasia. Squamous carcinoma is known to be associated with calculi and chronic infection, but may also arise de novo from the transitional epithelium. Macroscopically, they are usually flat and infiltrative, and carry a poor prognosis.

URETERS

Normal structure and function

The ureters form in continuity with the calyceal system and collecting ducts from an outgrowth of the Wolffian duct. Urine is conveyed to the bladder by peristaltic activity; this activity is reduced in pregnancy, predisposing to stasis and infection.

The lumen is lined by urothelium; the muscle layer is predominantly circular with a thin, inner longitudinal layer, and is invested in a fibrous adventitia. The ureteric orifice is slit-like, and the course of the terminal part of the ureter through the bladder wall is oblique to form a valve (Fig. 21.16).

Congenital lesions

Congenital lesions include *double or bifid ureters* which may be associated with structural abnormalities of the pelvicalyceal system. These usually have no consequences for renal function. However, a congenitally short terminal segment of the ureter, which is not oblique, results in vesico-ureteric reflux, an important cause of renal infection and scarring. *Hydroureter* is dilatation and often tortuosity of the ureter; this condition may occur as a congenital lesion, when it is thought to reflect a neuromuscular defect. The most frequent causes of hydroureter in the adult are low urinary obstruction and pregnancy.

Inflammation

The ureter may become inflamed due to a urinary tract infection, and chronic inflammation may supervene. In some patients with chronic inflammation, a condition called *ureteritis cystica* develops, in which epithelial cell nests become trapped by fibrosis and subsequently develop into thin-walled cysts.

Obstruction

Obstruction of the ureter is the most frequent problem requiring clinical attention. Acute ureteric obstruction causes intense pain known as renal colic. The consequences of chronic ureteric obstruction are hydroureter and hydronephrosis. In both acute and chronic ureteric obstruction there is an increased risk of ascending infection, causing pyelonephritis.

Ureteric obstruction may be either intrinsic or extrinsic. *Intrinsic lesions* are within the ureteric wall or lumen; the most common is a urinary calculus. Calculi become impacted where the ureter is nor-

mally narrowed, that is at the pelvi-ureteric junction, where it crosses the iliac artery, and where it enters the bladder. Strictures may be congenital, when they occur at the pelvi-ureteric junction or in the transmural terminal segment of the ureter. Acquired strictures occur as a result of trauma and involvement by adjacent inflammatory conditions such as diverticulitis and salpingitis. Severe haematuria may cause obstruction due to blood clot.

Extrinsic factors cause pressure from without, and include tumours of the rectum, prostate and bladder. Aberrant renal arteries may compress the ureter. Retroperitoneal fibrosis causes narrowing and medial deviation of the ureters and may be due either to drugs, such as methysergide, or be idiopathic.

Primary tumours of the ureter are usually transitional cell carcinomas. They may be multiple and are associated with urothelial tumours in the urinary pelvis and bladder.

BLADDER

Normal structure and function

The urinary bladder is a cavity lined by transitional cell epithelium — the *urothelium*, surrounded by connective tissue — the *lamina propria*, and smooth muscle. Histologically, the normal bladder urothelium is 7–8 cells thick and has three zones: basal, intermediate and a highly specialised surface layer. The smooth muscle is arranged in bundles which interlace rather than form defined layers. Urine drains into the bladder from the kidneys, via the ureters, for storage until a convenient time and place is found for its discharge through the urethra.

The bladder responds to obstruction to the outflow by undergoing muscular hypertrophy.

The proximity of the bladder to the genital tract in females, to the prostate in males, and to the bowel in both sexes, means that it is often invaded by tumours arising in these other organs.

Diverticula

Diverticula are outpouchings of the bladder mucosa. Bladder diverticula are either congenital or acquired. They are clinically important because urinary stasis within them predisposes to calculus formation and infection.

Congenital diverticula are usually solitary. They arise from either a localised developmental defect in the muscle or urinary obstruction during fetal life.

Acquired diverticula are small and multiple. They are most often associated with outflow obstruction, and the high incidence in elderly males correlates with prostatic enlargement. They occur between the bands of hypertrophic muscle, known as trabeculae, which form in response to obstruction.

Congenital lesions

Exstrophy of the bladder is a serious developmental defect affecting the anterior abdominal wall, bladder and, in some cases, the symphysis pubis. The bladder opens directly on to the external surface of the lower abdomen. Infection and pyelonephritis, together with a predisposition to adenocarcinoma, are important sequelae.

Vesico-ureteric reflux (VUR) is an important consequence of a developmental abnormality of the terminal part of the ureter, which appears to correct itself as the patient matures. However, during early childhood reflux occurs, which results in substantial scarring of the renal parenchyma. This condition is an important cause of renal impairment and infection in adult life (p. 646).

Persistence of the urachus may be partial or complete. Retention of the entire structure results in a fistula connecting the bladder with the skin at the umbilicus. Partial retention results in a diverticulum arising from the dome of the bladder. Alternatively the central area may persist and present as a cyst. Adenocarcinomas develop in these urachal remnants.

Cystitis

Inflammation of the bladder (cystitis) is a common occurrence as part of a urinary tract infection.

Aetiology. The causative organism is usually derived from the patient's faecal flora. Unusual organisms do occur: for example, *Candida* is seen in patients on prolonged antibiotic therapy, and tuberculous cystitis almost always reflects tuberculosis elsewhere in the urinary tract. Radiation and trauma due to instrumentation cause cystitis which is often sterile.

Clinical features. Cystitis presents with frequency, lower abdominal pain and dysuria (scalding or burning pain on micturition), and occasionally haematuria. In some patients there is general malaise and pyrexia. Cystitis usually responds readily to treatment. However, its clinical importance lies in the predisposition to pyelonephritis, a serious complication.

Pathological forms
Several different forms of cystitis occur, each expressing increasing severity. The initial hyperaemia may

be excessive, causing *haemorrhagic cystitis*. When there are areas of yellow fibrinous exudate, *exudative cystitis* is present. In some patients, the exudate is mixed with necrotic mucosa, and the term *membranous cystitis* applies. Finally, ischaemia results in black necrotic mucosa, which is termed *gangrenous cystitis*.

When chronic cystitis is due to urea-splitting organisms, the alkalinity of the urine encourages precipitation of calcium ammonium phosphate crystals on the surface of the bladder and as calculi in the lumen.

Cystitis cystica occurs as a result of nests of urothelial cells becoming trapped in inflammatory fibrous tissue in patients with chronic cystitis. Sometimes these cells undergo glandular metaplasia; this is *cystitis glandularis*. The presence of lymphoid follicles in the lamina propria of patients with chronic cystitis is termed *cystitis follicularis*.

Malakoplakia is an uncommon variant of importance because it can mimic a tumour. Broad flat yellow plaques form in the mucosa, which may subsequently ulcerate. The plaques comprise a mixture of chronic inflammatory cells, including characteristic macrophages; these contain calcified granules known as Michaelis–Gutmann bodies. The granules are composed of bacterial debris, and they are thought to reflect defective macrophage function.

Tuberculous cystitis nearly always implies tuberculosis elsewhere in the renal tract. The organisms enter the mucosa from the urine and stimulate the usual granulomatous response causing small tubercles which subsequently ulcerate. The tubercles form around the ureteric orifices and in the region of the bladder base. Eventually the bladder wall may become thickened, contracted and fibrous, and lined by caseous material.

Schistosomiasis also causes a granulomatous cystitis, in which the parasites are demonstrable, and is notable for the increased risk of squamous cell carcinoma.

Obstruction

Obstruction to the urinary outflow from the bladder has serious repercussions on the kidneys as well as causing changes in the bladder wall. Most cases are due to:

- prostatic disease in elderly men (Ch. 20)
- prolapse in elderly women, when part of the bladder protrudes into the vagina producing a pouch
- calculi
- bladder tumours (see below)

- urethral strictures
- neurological damage.

The bladder wall becomes thickened due to hypertrophy of the muscle bundles, causing the characteristic interlacing ridges — trabeculae — between which small diverticula may develop.

Bladder calculi

Diverticula, obstruction and inflammation are all important in the development of stones within the bladder. Alternatively, calculi may be passed down the ureter from the kidney. Bladder stones may be asymptomatic, but eventual chronic irritation and infection lead to frequency, urgency, dysuria and sometimes haematuria. There is an increased risk of bladder carcinoma; this is often of squamous type arising from metaplastic squamous epithelium.

Fistulae

Fistulae between the bladder and adjacent structures occur as a result of:

- invasion by a malignant neoplasm
- radiation necrosis
- inflammatory bowel lesions (diverticulitis of the colon, Crohn's disease)
- surgical complications.

Vesico-vaginal and vesico-uterine fistulae, presenting with urine draining through the vagina, result from carcinoma of the cervix and uterus respectively. Vesico-enteric fistulae cause turbid urine with bacterial contamination and inflammation, and in some cases faecal material in the urine.

Tumours of the bladder

> ▶ Most bladder tumours are transitional cell carcinomas
> ▶ Squamous cell carcinomas and adenocarcinomas are less common
> ▶ Sarcomas are rare
> ▶ Aetiological factors for transitional cell carcinoma include smoking and occupational exposure to dyes
> ▶ Aetiological factors for squamous cell carcinoma include calculi and schistosomiasis

Epithelial tumours of the bladder are common; sarcomas are relatively rare. The majority are transitional cell carcinomas; a small proportion are squamous. Adenocarcinoma of the bladder is uncommon.

Aetiology

The strong association of bladder tumours with certain chemicals (Ch. 11) has resulted in measures in industrial processes to reduce the level of risk to the employees. Bladder carcinogens include some dyes in textiles and printing, and reagents in the rubber, cable and plastics industries. The carcinogenic substances are intermediate metabolites of aniline compounds; these are excreted in combination with glucuronic acid, and are subsequently released in the bladder by the action of β-glucuronidase which is facilitated by the acidity of the urine. An increased incidence of urothelial tumours is also seen in heavy smokers and analgesic abusers. Schistosomiasis is an important cause of squamous cell carcinoma of the bladder.

Transitional cell carcinoma

Transitional cell carcinomas arise from the urothelium and are frequently multiple. The multifocal origin suggests that the entire urothelium may be unstable as a result of exposure to a carcinogen. Carcinoma is often preceded by dysplasia.

Painless haematuria is the commonest presenting feature, with dysuria, frequency and urgency occurring in some patients. When the tumour is near a ureteric orifice, obstruction causes unilateral pyelonephritis or hydronephrosis. Many of these tumours are papillary and tumour cells are frequently shed into the urine where they can be detected by cytology.

Morphology

Most bladder tumours are papillary, the delicate fronds of which are best appreciated cystoscopically. The fronds are covered by an abnormally thick layer of urothelium, with atypical cytological features (Fig. 21.20). In some lesions, the cells closely resemble normal urothelium and there is no evidence of invasion. With increasing cytological abnormalities, however, the likelihood of invasion of the lamina propria increases. When the deep muscle of the bladder wall is invaded, the tumour becomes fixed clinically. Poorly differentiated transitional cell carcinomas are solid, usually invasive, and display severe cytological atypia.

A significant proportion of transitional cell carcinomas show microscopic foci of squamous, or more rarely, glandular metaplasia. Such areas form a substantial part of the tumour in about 5% of transitional carcinomas, which are then termed mixed tumours.

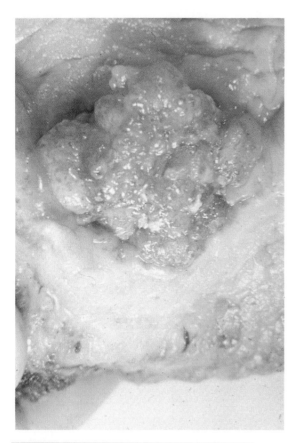

Fig. 21.20   Transitional cell carcinoma of the bladder

These common tumours usually initially project into the bladder lumen before invading the underlying bladder wall.

Staging and grading
Transitional cell carcinomas are graded I–III according to the degree of cytological atypia; this is a guide to prognosis. Staging is also used to judge prognosis; the TNM system is used (Ch. 11). There is good correlation between grade and stage, since the majority of papillary growths are grade I and are non-invasive. In contrast, grade III lesions are usually flat, ulcerated and invasive, and carry a poor prognosis.

Carcinoma in situ
Carcinoma in situ of the urothelium is often found as a multifocal change in areas between tumours, and in some bladders in which no obvious tumours are present. It is a precursor of invasive carcinoma.

Squamous cell carcinoma

Squamous cell carcinomas arise from metaplastic squamous epithelium; this change occurs most often in association with calculi and with schistosomiasis. They are usually solid invasive tumours. The prognosis is not as good as for transitional carcinoma, but depends on the grade and stage of the individual tumour. A similar histological appearance is produced by involvement of the bladder by a squamous carcinoma of the cervix; this sometimes causes diagnostic confusion.

Adenocarcinoma

Adenocarcinoma of the bladder is uncommon. It can arise from:

- urachal remnants at the bladder apex
- cystitis cystica
- glandular metaplasia in a transitional carcinoma
- periurethral and periprostatic glands.

Mesenchymal tumours

Benign and malignant mesenchymal tumours occur in the bladder, but uncommonly. Benign tumours reflect the range of cell types in the wall:

- leiomyoma
- rhabdomyoma
- haemangioma
- neurofibroma.

Malignant mesenchymal tumours are usually rhabdomyosarcomas and occur in both adults and children. The appearance in the two groups is distinctive and merits comment. Rhabdomyosarcomas in adults occur in patients over 40 years, and are usually solid growths, histologically resembling the rhabdomyosarcoma seen in striated muscle. In children, the tumours are large and composed of polypoid clusters resembling bunches of grapes, typical of a sarcoma botryoides or embryonal rhabdomyosarcoma.

Secondary tumours

Secondary tumours of the bladder usually occur by direct extension, most often from the cervix, prostate or rectum. Haematogenous and lymphatic spread may occur from carcinomas in distant primary sites, e.g. lung.

FURTHER READING

Hill G S 1989 Uropathology. Churchill Livingstone, New York
Rosen S (ed) 1983 Pathology of glomerular disease.
    Churchill Livingstone, New York

Young R H (ed) 1989 Pathology of the urinary bladder.
    Churchill Livingstone, New York

Lymph nodes, thymus and spleen

LYMPH NODES

NORMAL STRUCTURE AND FUNCTION

Lymph nodes are discrete encapsulated structures, usually ovoid and ranging in diameter from a few millimetres to several centimetres. They are situated along the course of lymphatic vessels and are more numerous where these vessels converge (e.g. roots of limbs, neck, pelvis and mediastinum).

Micro-architecture and functional anatomy

Lymph nodes are surrounded by a connective tissue capsule, with trabeculae which extend into the substance of the node and provide a framework for the contained cellular elements. Beneath the capsule is a slit-like space, the subcapsular sinus, into which the afferent lymphatics drain after penetrating the capsule. Lymph from the subcapsular sinus passes via the medullary cords to the hilum of the lymph node from which the efferent lymphatic drains.

Three distinct micro-anatomical regions can be recognised within normal lymph nodes (Ch. 9). These regions are:

- the *cortex*, which contains nodules of B-lymphocytes either as primary follicles or as germinal centres
- the *paracortex* or *deep cortex*, which is the T-cell-dependent region of the lymph node
- the *medulla*, containing the medullary cords and sinuses which drain into the hilum.

The micro-anatomical regions of the lymph nodes are populated by a variety of specialised cells with different functional characteristics.

Germinal centres

The germinal centre is the principal site of B-cell activation in response to antigenic challenge. Antigen entering the lymph node via the afferent lymphatics is trapped upon the surface of specialised antigen-presenting cells called *dendritic reticulum cells* (DRC) which are restricted to B-cell areas. DRCs are binucleate cells with long cytoplasmic processes linked by desmosomes which form a network throughout the germinal centre. Antigen trapped upon the surface of the DRC is presented to 'virgin' B-lymphocytes in the presence of T-helper cells

(T-cell co-operation) and these B-cells subsequently undergo a series of morphological and functional changes (Table 22.1). The exact sequence of morphological changes undergone by the germinal centre B-cells is controversial. However, most evidence favours that, after antigenic challenge, the initial step in B-cell transformation is the formation of the *centroblast*, which then develops into a *centrocyte* (Fig. 22.1B).

The function of germinal centres is to generate immunoglobulin-secreting plasma cells in response to antigenic challenge. Within the lymph node, plasma cells are located principally within the *medullary cords*.

Table 22.1   Characteristics and nomenclature (Kiel scheme) of follicle-centre cells and therefore B-cell lymphomas derived therefrom

Cell features	Nomenclature
Small lymphocyte with round nucleus	**Lymphocyte**
Small or large cell with indented nucleus	**Centrocyte**
Large cell with round nucleus and usually multiple nucleoli	**Centroblast**
Large cell with round nucleus and large nucleolus	**Immunoblast**

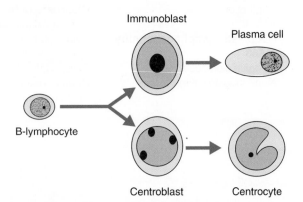

Fig. 22.1   Morphological changes of the germinal centre B-cell

Schematic diagram of hypothetical follicle centre B-cell transformation. The virgin B-lymphocyte has two activation pathways. The first involves direct transformation to an immunoblast following exposure to an antigen, with subsequent differentiation to an immunoglobulin-secreting plasma cell; this pathway is independent of the germinal centre. The second pathway occurs within the germinal centre and involves the generation of a centroblast as the initial reaction to antigen exposure, with subsequent differentiation to a centrocyte.

The fully formed germinal centre is seen histologically as a rounded, pale structure in the cortex of the lymph node, surrounded by a rim of small, round lymphocytes termed the *mantle zone*. Distinct zonation may be seen within the germinal centre: a pale zone faces towards the subcapsular sinus and is rich in centrocytes and T-cells and contains the greatest density of DRCs; at the opposite pole of the germinal centre is a dark zone rich in rapidly dividing centroblasts mixed with tingible body macrophages which phagocytose the cellular debris generated by apoptosis (Fig. 22.2).

Paracortex

The paracortex is the T-cell-dependent region of the lymph node and accordingly contains large numbers of T-lymphocytes with a predominance of the helper/inducer subset (CD4 positive). The cluster of differentiation (CD) 4 antigen is expressed by helper/inducer T-cells. As in the germinal centre, specialised antigen-presenting cells are present in the paracortex; these are called *interdigitating reticulum cells* (IDC) and are different morphologically and functionally from the DRCs. IDCs possess abundant cytoplasm with complex membrane profiles which interdigitate with surrounding T-cells. Large amounts of class II HLA substances are expressed on the surface of the IDC and this is important for interactions between immune cells, especially in antigen presentation to T-cells (particularly the helper T-cells).

Medulla

Lymph enters the marginal sinus of the node and drains to the hilum through sinuses which converge in the medullary region. The sinuses are lined by macrophages which phagocytose particulate material within the lymph. Between the sinuses in the medulla lie the medullary cords which contain numerous plasma cells and are one of the main sites of antibody secretion within the lymph node.

LYMPH NODE ENLARGEMENT

▶ Localised or generalised
▶ Diagnosis often requires lymph node biopsy
▶ May be due to inflammatory, reactive or neoplastic disorders
▶ Neoplastic disorders may be primary (e.g. lymphoma) or secondary (e.g. metastatic carcinoma)

Pathological basis of signs and symptoms attributable to the lymphoreticular system	
Sign or symptom	Pathological basis
Enlarged lymph nodes	Neoplastic infiltration • primary (lymphoma) • secondary (metastases) Specific infections (e.g. tuberculosis, toxoplasmosis, infectious mononucleosis) Reactive hyperplasia
Enlarged spleen	Congestion (heart failure, portal hypertension) Storage disorder Neoplastic infiltration (leukaemia, lymphoma)
Susceptibility to infection	Immune deficiency • congenital • acquired (lymphoma, leukaemia, AIDS, iatrogenic)
Weight loss/ pyrexia	Interleukins produced by inflammatory or lymphomatous (i.e. type B symptoms) tissue acting on thermoregulatory centre in hypothalamus
Muscle weakness (myasthenia gravis)	Thymic hyperplasia or neoplasia
Howell–Jolly inclusions in red cells	Persistence of DNA fragments in red cells due to splenic atrophy

Lymph node enlargement (lymphadenopathy) may be localised or widespread and is a common clinical problem which frequently requires a biopsy to establish a diagnosis. The causes of lymphadenopathy are varied and include:

• infection (both local and systemic)
• autoimmune disorders
• neoplasms (either primary or metastatic).

NON-NEOPLASTIC LYMPHADENOPATHY

Lymph nodes respond to a wide variety of inflammatory stimuli by cellular proliferation which leads to node enlargement. The cell type which proliferates is dependent upon the antigenic stimulus, which may elicit:

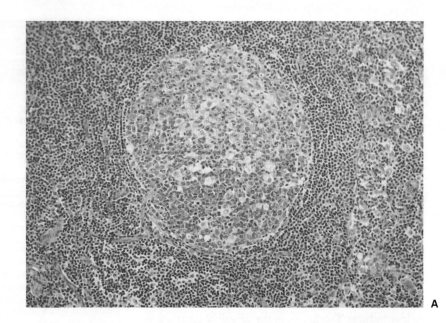

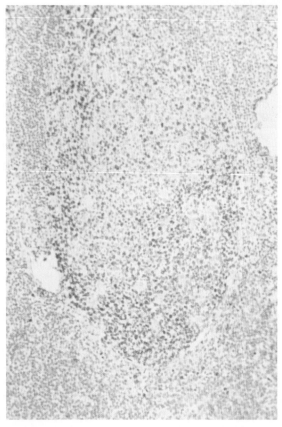

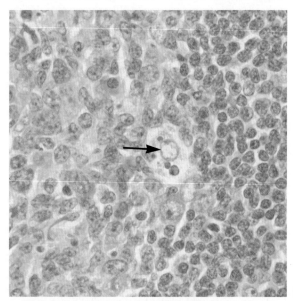

Fig. 22.2   Lymph node germinal centre

A. Normal germinal centre showing distinct zoning, the lower half containing closely packed and rapidly dividing centroblasts. **B.** A germinal centre stained with monoclonal antibody to proliferating cells (Ki-67). Numerous dividing cells (brown nuclei) are seen in the lower, centroblast rich, region of the germinal centre. **C.** High-power view of phagocytic or 'tingible body' macrophage (arrowed) engulfing apoptotic lymphoid cells. These are concentrated in the most proliferative part of the germinal centre.

- a predominantly *B-cell response* with germinal centre hyperplasia
- a predominantly *T-cell response* with paracortical expansion
- a *macrophage response* which is associated with sinus hyperplasia
- most commonly, a *mixed response* in which all the cellular elements of the lymph node are activated and proliferate.

Non-specific reactive hyperplasia

The pattern of cellular proliferation within a lymph node may give some clue to the aetiology of the lymphadenopathy (see below); however, in many instances these clues are absent and the features are termed *non-specific reactive hyperplasia*. On occasions the node enlargement may reach a considerable size (rarely, up to 100 mm in diameter) and be difficult to distinguish clinically and macroscopically from neoplastic disorders. Microscopically, numerous enlarged germinal centres are seen which may be present throughout the node and are not restricted to the outer cortex as in the normal state. The germinal centres are active, with a predominance of large blast cells, a high mitotic rate, and often contain numerous tingible body macrophages. The paracortex usually shows some degree of hyperplasia characterised by the presence of transformed, large lymphoid cells and vessels lined by large endothelial cells (high endothelial venules). The sinuses often show hyperplasia of the lining macrophages termed *sinus histiocytosis*.

Non-specific reactive hyperplasia may occur in lymph nodes draining sites of infection and, in some cases, pathogenic organisms may cause inflammatory changes within the substance of the node, termed *lymphadenitis*, which may progress to abscess formation.

Specific disorders

Some types of non-neoplastic lymphadenopathy exhibit histological features which allow the pathologist to make an exact diagnosis. These may be grouped into the following categories:

- granulomatous lymphadenitis
- necrotising lymphadenitis
- sinus histiocytosis
- paracortical hyperplasia.

Granulomatous lymphadenitis

Granulomatous lymphadenitis can occur in a variety

of clinical settings such as mycobacterial infection (Ch. 14), sarcoidosis (Ch. 14) and Crohn's disease (Ch. 15). These are described elsewhere and will not be detailed here.

Infection with *Toxoplasma gondii*, a protozoal organism, in the immunocompetent host produces a flu-like illness of short duration and localised lymphadenopathy, usually occipital or high cervical, which persists for some weeks. The affected lymph node is enlarged and shows germinal centre hyperplasia with formation of ill-defined granulomas adjacent to them. In addition, the node sinuses are distended with medium-sized, monomorphic B-cells called monocytoid B-cells. This histological triad of follicular hyperplasia with adjacent granulomas and sinus distension by monocytoid B-cells suggests a diagnosis of toxoplasmic lymphadenitis which should be confirmed serologically (Fig. 22.3).

Lymph nodes draining tumours occasionally show a granulomatous reaction in the absence of metastatic involvement, possibly a reaction to tumour antigens. It is particularly common in Hodgkin's disease. Lymph nodes may develop a granulomatous response to foreign, particulate material; this most often occurs as a response to silicone compounds used in plastic surgery and joint replacement.

Necrotising lymphadenitis

A variety of diseases caused by infectious agents may lead to necrosis within lymph nodes. Examples are lymphogranuloma venereum and cat scratch disease. *Lymphogranuloma venereum* is a sexually transmitted chlamydial disease and most commonly affects the groin nodes. *Cat scratch disease* follows a bite or scratch from an infected cat. Days to weeks later, tender lymphadenopathy develops in the cervical or axillary regions; the groin is less commonly affected. The organism responsible for cat scratch disease is a recently described extracellular, pleomorphic coccobacillus (*Afipia felis*). Both diseases show histological similarities, with formation of stellate abscesses within the lymph node, surrounded by palisaded histiocytes (Fig. 22.4).

A rare form of necrotising lymphadenitis is *Kikuchi's disease*, in which tender cervical or occipital lymphadenopathy develops most commonly in young adult women. The aetiology is unknown.

Sinus histiocytosis

Sinus histiocytosis with massive lymphadenopathy (SHML or Rosai–Dorfman syndrome) is a rare condition of unknown aetiology which is more common

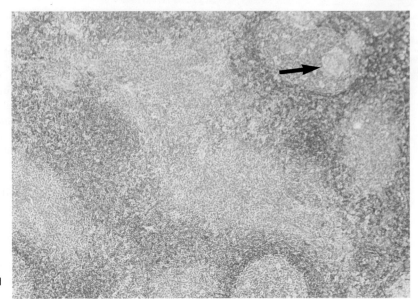

Fig. 22.3 Toxoplasmic lymphadenitis

There is follicular hyperplasia with epithelioid granulomas adjacent to germinal centres. A perifollicular proliferation of uniform B-cells, termed monocytoid B-cells, is also present.

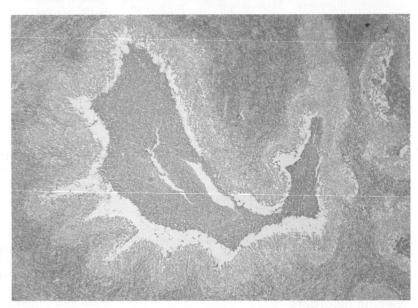

Fig. 22.4   Cat scratch disease

Lymph node showing central abscess formation surrounded by palisaded histiocytes.

in blacks than in other races. It presents typically with bulky cervical lymphadenopathy in the first decade of life and may persist for several years. SHML may however affect any age and any organ. Histologically, the lymph node sinuses are grossly distended by an infiltrate of large histiocytic cells whose morphology is quite distinctive; admixed with these cells are lymphocytes and plasma cells, which are often seen in the cytoplasm of the histiocytes. The disease often follows a benign course and may regress spontaneously.

Langerhans' cell granuloma (histiocytosis X) may affect lymph nodes and characteristically involves the sinuses initially, where clusters of typical, pale Langerhans' cells with folded nuclei may be seen among giant cells and eosinophils.

Paracortical hyperplasia

Paracortical hyperplasia is a prominent feature in many cases of lymphadenopathy. Two entities deserve special mention: dermatopathic lymphadenopathy and infectious mononucleosis.

Patients with exfoliative chronic skin conditions

such as severe eczema or psoriasis, and patients with cutaneous T-cell lymphoma, quite commonly develop enlarged lymph nodes in the groin and axilla. This condition is *dermatopathic lymphadenopathy*. The enlarged lymph nodes may have a yellow or brown cut surface and, microscopically, the paracortex is expanded by pale histiocytes with the cytological features of interdigitating reticulum cells and Langerhans' cells; lipid droplets and melanin pigment may also be apparent.

Infectious mononucleosis is due to Epstein–Barr virus. This causes widespread lymphadenopathy and is characterised, certainly in the later stages, by paracortical hyperplasia with numerous, large transformed T-cells. The histological picture may be mistaken for high-grade non-Hodgkin's lymphoma or Hodgkin's disease by the unwary pathologist.

Human immunodeficiency virus infection

The human immunodeficiency virus (HIV) specifically binds to the cluster of differentiation (CD) 4 antigen, which is expressed by helper/inducer T-cells and by cells of the mononuclear phagocytic system. The destruction of cells bearing the CD4 antigen causes a severe immune dysregulation, which ultimately leads to a profound immunodeficiency state called the *acquired immunodeficiency syndrome* (AIDS).

Lymphadenopathy is extremely common in HIV infection and may be observed in association with systemic symptoms in the AIDS-related complex (Ch. 9) and in the persistent generalised lymphadenopathy (PGL) syndrome (defined as persistent, extra-inguinal lymphadenopathy, in two or more non-contiguous sites, of greater than 3 months duration and of no known aetiology other than HIV infection).

Morphology
Lymph node biopsies from patients infected with HIV show a spectrum of appearances which, although not absolutely specific, are virtually diagnostic in the appropriate clinical setting. Initially the follicles are hyperplastic and often markedly irregular in shape. Ultrastructurally, a proliferation of dendritic reticulum cells is observed, with complex branching of their processes. In between the DRC processes, retroviral particles can be identified. In some follicles there is focal destruction of the DRC meshwork; this is associated with an implosion of mantle zone lymphocytes and focal haemorrhage into the germinal centres ('follicular lysis'). The paracortical reaction is usually disproportionate to the degree of follicular activation and only scattered immunoblasts and transformed lymphocytes are observed. There is also a reversal of the normal CD4/CD8 ratio of T-cells, often with a preponderance of CD8 positive cells. The sinuses may be filled with monocytoid B-cells.

In the later stages of HIV infection, involutional changes are apparent. There is loss of germinal centre B-cells and depletion of paracortical T-cells; sinus histiocytosis may be prominent. These involutional changes are a poor prognostic sign and portend the development of AIDS.

Complications
Lymphadenopathy in HIV infection may not be due solely to immune dysregulation and aberrant lymphocyte proliferation; a variety of neoplastic and infective conditions may also affect the lymph node. Lymphadenopathic Kaposi's sarcoma and high-grade B-cell non-Hodgkin's lymphoma (often with Burkitt-like morphology) are common. A wide variety of infectious agents may cause lymph node enlargement, of which atypical mycobacterial infection is frequently encountered (Fig. 22.5).

NEOPLASTIC LYMPHADENOPATHY

Neoplastic lymph node enlargement may occur in:

- malignancies of the immune system (Hodgkin's disease and the non-Hodgkin's lymphomas)
- metastatic spread of solid tumours and involvement by leukaemia.

Hodgkin's disease

> ▶ A type of lymphoma characterised by the presence of Reed–Sternberg cells
> ▶ One-third of patients have systemic symptoms, notably weight loss and pyrexia
> ▶ Classified according to Rye system: nodular sclerosis, lymphocyte-predominant, mixed cellularity, lymphocyte-depleted

Although described over 150 years ago by Thomas Hodgkin, Hodgkin's disease is still an enigma. The precise identity of the malignant cells remains obscure and, unlike other neoplasms, they form only a small percentage of the total population within affected tissue, the bulk of which is composed of reactive lymphocytes, plasma cells, histiocytes and eosinophils. Hodgkin's disease appears to arise in

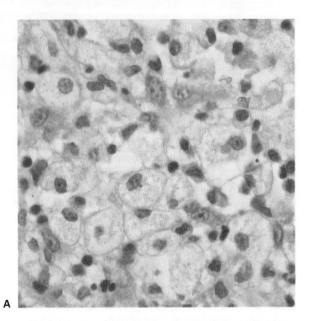

A

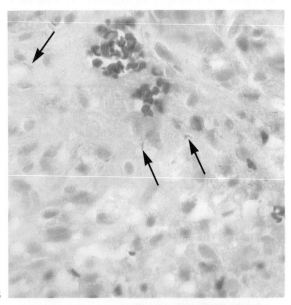

B

Fig. 22.5   Mycobacterial infection of a lymph node in AIDS

A. Aggregates of large histiocytes with foamy cytoplasm.
B. A similar area stained for acid-fast bacilli (Ziehl–Neelsen stain), demonstrating numerous mycobacteria (stained red; arrowed).

lymph nodes or the thymus, and spreads, certainly in its early stages, via the lymphatics in a contiguous and predictable fashion. Involvement of the liver and bone marrow is rarely seen in the absence of splenic

involvement and thus the spleen appears to be the key to haematogenous dissemination.

Clinical features

Hodgkin's disease shows a peak incidence in the third and fourth decades and is relatively rare in childhood and old age.

The commonest clinical presentation is one of lymphadenopathy, most often in the upper half of the body, with involvement of cervical and/or axillary lymph nodes. The enlarged nodes are typically rubbery, discrete and mobile and may achieve a considerable size. Radiological evidence of mediastinal involvement is present in over 40% of patients and on occasion may be massive, causing respiratory embarrassment. A third of patients with Hodgkin's disease have systemic symptoms (weight loss greater than 10%, unexplained pyrexia of 39°C or more, and drenching night sweats) and in a small proportion the clinical picture will be dominated by these symptoms.

Stage is an important determinant in the treatment and prognosis of patients with Hodgkin's disease; the staging system currently used is that proposed at the Ann Arbor workshop in 1971:

- *Stage I*. Involvement of a single lymph node region (I) or of a single extralymphatic organ or site (Ie).
- *Stage II*. Involvement of two or more lymph node regions on the same side of the diaphragm (II) or localised involvement of an extralymphatic organ or site and of one or more lymph node regions on the same side of the diaphragm (IIe).
- *Stage III*. Involvement of lymph node regions on both sides of the diaphragm (III) which may also be accompanied by splenic involvement (IIIs) or by localised involvement of an extralymphatic site (IIIe) or both (IIIse).
- *Stage IV*. Disseminated involvement of one or more extralymphatic organs such as liver, lung and bone marrow with or without lymph node involvement.

The absence or presence of the systemic symptoms described above is indicated by the suffix A or B respectively. The survival of patients with Hodgkin's disease declines with advancing stage and the presence of systemic (B) symptoms.

Hodgkin's disease is also associated with a variety of haematological and biochemical abnormalities such as anaemia, lymphocytopenia, a raised erythrocyte sedimentation rate (ESR) and a low serum albumin. These abnormalities are also indicators of a reduced survival.

Morphology

Hodgkin's disease is principally a disease of lymph nodes. A lymph node biopsy is usually done to establish the diagnosis.

Macroscopically, affected lymph nodes are enlarged, with a smooth surface. Hodgkin's disease, unlike the non-Hodgkin's lymphomas, rarely breaches the lymph node capsule, a fact which accounts for the discrete nature of the lymphadenopathy upon palpation. The cut surface is usually homogeneously white (Fig. 22.6), although in some histological subtypes a nodular or fibrotic appearance may be present.

Microscopically, affected lymph nodes show a partial or complete effacement of their normal architecture by a mixed infiltrate containing lymphocytes, histiocytes, plasma cells and eosinophils as well as the malignant cells of Hodgkin's disease: these are large cells and take the form of mononuclear Hodgkin's cells or of Reed–Sternberg cells which have a large, pale multilobed nucleus and a prominent eosinophilic nucleolus about the size of a red blood cell (Fig. 22.7).

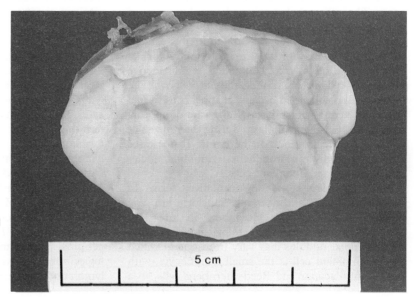

Fig. 22.6 Mixed cellularity Hodgkin's disease

Macroscopic appearances of an axillary lymph node from a 32-year-old man with mixed cellularity Hodgkin's disease. There is a homogeneous white cut surface. The capsule is not involved and there is no infiltration of surrounding fat.

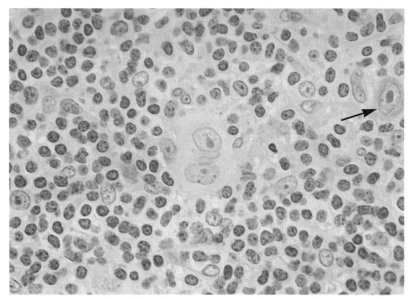

Fig. 22.7 Hodgkin's disease

A classical Reed–Sternberg cell shows the typical binucleate appearance with prominent nucleoli. A mononuclear Hodgkin's cell is present (arrowed).

The almost universally accepted histological classification of Hodgkin's disease is the Rye modification of the Lukes and Butler classification. This contains four subtypes:

- nodular sclerosis
- lymphocyte-predominant
- mixed cellularity
- lymphocyte-depleted.

Nodular sclerosis

The term nodular sclerosis describes many of the histological features of this subtype of Hodgkin's disease. The normal lymph node architecture is replaced by cellular nodules which are separated by bands of collagen (Fig. 22.8). Within the cellular nodules is a mixed infiltrate similar to other types of Hodgkin's disease but containing a distinctive Hodgkin's cell variant termed the *lacunar cell*. The lacunar cell is so named because it appears to sit in a space or 'lacuna' which is caused by the disappearance of its lipid-rich cytoplasm during the process of creating a paraffin block of the tissue. It possesses the large nucleus and prominent eosinophilic nucleolus seen in other Hodgkin's cells.

Nodular sclerosis is a distinctive form of Hodgkin's disease and does not transform into any of the other subtypes described in the Rye classification. However, the cytological composition of the cellular nodules may vary from one in which the predominant cell is the small lymphocyte, with only scanty lacunar and Reed–Sternberg cells, to a histological picture which is dominated by Hodgkin's cells with depletion of lymphocytes. This latter form has been correlated with an aggressive natural history and is termed grade II nodular sclerosis; all other histological subtypes are classified as grade I nodular sclerosis.

Nodular sclerosis displays distinct clinical differences from other subtypes of Hodgkin's disease, having an almost equal sex ratio (most forms of Hodgkin's disease show a marked male predominance), a striking propensity for mediastinal involvement at presentation (50% of patients) and an association with the bizarre syndrome of alcohol intolerance (5% of patients).

Lymphocyte-predominant

Histologically, lymphocyte-predominant Hodgkin's disease is characterised by a paucity of typical Hodgkin's and Reed–Sternberg cells and abundant lymphocytes, sometimes admixed with bland histiocytes. Most commonly there is a nodular growth pattern but occasionally it is diffuse. Collagen band formation is not a feature. As in nodular sclerosis, lymphocyte-predominant Hodgkin's disease contains a distinctive Reed–Sternberg cell variant which is called the 'popcorn' cell because of its excessively lobulated nucleus. Much evidence has accumulated to suggest that, particularly in its nodular form, lymphocyte-predominant Hodgkin's disease is derived from germinal centres and thus, unlike all the other histological subtypes (which start in the T-cell region of the lymph node), appears to be a disease of B-cells.

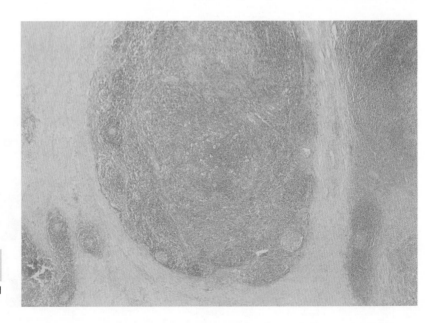

Fig. 22.8 Nodular sclerosing Hodgkin's disease

The cellular nodules are surrounded by thick collagen bands.

Patients with lymphocyte-predominant Hodgkin's disease are at greatly increased risk of developing secondary, high-grade non-Hodgkin's lymphoma; 4% of these patients will develop NHL within 20 years. These 'secondary' NHLs are usually of B-cell lineage and may represent a form of tumour progression in lymphocyte-predominant Hodgkin's disease.

Lymphocyte-predominant Hodgkin's disease is more common in males (>80% of patients), tends to present with localised, asymptomatic high cervical or inguinal lymphadenopathy, and has an excellent survival.

Mixed cellularity

Mixed cellularity is the second commonest subtype of Hodgkin's disease (18% of cases). As the name suggests, the histological picture is an admixture of lymphocytes, histiocytes, plasma cells, eosinophils, Hodgkin's cells and Reed–Sternberg cells; the latter are relatively abundant compared to lymphocyte-predominant Hodgkin's disease.

Mixed cellularity is a rather aggressive form of Hodgkin's disease when compared to lymphocyte-predominant and grade I nodular sclerosis: it presents at an advanced stage relatively frequently (stages III and IV >50% of patients) and with systemic (B) symptoms (35% of patients) and a poor overall survival.

Lymphocyte-depleted

Two histological subtypes of lymphocyte-depleted Hodgkin's disease may be recognised:

- reticular, which is characterised by numerous Hodgkin's and Reed–Sternberg cells with depletion of lymphocytes
- diffuse fibrosis, where the lymph node architecture is replaced by a hypocellular infiltrate containing bizarre Reed–Sternberg cells and associated with non-collagenous fine fibrosis.

These two patterns of lymphocyte depletion may co-exist in the same lymph node and are closely allied conditions. Extensive necrosis is common in both subtypes.

Lymphocyte depletion is rare (2% of all cases of Hodgkin's disease) and carries the worst prognosis. Patients often present acutely with systemic (B) symptoms and usually at an advanced stage, with a high frequency of involvement of liver (60% of patients) and bone marrow (40% of patients).

Survival in Hodgkin's disease

The overall survival figures for Hodgkin's disease vary between different treatment centres, but results from a British multi-centre trial show that approximately 75% of patients were still alive 5 years after diagnosis (Fig. 22.9). As relapse tends to occur early in the course of the disease (usually within 2 years) the majority of these patients are probably cured.

Factors which adversely affect survival are:

- advanced age
- systemic (B) symptoms
- advanced stage
- abnormal haematological parameters at presentation
- aggressive histopathological subtype.

Non-Hodgkin's lymphomas

▶ Lymphomas other than Hodgkin's disease
▶ Classified according to anatomical origin (central, peripheral), histological architecture and predominant cell: follicular or diffuse; centrocytic; centroblastic; immunoblastic; etc.
▶ Majority are of B-lymphocyte origin
▶ T-cell lymphomas are less common; two types involve the skin: mycosis fungoides and Sézary syndrome

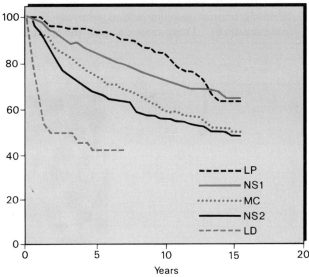

Survival (%)

Fig. 22.9 Actuarial survival of patients with Hodgkin's disease

The data are subdivided according to a modified Rye histological classification with subdivision of nodular sclerosis (NS) into grades 1 and 2. (LP = lymphocyte-predominant; MC = mixed cellularity; LD = lymphocyte-depleted.) Data from the British National Lymphoma Investigation.

The non-Hodgkin's lymphomas (NHL) are malignant tumours of the immune system other than Hodgkin's disease. The vast majority are derived from lymphoid cells; solid tumours of the mononuclear phagocytic system (termed histiocytic lymphoma) are extremely rare.

NHLs form a wide spectrum of disease both clinically and biologically, ranging from slowly progressive neoplasms to rapidly growing destructive tumours. This diversity of clinical behaviour is reflected in the wide range of histological appearances exhibited by NHLs. Classification of non-Hodgkin's lymphoma is based on the cell lineages in the normal immune system in which precursor lymphoid cells are processed in the thymus and bursa equivalent tissue into lymphoid cells which are located in peripheral sites such as lymph nodes, spleen and mucosa-associated lymphoid tissue; these are termed peripheral T and B cells respectively.

Precursor lymphoid neoplasms

These are high-grade non-Hodgkin's lymphomas composed of diffuse sheets of medium-sized lymphoid cells possessing a high nucleo-cytoplasmic ratio. They may be of T-cell or B-cell lineage and commonly express the nuclear antigen TDT (terminal deoxynucleotidyl transferase; an enzyme enabling immunoglobulin or antigen receptor gene rearrangement). These tumours form the spectrum of disease termed *lymphoblastic lymphoma* and *lymphoblastic leukaemia*.

Lymphoblastic lymphomas are commonest in childhood but also occur in adults. Bone marrow infiltration is frequent and a leukaemic phase is often seen; this presents difficulties in separating acute lymphoblastic leukaemia (ALL) from lymphoblastic lymphoma. An arbitrary subdivision is made on the percentage of lymphoblasts present in the bone marrow (<25% is lymphoma; >25% is ALL).

Precursor T-cell lymphomas tend to involve the mediastinum of adolescent boys; histologically, the lymphoblasts have a distinct convoluted nuclear morphology (Fig. 22.10). Precursor B-cell lymphomas may present in leukaemic phase or have solid tumour deposits involving nodal and extranodal sites.

Peripheral non-Hodgkin's lymphoma

Unlike the precursor or lymphoblastic lymphoma, the peripheral non-Hodgkin's lymphomas form a heterogeneous group of neoplasms with a wide range of histological appearances. They may be conveniently subdivided into the following groups:

- lymphocytic lymphoma
- follicular lymphoma
- mantle cell lymphoma
- diffuse large B-cell lymphoma
- Burkitt's lymphoma

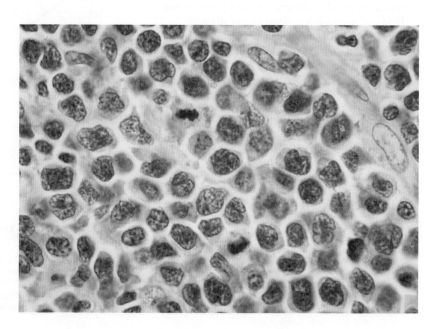

Fig. 22.10   T-cell lymphoblastic lymphoma

Medium-sized cells with a high nucleo-cytoplasmic ratio and convoluted nuclear morphology are shown.

- peripheral T-cell lymphoma
- anaplastic large cell lymphoma.

Lymphocytic lymphoma

Lymphocytic lymphomas are tumours of immature small round lymphocytes. Most are of B-cell lineage; the remainder are T-cell in origin. The borderline between lymphocytic lymphoma and chronic lymphocytic leukaemia is blurred; there is close morphological and immunophenotypic homology between the neoplastic cells of the two conditions. The two conditions are so similar that some regard B-cell lymphocytic lymphoma as a tissue manifestation of B-cell CLL.

Affected lymph nodes are enlarged and usually smooth surfaced with a homogeneous white cut surface. In B-cell lymphocytic lymphoma the normal nodal architecture is replaced by a monotonous infiltrate of small lymphocytes with scattered larger cells (called prolymphocytes) which may form aggregates termed pseudofollicles.

The disease is almost invariably disseminated with a high frequency of splenic, liver and bone marrow infiltration. In the rare T-cell CLL there is a high frequency of cutaneous and mucosal infiltration.

Lymphocytic lymphoma is almost exclusively a disease of adults. It runs an indolent course, with many patients dying of unrelated causes. As the disease progresses it may cause death by extensive bone marrow infiltration and bone marrow failure. In 5–10% of patients the disease will transform into a high-grade pleomorphic large cell lymphoma (*Richter's syndrome*) which is refractory to treatment and has a poor prognosis. Patients with B-cell lymphocytic lymphoma are frequently hypogammaglobulinaemic and are particularly susceptible to bacterial infections.

Follicular lymphoma

Follicular lymphomas are tumours derived from (or differentiated towards) germinal centre B-cells. These lymphomas contain an admixture of centroblasts and centrocytes and may have a purely follicular growth pattern or may have a mixed pattern with follicular and diffuse areas. In addition to the neoplastic B-cells, non-neoplastic T-lymphocytes and dendritic reticulum cells are also present within the neoplastic follicle having been recruited by the neoplastic B-cell clone.

Important in the pathogenesis of follicular lymphoma is a specific chromosomal translocation involving the immunoglobulin heavy chain promoter region on chromosome 14 and the anti-apoptotic gene *bcl 2* on chromosome 18 (t(14;18)(q32;q21)).

This translocation causes the constitutive overexpression of *bcl 2* protein, rendering follicular lymphoma cells relatively resistant to apoptosis.

Lymph nodes replaced by follicular lymphoma are usually enlarged and smooth surfaced. Cut surfaces are homogeneous grey/white with occasional areas of haemorrhage and necrosis. A faintly nodular pattern may be seen with a magnifying glass. Microscopically, the normal lymph node architecture is replaced by closely packed neoplastic follicles often extending through the lymph node capsule into perinodal fat (Fig. 22.11); diffuse areas may also be present. The neoplastic follicles contain a mixture of centroblasts and centrocytes; the relative proportion of these cells forms the basis of grading these lymphomas. Tumours with relatively large numbers of centroblasts have a worse prognosis.

Follicular lymphoma is one of the commonest types of non-Hodgkin's lymphoma and is a disease of late adult life with a peak age incidence in the sixth and seventh decades. It is exceptionally rare in children and young adults. Most patients with follicular lymphoma will present with painless, slowly progressive lymphadenopathy, usually with disseminated disease (stages III and IV); 40% of patients will have systemic symptoms.

Involvement of bone marrow, spleen and liver is common in follicular lymphoma. The earliest morphological manifestations of marrow infiltration are localised collections of irregular small lymphoid cells adjacent to bone trabeculae (termed paratrabecular infiltration). Extensive bone marrow replacement may occur with consequent marrow failure. A leukaemic phase of follicular lymphoma is seen in a significant percentage of patients, when neoplastic B-cells may be found in peripheral blood.

Splenic involvement may be either minimal or cause massive splenomegaly with hypersplenism. The neoplastic cells of follicular lymphoma maintain some degree of physiological homing function and selectively infiltrate the B-cell areas of the white pulp of the spleen, progressively replacing and expanding these structures such that the cut surface of the organ may be seen to contain numerous discrete white nodules separated by normal red pulp.

Follicular lymphoma is an indolent disease but it is generally regarded as incurable when disseminated, and the majority of patients die as a direct result of their lymphoma. The exact mode of death is sometimes difficult to determine but in at least 20% of patients the disease will transform into a diffuse large B-cell lymphoma. This lymphoma behaves aggressively and is usually refractory to treatment. In

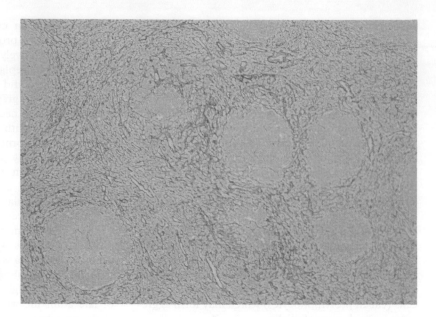

Fig. 22.11 Follicular lymphoma

Numerous rounded lymphoid aggregates are seen throughout the lymph node. Staining for reticulin highlights the rounded structure and expansile growth of the neoplastic follicles.

the remainder, following a clinical course of multiple remissions and relapses, the tumour becomes unresponsive to further chemotherapy with a progressively increasing tumour burden leading to death.

Although it is difficult to determine prognosis for an individual patient with follicular lymphoma, factors which are associated with a reduced survival are rapid disease progression, the presence of systemic (B) symptoms and infiltration of vital organs.

Mantle cell lymphoma
Mantle cell lymphoma is the term currently used to describe a low-grade B-cell lymphoma which is derived from or differentiates towards the mantle zone of the germinal centre. The term encompasses entities such as centrocytic lymphoma and intermediately differentiated lymphocytic lymphoma.

Mantle cell lymphoma may have a nodular or diffuse architecture and is composed of a mixture of irregular small B-cells, follicular dendritic cells and T-cells; the B-cell component is monoclonal.

Mantle cell lymphoma has a distinctive chromosomal translocation—t(11;14)(q13;q32). This leads to the deregulation of the PRAD-1 gene with subsequent overexpression of the important cell cycle control protein cyclin D1.

Mantle cell lymphoma is relatively rare (<5% of all NHLs) and has a peak age incidence in the seventh decade. It is generally regarded as a low-grade lymphoma but its natural history appears to be more aggressive than other low-grade NHLs and it has the ability to transform into a 'blastoid' from which has a

very poor survival. The disease usually presents with lymphadenopathy but a distinctive pattern is seen in the gastrointestinal tract where it is termed *lymphomatous polyposis*. Most patients have advanced stage symptomatic disease. Leukaemic overspill is quite common.

Diffuse large B-cell lymphoma
Diffuse large B-cell lymphoma forms the commonest type of high-grade NHL; it may arise de novo or as a result of the transformation of a low-grade B-cell lymphoma (usually follicular lymphoma). As the name implies, this lymphoma is characterised by a diffuse outgrowth of large B-cells which may display centroblastic or immunoblastic cytology (Fig. 22.12).

Diffuse large B-cell lymphoma is usually a disease of adults but may occur in childhood. The majority of patients present with rapidly progressive nodal disease but extranodal involvement is common; involvement of the gastrointestinal tract and Waldeyer's ring is most frequent.

Unlike the low-grade lymphomas, diffuse large B-cell lymphoma is frequently localised (stages I and II in 45% of patients) and curable even when advanced (5-year survival for patients with stage III and IV disease is approximately 35%). A variety of cytogenetic abnormalities are seen in diffuse large B-cell lymphoma; the commonest is the t(14;18) translocation resulting in deregulation of the *bcl 2* gene and translocations involving the 3q27 breakpoint with overexpression of the *bcl 6* gene.

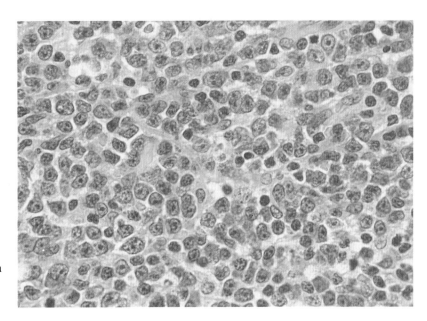

Fig. 22.12 Diffuse large B-cell lymphoma

The majority of the cells, growing in a diffuse pattern, are large B-cells (centroblasts) with multiple nucleoli often peripherally located.

Burkitt's lymphoma

Burkitt's lymphoma is a distinctive type of B-cell lymphoma, regarded as lymphoblastic in some classifications, which is endemic in para-equatorial Africa and New Guinea and occurs much less commonly in other regions. The disease affects children and adolescents, is associated with Epstein–Barr virus infection and malaria (Ch. 11) and involves extranodal sites, particularly the jaw, gastrointestinal tract and gonads. The histological appearances are distinctive, with tightly packed lymphoblasts interspersed with phagocytic macrophages which impart a 'starry sky' appearance to histological sections.

Peripheral T-cell lymphoma

T-cell lymphomas are relatively uncommon in Europe and America, making up no more than 10% of NHL cases. In Japan and the Caribbean region it is much commoner. This increased disease prevalence is due to the presence of an endemic retrovirus, the human T-cell leukaemia/lymphoma virus (HTLV I), which appears to be a causative agent in some forms of T-cell malignancy.

The spectrum of T-cell NHL appears as broad as that of B-cell tumours and complicated classification schemes have been proposed. More recently it has been appreciated that the histological recognition of different subtypes of nodal peripheral T-cell lymphoma is difficult to perform reliably and that morphology is not a good indicator of clinical behaviour. For this reason the majority of these tumours have been categorised as *peripheral T lymphoma unspecified*. Within this group of tumours there is wide variation in the size and shape of the neoplastic T-cells and they are frequently mixed with other non-neoplastic components of the paracortex, such as interdigitating reticulum cells and high endothelial venules; aggregates of epithelioid histiocytes and an eosinophil infiltrate may also be prominent.

Within the heterogeneous group of T-cell lymphomas there are several distinctive clinicopathological entities:

- cutaneous T-cell lymphomas (CTCL; mycosis fungoides and Sézary syndrome)
- adult T-cell lymphoma/leukaemia (ATLL)
- angioimmunoblastic T-cell lymphoma (AILD)
- anaplastic large cell lymphoma (ALCL).

Mycosis fungoides (MF) and *Sézary syndrome* are closely allied cutaneous T-cell lymphomas. The neoplastic T-cells usually have a 'helper' cell phenotype (CD4) and form a band-like upper dermal infiltrate with a moderate degree of epidermal infiltration, often forming small aggregates of cells within the epidermis (termed *Pautrier's microabscesses*) usually in association with epidermal Langerhans' cells. The neoplastic T-cells are larger than normal lymphocytes and usually have a markedly irregular nuclear profile imparting a cerebriform appearance.

Cutaneous T-cell lymphoma is a disease of adult life with a tendency to involve older age groups.

Mycosis fungoides clinically progresses through three stages:

- the *patch stage*, characterised by erythematous macules usually occurring on areas not exposed to sunlight
- the *plaque stage*, with elevated scaly plaques which may be pink or red/brown and are often intensely pruritic
- the *tumour stage*, with dome-shaped firm tumours which may ulcerate.

The density of the lymphoid infiltrate increases from the patch to the tumour stage and in some cases of tumour stage MF there may be transformation to a large-celled cytological pattern. Although MF is initially confined to the skin, lymph node and visceral organ involvement become clinically apparent later in the course of the disease and are particularly common in the tumour stage. This is a bad prognostic feature with a median survival of only 2.5 years compared to a 12-year median survival for patients with limited extent cutaneous disease.

The Sézary syndrome variant of CTCL is characterised by the presence of generalised erythroderma, lymphadenopathy and at least 10% of peripheral blood mononuclear cells having an atypical cerebriform morphology. The prognosis of patients with the Sézary syndrome is poor.

Adult T-cell leukaemia/lymphoma is one of the few human malignancies for which there is strong evidence of a viral aetiology. The disease is endemic in the islands of southern Japan, the Caribbean basin, the tropical islands of the Pacific Ocean and in the Seychelles. Outside endemic areas the majority of affected patients have been black. The disease is associated with the retrovirus *HTLV 1*. The disease presents with lymphadenopathy and a leukaemic blood picture, often associated with cutaneous infiltration and hypercalcaemia (secondary to the production of parathormone-related peptide). Low-grade and chronic forms of ATLL have a more indolent course. The affected lymph nodes are infiltrated by a pleomorphic T-cell proliferation, indistinguishable from other non-virus-associated T-cell lymphomas. The disease has a poor prognosis, with a median survival of less than one year; most patients die of opportunistic infection due to severe immunosuppression.

Angioimmunoblastic T-cell lymphoma is a rare but distinctive form of T-cell lymphoma. Although originally it was not thought to be neoplastic the demonstration of T-cell receptor gene rearrangement in the majority of cases studied has indicated that this lesion should be regarded as a lymphoma. Patients usually present with widespread lymphadenopathy, systemic symptoms, skin rashes, polyclonal hypergammaglobulinaemia and evidence of immunosuppression. The prognosis for angioimmunoblastic T-cell lymphoma is poor, although occasional spontaneous or steroid-induced remissions are described.

Anaplastic large cell lymphoma (ALCL) is a recently described high-grade NHL that is often of T-cell lineage, less commonly of B-cell origin. ALCL may arise de novo or may be a high-grade transformation of a low-grade NHL. Primary ALCL shows a bimodal age distribution with a peak in childhood and a second peak in the seventh decade. The disease may be nodal or extranodal; common sites of extranodal disease include the skin, gastrointestinal tract and Waldeyer's ring.

Histologically, ALCL is characterised by a pleomorphic large cell population of neoplastic lymphoid cells, some bearing a resemblance to Hodgkin's cells. The tumour cells tend to involve lymph node sinuses and to preferentially invade blood vessels. (Fig. 22.13).

ALCL is associated with a particular chromosomal translocation, t(2;5)(p23;q35), which leads to the aberrant expression of a newly described membrane-bound kinase called *anaplastic lymphoma kinase* (ALK).

Despite its very aggressive histological appearance, primary ALCL has a relatively good overall survival (approximately 70% of patients alive at 5 years) particularly when extranodal disease predominates.

Extranodal lymphoma

Extranodal lymphoid tissue is widely distributed in the body, often located adjacent to mucosal surfaces (e.g. Peyer's patches in the terminal ileum). The structure of this mucosa-associated lymphoid tissue (MALT) differs from that in peripheral lymph nodes and there are differences in function and patterns of lymphocyte recirculation. Many extranodal lymphomas show features in common with MALT and it is now clear that these are distinctive forms of NHL.

Extranodal lymphomas make up at least a quarter of all NHLs and occur most commonly in the gastrointestinal tract (Ch. 15); other common sites include skin, salivary gland, thyroid and orbit. Most extranodal lymphomas occur in sites normally devoid of lymphoid tissue; the acquisition of lymphoid tissue as the result of either an autoimmune (such as Hashimoto's thyroiditis) or infective (as seen in *Helicobacter* gastritis) process is the essential

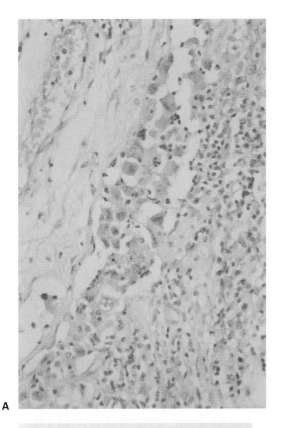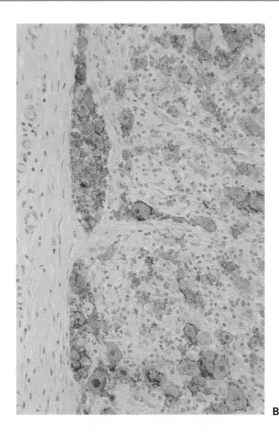

Fig. 22.13 Anaplastic large cell lymphoma

A. Pleomorphic large cells are localised to and distend the sinus of the lymph node. **B.** Stained for CD30 showing strongly positive cells preferentially localised to the sinus.

forerunner to the development of lymphoma in these locations.

Extranodal lymphomas of MALT type share common histological and cytogenetic features wherever they occur. Histologically, they are characterised by the presence of reactive germinal centres surrounded by a population of neoplastic B-cells which bear some cytological similarities to the marginal zone B-cell and are called centrocyte-like cells. These centrocyte-like cells infiltrate epithelial structures to form *lympho-epithelial lesions* which are characteristic of MALT lymphomas (Fig. 22.14). These lymphomas often show impressive degrees of plasma cell differentiation usually adjacent to the mucosal surface. Many MALT lymphomas are low-grade but some show features of high-grade lymphoma, usually of diffuse large B-cell type. These high-grade MALT lymphomas may arise de novo or be associated with a low-grade component.

MALT lymphomas lack the common cytogenetic abnormalities seen in nodal lymphomas (t(14;18) and t(11;14)) and are associated with novel karyotypic changes such as trisomy 3, t(2;7) and t(1;14).

There are marked differences in the clinical behaviour of MALT lymphomas compared to nodal lymphomas. They appear to remain localised for long periods and have an indolent natural history, often with a very good prognosis. The pattern of relapse is also different with a tendency to recur in extranodal locations.

The remarkable similarities in histology, cytogenetics and clinical course of extranodal lymphomas from different sites strongly suggests they represent a common biological entity. The recognition and characterisation of the MALT lymphoma group is an important advance in lymphoma pathology.

Not all extranodal lymphomas correspond to the MALT pattern; some are identical to nodal lymphomas and some are distinctive clinicopathological entities which present in extranodal locations.

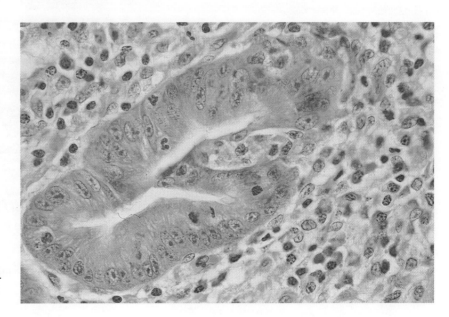

Fig. 22.14 Low-grade MALT lymphoma of the stomach

Centrocyte-like cells infiltrate a gastric gland and form a lympho-epithelial lesion characteristic of low-grade MALT lymphoma.

Lymphomatous polyposis is a manifestation of mantle cell lymphoma in the gastrointestinal tract. It is characterised by the presence of multiple mucosal polyps throughout the alimentary system; these may range in size from half a millimetre to many centimetres in diameter and tend to centre around the ileocaecal valve (Fig. 22.15). This is an aggressive lymphoma which frequently becomes leukaemic at some point in its natural history.

Enteropathy-associated T-cell lymphoma (EATL) is a pleomorphic T-cell lymphoma which develops in some patients with coeliac disease. EATL has a predilection for jejunal involvement where it often presents as multifocal lesions — ulcers, fissures and perforation. This is an aggressive lymphoma with a poor survival.

Classification of the non-Hodgkin's lymphomas

The ideal classification should provide good clinicopathological correlation and be easy and reproducible to apply; the terminology should accurately reflect the biology of the disease. Although many classifications exist, none fulfils these exacting requirements.

In a recent attempt to describe lymphoma entities which lymphoma pathologists recognise, a group of European and American pathologists have proposed a new classification termed the Revised European American Lymphoma (REAL) classification. It is hoped that this will provide a useful framework for a unified approach to diagnosis and treatment of the NHLs. The fundamental point is the recognition of B-cell and T-cell lineage. The distinction between low- and high-grade forms of the disease is also of major clinical importance (Fig. 22.16).

THYMUS

NORMAL STRUCTURE AND FUNCTION

The thymus develops from the third and occasionally the fourth pharyngeal pouches. It is a pyramidal, bilobed, encapsulated organ situated in the anterior superior mediastinum. The relative weight of the thymus in comparison to body weight is greatest in the neonate (20–30 g). The absolute thymic weight peaks around puberty (40–50 g) and thereafter declines such that in the elderly adult the thymus is atrophic and composed largely of adipose tissue. The significance and the mechanisms of thymic atrophy are largely unknown.

The lobes of the thymus are divided into lobules by connective tissue septa which grow in from the fibrous capsule. Subdivision of the thymus into an outer, dark cortex and inner, pale medulla is apparent macroscopically.

The thymus is a central lymphoid organ and is

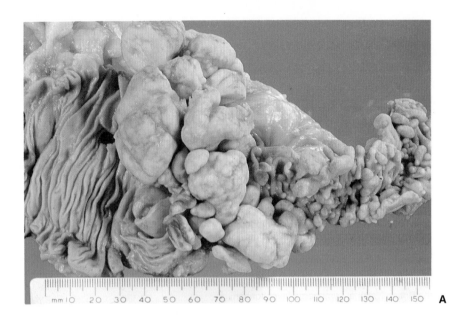

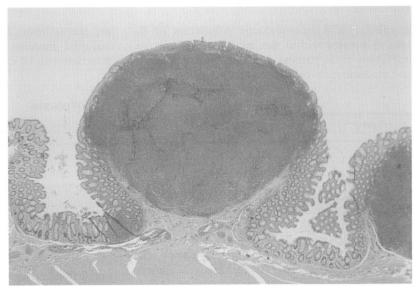

Fig. 22.15 Multiple lymphomatous polyposis of gut (mantle cell lymphoma)

A. The terminal ileum (right) and ascending colon are affected. These are characteristic macroscopic appearances with multiple mucosal polyps increasing in size towards the ileo-caecal valve. **B.** Low-power histology showing nodular infiltration of the lamina propria by mantle cell lymphoma.

responsible for the induction of cell-mediated immune function in developing lymphoid cells (Ch. 9). Most of this inductive activity appears to be located in the cortex, which contains densely packed medium-sized lymphoid cells, scattered epithelial cells and abundant interdigitating reticulum cells. The precise function of the thymic epithelial cells is unknown, but they may be responsible for the secretion of thymic hormones such as thymosin and thymopoietin which are ne-

cessary for T-cell maturation. During the acquisition of immunocompetence the cortical lymphoid population is rapidly dividing, but many cells die in situ and relatively few migrate to the medulla and then to peripheral lymphoid organs. The thymic medulla is far less cellular than the cortex. In addition, the thymic medulla contains structures termed *Hassall's corpuscles*, which are concentrically arranged squamous epithelial cells with central keratinisation; their function is unknown. A small and

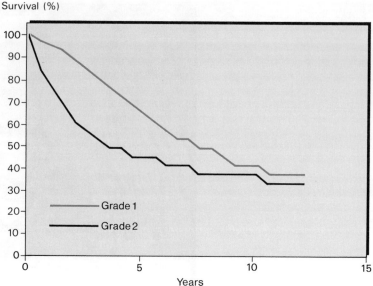

Survival (%)

Fig. 22.16 Actuarial survival of patients with non-Hodgkin's lymphoma

The graph is subdivided into low-grade (grade 1) and high-grade (grade 2) forms of the disease. Patients with high-grade lymphoma have an initial high death rate but the survival curve forms a plateau at 5 years, indicating that a significant proportion of patients are cured of their disease. Low-grade lymphomas, although having an indolent initial course, show a continuing death rate after 5 years and appear to be incurable with current therapies. By 10 years the survival rates of low- and high-grade lymphoma are similar. Data from the British National Lymphoma Investigation.

morphologically inconspicuous population of B-cells is present within the medulla and may be important in the pathogenesis of myasthenia gravis and mediastinal B-cell lymphoma.

DISORDERS OF THE THYMUS

Agenesis and hypoplasia

Agenesis and hypoplasia may occur because of a failure of either the epithelial or the lymphoid component of the thymus to develop properly.

In the *Di George* and *Nezelof syndromes*, there is defective development of the epithelial component of the thymus from the third pharyngeal pouch. The Di George syndrome has, in addition, defective development of the fourth pharyngeal pouch, which results in an absence of the parathyroid glands. The thymus is either completely absent in these two syndromes or is represented by a fibrous streak.

Abnormalities of lymphoid colonisation of the thymus occur in the severe combined immune deficiency syndromes, *ataxia-telangiectasia* and *reticular dysgenesis*. In reticular dysgenesis the thymus is small, weighing little more than a few grams, and is composed of disordered aggregates of epithelial cells.

Acquired hypoplasia may be seen as a natural age-

ing phenomenon, as a response to stress and in the acquired immune deficiency syndrome following infection with HIV.

Hyperplasia

Thymic hyperplasia is strongly associated with autoimmune disease (in particular, *myasthenia gravis*). Hyperplasia is difficult to diagnose from the thymus size or weight alone, owing to extreme variation in these indices in the general population. The most reliable criterion is the formation of germinal centres within the thymus. The germinal centres are located principally in the medulla, from which they expand and may cause cortical atrophy. They are identical to the germinal centres in peripheral lymphoid sites.

Neoplasms

A wide variety of neoplasms occur within the thymus:
- epithelial — benign thymoma; malignant thymoma, thymic carcinoma
- lymphoid — Hodgkin's disease; non-Hodgkin's lymphoma
- germ cell — seminoma; teratoma
- stromal — thymolipoma
- others — thymic carcinoid; oat cell (small cell) carcinoma.

Thymomas

Only those neoplasms in which the neoplastic cell is derived from thymic epithelium are termed thymomas. The vast majority of thymomas arise within the thymus, but thymomas from ectopic thymus tissue have been described in the soft tissues of the neck, hilum of the lung, other sites within the mediastinum and, rarely, the thyroid.

In addition to the neoplastic epithelial component, thymomas contain variable numbers of lymphoid cells; those that contain large numbers are termed 'lymphocyte-rich' and those with scanty numbers are termed 'lymphocyte-poor'. The lymphocyte-rich thymomas to some extent recapitulate the structure of the cortical thymus in their microscopic appearances and the phenotype of the lymphoid cells present. Conversely, the lymphocyte-poor thymomas show similarities with the thymic medulla. In addition to variations in the degree of lymphocytic infiltration, there are also variations in the cytological appearances of the neoplastic epithelial cells, which may range from round to spindle shaped.

Many thymomas are asymptomatic and are detected by chest X-ray performed for other reasons; some present with signs of local disease such as dyspnoea, cough and stridor, and the remainder present with autoimmune disease. The majority of thymomas (60–80%) are benign and complete surgical excision is curative. The remaining cases are termed malignant thymomas. There is a good correlation between survival and the extent of spread or presence of metastases in malignant thymomas.

Thymomas may be associated with a variety of disorders including myasthenia gravis, pure red cell aplasia, neutropenia, thrombocytopenia, hypogammaglobulinaemia and systemic lupus erythematosus.

Other thymic neoplasms

Thymic involvement by *Hodgkin's disease* is relatively common and occurs particularly in the nodular sclerosing subtype.

Non-Hodgkin's lymphomas originating in the thymus tend to be high-grade tumours of either T-lymphoblastic or large B-cell types. The T-lymphoblastic lymphomas of the thymus occur in young and adolescent boys, often possess a characteristic convoluted nuclear morphology, and usually develop a leukaemic phase. Their phenotype shows similarities to the cortical thymic lymphoid cell. The large B-cell lymphomas of the thymus tend to occur in women in the second and third decades of life. It has been postulated that they arise from thymic medullary B-cells. These are aggressive tumours with a high rate of local and distant relapse and a relatively poor survival. Low-grade NHLs with histological features of MALT lymphoma also occur in the thymus.

The same spectrum of *germ cell neoplasia* is apparent in the thymus as in the gonad. These neoplasms are thought to arise from primitive germ cells which have become misplaced during migration to the developing gonadal anlage. Mediastinal germ cell tumours are also rarely associated with haemopoietic neoplasms with features of malignant histiocytosis.

Thymolipomas are circumscribed stromal tumours composed of an admixture of mature fat and thymic tissue. They are benign but may reach a substantial size, often weighing over half a kilogram.

Thymic carcinoids and *oat cell carcinomas* are rare neoplasms thought to arise from neuro-endocrine cells scattered in the organ. About a third of thymic carcinoids are associated with Cushing's syndrome. Both thymic carcinoids and oat cell (small cell) carcinomas are aggressive malignant neoplasms.

SPLEEN

NORMAL STRUCTURE AND FUNCTION

The spleen is an encapsulated organ normally weighing 100–150 g in the adult and situated in the left upper quadrant of the abdomen, mostly concealed by the lower ribs. The spleen has two functions: it is a lymphoid organ and it has a great capacity for phagocytosing particulate material in the circulation and culling senescent red cells. These two functions of the spleen are architecturally distinct; the lymphoid function occurs in the *white pulp* and the phagocytic activity resides in the *red pulp*.

White pulp

The splenic artery enters the spleen at the hilum, then branches and follows the trabeculae of the fibrous capsule into the substance of the organ. Leaving the trabeculae as central arteries and arterioles, these branches become ensheathed in lymphoid cells. These aggregates of lymphoid cells are termed the white pulp and can be seen on the cut surface of the spleen as 1–2 mm diameter white nodules in the deep-red background of the red pulp. As in lymph nodes, the lymphocytes within the white pulp of the spleen show distinct micro-architectural segregation of different functional subsets. T-cells are found in the immediate vicinity of the central arterial vessel of the white pulp and are termed the *peri-arteriolar lymphoid sheath*. The B-cell follicle is eccentrically placed within the white pulp and may be composed predominantly of small lymphocytes, or may form a germinal centre when stimulated. At the junction of the red and white pulp and surrounding the peri-arteriolar lymphoid sheath and the B-cell follicle, is a group of specialised B-cells termed marginal zone lymphocytes; their precise function is unknown. The white pulp is a major site of antibody production.

Red pulp

Most of the spleen is occupied by the red pulp, whose main function appears to be destruction of senescent red cells and phagocytosis of particulate material. The red pulp has a dual circulation, with a 'closed' sinusoidal pathway and an 'open' system through the splenic pulp cords.

The splenic arterial supply, having traversed the white pulp, flows through the penicillary arteries into the splenic sinuses or pulp cords. The sinuses are narrow channels with a discontinuous endothelial lining which allows adjacent macrophages access to the red cells as they traverse sinuses and drain into the trabecular veins. The open pulp-cord circulation places the red cells in prolonged intimate contact with serried ranks of macrophages before entering the splenic sinuses. Within the pulp cords, macrophages remove any intracytoplasmic inclusions (such as Howell–Jolly bodies—a process termed pitting) and excess surface membrane from the red blood cells. The environment within the pulp cords is hostile and the red cells must possess marked deformability and intact metabolic machinery to survive. Those cells that do not survive are phagocytosed and broken down.

DISORDERS OF THE SPLEEN

Congenital abnormalities

Congenital abnormalities in the form of accessory

spleens or splenunculi are relatively common, occurring in about 10% of the population. They are rounded, encapsulated structures up to several centimetres in size and usually located near the spleen. Congenital asplenia and polysplenia are rare and often associated with other congenital malformations, particularly of the cardiovascular system.

Hypersplenism

The term 'hypersplenism' is applied to the association between a peripheral blood pancytopenia and splenic enlargement. It may be primary or secondary to a wide variety of pathological processes.

Primary hypersplenism is a poorly understood condition of unknown aetiology, characterised by marked and often massive splenomegaly and pancytopenia, in which leukopenia is particularly pronounced. Within the spleen there is marked lymphoid hyperplasia. The haematological response to splenectomy is excellent, though some patients may remain leukopenic.

Secondary splenomegaly (see below) may also be associated with hypersplenism.

Splenomegaly

> ▶ Many causes including vascular congestion, inflammatory and reactive disorders, leukaemias and lymphomas, and storage disorders
> ▶ Enlarged spleen may rupture after only minor trauma
> ▶ Secondary splenomegaly (due to above causes) may result in hypersplenism

The causes of secondary splenomegaly are numerous and include the following basic pathological processes:

- congestion
- infection
- immune disorders
- primary or metastatic neoplasms
- storage disorders
- amyloidosis (Ch. 7).

Congestive splenomegaly

Conditions which lead to a persistent elevation of splenic venous blood pressure are capable of causing splenomegaly. The splenic venous pressure may be raised due to pre-hepatic, hepatic and post-hepatic causes.

Pre-hepatic causes include thrombosis of the

extrahepatic portion of the portal vein or of the splenic vein.

Very marked splenomegaly occurs in longstanding portal hypertension associated with cirrhosis (Ch. 16).

Post-hepatic causes of congestive splenomegaly are associated with a raised pressure in the inferior vena cava, which is transmitted to the spleen via the portal system. These are usually associated with ascites and hepatomegaly. Decompensated right-sided heart failure and pulmonary or tricuspid valve disease are the usual post-hepatic causes of congestive splenomegaly.

The spleen in congestive splenomegaly is variably enlarged and may reach a massive size, weighing a kilogram or more. The capsule may be thickened and fibrotic, but it is in the red pulp that the major pathological alterations occur. The cut surface of the spleen has a beefy-red colour with an inconspicuous white pulp, often containing scattered, firm brown nodules; these are Gamna–Gandy nodules and represent areas of healed infarction, composed of fibrous and elastic tissue with abundant haemosiderin and dystrophic calcification. In the early stages of congestive splenomegaly, the sinusoids are distended with red cells. Later, fibrosis occurs around the sinusoids, which appear ectatic and empty. Foci of extramedullary haemopoiesis may be seen and it is postulated that these are secondary to local hypoxia within the spleen.

Infection

Systemic infection may cause moderate splenomegaly characterised by congestion and macrophage hyperplasia within the red pulp. The white pulp is usually prominent macroscopically and shows reactive changes microscopically, often with germinal centre formation.

Some viral diseases, in particular infectious mononucleosis, may produce more severe splenomegaly. In addition to the changes described above, the splenomegaly may also show immunoblastic infiltration of the red pulp. In infectious mononucleosis, the spleen is susceptible to rupture (Fig. 22.17).

Chronic malarial infection may lead to massive splenomegaly. The splenic capsule is thickened and fibrotic and the cut surface has a slate-grey coloration due to the abundant, iron-containing malarial pigment. Microscopically, there is pronounced red pulp macrophage hyperplasia containing malarial parasites.

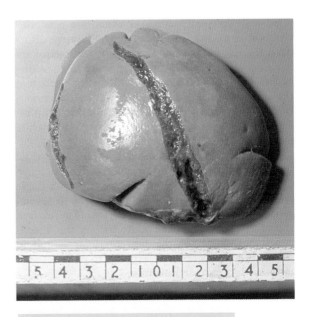

Fig. 22.17 Splenic rupture in infectious mononucleosis

This spleen was removed from an adolescent with infectious mononucleosis who sustained minor abdominal trauma.

Immune disorders

A variety of immune disorders may lead to splenomegaly, in particular rheumatoid disease and systemic lupus erythematosus. Hypersplenism may ensue, and, in the case of rheumatoid disease in adults, is called Felty's syndrome.

Neoplasms

Splenic infiltration is a common feature of a wide variety of haematological neoplasms including:

- acute and chronic leukaemias
- myeloproliferative disorders
- Hodgkin's disease
- non-Hodgkin's lymphomas.

The pattern of splenic involvement is characteristic of each group of neoplasms.

Acute leukaemias preferentially infiltrate the red pulp, although minor degrees of white pulp involvement may be seen, particularly in acute lymphoblastic leukaemia. The splenic red pulp cords and sinuses are filled with numerous primitive haemopoietic blast cells.

Chronic myeloid leukaemia (CML) and the myeloproliferative syndromes may lead to massive degrees of splenomegaly. In CML, the red pulp is filled with myeloid precursors which are predominantly mature and, in the myeloproliferative disorders, the red pulp contains areas of extramedullary haemopoiesis. The red pulp expansion in these disorders gradually effaces the white pulp such that the cut surface of the spleen has a homogeneous brick red appearance. In contrast, chronic lymphocytic leukaemia infiltrates both the red and white pulp.

Hodgkin's disease preferentially invades the white pulp and forms expansile nodules which encroach upon the red pulp. These may be single or multiple and range in size from a few millimetres to several centimetres in diameter (Fig. 22.18). The earliest site of involvement in the white pulp is the T-cell-dependent region of the peri-arteriolar lymphoid sheath which progressively expands to obliterate the normal white pulp architecture.

Non-Hodgkin's lymphomas (NHLs) also princi-pally affect the white pulp, but their pattern of disease varies. The low-grade lymphomas form multiple small and medium-sized nodules which expand and replace the normal white pulp; the cut surface of the spleen is seen to be studded with numerous relatively even-sized nodules (Fig. 22.19). In contrast, high-grade lymphomas form small numbers of large destructive nodules. These differences in the pattern of splenic involvement by low- and high-grade NHLs are probably due to the physiological homing of the recirculating lymphoid cells of low-grade lymphomas to their natural milieu within the white pulp.

Although haemopoietic malignancies frequently involve the spleen, other tumours rarely metastasise to the spleen, and then only as part of a widely disseminated malignancy. Primary tumours of the spleen are rare and include hamartomas, benign and malignant vascular tumours and occasionally other mesenchymal neoplasms.

Storage disorders

Several storage disorders may cause splenomegaly: these include Niemann–Pick disease, Gaucher's disease and the mucopolysaccharidoses (Ch. 7). Characteristically, there is marked red pulp expansion by macrophages whose cytoplasm is distended with the abnormal storage product (Fig. 22.20).

Splenic infarction

Splenic infarction follows occlusion of the splenic artery or its branches and is usually secondary to emboli that arise in the heart (Ch. 8). Occasionally, splenic infarction may be due to local thrombosis as in sickle cell disease, myeloproliferative disorders and malignant infiltrates.

Splenic infarcts are macroscopically pale and wedge-shaped with the base adjacent to the splenic capsule. They may be single or multiple, and heal forming depressed scars.

Rupture of the spleen

Rupture of the spleen is usually caused by blunt abdominal trauma, particularly automobile accidents. Massive, life-threatening intraperitoneal haemorrhage may follow splenic rupture, necessitating emergency splenectomy.

Spontaneous rupture of the spleen may occur, particularly in infectious mononucleosis and in spleens enlarged by haemopoietic proliferations such as myelofibrosis.

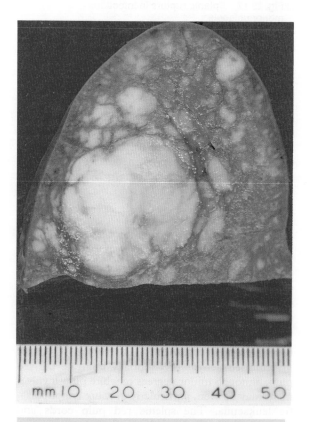

Fig. 22.18 Spleen infiltrated by Hodgkin's disease

Note the discrete white nodules of tumour ranging in size from a few millimetres to several centimetres. The appearances have been likened to toffee containing Brazil nuts and are sometimes termed 'hard bake spleen'.

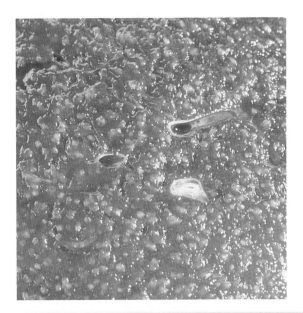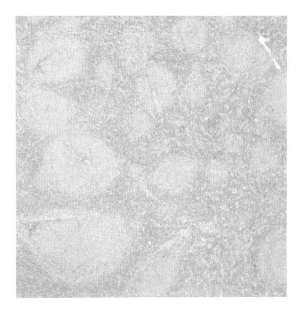

Fig. 22.19   Spleen infiltrated by low-grade non-Hodgkin's lymphoma

A. Macroscopic appearance. The cut surface is studded by small white nodules which stand out against the red pulp. **B.** Low-power view showing numerous lymphoid aggregates with adjacent unaffected red pulp.

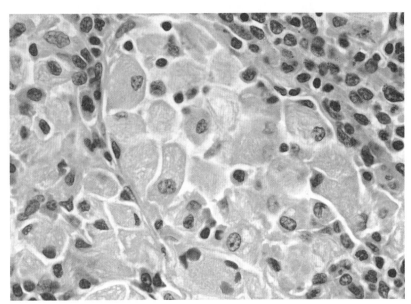

Fig. 22.20   Gaucher's disease

Characteristic histiocytes of Gaucher's disease contain abundant glucocerebroside which accumulates due to a deficiency of the enzyme glucocerebrosidase.

Splenic atrophy

Splenic atrophy may occur in association with intestinal malabsorption states such as coeliac disease. In splenic atrophy, the spleen is small and weighs less than 50 g. There is evidence of hyposplenism with numerous target cells and Howell–Jolly inclusion bodies in red cells.

Patients with sickle cell disease suffer multiple splenic infarcts and the spleen is greatly reduced in size and function.

FURTHER READING

Harris N L, et al. 1994 A revised European-American classification of lymphoid neoplasms: a proposal from the international lymphoma study group. Blood 84: 1361–1392

Isaacson P G, Norton A J 1994 Extranodal lymphomas. Churchill Livingstone, Edinburgh

Jaffe E S (ed) 1995 Surgical pathology of the lymph nodes and related organs. 2nd edn. Saunders, Philadelphia

Wolf B C, Neiman R S 1989 Disorders of the spleen. Saunders, Philadelphia

Wright D H, Isaacson P G 1983 Biopsy pathology of the lymphoreticular system. Chapman and Hall, London

23

Blood and bone marrow

COMPOSITION, PRODUCTION AND FUNCTIONS OF BLOOD

Blood is a unique organ: it is fluid and comes into contact with almost all other tissues. The blood cells are non-cohesive and supported in the fluid medium of blood — the plasma. The blood cells comprise the non-nucleated erythrocytes and platelets, and the nucleated cells or leukocytes.

In addition to primary disease of the blood-forming organ — the bone marrow — many disease states produce secondary changes in the blood. For this reason, the counting and morphological examination of blood cells is routine in the clinical assessment of disease, frequently providing valuable diagnostic information.

CELLULAR COMPONENTS

The peripheral blood is investigated by microscopy of a droplet spread evenly over the surface of a glass slide — the blood film. Routinely, the blood film is stained by the Romanowsky technique, a combination of stains allowing identification of nuclear and cytoplasmic detail.

Quantitation of blood cells is essential; in modern laboratories this is routinely performed by automated cell-counting equipment. The size and concentration of erythrocytes, and the leukocyte and platelet concentrations are measured. Haemoglobin is automatically measured. Also, the proportion of leukocytes of each category — the differential white cell count — is measured from cell size and granule content.

Erythrocytes

Erythrocytes (red blood cells) are deformable, non-nucleated and biconcave discs (Fig. 23.1). They are the most abundant blood cell. When blood is separated, by centrifugation, into cellular and plasma components, the red cell portion is approximately 45% of the total volume: this is the 'packed cell volume' or *haematocrit*.

The erythrocyte is a special oxygen-carrying cell because it is rich in haemoglobin. The cell membrane is composed of a phospholipid bilayer with integral proteins. The shape of the cell is maintained by structural proteins which form a cytoskeleton. Enzyme systems protect the haemoglobin from irre-

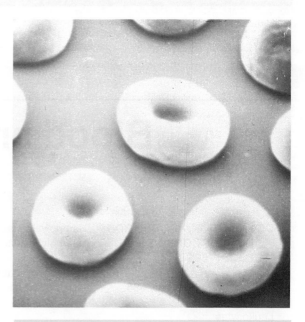

Fig. 23.1 Scanning electron micrograph of red cells

versible oxidation. The mature erythrocyte has no nuclear material, so new protein cannot be synthesised.

Absolute values

The absolute values are measures of red cell size and haemoglobin content which provide valuable information in the assessment of anaemia. They are calculated from the red cell concentration, haemoglobin concentration and haematocrit as follows:

Mean corpuscular volume (MCV) in femtolitres (fl) =

$$\frac{\text{Haematocrit (l/l)}}{\text{Red cell concentration (per litre)}}$$

Mean corpuscular haemoglobin (MCH) in picograms (pg) =

$$\frac{\text{Haemoglobin concentration (g/dl)}}{\text{Red cell concentration (per litre)}}$$

Mean corpuscular haemoglobin concentration (MCHC) in grams per decilitre (g/dl) =

$$\frac{\text{Haemoglobin concentration (g/dl)}}{\text{Haematocrit (l/l)}}$$

Morphology

The biconcave erythrocyte shape provides a large surface area for oxygen diffusion. By light microscopy erythrocytes appear as uniform round cells with central pallor. Up to 1% of cells stain with a purplish tinge and are of rather greater diameter. These are polychromatic cells; this purple staining is due to the residual ribonucleic acid (RNA) of the immature erythrocyte. These young cells become indistinguishable from the mature red cell population after 48 hours in the blood. When stained with a supravital stain (such as methylene blue) polychromatic cells are more easily identified by the presence of characteristic inclusions; they are then termed *reticulocytes*. The inclusions are remnants of RNA. When bone marrow production of erythrocytes is increased, the proportion of polychromatic cells, or reticulocytes, in the peripheral blood becomes greater than 1% or $100 \times 10^9/1$.

Changes in disease

Anaemia is present when the haemoglobin concentration is less than 13.0 g/dl in a male or 11.5 g/dl in a female (Table 23.1); the haematocrit is also reduced. An increased red cell concentration is referred to as *polycythaemia*; it is usually accompanied by a raised haemoglobin concentration and haematocrit.

Anaemias may be simply classified according to red cell size (MCV) and haemoglobin content (MCH). This classification is of great diagnostic value in most common types of anaemia (Table 23.2). Further diagnostic information is obtained by examination of the red cell morphology. Disease of the blood is frequently associated with increased variation in red cell size — *anisocytosis* — and the presence of erythrocytes of abnormal shape — *poikilocytosis* (Fig. 23.2). Increased erythrocyte anisocytosis and poikilocytosis are non-specific abnormalities present in many haematological and systemic disorders.

In the absence of a functioning spleen, due to surgical removal or secondary to disease, there are characteristic changes of red cell morphology. Howell–Jolly bodies (Fig. 23.3) are remnants of nuclear material from the developing erythrocytes (called normoblasts) which would normally be removed by a process, termed pitting, within the spleen. The occasional poikilocytes formed in normal individuals are removed by the spleen but they continue to circulate when splenic function is impaired or absent; poikilocytosis in the presence of normal splenic function denotes a haematological abnormality.

Table 23.1 Normal red cell values

Value	Male	Both sexes	Female
Haemoglobin (g/dl)			
Adult	13.0–17.0		11.5–16.0
Newborn		13.5–19.5	
3 months		9.5–13.5	
12 months		10.5–13.5	
Haematocrit (l/l)	0.39–0.50		0.34–0.47
Red cell count ($\times 10^{12}/l$)	4.3–5.7		3.9–5.1
MCH (pg)		26–33	
MCV (fl)		78–98	
MCHC (g/dl)		30–35	

These values will vary slightly between laboratories. All laboratory ranges include values for 95% of the normal population. 5% of normal subjects will therefore have values slightly outside the range quoted. (MCH = mean corpuscular haemoglobin; MCV = mean corpuscular volume; MCHC = mean corpuscular haemoglobin concentration)

Table 23.2 Morphological classification of anaemia

Morphology	Absolute values		Common causes
Microcytic **Hypochromic**	MCV <78 MCH <26		Iron deficiency Thalassaemia
Macrocytic	MCV >98		Megaloblastic anaemias
Normocytic **Normochromic**	MCV MCH	Normal	Acute blood loss Most haemolytic anaemias Anaemia of chronic disorders* Bone marrow failure

*There may be slight microcytosis.

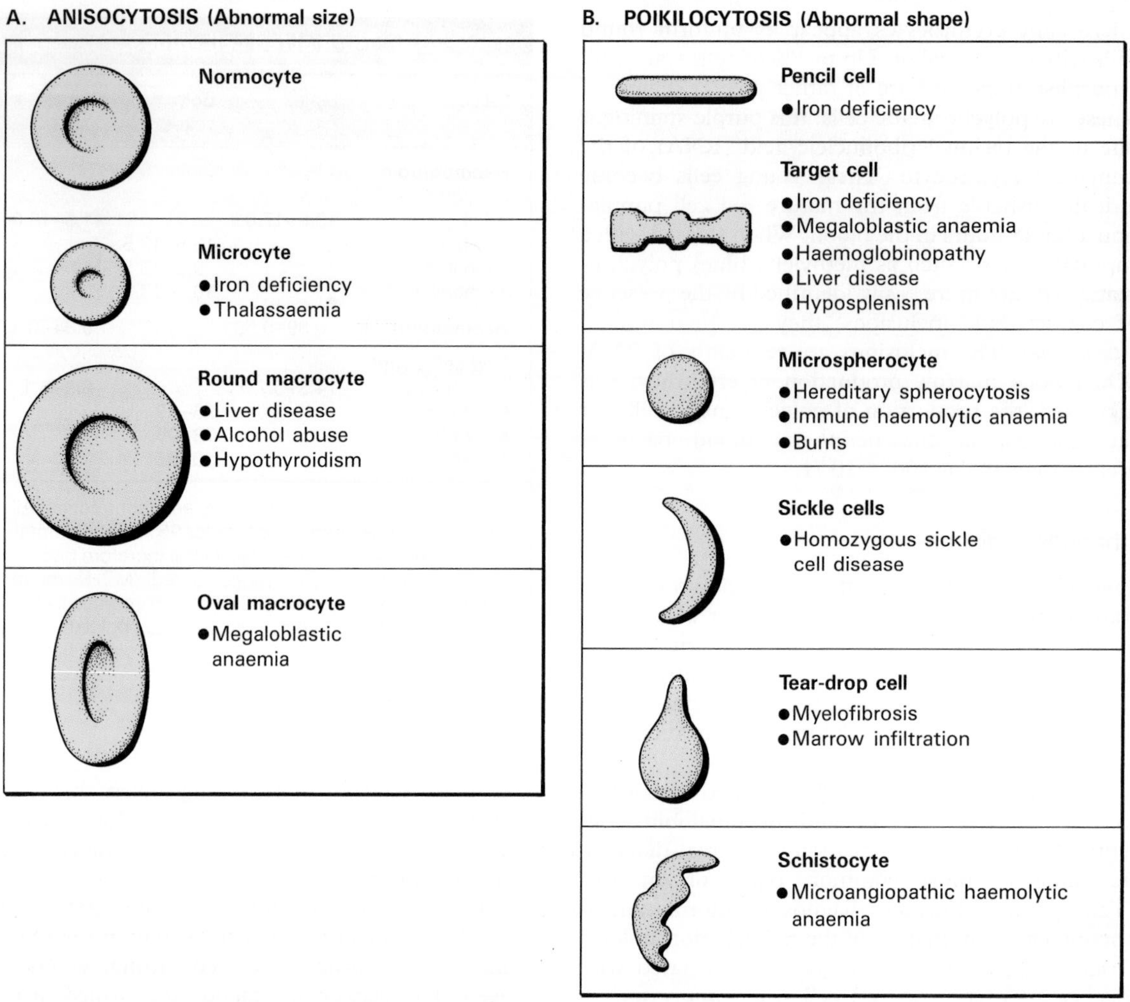

A.   ANISOCYTOSIS (Abnormal size)

Normocyte

Microcyte
- Iron deficiency
- Thalassaemia

Round macrocyte
- Liver disease
- Alcohol abuse
- Hypothyroidism

Oval macrocyte
- Megaloblastic anaemia

B.   POIKILOCYTOSIS (Abnormal shape)

Pencil cell
- Iron deficiency

Target cell
- Iron deficiency
- Megaloblastic anaemia
- Haemoglobinopathy
- Liver disease
- Hyposplenism

Microspherocyte
- Hereditary spherocytosis
- Immune haemolytic anaemia
- Burns

Sickle cells
- Homozygous sickle cell disease

Tear-drop cell
- Myelofibrosis
- Marrow infiltration

Schistocyte
- Microangiopathic haemolytic anaemia

Fig. 23.2   Abnormalities of red cell size and shape
A. Increased variation in size: anisocytosis. **B.** Variation in shape: poikilocytosis.

In addition to Howell–Jolly bodies, red cells may contain other inclusions (Fig. 23.3) under certain circumstances. The basophilic stippling of the 'stipple cell' is due to the presence of residual RNA; stipple cells may be present in several anaemias, especially thalassaemia. Siderotic granules contain iron and may occur in states of iron overload. Occasionally, nucleated red cell precursors may escape into the peripheral blood; when these normoblasts are accompanied by immature neutrophil leukocytes the film is described as *leukoerythroblastic*. A leukoerythroblastic blood film results from gross marrow disturbance such as infiltration by malignancy, myelofibrosis or severe megaloblastic anaemia.

Supravital staining is used to detect the presence of reticulocytes, as described above, and also to demonstrate the presence of denatured haemoglobin — Heinz bodies — in certain haemolytic anaemias, especially those due to a deficiency in the protective enzyme systems.

Leukocytes

The nucleated cells of the peripheral blood are termed white blood cells or leukocytes. Their primary role is protection against infection or infestation of the body. Morphologically, on a Romanowsky-stained blood film, five varieties of leukocyte are identified.

A. Visible on a Romanowsky-stained film

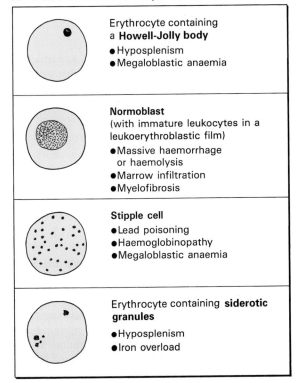

Erythrocyte containing
a **Howell-Jolly body**
● Hyposplenism
● Megaloblastic anaemia

Normoblast
(with immature leukocytes in a
leukoerythroblastic film)
● Massive haemorrhage
  or haemolysis
● Marrow infiltration
● Myelofibrosis

Stipple cell
● Lead poisoning
● Haemoglobinopathy
● Megaloblastic anaemia

Erythrocyte containing **siderotic
granules**
● Hyposplenism
● Iron overload

B. Visible only after supravital staining

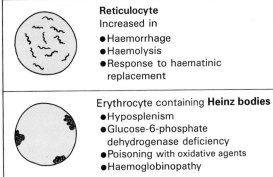

Reticulocyte
Increased in
● Haemorrhage
● Haemolysis
● Response to haematinic
  replacement

Erythrocyte containing **Heinz bodies**
● Hyposplenism
● Glucose-6-phosphate
  dehydrogenase deficiency
● Poisoning with oxidative agents
● Haemoglobinopathy

Fig. 23.3   Red cell inclusions

Normal white cell concentrations in the older child and adult are:

- Neutrophil granulocytes $2.0–7.5×10^9/l$
- Lymphocytes $1.0–3.0×10^9/l$
- Monocytes $0.15–0.6×10^9/l$
- Eosinophil granulocytes $0.05–0.35×10^9/l$
- Basophil granulocytes $0.01–0.10×10^9/l$

The granulocytes and monocytes are phagocytic leukocytes produced from precursor cells in the bone marrow. The lymphocytes are part of the immunologically competent series, which includes immunoglobulin-producing plasma cells; they are produced initially in the bone marrow and thymus, and later develop in the lymphoid tissue of the body.

Neutrophil granulocytes
Neutrophils are the most numerous leukocytes in the blood of the healthy adult. The nucleus of the neutrophil granulocyte is characteristically segmented into up to five lobes and the nuclear chromatin stains densely. The abundant cytoplasm stains pink and contains characteristic granules. Within the granules are enzymes, including myeloperoxidase and alkaline phosphatase, and lysozyme. Neutrophils have a scavenging function and are of particular importance in the defence against bacterial infection.

Neutrophil precursors and neutrophils spend 14 days in the bone marrow, whereas the half-life of neutrophils in the blood is only 6–9 hours. Peripheral blood counts therefore measure less than 10% of the total body neutrophils. Within the circulation the cells move between a circulating and a 'marginating' pool, margination being attachment to vascular endothelial cells. To perform their scavenging function granulocytes irreversibly enter the tissues by penetrating endothelial cells modified by inflammatory mediators. Cytokine-stimulated endothelial cells present adhesion molecules which interact with neutrophils: one such is ICAM-l (intercellular adhesion molecule-l).

Lymphocytes
The peripheral blood lymphocytes are small leukocytes with a round or only slightly indented nucleus

and scanty sky-blue-staining cytoplasm which may contain an occasional pink- or red-staining granule. A small proportion of lymphocytes may be larger with abundant cytoplasm, sometimes referred to as 'activated' lymphocytes. These are believed to represent cells which have been stimulated, perhaps by foreign antigen. A more complete description of the classification and role of lymphocytes is to be found in Chapter 9.

Monocytes
Monocytes are the largest blood cells. The nucleus is oval or reniform but not lobed. The abundant cytoplasm stains pale blue and often contains pink granules; vacuoles are often present. The function of monocytes is similar to that of neutrophil granulocytes: they enter the tissues and are responsible for the phagocytosis and digestion of foreign material and dead tissue.

Eosinophil granulocytes
Eosinophil granulocytes contain much larger and red-staining granules. The nucleus is lobulated, but usually only two or three lobes are seen. The eosinophil is important in the mediation of the allergic response and in defence against parasitic infestation.

Basophil granulocytes
Basophil granulocytes are the least frequent leukocytes in normal blood. The granules are large, blue–black and obscure the bilobed nucleus; they contain heparin and histamine. Basophils are closely related to tissue mast cells but their function has not been determined precisely. They appear to be key mediators of immediate hypersensitivity reactions, involving release of histamine.

Changes in disease

Changes may be *quantitative* or *qualitative*; the former are more important and often of diagnostic value. A knowledge of the causes of increased numbers of the various leukocytes in the peripheral blood is especially useful.

Quantitative changes
Leukocytosis means an increase in numbers of circulating white blood cells. Depending on the cause, there may be a polymorphonuclear leukocytosis (neutrophilia — increased neutrophil leukocytes), monocytosis, eosinophil leukocytosis (eosinophilia), basophil leukocytosis (basophilia) or lymphocytosis.

Causes of reactive neutrophil leukocytosis include:

- sepsis (e.g. acute appendicitis, bacterial pneumonia)
- trauma (e.g. major surgery)
- infarcts (e.g. myocardial infarction)
- chronic inflammatory disease (e.g. systemic lupus erythematosus (SLE), rheumatoid disease)
- malignant neoplasms
- steroid therapy
- acute haemorrhage or haemolysis.

Monocytosis may be reactive to:

- sepsis
- chronic infections (e.g. tuberculosis)
- malignant neoplasms.

Eosinophil leukocytosis may be reactive to:

- allergy (e.g. asthma)
- parasites (e.g. tapeworm infestation)
- malignant neoplasms (e.g. Hodgkin's disease)
- miscellaneous conditions (e.g. polyarteritis nodosa).

Lymphocytosis is most commonly associated with an infection such as infectious mononucleosis, tuberculosis, etc. However, in addition to these causes of a reactive leukocytosis, increased white cell counts may occur in primary disease of bone marrow, particularly the leukaemias.

In some disorders the leukocytosis may be extreme (for example $100 \times 10^9/l$), particularly in children. There may also be a tendency for immature leukocytes, particularly myelocytes and metamyelocytes, to appear in the peripheral blood. Severe bacterial infection may result in such an extreme reactive picture, which has in the past been referred to as a 'leukaemoid reaction' because of the similarity of the blood picture to that of chronic myeloid leukaemia. Occasionally, the lymphocyte series may be involved in such an extreme reactive process, especially during childhood viral infection.

A characteristic leukocytosis composed of 'atypical' lymphocytes is a feature of *infectious mononucleosis* (glandular fever). The infection is common in young adults and often manifests as a sore throat with enlarged lymph nodes and spleen and skin rash. It is due to infection with Epstein–Barr (EB) virus and is common between 15 and 25 years of age. The major features are:

- infection of B-lymphocytes with EB virus
- T-lymphocytosis
- blood lymphocytosis with atypical forms
- lymph node enlargement
- splenomegaly
- hepatitis often present

- development of antibodies reactive with non-human erythrocytes (heterophile antibodies)
- development of antibodies to EB virus.

The atypical cells in peripheral blood are recognisable as lymphocytes but are much larger and with abundant cytoplasm and nuclear irregularities (Fig. 23.4). They are probably reactive T-lymphocytes responding to B-lymphocytes containing the virus, are detectable in blood about 7 days after the onset of illness and may persist for 6 weeks or more. Apparently fortuitously, but usefully, antibodies reactive against horse, sheep and ox red cells (heterophile antibodies) typically develop during the second week and may persist for a few months; they are detected in the Paul–Bunnell test or by more convenient commercial screening slide tests such as the 'Monospot' test, and are of diagnostic value. A very similar clinical and haematological (but not serological) picture can develop as a result of other infections, especially with human immunodeficiency virus (HIV), cytomegalovirus and toxoplasma.

A reduction in circulating leukocytes is termed *leukopenia*. Most important is a deficiency of neutrophil granulocytes — neutropenia. Lymphopenia is less common and usually due to therapy with the cytotoxic drugs used in malignant disease, or to irradiation; it is also a feature of infection with the human immunodeficiency virus. Neutropenia is commonly seen in association with a reduction in other blood cells, that is, as part of a pancytopenia. Important causes of pancytopenia are:

- bone marrow failure (e.g. hypoplastic anaemia; marrow infiltration with leukaemia or carcinoma; due to cytotoxic drug therapy; due to irradiation)
- megaloblastic anaemia
- hypersplenism.

Important causes of selective neutropenia are:

- overwhelming sepsis (e.g. septicaemia, miliary tuberculosis)
- racial (in African races)
- autoimmune (e.g. due to auto-antibody, often in association with other autoimmune disease such as rheumatoid arthritis)
- drug-induced (as an idiosyncratic reaction)
- cyclical.

In cyclical forms the neutropenia is temporary and recurrent, often with a periodicity of 3–4 weeks.

Neutropenia with counts of less than $0.5 \times 10^9/l$ may result in severe sepsis, especially of the mouth, pharynx (Fig. 23.5) and perianal regions, and also in disseminated infection. This clinical picture is now most commonly seen in patients receiving drug or irradiation therapy for malignant disorders, especially leukaemias and lymphomas.

Qualitative changes

Qualitative leukocyte changes are less important than quantitative abnormalities. Defects of phagocytic cell function resulting in an increased tendency to bacterial infection are recognised, particularly as acquired defects after splenectomy, in leukaemic disorders and due to corticosteroid therapy. Congenital abnormali-

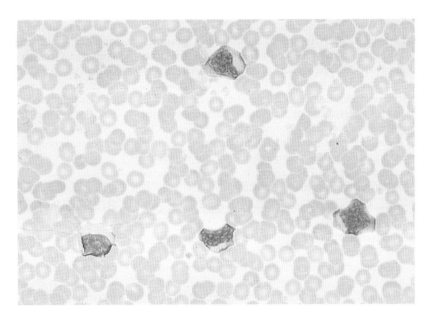

Fig. 23.4 Atypical mononuclear cells in infectious mononucleosis

These large T-lymphocytes have copious basophilic cytoplasm with irregular cell outline.

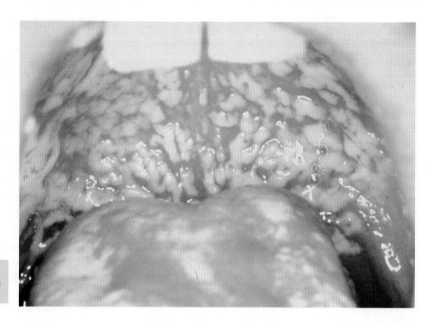

Fig. 23.5   Oral infection with *Candida albicans* ('thrush') in a neutropenic patient

ties of leukocyte function are uncommon. 'Atypical' lymphocytes in infectious mononucleosis have been described earlier. Other abnormalities of neutrophil morphology are also recognised (Fig. 23.6).

Platelets

On a stained blood film platelets appear as non-nucleated fragments of granular cytoplasm, approximately one-fifth the diameter of erythrocytes and in a concentration of 150–400 × 10⁹/l. Electron microscopy reveals the presence of cytoskeletal elements which maintain the discoid shape of the resting platelet, and numerous intracellular granules. Platelets are contractile and adhesive cells, the function of which is the maintenance of vascular integrity; exposure of vascular subendothelial structures results in rapid adhesion of platelets to the exposed area and aggregation of platelets to each other in the formation of a primary haemostatic plug (Fig. 23.7).

A deficiency of blood platelets is termed *thrombocytopenia*, the causes and consequences of which are described on page 734. *Thrombocytosis*, or increased platelet numbers, is usually reactive to:

- acute and chronic blood loss (e.g. from peptic ulcer, menorrhagia)
- iron deficiency (e.g. dietary deficiency, chronic blood loss)
- chronic inflammatory disease (e.g. rheumatoid arthritis)
- neoplastic disease (e.g. bronchial carcinoma, lymphoma)

- tissue trauma (e.g. post-operative state, especially splenectomy).

Thrombocytosis may also occur in primary disorders of bone marrow—the myeloproliferative diseases. Morphological platelet abnormalities are of minor importance, although 'giant' platelets, with a diameter exceeding that of an erythrocyte, are a feature of the myeloproliferative disorders.

Blood count and morphology in disease

Changes in the blood are present in a wide range of diseases of other organs. These changes are most commonly reactive or secondary but may be useful in providing a clue to the presence of the underlying, often occult, disease, e.g. polymorphonuclear leukocytosis in bacterial sepsis; eosinophilia in some parasitic infections. In other cases the abnormalities of cell number and morphology are due to a primary haematological disorder.

BLOOD PLASMA

Plasma amounts to greater than 50% of blood volume. While changes in the innumerable constituents of plasma are outside the scope of this text, consideration of certain major plasma proteins is necessary for an understanding of the pathology of some blood and systemic disorders.

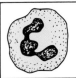

	Normal 'mature' neutrophil leukocyte
	'Band' cell or 'stab' cell. An immature form. Present in increased proportion in the presence of bacterial sepsis.
	Hypersegmented form. A large cell with an increased number of nuclear lobes. Present in megaloblastic anaemia.
	Pelger form. Majority of neutrophils have bilobed nucleus. Present in myelodysplasia or as a congenital variant.
	'Toxic' granulation. Coarse, increased granulation. Often with neutrophil leukocytosis, in bacterial sepsis. A Döhle body (bluish, peripheral inclusion body) is also often present.
	Hypogranular form. Present in myeloid leukaemias and myelodysplasia.
	Blast cell. Present in acute leukaemias.

Fig. 23.6   Abnormalities of neutrophil morphology

Blood coagulation

For normal homeostasis it is essential that blood remains fluid; however the capacity to minimise loss of blood through breaches of the vascular system is an essential requirement. Rapid plugging of defects in small vessels is the function of platelets (Fig. 23.7); however, a more permanent and secure seal results from the generation of insoluble fibrillar fibrin from its soluble plasma protein precursor fibrinogen in the process of blood clotting. Failure of primary haemostasis, due to platelet disorders, or of coagulation, can each result in life-threatening haemorrhage. In contrast, inappropriate activation of platelets or blood clotting may result in vascular occlusion, ischaemia and tissue death. A complex system of activators and inhibitors in plasma has therefore evolved (Fig. 23.8). In health, these are finely balanced in order to allow normal haemostatic responses whilst preventing pathological thrombosis. The inhibitor antithrombin III requires glycosaminoglycan 'heparans', present on the vascular endothelial cell surface, for full inhibitory activity. Heparin is a major anticoagulant drug, also a glycosaminoglycan, which acts through antithrombin III. Another important inhibitor, protein C, requires activation by thrombin in a negative feedback loop before it can, in association with protein S, act as a coagulation inhibitor.

Almost all of the coagulation factors and inhibitors are synthesised in the liver. They form part of a biological amplification system: thus 1 mole of activated XIa generates over 10^8 moles of fibrin. Factors II, VII, IX, X, XI and XII are serine proteases, that is enzymes in which the presence of serine at the active site is necessary for their action in hydrolysing peptide bonds. Factors II, VII, IX and X and inhibitors protein C and S require vitamin K for synthesis in their completed form.

Several components of the fibrinolytic system (Fig. 23.8) also originate in the liver; tissue plasminogen activator is, however, a product of vascular endothelial cells.

The intrinsic coagulation pathway is activated by exposed collagen and progresses slowly. The extrinsic system depends upon release of tissue factors (lipoproteins) by tissue injury and proceeds more rapidly. While subdivision of this complex process into intrinsic, extrinsic and fibrinolytic systems is convenient, it is undoubtedly an oversimplification; there are points of interaction between the components. Of importance are activation of factor IX by VIIa (Fig. 23.8), feedback loops involving activation of factors VII and V by thrombin, and, intriguingly, the requirement for thrombin in the activation of protein C as described above. Also, platelet activation provides phospholipid for thrombin generation, and products of the coagulation cascade, including thrombin, are potent platelet activators.

The pathology and consequences of deficiency of the components of the coagulation and fibrinolytic system are described on page 737.

Rheological considerations

Blood is a viscous fluid and changes in its physical properties accompany some diseases. The unique

A. Platelet adhesion

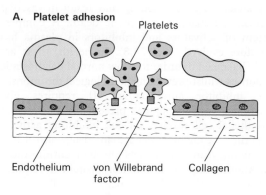

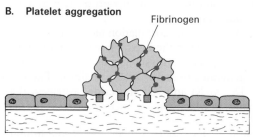

Platelets

Endothelium   von Willebrand   Collagen
factor

B. Platelet aggregation

Fibrinogen

C. Fibrin generation

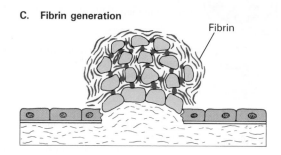

Fibrin

Fig. 23.7 The physiology of primary haemostasis

A. Platelet adhesion. Exposure of subendothelial material causes activation of platelets, which change shape and produce pseudopodia, and rapidly adhere to the area via receptor sites which interact with *von Willebrand factor* (vWF). vWF is a multimeric protein synthesised by endothelial cells and megakaryocytes. It associates with a coagulation factor, factor VIII, in plasma. **B. Platelet aggregation.** Platelets interact with each other via receptor sites which use *fibrinogen* as an intercellular bridge. Platelets contract and release granules which contain pro-aggregatory substances which promote the aggregation response. These include ADP, 5-hydroxytryptamine, fibrinogen and vWF. Metabolism of arachidonic acid, a fatty acid of the cell membrane, to the prostaglandin-like metabolite thromboxane A_2 also promotes aggregation and, in addition, vasoconstriction. **C. Fibrin generation.** The exposed surface also causes activation of the intrinsic coagulation system and release of tissue factor activation of the extrinsic system. *Thrombin* generation augments the platelet activation and activated platelets provide phospholipid, which is an essential co-factor at several points in the coagulation cascade.

composition of the blood—a suspension of deformable cells in a protein-rich solution—results in complex physical characteristics: it behaves in a non-Newtonian fashion. Within the major vessels, shear rates (i.e. velocity differences between fluid layers) are very high adjacent to the walls of large arteries; in contrast, low rates of shear exist in small veins. The non-Newtonian behaviour is due to aggregation of red cells at low shear rates and their ability to deform at high shear rates.

The major determinant of blood viscosity is *haematocrit*. Numbers of leukocytes and platelets make a negligible contribution in health. However, when leukocyte counts exceed $300 \times 10^9/l$, usually in leukaemia, viscosity may be influenced and a *hyperviscosity state* ensues. This state is associated with stasis within the microcirculation and tissue

anoxia. Cerebral dysfunction, with headache, visual disturbance and drowsiness progressing to coma may result.

The plasma *fibrinogen* concentration is the major determinant of the red cell aggregation occurring at low rates of shear and is second only to haematocrit as a factor in determination of blood viscosity. An increase in plasma fibrinogen of 1 g/l doubles whole blood viscosity at low shear rates (normal plasma fibrinogen concentration is around 2–3 g/l). Other plasma protein molecules tend to be smaller and more symmetrical than fibrinogen and consequently have a much lesser effect on viscosity. However, when they are present in increased concentrations, blood viscosity may be affected. Again, this may result in a hyperviscosity syndrome. Very high plasma immunoglobulin concentration, which is a common

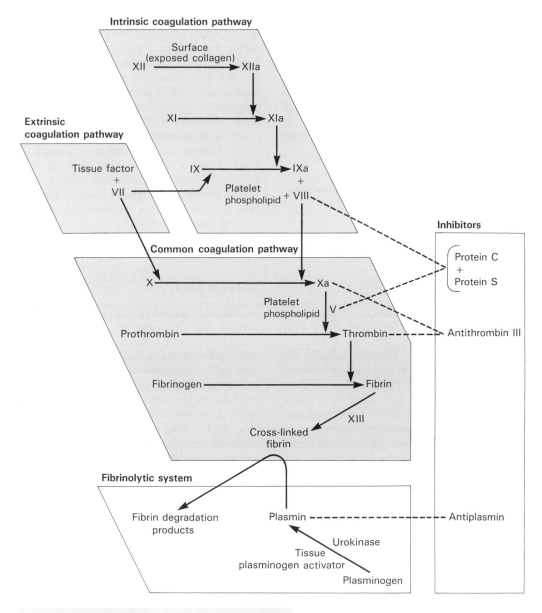

Fig. 23.8 The coagulation and fibrinolytic systems

feature of the malignant disorders multiple myeloma and macroglobulinaemia, is a common cause of the hyperviscosity syndrome.

The hyperviscosity syndromes represent extreme abnormalities of blood flow producing organ dysfunction. However, epidemiological studies suggest that even minor increases in blood viscosity, due to increased haematocrit or fibrinogen concentration, may result in a tendency to vascular occlusion, manifesting as an increased incidence of myocardial

infarction and cerebral infarction. The concentration of plasma fibrinogen is a risk factor for arterial occlusive disease which is at least as potent as the level of serum cholesterol. The interplay between rheological and haemostatic changes in thrombotic disease is not yet fully understood.

Erythrocyte sedimentation rate

The erythrocyte sedimentation rate (ESR) measures the rate at which red cells sediment by gravity in plasma in one hour and is a widely used laboratory test. Increased aggregation and sedimentation occur in the presence of high concentrations of immunoglobulin and fibrinogen. As the latter is an acute phase reactant, the ESR is increased in a wide variety of inflammatory and neoplastic conditions. It is an entirely non-specific test and a normal value for ESR can never be used to exclude the presence of significant disease. Measurement of plasma viscosity provides equally useful data.

HAEMOPOIESIS AND BLOOD CELL KINETICS

Haemopoiesis is the formation of blood cells.

Sites of haemopoiesis

In the adult all blood cells are produced in the red marrow, which is restricted to the bones of the axial skeleton — vertebrae, ribs, sternum, skull, sacrum, pelvis and proximal femora. In these regions the bone marrow is composed of approximately 50% fat, within adipocytes, and 50% blood cells and their precursors (Fig. 23.9). The fatty marrow of other bones is capable of haemopoiesis when requirements for blood cells are increased in some diseases.

In the infant and young child, practically all of the bones contain haemopoietically active marrow.

In fetal life the liver and spleen are the major haemopoietic organs between about 6 weeks' and 6–7 months' gestation; the yolk sac is the main site before 6 weeks. In disease, the liver and spleen can again become haemopoietic organs, even in adult life; this development is referred to as *extramedullary haemopoiesis* and is particularly associated with the progressive fibrosis of bone marrow seen in the myeloproliferative disorders.

The bone marrow is examined histologically in two ways. Marrow can be aspirated through a needle inserted into a marrow cavity (usually sternum or pelvis), smeared on a slide and stained in a method similar to that for peripheral blood. Further information, particularly on the structure and cellularity of the marrow, can be obtained by preparation of sections of a marrow trephine biopsy: this is a core of tissue obtained using a wide-bore needle (Fig. 23.9).

Stem cell theory

Studies of bone marrow in culture lead to the conclusion that erythrocytes, leukocytes (including lymphocytes) and platelets are derived from a common, self-replicating precursor cell or 'pluripotent stem cell'. By a series of cell divisions, cells committed to each line are produced and further divisions result in mature cells — erythrocytes, granular leukocytes, megakaryocytes and T- and B-lymphocytes (Fig. 23.10). The pluripotent stem cells possess the ability to renew in addition to the capacity to differentiate. They have not been definitely identified morphologically. The development and preferential

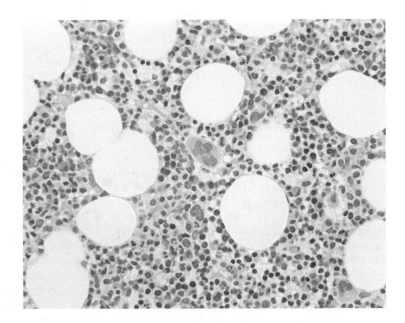

Fig. 23.9   Normal bone marrow
From a section of a bone marrow biopsy from the pelvis. Marrow cells are interspersed between fat spaces.

survival of a malignant clone of haemopoietic cells explains the pathological features of the leukaemias and dyserythropoietic anaemias.

If human bone marrow is infused intravenously into a subject without functioning marrow, as during bone marrow transplantation treatment, normal blood cell production returns after a period of several weeks. This finding confirms the presence of pluripotent stem cells in bone marrow and also indicates that the microenvironment of the bone marrow is central to normal blood production; stem cells do not tend to thrive in other sites, and blood production resumes only in the marrow cavities after marrow infusion. Stem cells can be made to circulate in the peripheral blood. This is most conveniently achieved by the administration of one of the cytokines responsible for stimulation of haemopoiesis—the colony stimulating factors (p. 697). Using an extracorporeal centrifugation technique these cells can be harvested and used as an alternative to bone marrow cells in transplantation therapy—a peripheral blood stem cell transplant.

Erythropoiesis

The pronormoblast is the earliest red cell precursor that can be identified in the bone marrow. It is a large cell with prominent nucleoli within the nucleus. By a series of four cell divisions a fully haemoglobinised, non-nucleated erythrocyte is produced. During differentiation the nucleus becomes increasingly condensed or pyknotic and the cytoplasm contains increasing amounts of haemoglobin and less RNA; the early (basophilic), intermediate (polychromatic) and late (pyknotic) normoblasts can be identified morphologically (Fig. 23.11). The pyknotic nucleus is eventually extruded, leaving a 'polychromatic' erythrocyte which remains in the marrow for a further 48 hours; it then circulates and matures in the spleen for approximately 48 hours, at which point it becomes a mature erythrocyte.

Only polychromatic erythrocytes and mature erythrocytes normally circulate. However, nucleated red cell precursors are present in the peripheral blood in the presence of some marrow disorders.

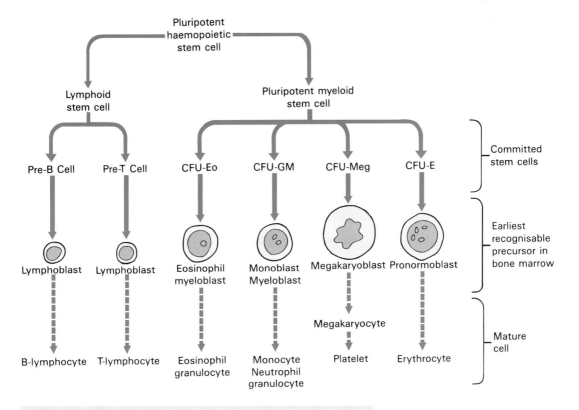

Fig. 23.10 Blood cell differentiation: normal haemopoiesis

The term 'CFU' (colony forming unit) is derived from marrow culture studies. Progenitor cells form colonies of cells with identifiable characteristics in culture.

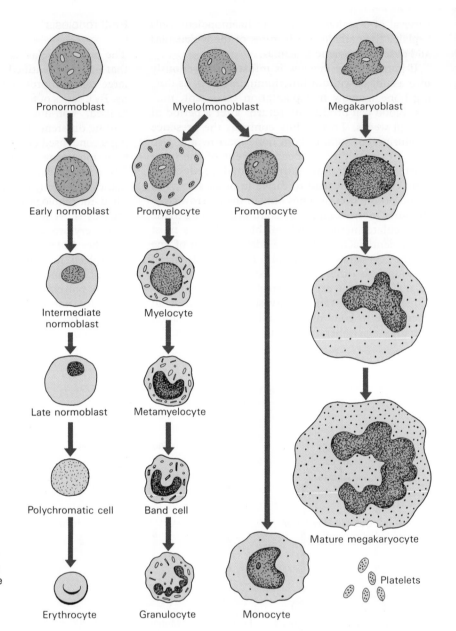

Fig. 23.11   Haemopoiesis

A schematic representation of the stages of erythrocyte, megakaryocyte and myeloid cell development.

Leukopoiesis

The normal bone marrow contains many more myeloid than nucleated erythroid cells (around 5:1). In the granulocyte series these include the myeloblast, promyelocyte and myelocyte, which are capable of cell division, and the metamyelocyte and band cell which are undergoing maturation without further division (Fig. 23.11). Maturation of granulocytes from myeloblast to band cell involves a reduction in cell size, development of cytoplasmic granules, increased condensation of nuclear chromatin, and irregularity of nuclear outline.

Monoblasts cannot easily be distinguished from myeloblasts. They mature in the bone marrow to monocytes via a promonocyte stage. Leukocyte precursors do not normally circulate but, as previously mentioned, may do so in the presence of severe infection or bone marrow disease.

Megakaryocytopoiesis

Megakaryocyte maturation is unique. The earliest identifiable precursor, the megakaryoblast, is a large cell which undergoes nuclear replication without cell division, the cytoplasmic volume increasing as the nuclear material increases, in multiples of 2, up to 32N (Fig. 23.11). Cytoplasmic maturation occurs, often at the 8N stage, and platelets are released by an unknown mechanism, possibly by fragmentation of the cytoplasm of circulating megakaryocytes in the lung. Megakaryocytes are not seen in peripheral blood by routine methods.

Blood cell kinetics

Erythrocytes circulate for an average of 120 days and are then destroyed, predominantly in the bone marrow, but also in liver and spleen. The relative contribution of liver and spleen to erythrocyte breakdown may increase considerably in some diseases, especially the haemolytic anaemias. There is no significant storage pool of erythrocytes in man. In contrast, some ten times more granulocytes are present in the bone marrow than in the peripheral blood, constituting a storage pool of leukocytes which can be mobilised rapidly in response to some stimulus, such as infection or tissue damage. Granulocytes spend only a few hours in the circulation before they enter the tissues, where they act as phagocytes, surviving for several days under normal circumstances. Monocytes also spend a limited time in the circulation, after which they enter the tissues and become tissue macrophages; they may survive for many months.

Platelets circulate for approximately 10 days. The spleen acts as a reservoir of reserve platelets; some 30% are present in the spleen at any time.

Control of haemopoiesis

Peripheral blood cell counts are normally maintained within close limits. However, the ability of each cell line to respond appropriately to increased requirements is exemplified by the increased red cell production after haemorrhage, granulocyte leukocytosis in response to sepsis and enhanced platelet production which results from chronic bleeding.

Erythropoietin is a glycoprotein hormone produced by the kidney, which, with a plasma protein cofactor, increases erythropoietic activity. The production of erythropoietin is increased in response to a reduced oxygen tension in the blood reaching the kidney. It results in an increase in the number of cells committed to the erythroid line, reduced maturation time and early release of erythrocytes from the bone marrow. Erythropoietin mediates the physiological response of the bone marrow to anaemia or hypoxia. In pathological states, failure of erythropoietin production is a major contributor to the anaemia of chronic renal failure and this can be corrected by erythropoietin administration; inappropriate excessive erythropoietin production results in polycythaemia secondary to some renal cysts and tumours.

Advances in molecular biology have recently allowed the identification of a group of compounds which can stimulate production of leukocytes and megakaryocytes; these are known as *colony stimulating factors*. They include granulocyte- and granulocyte/monocyte-colony stimulating factors (G-CSF and GM-CSF). These cytokines are now in therapeutic use, particularly in cancer chemotherapy, where the duration of drug-induced neutropenia can be limited by cytokine administration. Thrombopoietin, capable of the stimulation of platelet production, has recently been identified and will also have therapeutic applications.

Haemoglobin

Structure, synthesis and metabolism

Some knowledge of haemoglobin structure and metabolism is necessary for an understanding of the pathology of the anaemias.

By 1 month of age red cell precursors synthesise predominantly haemoglobin A, composed of haem (Fig. 23.12) and four polypeptide (globin) chains, of which two molecular forms are present: α and β chains. Haemoglobin A thus has the structure $\alpha_2\beta_2$. Up to 2.5% of the haemoglobin in adults has δ chains ($\alpha_2\delta_2$) — haemoglobin A_2, and up to 1% of the haemoglobin in adults has γ chains ($\alpha_2\gamma_2$) — haemoglobin F. Adult blood therefore has predominantly haemoglobin A with some A_2 and F (Table 23.3).

In later fetal and early neonatal life haemoglobin F predominates. In early fetal life three other haemoglobins are present: Gower 1, Gower 2 and Portland (Table 23.3). In the congenital disorders collectively known as *haemoglobinopathies* the rate of synthesis of one globin chain type is defective (the *thalassaemias*) or an abnormal chain is synthesised (the *sickle haemoglobinopathies* and other haemoglobin variants).

Each globin chain has its own oxygen-carrying haem group (Fig. 23.12), composed of a protoporphyrin ring structure with an iron atom. The whole haemoglobin molecule is thus composed of a tetramer of globin chains each with a haem group. The complex structure of the molecule is responsible for its

A

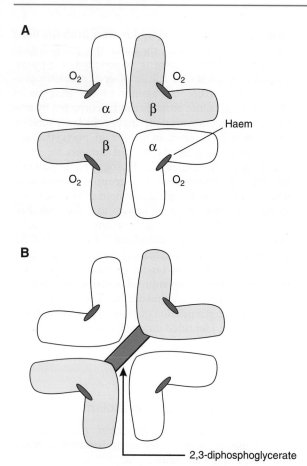

B

2,3-diphosphoglycerate

Fig. 23.12 Oxygenated (A) and deoxygenated (B) adult haemoglobin

Uptake and release of oxygen (O_2) is associated with movement of the globin chains. On release of O_2 the β chains are moved apart, allowing entry of 2,3-DPG and a reduction in the affinity of the haemoglobin molecule for O_2.

Table 23.3 Human haemoglobins

Type	Chains	Nomenclature	
Adults	$\alpha_2\beta_2$	A	
	$\alpha_2\sigma_2$	A_2	
Fetal	$\alpha_2\gamma_2$	F	
Embryonic	$\alpha_2\epsilon_2$	'Gower 2'	Present in
	$\zeta_2\epsilon_2$	'Gower 1'	early fetal
	$\zeta_2\gamma_2$	Portland	life only

After 1 year of life and in the adult less than 1% haemoglobin is F and less than 2.5% A_2.

oxygen (O_2) binding characteristics, the globin chains moving against each other during transfer of O_2. The affinity of the haemoglobin molecule for O_2 is also controlled by its ability to bind the metabolite 2,3-diphosphoglycerate (2,3-DPG). When 2,3-DPG enters the haemoglobin molecule as the β chains pull apart during release of O_2, the affinity for O_2 of the haemoglobin–2,3-DPG complex is reduced, allowing O_2 to be given up more readily. Haemoglobin F cannot bind 2,3-DPG and thus has a relatively high O_2 affinity, facilitating O_2 transfer from maternal blood across the placenta. Certain rare haemoglobin variants behave similarly: the high O_2 affinity results in relative tissue hypoxia, increased erythropoietin production and polycythaemia.

At the end of the erythrocyte life-span haemoglobin is metabolised, with conservation of iron and amino acids. Iron is carried by plasma transferrin to the bone marrow and utilised in the synthesis of haem. Globin is degraded to its constituent amino acids, which enter the general pool. Liver, gut and kidneys are all involved in excretion of products of haem breakdown as derivatives of bilirubin.

FUNCTIONS OF THE BLOOD: SUMMARY

From a consideration of the preceding sections the functions of blood and the major pathological consequences of blood and marrow disease will be apparent.

O_2 transport is the primary function of the red blood cells. Failure of red cell production, or loss or dysfunction thereof, results in tissue hypoxia affecting the metabolism of all organs.

The cells responsible for host defence against infection are carried, in the blood, from the bone marrow to sites of infection. Infections with bacteria, viruses and fungi are the predictable results of a failure to produce normal leukocytes in adequate numbers, especially when, as is often the case in haematological disease, treatment of the disorder also results in immunosuppression.

The primary haemostatic and coagulation mechanisms allow the transport functions of blood to operate without risk of exsanguination from breaches of the vascular compartment. Failure of these leads to spontaneous haemorrhage, whereas a defect in the control mechanisms can result in inappropriate thrombosis and vascular occlusion.

The diseases which interfere with the function of the blood and their pathological consequences are now described.

Pathological basis of haematological signs and symptoms

Sign or symptom	Pathological basis
Tiredness, dyspnoea	Reduced oxygen-carrying capacity of blood due to anaemia
Mucosal pallor	Anaemia
Glossitis (Sore mouth, smooth tongue)	Mucosal effects of haematinic deficiency
Spoon-shaped nails	Due to iron deficiency
Jaundice	Bilirubin accumulation from haemolysis
Abnormal tendency to infections	Neutropenia, e.g. in leukaemia or hypoplastic anaemia Immune deficiency, e.g. in myeloma, and due to chemotherapy in leukaemia and lymphoma
Splenomegaly	Myeloid metaplasia in myeloproliferative disorders, red cell pooling and destruction in haemolytic anaemias, infiltration in leukaemias and lymphomas. Also non-haematological causes, e.g. portal hypertension
Lymphadenopathy	Infiltration with leukaemia or lymphoma. Non-neoplastic causes, e.g. infectious mononucleosis
Bone pain and fractures	Osteoclast activation in myeloma
Purpura, bruising, mucosal or traumatic bleeding	Thrombocytopenia or severe platelet dysfunction
Bruising, muscle and joint bleeding and traumatic bleeding	Severe coagulation factor deficiency

ANAEMIAS

► Defined as when the haemoglobin is less than 13 g/dl in a male or 11.5 g/dl in the female adult
► Usually represent a reduction in the body red cell mass, except in the dilutional 'physiological anaemia' of pregnancy
► Result in tissue hypoxia
► Are due to failure of erythrocyte production or loss or destruction of erythrocytes

Anaemia is present when the haemoglobin falls below 13.0 g/dl in a male or 11.5 g/dl in a female. The different lower limits of normal haemoglobin concentration for neonates, infants and children should be noted (Table 23.1).

A low haemoglobin concentration usually reflects a reduction in the body red cell mass. An important exception is pregnancy, when both red cell mass and plasma volume increase, but the latter to a greater degree. This process results in a haemoglobin concentration in blood which is lower than in the non-pregnant state in the presence of a relatively increased red cell mass and overall oxygen-carrying capacity; this condition is often referred to as the physiological 'anaemia' of pregnancy, an essentially dilutional phenomenon. The increased red cell mass during pregnancy is necessary to support the increased metabolic requirement of the mother and fetus. The reason for the expansion of the plasma compartment is obscure, but it may be explained in part by a need for increased skin perfusion for heat loss due to the increased metabolic rate.

Expansion of the plasma volume, resulting in dilutional anaemia, may also occur when the spleen is pathologically enlarged. (The spleen appears to exert a controlling influence on plasma volume.) Other mechanisms also operate in this situation, however, as described under hypersplenism.

The consequences of anaemia are dependent upon the speed of onset. Thus the rapid loss of 10% or more of the circulating blood volume through haemorrhage will result in shock, that is the failure of adequate perfusion of all tissues and organs, with consequent hypoxia. In this situation the subject may not initially be anaemic, as both red cells and plasma are lost through haemorrhage. The plasma component is more rapidly replaced, however, and anaemia will be present after several hours have elapsed.

Anaemia which develops more gradually is better tolerated. A haemoglobin concentration as low as 2 g/dl may be consistent with survival if it develops over a protracted period. The inevitable result of anaemia, however, is a reduction in the oxygen-carrying capacity of the blood and thus chronic tissue hypoxia.

The general consequences of anaemia are due to the tissue hypoxia, which can result in fatty change, especially in the myocardium and liver, and even infarction. Lethargy and increased breathlessness on exertion are typical clinical features. Breathlessness at rest implies the development of heart failure, a result of severe anaemia. Expansion of the red marrow is present in those anaemias where a marrow response is possible — generally the haemolytic anaemias. Other features are specific to anaemias resulting from a particular mechanism, such as the jaundice of haemolytic anaemias, or are specific to anaemia of a particular type, such as the nail changes of iron deficiency anaemia. Such pathological features are described in the relevant sections.

Classification

Table 23.4 outlines a classification of anaemias. Anaemias are divided into two categories: those where anaemia is due to failure to produce erythrocytes, and those in which erythrocyte loss is increased but production is normal (or usually increased, in response to the anaemia). While useful, this categorisation is an oversimplification, as both mechanisms are present in some anaemias. Thus, in the megaloblastic states, cell production is defective due to lack of vitamin B_{12} or folic acid for nucleic acid synthesis but, in addition, the erythrocytes which are produced are

abnormal and of diminished survival. In thalassaemia, cell production is not optimal: ineffective erythropoiesis is present as well as increased erythrocyte destruction. Ineffective erythropoiesis is associated with destruction of developing erythroblasts and erythrocytes before they leave the bone marrow.

The myeloid and megakaryocytic lines are also involved in some anaemias due to failure of haemopoiesis (megaloblastic anaemia, hypoplastic anaemia) but not others (iron deficiency anaemia).

Despite these qualifications, the classification described is useful as an aid to determining the cause of the anaemia.

PRODUCTION FAILURE ANAEMIAS

The most commonly encountered anaemias are in the production failure group.

Haematinic deficiency

Haematinics are dietary factors essential for either haemoglobin synthesis or erythrocyte production.

Iron deficiency

▶ A production failure anaemia
▶ The commonest cause of anaemia
▶ Results in a microcytic hypochromic blood picture
▶ Usually indicative of chronic blood loss
▶ Frequently indicative of an occult, bleeding lesion of the gastrointestinal tract

Iron deficiency is the commonest cause of anaemia world-wide. It is particularly common relative to other anaemias in the United Kingdom, where congenital disorders producing anaemia such as thalassaemia, and infections such as malaria, are uncommon.

Iron deficiency is the commonest cause of a microcytic hypochromic blood picture, the others being thalassaemias and (rarely) sideroblastic anaemias.

Iron metabolism
Iron is an essential requirement. It is also one of the commonest elements present in the earth's crust. Excessive iron deposited in the tissues is, however, toxic, causing damage to the myocardium, pancreas and liver in particular (Ch. 16). As the body has no active method for iron excretion, iron status is controlled largely by its absorption; the capacity to absorb iron is, however, limited and any tendency to increased loss of iron, due to haemorrhage, is highly

Table 23.4	A classification of anaemias
Type	Cause
Production failure anaemia	
Haematinic deficiency	Iron Vitamin B_{12} or folic acid
Dyserythropoiesis	Sideroblastic anaemia 'Refractory' anaemias Anaemia of chronic disorders
Hypoplasia	
Marrow infiltration	In leukaemias In myeloproliferative states In non-haematological malignancies Miscellaneous infiltrates
Increased red cell loss, lysis or pooling	
Acute blood loss	

Haemolysis due to red
cell abnormality
	Membrane defects, e.g.
	    hereditary spherocytosis
	Enzyme defects, e.g. pyruvate
	    kinase deficiency
	Haemoglobinopathies,
	    e.g. thalassaemia, sickle
	    disorders
	Paroxysmal nocturnal
	    haemoglobinuria

Haemolysis due to abnormality outside the red cell	Immune haemolytic anaemias Microangiopathic haemolysis Drugs, toxins and chemicals Parasites
Hypersplenism	

likely to result in a negative iron balance and iron deficiency. These factors explain the high prevalence of iron deficiency.

Normally, at least 60% of the body iron is in the haemoglobin of erythroid cells. Approximately 30% is stored within the reticulo-endothelial system, especially in the bone marrow, as *ferritin* and *haemosiderin*. A small proportion of total body iron is present in other tissues, especially muscle and iron-containing enzymes. This tissue iron is relatively conserved during states of iron deficiency. Only a small fraction of the total body iron is in transport, attached to the carrier protein *transferrin*.

Ferritin is a protein-iron complex. The protein — apoferritin — is a shell made up of 22 subunits. The core is composed of ferric oxyhydride. Haemosiderin consists of partially degraded ferritin aggregates. Ferritin is present in all tissues, but especially in the macrophages of the bone marrow and spleen and in hepatocytes. A small amount is detectable in plasma and, as it is derived from the storage pool of body iron, its plasma concentration is an accurate indicator of body iron stores.

Ferritin is water-soluble and not visible by light microscopy; haemosiderin is insoluble and forms yellow granules. When exposed to potassium ferrocyanide (Perls' stain) the granules are blue–black. When iron stores are normal, only small amounts of haemosiderin are visible, mainly in marrow reticulo-endothelial cells. In iron overload, most of the iron is in the form of haemosiderin.

Transferrin is an iron-binding β-globulin responsible for iron transport and delivery to receptors on immature erythroid cells. Each molecule of transferrin can bind two atoms of iron, but normally the transferrin is only one-third saturated (thus the serum iron concentration is normally one-third of the total serum iron-binding capacity). Transferrin is reutilised after delivering its iron.

In order to maintain iron balance, sufficient iron must be absorbed to replace that lost from the urinary and gastrointestinal tracts as shed cells and in sweat, together with any extra requirements.

Daily iron requirements are:

- adult male   1.0 mg
- child   1.5 mg
- pregnant female   1.5–3 mg
- menstruating female   2.0 mg

Thus, requirements vary with circumstances, extra iron being required for growth during childhood, for the fetus and placenta and expansion of maternal red cell mass during pregnancy and to compensate for menstrual loss of women of child-bearing age.

As a Western diet contains only 10–20 mg of iron per day and only a maximum of one-third of this can be absorbed, excess losses of iron of just a few milligrams will inevitably result in negative iron balance and eventual depletion of iron stores. One millilitre of blood contains 0.5 mg iron. Thus, loss of 10 ml of blood daily will inevitably exceed the capacity to absorb sufficient iron, even from a good diet. This explains the finding of some degree of iron depletion in 25% or more menstruating women.

Iron absorption takes place in the duodenum and upper jejunum. Haem iron is present in meat and readily absorbed, with little effect from other dietary components. Inorganic iron in vegetables and cereals is mostly trivalent and may be complexed to amino acids and organic acids, from which it must be released and reduced to the divalent state for absorption. HCl produced by the stomach and ascorbic acid in food favour its absorption. In contrast, phosphates and phytates form precipitates and prevent absorption.

Mechanisms controlling the rate of iron absorption are incompletely understood. Major influences are the total body iron stores and rate of erythropoiesis. Thus, if iron stores are replete a smaller proportion of available iron is absorbed; when erythropoiesis is active, extra iron is absorbed even though total stores may be high. This is a feature in thalassaemia and iron overload may ensue. At the cellular level some control is exerted at the brush border of the mucosal cell by an unknown mechanism. In addition, excess iron entering the cell is not absorbed but becomes bound to apoferritin and remains within the mucosal cell as ferritin, being subsequently shed with the cell into the gut lumen when the tip of the villus is reached.

Mechanisms of iron deficiency

In the UK, iron deficiency in the non-pregnant adult most frequently results from chronic blood loss, often from the gastrointestinal tract. As it is possible to lose several millilitres of blood daily into the gut lumen without marked change in appearance of the stool, such blood loss is frequently occult. Iron deficiency anaemia is thus commonly a presenting feature of lesions within the gastrointestinal tract (Fig. 23.13).

Causes of iron deficiency are:

- chronic blood loss (e.g. peptic ulcer; carcinoma of stomach, caecum, colon, rectum or urinary tract; haemorrhoids; menorrhagia)
- increased requirements (e.g. in childhood and pregnancy)

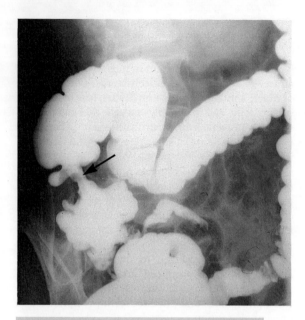

Fig. 23.13   Carcinoma of caecum causing iron deficiency anaemia

An annular carcinoma can be seen as a lesion which causes narrowing of the barium-filled bowel (arrowed) and from which blood loss has occurred.

- malabsorption (due to gastrectomy, coeliac disease, phytates in food)
- malnutrition.

More than one factor may operate. Thus a poor-quality vegetarian diet is highly likely to induce iron deficiency in a menstruating female. In a male or post-menopausal female, failure to ingest or absorb any iron would result in complete depletion of iron stores only after 3 or more years (1 mg/day). Malnutrition or malabsorption is thus rarely the sole cause of iron deficiency, although it may be an important contributory factor.

The microcytic hypochromic anaemia is a late stage in iron deficiency; it does not occur until iron stores are severely depleted. The microcyte results from an extra cell division, in addition to the normal four, during red cell production. Increasing cytoplasmic haemoglobin concentration normally acts as an inhibitor of normoblast division. The failure of haemoglobin synthesis which results from iron deficiency therefore allows extra mitoses to occur, with the production of small erythrocytes. The same mechanism is responsible for the microcytes in thalassaemia, another disorder of haemoglobin synthesis.

Blood and bone marrow changes
The typical blood picture is one of microcytic,

hypochromic red cells, with increased anisocytosis and poikilocytosis; elongated 'pencil' or 'cigar' cells are typically present (Figs 23.2 and 23.14). The proportion of polychromatic cells (or reticulocytes) is low for the degree of anaemia, indicating an inability of the bone marrow to respond due to lack of iron for haemoglobin synthesis. The platelet count is often raised, especially if chronic bleeding is present. The leukocytes are typically normal.

Occasionally, a mixture of microcytic, hypochromic erythrocytes and macrocytic cells is seen. This is termed a dimorphic picture and occurs in mixed deficiency of iron and folic acid or vitamin B_{12}. The MCV and MCH may be misleadingly normal.

A mixture of microcytic, hypochromic cells and normocytes is present in iron deficiency responding to iron replacement or after transfusion (Fig. 23.15). In the former circumstance, mildly increased polychromasia (and reticulocytosis) may be present.

Abnormalities are also present in the bone marrow. The nucleated red cell precursors are small in diameter and the cytoplasm is frequently ragged—micronormoblastic erythropoiesis. Staining for haemosiderin (Perls' stain) reveals its absence from macrophages and normoblasts.

Important biochemical changes in the blood are a fall in serum iron and increase in total iron-binding capacity (representing a compensatory increased transferrin concentration). Saturation of iron-binding capacity is thus reduced to 10% or less, from the normal 33%. The serum ferritin is markedly reduced, corresponding to severely depleted body iron content. This situation contrasts with the anaemia associated with chronic inflammatory disease or neoplasia ('anaemia of chronic disorders'; where serum iron may also be low but iron stores are normal; total iron-binding capacity is usually also reduced, in contrast to the situation in iron deficiency. Also, serum ferritin may be raised in the presence of inflammation and some malignancies, even in the presence of tissue iron depletion; these biochemical markers of iron deficiency are therefore unreliable in such situations.

Changes in other organs and tissues
In addition to the manifestations of chronic anaemia, a variety of epithelial changes may be present in chronic iron deficiency:

- angular cheilitis
- atrophic glossitis
- oesophageal web
- gastric achlorhydria
- brittle nails
- koilonychia.

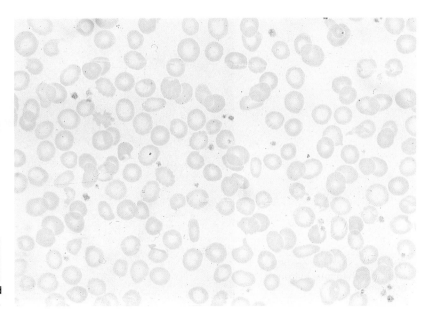

Fig. 23.14   The blood in iron deficiency: microcytic hypochromic anaemia

Marked poikilocytosis with elongated ('cigar' or 'pencil') red cells is typical.

The cause is unknown. Angular cheilitis (Fig. 23.16), painful fissuring of the mouth corners, is common but not specific: it occurs in dental malocclusion, most often due to poorly fitting dentures. Smooth tongue is also common (Fig. 23.16). Gastric achlorhydria appears to be an occasional result, as well as a contributory cause, of iron deficiency.

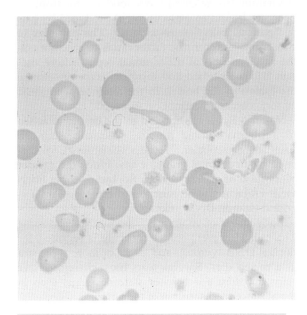

Fig. 23.15   A dimorphic blood film in iron deficiency anaemia responding to oral iron therapy

Microcytes and normocytes are present.

Dysphagia (difficulty in swallowing) due to the presence of a web or fold of mucosa in the post-cricoid region is an uncommon association of iron deficiency. The combination has been termed Paterson–Kelly or Plummer–Vinson syndrome and is important mainly because the mucosal abnormality is premalignant, carcinoma occasionally developing at the site.

Koilonychia (spoon-shaped nails) of chronic tissue iron depletion are typical but only rarely seen.

The pathological changes of iron deficiency are reversed by adequate replacement therapy.

Vitamin B$_{12}$ and folate deficiency

- ▶ Result in a macrocytic anaemia with marrow megaloblasts
- ▶ Nucleic acid synthesis for cell division is defective
- ▶ B$_{12}$ deficiency is most commonly due to Addisonian pernicious anaemia
- ▶ Folate deficiency is most commonly due to poor diet or increased requirements
- ▶ Pancytopenia is common
- ▶ Neurological involvement (subacute combined degeneration of the spinal cord, peripheral neuropathy) in B$_{12}$ deficiency only

Vitamin B$_{12}$ and folic acid are essential co-factors for blood cell production. Deficiency of either results in macrocytic anaemia with characteristic pathological appearances in the bone marrow described as *megaloblastic haemopoiesis*. Megaloblastic anaemias are

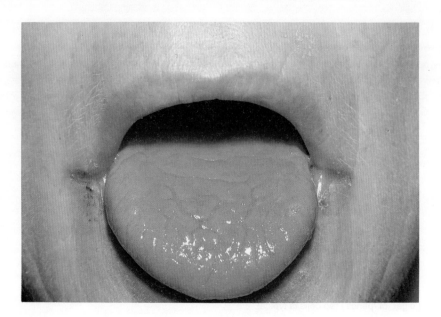

Fig. 23.16 Angular cheilitis and smooth tongue in iron deficiency

common, being second in incidence only to iron deficiency and the so-called anaemia of chronic disorders among production failure anaemias. Some other disorders may be associated with macrocytosis (Fig. 23.2) but megaloblastic haemopoiesis is most commonly due to deficiency of vitamin B_{12} or folate.

Vitamin B_{12} deficiency

Vitamin B_{12} metabolism

Vitamin B_{12} is necessary for DNA synthesis. Deoxyadenosylcobalamin is the main form of vitamin B_{12} in tissues and methylcobalamin is the main form in plasma. These forms differ only in the type of chemical group (deoxyadenosyl- or methyl-) attached to the cobalt atom which is located at the centre of a corrin ring, to which a nucleotide portion is attached. (The corrin ring is similar to the porphyrin ring of haem). The vitamin is known to be a coenzyme in the methylation of homocysteine to methionine and also in conversion of methylmalonyl CoA to succinyl CoA. During the former reaction, methylcobalamin loses its methyl group and this is replaced from methyltetrahydrofolic acid, the principal form of folic acid in plasma. The tetrahydrofolic acid is essential for the generation of deoxythymidine monophosphate, a precursor of DNA. Metabolism of vitamin B_{12} and of folate are thus closely related and essential for nucleic acid production.

Vitamin B_{12} is present in foods of animal origin. It cannot be synthesised by higher animals but is produced by micro-organisms. Animals obtain the vitamin from bacterially contaminated foods. Cereals, fruit and vegetable foods contain no vitamin B_{12} unless they have undergone bacterial contamination. Milk and eggs contain sufficient vitamin B_{12} for man's needs (1–2 μg daily) and thus dietary deficiency can occur only if a strictly vegetarian (vegan) diet is consumed. Nutritional vitamin B_{12} deficiency (in contrast to dietary folate deficiency) is thus rarely encountered.

Vitamin B_{12} released from food in the stomach becomes bound to a glycoprotein produced by gastric parietal cells—*intrinsic factor*. The complex of cobalamin and intrinsic factor binds to receptors on the mucosal cells of the terminal ileum, where vitamin B_{12} is absorbed and intrinsic factor remains in the lumen of the bowel. In the absence of intrinsic factor, cobalamin cannot be absorbed.

Vitamin B_{12} is transported to the tissues attached to a plasma-binding protein—transcobalamin II. Another transcobalamin (transcobalamin I), synthesised by neutrophil granulocytes, binds the greater proportion of plasma vitamin B_{12} but does not liberate it efficiently. The function of transcobalamin I-bound vitamin B_{12} is unknown.

Body stores of vitamin B_{12} amount only to some 2–3 mg. However, only 1 μg daily is required for normal DNA synthesis and 20 μg or more is present in a mixed diet. Several years must therefore have elapsed before a deficiency state develops, even in the absence of absorption of the vitamin.

Mechanisms of vitamin B_{12} deficiency

Causes of vitamin B_{12} deficiency are:

- pernicious anaemia due to lack of intrinsic factor

- gastrectomy resulting in lack of intrinsic factor
- congenital due to lack of intrinsic factor
- blind-loop syndrome due to bacterial overgrowth competing for vitamin B_{12}
- ileal resection resulting in lack of absorption site
- Crohn's disease resulting in lack of absorption site
- tropical sprue
- malnutrition (e.g. dietary deficiency of vitamin B_{12} in veganism).

Addisonian pernicious anaemia accounts for the majority of cases of megaloblastic anaemia due to deficiency of vitamin B_{12}. Most other cases occur after gastric resection, usually total gastrectomy. Blind loops of bowel have previously been the result of gastric surgery and this is now a rare cause of vitamin B_{12} deficiency, with improvements in the medical and surgical management of gastric and duodenal disease.

Addisonian pernicious anaemia is a common disorder in which chronic atrophic gastritis and failure of intrinsic factor synthesis lead to malabsorption of vitamin B_{12} and, after several years, the development of megaloblastic anaemia. Untreated, this was severe and eventually fatal; the condition was indeed 'pernicious' but is now easily corrected by injections of vitamin B_{12}.

It is likely that pernicious anaemia is due to an autoimmune process, resulting in atrophy of the chief and parietal glands of the stomach, with consequent failure of acid and intrinsic factor production. An auto-antibody to parietal cells is present in the serum in the majority of cases, but is not specific to this disorder. Antibodies to intrinsic factor are often present and virtually specific to pernicious anaemia. These latter antibodies are of two types: one inhibits binding of vitamin B_{12} to intrinsic factor, and the second inhibits ileal binding.

The disease is rather more common in females and rarely presents before 30 years of age, although an uncommon childhood form is occasionally seen. The patient may have another autoimmune disorder such as thyroid disease or vitiligo. There is an association with blue eyes and premature greying of hair.

Blood and bone marrow changes

In contrast to iron deficiency, the defect in DNA synthesis affects all cell lines, and pancytopenia is frequently present. The reduction in leukocyte and platelet count is usually modest; however, the MCV is high, and oval macrocytes are visible on the blood film (Figs 23.2 and 23.17). In megaloblastic anaemia, a reduction in the number of mitoses during red cell development, due to impaired DNA synthesis with normal RNA and protein synthesis, results in the production of macrocytes. The degree of polychromasia on the blood film is not appropriate to the severity of anaemia, because the marrow is unable to respond to the anaemia.

A proportion of neutrophil leukocytes have exaggerated lobulation of the nucleus and are often large (neutrophil hypersegmentation). Rarely, the blood picture is leukoerythroblastic.

The bone marrow is hypercellular and the stained

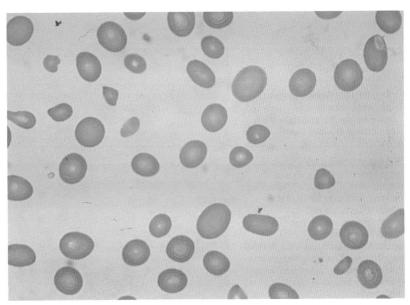

Fig. 23.17 A macrocytic blood film in megaloblastic anaemia

Oval macrocytes and neutrophil nuclear hypersegmentation (Fig. 23.6) are typical.

smears reveal the characteristic megaloblastic change of the developing red cells (Fig. 23.18): the red cells are larger than normal at each stage of development; nuclear chromatin has a very open appearance, with little condensation, and nuclear development lags behind that of the cytoplasm; thus well-haemoglobinised cells with an immature nucleus are a feature. Multilobed polymorphonuclear leukocytes may be seen, as well as particularly large metamyelocytes and band cells. Megakaryocytes may also appear abnormal.

Biochemical abnormalities detectable in the serum include unconjugated hyperbilirubinaemia and increased concentration of lactic dehydrogenase. These changes are due to increased cell breakdown within the marrow, ineffective erythropoiesis, and the breakdown of macrocytes, which may have a diminished survival time, in the reticulo-endothelial system. The serum concentration of vitamin B_{12} is reduced.

Changes in other organs and tissues

Lesions of the nervous system are a frequent feature of vitamin B_{12} deficiency from any cause. Myelin degeneration of the posterior and lateral columns of the spinal cord is typical and often associated with a peripheral neuropathy affecting sensory neurones. This *subacute combined degeneration of the cord* may be present despite normal haemoglobin levels, although the megaloblastic erythropoiesis is always detectable. Conversely, extreme megaloblastic change and profound anaemia may be present without evidence of damage to the nervous system from vitamin B_{12} deficiency. Optic atrophy and central changes resulting in psychiatric disease are less common accompaniments of deficiency of vitamin B_{12}. The cause may be failure of synthesis of S-adenosyl methionine necessary for myelin formation. Deficiency of folate is *not* associated with the neurological features of cobalamin deficiency.

Mucosal abnormalities may be present. Atrophic glossitis is a common feature. In pernicious anaemia there is atrophy of the glands of the gastric body affecting chief cells and parietal cells; there is replacement by mucus-secreting goblet cells. The intestinal epithelial cells are often larger than normal, reflecting megaloblastic change akin to that in the bone marrow.

In addition to the above, changes may be present in the heart and elsewhere due to the chronic hypoxia of severe anaemia. Cardiomyopathy is a particularly important feature; transfusion is tolerated badly due to volume overload and may result in fatal cardiac failure.

The clinical features of B_{12} deficiency are explained by the pathology, although it is unusual for all features to be present together:

- lethargy, breathlessness and cardiac failure due to megaloblastic erythropoiesis with anaemia
- bruising and mucosal haemorrhage due to thrombocytopenia in severe cases
- weight loss due to malabsorption resulting from mucosal changes
- sore mouth due to mucosal changes

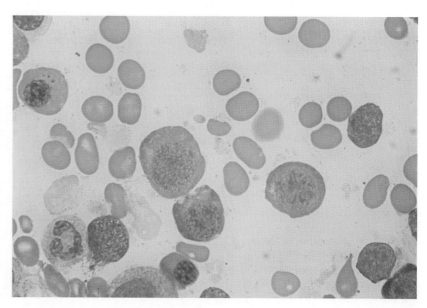

Fig. 23.18 Bone marrow appearances in megaloblastic anaemia from a vitamin B_{12} deficient patient

The megaloblasts are extremely large red cell precursors and the nucleus has a very open, speckled pattern. Although some of the megaloblasts are well haemoglobinised the nucleus is still present suggesting nuclear/cytoplasmic developmental asynchrony. The more mature non-nucleated red cells are also large and oval in shape — oval macrocytes.

- sensory impairment in the feet, altered gait, visual disturbance and dementia due to demyelination and axonal degeneration.

The haematological abnormalities are completely reversed by vitamin B_{12} replacement. However the neuropathology and associated clinical features may only be partly corrected. The gastric atrophy and achlorhydria are primary features in pernicious anaemia, not secondary to the deficiency state, and as such do not reverse on treatment of the deficiency. There is a life-long slightly increased risk of carcinoma of the stomach.

The haematological response is manifested by marked increase in the reticulocyte count from 2–3 days after administration of vitamin B_{12} and maximal at 7 days; the rise is proportional to the severity of the anaemia. White cell and platelet count recover within several days and haemoglobin increases at about 1 g/dl each week, with an accompanying fall in the MCV to normal values. Erythropoiesis is already normoblastic within 48 hours of starting replacement therapy.

Folic acid deficiency

Deficiency of folic (pteroylglutamic) acid, the parent compound of folates, causes a macrocytic anaemia with megaloblastic haemopoiesis identical to that resulting from deficiency of cobalamin.

Folate metabolism
Folates are required for DNA synthesis. Folate polyglutamates (pteroylglutamic acid with extra glutamic acid residues) are the main intracellular forms. However, all dietary folates are metabolised to the monoglutamate methyltetrahydrofolate during absorption from the gut and are transported in this form. Folates are necessary for single carbon unit transfer reactions in amino acid interconversions, in purine synthesis and, crucially, in the thymidylate synthetase reaction.

Man cannot synthesise folates *de novo*. Vegetables and fruits are especially rich in folates as polyglutamate conjugates, but most foods contain some folate. Absorption occurs in the proximal jejunum. Dietary polyglutamates are, however, very sensitive to heat, and cooking can markedly deplete foods of their available folate.

Body stores of folate, mainly in the liver, are modest, amounting to some 10 mg. As up to 200 μg is required daily, a deficiency state can develop within weeks, in contrast to deficiency of vitamin B_{12}. Furthermore, folate requirements are markedly increased in pregnancy and in some diseases associated with increased cell turnover, such as chronic haemolysis.

Mechanisms of folic acid deficiency
Causes of folate deficiency are:

- malnutrition (e.g. poor diet, overcooking of food, alcoholism)
- malabsorption (e.g. coeliac disease, tropical sprue, Crohn's disease)
- increased requirements (e.g. pregnancy and lactation, haemolytic anaemias, myelofibrosis, malignancy, extensive psoriasis or dermatitis)
- drugs (e.g. anti-convulsants).

Whereas malnutrition is an unusual cause of deficiency of vitamin B_{12}, it is the most common mechanism of folate deficiency. It is most prevalent in the elderly. Overcooking of food and lack of fresh foods contribute. Nutritional deficiency in combination with increased folate requirements is likely to lead to rapid depletion of folate stores.

During pregnancy, folate and iron deficiency may occur if no supplements are given. In contrast, vitamin B_{12} deficiency is almost unknown, as fertility is impaired in vitamin B_{12} deficiency and the commonest cause, pernicious anaemia, is a disease of late middle age and after.

In some disorders the folate deficiency is likely to be multifactorial, as in malignant disease, where lack of appetite with resultant malnutrition may aggravate folate deficiency secondary to increased utilisation of folate by the malignant tissues.

Phenytoin and phenobarbitone used long-term as anti-convulsants probably impair folate absorption and may interfere with folate metabolism.

Some anti-cancer drugs act as folic acid antagonists. Methotrexate inhibits the enzyme dihydrofolate reductase, thus depleting tetrahydrofolate. The antimalarial pyrimethamine acts similarly. Trimethoprim acts as a folate inhibitor in bacteria but is ineffective as an inhibitor in man.

Blood and bone marrow
In folic acid deficiency, blood and bone marrow changes are indistinguishable from those in vitamin B_{12} deficiency. The concentration of folic acid in serum and erythrocytes (red cell folate) is reduced.

Changes in other organs and tissues
Peripheral neuropathy and lesions of the central nervous system do not occur in folate deficiency. Also, the gastric changes typical of pernicious anaemia are not present, although megaloblastic changes in the

mucosal cells of the gastrointestinal tract may be apparent.

Oral folic acid supplements result in a complete reversal of the pathological features. Even in malabsorption states, sufficient folate can be absorbed from pharmacological doses. The time course of the response is identical to that in vitamin B_{12} deficiency.

Contrasting features of vitamin B_{12} and folate deficiency are listed in Table 23.5.

Megaloblastic anaemia is the result of deficiency of vitamin B_{12} or folate in the vast majority of instances. However, other causes include drugs and congenital defects. Prolonged anaesthesia with N_2O causes inactivation of vitamin B_{12} by oxidising the cobalt moiety and has resulted in pancytopenia with megaloblastic erythropoiesis. Cases of congenital deficiency of enzymes involved in cobalamin or folate metabolism or purine or pyrimidine synthesis are extremely rare. However, several anti-neoplastic drugs act by inhibition of synthesis of purine or pyrimidine (hydroxyurea, cytosine arabinoside) and subsequently can cause a reversible marrow pathology similar to megaloblastic haemopoiesis.

Dyserythropoietic anaemias

The term dyserythropoietic anaemias is used to describe some incompletely understood disorders where anaemia is at least in part due to production failure, but haematinic deficiency is not present and marrow cellularity is normal or increased.

Anaemia of chronic disorders

Anaemia of chronic disorders is one of the most common anaemias. It is found in association with a range of chronic inflammatory diseases, especially connective tissue disorders, chronic infections such as osteomyelitis or tuberculosis, and malignancies such as carcinoma and lymphoma. Anaemia is not severe; the haemoglobin concentration is 8 g/dl or greater and the red cells normocytic and normochromic. A degree of microcytosis and hypochromia may be present, but never to the degree seen in iron deficiency. Bone marrow iron is plentiful but no iron is seen in developing normoblasts. Serum iron and iron-binding capacity are typically both reduced, but serum ferritin concentration is normal or increased. If the underlying chronic disorder remits, the anaemia resolves.

The disorder may represent a failure of transfer of iron from reticulo-endothelial cells to normoblasts. A minor haemolytic component may also be present. This type of anaemia occurs in disorders frequently associated with other types of anaemia, resulting in a complicated picture, for example in rheumatoid arthritis, where iron and folate deficiency are common and hypersplenism and immune haemolytic anaemia may also be present.

Sideroblastic anaemias

The term sideroblastic anaemias describes a rather diverse and uncommon group of anaemias in which a defect of haem synthesis is present and a characteristic cell is seen in the bone marrow — the *ring sideroblast*. This cell is a nucleated red cell precursor which has granules of haemosiderin surrounding the nucleus, visible on staining with Perls' reagent. Causes include:

Table 23.5 Comparison of features of vitamin B_{12} and folic acid deficiency states

Feature	Cobalamin (vitamin B_{12}) deficiency	Folate deficiency
Nutritional deficiency	Uncommon	Common
Onset	Slow (years)	More rapid (weeks)
Revealed by increased demands	Never	Frequently
Absorption	In terminal ileum as a complex with intrinsic factor. Gastric and terminal ileal disease (e.g. autoimmune gastritis, Crohn's disease) may cause deficiency.	In jejunum. Jejunal disease (e.g. coeliac disease) may cause deficiency.
Drug-related	Never	May be due to anti-convulsant therapy. Anti-metabolites induce a similar deficiency.
Neurological lesions	Frequent	None

- primary acquired sideroblastic anaemia in the middle-aged or elderly due to somatic mutation/clonal abnormality of erythroid cells
- secondary in patients with a bone marrow malignancy (e.g. myeloma, myeloid leukaemia, etc.)
- due to drugs and toxins (e.g. vitamin B_6 antagonism by isoniazid; lead poisoning which inhibits synthesis of haem; alcoholism)
- hereditary due to enzyme defect in haem synthesis.

Although deficiency of vitamin B_6 (pyridoxine) causes a similar anaemia in animals, it is never the cause in man. However, vitamin B_6 antagonism can result from antituberculous therapy, and other sideroblastic anaemias occasionally respond partially to pharmacological doses of vitamin B_6.

Primary acquired sideroblastic anaemia can also be classified among the 'refractory' anaemias or 'pre-leukaemic' states.

Refractory anaemias

Refractory anaemias, which in some cases are clearly 'pre-leukaemic' (acute myeloid leukaemia supervening), are also known as the *myelodysplastic syndromes*. The common feature is the presence of qualitative (morphological) and quantitative abnormalities in the erythroid series, often accompanied by such abnormalities in the myeloid and megakaryocyte series. They are due to the development of a clone of abnormal marrow cell precursors which give rise to defective cells.

The blood changes are therefore of anaemia, usually normocytic or macrocytic, with leukopenia and thrombocytopenia, often with abnormal forms such as hypogranular neutrophils (Fig. 23.6).

The bone marrow is usually cellular and morphological abnormalities may be present, including changes similar to those in megaloblastic marrow (but unresponsive or 'refractory' to vitamin B_{12} or folate), ring sideroblasts, abnormalities of developing white cells (hypogranularity) and megakaryocytes. Marrow chromosomes may be abnormal, consistent with the malignant and clonal nature of these disorders. The refractory anaemias can be subclassified depending on the presence of ring sideroblasts and the proportion of leukaemic-type 'blast cells' in the bone marrow.

The refractory anaemias are commonest in the middle-aged and elderly. The clinical features are, predictably, those of anaemia together with infections and mucosal haemorrhage. Splenic enlargement is unusual. Progression to a frank leukaemia, usually myeloid, is common. Treatment is largely supportive, by blood transfusion and treatment of infection. Survival is variable, but may be for years.

Hypoplastic anaemia

Hypoplastic (aplastic) anaemia is pancytopenia (anaemia, neutropenia and thrombocytopenia) resulting from bone marrow hypoplasia of variable severity. Hypoplastic anaemia probably results from failure or suppression of pluripotent stem cells. Very occasionally, the defect appears to affect cells committed to the erythroid series only, when 'pure red cell aplasia' results.

In the majority of cases, the cause is unknown. However it is occasionally congenital or due to poisoning or to iatrogenic causes. Thus, hypoplastic anaemia may be:

- idiopathic
- due to chemical agents (e.g. benzene, cytotoxic drugs, chloramphenicol)
- due to ionising radiation
- due to infection such as hepatitis viruses and parvovirus
- congenital.

Most cases caused by anti-neoplastic drugs are reversible. Aplasia is also often a feature of the rare disorder paroxysmal nocturnal haemoglobinuria (PNH). PNH (p. 718) is thought to be a clonal disorder of bone marrow. The development of a clone with poor capacity for differentiation may explain the aplasia which occasionally develops in this disorder.

In idiopathic forms of hypoplastic anaemia there is evidence that T-lymphocytes are involved in the suppression of stem cell development. Immunosuppressive therapy is occasionally successful. Although a defect of marrow micro-environment has been postulated, the high success rate of marrow transplantation, in which healthy human donor marrow is infused intravenously into the recipient with aplastic anaemia, suggests that this is not commonly the underlying cause.

The reason for an idiosyncratic response to some drugs is unknown. Chloramphenicol, an antibiotic, and gold, used in treatment of rheumatoid arthritis, are especially likely to produce marrow aplasia, often irreversible. Infection with parvovirus causes a transient suppression of erythropoiesis; this suppression is brief and clinically insignificant in otherwise healthy subjects. However, where red cell survival is markedly shortened, as in sickle cell disease, such infection may cause a catastrophic fall in haemoglobin. 'Aplastic' anaemia is a rare late complication of viral hepatitis.

There is anaemia (normocytic or slightly macrocytic), leukopenia (including lymphopenia in severe cases) and thrombocytopenia. There is reduced polychromasia, especially in relation to the degree of anaemia, and the reticulocyte count is very low. Morphologically abnormal cells are not a feature.

Marrow aspiration often fails. Trephine biopsy reveals increased fat spaces and little residual marrow activity, although a few small clusters of haemopoietic cells occasionally remain.

Clinically, anaemia, infections and bleeding due to thrombocytopenia occur. Splenomegaly and lymphadenopathy are absent. Without successful treatment of the aplasia, severe forms are fatal. Spontaneous remission occasionally occurs. Bone marrow transplantation can be curative.

Anaemia due to bone marrow infiltration

Not infrequently, carcinoma and lymphoma involve the bones and bone marrow (Fig. 23.19). A leuko-erythroblastic blood picture may result. In carcinomatosis, numerous other factors are likely to be contributory to the anaemia, such as bleeding from carcinoma of the gastrointestinal tract, folate deficiency and chemotherapy.

The marrow is replaced by reticulin and collagen in myelofibrosis. Fibrosis of the marrow is also a feature of other myeloproliferative disorders and some other malignant marrow infiltrates.

Other causes of marrow infiltration are very uncommon, e.g. Gaucher's disease, a metabolic defect where glucocerebroside accumulates in the reticulo-endothelial cells of many organs (Ch. 7).

ANAEMIAS DUE TO INCREASED CELL LOSS, LYSIS OR POOLING

The haemolytic states are the main members of the group of anaemias due to increased cell loss, lysis or pooling. However, anaemia due to acute blood loss and the pancytopenia of hypersplenism are also conveniently included.

A fall in haemoglobin of much greater than 1 g/dl per week must indicate the presence of haemorrhage or haemolysis, as complete cessation of erythropoiesis would result in a rate of fall of no more than 1 g/dl per week. An exception is the rapid fall in haematocrit due to infusion of cell-free fluids in a dehydrated subject.

Acute blood loss anaemia

Chronic haemorrhage, usually gastrointestinal, causes anaemia by depletion of iron stores. Acute blood loss may result initially in a state of cardiovascular collapse, as described in an earlier section. Following adjustment to the plasma volume over a

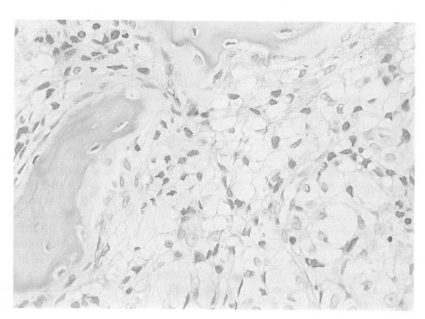

Fig. 23.19 Carcinoma cells infiltrating bone marrow

Sheets of non-haemopoietic carcinoma cells replace normal bone marrow.

period up to 48 hours, anaemia will be apparent. The blood picture is normocytic and normochromic, and an increased number of polychromatic erythrocytes and reticulocytes in the days following a brisk haemorrhage reflects increased haemopoiesis. Transient leukocytosis and thrombocytosis commonly occur.

Haemolytic anaemias

> ▶ Characterised by a reduction in red cell life-span
> ▶ Can be classified into hereditary red cell disorders and acquired haemolytic states due to a defect outwith the red cell
> ▶ Important hereditary haemolytic disorders include sickle cell disease, thalassaemias and spherocytosis
> ▶ Important acquired haemolytic disorders include autoimmune haemolytic anaemias, malaria and microangiopathic haemolytic anaemias
> ▶ Normocytic anaemia with increased reticulocytes and hyperbilirubinaemia is typical
> ▶ Splenomegaly is commonly present

The haemolytic anaemias are those in which a major feature is a reduction in red cell life-span. In severe haemolysis red cell survival may be reduced from the normal 120 days to less than 10 days. Although erythropoiesis will increase, anaemia is inevitable under such circumstances. Even in the presence of normal marrow function and adequate supplies of haematinics, the maximum potential increase in red cell production is some 6 times the normal rate. In the presence of a defect of red cell production, as in folate deficiency or thalassaemia major, the severity of the anaemia is increased in relation to the degree of shortening of red cell survival.

Classification and incidence

Haemolytic anaemias can be divided usefully into those due to a defect of the red cell itself and those due to an abnormality outside the red cell (Table 23.4). Almost all the former are hereditary; an exception is the uncommon acquired disease paroxysmal nocturnal haemoglobinuria (PNH). Those due to mechanisms 'outside' the red cell are acquired disorders.

The relative incidence of haemolytic anaemias is highly variable geographically. In the United Kingdom the acquired haemolytic states, especially autoimmune haemolytic anaemias, are relatively common disorders. Worldwide, however, thalassaemia, sickle cell disease and malaria are of major importance.

Consequences of haemolysis

In addition to the particular pathological and clinical features of the various haemolytic diseases, certain consequences of the haemolytic process and the response to it are common to all types of haemolytic disorder. These consequences are:

- raised serum bilirubin (unconjugated) resulting in the formation of pigment gallstones
- raised urine urobilinogen
- raised faecal stercobilinogen
- absent serum haptoglobin, which binds haemoglobin; the complex is removed by the liver
- splenomegaly
- reticulocytosis in peripheral blood
- erythroid hyperplasia in bone marrow, causing bone deformity in children in extreme cases, especially thalassaemia.

Red cell destruction occurs predominantly in the reticuloendothelial tissues of the spleen and liver. Splenomegaly is therefore common in chronic haemolytic anaemia and hepatomegaly may also be present. Within the spleen there is congestion within the cords and deposition of haemosiderin.

Less commonly, the red cells are destroyed within the circulation. Examples are haemolysis following major blood group mismatch, and that due to the presence of a foreign surface such as a (malfunctioning) artificial heart valve, malaria and glucose-6-phosphate dehydrogenase deficiency. Particular features of intravascular haemolysis are the presence of free haemoglobin in plasma and urine (haemoglobinaemia, haemoglobinuria), of methaemalbumin in plasma (oxidised haem bound to albumin) and of haemosiderin in urine (in shed renal tubular cells which have reabsorbed haemoglobin from the tubular contents; the haem is incorporated into haemosiderin).

Haemolytic anaemia due to red cell defects

The major components of the erythrocyte are haemoglobin, enzymes involved in protection of haemoglobin from oxidant stress, and the plasma membrane. Abnormalities of each of these components can be a cause of chronic haemolytic anaemia.

Defects of the red cell membrane

Hereditary spherocytosis and *hereditary elliptocytosis* include several disorders in which diminished red cell survival is due to a defect in the structural proteins of the erythrocyte membrane. Involvement of the major erythrocyte skeletal protein *spectrin* appears to be most common, although the precise defect is not known. Inheritance is dominant. Spherocytosis is the most common cause of hereditary haemolytic anaemia among Caucasians in the UK.

The erythrocytes are of reduced deformability, which causes difficulties when traversing the splenic microcirculation. The cells are retained for long periods in the splenic cords. They become metabolically stressed by glucose lack and acidosis, and are eventually prematurely phagocytosed. The abnormal red cells in these disorders are more sensitive than normal to lysis under osmotic stress. This increased osmotic fragility is of diagnostic value.

Anaemia is usual but varies in severity between affected kindreds. The blood film has many spherocytes (Fig. 23.20); they appear smaller than normocytes and more dense, with loss of the central pallor. Polychromatic cells are increased. General features of chronic haemolysis are also present. Haemolysis tends to be less severe in elliptocytosis. (Spherocytes are not confined to hereditary spherocytosis but are also present in the blood film in immune haemolytic anaemia.)

The clinical features are variable and are those of chronic extravascular haemolysis. Pigment gallstones commonly develop. The disorder can be subclinical. Occasionally, transient red cell aplasia

secondary to parvovirus infection can develop, when several family members may be affected by aplasia simultaneously.

Removal of the spleen results in resolution of the anaemia, confirming the role of the spleen in the haemolytic process.

Defects of red cell enzymes

Defects of red cell enzymes render the erythrocyte susceptible to damage by oxidant compounds. The generation of reduced glutathione by the metabolic activity of the red cell normally inactivates oxidants. Reduced glutathione is generated by the hexose monophosphate shunt of the Embden–Meyerhof glycolytic pathway, which is the source of: energy, as ATP, necessary for maintenance of red cell shape, volume and flexibility; NADH for reduction of oxidised haemoglobin; and 2,3-diphosphoglycerate (2,3-DPG) for the regulation of the oxygen affinity of haemoglobin.

Deficiency of several of the enzymes involved in these reactions has been identified. Only two are of pathological and major clinical significance: glucose-6-phosphate dehydrogenase deficiency and pyruvate kinase deficiency.

Glucose-6-phosphate dehydrogenase deficiency
Inherited G6PD deficiency is an uncommon cause of anaemia in the UK but is amongst the most common genetic disorders worldwide. It is a sex-linked disorder: female heterozygotes are usually asymptomatic

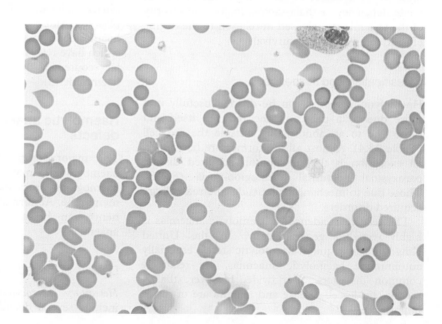

Fig. 23.20 Hereditary spherocytosis

Densely staining spherocytic erythrocytes predominate.

and may have some protection from falciparum malaria; this probably explains the high prevalence of the disorder in many parts of the world, the commoner varieties existing as balanced polymorphisms.

The common isoenzymes are traditionally designated 'Type B', the most common, 'Type A' and 'Type A-minus', found among American blacks (30% and 11% respectively). Type A differs from Type B by a single amino acid substitution and is functionally normal. Type A-minus has an additional amino acid substitution resulting in decreased red cell enzyme activity and disease. Typically there is a tendency to the development of an acute haemolytic episode associated with the ingestion of an oxidant drug (for example some anti-malarials and antibiotics) and with other stresses such as surgery or infection. Clinically, a self-limiting episode of anaemia and jaundice develops.

A further variant is found in Mediterranean populations and is associated with the acute haemolytic tendency known as *favism*, where ingestion of the fava (broad) bean results in acute haemolysis. The responsible oxidant compound has not yet been identified. Again, oxidant drugs, surgical stress and infections may also lead to haemolysis.

Many other less common genetic variants have been recognised. Some result in a more chronic haemolytic state or neonatal jaundice.

The blood picture during haemolytic crisis includes increased poikilocytosis with contracted red cells, 'bite' cells and 'blister' cells (poikilocytes with bite-shaped defects or surface blebs). Oxidised, denatured haemoglobin is seen as red-cell inclusions (Heinz bodies) attached to the cell membrane, when blood is stained supravitally as in the reticulocyte preparation. Haemolysis is generally self-limiting because of the rapid outpouring of new red cells, with higher G6PD content, from the marrow in response to the falling haemoglobin. The blood picture is normal between haemolytic episodes.

Treatment consists essentially of avoidance of known precipitating factors for haemolysis. Health is generally good between haemolytic episodes.

Pyruvate kinase deficiency
Pyruvate kinase (PK) deficiency results in congenital chronic haemolytic anaemia. The blood film has increased poikilocytosis. The chronic anaemia is associated with increased erythrocyte 2,3-DPG because of the site of the metabolic block. This situation results in reduced oxygen affinity of haemoglobin and increased oxygen delivery to the tissues; the anaemia is thus less symptomatic than would be expected from its severity. No specific treatment is available.

Haemoglobinopathies — abnormal haemoglobins

Abnormal haemoglobins are caused by a single point mutation in the genetic code resulting in an amino acid substitution in the α or β globin chain of haemoglobin A. Variant haemoglobins can be readily identified by their electrophoretic mobility (Fig. 23.21). Several hundred variant haemoglobins have been identified but few are clinically significant and almost all of those involve β chain substitutions. Depending on the site of the substitution four main types of functional defect result:

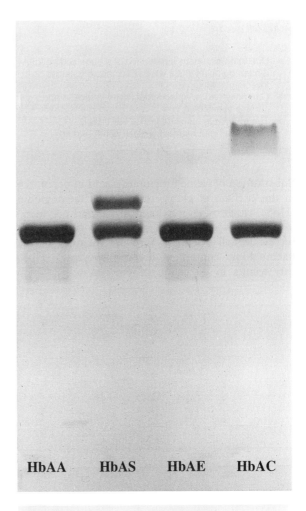

HbAA   HbAS   HbAE   HbAC

Fig. 23.21   An example of haemoglobin electrophoresis: acid haemoglobin electrophoresis (pH 6.0)

This procedure clearly separates haemoglobins S and C from A. The carrier for haemoglobin E cannot be distinguished from AA but would be by performing the procedure at alkaline pH.

- a haemoglobin which becomes crystalline at low oxygen tension, e.g. HbS, causing haemolysis and microvascular occlusion
- an unstable haemoglobin causing chronic haemolysis with Heinz bodies (red-cell inclusions composed of denatured haemoglobin)
- a haemoglobin of increased oxygen affinity causing polycythaemia
- a haemoglobin which tends to the oxidised state (methaemoglobin) causing cyanosis.

The first defect is the most common. HbS is very common worldwide as are three related haemoglobins: C, D and E.

Sickle cell disease

> ▶ Due to homozygous inheritance of a gene coding for a haemoglobin variant which becomes crystalline at low oxygen tensions
> ▶ Characterised by episodes of tissue infarction and chronic haemolysis
> ▶ The heterozygous state (sickle cell trait) is associated with normal full blood count and no symptoms

Substitution of valine for glutamic acid in position 6 in the β chain of globin results in a haemoglobin (HbS) which undergoes aggregation and polymerisation at low oxygen tensions. In the homozygote for sickle cell disease, where the majority of the haemoglobin content of the erythrocytes is HbS, this results in distortion of the red cells, which acquire a sickle shape. The consequence of this distortion and the predominant features of sickle cell disease are a chronic haemolytic anaemia and microvascular occlusion, causing ischaemic tissue damage. The results of the latter dominate the clinical picture.

The gene for HbS is common in the West and Central African populations, the Mediterranean, Middle East and some parts of the Indian subcontinent. Carriage of the gene may confer some protection against falciparum malaria. The gene is carried by 8% of black Americans and 30% of black Africans. The heterozygous state, or *sickle cell trait*, results in less than 40% HbS, the remainder being mostly normal HbA; the carrier is clinically and haematologically essentially normal, sickling occurring very uncommonly and only under conditions of severe hypoxia. Hypoxic sickling in such patients is an avoidable risk of general anaesthesia. Haematuria may, however, be a feature. Two major bands are present on electrophoresis of haemoglobin: one corresponding to HbS and one to HbA.

In the homozygote the haemoglobin concentration is low (7–9 g/dl). Sickle cells and target cells are present on the blood film, as are features of hyposplenism in the adult (Fig. 23.22). (Splenomegaly due to chronic haemolysis is present during childhood but the spleen shrinks progressively due to microvascular occlusion and infarction.) The bone marrow is hyperplastic with erythroid hyperplasia. Extramedullary erythropoiesis in the liver and, occasionally, other sites is a minor feature. Pathological

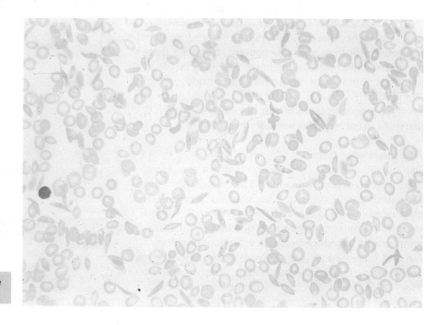

Fig. 23.22   Sickle cell disease (homozygous)

changes in other organs result from the effects of local ischaemia (Fig. 23.23). Haemoglobin electrophoresis reveals a characteristic single band of HbS.

Clinical features. These are predictable from the above. Sickle 'crises' of various clinical types appear after the age of 1–2 years, when HbF levels have fallen and the proportion of HbS has increased. Vascular occlusion with resultant ischaemia causes severe pain, often in the long bones, abdomen or chest. Acute sequestration of sickle cells in the liver or (in children) spleen may cause pain and acute exacerbation of anaemia. Between episodes of crisis, health may be good. Cholecystitis, due to the presence of pigment stones, is a frequent occurrence. As in pyruvate kinase deficiency, oxygen affinity of the haemoglobin is low and symptoms of anaemia mild, due to the relatively enhanced O_2 delivery to tissues. Premature death, often from respiratory complications, may occur in early middle age, but longer survival is a feature in some populations.

Treatment. This is essentially conservative, with avoidance of factors known to precipitate crises, especially hypoxia, and provision of warmth and rehydration during crises. Pregnancy may be particularly hazardous.

Haemoglobin C, D and E. These are also the result of point mutations in the β chain gene. In the homozygous state they produce mild chronic haemolysis with splenomegaly but without the occlusive manifestations of sickle cell disease. They are commonly found in West Africa, India and South-East Asia respectively. Due to their geographical distribution, the gene for HbC is often inherited with that for HbS. HbS-C disease behaves as a mild sickle disease with a particular tendency to venous thrombosis.

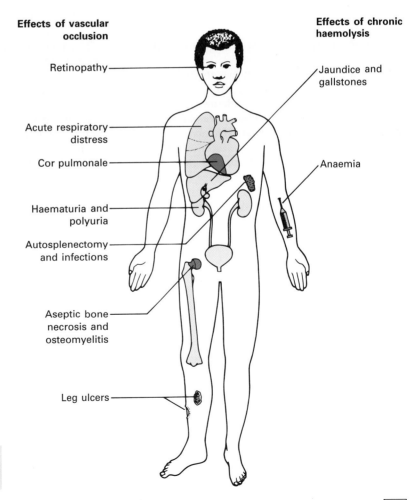

Effects of vascular occlusion

Retinopathy

Acute respiratory distress

Cor pulmonale

Haematuria and polyuria

Autosplenectomy and infections

Aseptic bone necrosis and osteomyelitis

Leg ulcers

Effects of chronic haemolysis

Jaundice and gallstones

Anaemia

Fig. 23.23   The pathogenesis and clinical consequences of sickle cell disease

Thalassaemias

> ▶ Due to abnormalities of (α or β) globin chain synthesis
> ▶ Characterised by a microcytic, hypochromic blood picture
> ▶ β-Thalassaemia major results in severe anaemia from infancy, splenomegaly, marrow expansion with bony deformities and premature death
> ▶ β-Thalassaemia minor is clinically mild
> ▶ α-Thalassaemias include disorders resulting in intra-uterine death from severe anaemia and heart failure and those producing clinically insignificant disease

In contrast to the abnormal haemoglobin states described above, where a structurally abnormal globin is synthesised but at a normal rate, in thalassaemia the globin chains are of normal composition, but the rate at which the globin chain (α or β) is synthesised is reduced. In α-thalassaemia the α globin chain synthesis is so affected; in β-thalassaemia the β chain is affected. Accumulation of an excess of the unaffected globin chains results in damage to the developing and mature erythrocytes.

Again, in contrast to 'variant haemoglobin' conditions (such as sickle cell disease) where point mutations affecting coding regions underlie the disorders, in thalassaemias the genetic lesions are of a regulatory nature, affecting the normal *expression* of the globin structural genes.

Each chromosome 16 has a pair of α globin genes, thus each cell has four genes coding for α globin, all of them functional. The genes for β globin, as well as those for γ and δ are located in close linkage on chromosome 11.

In the α-thalassaemia syndromes there is deletion of all four genes or of three of the four. In α-thalassaemia trait, there is deletion of two or only one gene (Table 23.6).

More than 40 genetic defects responsible for β-thalassaemia have now been described. The type of defect tends to vary between racial groups. Some defects result in an absence of chain synthesis (β^0); in others, chain synthesis is severely restricted but present (β^+).

α-Thalassaemia. This is an uncommon cause of anaemia in the UK. Haemoglobin H disease (Table 23.6) is seen mainly in Asian populations. HbH is identifiable on electrophoresis in the 3-gene deletion disorder. Electrophoresis is normal in α-thalassaemia trait and the conditions can be confirmed only by direct measurement of rate of synthesis of α and β chains.

β-Thalassaemia major (Mediterranean or Cooley's anaemia). This is a severe disorder due to the inheritance of two genes for β-thalassaemia —β^+/β^+, β^0/β^0 or occasionally β^+/β^0. The β-thalassaemia genes are most frequent in Mediterranean countries and parts of Africa and South-East Asia.

The blood picture is that of a severe microcytic, hypochromic anaemia (haemoglobin concentration 3–6 g/dl) developing from 3 to 6 months of age (when β-chain production should have completely taken over from that of the γ chains).

In response to the defective haemoglobin synthesis and haemolysis the red bone marrow is dramatically expanded with gross erythroid hyperplasia. As a result cortical bone is thinned and new bone deposits on the outer aspect, especially in the skull vault, maxilla and frontal facial bones (Fig. 23.24). Cortical thinning and fractures may develop in the long bones, vertebrae and ribs. The spleen is grossly enlarged, with expansion of the reticulo-endothelial

Table 23.6	The α-thalassaemia disorders	
Number of globin genes deleted	Syndrome	Clinicopathological features
4	**Hydrops fetalis**	Death in utero. Congestive cardiac failure secondary to an extreme degree of anaemia
3	**Haemoglobin H disease**	Free β chains form tetramers: HbH (Hb Bart's — γ_4 in fetal life). Moderate microcytic, hypochromic anaemia. HbH inclusions visible in erythrocytes on supravital staining. Splenomegaly
2	*α*-Thalassaemia trait	Normal haemoglobin concentration. Low MCV and MCH. Occasional HbH inclusion visible. A subclinical disorder, resembling β-thalassaemia minor
1	**Thalassaemia trait**	Normal haematology or slightly reduced MCV

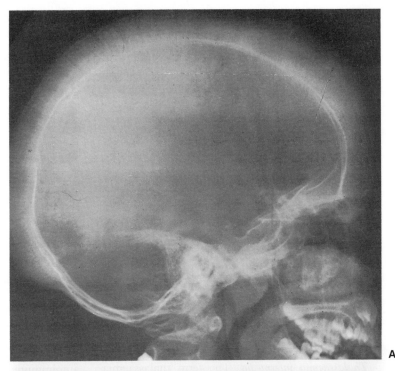

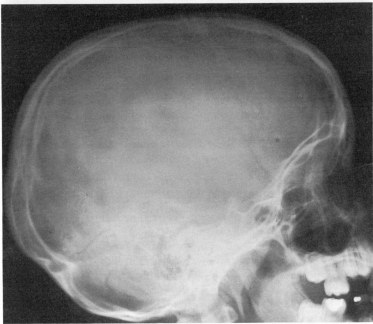

Fig. 23.24 X-ray appearances of the skull in β-thalassaemia major

A. Characteristic 'hair-on-end' appearances of the skull vault due to marrow expansion.
B. Normal subject.

elements and extramedullary erythropoiesis. The liver is similarly affected. Iron overload is apparent and often gross.

Haemoglobin electrophoresis reveals absent or markedly reduced haemoglobin A. Small (normal) amounts of haemoglobin A_2 are present and the remainder of the haemoglobin is F.

Predictably, the clinical features are those of

severe anaemia, including growth retardation, and haemosiderosis. The latter may result in failure of sexual development due to iron deposition in endocrine organs and gonads, as well as heart failure. Facial deformities result from the bone changes. Death often occurs, even with transfusion support, in childhood or early adult life. The situation may be improved by iron chelation therapy to reduce tissue iron. Bone marrow transplantation has been curative.

β-Thalassaemia minor. This is mild and most commonly subclinical. The characteristic pathology is gross microcytic and hypochromic change on the blood film with normal or slightly raised red cell count and normal haemoglobin concentration. Mild anaemia may be present during pregnancy, when the condition is often first diagnosed. The blood picture is very similar to that of iron deficiency but the MCV and MCH are disproportionately low for the level of haemoglobin. Iron stores are normal or high. Bone changes and hepatosplenomegaly are absent. Haemoglobin electrophoresis reveals raised haemoglobin A_2 concentration (>2.5%).

Thalassaemia intermedia. The term thalassaemia intermedia describes disease of intermediate severity, often not requiring transfusion and compatible with prolonged survival. Hepatosplenomegaly and iron overload are present. It is genetically heterogeneous, some cases being severely affected heterozygotes, others homozygotes with an unusually mild β-chain deficiency.

Occasional patients are doubly heterozygous for β-thalassaemia and HbS. These patients may have either a mild variant of sickle cell disease or show the full clinical picture.

Paroxysmal nocturnal haemoglobinuria

Paroxysmal nocturnal haemoglobinuria is an acquired disorder in which chronic haemolysis is due to a clonal abnormality of erythrocytes which renders them abnormally sensitive to complement lysis. It is rare and often chronic. Aplastic anaemia, chronic haemolytic anaemia and venous thrombosis in the portal, hepatic or cerebral veins are major features. Haemoglobinuria occurring at night or in early morning is not a common feature, despite the name (nocturnal) of the disorder.

The presence of haemosiderinuria and tendency of erythrocytes to lyse at low pH (acid lysis or Ham test) are useful diagnostically. Treatment is supportive and death is often ultimately due to sepsis or thrombosis.

Haemolytic anaemia due to a defect outside the red cell

Haemolytic anaemias due to a defect outside the red cell are all acquired disorders.

Immune haemolytic anaemias

> ► Red cell damage is immune-mediated
> ► Direct antiglobulin (Coombs') test is positive, indicating erythrocyte sensitisation with immunoglobulin or complement
> ► In the autoimmune types an auto-antibody causes haemolysis and the clinical features depend on the thermal characteristics of the antibody ('warm' or 'cold' reacting); the disorder may be idiopathic or symptomatic of underlying disease
> ► In mismatched blood transfusion and in haemolytic disease of the newborn an allo-antibody causes haemolysis

Immune haemolytic anaemias are due to red cell damage by an antibody. The phenomenon may be *autoimmune,* as in idiopathic and drug-induced autoimmune haemolytic anaemias and cold antibody disorders, or *alloimmune* (where the antibody forms to an antigen foreign to that individual) as in haemolysis due to mismatched blood transfusion and that in haemolytic disease of the newborn (Table 23.7). In all cases the presence of antibody or complement on the red cell surface is confirmed by the direct antiglobulin (or Coombs') test which uses antibodies to human immunoglobulin or complement raised in an animal to cause in vitro agglutination of red cells sensitised with antibody or complement in vivo (Ch. 9).

In some (the more common) instances of autoimmune haemolysis the auto-antibody is IgG and most reactive at 37°C — 'warm antibody' autoimmune disorders. In 'cold antibody' autoimmune disorders an IgM antibody is active at 4°C, becoming less active at higher temperatures, but is still able to bind complement and agglutinate red cells at the temperature (c. 30°C) of the peripheral tissues (hands, feet, nose, ears).

Antibody-coated cells bind to macrophages of the reticulo-endothelial system via Fc receptors. Partial phagocytosis results and the erythrocyte loses some membrane. In order to maintain cellular integrity after this reduction of surface area, a sphere is formed. Such spherical red cells are less deformable than normal; they eventually become trapped in the spleen and are removed by phagocytosis.

Table 23.7   The immune haemolytic anaemias

Autoimmune		Alloimmune
'Warm antibody'	'Cold antibody'	
Idiopathic Autoimmune haemolytic anaemia	**Idiopathic** Chronic haemagglutinin disease	Mismatched blood transfusion
Secondary Chronic lymphatic leukaemia Lymphoma Systemic lupus erythematosus and other autoimmune disorders	**Secondary** Infectious mononucleosis Mycoplasma pneumonia Lymphoma Carcinoma	Haemolytic disease of the newborn
Drug-related e.g. methyl dopa		

'Warm antibody' immune haemolytic anaemia

In 'warm antibody' immune haemolytic anaemia, the auto-antibody is usually IgG and may or may not bind complement. Red cell destruction occurs in the cells of the reticulo-endothelial system, especially the spleen. Most cases are idiopathic, occurring in adult life; there may be a family history of autoimmune disease. In about one-third of instances the process is initiated by a drug or it occurs in association with some other disease, particularly a lymphoproliferative disorder, or collagen vascular disease such as systemic lupus erythematosus or rheumatoid arthritis (Ch. 25).

Drugs can cause the disorder by one of three mechanisms (Fig. 23.25). Withdrawal of the drug results in resolution of the disorder.

The blood picture in 'warm antibody' haemolysis is that of a chronic anaemia with microspherocytes and increased polychromasia (and reticulocytosis). The degree of anaemia is very variable within and between cases but may be extremely severe. Erythroid hyperplasia is marked in the bone marrow; megaloblastic erythropoiesis may supervene as in all haemolytic anaemias, due to increased folate requirements. The spleen is moderately enlarged and congested. Features of an underlying disorder, such as lymphoma, may also be present.

Clinical features and treatment. The clinical features are those of haemolytic anaemia — pallor, jaundice and splenomegaly. In those instances where a drug cannot be implicated, treatment by immunosuppression or splenectomy may be successful.

'Cold antibody' immune haemolytic anaemias

In 'cold antibody' immune haemolytic anaemias, the IgM antibody attaches to red cells in the peripheral circulation and complement is bound. On re-entering the central circulation the IgM antibody may become detached, but complement activation leads to red cell destruction in the reticulo-endothelial system. The main consequences of this sequence of events are agglutination of erythrocytes in cooler areas, which causes sluggish flow and reduced oxygen saturation, and chronic haemolysis. Severity relates particularly to the thermal amplitude of the antibody, that is its activity at temperatures up to 30°C.

The pathological features are those of chronic haemolysis with a tendency to marked agglutination of red cells on the blood film. If the film is prepared at 37°C the agglutination is no longer present. The reticulocyte count is increased.

Clinical features and treatment. The clinical features are of anaemia and of blueness and coldness of the fingers, toes, nose and ears, occasionally progressing to ischaemia and ulceration. Many cases occur spontaneously in older adults. The disorder is chronic and often mild. It occurs as an unusual complication of lymphoma, and also, rarely and transiently, in infectious mononucleosis or mycoplasma pneumonia.

The degree of haemolysis can be reduced by maintenance of a warm environment. Splenectomy is rarely successful, probably because complement-sensitised cells tend to be destroyed at other sites, especially the liver.

Haemolytic disease of the newborn

Haemolytic disease of the newborn, a previously common disorder, is due to passage across the placenta of maternal IgG antibodies which are reactive against, and cause destruction of, the fetal red cells.

A

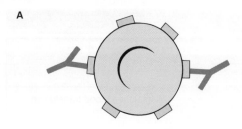

☐ Drug attached to membrane, e.g. penicillin

B

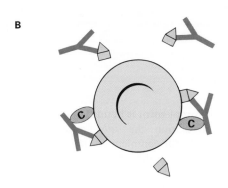

☐—— Drug, e.g. quinidine, forming a complex with:

△———— a plasma protein, which induces:

formation of an immune complex. The immune complex attaches to the cell and dinds complement ⓒ

C

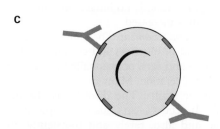

The drug e.g. methyl dopa, induces an auto antibody against a rhesus blood group antigen

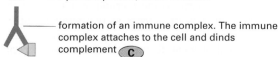

Fig. 23.25   Three mechanisms of drug-induced immune haemolysis

A. The drug acts as a hapten. **B.** The drug forms an immune complex which attaches non-specifically to red cells. **C.** The drug induces an auto-antibody.

This disorder requires the inheritance by the fetus of a red cell antigen from the father which is not present on the maternal red cells, thus provoking antibody development in the mother. Antibodies against the D antigen of the rhesus blood group system are most commonly implicated, but with improvements in management classical rhesus haemolytic disease is now much less common and an increased proportion of cases are due to antibodies to other antigens in the rhesus system, the A antigen of the ABO system or occasionally other antibodies.

Approximately 15% of the population are negative for the rhesus D antigen and can become sensitised to produce anti-D. Passage of fetal red cells into the maternal circulation occurs normally at delivery or as a result of miscarriage or operative intervention during pregnancy and these D-positive cells sensitise a D-negative mother. Further stimulation of antibody production occurs in subsequent pregnancies with a D-positive fetus. Antibody then crosses the placenta from mother to fetus and causes immune destruction of fetal red cells. Thus, the disorder does not manifest in the first pregnancy. The pathogenesis is similar for other antibodies; however, the fetus may be affected in the first pregnancy in ABO haemolytic disease of the newborn.

Clinicopathological features. The pathological features are those of a haemolytic anaemia of variable severity occurring in utero. In the most severe cases, associated with a high titre of anti-D, the result is death in utero from 'hydrops fetalis': the fetus is extremely pale and oedematous and has gross hepatosplenomegaly, the result of severe anaemia with cardiac and hepatic failure and increased extramedullary erythropoiesis. In less severe examples the neonate is pale and jaundiced at birth, with hepatosplenomegaly.

The blood picture is that of anaemia, polychromasia with increased reticulocytes and often nucleated red cells in the peripheral blood. The direct antiglobulin test on the neonatal red cells is positive, indicating that they are coated with antibody. When unconjugated bilirubin levels are very high, bile pigment becomes deposited in the central nervous system, especially the basal ganglia, causing severe damage, known as *kernicterus*. The bilirubin levels rise rapidly after birth due to immaturity of the liver, with further central nervous system damage. Spasticity and mental retardation may be the clinical consequences of this damage.

In some cases of haemolytic disease of the newborn due to anti-D, and most due to anti-A, the disease is mild, with neonatal anaemia and mild jaundice.

Management. The incidence of the disorder has been reduced by the prophylactic removal of fetal cells entering the maternal circulation before sensitisation can occur, by injection of anti-D into the mother.

Management of the affected fetus centres around provision of unsensitised red cells by intra-uterine transfusion and removal of bilirubin by exchange blood transfusion postnatally.

Haemolysis due to mismatched blood transfusion
Haemolytic transfusion reaction constitutes a second type of alloimmune haemolysis. Severe reactions result from transfusion of red cells possessing an antigen, e.g. ABO group antigens to which the recipient possesses complement binding antibody of IgG or IgM class (see p. 744).

Microangiopathic haemolytic anaemia

The term microangiopathic haemolytic anaemia describes the dramatic haematological picture which occurs when haemolysis is caused by physical trauma to erythrocytes as they are forced through narrow areas in the microvasculature (Fig. 23.2). Characteristic cells are present on the blood film: schistocytes, helmet cells and crenated cells. This type of process is commonly present in disseminated intravascular coagulation (see p. 740); the erythrocytes are damaged on fibrin strands deposited in small blood vessels. It is also a feature of the haemolytic–uraemic syndrome, thrombotic thrombocytopenic purpura (p. 736), malignant hypertension and of the extensive vasculitis in systemic lupus erythematosus. In many of these conditions, thrombocytopenia is also present.

Similar erythrocyte damage without microvascular lesions occurs in march haemoglobinuria, originally described in soldiers after prolonged marching; red cell damage presumably occurs in the feet. An analogous situation has been described in marathon runners, bongo drummers and exponents of karate!

Finally, schistocytes and haemolysis, sometimes catastrophic, are occasionally the result of red cell injury from an artificial heart valve or other vascular prostheses. With modern materials this occurrence is unusual.

In most of these situations the haemolysis is not chronic, and splenomegaly and other features of chronic red cell destruction are absent. The direct antiglobulin test is negative, as antibody is not involved in the pathogenesis.

Other causes of haemolytic anaemia

Extensive burns are associated with haemolysis, in part due to direct heat damage of erythrocytes in blood vessels of the burned areas, and in part due to a microangiopathic mechanism. Snake bites, spider bites and chemicals are occasional causes.

Infection with clostridia is a rare cause of haemolysis. Malarial infection is common and results in haemolytic anaemia (Fig. 23.26). Schizonts escape by rupturing the erythrocytes in which they have matured. In chronic malarial infection, extreme splenomegaly is often present. Histologically, there

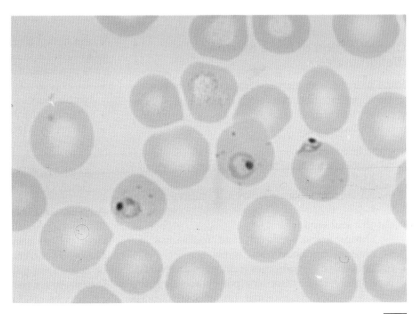

Fig. 23.26   The blood in falciparum malaria

Ring forms of the parasite are visible in several of the erythrocytes.

is marked congestion and expansion of reticulo-endothelial cells: macrophages contain parasites and red cells, and are laden with malarial pigment.

Hypersplenism

Hypersplenism is defined as anaemia (often accompanied by leukopenia and thrombocytopenia) secondary to splenic enlargement (Ch. 22). This anaemia is in part due to a haemolytic component, presumed to be due to increased red cell sequestration in the enlarged spleen, with enhanced phagocytosis by macrophages. However, other mechanisms contribute: the plasma volume increases in proportion to the degree of splenic enlargement, resulting in a dilutional anaemia, and pooling of blood cells also occurs within the spleen.

Hypersplenism is associated with splenomegaly from any cause, such as portal hypertension and collagen vascular disease. Hypersplenism in rheumatoid arthritis has the eponym *Felty's syndrome*; in this condition, however, other mechanisms are also likely to contribute to the pancytopenia, including autoantibody production against blood cells and folate deficiency.

The blood picture in hypersplenism is that of a pancytopenia with no specific features. The haemoglobin concentration would rarely be less than 8 g/dl and the platelet count less than 60×10^9/l due to hypersplenism alone.

NEOPLASTIC DISORDERS OF THE BONE MARROW

Classification of bone marrow malignancies

Bone marrow malignancies are classified according to their presentation (acute or chronic, and with or without leukaemia) and their histogenesis (e.g. myeloid, lymphoid):

- acute leukaemias
  — acute myeloblastic leukaemia (subtypes M_1 to M_7)
  — acute lymphoblastic leukaemia (subtypes L_1 to L_3)
- chronic leukaemias
  — chronic granulocytic (myeloid) leukaemia
  — chronic lymphocytic leukaemia
- myelodysplastic syndromes (refractory anaemias)
- myeloproliferative disorders (polycythaemia rubra vera, myelofibrosis, essential thrombocythaemia)

- lymphoproliferative disorders (Hodgkin's and non-Hodgkin's lymphomas)
- plasma cell neoplasms (multiple myeloma, solitary plasmacytoma, Waldenström's macroglobulinaemia).

Chronic granulocytic leukaemia is also regarded as a myeloproliferative disorder, and chronic lymphocytic leukaemia has features in common with lymphoproliferative disorders.

The lymphomas are described in Chapter 22. The myelodysplastic syndromes have already been described on page 709.

LEUKAEMIAS

Leukaemias are neoplastic proliferations of white blood cell precursors. This proliferation results in the common features of leukaemia:

- diffuse replacement of normal bone marrow by leukaemic cells with variable accumulation of abnormal cells in the peripheral blood
- infiltration of organs such as liver, spleen, lymph nodes, meninges and gonads by leukaemic cells.

Bone marrow failure with anaemia, neutropenia and thrombocytopenia is the most important consequence, particularly in the acute leukaemias.

In the majority of cases the cause is unknown. It seems likely that several predisposing factors acting together trigger the onset of the disease in most cases. However, certain factors are known to initiate leukaemic transformation:

- irradiation (e.g. atomic bomb survivors, spinal irradiation in ankylosing spondylitis, ^{32}P therapy in myeloproliferative disease)
- drugs (e.g. alkylating agents in treatment of lymphomas)
- other chemicals (e.g. benzene exposure)
- viruses (e.g. leukaemia in some animals; human T-leukaemia virus in T-cell leukaemia of Japanese)
- genetic factors (e.g. increased incidence in Down's syndrome).

All leukaemias represent neoplastic monoclonal proliferations of haemopoietic stem cells. The variety of stem cell in each type has not been determined. However, current evidence suggests that most cases of acute lymphoblastic leukaemia (ALL) involve a very primitive B-cell which has not yet developed the capacity to produce immunoglobulin; most cases of chronic granulocytic leukaemia (CGL), where megakaryocytes and erythroid cells are involved as well as leukocytes, presumably derive from a pluripotent stem cell; acute myeloid leukaemia (AML) of a variety of types appears to develop from myeloid stem cells at several possible stages of differentiation. Most cases of chronic lymphocytic leukaemia (CLL) are of B-cell origin, but these cells are much more differentiated than those in ALL.

In acute leukaemia the typical cells — 'blast' cells — accumulate as a result of failure of maturation. In CGL the abnormal myeloid stem cells also accumulate, but maturation occurs in addition, with increased numbers of mature myeloid cells in blood and bone marrow, as well as blast cells.

Current evidence suggests that chromosomal rearrangements are important events in the development of leukaemia. The reciprocal translocation between chromosomes 22 and 9 known as the Philadelphia chromosome has long been recognised in 95% of cases of CGL. More recently, specific translocations (e.g. between chromosomes 8 and 21, and between 15 and 17) have been recognised in subtypes of AML, and chromosomal abnormalities are occasionally found in ALL. It is likely that subtle karyotypic defects are present in all cases of acute leukaemia. In the case of the Philadelphia chromosome it is now known that it results in the translocation of oncogenes between chromosomes 9 and 22. It has been speculated, therefore, that chromosomal changes in leukaemias may usually involve such oncogenes (Ch. 11), a proportion of which code for products regulating cell growth. On translocation, the oncogene may become activated and produce cell autonomy, in a marrow stem cell in the case of the leukaemias.

Acute leukaemias

> ▶ Occur in all age groups
> ▶ Have a rapidly progressive course characterised by bleeding, infection and anaemia due to bone marrow infiltration and failure
> ▶ Acute leukaemia in childhood is usually lymphoblastic; in adults it is usually myeloblastic

Acute leukaemia in childhood is usually lymphoblastic (ALL) and most common at 3–4 years of age. ALL is the commonest cause of cancer death in childhood. A second increase in incidence of ALL occurs around middle age, but most cases of adult leukaemia are myeloblastic (AML).

Recently, the classification of acute leukaemias has been aided by improved techniques. While myeloblasts can usually be distinguished morphologically from lymphoblasts (Fig. 23.27), special cytochemical stains (tests for enzymes specific to certain cell types), and use of immunological markers (e.g. monoclonal antibodies which identify specific ALL types such as 'common' ALL cells) have allowed precise classification. The disorder can also be classified according to the cytological features of the blast cells. In ALL, degree of uniformity of cell size and vacuolation determine three subtypes (L_1 to L_3). In AML, seven subtypes (M_1 to

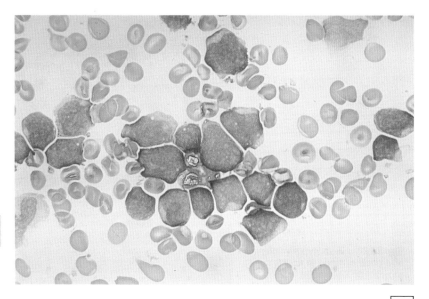

Fig. 23.27 Blast cells in acute lymphoblastic leukaemia

Blast cells are relatively large leukocytes with fine chromatin, nucleoli and basophilic cytoplasm.

M_7) are recognised with varying degrees of cytoplasmic granularity, monocytic differentiation or features suggestive of an erythroid or megakaryocytic cell line origin. Some subtypes of leukaemia have particular clinical associations although the major clinical and pathological features are common to all types.

Blood and bone marrow changes

In peripheral blood the white cell count is usually increased; counts of greater than $100 \times 10^9/l$ are not uncommon. Alternatively, leukopenia is an occasional feature, despite massive marrow infiltration with blast cells. The majority of nucleated cells are leukaemic blasts. In AML, cells containing diagnostic rod-like granular structures (Auer rods) may be present, as may hypogranular polymorphonuclear variants and pseudo-Pelger cells (Fig. 23.6). Anaemia is present, usually normocytic and normochromic. Thrombocytopenia is marked, particularly in AML.

Bone marrow cellularity is markedly increased. Blast cells constitute at least 30% of nucleated cells present and often greater than 80%. Extension into areas of previously fatty marrow may occur. Gross bone erosion with fractures is not generally a feature of acute leukaemia. Karyotype analysis reveals abnormalities in the leukaemic blasts, with gains and losses of whole chromosomes as well as translocations. Thus gain of chromosome 8 (trisomy 8) is present in 13% of cases of AML. Some changes are highly specific for subtypes of leukaemia and hence diagnostically useful, such as the rearrangement or translocation involving the long arms of chromosomes 15 and 17 in the promyelocytic variant (M_3) of AML.

Changes in other organs

Lymph nodes, liver and spleen may be infiltrated with leukaemic blast cells in all types of acute leukaemia. Lymph node enlargement is generally mild and nodes remain discrete, although in some cases of ALL massive involvement of mediastinal lymph nodes is a feature. Splenic enlargement, where present, is also minor in contrast to that in chronic leukaemias. Histologically, there is effacement of normal node architecture by sheets of leukaemic blasts and focal or diffuse infiltration of the spleen.

A diffuse infiltrate of leukaemic cells may also be present in most other organs. Evidence of bacterial, fungal or viral infection may be apparent, as may haemorrhage secondary to thrombocytopenia.

Meningeal infiltration in ALL is an important feature. Leukaemic blasts within the CNS are protected from chemotherapeutic agents by the blood–brain barrier. Perivascular aggregates of blast cells later form diffuse lesions and plaques which may result in compression of adjacent nerve tissue.

Infiltration of the gums (Fig. 23.28) and skin is a peculiar feature of the monocytic types of AML (M_4 and M_5).

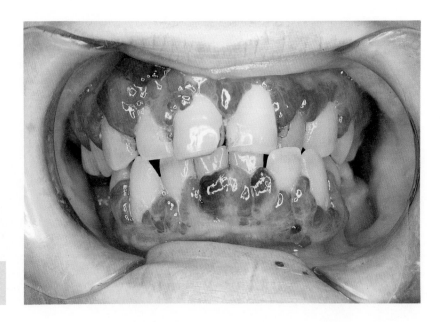

Fig. 23.28 Gum hypertrophy and haemorrhage in acute monocytic leukaemia

Severe, life-threatening coagulation failure occurs in the promyelocytic form of AML (M_3), probably due to coagulation activation and consumption of clotting factors by activators released from the granules of the leukaemic promyelocytes.

Clinical course

The onset is often very rapid and progression to death from anaemia, haemorrhage or infection occurs within weeks if no treatment is given. The features are those of marrow failure.

The course is typified by a series of overwhelming infections—bacterial, viral and fungal—and mucosal haemorrhage (Figs 23.5 and 23.29). The situation may be exacerbated, especially in AML, by transient aplasia induced by highly myelotoxic chemotherapeutic agents. The clinical course is, however, often less catastrophic in childhood ALL.

Treatment
Treatment is by chemotherapeutic agents in combination to clear the blood, bone marrow and other sites of leukaemic blasts as far as is possible, then further therapy to maintain this state of remission. Intensive support by transfusion of blood products and use of antibacterial and antifungal agents is necessary. Bone marrow transplantation is sometimes useful. Survival is months or a few years in adults, with an increasing proportion of long-term survivors with advances in therapy. The outlook is much better in childhood ALL, where significant cure rates are now achieved.

Chronic leukaemias

Chronic granulocytic leukaemia

> ▶ Occurs in all age groups
> ▶ Often pursues a more protracted course
> ▶ Associated with a chromosomal rearrangement ('Philadelphia' chromosome) in marrow cells, massive splenomegaly and a terminal acute leukaemia-like illness

Although a 'chronic' leukaemia, CGL is a fatal disorder with a mean survival of about 3 years. It occurs in all age groups. Normal bone marrow is replaced by an abnormal myeloid clone which in the majority of cases is characterised by the presence of a karyotypic abnormality, the Philadelphia chromosome (reciprocal translocation of part of the long arm of chromosome 22 to another chromosome, usually 9). Erythroid, megakaryocytic and B-lymphocyte cell lines all carry the defect, as well as the granulocytic series. In most cases the disease eventually enters a more aggressive phase due to the emergence and dominance of a more malignant clone of myeloid cells. The disease then bears a close resemblance to AML (or rarely ALL) and is rapidly fatal.

Blood and bone marrow changes
Leukocytosis is a uniform feature, with occasional cell counts in excess of 300×10^9/l. The cell picture in the blood can superficially resemble that in a bone marrow aspirate, with myelocytes, promyelocytes,

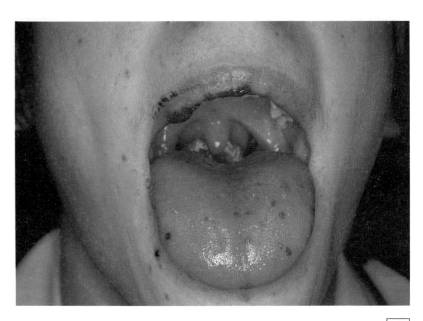

Fig. 23.29 Mucosal haemorrhage due to severe thrombocytopenia in acute leukaemia

myeloblasts and normoblasts present as well as large numbers of band cells and mature polymorphonuclear granulocytes (Fig. 23.30). Basophilia is common. Platelets are increased (sometimes over 1000×10^9/l), normal or reduced. A normochromic anaemia is often present.

The leukocytes are abnormal, as exemplified by an absence or severe reduction of their content of alkaline phosphatase, a feature unique to CGL and of diagnostic value. Serum vitamin B_{12} is elevated due to production of binding protein by the granulocyte series.

The bone marrow is hypercellular with marked reduction of fat spaces; granulocytopoiesis predominates. In the acute, terminal phase increased numbers of blast cells become evident in blood and bone marrow, and anaemia and thrombocytopenia are more marked.

Changes in other organs
The spleen is enlarged, often massively, due to infiltration by CGL cells (Fig. 23.31); it may fill the abdominal cavity and extend into the pelvis. Areas of infarction are present due to the rapid enlargement outstripping the available blood supply. Hepatomegaly is also frequently present. Infiltration in other organs is an occasional feature. Infection and bleeding are not common in the chronic phase.

Clinical course
Symptoms may be mild in the chronic phase and are essentially those of anaemia and massive spleno-megaly (abdominal fullness and pain from splenic infarction). Rarely, a hyperviscosity state may develop when the white count is greater than 300×10^9/l. In the acute phase the clinical features are those of acute leukaemia.

Treatment. In the chronic phase, treatment is by use of alkylating agents or hydroxyurea (anti-neoplastic drugs which inhibit cell division) to control the blood count and symptoms. Interferon treatment occasionally results in disappearance of the leukaemic clone, and thus of the Philadelphia chromosome, and improves survival. Bone marrow transplantation offers hope of cure. Mean duration of survival is 4 years, but may be over 10 years.

Chronic lymphocytic leukaemia

▶ Occurs in older age groups
▶ Slowly progressive, with lymphoid infiltration of nodes, liver, spleen and bone marrow

CLL is a chronic lymphoproliferative disorder with features similar to a low-grade lymphoma but with predominant blood and marrow involvement. It is a considerably less aggressive disorder than are the other leukaemias. It is a disease of the elderly. It is slowly progressive, usually following a predictable clinical course over a period of years (Fig. 23.32), as lymphocytes slowly accumulate in blood, marrow, liver and spleen until the total lymphoid mass is expanded up to a hundred-fold. The turnover of cells

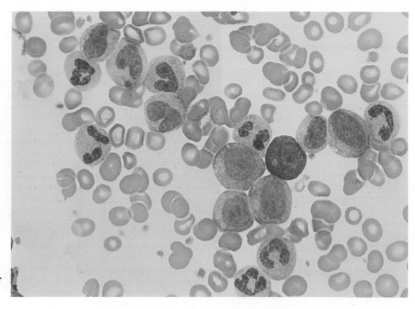

Fig. 23.30 The blood in chronic granulocytic leukaemia

Myelocytes and metamyelocytes enter the circulation.

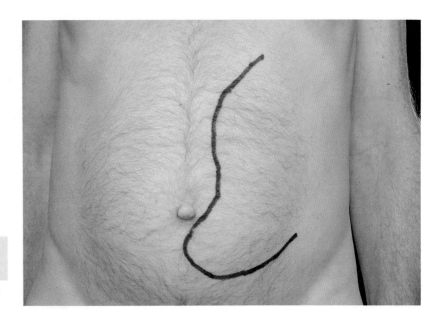

Fig. 23.31 Massive splenomegaly in chronic granulocytic leukaemia

The palpable margins of the spleen are indicated.

is extremely slow; the leukaemic cells are non-functional immunologically and of prolonged life-span.

Blood and bone marrow changes

Leukocytosis is present; up to 99% of nucleated cells are small lymphocytes (Fig. 23.33) of B-cell origin in most instances. The lymphocyte count is between 5×10^9/l and more than 300×10^9/l. The CLL cells tend to fragment during preparation of the blood film, producing many 'smear cells' (Fig. 23.33). Anaemia (normocytic) and thrombocytopenia are late developments (Fig. 23.32). However, in up to 10% of cases a secondary autoimmune haemolytic anaemia develops, with reticulocytosis and microspherocytes and positive direct antiglobulin test. Serum immunoglobulins are low in the later stages of the disease.

The bone marrow is hypercellular, with progressive replacement of normal tissue by small lymphocytes, resulting eventually in anaemia and thrombocytopenia.

Advanced stage non-Hodgkin's lymphoma may result in blood and marrow involvement superficially resembling CLL. However, extensive involvement usually occurs late in the course of the disease and the lymphoma cells are morphologically distinct from the lymphocytes of CLL.

Changes in other organs

The lymph nodes, liver and spleen are characteristically involved. In nodes and spleen the normal architecture becomes completely effaced by the infiltrate of monomorphic small lymphocytes, and similar cells are present in the portal tracts of the liver.

Clinical course

The clinical course is protracted; it is summarised in

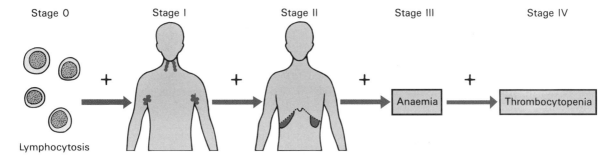

Fig. 23.32 The clinical course and staging of chronic lymphocytic leukaemia

Five stages are recognised in the 'Rai' classification.

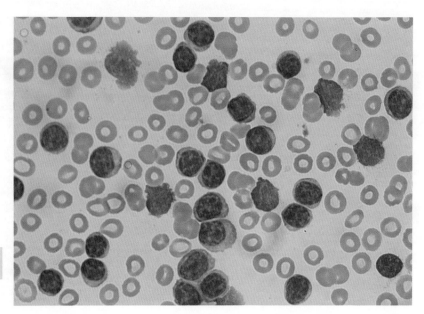

Fig. 23.33 The blood in chronic lymphocytic leukaemia

Numerous small lymphocytes and 'smear' cells are characteristic.

Figure 23.32. The protracted course means that many cases are diagnosed as a result of routine blood tests or clinical examination for some other reason.

Survival for 10 years or more from diagnosis is not uncommon. CLL being a disease of the elderly, death is often from an unrelated cause. Anaemia, haemorrhage and infection become life-threatening in the later stages. The disease often responds well to alkylating agents but may require no treatment in the early stages.

Occasionally, CLL develops in younger subjects and pursues a more aggressive course, with massive glandular enlargement and severe infections secondary to immune paresis (failure of immunoglobulin production).

Other leukaemias

The *prolymphocytic variant of CLL* is more aggressive and responds poorly to therapy. Splenomegaly is massive. The leukaemic cells in blood and bone marrow are larger and of more primitive appearance than is the case in CLL. *T-CLL* occurs in younger subjects than does the more common B-cell CLL described above. Skin involvement is common.

Hairy-cell leukaemia is a rare B-cell leukaemia of the middle-aged and elderly. The characteristic cells in the blood have cytoplasmic projections or 'hairs'. Pancytopenia is typical as is splenomegaly, which may be gross. The marrow is diffusely infiltrated by the malignant cells and marrow fibrosis is present.

The disorder may run a chronic course and is of particular interest as treatment with interferon is often effective. Splenectomy is also useful in management.

MYELOPROLIFERATIVE DISORDERS

▶ Malignant proliferations of myeloid cells with differentiation to mature forms
▶ In polycythaemia rubra vera, a pancytosis is accompanied by splenomegaly and hyperviscosity
▶ In essential thrombocythaemia, thrombocytosis is accompanied by splenomegaly or hyposplenism and by bleeding or thrombosis
▶ In myelofibrosis, anaemia and marrow fibrosis are accompanied by massive hepatosplenomegaly due to extramedullary haemopoiesis

The myeloproliferative disorders are listed in Table 23.8. This list is something of an oversimplification as intermediate forms exist. More importantly, progression in an individual from one such disorder to another within the group is common (Fig. 23.34).

Each myeloproliferative disorder represents a neoplastic proliferation of a marrow myeloid stem cell with differentiation to the mature form(s) (in contrast to the acute myeloid leukaemias, where maturation is very limited). The normal control mechanisms governing the cell line(s) involved are no longer active, allowing accumulation of erythrocytes, platelets or leukocytes. Proliferation of mega-

Table 23.8 The myeloproliferative diseases

Disorder	Morphology of bone marrow	Clinical features
Myelofibrosis	Increased reticulin/collagen	Leukoerythroblastic blood picture Anaemia with tear-drop poikilocytes Gross hepatosplenomegaly due to myeloid metaplasia
Chronic granulocytic leukaemia	Increased cellularity, particularly of the myeloid series Philadelphia chromosome	Leukoerythroblastic blood picture Anaemia, neutrophilia with immature forms Basophilia Splenomegaly, often gross
Polycythaemia rubra vera	Increased cellularity, particularly of the erythroid series	Erythrocytosis, often neutrophilia and thrombocytosis Plethora Pruritus Thrombosis or haemorrhage Splenomegaly
Essential thrombocythaemia	Increased megakaryocytes	Thrombocytosis Thrombosis or haemorrhage Sometimes splenomegaly

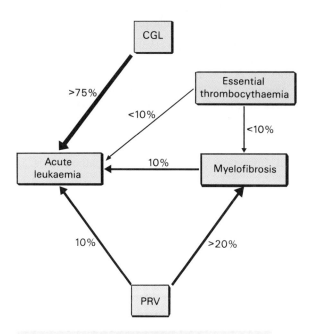

Fig. 23.34 The natural history of the myeloproliferative disorders

Acute myeloid leukaemia never transforms to chronic myeloproliferative disease. The acute 'blast crisis' in chronic granulocytic leukaemia (CGL) is occasionally lymphoid. The progression to acute leukaemia in polycythaemia rubra vera (PRV) may be influenced by prior treatment with alkylating agents.

karyocytes produces growth factors causing a secondary overgrowth of fibroblasts (myelofibrosis).

Chronic myeloid leukaemia behaves as a myeloproliferative disorder and can be usefully regarded as such, along with the non-leukaemic myeloproliferative disorders polycythaemia rubra vera (PRV), essential thrombocythaemia and myelofibrosis. The main features of these conditions are summarised in Table 23.8 and described below. Non-myeloproliferative causes of polycythaemia are also considered here.

Polycythaemia rubra vera

Polycythaemia is an increase in the concentration of red cells above normal, usually with a corresponding increase in haemoglobin concentration and haematocrit. In polycythaemia rubra vera it is an idiopathic, primary condition.

The body red cell mass and plasma volume can be accurately assessed by isotopic labelling techniques. Normal ranges are 25–35 ml/kg for red cell mass (22–32 ml/kg in females) and 35–45 ml/kg for plasma volume.

Blood and bone marrow changes

The haemoglobin concentration is raised, often to 20 g/dl or more, with haematocrit values of up to 75%. Red cell mass may be as high as 80 ml/kg. However, iron deficiency is not uncommon, partly due to increased requirements and partly to a bleeding tendency with chronic gastrointestinal blood loss due to production of functionally abnormal platelets. In such circumstances of iron-deficient polycythaemia, haemoglobin and haematocrit may be normal or even low, but the red cell count is still high.

Thrombocytosis and neutrophil leukocytosis are present in up to 50% of cases. The serum vitamin B_{12} and uric acid are increased, the former due to production of binding protein by myeloid cells, the latter due to increased cell turnover. The bone marrow is hypercellular. Erythroid hyperplasia is present. Megakaryocytes may be prominent and increased reticulin deposition is common.

Changes in other organs

The spleen is enlarged in 75% of cases, usually to a moderate extent. Splenic sinuses are engorged. Extramedullary haemopoiesis may be present: normoblasts and cells of the developing myeloid series are present in the spleen and often the liver. Infarction of heart, brain and spleen is common due to the high blood viscosity and poor flow.

Haemorrhagic lesions may be a feature, especially in the gastrointestinal tract. Peptic ulceration is common in PRV, for unknown reasons.

Clinical features

Clinical features correspond to the pathological changes described above. The skin is plethoric and cyanosis is common. Itching is typical and usually exacerbated by changes in temperature, as after bathing. The conjunctival vessels appear congested, as are retinal vessels. Hyperviscosity results in headache and lethargy. The spleen is palpable. Acute gout may be a presenting feature. Evidence of mucosal bleeding or of thrombosis (particularly arterial) may be present.

Treatment is by venesection or myelosuppression by alkylating agents, hydroxyurea or use of radiophosphorus (^{32}P). Survival is for many years. Progression to a myelofibrotic state is common and transformation to acute myeloid leukaemia may occur, especially following ^{32}P treatment. Myeloproliferative polycythaemia (rubra vera) must be distinguished from other causes of polycythaemia, in which splenomegaly and pancytosis are not features.

Secondary and relative polycythaemias

Most cases of polycythaemia are not due to polycythaemia rubra vera, but are due to:

- high altitude
- cyanotic heart disease
- respiratory disease
- smoking
- haemoglobinopathy.

Any disorder resulting in chronic hypoxia results in stimulation of erythropoietin production and secondary polycythaemia, as in severe chronic bronchitis, emphysema or alveolar hypoventilation for any reason. Congenital heart disease in which a right-to-left shunt is present is a potent cause; haemoglobin concentrations of 20 g/dl are not uncommon. Cigarette smokers have a higher haematocrit than non-smokers, due in part to the carbon monoxide in tobacco smoke. In these situations the polycythaemia is frequently not symptomatic and the blood and bone marrow are otherwise normal. Treatment is rarely necesary.

The following renal disorders and tumours are (very uncommonly) associated with inappropriate erythropoietin production and polycythaemia:

- renal carcinoma or cysts
- renal artery stenosis
- massive uterine fibroids
- hepatocellular carcinoma
- cerebellar haemangioblastoma.

Polycythaemia may also result from a contraction of the plasma volume with normal red cell mass. This situation occurs chronically in so-called *stress polycythaemia*, also known as Gaisbock's syndrome, where the plasma volume may be 30 ml/kg or less. It is a common disorder, especially in middle-aged, overweight male heavy smokers. It is associated with increased risk of arterial occlusion causing myocardial infarction and stroke. The pathogenesis is obscure.

Myelofibrosis

Also known as myelosclerosis, myelofibrosis is characterised by the predominant features of gross marrow fibrosis with massive extramedullary haemopoiesis in liver and spleen. The fibrosis is reactive (a polyclonal proliferation of fibroblasts is present). Factors released from pathological megakaryocytes which proliferate in the bone marrow are thought to be the stimulus to the fibroblastic response. It is a chronic disorder of late middle age and beyond.

Blood and bone marrow changes

Anaemia is usually present; platelets and leukocytes

are often increased, but become subnormal eventually. The blood film is typically leukoerythroblastic. Characteristic poikilocytes with a tear-drop shape are a consistent finding (Fig. 23.2).

Bone marrow cannot be aspirated. Trephine biopsy reveals variable cellularity with increased reticulin, progressing to massive deposition of collagen. Megakaryocytes are often increased. Bony trabeculae may be expanded.

Changes in other organs

The spleen is invariably enlarged, often to a massive degree. Lymphoid follicles are preserved but the red pulp is expanded with diffuse areas of extramedullary haemopoiesis. The liver is often enlarged, with obvious foci of haemopoiesis present. Occasionally, lymph nodes are also involved. The liver involvement may result in portal hypertension, causing oesophageal varices and ascites.

Clinical features

Symptoms are caused by the anaemia and massive splenomegaly. Symptoms of hypermetabolism may also be present, especially weight loss and night sweats. Sclerosis of bones may be apparent on X-ray examination. Many patients have a history of polycythaemia rubra vera or essential thrombocythaemia (Fig. 23.34); in others, the onset is insidious. With supportive therapy (blood transfusion), survival is often a few years. If the enlarged spleen is troublesome, splenectomy can be safely performed, surprisingly without exacerbation of the anaemia.

Essential thrombocythaemia

Essential thrombocythaemia, a myeloproliferative disorder, is an important cause of thrombocytosis. The diagnosis is being made more frequently as an incidental finding now that automated cell counters are routinely used.

Blood and bone marrow changes

The platelet count is raised, often to $1000 \times 10^9/l$ and even to $3000 \times 10^9/l$. Neutrophil leukocytosis may also be a feature. 'Giant' platelets and megakaryocyte fragments may be present. Anaemia, when present, is due to iron deficiency from chronic blood loss. Howell–Jolly bodies and other features of hyposplenism may be apparent due to splenic infarction. Bone marrow cellularity is normal or increased,

megakaryocytes predominate and some increase in marrow reticulin is common.

Changes in other organs

The spleen may be enlarged but is usually normal or reduced in size due to infarction. Ischaemic changes in the area supplied by digital arteries may be present, as may evidence of infarction in other organs. Paradoxically, haemorrhagic lesions also occur, often in the gastrointestinal tract.

Clinical features

The disorder may be asymptomatic for many years. Painful ischaemic lesions of the digits are an occasional feature. Paradoxical haemorrhage, which may be serious, occurs particularly in association with platelet counts over $1000 \times 10^9/l$. Treatment with alkylating agents or hydroxyurea is effective and survival prolonged. Progression to myelofibrosis may occur.

PLASMA CELL NEOPLASMS

Plasma cells are the immunoglobulin-producing cells and are normally identifiable in the bone marrow. Diffuse neoplastic, monoclonal proliferation of plasma cells throughout the red marrow is characteristic of the disorder *multiple myeloma*. When the proliferation is more localised an apparently discrete plasma cell tumour develops, usually in bone—*solitary plasmacytoma*. Monoclonal proliferation of IgM-producing plasma cells and lymphoplasmacytoid cells in the reticulo-endothelial organs, bone marrow, liver and spleen is present in a third type of plasma cell neoplasm—Waldenström's macroglobulinaemia.

Multiple myeloma

▶ Malignant proliferation of plasma cells in bone marrow
▶ Occurs in older age groups
▶ Usually associated with the accumulation of a monoclonal immunoglobulin or light chains (Bence Jones protein) in plasma
▶ Often causes renal failure
▶ Results in bone destruction in the axial skeleton, with pain and fractures

Multiple myeloma is a common neoplastic disease affecting especially the elderly: almost all cases occur

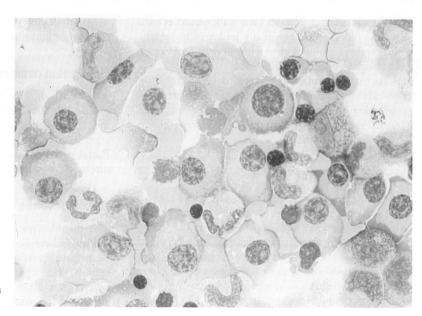

Fig. 23.35 The bone marrow in multiple myeloma

An infiltrate of atypical plasma cells is a major diagnostic criterion.

after the age of 40 years. Multifocal plasma cell tumours erode the bones of the axial skeleton; the plasma cells synthesise a monoclonal immunoglobulin or light chain, referred to as the *M-component* or paraprotein in plasma. The M-component is present in over 99% of cases of multiple myeloma; it is most commonly IgG (60% of cases) but may be IgA or immunoglobulin light chains only (kappa or lambda). IgD and IgE M-components are unusual and IgM types are much more commonly a feature of Waldenström's macroglobulinaemia. In two-thirds of cases of IgG and IgA myeloma, monoclonal free light chains are produced in addition to the complete immunoglobulin molecule, presumably due to a functional defect in the malignant plasma cells. While immunoglobulins cannot pass the glomerular filter, free light chains are small enough to enter the urine, where they are called *Bence Jones protein*. The plasma concentration of the unaffected immunoglobulins is often markedly suppressed ('immune paresis').

Paraprotein formation is not unique to multiple myeloma; a monoclonal immunoglobulin is present occasionally in CLL and lymphomas and, rarely, in carcinomatous disease. Furthermore, a proportion of elderly subjects are found to have a stable paraprotein without immune paresis and without the other features of multiple myeloma or lymphoproliferative disease — so-called 'benign monoclonal gammopathy'.

Blood and bone marrow changes

Anaemia is common. The blood film often has rouleaux formation: a tendency for the erythrocytes to adhere to each other and form columns one cell across in the blood film, due to the presence of a high concentration of immunoglobulin. The anaemia is normocytic, but automated cell counters may suggest a high MCV, probably due to rouleaux formation. In advanced disease, pancytopenia is present. Abnormal plasma cells are only occasionally seen in the peripheral blood.

The marrow is hypercellular; 15–90% of the cells are morphologically abnormal plasma cells, including multinucleate forms (Fig. 23.35). Increased numbers of osteoclasts actively resorbing bone may be seen on trephine biopsy; they are stimulated by activating factors produced by the malignant plasma cells, including interleukins.

The plasma cell infiltrate and discrete tumours are present in those bones normally containing red marrow, especially the skull, ribs, vertebrae and pelvis (Fig. 23.36). The distal long bones and those of the extremities are rarely involved. Generalised osteoporosis is common.

Changes in other organs

Renal involvement is present in over half of the

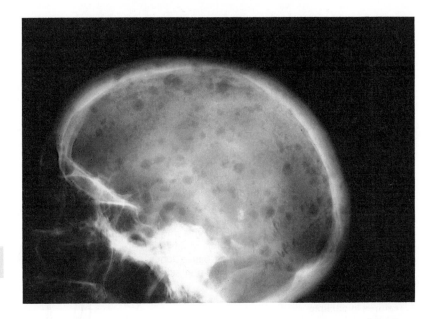

Fig. 23.36 Skull radiograph in multiple myeloma

There are numerous osteolytic bone lesions.

cases. The most common abnormality is the presence of protein casts in the distal convoluted and collecting tubules with surrounding giant cells and atrophy of tubular cells — 'Bence Jones or myeloma kidney'. Metastatic calcification, changes of pyelonephritis and primary amyloid may also be present in the kidneys. Systemic amyloidosis (Ch. 7) is present in 10% of cases, particularly in the tongue, heart and peripheral nerves, as well as the kidneys.

Clinical features

The clinical features in multiple myeloma are outlined in Figure 23.37. Not all are present in every case. Bone pain is present in the majority and is often severe. Renal failure is common and prognostically sinister. Hyperviscosity is especially associated with IgA paraproteins because of the physical characteristics of IgA.

Treatment involves alkylating agents and radiotherapy. Survival is 2–3 years in most cases.

Solitary plasmacytoma

Solitary tumours composed of malignant plasma cells identical in morphology to those in multiple myeloma occasionally arise in bone or extra-osseous sites. A paraprotein may be synthesised by the cells of the tumour. Solitary plasmacytoma of the bone may progress to multiple myeloma.

Waldenström's macroglobulinaemia

In Waldenström's macroglobulinaemia the marrow, lymph nodes, liver and spleen are infiltrated by cells with morphology between lymphocytes and plasma cells, which synthesise a monoclonal IgM. The disorder is uncommon and tends to occur in the later years. It behaves as a low-grade lymphoma (moderate lymph node enlargement and hepatosplenomegaly) and does not produce the characteristic osteolytic bone lesions and hypercalcaemia of multiple myeloma. Hyperviscosity is common and occurs at lower paraprotein concentrations than is the case in myeloma, due to the physical characteristics of the IgM molecule. Visual deterioration, lethargy, bleeding tendency and disturbance of consciousness result.

Survival for many years follows treatment with alkylating agents.

DISORDERS OF BLOOD COAGULATION AND HAEMOSTASIS

The components of the haemostatic system are described on page 691. Although it is convenient to describe separately the intrinsic and extrinsic pathways of blood coagulation, platelet adhesion and aggregation, and activation of the fibrinolytic system, there are numerous points of interaction.

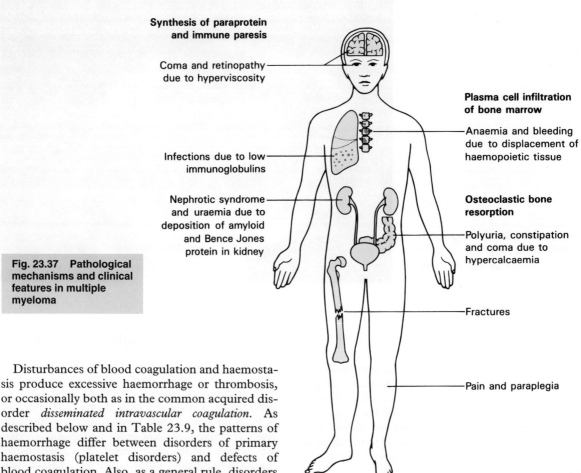

Fig. 23.37 Pathological mechanisms and clinical features in multiple myeloma

Synthesis of paraprotein and immune paresis

Coma and retinopathy due to hyperviscosity

Infections due to low immunoglobulins

Nephrotic syndrome and uraemia due to deposition of amyloid and Bence Jones protein in kidney

Plasma cell infiltration of bone marrow

Anaemia and bleeding due to displacement of haemopoietic tissue

Osteoclastic bone resorption

Polyuria, constipation and coma due to hypercalcaemia

Fractures

Pain and paraplegia

Disturbances of blood coagulation and haemostasis produce excessive haemorrhage or thrombosis, or occasionally both as in the common acquired disorder *disseminated intravascular coagulation*. As described below and in Table 23.9, the patterns of haemorrhage differ between disorders of primary haemostasis (platelet disorders) and defects of blood coagulation. Also, as a general rule, disorders which allow the unchecked generation and deposition of fibrin tend to be associated with thrombosis in the venous circulation (red thrombus), whereas excessive platelet activation tends to result in vascular occlusion in arteries and arterioles (white thrombus), although this is by no means a rigid distinction.

DISORDERS OF PRIMARY HAEMOSTASIS

Theoretically, primary haemostasis could be defective as a result of platelet abnormalities or defects of the small blood vessels. In fact, vascular disease is rarely the cause of clinically important haemorrhage. Bleeding due to primary haemostatic defects is most commonly secondary to acquired platelet disorders such as thrombocytopenia or disturbance of platelet function.

In bleeding due to disorders of primary haemostasis the skin and mucous membranes are especially involved (Table 23.9 and Fig. 23.29).

Thrombocytopenias

▶ Cause spontaneous bleeding when the blood platelet count falls below $20 \times 10^9/l$
▶ Due to failure of platelet production or increased destruction/sequestration
▶ When due to production failure, thrombocytopenia is usually accompanied by anaemia and leukopenia or leukocytosis
▶ When due to increased destruction, immune mechanisms and disseminated intravascular coagulation are common causes

While a bleeding tendency may be associated with

Table 23.9 Features which may distinguish bleeding in coagulation defects from that in platelet disorders*

Feature	Platelet defect	Severe coagulation defect
Purpura	Very common	Absent
Mucosal bleeding	Common from mouth and gut	Relatively uncommon except from urinary tract
Joint bleeding	Absent	Very common in severe congenital factor deficiencies
Muscle haematomas	In response to trauma	Spontaneous
Bleeding after surgery	Immediate	Often delayed several hours

*Severe thrombocytopenia and severe haemophilia are taken as examples

the thrombocytosis of myeloproliferative disorders, a quantitative platelet abnormality causing haemorrhage is most commonly due to the presence of reduced platelet numbers. No clinical defect of primary haemostasis occurs with platelet counts greater than $80 \times 10^9/l$ if they function normally. Increased bleeding after trauma is present with counts of $40–50 \times 10^9/l$ but spontaneous skin and mucosal haemorrhage occur only when platelet counts fall to $20 \times 10^9/l$. The skin bleeding time increases progressively as the platelet count falls below $80 \times 10^9/l$ and, when performed in a standardised manner, is a good test of primary haemostasis. The bleeding time is not affected by disorders of coagulation.

Classification

Thrombocytopenia can be conveniently classified according to pathogenesis:

- Failure of platelet production
  - megaloblastic anaemia
  - leukaemia
  - myelofibrosis
  - other marrow infiltration, e.g. carcinoma, lymphoma, myeloma
  - hypoplastic anaemia
  - chemotherapeutic agents and occasionally other drugs, e.g. thiazides

  - alcohol
  - viral infections
  - congenital absence of megakaryocytes
- Increased platelet destruction
  - acute and chronic autoimmune thrombocytopenic purpura
  - drug-induced immune thrombocytopenia
  - neonatal and post-transfusion purpura (alloimmune)
  - massive blood loss and transfusion
  - disseminated intravascular coagulation
  - thrombotic thrombocytopenia/ haemolytic–uraemic syndrome
- Platelet sequestration
  - hypersplenism.

Where thrombocytopenia is an isolated finding, with normal haemoglobin and white cells, increased platelet destruction is most likely. Failure of platelet production due to a bone marrow abnormality is most commonly associated with a pancytopenia, or a leukocytosis, in the leukaemias.

Of the causes of thrombocytopenia due to platelet production failure, those due to thiazides, viral infection and congenital megakaryocyte abnormalities are very uncommon. The other disorders resulting in marrow failure have been described earlier.

Autoimmune thrombocytopenic purpura and disseminated intravascular coagulation are the most common disorders in which thrombocytopenia is due to increased destruction/utilisation of platelets.

Autoimmune thrombocytopenic purpura

In autoimmune thrombocytopenic purpura platelets are destroyed in the reticulo-endothelial system, especially the spleen, due to coating with auto-antibody. The disorder is analogous to autoimmune haemolytic anaemia. It occurs in an acute, spontaneously remitting form in children, as a chronic idiopathic state in adults and as a drug-induced phenomenon. The acute childhood variety may follow an infection such as measles. The chronic type is occasionally symptomatic of a disorder such as chronic lymphocytic leukaemia, or lymphoma, or may occur in association with other autoimmune disease such as rheumatoid arthritis. Drugs associated with idiopathic thrombocytopenic purpura (ITP) include quinine, heparin and sulphonamides; in most cases, an immune complex mechanism is involved, similar to that in some cases of drug-induced immune haemolytic anaemia.

Blood and bone marrow changes
Thrombocytopenia is present; severity is variable. Platelet counts of less than $10 \times 10^9/l$ are not uncommon. Erythrocytes and leukocytes are usually normal. Iron deficiency anaemia may be present due to chronic mucosal bleeding. In the bone marrow there is a non-specific increase in megakaryocyte size and number. It may be possible to detect the auto-antibody in serum by tests analogous to the antiglobulin test used in the investigation of haemolytic anaemias. The skin bleeding time is prolonged.

Changes in other organs
Changes in other organs are those of haemorrhage. Bleeding into the skin in the form of purpura is common (Fig. 23.29). Purpura (petechiae) of thrombocytopenic type is due to apparently spontaneous leakage of red cells from capillaries and arterioles in the skin. It is usually most prominent in the skin of the lower legs and feet, suggesting that hydrostatic pressure may play a role. Areas of skin trauma may also be affected. Histological evidence of capillary bleeding may also be present in the serosal linings, mucosae of gastrointestinal and urinary tract and the central nervous system. The spleen is usually of normal size or only moderately enlarged, not extending below the costal margin. The sinusoids are congested and splenic follicles reactive. Megakaryocytes may be present in the spleen, a response to the increased platelet turnover.

Clinical features
Clinical features are restricted to excessive haemorrhage. Purpuric rash, epistaxis, menorrhagia and gastrointestinal haemorrhage are common. The acute form in childhood is transient and often requires no treatment. Drug-induced ITP responds to withdrawal of the offending medication. Chronic 'idiopathic' ITP often responds to immunosuppression with corticosteroids or to splenectomy. Prognosis is good; the main risk is fatal cerebral haemorrhage.

Other immune thrombocytopenias

Thrombocytopenia is a frequent manifestation of AIDS and, in some cases, has an autoimmune pathogenesis. Neonatal thrombocytopenia due to placental transfer of the platelet-reactive IgG auto-antibody can occur in infants of women with chronic ITP. Also, a condition analogous to rhesus haemolytic disease, due to transplacental passage of an antibody, is occasionally recognised as a cause of neonatal thrombocytopenia. The pathogenesis is comparable to that of haemolytic disease of the new-born, the fetus possessing a platelet antigen lacking in the mother.

Post-transfusion purpura is a very uncommon immune thrombocytopenia in women following blood transfusion.

Thrombotic thrombocytopenic purpura and haemolytic–uraemic syndrome

Thrombotic thrombocytopenic purpura (TTP) and haemolytic–uraemic syndrome (HUS) are probably manifestations of a common but poorly understood pathogenetic mechanism. The dominant features are thrombocytopenia due to platelet consumption in microvascular occlusive platelet plugs and a microangiopathic haemolytic anaemia (Fig. 23.2). Glomerular lesions are characteristic (Ch. 21), but vascular lesions in other organs, especially the central nervous system, may be a feature. In children, HUS may occur in epidemics, suggesting an infectious origin: toxins produced by *E. coli* have been implicated. The cause of the platelet activation is unknown but a variety of vascular endothelial cell abnormalities have been postulated.

Clinically, haemorrhage and organ dysfunction due to the microvascular lesions predominate. Renal failure is present. Transient neurological abnormalities characterise TTP and distinguish it from HUS. The disease runs a subacute or chronic course. Spontaneous remission is not uncommon in the childhood form, but chronic renal impairment may result.

Qualitative disorders of platelets

Disorders of platelet function result in excessive bleeding of platelet type and prolonged skin bleeding time in the presence of normal platelet numbers.

Acquired disorders of platelet function

Acquired disorders of platelet function are due to:

- drugs (e.g. aspirin, anti-inflammatory drugs, high dose penicillin)
- metabolic disorders (e.g. uraemia, hepatic failure)
- myeloproliferative disorders (essential thrombocythaemia, polycythaemia rubra vera)
- plasma cell disorders (e.g. multiple myeloma, Waldenström's macroglobulinaemia).

Aspirin and anti-inflammatory drugs block the cyclo-oxygenase enzyme necessary for platelet synthesis of pro-aggregatory thromboxane. The bleeding tendency is mild, with increased skin bruising and bleeding after surgery. Gastric haemorrhage from acute mucosal erosions may be life-threatening. In uraemia and liver failure, platelet interactions with subendothelium are abnormal and bleeding may be severe. In myeloproliferative disease, the clonal defect gives rise to functionally abnormal platelets, and in myeloma platelets become coated with immunoglobulin which blocks surface receptors and prevents platelet aggregation.

Congenital disorders of platelet function

Hereditary platelet disorders causing life-threatening haemorrhage such as those where the platelet glycoprotein receptors for von Willebrand factor (Fig. 23.8) (Bernard–Soulier syndrome) or fibrinogen (Glanzmann's disease) are absent are extremely rare diseases. Mild defects of platelet function, causing easy bruising and bleeding after trauma, are more common. In some, a familial pattern is apparent. Various metabolic disturbances of platelets may be responsible, such as a deficiency of adenine nucleotides (platelet storage pool deficiency). Prolongation of skin bleeding time is a common feature of these qualitative platelet disorders.

Bleeding due to vascular disorders

Vascular disorders do not usually cause serious bleeding. Skin haemorrhage and occasional mucosal haemorrhage may occur. In some disorders, the collagen which supports vessel walls is abnormal. This mechanism probably accounts for the bruising of Cushing's syndrome and the bruising, mucosal bleeding and perifollicular skin haemorrhages of scurvy (Ch. 7).

Henoch–Schönlein or anaphylactoid purpura

Henoch–Schönlein purpura is an immune complex hypersensitivity reaction, usually in children. A rash, superficially similar to thrombocytopenic purpura but with localised oedema causing the lesions to be raised above the skin level, is present on buttocks and lower legs. Arthralgia, abdominal pain and haematuria may occur. It is usually self-limiting. Although the skin rash resembles thrombocytopenic purpura, the platelet count and bleeding time are normal and a generalised bleeding tendency is not present.

Hereditary haemorrhagic telangiectasia

Telangiectases (microvascular dilatations) accumu-

late from childhood on mucous membranes, in liver and lungs and on the skin of hands and face (Fig. 23.38). It is inherited as an autosomal dominant trait. Nosebleeds and gastrointestinal bleeding may be severe.

In these vascular conditions, platelet numbers and skin bleeding time are normal.

Platelet disorders causing thrombosis

HUS and TTP have been described; however, the abnormality causing increased platelet reactivity probably does not lie within the platelet itself but with the vascular endothelium. Thrombosis is a feature of myeloproliferative disease with thrombocytosis, especially essential thrombocythaemia and polycythaemia rubra vera. Laboratory evidence for increased platelet reactivity can be found in subjects with coronary thrombosis, cerebral thrombosis, diabetes mellitus and other disorders, but the precise role of platelet hyperactivity in occlusive events in these conditions is unknown.

Paradoxically, the heparin-induced immune thrombocytopenia which occasionally develops on exposure to this anticoagulant drug may be associated with extensive arterial and venous thrombosis, due to platelet activation by the auto-antibody.

In contrast to the situation in the coagulation system, no familial abnormality of primary haemostasis causing a thrombotic tendency has yet been described.

DISORDERS OF BLOOD COAGULATION

▶ Can be congenital or acquired
▶ Congenital disorders are uncommon, the most important being von Willebrand's disease and haemophilia
▶ Acquired disorders are common, due to anticoagulant drugs, vitamin K deficiency, liver disease, and disseminated intravascular coagulation

Diseases of the coagulation/fibrinolytic system causing thrombosis as well as those causing haemorrhage are recognised. In practice, the majority of bleeding disorders are acquired and due to anticoagulant drugs or to liver disease, or to clotting factor consumption in disseminated intravascular coagulation. The severe congenital haemorrhagic diatheses are uncommon but clinically important disorders due to an inherited defect of production of a coagulation factor.

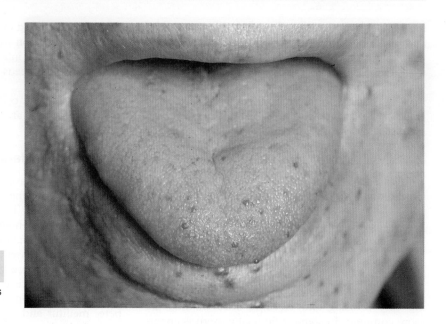

Fig. 23.38 Hereditary haemorrhagic telangiectasia

Typical vascular lesions on the lips and facial skin.

Congenital clotting factor deficiencies

Deficiencies of most of the coagulation factors have been described but deficiency of factor VIII (haemophilia A) and factor IX (haemophilia B or Christmas disease), and of von Willebrand factor (von Willebrand's disease) are the only relatively common disorders in the group.

Factor VIII coagulation protein is a co-factor for fibrin generation in the intrinsic coagulation pathway (Fig. 23.8); it is probably synthesised predominantly by hepatocytes. In order to circulate in plasma with a normal half-life of 12 hours it requires a carrier protein — von Willebrand factor (vWF) (Fig. 23.39). vWF is a large multimeric protein synthesised and assembled by vascular endothelial cells and megakaryocytes. It has no role in the coagulation cascade but is an essential co-factor for interaction of platelets with exposed subendothelium in primary haemostasis (Fig. 23.7).

Factor VIII production is controlled by a gene on the X chromosome. vWF synthesis is under autosomal control.

Haemophilia

Haemophilia A and B are identical clinically and pathologically, differing only in the deficient factor. In each case the disorder is due to sex-linked recessively inherited deficiency of the clotting factor, or synthesis of a defective clotting factor. Males are affected. Female carriers have approximately 50% of the normal factor level and may occasionally be mildly clini-

cally affected. Mild, moderate and severe forms are recognised, depending on the residual clotting factor activity (Table 23.10); degree of severity is constant within a kindred. The blood clotting time is prolonged. In severe disease, the blood is incoagulable.

The bleeding is of the coagulation deficiency type (Table 23.9). Purpura is not a feature. In severe disease, bleeding from wounds persists for days or weeks. Control can be achieved by clotting factor replacement by the intravenous route.

Molecular genetics

Molecular genetic studies have recognised a variety of defects in haemophilia, including partial and complete deletions of the factor VIII gene, as well as single base changes, which create either a translational stop signal (so-called nonsense mutations) with the consequent synthesis of a truncated protein which is ineffective functionally and rapidly degraded, or single amino acid substitutions which alter the stability and function of the proteins. Mutations occurring de novo account for a substantial proportion of affected subjects (around 30%). Comparable defects in the factor IX gene are seen in haemophilia B.

Clinical features and treatment

Apparently spontaneous haemorrhage into a major joint, especially knees, hips, elbows and shoulders, occurring several times each month is typical of the severe disease. Without factor replacement therapy bleeding continues until the intra-articular pressure rises sufficiently to prevent further haemorrhage.

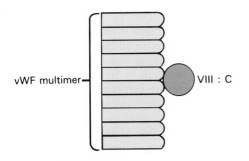

Fig. 23.39 Schematic representation of the factor VIII:von Willebrand factor (vWF) complex in plasma

Each unit has antigenic properties identifiable as vWF antigen or 'factor VIII-related antigen' but only the multimeric structure possesses the ability to bind platelets to subendothelium.

Table 23.10	Classification of haemophilia A		
Category	Factor VIII % of normal	Features	
Severe	0–1	Frequent and spontaneous haemorrhage into joints and soft tissues from birth Degenerative joint disease	
Moderate	1–3	Bleeding after trauma, including dental and other surgical trauma Bruising	
Mild	>3	Bleeding after trauma only May be subclinical in mildest form	

Slow resolution of this acute haemarthrosis then occurs. Recurrent bleeds within a joint produce massive synovial hypertrophy, erosion of joint cartilage and para-articular bone and changes of a severe osteoarthritis (Ch. 25).

Bleeding into muscles (Fig. 23.40), retroperitoneal tissues and the urinary tract also occurs. Pressure necrosis of adjacent structures such as peripheral nerves may result.

The clinical picture in severe haemophilia is one of recurrent spontaneous haemarthrosis and soft tissue haemorrhage from birth. External bleeding from the urinary tract and epistaxis are also common.

Replacement therapy with clotting factor concen-trates has led to other pathology in subjects receiving such treatment due to virus transmission in these blood products. Liver disease is universal; hepatitis C is a particular problem (Ch. 16). This disease may be progressive, with changes of cirrhosis eventually ensuing in a large proportion of patients. Death from liver failure may occur.

Approximately one-third of the UK haemophiliacs are infected with HIV. Many have developed the pathological features of the acquired immune deficiency syndrome (AIDS), including *Pneumocystis carinii* pneumonia, toxoplasmosis and systemic candidiasis. Modern heat-treated factor concentrates appear to be free of hepatitis viruses and HIV.

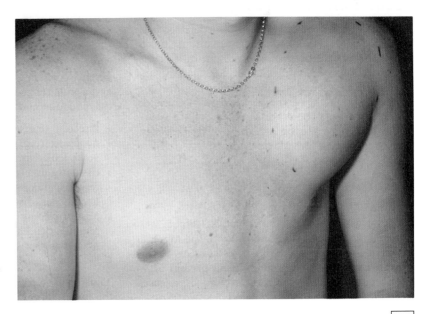

Fig. 23.40 Muscle haematoma in severe haemophilia

The left pectoral muscle is the site of haemorrhage which developed spontaneously.

Von Willebrand's disease

Von Willebrand's disease (vWD) is a moderate to mild bleeding disorder due to synthesis of vWF in reduced amounts or production of functionally abnormal vWF. It is transmitted as an autosomal dominant disorder in most kindred, and epidemiological studies suggest it may be common in mild or subclinical form.

The majority of cases have a quantitative deficiency of vWF (Type 1), but in around 20% a dysfunctional vWF is synthesised and in these the multimeric structure of vWF (Fig. 23.39) is abnormal, with a reduction in the large multimers (Type 2). Because of the size of the vWF gene and the molecular complexity of the protein relatively little is known of the genetic abnormalities responsible for the disease. The homozygous disease (Type 3) is a serious bleeding diathesis but is extremely uncommon. In the more usual heterozygous form the main manifestations are easy bruising, bleeding after trauma and menorrhagia in females. Haemarthrosis and muscle haematomas are not common features of vWD. The plasma concentration of vWF is reduced, and, because of the requirement for vWF as a carrier protein, VIII activity is reduced in parallel; levels of less than 10–20% of normal are unusual, however. The bleeding time is prolonged, as is the blood clotting time due to the reduced VIII. Although the platelet count is usually normal, platelet interaction with subendothelium is defective due to the deficiency of vWF.

Acquired disorders of coagulation

Bleeding due to acquired platelet disorders has been described above. A haemorrhagic diathesis due to coagulation factor deficiency is present in liver disease, disseminated intravascular coagulation, and vitamin K deficiency due to immaturity (haemorrhagic disease of the newborn), obstructive jaundice, pancreatic or small bowel disease.

Bleeding may also be a feature of therapy with anticoagulant and fibrinolytic drugs.

Vitamin K deficiency

Vitamin K is obtained from green vegetables and by bacterial synthesis in the gut. It is a fat-soluble vitamin and requires bile for its absorption. Vitamin K is essential for the γ-carboxylation of clotting factors II, VII, IX and X (and protein C and protein S); in the absence of vitamin K, these factors are released from the liver in an incomplete and inactive form.

A coagulopathy due to vitamin K deficiency occurs when absorption is defective, particularly in obstructive jaundice. In addition, the neonate tends to vitamin K deficiency due to lack of gut bacteria and low concentrations of the vitamin in breast milk. This exacerbates the inefficient coagulation due to low levels of clotting factors secondary to liver immaturity and may produce life-threatening haemorrhage during the first week of life — *haemorrhagic disease of the newborn*. Vitamin K supplementation corrects the defect.

The oral anticoagulant drug warfarin is a vitamin K antagonist and acts by inhibition of the complete synthesis of coagulation factors II, VII, IX and X. Its use is therefore associated with an increased risk of haemorrhage.

Liver disease

Liver disease, other than obstructive jaundice, is commonly associated with coagulation defects due to failure of clotting factor synthesis and production of abnormal fibrinogen — dysfibrinogenaemia. This is often compounded by thrombocytopenia due to hypersplenism and a qualitative platelet disorder. Life-threatening haemorrhage may result, particularly from oesophageal varices.

Disseminated intravascular coagulation

Disseminated intravascular coagulation (DIC) is a common state in which a combination of haemorrhage and thrombosis complicates another disorder. Activation of coagulation leads to the formation of microthrombi in numerous organs and to the consumption of clotting factors and platelets in the process of clot formation, in turn leading to a haemorrhagic diathesis. There are several potential triggers to coagulation activation in DIC (Fig. 23.41) and a wide range of disorders can be complicated by this phenomenon:

- infection (e.g. septicaemia, malaria)
- neoplasm (e.g. mucin-secreting adenocarcinoma, acute leukaemia)
- tissue trauma (e.g. burns, major accidental trauma, major surgery, shock, intravascular haemolysis, dissecting aortic aneurysm)
- obstetric complications (e.g. abruptio placentae, retained dead fetus, amniotic fluid embolism, toxaemia)
- liver disease.

Thus, in obstetric disorders, tissue factor release into the maternal circulation from the placenta or fetus,

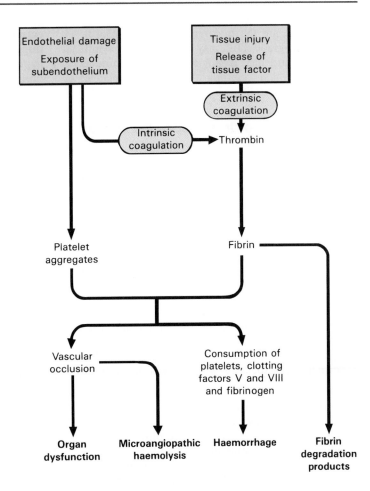

Fig. 23.41   The pathogenesis of disseminated intravascular coagulation

or in amniotic fluid, may trigger coagulation. Many tumours are also rich in procoagulant substances. Septicaemia may cause coagulation activation by damage to vascular endothelium.

The fibrinolytic system is activated in DIC and plasmin generated. This plasmin may attack fibrinogen and coagulation factors V and VIII as well as fibrin. Digestion of fibrin and fibrinogen generates split products (fibrinogen and fibrin degradation products; FDP) which themselves have an anticoagulant and anti-platelet effect and contribute to the haemorrhagic diathesis (Fig. 23.41).

Thrombi, composed of platelets and fibrin, may be found in the microvasculature of brain, lungs, kidneys, heart, spleen and liver. Other organs may also be affected. The distribution of affected organs is variable. Micro-infarcts or more major areas of infarction such as renal cortical necrosis or hepatic necrosis may result. Areas of haemorrhage may also be apparent histologically and on gross examination; any organ may be affected.

The blood platelet count is often low and the clotting times prolonged. Fibrinogen concentration is reduced. Coagulation factors V and VIII are consumed during fibrin generation and also attacked by plasmin, and plasma levels may be severely reduced. FDP are present in high concentration. Red cells become damaged as they are forced through partially occluded small vessels, and the blood changes of a microangiopathic haemolytic anaemia may be present. The above changes are present in florid DIC. In some cases the course is more chronic and the blood changes considerably more subtle.

Clinical features. These include haemorrhage, which may be torrential, organ dysfunction due to ischaemia, and haemolytic anaemia. Bleeding is from mucous membranes, and into skin, serosal cavities and internal organs. Organ dysfunction may manifest as hepatic or renal failure, neurological disturbance or cardiac and respiratory failure. In some cases a predominantly haemorrhagic picture dominates; in others, thrombotic peripheral ischaemia and gangrene are the major features (Fig. 23.42). Chronic 'low-grade' DIC may be only mildly symptomatic. Treatment is largely removal of the underlying cause and clotting factor and platelet replacement. Mortality is high in severe cases.

Coagulation disorders associated with a thrombotic tendency

Control mechanisms for the prevention of inappropriate fibrin deposition are an important feature of the coagulation system. These mechanisms include the rapid lysis of fibrin by plasmin generated at the site of a thrombus, neutralisation of thrombin by antithrombin III, and inactivation of factors V and VIII by protein C with its co-factor, protein S (Fig. 23.8). Hereditary defects of these control mechanisms have been described which lead to a life-long tendency to thrombosis—*thrombophilia*. The thrombosis is usually in the venous system: deep venous thrombosis of the limbs and pulmonary embolism. Thrombotic events rarely manifest before adulthood. The recognised familial abnormalities associated with such a thrombotic tendency are:

- *antithrombin III deficiency* resulting in failure of thrombin neutralisation
- *protein C and protein S deficiency* resulting in failure of neutralisation of activated V and VIII
- *activated protein C resistance*, where a point mutation in the factor V gene leads to synthesis of a factor V variant which has normal procoagulant activity but which is not inhibited by activated protein C; this is the commonest

currently identified cause of familial thrombophilia
- *dysfibrinogenaemia* resulting in abnormal fibrinogen.

Individuals with antithrombin III deficiency are usually heterozygous for the defect. Over 30 mutations leading to deficiency of the protein have been discovered, mostly caused by frameshifts or base changes resulting in a protein that is not secreted or is rapidly removed from the circulation. This type of deficiency is designated 'Type 1'. In Type 2 a dysfunctional protein is produced due to one of several single base changes which alter the amino acid sequence of the synthesised antithrombin III.

Subjects deficient in protein C and protein S are also heterozygous, the homozygous condition producing a severe thrombotic disease often manifesting in the neonate. Type 1 and Type 2 (dysfunctional) defects are also found in protein C deficiency. Point mutations in the gene for protein C have been identified.

Acquired coagulation disorders causing thrombosis are also recognised. In systemic lupus erythematosus (SLE) a predisposition to arterial and venous thrombosis is associated with a paradoxical prolongation of clotting times in vitro, apparently due to the development of auto-antibodies which interact with phospholipid-bound proteins involved in coagulation activation (anti-phospholipid antibodies). These antibodies are also occasionally associated with major thrombotic disease in subjects without other evidence of SLE. Women with such antibodies are prone to pregnancy failure due to recurrent miscarriage, possibly secondary to placental thrombosis. The term

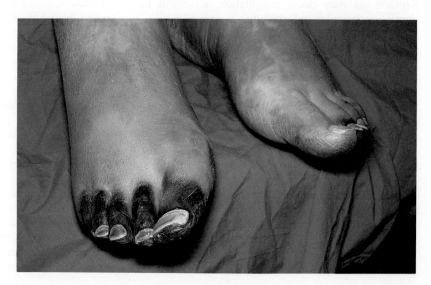

Fig. 23.42 Disseminated intravascular coagulation

There is peripheral gangrene due to small vessel thrombosis.

'*antiphospholipid syndrome*' describes these patients with thrombosis or pregnancy failure associated with antiphospholipid antibody.

ANTENATAL DIAGNOSIS OF BLOOD DISORDERS

Several of the more serious haematological disorders can be diagnosed in the fetus. Fetal blood can be obtained from the placenta or umbilical vein with imaging using ultrasound scanning techniques. This material can be used for detection of abnormalities of red cells, white cells or platelets and for diagnosis of clotting factor deficiencies. For example, thalassaemia can be identified by measuring relative rates of globin chain synthesis. Alternatively amniotic fluid cells can be obtained by aspiration of the amniotic fluid, and techniques have been developed by which fetal material can be safely obtained by biopsy of chorionic villi, this being performed as early as 9–11 weeks' gestation.

Fetal DNA can be analysed by restriction endonuclease mapping and RFLP linkage analysis. More recently the application of PCR technology and use of oligonucleotide probes has allowed the very early and rapid diagnosis of haematological disorders. Using these techniques first-trimester prenatal diagnosis of β-thalassaemias and of haemophilia has become possible. Gene probes for the diagnosis of red cell enzyme defects are also becoming available.

BLOOD TRANSFUSION

Donor blood, or fractions of blood, can be safely and beneficially administered intravenously. Transfusion of red cells is valuable in the management of some anaemias and in resuscitation after acute haemorrhage and is essential for the safe performance of many surgical procedures. Other cellular components of blood, especially platelets, can be usefully transfused, for example to treat bleeding in severely thrombocytopenic subjects. Blood plasma is fractionated to provide albumin, immunoglobulin and coagulation factors.

In red cell transfusion it is essential that compatibility is ensured between antigens on the donor erythrocytes and antibodies present in the recipient's plasma in order to avoid acute haemolysis of the donor cells which may be fatal. The cross-match procedure is used to determine compatibility.

Red cell antigens and antibodies

Although there are about 400 red blood cell antigens, most inherited in Mendelian dominant fashion, only a minority are clinically important. An individual lacking a particular antigen may develop an antibody after exposure to red cells carrying the antigen. Exposure occurs by transfusion of red cells or by passage of fetal red cells into the maternal circulation during pregnancy, the fetal cells carrying paternal antigens foreign to the mother. The clinical consequences of the development of such an 'immune' antibody are the development of a *haemolytic transfusion reaction* on further exposure to red cells carrying the antigen, and *haemolytic disease of the newborn* due to transplacental passage of maternal IgG antibody against fetal red cell antigens (p. 719).

The most important '*immune*' antibody is anti-D, an antibody to the major antigen of the rhesus blood group system (Table 23.11). It is a major cause of haemolytic disease of the newborn.

Table 23.11 The rhesus blood group system

Allelic genes at closely linked loci code for paired antigens designated C and c, E and e and D. Absence of D is termed d. A set of genes and hence antigens is inherited from each parent and the presence of D determines rhesus 'positivity'.

Genotype	Rhesus status	% Frequency (UK)
cde\cde	Negative	15
CDe\cde	Positive	32
CDe\CDe	Positive	17
cDe\cde	Positive	13
CDe\cDE	Positive	14
Others	Positive	9

Table 23.12 The ABO blood group system

There are three allelic genes: A, B and O. A and B genes control the synthesis of enzymes which modify the red cell membrane glycolipid. The unmodified molecule is known as H substance and is not modified in the presence of the O gene alone, which is an amorph. Thus there are 6 genotypes and 4 phenotypes.

Genotype	Phenotype	Natural antibodies	% Phenotypic frequency (UK)
OO	O	Anti-A, -B	46
AA or AO	A	Anti-B	42
BB or BO	B	Anti-A	9
AB	AB	None	3

As well as 'immune' antibodies, '*naturally occurring*' antibodies to red cell antigens are also important. In contrast to the IgG immune antibodies, they are predominantly IgM and require no previous red cell antigen exposure. They occur in the ABO blood group system, where naturally occurring anti-A and anti-B are present in subjects whose red cells lack the corresponding antigen (Table 23.12).

In addition to the ABO and rhesus blood group systems the major red cell antigen systems of clinical importance are Kell, Duffy and Kidd as, with ABO and rhesus, their antibodies are responsible for most cases of haemolytic transfusion reaction and haemolytic disease of the newborn.

Haemolytic transfusion reactions

Immediate reactions

Massive intravascular haemolysis occurs when complement-activating antibodies, such as anti-A and anti-B, interact with the relevant antigen on transfused red cells. There is typically collapse, with hypotension and pain in the lumbar region. Haemoglobin-stained urine may be passed and oliguric renal failure may ensue. Red cells lysis may trigger disseminated intravascular coagulation. This clinical scenario can develop after transfusion with only a few millilitres of incompatible red cells. Treatment includes immediate interruption of the transfusion, resuscitation with intravenous fluid, immunosuppression with corticosteroid therapy and management of the renal failure. Fatalities still occur.

Because antibodies to the rhesus system are not complement-fixing, cell lysis occurs in the reticuloendothelial system and reactions are generally milder, although they can still be life-threatening.

Delayed reactions

Occasionally a low titre antibody is too weak to be detectable in the cross-match and is unable to cause lysis at the time of transfusion. Transfusion of red cells carrying the relevant antigen leads to a gradual increase in the titre of the antibody, developing over a period of a few days. Delayed, gradual red cell lysis occurs producing anaemia and jaundice; this is a delayed transfusion reaction.

The risk of development of a haemolytic transfusion reaction is minimised in practice by matching the ABO and rhesus D type of donor and recipient and the performance of a *cross-match procedure* to detect antibody in the recipient serum. Red cells from each donor unit are tested for agglutination when incubated with the serum of the recipient. A range of techniques is used to maximise the chance of detection of a potentially dangerous antibody:

- incubation of cells in saline and test serum at 37°C: detects clinically significant IgM antibodies — anti-A, anti-B
- prior treatment of the cells with a proteolytic enzyme, e.g. papain, and incubation at 37°C: detects clinically significant IgM antibodies — anti-A, anti-B
- incubation of cells with a low ionic strength saline and test serum at 37°C: detects immune (mainly IgG) antibodies
- performance of an indirect antiglobulin test at 37°C: detects immune (mainly IgG) antibodies

Enzyme treatment and use of a low ionic strength saline improve the sensitivity for detection of some antibodies. The *indirect antiglobulin test* utilises an antihuman immunoglobulin (AHG) reagent prepared by immunising an animal (goat, sheep or rabbit) with human immunoglobulin or complement. A reagent with anti-IgG and anti-C_3d activity is generally employed in the test, which is in two parts. Initially donor red cells are incubated with recipient serum; they are then thoroughly washed and exposed to the AHG. The presence of agglutination at this stage indicates that the cells have become coated with an antibody or complement present in the recipient's serum which is not capable of causing agglutination. The AHG results in cross-linking of immunoglobulin or complement molecules and visible agglutination in the test. The indirect antiglobulin test is thus an essential, sensitive part of the cross-match procedure.

Other adverse effects of transfusion

Most nucleated cells, including leukocytes, carry antigens of the HLA (human leukocyte antigen) or major histocompatibility complex system. Prior exposure to HLA antigens by transfusion or pregnancy may lead to development of antibody capable of causing fever and rigors on subsequent exposure to the antigens present on leukocytes in transfused blood. This can be avoided by using filters to remove donor leukocytes prior to transfusion. Such *non-haemolytic transfusion reactions* are unpleasant but rarely dangerous. Allergic reactions may also develop in a recipient because of hypersensitivity to a protein present in the donor plasma. Fever, urticaria and oedema may result.

Virus transmission by blood transfusion remains a

significant problem. Transmission of hepatitis B, C, other non-A, non-B hepatitis viruses, as well as human immunodeficiency viruses, Epstein–Barr virus and cytomegalovirus can occur. Careful donor selection and screening of donations for antibodies to the viruses have considerably reduced the risk. Some other transmissible infections are syphilis and malaria.

Circulatory overload may result from transfusion of excessive volume. Because bank blood is devoid of functioning platelets, transfusion of large volumes can cause thrombocytopenia and haemorrhage.

Repeated red cell transfusion without blood loss, usually in the management of chronic anaemias such as thalassaemia, inevitably leads to *tissue iron overload*. A unit of blood contains 200 mg of iron, in haemoglobin. Although, initially, deposition occurs in reticulo-endothelial tissues without toxic results, iron later accumulates in skin, liver, myocardium and pancreas. Pigmentation, liver cirrhosis (Ch. 16), heart failure and diabetes mellitus are the consequences. An iron chelating compound, desferrioxamine, is administered by subcutaneous infusion to minimise iron accumulation in tissues.

FURTHER READING

Hoffbrand A V, Lewis S M (eds) 1989 Postgraduate haematology, 3rd edn. Heinemann, Oxford

Hoffbrand A V, Pettit J E (eds) 1993 Essential haematology, 3rd edn. Blackwell Scientific Publications, Oxford

Skin

NORMAL STRUCTURE AND FUNCTION

The two major layers of the skin—the epidermis and dermis—are derived from different embryonic components and retain a radically different morphology (Fig. 24.1). The epidermis is highly cellular, avascular, lacks nerves, sits on a basement membrane and shows marked vertical stratification (Fig. 24.2). It produces a highly complex mixture of proteins collectively termed *keratin*. A series of highly specialised *adnexa* extend from the epidermis into the dermis. The density of these adnexa varies from site to site on the body as does the thickness of the epidermis and the structure of the keratin layer. This site-to-site variation means that the histological interpretation of diagnostic biopsies has to take into account the area of the body from which the biopsy originally came; what may constitute severe hyperkeratosis (excess keratin) on the forehead may be normal for the sole of the foot.

Although the epidermis consists mostly of epithelial cells in various stages of maturation, from the mitotic pool in the basal layer through the various post-mitotic squamous cells to fully-formed keratin, there are other, non-epithelial, cells present. Some of these cells are dendritic, like the melanocytes described below, but they contain no melanin; indeed, these cells—

Langerhans' cells—were for a long while thought to be exhausted melanocytes. Their function is to present antigen to lymphocytes; they are probably members of the monocyte/macrophage series. They contain a sub-cellular organelle found in no other cell—the Birbeck granule—and similar cells are found in the lymph node presenting antigen to T-lymphocytes, and in the thymus, also in intimate contact with lymphocytes. Indeed, there are many similarities between skin and thymus: the thymus contains keratinised structures and Hassall's corpuscles, and the same mutation that results in athymic mice also renders them hairless ('nude' mice).

The *dermis* is relatively acellular and is recognisably divided into two zones: the outer zone consists of those areas which extend upwards between the downward projecting rete ridges ('pegs') of the epidermis and is called the *papillary dermis*; beneath this zone is the *reticular dermis*. Both regions of the dermis contain blood and lymph vessels as well as nerves. The intervening connective tissue consists of the characteristic dermal proteins collagen and elastin, together with various glycosaminoglycans. These proteins and complex carbohydrates are secreted by the principal cells of the dermis, the fibroblasts. Although the proteins of the dermis appear to be arranged in an haphazard fashion when viewed in standard histological preparations, they

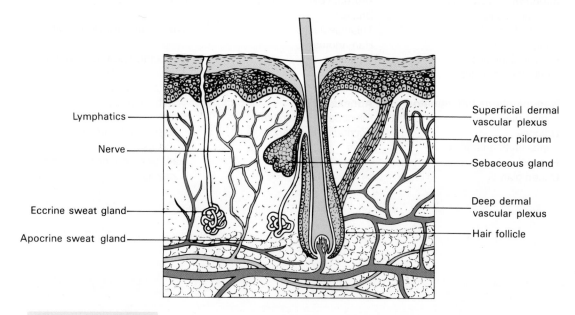

Lymphatics

Nerve

Eccrine sweat gland

Apocrine sweat gland

Superficial dermal vascular plexus

Arrector pilorum

Sebaceous gland

Deep dermal vascular plexus

Hair follicle

Fig. 24.1 Normal skin

There are two main regions: the cellular epidermis with adnexal extensions into the relatively acellular dermis. Notice that there are no blood vessels, lymphatics or nerves in the epidermis.

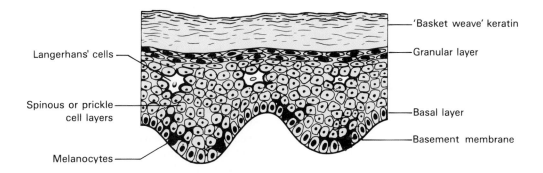

Fig. 24.2 Normal epidermis

The cells in the basal layer divide and a daughter cell progresses through the epidermis and eventually dies and contributes to the outer, keratin layer. At the base there are dendritic melanocytes producing and donating pigment to surrounding epidermal cells. Scattered through the epidermis are dendritic Langerhans' cells which are part of the antigen-presenting system of the body.

are in fact arranged in specific patterns that are characteristic of different sites in the body; these patterns are the *Langer's lines*. The significance of this knowledge is that if incisions are made in the skin along the long axis of the dermal collagen fibres then little permanent scarring will occur. If, however, incisions are made across the fibres and disrupt them, then in the effort to repair the damage scarring is bound to result. A considerable part of the surgeon's skill relies on knowing the characteristic orientation of these fibres and in making incisions that generate the minimum risk of permanent scars. Scattered within the dermis and often clustered about blood vessels are the *mast cells*. The nerves of the dermis approach close to the epidermis and often end in specialised sensory structures such as *Paccinian corpuscles*. Similarly, the dermal blood vessels run close to the underside of the epidermis although they are organised into two recognisable structures — the *superficial* and *deep vascular plexuses*.

At the dermo-epidermal junction are pigmented dendritic cells — the *melanocytes*. There is about one to every six basal epithelial cells, regardless of race or degree of pigmentation. On electron microscopy, their dendritic processes can be seen to be closely applied to the surrounding basal cells, to which they transfer packets of pre-formed *melanin*. The melanin forms a cap over the nucleus, protecting it from damage by sunlight.

Below the dermis is a layer of fat (panniculus adiposus) and in most mammals, but not in man, there is also a layer of muscle (panniculus carnosus). In man, the only remnants of this are the platysma muscle in the neck and the dartos muscle in the scrotum; strangely, the former is a voluntary skeletal muscle whilst the latter is an involuntary muscle.

The function of these muscles is to move the skin. The only other muscles found in human skin are those associated with hair follicles — the *arrector pili*.

Skin as a barrier

The most important function of the skin is to serve as a barrier between the individual and the external environment. It is this barrier that some parasites must overcome if they wish to gain access to the individual's internal environment, and it is this barrier that has been breached when the contents of the body leak out following penetrating wounds. But the barrier has more subtle properties. It is possible to measure so-called insensible perspirations (the inapparent water loss that occurs continuously across the skin) and to follow this perspiration as successive layers are stripped off. This experiment can be done by pressing adhesive tape onto the skin surface and pulling it off again; this process progessively removes the surface layers of the skin without doing any other damage. As successive layers are stripped off, the insensible perspiration increases slowly, but at a certain point there is a sudden sharp rise in water loss as the functional water barrier is breached. This result shows that there is a discrete water barrier within the epidermis and that transepidermal water loss is not just a function of the thickness of the stratum corneum as a whole. This finding is important because burns victims die of their loss of barrier function through water loss and bacterial invasion.

The other way in which the barrier is often breached is at the weak points where there are natural holes in the barrier, such as the sweat glands and hair ducts. Organisms may use these portals of entry, just as the large-scale communications between the inside and outside (such as the mouth, anus, genital and urinary orifices) provide common routes of entry for infection.

Eczema and immersion: failure of the barrier

The barrier function of the skin can be either damaged (resulting in eczema) or overwhelmed (by immersion).

Eczema

> ▶ A reaction pattern, not a disease
> ▶ Many causes
> ▶ Varied clinical patterns
> ▶ Characterised histologically by inflammation and spongiosis

The word *eczema* comes from the Greek meaning to 'bubble up'; this meaning conveys well the clinical development of the lesions. The skin becomes reddened and tiny vesicles may develop (pompholyx); the surface develops scales, and cracking and bleeding can cause great discomfort (Fig. 24.3). The skin becomes tender and secondary infection may occur. The clinical pattern is very varied and there are many different types of eczema. Sometimes the variation is due to the cause of the eczema, such as contact with a toxic or allergenic material; sometimes the site of the lesion or the age of the patient is sufficient to make the disease a clinical entity. For example, chromate hypersensitivity causes eczema in cement workers and infantile eczema occurs in atopic babies. Whatever the cause, the underlying pathological processes are recognisably similar and can be seen as a stereotyped reaction pattern to a variety of different stimuli.

The earliest histological change in eczema is swelling within the epidermis (Fig. 24.4). This swelling is due to separation of the keratinocytes by fluid accumulating between them. Since the keratinocytes are held together by desmosomes, the connections are stressed and the prickles in the prickle cell layer become more obvious. This appearance is known as *spongiosis*. Later, there may be hyperkeratosis (an increase in the volume of the stratum corneum), which gives rise to the clinical scales, and various degrees of inflammation, which give rise to the classical inflammatory signs and symptoms (Ch. 10). In severe cases the intra-epidermal oedema may be sufficiently pronounced for the desmosomes to give way in some areas; the intercellular oedema can then join up to form foci of fluid within the epidermis recognised clinically as 'water blisters' or *pompholyx* (Fig. 24.5).

In all forms of eczema the barrier is destroyed and water loss can occur, but material can also pass the other way and allergens may enter the skin, elicit an allergic response and produce a superimposed allergic eczema. People with longstanding eczema commonly have hypersensitivities to numerous materials which the eczema has allowed to penetrate, particularly medicaments which have been used to treat it!

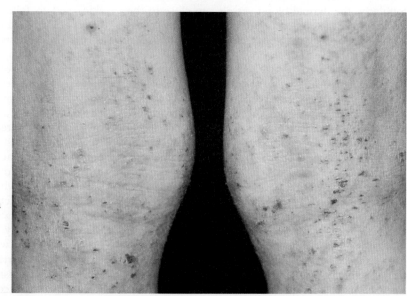

Fig. 24.3 Eczema

This scaly skin eruption can occur as a reaction to many triggering factors. There is marked oedema within the epidermis and the lesions are often very itchy. This is a case of atopic eczema, in which there is an inherent predisposition to eczema as well as to allergic rhinitis and asthma.

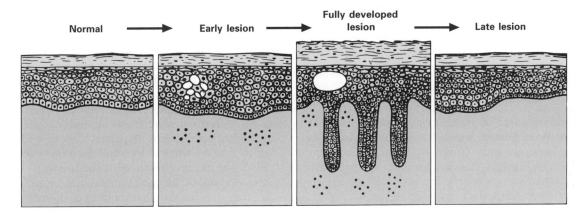

Fig. 24.4 Eczema

This inflammatory skin condition may have a great variety of precipitating factors. The progression from normal skin to healed lesion is shown diagrammatically from left to right.

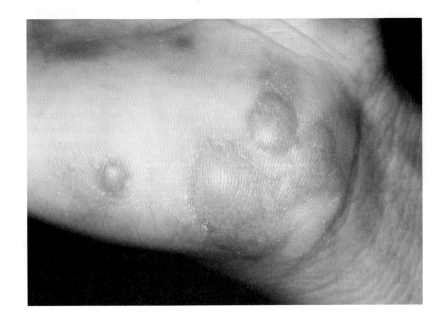

Fig. 24.5 Pompholyx

The extreme form of epidermal oedema (spongiosis) can express itself as intra-epidermal blisters.

Immersion

► Prolonged immersion may overwhelm the barrier
► May be used for topical therapy

The barrier function of the skin, although efficient, can be overwhelmed; this occurs after prolonged immersion. The extreme form of this can be seen in corpses recovered from water, in which the bloating due to decomposition is added to by the influx of water due to osmotic forces when the skin breaks down. Localised swelling can be seen following occlusive dressings for burns or under surgical dressings. Use is made of this phenomenon of breakdown of the skin barrier in the use of topical pharmacological agents beneath occlusive dressings which aid penetration.

Various groups of patients are occupationally exposed to immersion; the most common are housewives. They are in daily skin contact with large amounts of water, often containing agents capable of removing the skin barrier, such as detergents. This situation has led to the development of numerous synthetic barrier creams, containing water repellents such as silicone, which mimic the action of the physiological barrier.

CLINICAL ASPECTS OF SKIN DISEASES

Any component of the skin can be affected by any category of disease, whether it be inflammatory or neoplastic, but some components are affected more often and more characteristically by particular processes than are others. For instance, the epidermis frequently produces tumours of various degrees of malignancy, whilst a malignant tumour of the sweat glands is a rarity. Similarly, with age, some diseases are more likely than others: blisters in the young are likely to be infective, in the adult they are likely to be dermatitis herpetiformis, while in the elderly they are more likely to be pemphigoid. However, mere statistics are no substitute for proper pathological evaluation and it is with this evaluation that the subsequent sections in this chapter are concerned.

There are several reasons why the skin seems to produce such a wide variety of pathological conditions. One reason is that it is so visible: conditions that cause no actual disability would, if they occurred in the liver for instance, never cause a patient to present to their doctor, but are apparent and significant on the skin. Benign blemishes of the skin may be a source of great social distress and stigma, and may drive patients to commit suicide over a painless, non-progressive lesion of merely academic pathological significance. A person's appearance is often all that we know of him and the quality of the skin is a major contribution to his appearance.

A second reason for the complexity and variety of skin diseases is the fact that the skin comprises two distinct organs welded together, so that there are diseases of the epidermis, diseases of the dermis and diseases of the relationship between the two organs.

Added to all of this are the effects of the mechanical, chemical, thermal, radiant, parasitic, cosmetic and therapeutic environments. The skin is routinely beaten, burned, painted, tattooed and injected in a way that no other organ would, or could, tolerate. Its appendages are dyed, permed, deodorised and varnished in accordance with fluctuations in fashion; new generations of micro-organisms attack it daily and it is torn and plundered in the surgeon's incessant hunt for internal disease.

The great advantages of the skin from the pathologist's point of view are that the gross pathology is always visible and does not have to be inferred from stethoscopes, X-rays or ultrasound, and that its accessibility means that it can be readily biopsied.

Incidence of skin diseases

Skin diseases, like all diseases, vary in their distribution according to a wide range of factors (Table 24.1), but they also vary markedly in the experience of particular doctors. A hospital dermatologist running a pigmented skin lesion clinic will see many melanomas in a year, depending on the population make-up of the catchment area and its size, whereas a community physician in the same area may expect to see only one every two years. A dermatologist will see only exceptional cases of acne and very occasional cases of pityriasis rosea but a community physician will see numerous cases of both. With these reservations in mind, skin diseases can be categorised according to their frequency:

- common — acne, psoriasis, eczema, varicose leg ulcers, basal cell carcinoma, squamous cell carcinoma

Pathological basis of dermatological signs and symptoms	
Clinical sign	Pathological basis
Scaling	Hyperkeratosis, parakeratosis
Erythema	Dilatation of skin vessels
Blisters	Separation of layers of the epidermis or epidermis from dermis
Bruising	Leakage of blood into dermis
Pigmentation	Increased activity of melanocytes Increased numbers of melanocytes Endogenous pigment, e.g. ochronosis Exogenous pigment, e.g. tattoo
Plaques	Increase in epidermal thickness
Nodules	Epidermal tumours Adnexal tumours Dermal tumours (fibroblasts, vessels, etc.)
Rashes restricted to exposed areas	Photosensitivity Contact eczema
Nail abnormalities	Trauma to nail bed Psoriasis Systemic poisons

Table 24.1 Incidence of skin diseases

Variable	Associations
Age	Impetigo in children Acne in adolescence Pemphigus in old age
Sex	Acne commoner in boys Bullous pemphigoid of pregnancy ('herpes gestationis')
Anatomical site	Psoriasis and dermatitis herpetiformis common on elbows and knees Atopic eczema (lichenified) antecubital fossae Scabies in finger webs
Geography	Parasites in developing world Psoriasis in Faroe Islands (inbred community)
Exposure	Basal cell carcinoma and squamous cell carcinoma common on sun-exposed sites Basal cell carcinoma in arsenic exposure common on covered sites
Race	Basal cell carcinoma and squamous cell carcinoma and melanoma rare in blacks (protected by pigmentation)

- uncommon — pemphigoid, pemphigus, melanoma, scabies
- rare — xeroderma pigmentosum, dermatitis artefacta, mycosis fungoides.

DISORDERS INVOLVING INFLAMMATORY CELLS

Many of the characteristics of inflammation (Ch. 10) were first observed and studied in the skin. The various phases and types of inflammation are characterised by a particular spectrum of cells which mediates the inflammatory response. Because the types of cells in a particular lesion are there in response to the initiating factor, then a careful analysis of the composition of a particular lesion will significantly narrow down the differential diagnosis. Thus, cuffing of vessels by plasma cells would strongly suggest syphilis; the presence of granulomas with caseous centres would suggest tuberculosis, even if the clinical picture strongly suggested eczema; all three lesions are inflamed clinically.

Because inflammatory cells must enter tissues from the blood stream, the epidermis, which lacks blood vessels, must receive its inflammatory infiltrate

secondarily from the dermis. The only cells that are an exception in this situation are the Langerhans' cells — dendritic epidermal cells related to the monocyte/macrophage series and first described by Paul Langerhans when a medical student. These antigen-presenting cells are normally resident in the epidermis. Obviously, in the epidermis they are in a prime position to encounter new antigens and it is believed that Langerhans' cells are intimately involved in the development of those contact hypersensitivities whose clinical expression is eczema.

In most cases, the presence of inflammatory cells in the skin in significant numbers has the usual significance of inflammation; namely, there is some foreign substance or organism present that the body is reacting to and attempting to eliminate. However, as in most other body sites, there can also be an aberrant response by the body where an inflammatory reaction occurs without apparent justification, as in the case of autoimmunity. In other cases, there is inflammation with no foreign material and no evidence of autoimmunity, as in psoriasis. In other cases, the inflammatory cells themselves may become abnormal and the skin may become the site for neoplastic lesions composed of these cells.

Polymorph infiltrates

- ▶ Pustules contain polymorphs and debris
- ▶ May contain organisms (impetigo)
- ▶ May be sterile (psoriasis)

Neutrophil polymorphs can accumulate in the skin in response to infection by pyogenic bacteria (e.g. *Staphylococcus aureus*) as in *impetigo* (p. 755).

Several conditions are characterised by polymorph infiltrations although no infective process can be identified. *Psoriasis* is a very common disease which is thought to be a disorder of epidermal maturation and keratin formation and is considered fully below (p. 758). However, psoriasis is also characterised by neutrophil migration from dilated superficial dermal vessels in such numbers that the disease may sometimes be dominated by the presence of numerous sterile pustules within the epidermis (pustular psoriasis).

Some diseases, such as *Sweet's disease* and *pyoderma gangrenosum* (skin lesions which may occur in association with various internal diseases such as chronic inflammatory bowel diseases; Ch. 15), show massive infiltration by polymorph neutrophils in the dermis with no clue as to what attracts them there.

In some cases, polymorphs are attracted by the

deposition of auto-antibodies (Ch. 9) and in these cases the resulting damage often causes blistering, or bullae. Antibodies to the basement membrane on which the epidermis sits and to the desmosome complexes that hold epidermal cells to one another cause *dermatitis herpetiformis* and *pemphigus* respectively (see below). The presence of one type of polymorph rather than another suggests different aetiological processes and dermatitis herpetiformis can sometimes be distinguished from bullous pemphigoid by the relative excess of neutrophil polymorphs in the former and eosinophil polymorphs in the latter.

Very rarely, deposits of leukaemia cells may occur in the skin, but the cells are immature and generally do not resemble those seen within inflammatory pustules.

Lymphocytic infiltrates

> ▶ Most chronic skin lesions contain lymphocytes
> ▶ Eczema is characterised by lymphocytes
> ▶ Neoplastic lymphoid lesions can be primary or secondary

Any chronic inflammation of the skin will eventually come to be dominated by lymphocytes, but there are many skin conditions that are primarily due to lymphocyte accumulation and whose distinctive clinical character is due to the disposition and behaviour of these cells.

In *eczema* the epidermis is penetrated by lymphocytes that eventually can accumulate in sufficient numbers to form an intra-epidermal abscess. In *lupus erythematosus* the lymphocytes cluster about the hair follicles and the base of the epidermis and nibble them away, resulting in atrophy of the skin and scarring alopecia (baldness). In other cases, such as *lichen planus*, the attack on the base of the epidermis can be so aggressive that it begins to separate from the dermis, causing blistering. Sometimes the lymphocytes occur in diffuse patches or in dense nodules and the clinical appearance is of a nodular rash or of intradermal tumours. This last group is very difficult to classify and includes a number of initially benign conditions which have a fairly high rate of conversion into lymphomas.

Cutaneous lymphomas

Secondary deposits of systemic lymphomas and primary lymphomas may arise within the skin. Both are relatively rare. Any of the lymphomas and leukaemias that occur systemically (Ch. 22) can give secondary deposits in the skin, but usually only in advanced cases. The primary lymphomas include *mycosis fungoides* which is a T-cell lymphoma and which, as it develops, can spill over into the blood to give an associated T-cell leukaemia, the association being called the *Sézary syndrome*.

Mycosis fungoides provides a good example of the progression of a malignant lymphoid condition. Initially, the infiltrate is sparse and the only clinical sign is a reddening of the skin, mainly due to the dilated vessels. This reddening gives the clinical picture that used to be called 'l'homme rouge' (the red man). As the lymphocytes begin to accumulate, raised plaques become visible on the skin. These become more and more pronounced until they form frank, ulcerating tumour nodules.

INFECTIONS

Infections must penetrate the skin surface or come from within the body. The clinical appearance depends on:

- site within the skin
- nature of the organism
- nature of the body's response to the organism.

There are two routes by which infection may arrive in the skin:

1. internally via some route such as the blood stream
2. externally by penetrating the skin barrier.

In practice, most infections arise via the latter route. Another possible mechanism whereby infections can cause skin lesions is where the organism infects some other part of the body and produces a skin rash in which it is impossible to identify any organisms; this mechanism occurs in acute rheumatic fever for instance and is parallel to the effects on the heart also seen in this condition (Ch. 13).

Infections may be due to a variety of different organisms — fungi, viruses, bacteria, protozoa and various metazoa. Many organisms live on or even in the skin but cause no harm to the host: these are called *commensals*, or, if they merely consume dead material, they may be called *saprophytes*.

The precise clinical nature of an infective skin disease depends not only on the nature of the infecting organism, but also on the precise nature of the host response to it; such a response has usually evolved over millions of years and represents some balance of survival strategies that permits the disease to continue without either of the partners in the relationship becoming extinct. Old diseases tend to be chronic and endemic; new ones are often fulminant and epidemic.

Viral infections

Viruses are obligate intracellular parasites that usurp the replicative processes of the cell for their own replication. In the skin, they tend to parasitise the metabolically active basal cells of the epidermis which are producing new DNA and RNA; these processes are taken over by the virus for its own reproduction. The actual assembling and packaging of total virions occurs higher in the epidermis and this process is complete by the time they reach the surface, where they are released to be passed on to another host. Consequently, they are easiest to detect in the upper layers of the epidermis where they are fully formed and present in large numbers.

- *Human papillomavirus* (HPV) (a DNA virus of which there are more than 30 subtypes so far described) has attracted a lot of attention because of its role in the production of cancers of the skin in lower animals and its possible role in the development of cervical cancer in the human (Chs 11 and 19). In human skin these viruses are responsible for the various warts or *verrucae*. The precise clinical appearance of the wart depends on the particular HPV type concerned and the body site involved. The keratotic, exophytic growths of *verrucae vulgaris* may occur anywhere on the skin or oral mucosa while the flat *verruca plana* occurs more commonly on the face and the backs of hands. Another form, *verruca palmaris* or *plantaris* is much deeper and causes the bothersome lesions on the soles of the feet of children and of industrial workers who share communal washing facilities. Genital warts are large, fleshy polyps called *condyloma acuminatum* and are located at those sites where person-to-person contact is most likely to promote effective spread. So far no HPV has been firmly implicated in human skin cancers although such mechanisms are well established in other mammals.
- *Molluscum contagiosum* is a very characteristic umbilicated lesion produced by a DNA pox virus.
- *Herpes viruses* are DNA viruses responsible for a vast range of systemic diseases, of which several are classically viewed as skin diseases. Herpes zoster virus is responsible for the relatively benign infectious disease of childhood known as *chickenpox*, but it can also take refuge in the dorsal root ganglia and lie dormant for many years. As the patients become older and develop some degree of

immune paresis, or if they develop some disease that produces or is treated by immunosuppression, the virus may escape its host restraints, travel down the nerves and manifest as *shingles*. This is a rash of herpetic blisters in a single nerve root distribution with a severe pain and discomfort that may persist even after the blisters have healed and the viruses returned to their ganglionic hiding place.
- Other herpes viruses are responsible for *cold sores* (HSV1) and for *genital herpes* (HSV2). The great problem with these kinds of herpetic infections is that they are infections for life.

Bacterial infections

Bacteria are responsible for a wide range of skin infections.

- *Impetigo* is a staphylococcal infection in young children but is more commonly streptococcal in older patients. The organisms penetrate only a little way into the epidermis and form subcorneal pustules (collections of pus just beneath the stratum corneum). Underneath the epidermis, the dermal vessels are dilated and the upper dermis contains some polymorphs migrating from the oedematous (spongiotic) deep epidermis on their way to the site of the action. Because the pustules are so superficial, they rupture rapidly and the clinical picture of impetigo is a mixture of yellow pustules and crusted lesions, usually in a child. A complication in the streptococcal lesions is an immune reaction resulting in glomerulonephritis about 3 weeks after the onset of the skin rash. This reaction is thought to be the body's antibody response to an antigen in the kidney that cross-reacts with a streptococcal antigen.
- *Cellulitis* is often caused by *Streptococcus pyogenes* and its particular mode of spread within the superficial dermis results from its production of a 'spreading factor' (hyaluronidase) that enzymatically breaks down the connective tissue of the dermis and allows the organism to spread. The affected area is diffusely swollen, red and painful, thus demonstrating the cardinal features of acute inflammation (Fig. 10.1, Ch. 10). The rapidly progressive and often fatal condition of *necrotising fasciitis* is due to mixed synergistic bacterial infections.
- *Abscesses* of various sorts occur in the skin as elsewhere, but their clinical picture often depends upon the adnexa involved; a *furuncle* is a deep abscess of a single hair follicle, often with extensive necrosis, while a *carbuncle* involves several contiguous hair follicles. Obviously, the hair follicle

is an effective hole in the skin barrier and so it comes as no surprise that bacteria may use it as a portal of entry into the skin.

- *Tuberculosis* of the skin ('lupus vulgaris') is uncommon in developed countries but still occurs. Often the presentation is atypical and unsuspected, resulting in misdiagnosis. The offending organism may be either the human form of *Mycobacterium tuberculosis* or the bovine organism *Mycobacterium bovis*. A classical presentation is involvement of the overlying skin from a subcutaneous tuberculous lymph node, a condition which glories in the name of *scrofuloderma*. The basic pathology is of typical caseous granulomas as described in Chapter 10.
- *Leprosy* is still a cause of considerable morbidity worldwide: estimates suggest about 10 million patients in total. In developed countries the disease is very rare and usually imported. It is caused by *Mycobacterium leprae* and a variety of clinical forms are described. The differences between these clinical forms are determined by the host immune response. In *lepromatous leprosy* the host seems to mount little response to the infection and bacteria are numerous in the skin and in nasal secretions. In the *tuberculoid* form the host develops a strong immunological reaction and the lesions tend to contain very few organisms and eventually heal spontaneously. The lepromatous form is often progressive and lethal since the host is not mounting an effective response. However, in the tuberculoid form, it is the immune response itself which destroys tissues and nerves to produce the classical, mutilated leonine facies and auto-amputations of digits that have caused lepers to be so feared and shunned.

Fungal infections

Various fungi attack the skin, usually living in the upper keratinised layers and spreading outwards in a ring of erythematous scaling dermatitis that is commonly known as *ringworm*. In other sites the lesions are somewhat different in appearance: between the toes the lesions appear as *athlete's foot*, and in the groins as *tinea cruris*. The organisms responsible for these infections vary but the commonest are various *Trichophyton* species.

Pityrosporum species are responsible for various superficial fungal infections of the skin; the most common is *tinea versicolor* in which pigment changes are very characteristic.

A different type of organism, *Candida*, which is a yeast, is responsible for another group of fungal infestations, most commonly of mucosal and adjacent areas. This infection causes the clinical condition of *thrush*, commonly seen in babies' mouths and in the vagina. When the infection spreads on to the adjacent skin it can produce a painful blistering eruption not immediately recognisable as a fungal rash. Somewhat more rarely, candida can affect the nails, where it causes considerable deformity and is very difficult to eradicate.

Fungal lesions are rarely biopsied because they are usually diagnosed clinically. Histologically, they often present a very bland appearance with routine stains; the fungi are revealed only when stains that react with their cell walls are used, such as silver stains or stains for neutral polysaccharides (periodic acid Schiff: PAS). Under these circumstances the diagnosis is achieved only when the pathologist is alerted by the clinical history, illustrating the importance of providing full clinical details with all biopsies.

Deeper fungal infections tend to cause chronic abscesses, often with severe destruction. They are common in tropical conditions but are also seen particularly as opportunistic infections in the immunosuppressed. Blastomyces, actinomyces and nocardia may all be encountered now outside their traditional endemic areas due to foreign travel and immunosuppression.

Protozoal infections

Protozoal infections are rare in temperate climates, but worldwide *amoebiasis, trypanosomiasis, leishmaniasis* and *toxoplasmosis* account for a formidable volume of suffering and in some areas of the world will be the predominant dermatological conditions encountered by physicians. Many of these conditions, like many other tropical diseases, are spread by arthropod parasites and the most effective means of control has proven to be elimination of the vector rather than treatment of the disease.

Leishmaniasis is an infection caused by *Leishmania tropica* which is transmitted by sandflies. The organisms have developed a mechanism for subverting the body's defences and can be found living in abundance within the host macrophages.

Metazoan parasites

Metazoan parasites are mainly worms or arthropods; the former tend to invade and parasitise, while the latter are more common as 'predators'. The worms are again a tropical problem primarily and *onchocerciasis, larva migrans, strongyloidiasis, ancylostomiasis, filariasis* and *schistosomiasis* have often determined where man and his livestock can and cannot survive in many tropical regions. Again, the skin presentations of these lesions may be spectacular and may form a dominant proportion of tropical dermatological practice.

Apart from the arthropod vectors of disease, many of these ubiquitous animals live in intimate contact with human hosts; fleas, bedbugs and lice have generated a huge technical and popular literature. There are poems, operatic songs and books of philosophical speculation devoted to the flea, not to mention the blame for spreading the Black Death; other pests are only slightly less celebrated. The louse lives on its human host and attaches its eggs to the hair, where they are seen as small bead-like 'nits'. The scabies mite is recorded in Anglo-Saxon poetry and burrows into the skin, leaving a little track by which its progress can be observed; when a pin is stuck into the end of the track the mite clings to the tip and can be extracted to demonstrate the infestation, a performance which never fails to enliven a dermatology clinic. Some little mites (*Demodex folliculorum*) have adapted so well to living within the hair follicle that they can be found in the majority of the normal population living as simple commensals and, as far as we know, causing no host response and therefore no disease. The house dust mite, on the other hand, lives free in our bed linen in even the cleanest homes and ekes out a blameless existence consuming shed keratin skin flakes. However, the end products of this diet are excreted into our environment and, in susceptible individuals, produce the chronic skin rash of atopic dermatitis mediated by a hypersensitivity response.

However, man and arthropods have been co-existing for many millions of years and although these creatures are responsible for a great volume of human misery, it is not in their interests to kill us off; the same is not necessarily true of our attitudes towards them, or indeed to any of the organisms which parasitise us.

NON-INFECTIOUS INFLAMMATORY DISEASES

Many skin diseases are characterised by inflammatory reactions without an identifiable causative agent. These conditions could be due to micro-organisms but they have so far resisted identification; currently their causes are obscure. Some of these diseases, such as lupus erythematosus, have a well-established autoimmune component, while others are known to arise as a result of drug sensitivities or insect bites

(urticaria). Why some individuals develop these diseases and others do not, even when exposed to the same stimuli, remains a mystery.

Yet other conditions, such as lichen planus and psoriasis, remain complete enigmas with no real clues to their aetiology despite intensive investigations over many years.

Urticaria

> ► Urticaria (hives or nettle rash) is a reaction pattern
> ► The basic lesion is oedema of the dermis
> ► Characterised clinically by itching and swelling

When classified according to their causes there are many types of urticaria, but the final common pathway of expression in this condition is always the same. An urticarial lesion results from a sudden marked increase in the permeability of small vessels, resulting in oedema of the dermis or subcutis and the production of a clinically erythematous and/or oedematous papule. The classical lesion is seen in nettle rash or hives. Extreme forms involving the mouth and upper respiratory passages may follow insect stings in these areas and may be life threatening; it is one of the few indications for emergency tracheostomy.

Histologically, the collagen bundles of the dermis are separated by the oedema and a sparse infiltrate of polymorphs, often including eosinophils. Sometimes, there are increased numbers of mast cells, or changes in the granules may be seen, but often they are normal in numbers and appearance.

The commonest mediator of this process is histamine but other substances such as kinins and various circulating globulins, mainly IgE, may play a role (Ch. 10). Many factors are involved in the production of urticaria in susceptible individuals: the relative lability of mast cells; the responsiveness of the microvasculature to the released mediators; the rate of destruction of the mediators; and the patient's idiosyncratic sensitivity to the precipitating agents. These agents include:

- plant and animal toxins
- physical stimuli such as pressure or heat or cold
- various drugs (including aspirin).

Lupus erythematosus

> ► Autoimmune disease affecting connective tissue
> ► Systemic form involves kidneys
> ► Skin lesions also involve epidermis and adnexa

Lupus erythematosus (LE) is a failure in immune self tolerance. This failure results in the production of a large range of auto-antibodies directed at a wide variety of tissue components; the disease is, therefore, an autoimmune disease.

Clinicopathological features

Clinically, LE is a multisystem disease which may present with symptoms associated with almost any organ; in practice, skin and renal (Ch. 21) involvement are among the commonest. In many cases the skin appears to be the only organ involved and the disease is then called *discoid* LE. The systemic variant may or may not involve the skin but in any case is called *systemic* LE. Some doubt arises as to whether or not the form limited to the skin is true LE. However, the fact that the lesions in discoid and systemic cases are often indistinguishable and the occurrence of serological abnormalities of the systemic type in many pure discoid cases suggest that the relationship is close.

The skin lesions are erythematous, scaly and indurated in the acute forms and slowly progress to atrophic scarred patches, often with hyperpigmented edges in the older lesions. They are often symmetrical on the face in a butterfly distribution over the nose and cheeks, and on the scalp may be associated with a scarring alopecia. The scales can often be picked off and are shaped like tin-tacks. These features are explained by the histology, which shows a dilatation of superficial vessels with a dense accumulation of lymphocytes around them, leading to the observed erythema. The infiltrate also involves the dermo-epidermal interface and damages the melanocytes. The melanocytes lose their melanin to dermal macrophages in which the pigment accumulates, accounting for the hyperpigmentation in older lesions. The persistent junctional inflammation results in damage to hair follicles, with the formation of follicular plugs (tin-tacks) and eventually atrophy of hair follicles and the epidermis itself.

Immunofluorescence reveals deposits of IgG and IgM at the epidermal basement membrane. This is the 'lupus band test', a helpful diagnostic feature in doubtful cases.

Psoriasis

▶ Inherited disease
▶ Silvery-grey scales of parakeratosis
▶ Polymorphs enter epidermis but abscesses are sterile

Psoriasis is a common, genetically determined disease associated with HLA haplotypes CW6, B13 and B17. The appearance of the disease is often triggered by environmental factors such as various drugs. It pursues a chronic course and, in 5–10% of cases, is complicated by a very destructive arthropathy.

Clinicopathological features

The lesions are commonest on the extensor surfaces (Fig. 24.6), such as the knees and elbows, and the first appearance may be in a site of trauma such as a

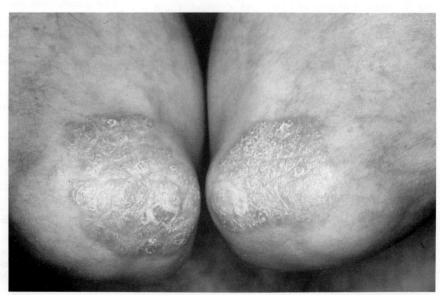

Fig. 24.6 Psoriasis

This inflammatory condition has a strong genetic tendency. It is characterised by silvery scales of parakeratosis and bleeds when scratched superficially. The lesions show a predilection for extensor surfaces and are uncommon on the face.

surgical wound—a phenomenon known as the *Koebner effect*. The individual lesions are covered with a silvery scale and scraping the scale off reveals a series of small bleeding points (*Auspitz's sign*). The loss of protein from the scales is pronounced and in an acute attack may be life threatening, although this is rare.

Histologically (Fig. 24.7), the normal pattern of rete ridges becomes accentuated and the dermal papillae are covered only by a thin layer of epidermis two or three cells thick. This accounts for the bleeding points seen when the scale is scratched off. The progress of the epidermal cells through the epidermis appears to be speeded up and maturation is incomplete. This is reflected in the accumulation of abnormal keratin with nuclear fragments (parakeratosis) in the form of the silvery scales. The maturation of the keratin is so disturbed that the normal granular layer of the epidermis is lost (Fig. 24.7). The erythema is caused by dilated vessels in the upper dermis and these can be seen to contain numerous polymorphs which migrate from the vessels into the epidermis, sometimes in sufficient numbers to form actual pustules. These sterile pustules may dominate the clinical picture in one variant of the disease and this presentation is often marked when the disease appears on the palms of the hands or soles of the feet.

Pathogenesis and treatment
There have been many theories regarding the cause and pathogenesis of psoriasis, but all that is certain is

that it is not contagious, that it is genetic and that the precise mechanism is not understood.

Some clue as to the cause of psoriasis can be found in the therapy of the disease. Almost anything that inhibits the growth of the epidermis will alleviate the disease; such therapies include coal tar, methotrexate and heavy-metal poisons such as arsenic. A very effective current therapy is with analogues of the retinoid subunit of vitamin A, overdose of which causes loss of the keratin layer of the normal skin. So from the therapeutic point of view it seems that psoriasis is a disease of epidermal proliferation and excess keratin production, a description that fits the clinical and histopathological observations very well.

The excessive epidermal proliferation appears to be driven by cytokines released from activated T-cells in the dermis.

Lichen planus

> ► Polygonal, itchy papules
> ► Band-like chronic inflammatory infiltrate
> ► Centred on dermo-epidermal junction

Lichen planus is a non-infectious inflammatory disease characterised by destruction of keratinocytes, probably mediated by interferon-γ and tumour necrosis factor from T-cells in the dermal infiltrate. Usually there is no precipitating factor but some drug eruptions may be indistinguishable. It affects the skin,

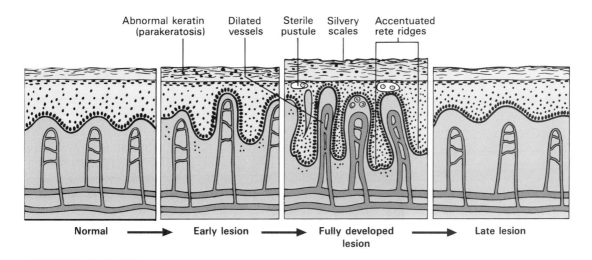

Fig. 24.7 Psoriasis

A common, inherited inflammatory condition of the skin, of unknown aetiology. The progression of the lesion from normal skin to the healed lesion is shown from left to right.

often the inner surfaces of the wrists (Fig. 24.8), and the mucosae, where it appears as a white lacy lesion. On the skin it presents as small, intensely itchy, polygonal, violaceous papules that may develop into blisters, particularly on the palms of the hands or soles of the feet (Fig. 24.9). As the eruption heals, which it usually does spontaneously, it may leave behind hyper- or hypo-pigmented patches.

Clinicopathological features
Histology reveals a lymphohistiocytic infiltrate in a band-like distribution at the dermo-epidermal junction. This finding explains the post-inflammatory pigmentary changes due to melanocyte disturbance at this site, similar to that seen in LE and any other inflammation affecting the dermo-epidermal junction. The basal layer of the epidermis comes under attack and foci of degeneration, apoptosis and regeneration are seen; this eventually gives the epidermis a characteristic saw-tooth profile. Little splits also occur at the junction and, rarely, these may coalesce to form bullae (Fig. 24.10). In contrast to psoriasis

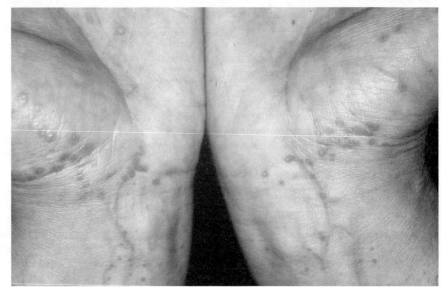

Fig. 24.8   Lichen planus

These intensely itchy lesions of unknown aetiology are most common on the palmar aspect of the wrists.

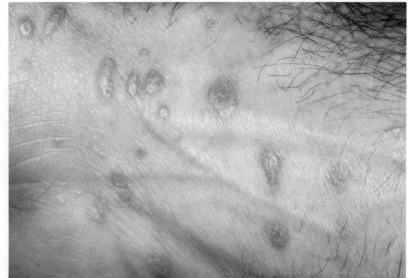

Fig. 24.9   Lichen planus

The lesions are violaceous, flat-topped and polygonal. White lines on the surface (Whickham's striae) are very characteristic.

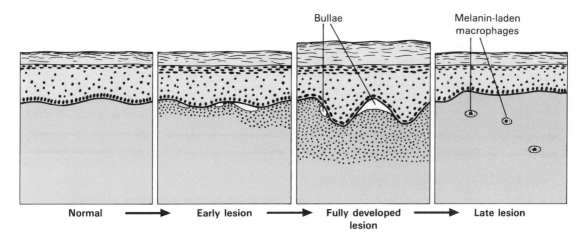

Fig. 24.10 Lichen planus

An inflammatory skin disease of unknown aetiology. The progression from normal skin to healed lesion is shown diagrammatically from left to right.

there is an increase in the granular layer; the scale is consequently different and presents as tiny white lines running over the papules. During the active phase of the eruption papules can be induced by minor trauma such as scratching. Treatment is with steroids, and in those cases in which a precipitating cause can be identified, this therapy can then be withdrawn.

EPIDERMAL CELLS

Normal structure and function

The epidermis consists of a stratified squamous epithelium resting on a basement membrane. The cells are recognisably different from each other in the various layers of the epidermis; at the base they are modified for attachment to the dermis via the basement membrane—this layer is called the *stratum basale* or *basal layer*. Cells in this layer and in the layer immediately above may often be seen in division and presumably provide the replicative pool of cells that regenerates the epidermis as cells grow up through it to form the overlying keratin layer. The cells in the mid zone of the epidermis are the recognisable squamous cells (keratinocytes) and they, like the rest of the epidermal cells, are held together by desmosomes. In histological preparations there is generally some shrinkage of the cells and the desmosomal bridges draw out small spines of cytoplasm from the cells, giving them their typical spinous or

prickle appearance, from which they derive their name of *stratum spinosum* or *prickle cell layer*. As the cells move up through the stratum spinosum they become simplified and their metabolism becomes totally directed to producing the components of the eventual horny layer. The last cellular layer contains many granules of pre-keratin called *keratohyaline granules*. Eventually, the cells die and leave a highly structured keratin layer behind—the *stratum corneum*.

Although the epidermis is secondarily involved in the pathogenesis of numerous diseases, such as lichen planus or eczema, the main diseases of significance that involve the epidermis primarily are disorders of keratinisation (such as ichthyosis and psoriasis) and various tumours, both benign and malignant. The range of epidermal neoplasms that have been described is very wide, but the majority are rare and of little clinical significance; those described below are common or important clinical problems (Fig. 24.11).

Benign tumours and tumour-like conditions

Skin tags

These pedunculated lesions with a fibrovascular core and a benign epidermal covering occur more frequently in the elderly and are common in the axillae. They may be a reaction to friction on the skin, acting primarily in the dermis. They have no clinical significance and they are probably not even true neoplasms.

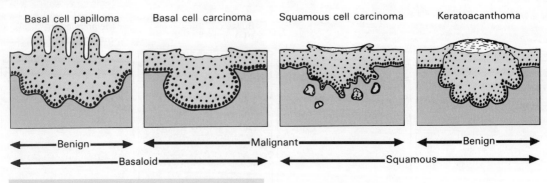

Basal cell papilloma Basal cell carcinoma Squamous cell carcinoma Keratoacanthoma

←——Benign——→ ←—————————Malignant—————————→ ←——Benign——→

←————————Basaloid————————→ ←————————————Squamous————————————→

Fig. 24.11 Common tumours of epidermal cells

Basaloid tumours (benign and malignant) are shown diagrammatically on the left and are compared with some squamous tumours (malignant and benign) shown diagrammatically on the right.

Basal cell papilloma

▶ Common in the elderly
▶ Benign
▶ Cells resemble those in the basal layer of the epidermis

Basal cell papillomas are much more common in the edlerly and are often called *seborrhoeic warts* although they have nothing to do with sebaceous glands and are not caused by wart virus (human papillomavirus) as far as we know. They are dark, greasy-looking (hence 'seborrhoeic') nodules with a craggy surface that may reach considerable sizes (Fig. 24.12). They can occur on most parts of the skin surface and are invariably benign. Histologically, they consist of a proliferation of cells with similar appearances to the basal cells of the epidermis. They have a very convoluted surface with keratin tunnels running deeply from the surface inwards. Mitoses are almost never seen. In some cases they may become inflamed, probably due to trauma, and the cells may become larger and clearer, but their essential benign nature remains unchanged. Although of no direct clinical significance, they are sometimes removed for cosmetic purposes, and in one very rare condition a sudden, widespread, pruritic crop of these lesions may be a sign of internal malignancy, usually in the gastrointestinal tract (the sign of Leser–Trélat).

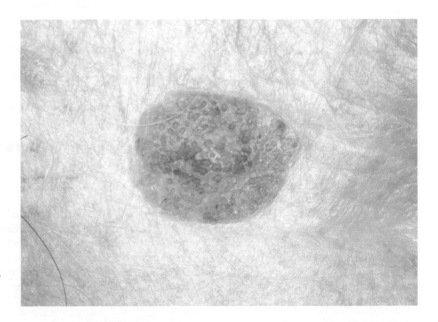

Fig. 24.12 Basal cell papilloma (seborrhoeic wart, seborrhoeic verruca)

A symmetrical, benign lesion. It may occur anywhere on the skin and is commoner in the elderly.

Squamous cell papilloma

There are many benign proliferations of cells resembling normal squamous cells, some of which can be given specific names such as viral warts, keratoacanthomas, etc. But some resist precise classification and are lumped together as squamous cell papillomas, by analogy with basal cell papillomas. However, these may not be separate entities but may simply reflect the inability of the pathologist to recognise their true identity.

Keratoacanthoma

> ▶ Benign, self limiting
> ▶ Can be confused with squamous carcinoma
> ▶ Crater-like symmetrical architecture
> ▶ Face is commonest site

This curious lesion appears, often on sun-damaged skin, grows very rapidly for up to 6 months and then regresses. The lesion is typically symmetrical and highly keratotic (Fig. 24.13) and may even develop a horn of keratin growing out of its centre. Histologically, it appears to have many of the features of a squamous cell carcinoma, but it never invades deeply and it never metastasises. One clue to the correct diagnosis is the crater-like architectural symmetry of the lesion, but this can be seen only in intact lesions and not in curettings or in punch or incisional biopsies. This strange lesion is of unknown aetiology, but because of its rapid and self-limiting growth pattern and accompanying inflammatory infiltrate, many people suspect a viral cause.

Cysts

> ▶ Classified from their linings
> ▶ Benign in almost all cases

Various benign cysts occur in the skin, the commonest being:

- *epidermal cysts*
- *pilar cysts*.

These are often incorrectly grouped together as 'sebaceous cysts'. They occur in the dermis and contain keratin, not sebum. The distinguishing feature is the nature of the cyst lining: in epidermal cysts, the lining is identical to normal epidermis; in pilar cysts, the lining is identical to the trichilemmal lining of the deep part of the hair follicle. Consequently, it is believed that epidermal cysts arise from the upper part of the hair follicle where it is lined by normal epidermis, and the pilar cysts arise from the deeper part of the hair follicle. It is not clear whether these structures are the results of trauma or whether they are true neoplasms, but in any case they are benign.

One variant that causes some problems is the *proliferating pilar tumour*. This tumour has been described as arising from a traumatised pilar cyst, but its behaviour is that of a low grade squamous carcinoma.

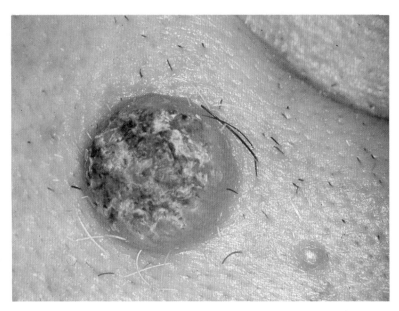

Fig. 24.13   Keratoacanthoma
This symmetrical, keratotic nodule usually occurs on sun-damaged skin. It generally grows for about 6 months and then regresses.

Malignant epidermal neoplasms

Basal cell carcinoma

> ▶ Very common skin malignancy
> ▶ Related to chronic sun exposure
> ▶ Occurs most commonly on the face
> ▶ Locally very invasive
> ▶ Metastasis extremely rare

Basal cell carcinomas are the commonest skin tumours and they are closely associated with chronic sunlight exposure. They are, therefore, most common on the face of elderly people. Clinically, they are often ulcerated irregular lesions, hence their common name of *rodent ulcers*, with a raised pearly border, often with tiny blood vessels visible on the border (Fig. 24.14).

Histologically, they are formed of clumps of small cells surrounded by a rim of cells whose nuclei line up like a picket fence (palisading). Mitoses are sometimes frequent and ulceration is common. The cells are very similar to those of the normal basal layer of the epidermis; the tumours are believed to arise from this layer and from hair follicles.

Their behaviour is interesting because, although they may be very invasive and locally destructive, they so rarely metastasise that when they do it casts doubt on the original diagnosis. Consequently they can be quite adequately treated by local excision or by radiotherapy.

Squamous cell carcinoma

> ▶ Common malignant skin neoplasm
> ▶ Associated with chronic sun exposure
> ▶ Locally invasive
> ▶ Metastasises late

Squamous cell carcinomas are also very common and are aetiologically related to chronic sunlight exposure or to chemical carcinogens such as arsenic, tar and machine oil. They also occur in the site of previous X-irradiation. They are much more common in the elderly on sun-exposed areas. Clinically, they may be roughened keratotic areas, ulcers or horns (Fig. 24.15). They are difficult to distinguish from keratoacanthomas except by their behaviour.

Histologically, they are composed of disorganised keratinocytes with typical malignant cytology. They also show foci of keratinisation within the tumour and sometimes in single cells; thus, they appear to echo the behaviour of the normal upper layers of the epidermis but in a disordered and malignant fashion.

Although they show obvious invasion, their behaviour is usually fairly indolent and metastasis, when it occurs, is a late and relatively uncommon complication. Treatment is by surgical excision, as they are much more resistant to radiation than are basal cell carcinomas.

Rarely, squamous cell carcinomas arise at the edge of chronic skin ulcers (Fig. 24.16).

Actinic keratosis and Bowen's disease
In situ malignant change within the epidermis can occur in both sun-exposed and protected skin. In the sun-exposed areas there is often an overlying mass of keratin and the lesion is referred to as an *actinic keratosis*; the dermis invariably shows elastosis (Ch. 7) due to actinic damage to dermal collagen. On non-light-exposed areas the lesions are generally less keratotic and are referred to as *Bowen's disease*. Invasive

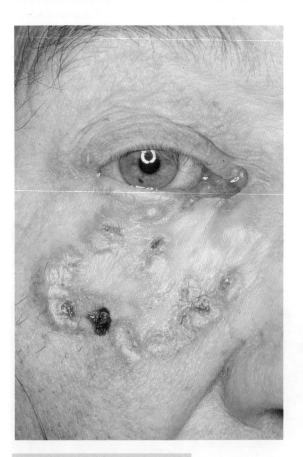

Fig. 24.14   Basal cell carcinoma

This highly invasive neoplasm occurs most commonly on the face. Note the raised border. Metastases are rare.

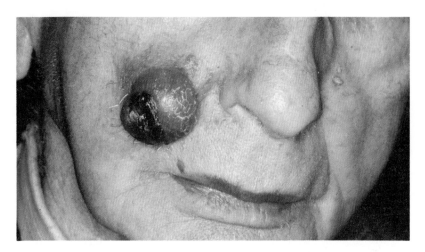

This asymmetrical lesion often occurs on sun-damaged skin. It grows slowly and metastasises late.

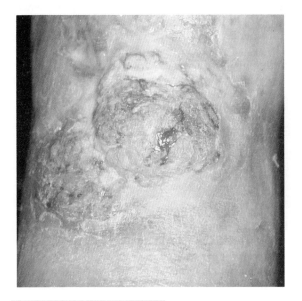

Fig. 24.16 Marjolin's ulcer

This is a squamous cell carcinoma which arises from chronic ulcers, typically varicose vein ulcers.

squamous carcinomas can develop in both lesions, but they usually remain in situ for a very long time.

Blisters (bullae)

Blisters or bullae are fluid-filled spaces within the skin due to separation of two layers of tissue and the leakage of plasma into the space. The most familiar form of blister is a friction blister, commonly on the heel, due to shearing forces set up within the skin as a result of poorly fitting footwear. Such blisters form at the dermo-epidermal junction but other blisters may form at any level within the skin and the precise site of blisters gives a very good clue as to their nature (Fig. 24.17). Many blisters form because a toxin, enzyme or antibody attacks some skin component that has a discrete distribution within the skin and this attack causes separation at that point. Subsequent damage to the blister roof causes it to be shed; the barrier function is lost and secondary infection may ensue.

There are several distinct mechanisms of blister formation:

1. The bonds between epidermal cells may be destroyed directly.

2. The cells may be forced apart by oedema fluid, as happens in eczema.

3. The cells themselves may be destroyed, leaving gaps, which is what happens in herpetic blisters.

4. The basement membrane or its attachments to the epidermis or dermis may be destroyed.

With care and the help of various immunofluorescent markers it is possible to recognise all of these types of blister formation histologically and even to distinguish subtypes among them (Table 24.2).

Many diseases (such as impetigo, eczema or sunburn) have blisters as an incidental part of their clinical presentation, but some conditions appear to be blistering disorders primarily and the more important of these are considered here.

Pemphigus

▶ More common in middle-aged to elderly people
▶ Fatal if untreated
▶ Intra-epidermal blister

Subcorneal

Impetigo

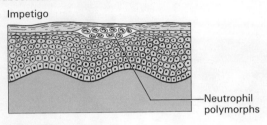

Neutrophil polymorphs

High intraepidermal

Pemphigus foliaceus

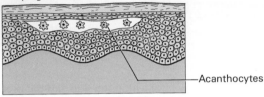

Acanthocytes

Low intraepidermal

Pemphigus vulgaris

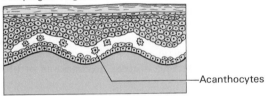

Acanthocytes

Subepidermal

Bullous pemphigoid   Dermatitis herpetiformis   Porphyria

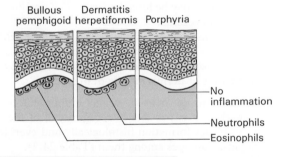

No inflammation

Neutrophils

Eosinophils

Fig. 24.17　Blistering conditions

Various diseases can have a blistering phase but in some the blister is the primary or only feature. The clinical presentation depends on the level in the skin at which the blisters form. The precise diagnosis often requires special diagnostic techniques such as immunofluorescence. (Porphyria is described in Ch. 7.)

Pemphigus is a disease of the middle-aged to elderly and, before the introduction of steroid therapy, most patients died within a year from the complication of serum electrolyte loss or from secondary infections.

Even now, it is a serious disease with a mortality of about 40%. The disease is caused by circulating auto-antibodies directed at components of the inter-cellular bridges (desmosomes) within the epidermis. The bridges are lysed and the epidermis falls apart, leaving loose keratinocytes within the blister cavity. These keratinocytes are no longer held in shape by the surrounding cells and consequently round up (acanthocytes); the whole process is known as *acan-tholysis*.

There are several varieties of the disease, depend-ing upon the precise site within the epidermis at which the blisters occur. Superficial blistering occurs in the subcorneal region in *pemphigus foliaceus* and more deeply in the more common form, *pemphigus vulgaris*. In the superficial form the blisters are so near the surface that their roof is very fragile and intact blisters are seldom seen. In vulgaris, where the split is located more deeply, the blisters are more persistent. In all varieties of the disease the skin is very fragile due to the weakening of the intercellular bridges and firm, sliding pressure on apparently normal skin will precipitate a blister (*Nikolsky's sign*).

Bullous pemphigoid

▶ More common in the elderly
▶ Self-limiting disease
▶ Blister forms at dermo-epidermal junction

This 'pemphigus-like' disease is more common than pemphigus, although still rare, and occurs mainly in the over-60-year age group (Fig. 24.18). It is gener-ally self-limiting but may be associated with a long period of pruritus even after the blisters have healed. In this disease the split occurs at the dermo-epider-mal junction and is due to circulating antibodies to the lamina lucida layer (immediately adjacent to the basal cells) of the epidermal basement mem-brane. Immunofluorescence reveals a linear deposi-tion of antibody, generally IgG, along the basement membrane. The antigen–antibody complex causes the release of various complement factors which can also be demonstrated by immunofluorescence and the whole reaction causes degranulation of mast cells. This accounts not only for the pruritus but also for the characteristic presence of eosinophils, which are the common accompani-ment of mast cell activation in any condition. Being deeper, the blisters are more persistent although the severe pruritus often results in them being destroyed by scratching.

Table 24.2 Clinicopathological features of bullous disorders

Disease	Location of bullae	Immune reactants	Clinical features
Pemphigus	Intra-epidermal	IgG on intercellular junctions	High mortality
Pemphigoid	Subepidermal	IgG on basement membrane	Elderly patients
Dermatitis herpetiformis	Subepidermal	IgA on basement membrane	Associated with coeliac disease

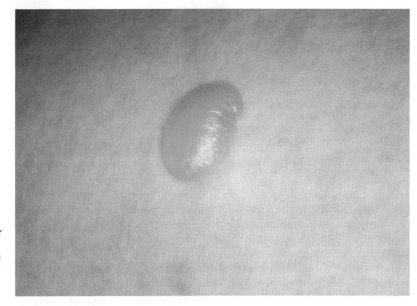

Fig. 24.18 Bullous pemphigoid

The junctional blisters are often larger and less itchy than dermatitis herpetiformis. There is no association with gluten-sensitive enteropathy and they show no particular site of predilection.

Dermatitis herpetiformis

> ▶ Most common in young adults
> ▶ Blister forms at dermo-epidermal junction
> ▶ May be associated with coeliac disease

This blistering condition is characterised by small, intensely itchy blisters occurring mainly on the extensor surfaces of knees and elbows of young adults (Fig. 24.19). The blisters are so pruritic that it is often difficult for the patient to keep one intact for the clinician to recognise. The blisters occur at the dermo-epidermal junction, but in this case the immunoglobulin deposit is granular rather than continuous in distribution and it is almost always IgA. Curiously, although the lesions are very pruritic, the characteristic inflammatory cell seen in the infiltrates is the neutrophil polymorph and not the eosinophil. The disease is also remarkable for the fact that the response to therapy with dapsone is usually so dramatic as to be diagnostic. A significant number of these patients are shown to have some degree of gluten sensitivity (coeliac disease; Ch. 15).

Ulcers

An ulcer is a defect in an epithelial surface. Ulcers in the skin are usually attributable to vascular insufficiency or trauma. In the elderly where there is often impaired blood flow, minor trauma can often result in severe, persistent ulceration requiring hospitalisation.

Venous ulcers

> ▶ Lower legs in the elderly
> ▶ Associated with varicose veins and varicose eczema
> ▶ Due to venous stasis

Venous ulcers commonly arise from chronic venous congestion in the lower legs of the elderly due to incompetence of the valves in the small veins connecting the deep and superficial venous systems of the leg.

Pathogenesis
The congestion results in the shunting of the deep

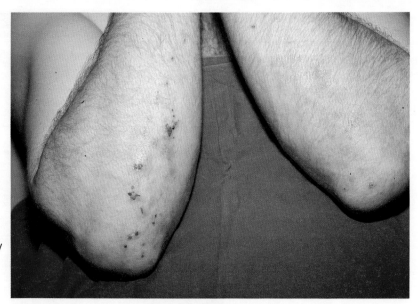

Fig. 24.19   Dermatitis herpetiformis

This is characterised by junctional, very itchy blisters that occur most commonly on elbows and knees. They are so pruritic that they are seldom seen intact. There is an association with gluten-sensitive enteropathy (coeliac disease).

venous pressure, generated by muscular contractions around veins, to the superficial veins which are not designed to withstand such high pressures. These veins dilate (*varicose veins*) and venous pooling occurs, resulting in venous stasis within the skin. This presents as a discoloured, often eczematous area of skin, frequently in the region of obvious varicose veins. Eventually, the venous drainage of the skin becomes too poor to support the metabolism of the epidermis, which dies and is sloughed off leaving a venous ulcer. This may happen spontaneously or be accelerated as a result of relatively minor trauma.

Treatment
Patients often attempt a variety of irrelevant topical medications (frequently with the help of their doctor!) and their ulcers are at least aggravated, and possibly maintained, by the superimposition of a wide range of topical hypersensitivities that perpetuate the local skin irritation with a mixture of venous and contact eczemas.

Mechanical therapies are the most favoured and include: compressive bandages, which prevent the pressure transfer to the skin, or surgical removal of incompetent vessels before ulceration occurs. Local grafting of the patient's own healthy epidermis into the ulcer with the leg elevated to reduce venous pressure is also effective.

However, all treatment is difficult in these cases as healing depends on a good circulation and that is what is defective in the first place.

Arterial ulcers

▶ On the legs, commonly in diabetics and patients with severe atheroma
▶ Usually associated with poor foot pulses and claudication

Arterial ulcers are more shallow, undermined and painful than their venous counterparts. They result from failure of the arterial supply to that region of skin. For this reason the common treatment used for venous ulcers, that of compressive bandaging, is a disaster since it reduces even further the arterial supply and large areas of skin may become necrotic before the error is appreciated.

Diabetic ulceration, like most of the long-term effects of diabetes, is mediated through the final common pathway of small artery damage.

Other ulcers

Many other conditions cause ulcers, in particular many tropical infections such as *yaws* and *leishmaniasis*, but ulcers can occur as non-specific lesions complicating conditions such as *herpes*. *Pyoderma gangrenosum* is a specific entity with violaceous, undermined ulcers that may present as a lesion complicating ulcerative colitis; in many cases an underlying monoclonal gammopathy can be demonstrated.

Behçet's syndrome is a rare condition, of unknown aetiology, with ulcers of the mucosae and a variety of systemic lesions. Opinion regarding its aetiology is fairly evenly split between those who favour a viral cause and those who believe that it is a disease of autoimmunity.

Persistent ulcers, which in practice generally means venous ulcers, provide a long-term irritation and a cause for continuous epithelial regeneration. In this sort of situation there is an increased tendency for malignant transformation to occur and squamous cell carcinoma may be a late complication of such ulcers. Such malignant ulcers are called *Marjolin's ulcers* (Fig. 24.16).

MELANOCYTES

Normal structure and function

At about the thirteenth week of embryonic life, cells migrate from the neural crest and come to lie at the dermo-epidermal junction. These cells become the pigmented melanocytes and are distributed among the cells of the epidermal basal layer. Within the cytoplasm of the melanocytes are organelles (melanosomes) which are specialised for the production of the black pigment melanin which is a condensation product of dihydroxyphenylalanine (DOPA).

The melanocytes transfer melanin to the basal keratinocytes where it comes to lie above the nucleus, protecting the nucleus from solar irradiation. The protective importance of melanin can be deduced from the high rate of skin cancers found in those people who lack melanin (albinos) and who

are exposed to levels of sunlight that do not cause cancer in normal subjects. The melanocyte system is very responsive to changes in exposure to sunlight and vast amounts of time and money are expended on driving these cells to the limits of their productiveness in pursuit of a "healthy" tan.

Although variations in skin colour are produced by variations in the activity of melanocytes and not by variations in their numbers, focal areas of increased activity may occur as a result of sun exposure in some individuals and these foci appear as *freckles* (ephelides).

It is a poignant fact that although the role of melanocytes is to protect the skin against the development of relatively benign skin cancers such as basal cell carcinomas and squamous carcinomas, the cancers that arise from melanocytes are amongst the most malignant of skin tumours.

Lentigo and melanocytic naevi

Lentigos are characterised by an increase in single melanocytes in the basal epidermis. Melanocytic naevi ('moles') are nests of melanocytes; the nest can lie:

- at the dermo-epidermal junction (*junctional naevus*)
- at the junction and in the dermis (*compound naevus*)
- in the dermis (*intradermal naevus*).

These clinical types of naevi are all believed to be stages in the evolution of the same pathological entity (Fig. 24.20). This is not to say that any one lesion

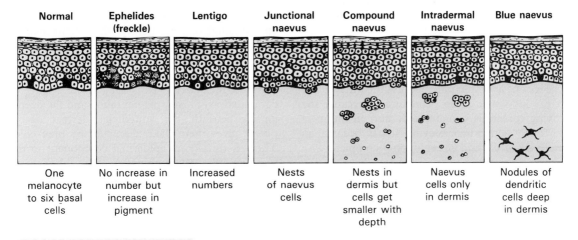

Normal	Ephelides (freckle)	Lentigo	Junctional naevus	Compound naevus	Intradermal naevus	Blue naevus
One melanocyte to six basal cells	No increase in number but increase in pigment	Increased numbers	Nests of naevus cells	Nests in dermis but cells get smaller with depth	Naevus cells only in dermis	Nodules of dendritic cells deep in dermis

Fig. 24.20 Naevocellular naevi

Normal melanocytes occur in the basal layer (about one melanocyte to six basal cells). The various patterns of abnormality are illustrated and are described in detail in the text.

must pass through all of these stages, for their development may cease at any point. However, we so frequently see forms that are intermediate in the progression that the temptation to unify is irresistible and therefore we describe these lesions as though this progression was an established fact.

Clinicopathological features

The earliest clinical feature is a small, pigmented macule (a flat skin lesion) caused by an increase in the number of individual melanocytes at the dermo-epidermal junction. At this stage the melanocytes appear completely normal; they are pigmented and dendritic and transfer their pigment to the surrounding keratinocytes, but because their numbers are increased the degree of skin pigmentation is increased. This lesion is called a *lentigo*.

In the next stage the melanocytes proliferate to form nests clustered at the dermo-epidermal junction. This clustering may cause the clinical lesion to become very slightly raised, but it is often impossible to distinguish this stage from the preceding one. The cells are still pigmented but are now losing their dendrites and becoming rounded, true 'naevus' cells. At this stage the lesion is termed a *junctional naevus* since all of the naevus cells remain at the dermo-epidermal junction.

With further development the junctional naevus cells seem to detach from the dermo-epidermal junction, become smaller and rounder and less metabolically active and lose the ability to divide (post-mitotic cells). The lesion now has two components histologically—a junctional component and an intradermal component—and is therefore called a *compound naevus* (Fig. 24.21). Clinically these are pigmented nodules and are so common as to be found in most normal subjects.

The last stage in the evolution of these naevi is reached when all of the junctional melanocytes have gone and only the intradermal naevus cells remain. These lesions are often pink because the intradermal cells produce little or no pigment and because the overlying epidermis contains only normal numbers of normally active melanocytes. It has become an *intradermal naevus* and its evolution is complete.

There seems to be some interaction between the naevus cells and the epidermis: in junctional and subsequent naevi there may be a very marked increase in the growth of the epidermis, either outwards to form a rough, papillary lesion, or inwards to form a highly reticulated naevus growth pattern. This pattern of growth involving both keratinocytes and melanocytes has led some pathologists to assert that melanocytic naevi are not benign neoplasms at

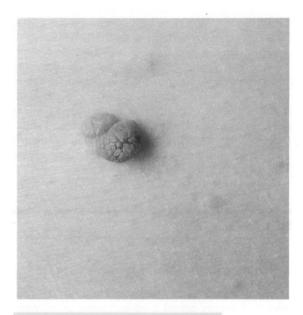

Fig. 24.21   Benign compound naevus

A collection of pigmented naevocellular naevus cells is situated in the dermis. There is no junctional component, the lesion is symmetrical and there is no risk of malignancy.

all, but are hamartomas, that is to say, congenital areas of malformation with the same genome as the rest of the individual's somatic cells.

Blue naevi

The blue naevus is a benign congenital lesion which occurs as a deep dermal nodule on any area of the skin and which, as its name suggests, often has a bluish tinge (Fig. 24.22). They rarely exceed 5 mm in diameter, although one unusual type that occurs mainly on the buttocks can be much larger. They are usually solitary and malignant transformation is very rare.

Histologically, they consist of deeply pigmented, dendritic melanocytes lying deep in the dermis. The combination of heavy pigmentation and the deep situation beneath the superficial dermal vascular plexus gives them their characteristic blue colour. There is usually no epidermal component to these tumours although combinations with other types of naevi can sometimes occur.

The fact that the cells of this tumour retain their dendrites and that they sit so deeply in the dermis has led to the attractive proposition that they are melanocytes arrested in their embryonic migration to the dermo-epidermal junction. This proposition would explain why they are so different from other pigmented naevi.

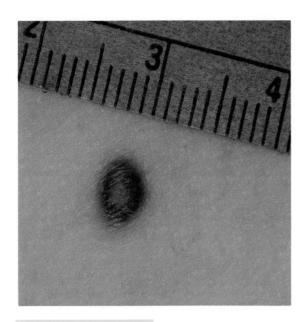

Fig. 24.22   Blue naevus

This is a congenital type of naevus that is symmetrical and occurs deep in the dermis and looks blue due to a combination of its pigmentation and overlying vasculature. They are usually benign, but rarely can be malignant.

Malignant melanoma

> ▶ Tumour is composed of malignant melanocytes
> ▶ Usually pigmented, but may be amelanotic
> ▶ Prognosis depends on thickness
> ▶ Aetiologically associated with fair skin and sunburn

The malignant tumours of melanocytic origin are called *melanomas*; more properly they should be called 'melanocarcinomas' since the term *melanoma* implies a benign tumour (Ch. 11) which these lesions certainly are not. In general, malignant melanomas are tumours of the skin, but since melanocytes may be found in central nervous sites such as the leptomeninges and the retina, primary malignant melanomas can arise there also.

The great clinical tragedy of malignant melanoma is that it is visible from its earliest stages and if excised before it has begun to invade the dermis it is totally curable. Nevertheless, each year many patients die of disseminated malignant melanoma and the incidence is increasing steadily.

Pathogenesis
The most important aetiological factor is UV light.

Melanomas occur most commonly in fair-skinned people (e.g. Caucasians) living in sunny climates (e.g. Australia).

Theoretically, malignant melanomas can arise from any melanocyte, whether it be one of the normal junctional melanocytes or a melanocyte present in a benign naevus. Statistically, we might expect at least some malignant melanomas to arise in benign naevi simply because they contain so many melanocytes. However, many of the cells in a benign compound naevus are post-mitotic, and all of those in an intradermal naevus are post-mitotic and we should not expect these cells to produce malignant melanomas. Clinical experience tends to bear this out: those melanomas that are thought to have arisen in pre-existing benign naevi do so only in those classes of naevi with an active junctional component. However, a large number of malignant melanomas appear to arise de novo and they may well pass through a stage where it is difficult to know whether or not they are true malignant melanomas, so the precise fraction that arise in naevi or de novo is difficult to determine.

Clinicopathological features
Broadly, the histological types of malignant melanomas parallel the benign lesions, although some may be unpigmented (amelanotic melanoma) and it is often only the cytological abnormalities or the presence of invasion that permits the pathologist to distinguish them. Clinicians recognise several clinical types of lesion with slightly differing prognosis, but in most cases the similarities are greater than the differences. In all cases, prognosis depends upon the thickness of the lesion at the time of excision; if it is less than 0.75 mm then the cure rate approaches 100%, but as the lesion thickens the prognosis worsens, until at 3.0 mm there are practically no cures to be expected.

Clinical variants
The main clinical variants of melanoma (Fig. 24.23) are:

- lentigo maligna
- acral lentiginous
- superficial spreading
- nodular malignant.

Lentigo maligna melanomas occur on the sun-damaged skin of the face in elderly people, and even when they become thick and nodular these lesions are thought to have a slightly more indolent course and a better prognosis than other malignant melanomas. However, the data on which this belief

Lentigo malignant melanoma

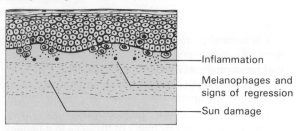

— Inflammation

— Melanophages and signs of regression

— Sun damage

Superficial spreading malignant melanoma

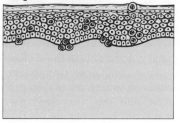

Nodular melanoma

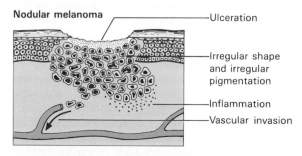

— Ulceration

— Irregular shape and irregular pigmentation

— Inflammation

— Vascular invasion

Fig. 24.23 Malignant melanoma (melanocarcinoma)

Three different types of lesion are shown and are discussed fully in the text.

is based are far from conclusive, since these are melanomas arising in an elderly population whereas all other melanomas arise in a much younger age group; it may just be that melanomas in the elderly are more indolent (as are most cancers) than those in younger people. The development of lentigo maligna melanoma occurs in a pre-existing lesion, lentigo maligna (Hutchinson's melanotic freckle), which is like the benign lentigos described above, but in which the lentigo cells appear cytologically atypical.

Acral lentiginous malignant melanoma arises on the palms and soles, most commonly at their junctions with the volar surfaces. These lesions are uncommon in Europeans, but are the commonest form of malignant melanoma in Japan.

The third type of thin lesion is the *superficial spreading malignant melanoma* and this is the commonest thin lesion in people of European descent. All three thin lesions are characterised by the proliferation of nests and single atypical melanocytes at the dermo-epidermal junction and their spread into the epidermis. This epidermal spread is the best diagnostic feature and produces a very recognisable pattern, variously described as pagetoid spread (so named because of the resemblance histologically to Paget's disease of the nipple) or, more colourfully, as 'buckshot scatter'. This phase persists for an unknown but variable time and may be many years in the case of lentigo maligna. But eventually dermal invasion occurs and the end stage of all superficial lesions is the development of a *nodular melanoma* (Fig. 24.24). Some nodular melanomas retain no features of a pre-existing superficial lesion and this has led some pathologists to suggest that at least some nodular malignant melanomas arise as nodules without a preceding superficial stage.

Clinical course

The final common pathway for malignant melanoma is metastatic spread. This occurs early in the development of the tumour; indeed, it occurs when the thickness of the original lesion exceeds 0.75 mm in many cases. It seems that the tumour cells have a great capacity for metastatic spread and begin to show this as soon as they come into contact with the superficial dermal vessels. The tumour spreads to all parts of the body, with a predilection for skin, brain and gastrointestinal tract. Currently, there is no effective therapy for widespread disease; the only effective treatment is early excision of the primary lesion.

Prevention

Because of the increasing incidence and the intractable nature of advanced disease a lot of emphasis has come to be placed on early diagnosis and on prevention. The main factor which seems to be associated with the development of the tumour is sunlight exposure. However, the pattern is not the same as for squamous cell carcinoma and basal cell carcinoma, which are associated with chronic sun exposure. With melanomas the most important factor appears to be episodic acute exposure with burning and, as might be expected therefore, the groups most at risk are pale-skinned individuals with blue eyes who always burn and never tan (so-called skin type 1 subjects). Several studies have shown a marked increase in thin melanomas in these individuals 2–3 years following very hot summers. The final

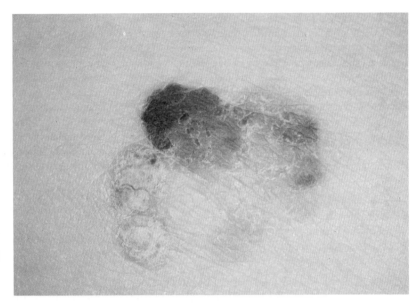

Fig. 24.24   Malignant melanoma

This asymmetrical lesion shows variable pigmentation and regression. The original lesion was a superficial spreading malignant melanoma and a nodule has now developed within it, giving it a significantly poorer prognosis.

irony is that these patients were trying to stimulate their melanocytes to protect them against sun exposure by sunbathing.

Dysplastic naevus syndrome

> ▶ Familial tendency to melanomas in some kindreds
> ▶ Possess atypical naevi
> ▶ High risk of developing melanoma

Recently it has become apparent that some families have a greater than normal frequency of malignant melanomas. These families are known as BK mole kindreds, the BK referring to the initials of the first recognised patients with this condition. Members of these families also have numerous atypical moles (*dysplastic naevi*) and it is from these naevi that their melanomas are thought to develop.

Clinically, the moles are irregular in outline and pigmentation and they alter in appearance as melanomas develop. Histologically, they look like benign naevi but show a lack of symmetry, some cytological atypia and are often inflamed as though the body recognises their malignant potential. What we see in these families is the missing link between benign naevi and malignant melanomas. Much effort has been expended on attempting to establish clinical and pathological criteria for recognising the dysplastic naevus with malignant potential. The assumption is that this will lead to more accurate early diagnosis in normal individuals who develop sporadic melanomas.

DERMAL VESSELS

The blood vessels of the dermis participate in inflammatory reactions; the details of this are identical to those seen in any organ of the body (Ch. 10). Discussed here are the phenomena affecting the skin vasculature which result in typical skin lesions. The skin lymphatics demonstrate a similar range of pathologies but these are much rarer and will not be discussed.

Bruises

Bruises are due to blood leaking from vessels into the dermis. Bruises can occur from:

- damaged vessels (trauma, vasculitis)
- changes in the blood (thrombocytopenia)
- changes in the dermis (old age, scurvy).

Bruises result when blood vessels are sufficiently damaged for red blood cells to escape into the surrounding connective tissue. The breakdown of this extravasated haemoglobin provides the attractive series of colour changes associated with the resolution of this common lesion; the initial bluish red of haemoglobin fades to the green of biliverdin then to the yellow of haemosiderin and finally disappears back to the body's general iron stores.

Bruises are commonly classified according to their sizes and causes and there are long clinical lists describing such minor variations as *petechiae*, *purpura* and *ecchymoses*. Bruises may arise due to blunt trauma of sufficient power to damage normal vessels, as a result of minor trauma to fragile vessels in the elderly or in patients on steroids, as a result of inadequacy of the clotting system as in liver failure or idiopathic thrombocytopenia, or because the supporting tissue has become defective due to vitamin C deficiency; the list is lengthy, but the end effect is the same.

Telangiectasia

Telangiectasia are dilatations of capillaries often seen:

- in irradiated skin
- in the elderly
- following prolonged steroid therapy
- in patients suffering from liver failure (when they are called *spider naevi*).

Histologically, the vessels are normal but dilated.

Naevus flammeus (port-wine stain) develops on the face in early infancy in histologically normal skin. The lesion is flat and in some cases is associated with an underlying meningeal vascular malformation (Sturge–Weber syndrome) which may bleed with catastrophic neurological results. Histologically, the overlying epidermis is normal and the vessels appear to be passively dilated with no evidence of endothelial proliferation, so although it is usually categorised as a naevus (see below) it is in fact telangiectasis occurring on the basis of congenitally abnormal vessels.

Hamartomas

Hamartomas are tumour-like malformations of tissues (Ch. 11). They consist of normal tissue elements in abnormal amounts and arrangements; in the skin, they are often called naevi or birthmarks. Naevi may contain any tissue element but in the skin the commonest are vascular naevi and pigmented naevi. The pigmented naevi derive from melanocytes; the vascular naevi are considered below.

Vascular naevi

There is one further problem in terminology: if vascular naevi are true hamartomas then their genetic make-up is the same as that of the rest of the patient's tissues, that is to say they are not truly neoplastic. Unfortunately, they are still commonly referred to in the clinical and pathological literature as 'haemangiomas', implying erroneously that they are true benign neoplasms.

Vascular naevi, present from birth or developing soon after, may be of any size and are very common. Their differences in appearance, clinical significance and prognosis depend upon their site and the calibre of vessels involved.

Capillary haemangiomas (strawberry naevi) appear in early infancy, but in contrast to the other vascular naevi they have a brief period of growth with endothelial proliferation followed by fibrosis and regression which may be total. Because of the vascular proliferation they are raised, often lobulated masses but they rarely give rise to anything other than cosmetic problems.

Cavernous haemangiomas lie in the deep dermis or subcutaneous tissues but may be associated with an overlying capillary haemangioma. The lesion consists of large, dilated thin-walled vessels that may contain so much blood with disturbed flow characteristics that, in rare cases, consumption coagulopathy can occur (Ch. 23).

Vasculitis

Vessels themselves may become inflamed and this results in a series of specific skin conditions, often with systemic symptoms. Conversely the classical systemic vasculitides frequently have skin manifestations. Several skin diseases such as lupus erythematosus and hypersensitivity reactions may have a vasculitic component. Then, they are characterised by purpura in addition to their normal clinical picture, because the vessel damage allows blood to leak into the dermis.

Other generalised vasculitides, such as polyarteritis nodosa and Wegener's syndrome, may cause skin lesions (Chs 12 and 25).

Tumours

Benign tumours

Benign tumours of blood vessels are rare and of little clinical or pathological importance. Most are small vascular proliferations that are often difficult to categorise as blood vascular or lymphatic and are collectively called *angiomas*. The only other benign lesion that is worthy of comment is the *glomus tumour*. This is a tiny, painful nodule which often occurs beneath the nail. They derive from the glomus apparatus, which is a contractile device governing flow in the cutaneous microvasculature. The tumours consist of groups of cells looking rather like epithelial cells around vascular spaces and can be shown to contain numerous nerve fibres as well as mast cells and fibroblasts.

Haemangiopericytomas arise from the pericytes surrounding blood vessels. These are rare tumours and there is a malignant variant.

Angiosarcoma

Malignant proliferations of blood vessels (or lymphatics) are called angiosarcomas. They are rare and many arise in sites of previous irradiation or in chronically oedematous limbs (following mastectomy with removal of axillary lymph nodes) or on the face or scalp of the elderly. The difficulty in separating malignant blood vessel tumours from malignant lymphatic tumours is due to the fact that abnormal anastomoses occur between the vessels, and blood cells can be found in both types of tumour.

Kaposi's sarcoma

Kaposi's sarcoma, a previously rare lesion, has recently assumed much more significance due to its association with AIDS (acquired immune deficiency syndrome), of which it can be one late manifestation. Kaposi's sarcoma presents most commonly as vascular lesions on the limbs. In non-AIDS cases, 90% are found in males. Prior to the AIDS outbreak they were seen in young Africans living around Lake Victoria, in elderly patients of Jewish or Mediterranean origin, and in some patients on long-term immunosuppression. The new risk groups — chiefly male homosexuals — are associated with venereally transmitted AIDS.

The lesions may be single or multiple, may resemble bruises or be raised nodules. Their histology resembles granulation tissue with proliferation of vessels with plump endothelial cells, extravasation of erythrocytes and interstitial inflammatory cells. The aetiology of the disease seems to be that of a viral-induced neoplasm.

ADNEXA

The skin adnexa — the *pilosebaceous system* and the *eccrine sweat glands* — are complex structures that develop from the epidermis and remain in continuity with it but reside in the dermis. Their distribution is characteristic of the anatomical site of the body and, consequently, the distribution of diseases related to them is also anatomically characteristic. They are metabolically highly active structures and very sensitive to toxic and hormonal influences; one only has to recall the induction of sweating by anxiety or the spectacular hair loss in patients subjected to chemotherapy to confirm this sensitivity.

One other set of adnexa actually protrude from the surface of the skin — the nails. These structures are also subject to a specific set of pathological conditions but, like the hair, they are non-living keratin and therefore only reflect metabolic events that happened as they were growing and which may later have ceased to operate.

In skin trauma, such as burns, the regrowth of the epidermis occurs from the viable edges of the wound but it can also occur from remnants of adnexa if the original destruction was not too deep (Ch. 6). If there is full thickness destruction including the adnexa, then epidermal regrowth will occur from the edges as usual but no adnexa will develop. This implies that the adnexal remnants have the ability to differentiate to produce epidermis but that epidermal cells have lost the ability to differentiate towards the highly specialised adnexal structures. This of course has implications for theories of the histogenesis of various skin tumours as well as for the more practical considerations of skin grafts.

Pilosebaceous system

Acne vulgaris

> ▶ Very common in adolescence
> ▶ Clinically consists of comedones and pustules
> ▶ Often heals with scarring
> ▶ Hormone dependent; more common in males

Acne vulgaris is so common among the adolescent population that it could be viewed as a normal variant, an attitude unlikely to win favour with those patients and pharmaceutical firms who spend so much on its treatment. Clinically, it is characterised by pilosebaceous units which are blocked by dark plugs or comedones (blackheads). These blocked follicles become infected and swell up to form the characteristic pustules which may discharge on to the skin surface or rupture into the dermis, with resultant scarring.

The development of acne is dependent on circulating testosterone which is converted to the active hormone by enzymes contained in the pilosebaceous system itself. Females also have significant levels of circulating testosterone, although generally at lower levels than in the male, which accounts for the lower incidence of acne in females; castrated males have no acne. Acne may also occur in pregnancy and with steroid therapy as well as a reaction to some halogens such as bromides and iodides and to various industrial oils. These secondary acnes suggest that the development of spontaneous acne vulgaris may be dependent on hormonal influences and perhaps on some toxic influences such as the products of bacterial breakdown of skin lipids. Currently, acne is very successfully treated by synthetic analogues of retinoids (a subunit of vitamin A) which modify keratin production, suggesting that the first step in the process may be the formation of a comedone in the form of a keratin plug.

The precise cause and pathogenesis of this common disease remains a problem, but at least there are now effective therapies available.

Alopecia

> ▶ Male pattern baldness due to irreversible loss of follicles
> ▶ Alopecia areata due to autoimmunity
> ▶ Lichen planus and lupus erythematosus can cause scarring alopecia

Hair loss for any reason is alopecia. The commonest form is *male pattern baldness*. This is an inherited trait which affects a large proportion of the adult male population and a much smaller proportion of the female population. It is characterised by a progressive loss of hair from the temples and from the crown of the head. The loss is permanent and occurs without any signs of inflammation. It is hormone dependent; eunuchs at least have the compensation of retaining their hair. Histologically, there is progressive loss of follicles and some sebaceous glands; such adnexa once lost are not recovered.

Another type of alopecia occurs as a result of autoimmune damage to the hair follicle: this is termed *alopecia areata*. Clinically, there is a circumscribed area of baldness with small exclamation-mark hairs regrowing within it. Histologically, there is a lymphocytic infiltrate around the deeper part of the follicle which is destroyed by the infiltrate. The upper part of the follicle remains so that the appearance is of a normal number of short, stubby follicles with deep inflammation.

Hair loss can also occur in inflammatory skin conditions in which there is epidermal damage such as *lichen planus* and *lupus erythematosus*. In these conditions there is usually obvious scarring of the scalp and signs of the disease in other sites. Histologically, there is the recognisable pattern of the disease involving the epidermis, but also spreading down the hair follicle. In distinction to alopecia areata, the inflammation affects the upper part of the follicle in continuity with the epidermis, and the end effect is to leave a thinned, atrophic skin with a diminished number of follicles.

Total hair loss can occur in some forms of systemic poisoning such as thallium intoxication, or from chemotherapy, in which the rapidly dividing hair cells are early victims of antimitotic agents (Ch. 5) in the same way as haemopoietic and intestinal epithelial cells.

Hirsutism

Unwanted hair is almost as much of a personal problem as baldness. Currently, our culture disapproves of facial, axillary and leg hair in women and a large amount of effort is directed towards its removal. Facial hair growth is a secondary sexual characteristic dependent upon circulating testosterone levels. It is not the testosterone that is active but a metabolite of it produced by enzymes within the hair follicle itself. There are then two factors involved: first, the level of circulating hormone, and second, the end organ sensitivity. In general it is not clear which of these is the important process in most cases of female hirsutism.

Facial hair also develops in the post-menopausal female as the small amount of testosterone produced by the adrenal glands is no longer counterbalanced by the ovarian oestrogens.

Facial hair may also develop as a result of various drug treatments and in response to virilising hormones (e.g. androgens) secreted by tumours (e.g. Cushing's syndrome).

Pilosebaceous tumours

There are a number of benign hair follicle tumours but these are not common or significant clinical problems. The commonest malignant tumour derived from the pilosebaceous system is the basal cell carcinoma (p. 764).

Eccrine sweat glands

A long period of evolution has provided land animals with an effective water-conserving kidney and an impermeable skin to prevent water and electrolyte loss. The value of this impermeable skin can readily be seen in the metabolic imbalance that develops in patients with severe burns. It is, therefore, rather curious that mammals have developed a system for pouring out water and electrolytes onto the skin in order to control their temperature. Long-distance athletes and newcomers to tropical climates find that they need to take in large amounts of water and salt in order to balance the losses due to eccrine gland thermal regulation. Another problem faced by unacclimatised dwellers in the tropics is that the eccrine gland pores swell up with the unaccustomed activity and block sweat excretion, causing 'prickly heat'.

Sweat gland tumours are even more esoteric an interest than the hair follicle tumours and, since eccrine glands do not give rise to basal cell carcinomas, they are even more rare.

Nails

The nails are affected in many general skin conditions such as psoriasis and fungal infections and may also be indicators of internal disease (p. 780). In the elderly, the great toenail may be disrupted by ill-fitting footwear or other trauma and develop into a startling hoof or horn-like protuberance (*onychogryphosis*) that is incapacitatingly difficult to deal with. In younger people, the direction of growth of the nail may be disturbed, from similar causes, resulting in *ingrowing toenail* which often needs ablation of the nail bed to cure it.

DERMAL CONNECTIVE TISSUES

The dermis contains the nerves and blood vessels that nourish and support the epidermis and its adnexa. In their turn, these dermal structures are supported by a matrix of proteins and complex sugars (glycosaminoglycans), collectively known as the connective tissue ground substance. This ground substance is secreted by fibroblasts and, to a lesser extent, by mast cells. The two characteristic proteins of the dermis are *collagen*, which provides the tensile strength of the skin, and *elastin*, which provides the elasticity. Together, these compounds make the skin tough, flexible and deformable but with the property of returning to its original shape once the deforming stresses are released. The complex sugars include *hyaluronic acid*, which binds water and provides the fluid environment in which the proteins can function. This substance seems to act as a selective filter and a barrier to the spread of organisms. Indeed, many organisms penetrate the dermis by producing an enzyme (hyaluronidase) that breaks down the hyaluronic acid. There are also various sulphated polysaccharides which act as a matrix on which the proteins are synthesised and organised three-dimensionally. These substances all seem to be synthesised by the *fibroblasts* — elongated cells scattered about

the dermis. The other cell type found in the dermis, usually around blood vessels, is the *mast cell*. These are not very obvious with routine histological stains, but special techniques reveal them to be cells containing numerous granules that can be shown to contain histamine and heparin, as well as a variety of other pharmacologically active substances.

The ground substance is not inert but is constantly, although slowly, being turned over and remodelled in response to the various forces acting upon it. Consequently, disturbances to the cell lineages within the dermis, or deficiencies in the enzyme systems concerned with the elaboration of the ground substance eventually result in considerable disturbance to skin structure and function.

Collagen and elastin

The normal effects of wear and tear on collagen and elastin are usually made good with no evidence being left that anything has happened. Eventually, however, because of the progressive accumulation of sun damage, the fibroblasts no longer secrete the ground substance in great enough quantities to repair the ravages of time and a lax, wrinkled poorly healing skin develops as one of the unmistakable signs of the ageing process. Sun damage seems to play a large part in this process, as can be seen by comparing, clinically or histologically, areas of skin from clothed or unclothed sites. Histologically, the collagen patterns in the upper dermis are disrupted and tangled and their staining properties change (elastosis — Ch. 12); the whole skin, including the epidermis, is thinned and many fibroblasts are lost. Old skin has great difficulty in healing, not only because of the failing circulation, but also because the dermis can no longer regenerate itself nor service the epidermis.

There are several inborn errors of metabolism involving the dermal proteins, the most spectacular of which results in folds of loose skin that can be hyperextended and which heal poorly (*Ehlers–Danlos syndrome*). Other organs are similarly affected and the patients may also have emphysema.

There is also a series of diseases in which collagen seems to be the subject of autoimmune attack by the body. *Granuloma annulare*, *necrobiosis lipoidica* and *rheumatoid nodules* are all characterised histologically by areas of degenerate collagen surrounded by an inflammatory infiltrate which seems to be causing the collagen destruction.

Another series of collagen diseases which are even more clearly autoimmune are the group including *dermatomyositis* and *scleroderma*. The latter disease occurs with a variety of other autoimmune phenomena and has recently come to light as one of the end effects of *graft-versus-host disease* when it involves the skin.

Glycosaminoglycans

The best known of the diseases involving the glycosaminoglycans (GAGs) are the range of conditions in which the enzymes involved in their breakdown are defective. Because these substances are usually being metabolised and resynthesised, when their enzymatic breakdown is inhibited, they slowly accumulate, causing monstrous deformities and a host of general body symptoms. The syndromes include Hunter's and Hurler's diseases (Ch. 7) which used to be lumped together as *gargoylism* in reference to the terrible physical effects that they produce.

Mast cells

The mast cells degranulate on stimulation to release histamine which is noxious to metazoan parasites. It also makes the skin itch and this probably results in the parasite being dislodged when the animal scratches. Histamine also causes the blood vessels to dilate, allowing the various elements of the immune response to escape into the tissue and also attack the invader (Ch.10).

Mast cells seem to be very labile in some individuals; these people seem to suffer from typical histamine-type responses to stimuli that would leave a normal individual unresponsive. Similarly, some individuals have a severe response to the release of histamine that can be life threatening. The classic histamine reaction is nettle rash where the nettle introduces its own histamine into the victim, but some subjects produce a nettle rash reaction to foods or drugs, and often no cause can be identified.

There are some proliferative mast cell diseases, the most notable of which is *urticaria pigmentosa*. This disease occurs in various clinical forms ranging from a benign rash in childhood that may regress completely, to a severe and systemic adult form with spill-over of mast cells into the blood and which may result in death from histamine shock.

Connective tissue tumours

Most dermal connective tissue tumours are benign. The most common is the *dermatofibroma* (Fig. 24.25);

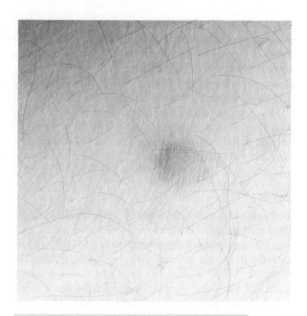

Fig. 24.25   Dermatofibroma (histiocytoma)
This benign tumour of dermal cells induces epidermal hyperplasia and pigmentation over it.

this lesion usually occurs on the legs. *Dermatofibrosarcoma protuberans* is a more aggressive variant characterised by high cellularity, mitotic activity and a protuberant surface; it has a marked tendency to recur locally.

Pyogenic granuloma

Pyogenic granuloma is a nodular profusion of granulation tissue that often protrudes from an area of damaged or ulcerated epidermis. This is the equivalent of the old surgical lesion called 'proud flesh' in which exuberant dermal regeneration prevents re-epithelialisation of a surgical incision. Pyogenic granulomas are similar lesions which have an intact or only focally ulcerated epidermal covering. These lesions may be idiosyncratic dermal responses to trauma. Their nomenclature is misleading because the lesions consist of granulation tissue, *not* granulomas, and they are only pyogenic (pus-forming) when secondarily infected.

ACCUMULATIONS

Various materials may accumulate in the skin for a variety of metabolic reasons. In general, the substances that accumulate do so for the same reasons that they accumulate in any other organ of the body.

In jaundice (Ch. 16), bile pigments accumulate in the blood and eventually diffuse into the tissue. All tissues are more or less stained (except for the brain in adults) but those tissues that contain the most elastin are the most heavily stained. Elastin specifically binds bile pigments and for this reason jaundice is very obvious in the skin and even more obvious in the sclera, which contain even higher amounts of elastin than does the skin.

For reasons that are mostly obscure many drugs, or their metabolites, accumulate in the skin. Some are visible, such as amiodarone, and the presence of some can only be implied because of their effects, such as the sweat gland damage seen in barbiturate overdose or the photosensitivity seen with chlorpromazine. Presumably, any drug which has a cutaneous side-effect (and there are many) is accumulating in the skin to some extent and not reaching the organ the pharmacologist intended.

Other accumulations affecting the skin include:

- amyloid
- calcification
- porphyrias.

The skin is involved in amyloidosis (Ch. 7) in the same way that other organs are affected. The skin shows raised, waxy plaques and depositions of the amorphous, eosinophilic material within the deeper dermis and subcutaneous tissue. In *localised cutaneous amyloidosis* there are several clinical variants, ranging from small discrete papules up to much larger, flat macules. The amyloid is located high in the skin, in the papillary dermis, and therefore causes the lesions to be more raised and to have sharper edges than those seen in systemic amyloidosis. The lesions are usually severely pruritic and therefore their appearance may be modified by the effects of scratching and rubbing. Recent studies have revealed that the amyloid in these lesions often contains modified keratin, which has presumably descended from the epidermis and been rendered inert and packaged as amyloid in the upper dermis.

Calcium tends to precipitate in many post-inflammatory situations (Ch. 7). Whilst pilar cysts often contain areas of calcification, epidermal cysts never do; similarly, calcified nodules arise fairly commonly in the scrotum but are almost never encountered in the vulva. Several distinct clinical entities of dystrophic calcium accumulation are known, such as *scrotal calcinosis, idiopathic calcinosis cutis, tumoral calcinosis* and *subcutaneous calcified nod-*

ules, in which no preceding cause can be identified. Other lesions, such as pilar cysts, scars and basal cell carcinomas, can have secondary deposits of calcium within them. One hair follicle tumour, the *calcifying epithelioma of Malherbe*, is highly specific and always calcifies eventually. In all of these examples, the deposits are chemically the same and consist of calcium and phosphate.

In porphyria (Ch. 7) the various porphyrins may accumulate in different organs of the body, resulting in a variety of curious metabolic diseases. When they accumulate in the skin, as in *porphyria cutanea tarda*, they are often capable of producing a photosensitivity. The reason is that these molecules are similar in structure to plant chlorophyll and can generate very reactive free radicals when excited by short-wave ultraviolet light.

CUTANEOUS NERVES

The epidermis contains no nerves; they all lie in the dermis. Many nerve fibres approach the epidermis; some terminate in specific structures which are specialised to subserve different functions, while others end as naked fibres, generally those that respond to painful stimuli. The significance of sensation to the skin itself can be seen in those rare conditions in which pain sensation is congenitally absent; such individuals generally do not survive since they are subject to continual wounds that are destructive but give no warning pain signals. A similar situation occurs when nerves are damaged by *diabetes* or *leprosy*. These patients develop skin ulcers and a variety of chronic infections in the distribution of the damaged nerves.

Tumours of cutaneous nerves

The majority of nerve tumours are benign. They are tumours of the various cells of the nerve sheath since mature nerves are post-mitotic and incapable of mitosis (Chs 12 and 26). The Schwann cells that support and insulate myelinated nerve fibres are capable of developing benign tumours (*schwannomas*). However, the other cells within the nerve sheath that seem to be more closely related to fibroblasts are the ones involved in *neurofibromatosis*, the congenital disease that has been identified as the cause of the Elephant Man's deformities. These tumours are usually multiple fleshy nodules that arise throughout life and which have significant eventual malignant potential.

BEHAVIOUR AND THE SKIN

The skin is the surface at which the world and the individual meet. Many individuals attempt to modify their relationship with the outside world by some manipulation of the aspect that is most visible. Much socially acceptable behaviour of this sort that is accepted as 'normal' occurs in the form of cosmetics in our society or ritual scarring in other societies. However, non-acceptable self-mutilation is usually an indication of severe emotional disturbance and it has recently been observed that 'body piercing' is a high risk activity for AIDS.

Tattoos

Tattooing is achieved by introducing stable, inert pigment into the upper dermis where it can be seen through the epidermis. This process can occur accidentally, in trauma cases where gravel and dirt enter wounds which subsequently heal, or in contact gunshot wounds where unburnt powder particles are driven into the skin, or deliberately as a decorative device. Clearly, any of these mechanisms is a potential route for infection, and the AIDS crisis has increased awareness of this problem. Some pigments that were formerly used were found to be less than ideally inert and cadmium pigments, used to produce yellow colours, were found also to produce the erythema of photosensitivity as an added bonus.

Dermatitis artefacta

There are a variety of self-inflicted skin disorders that come to the attention of dermatologists, and sometimes even pathologists. Curious patterns of baldness that do not conform to the usual clinical picture can be caused by patients habitually plucking hair (*trichotillomania*) as a nervous tic or as a more extensive behavioural activity. Curious patterns of rashes can be produced with the help of acids or caustic substances, only in the sites that can be reached by the patient and often with tell-tale drip marks. Strange stories of parasitic infestation backed up by various materials plucked from their own skins (including bits of adnexa, dermis and nerves) are offered by some patients with parasite phobias! The common feature of these conditions is the bizarre nature of the lesions, conforming to no known pattern of naturally occurring disease. The lesions occur only in the sites that the patient can reach, and the behaviour of the patient is abnormal. The pathologist is faced with an atypical clinical history and an

often very destructive lesion with no abnormality in the tissue itself and with no inflammation in the early lesion to explain its genesis.

TOXINS AND THE SKIN

Almost any rash can be the result of some drug or toxin either taken internally or applied to the skin surface. Such rashes may be directly toxic, where the skin is killed by contact with chemicals such as strong acids or other corrosives (Ch. 6). They may be photosensitive, where the actual substance does no harm until acted upon by specific wavelengths of light. They may be allergic rashes in which the compound itself, or a normal skin protein modified by the toxic compound, elicits an immune response. The compound may itself be inert but become toxic when modified by the body's own metabolic processes. Examples of all of these mechanisms are well known and have been mentioned in the appropriate places in the text.

The skin reactions themselves are often indistinguishable from the idiopathic lesions that they mimic. Thus, various drugs such as gold, antimalarials and photographic colour developers can produce very characteristic eruptions that are almost identical to lichen planus histologically. Contact dermatitis and photodermatitis are often impossible to distinguish histologically from a spontaneous eczema, and many drugs and toxins will produce blisters at all levels of the skin. Even malignant lymphomas may be mimicked by sandfly bites; often the only way to recognise the source of this lesion is to find the insect mouthparts in the skin.

In these situations the clinical history and the distribution of the lesions is a better guide to aetiology than the histological appearance.

SKIN MANIFESTATIONS OF INTERNAL DISEASE

Some skin conditions are pathognomonic of internal disorders, some are frequently associated with them and some are rare associations that may be no more than chance. Skin conditions are, however, very important clues that should be watched for with great attention. Nevertheless, they are mainly clinical diagnostic clues, and their histological appearance is often less dramatic than their clinical presentation. They are mentioned here for completeness and because the mechanisms by which they arise offer such fascinating speculations on pathological processes.

Skin lesions always associated with internal disease

Secondary deposits of tumour in the skin are, by definition, the manifestations of internal disease and the problem is to recognise that they are secondary deposits and not primary skin tumours. The skin is a relatively rare site for secondary tumour deposits, in particular before the primary lesion has declared itself, but it does happen and a biopsy can be of great diagnostic help. In general, secondary deposits retain the characteristics of the original tumour and a reasonable guess at its origins can be offered in most cases.

A more curious but fascinating phenomenon is the specific skin rash that accompanies the very rare tumour of the pancreas, glucagonoma. The skin lesion is a *necrotising migratory erythema* that is totally specific and seems to be due to some mechanism on the part of the tumour that deprives the skin of zinc.

Skin lesions sometimes associated with internal disease

This group is by far the largest and contains all of the classic skin lesions that suggest underlying disease such as:

- rashes associated with *arthritis* and with *chronic inflammatory bowel disease*

- dermatitis associated with myositis in the *dermatomyositis* complex
- dirty grey lesions of the armpits called *acanthosis nigricans* and sudden crops of *basal cell papillomas*, both of which signal gastrointestinal malignancies.

Perhaps the commonest rashes are those associated with diabetes, such as *necrobiosis lipoidica* which shows "necrotic" collagen surrounded by chronic inflammatory cells. Other common lesions are the *xanthomas* which often indicate an underlying hyperlipidaemia, and the *fingernail clubbing* which may be associated with a variety of internal diseases both inflammatory and malignant.

Rare associations with internal disease

Several infrequent associations have been reported. Their rarity renders them of little clinical use, or they represent two relatively common diseases in a group of patients, such as the elderly, and thus appear to be associated. A good example of this is the association between malignancy and pemphigus. Both diseases are more common in the middle-aged and elderly and they consequently have a relatively high chance of occurring together in this group, but the association seems to be no more than chance when the increased frequency of each is taken into account.

Acknowledgement

The author acknowledges the following for help in providing illustrations: Professor S S Bleehen, Dr A Messenger, Dr A Wright.

FURTHER READING

MacKie RM (ed) 1984 Milne's Dermatopathology. Edward Arnold, London
McKee P H 1989 Pathology of the skin. Lippincott, Philadelphia

Stevens A, Wheater P R, Lowe J S 1989 Clinical dermatopathology. Churchill Livingstone, Edinburgh

Osteoarticular and connective tissues

BONE

NORMAL STRUCTURE AND FUNCTION

The skeleton provides the structural support required by the body, both at rest and in motion. When this support is lost, as after a fracture, the subsequent pain and limitation of movement emphasise the importance of the intact skeletal system. The skull, and to a lesser extent the ribs, protect the brain and thoracic and upper abdominal organs from traumatic injury.

In the normal adult, bone is the sole site of haemopoietic marrow. In addition, the skeleton has an important metabolic function as the body's reservoir of calcium. Any abnormality of calcium metabolism, therefore, can affect the structure and integrity of the skeleton.

Bone is heavily mineralised by a calcium phosphate complex known as *hydroxyapatite*, deposited on the underlying matrix of proteins. Type 1 collagen is the major protein of bone but there are many other non-collagenous proteins, some with defined and others with less certain roles. Some of these are secreted by osteoblasts whilst others are absorbed from the circulation. These proteins have important roles in cell to cell interaction, calcium binding and bone mineralisation. Bone is also cellular and highly vascular, as demonstrated by the extensive haemorrhage which often accompanies fractures. The cells which form bone, *osteoblasts*, are derived from mesenchyme; their chief role is to synthesise bone matrix. The bone cells incorporated within the trabeculae are known as *osteocytes*. In contrast, *osteoclasts* are part of the monocyte/macrophage group of cells, are often multinucleated and have crucial roles in the breakdown and remodelling of bone. The exact mechanism by which bone is formed and mineralised is uncertain, but it is clear that osteoblasts are involved in both these processes. Because common bone diseases, such as osteoporosis, are major causes of morbidity and mortality, many research groups are studying the factors which influence osteoblast function. Some are attempting to unravel the complex system of protein signals (cytokines) that influence the functions of and interactions between osteoblasts and osteoclasts whereas others are studying genetic variation in the expression of receptors for vitamin D metabolites.

There are two types of mature bone—compact and cancellous. Both are composed of closely packed plates or *lamellae* which vary in thickness from 5–15 μm. In *compact bone*, for example the cortex of the limb bones, many lamellae are arranged concentrically around a central core which contains small arteries and veins; the central core is the *Haversian canal* and the entire concentric structure is the *Haversian system*. The spaces between the systems contain less regularly arranged lamellae and there are usually several concentric lamellae immediately beneath the periosteum. *Cancellous bone* is found in the medullary cavities of the limb bones and the vertebrae. In contrast to compact bone it is a meshwork of loosely arranged trabeculae. The thicker trabeculae also have fine canals containing blood vessels but they lack the organised structure of compact bone.

All bones have a dense outer connective tissue *periosteum* which retains an osteogenic capability throughout life. The medullary cavities are lined by an *endosteum* with similar functions. In the adult, the haemopoietic marrow is usually restricted to the ribs and vertebrae, the pelvic bones and the most proximal portions of the long bones of the limbs.

Development and growth of bones

Most tissues and organs grow as a result of a general increase in the number of their constituent cells. Because the proteinaceous matrix is so heavily calcified, a similar process is not possible in bone. Instead, when growth is necessary, new layers (lamellae) of bone are laid onto the surface of pre-existing trabeculae.

During development, bone is formed either directly in connective tissue, as in the skull (*intramembranous ossification*) or on pre-existing cartilage, as in the limb bones (*endochondral ossification*).

During intramembranous ossification the first bone that is laid down has a loose and rather haphazard arrangement. This 'woven bone' gradually matures into more organised and compact 'lamellar' bone.

Endochondral ossification is a much more complicated process during which a cartilagenous template is converted into a bony structure with capacity for further growth. In each bone, ossification occurs at particular sites or *centres of ossification* situated in the shaft (diaphyseal centres) or towards the ends of the bone (epiphyseal centres) (Fig. 25.1). Ossification proceeds at different, but predictable, rates in each particular bone. In long bones, a plate of epiphyseal cartilage persists into adolescent or early adult life; this allows a continual increase in bone length. The overall shape and size of bone changes during growth and, to some extent, in adult life. This involves both osteoclastic bone resorption and enlargement of pre-existing, or the formation of new, bony trabeculae. In order to preserve the strength and integrity of the

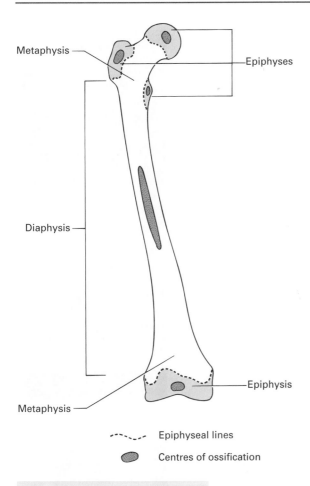

Metaphysis

Epiphyses

Diaphysis

Metaphysis

Epiphysis

- - - - - - Epiphyseal lines

⬭ Centres of ossification

Fig. 25.1 Structure of a long bone

Pathological basis of clinical signs and symptoms of bone disease	
Sign or symptom	Pathological basis
Pain	Stimulation of nerve endings in bone by: • inflammation • trauma (fracture) • tumour
Fracture after trivial injury	Bone weakening due to: • congenital disorders of bone integrity • metabolic bone disease • erosion of bone by tumour
Deformity	Bone weakening due to: • congenital disorders of bone integrity • metabolic bone disease Malunion of a fracture
Hypercalcaemia	Extensive bone erosion by tumour deposits Secretion of PTH by parathyroid adenoma

skeleton these processes are closely co-ordinated. If, as in osteoporosis (p. 788), these processes are imbalanced, the skeleton is weakened and liable to fracture.

FRACTURES AND THEIR HEALING

▶ Types of fracture: simple (clean break); comminuted (multiple bone fragments); compound (breaking through overlying skin); complicated (involving adjacent structures—blood vessels, nerves, etc.); stress fractures (small linear fractures)
▶ Pathological fracture: fracture of bone weakened by disease (e.g. tumours, osteoporosis, osteomalacia, Paget's disease)
▶ Healing requires immobilisation of approximated bone ends
▶ Healing may be impaired by movement, poor blood supply, interposition of soft tissue, infection, poor nutrition, steroid therapy

Causes of fractures

Fractures in normal bone are the result of substantial trauma, such as direct violence or a sudden unexpected fall. The precise site of fracture, the nature and direction of the fracture line and the speed of the subsequent repair process depend very much on the age of the patient, the particular bone involved and the precise pattern of injury (Fig. 25.2).

Repeated episodes of minor trauma, for example after marching, marathon running or training for sport, can produce small but often painful *stress fractures*. These usually occur in the long bones of the lower limbs but have also been described in the metatarsals, the upper limb, pelvis and spine. They usually heal satisfactorily after a short period of rest. Even professional athletes can develop these fractures.

Fractures often develop in bone which is structurally abnormal. They may occur after a trivial injury or minor fall or even spontaneously during normal activity. This is particularly common in patients with osteoporosis but also occurs in most forms of metabolic bone disease (e.g. in osteomalacia and rickets), in Paget's disease and in bone infiltrated by malignant tumours. Fractures in abnormal bone of any sort are called *pathological fractures*.

Fracture healing

The first stage in fracture healing is the formation of

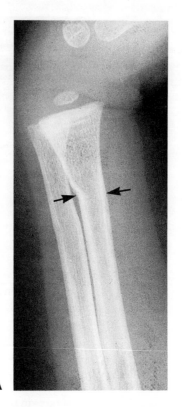

A

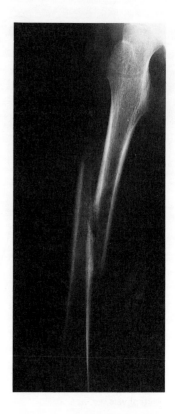

B

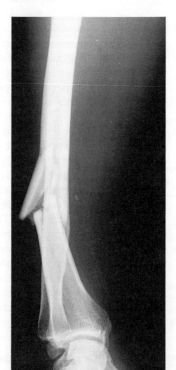

C

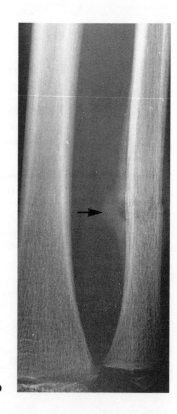

D

Fig. 25.2 Fracture types and fracture healing

A. A greenstick fracture of the distal radius in a young child (arrowed). **B.** A displaced spiral fracture of the femur in a child. **C.** A comminuted fracture of the tibia. One fragment of bone has almost separated from the shaft. **D.** A healing fracture of the ulna. The site of the break is just visible and is surrounded by callus (arrowed)

a bony bridge between the separated fragments. When this is formed, and some rigidity has been regained, remodelling and restructuring gradually restore the normal contours of the fractured bone. This process and the factors that can interfere with it are described in Chapter 6.

The major causes of delayed fracture healing are:

1. *Local factors*:
- excessive movement of fractured bone during healing
- extensive damage to fractured bone, i.e. bony necrosis in a comminuted fracture
- a poor intrinsic blood supply, e.g. lower tibia
- severe local soft tissue injury or impaired blood supply
- interruption of blood supply following fracture, e.g. head of femur, scaphoid
- infection — only if overlying skin surface is broken, as in compound fracture
- interposition of soft tissue in fracture gap, or wide separation of fracture ends.

2. General factors:
- elderly patients
- poor general health
- drug therapy, e.g. corticosteroids.

All of these are well recognised by orthopaedic surgeons, who modify the treatment in individual cases in line with the particular pattern of injury, and the age and general health of the patient. For example, a fracture through the neck of the femur usually deprives the head of its normal blood supply and satisfactory fracture healing is unlikely to occur. Surgical treatment, such as excision of the head and replacement by a metallic prosthesis, is therefore essential. Fractures in which the overlying skin surface is broken (compound fractures) are liable to infection, whereas this is extremely uncommon in closed fractures. Healing will be substantially delayed if a wound infection develops.

In many fractures, healing can be accelerated by prompt and appropriate surgical treatment using internal fixation by nails, plates and screws or external fixator devices to hold the fractured fragments in an appropriate position; this often allows early mobilisation. Primary callus does form but is reduced in amount. Small gaps are filled by new woven bone. Dead bone is gradually revascularised and new Haversian bone grows in.

Surgical treatment is sometimes necessary for fractures in which the healing process has been delayed. The object is to 'restart' the primary callus response. This can sometimes be achieved by lifting flaps of periosteum close to the fracture site. In addition, local 'grafting' with autogenous cancellous bone, usually taken from the iliac crest, can be effective. The exact mechanism by which these bone grafts induce the formation of callus is uncertain but there is no doubt that they are a potent local stimulus to new bone formation.

OSTEOPOROSIS AND METABOLIC BONE DISEASE

Normal calcium metabolism

The two major hormones that regulate calcium metabolism are *vitamin D* and *parathyroid hormone* (PTH). Vitamin D is not a vitamin in the strict sense of an essential dietary requirement, as it can also be synthesised photochemically in the skin. Vitamin D must be metabolised by the liver to 25-hydroxyvitamin D_3, and subsequently by the kidney to the active metabolite 1,25-dihydroxyvitamin D_3. A variety of other metabolites are also formed but these play no important physiological role in calcium metabolism. Receptors for vitamin D are present in a variety of cell types in the body; the physiological role of this vitamin may be much wider than is currently known. Expression of the receptors is subject to genetic variation within the population and may contribute to the individual differences in risk of developing metabolic bone disease. The combined effects of vitamin D and parathyroid hormone are:

- to stimulate bone calcium mobilisation
- to increase renal reabsorption of calcium in the distal tubule (chiefly PTH, but also vitamin D)
- to stimulate intestinal calcium and phosphate absorption (vitamin D).

The biological effects of 1,25-dihydroxyvitamin D_3 are initiated by the binding of this hormone to intracellular receptors present in the intestinal epithelium and the bone and, to a lesser extent, in many other tissues. It may well have an important role in regulating intracellular calcium concentrations throughout the body. There are important inter-relationships between PTH and vitamin D; for example, PTH stimulates the enzymatic hydroxylation of vitamin D precursors in the kidney. The major stimulus to PTH production is a reduced serum calcium level. In sites of new bone formation calcium and phosphate are maintained at a concentration that ensures supersaturation, otherwise bone mineralisation cannot proceed.

In contrast to PTH, *calcitonin*, a peptide hormone,

appears to lower serum calcium, but usually only when it is pathologically elevated. The stimulus to its secretion is an increase in the serum calcium concentration; it is produced in specialised parafollicular cells (C-cells) of the thyroid. Its exact physiological action is uncertain but it has an inhibitory effect on osteoclasts.

Although vitamin D, PTH and, to a lesser extent, calcitonin are the most important factors controlling calcium and phosphate concentrations, and therefore normal bone integrity, several other factors are also involved. Glucocorticoids have a role in the regulation of skeletal growth but prolonged corticosteroid therapy often induces osteoporosis. Thyroid hormone deficiency, as in cretinism, is associated with several skeletal abnormalities. Sex steroids accelerate the closure of epiphyses, and growth hormone has an effect on the development and maturation of cartilage.

Osteoporosis

> ▶ Reduction in total bone mass causing weakening
> ▶ Common in the elderly, particularly females
> ▶ Common predisposing cause of fractures, particularly neck of femur
> ▶ Complication of steroid therapy and Cushing's syndrome
> ▶ Follows any form of immobility
> ▶ Associated with alcoholism, diabetes, liver disease and smoking

In osteoporosis, the total mass of bone tissue is reduced but there are few other abnormalities. It results from the progressive imbalance between bone reabsorption and bone formation that is a feature of normal ageing. Some degree of osteoporosis is inevitable in all elderly patients. The disease assumes particular significance when complications such as fractures result.

Pathogenesis

In osteoporosis the total mass of bone tissue is reduced, but the bone that remains is normal, both histologically and biochemically. Throughout life all bones undergo a continual and carefully regulated process of remodelling. This occurs at focal points — bone remodelling units — and follows a cycle of changes lasting about 120 days. Small erosions are produced by osteoclasts and then repaired over a much longer period by osteoblasts. In osteoporosis it appears that osteoblastic repair in these erosions is incomplete, especially in trabecular bone. The ratio

of cortical to trabecular bone varies at different points in the skeleton and even within each bone. Towards the wrist, for example, the proportion of trabecular bone in the radius is more than 60% and this may explain why Colles' fractures are so common in osteoporosis. Bone loss in the cortex is less pronounced. Bone formation exceeds bone reabsorption at the periosteal aspect of long bones, but the opposite applies at the inner endosteal surface. As a result the total volume of long bones increases with age, but the thickness of the cortex decreases.

The total bone mass of an individual is influenced by factors such as body build, race, gender, physical activity and general nutrition. Osteoporosis is commoner in females than males and is less common in blacks, who have a greater skeletal mass than whites or Asians. Osteoporosis can be assessed radiologically or by techniques based on the ability of bone to absorb photons released by a γ-emitting isotope. These demonstrate a progressive loss of bone of 0.75–1% per annum in normal adults of both sexes from as early as 30 years of age. More importantly there is an accelerated phase of bone loss of up to 1–3% per year in females in the 5–10 years following the menopause.

Localised osteoporosis is inevitable after immobilisation of any part of the skeleton. Even young, healthy males confined to bed after a limb fracture show substantial bone loss. Painful joints in patients with rheumatoid arthritis restrict movement, and osteoporosis often develops in adjacent bones.

Complications

The major complications of osteoporosis are:

- skeletal deformity
- bone pain
- fracture.

The commonest clinical feature of osteoporosis is the progressive loss of height that occurs with age. This is a direct result of compression of vertebrae. Sudden collapse or unequal compression of individual vertebral bodies can cause severe localised back pain and deformities such as kyphosis or scoliosis (Fig. 25.3).

Wrist and hip fractures are common in elderly patients with osteoporosis. Although osteoporosis is the major underlying cause, other factors such as an increased tendency to fall and a loss of 'protective neuromuscular reflexes' (the ability to fall over safely) are also important. Hip fractures account for numerous hospital admissions and are a major

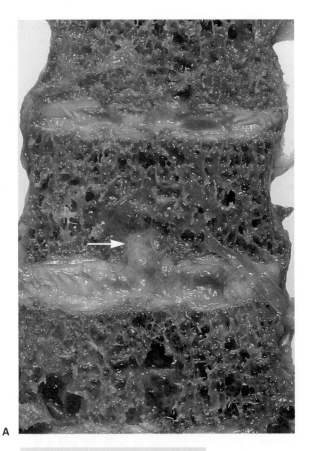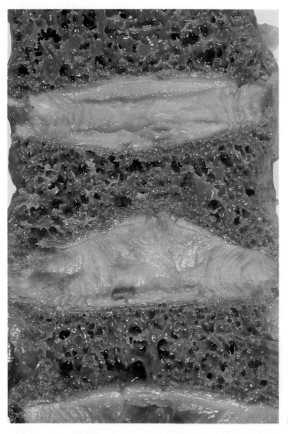

A

B

Fig. 25.3 Vertebral osteoporosis

A. The lower thoracic vertebrae, showing small protrusions of the intervertebral disc into the osteoporotic bone (arrowed).
B. The lumbar spine. The vertebral body in the centre has collapsed and has a typical biconcave shape.

source of disability, and a frequent cause of death in the elderly.

Prevention and treatment

Osteoporosis is a major social and economic problem in the elderly, and preventive measures should begin in the middle-aged. There is good evidence that osteoporosis is reduced in women treated with oestrogens from the time of the menopause (hormone replacement therapy — HRT). Disadvantages of this treatment include irregular vaginal bleeding, a slightly increased risk of venous thrombosis and a possible increase in carcinoma of the body of the uterus. Despite this, HRT is widely used in North America and Europe. Regular exercise and an increased dietary intake of calcium also have beneficial effects. The pharmaceutical industry is continually developing new agents that promote

bone formation and many of these are under clinical trial.

Rickets and osteomalacia

> ► Inadequate mineralisation of organic bone matrix
> ► Rickets occurs in children and is characterised by bone deformities
> ► Osteomalacia occurs in adults causing susceptibility to fracture but few deformities
> ► Due to deficiency of active metabolites of vitamin D
> ► Causes include nutritional deficiency of vitamin D, lack of sunlight, intestinal malabsorption, renal and liver disease

Osteomalacia is characterised by deficient mineralisation of the organic matrix of the skeleton. Rickets is the name given to osteomalacia affecting the growing skeleton of children; it results in characteristic deformities. Causes of osteomalacia, or rickets, include:

- dietary deficiency of vitamin D
- deficiency of vitamin D metabolites
- intestinal malabsorption
- renal disease.

Aetiology

In the past, nutritional deficiency of vitamin D was a common cause of rickets in children and, occasionally, of osteomalacia in adults. In most communities, this has been eliminated by improvements in diet and by the addition of vitamin D to foodstuffs. The disease still occurs in some Asian communities in the United Kingdom; skin pigmentation impairs photochemical synthesis of vitamin D, and a constituent of chapatti flour interferes with calcium and phosphate absorption in the gut.

Malabsorption of vitamin D from the intestine is the commonest cause of osteomalacia in adults. The underlying cause is often coeliac disease, but occasional cases result from Crohn's disease or extensive surgical resection of the small intestine. As the liver and kidney have important roles in the metabolism of vitamin D, renal and hepatic disorders may cause osteomalacia. This is uncommon in liver disease, but a complex pattern of bone disease which includes osteomalacia is seen in renal failure (p. 791). Occasional patients treated with anticonvulsants, such as phenytoin, develop osteomalacia. These drugs induce liver enzymes which degrade vitamin D to inactive metabolites.

Diagnosis

The characteristic clinical deformities of rickets include:

- bowing of the long bones of the leg
- pronounced swelling at the costochondral junctions
- flattening or 'bossing' of the skull.

Inadequate mineralisation of bone reduces its normal strength and allows deformities to develop, for example from pressure on the skull whilst lying in a cot or on the limbs as they begin to bear weight. Calcification of epiphyseal cartilage is an essential step in the normal process of ossification in long bone. When the levels of vitamin D metabolites are low, calcification cannot occur and cartilagenous proliferation continues. This accounts for the enlargement of long bones and the ribs at growth plates.

The characteristic pathological feature in adults with osteomalacia is spontaneous incomplete fractures ('Looser's zones') often in the long bones or pelvis. The main symptoms are bone pain and tenderness, and weakness of proximal limb muscles. Serum calcium levels may be reduced and a bone biopsy will demonstrate an increase in non-mineralised osteoid (Fig. 25.4).

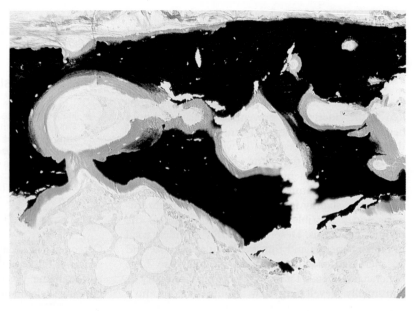

Fig. 25.4 Osteomalacia

Biopsy of the iliac crest from a 71-year-old female with longstanding malabsorption and osteomalacia. The black tissue is normally mineralised bone. The surrounding pink material is non-mineralised osteoid. In normal bone this would be hardly recognisable at this magnification.

Treatment and prevention

Uncomplicated rickets or osteomalacia will respond promptly to vitamin D treatment. Intramuscular injection can overcome problems associated with malabsorption, and underlying disorders, such as coeliac disease, should be treated appropriately. A normal balanced diet will prevent rickets or osteomalacia, but many foodstuffs are now artificially supplemented with vitamin D. The extension of supplementation to foodstuffs favoured by specific communities at risk for nutritional rickets has also been advocated.

Hyperparathyroidism and hypercalcaemia

► Hyperparathyroidism causes increased osteoclastic breakdown of bone
► Serum calcium is usually raised in primary hyperparathyroidism, but low or normal in secondary (reactive) hyperparathyroidism
► Bone lesions may be cystic and haemorrhagic ('brown tumours')

Persistent elevation of fasting blood calcium, after correction has been made for the serum albumin concentration, is an important indication for further investigation. The major pathological causes are:

• primary hyperparathyroidism
• secondary deposits in bone, i.e. metastases
• inappropriate secretion of PTH-like molecules by malignant tumours
• sarcoidosis
• renal failure
• immobility, thyrotoxicosis, thiazide diuretics, etc.

In many instances, hypercalcaemia is clearly secondary to either malignant disease or a systemic disorder such as sarcoidosis.

In hyperparathyroidism (Ch. 17), increased secretion of parathyroid hormone stimulates calcium absorption in the intestine, reabsorption in the kidney and osteoclastic breakdown of bone.

In *primary hyperparathyroidism* the usual cause is a parathyroid adenoma or, occasionally, diffuse hyperplasia of the parathyroid glands. In contrast, in *secondary hyperparathyroidism*, prolonged *hypocalcaemia* stimulates parathyroid hyperplasia and eventually produces parathyroid enlargement. This is usually the result of renal failure or malabsorption secondary to coeliac disease. In occasional patients, secondary hyperparathyroidism is associated with hypercalcaemia. This has been called *tertiary hyperparathyroidism* and usually results from inappropriately high

secretion of PTH by an adenoma arising in secondary hyperparathyroidism.

When obvious causes, such as malignant disease, sarcoidosis or drug therapy, have been excluded it must be suspected that an otherwise fit patient with hypercalcaemia has primary hyperparathyroidism (Table 25.1).

The advanced bone pathology associated with hyperparathyroidism is now rare. In the early stages there are subtle radiological changes such as subperiosteal reabsorption of phalangeal bone (Fig. 25.5) or characteristic changes around the teeth. As the disease progresses cystic bone lesions may develop — *osteitis fibrosa cystica (von Recklinghausen's disease of bone)*. These are sometimes referred to as 'brown tumours' although they are not neoplasms. The brown appearance is the result of haemorrhage and there is often a marked associated giant cell osteoclastic reaction.

Bone disease in renal failure (renal osteodystrophy)

Most patients with chronic renal failure have clinical, radiological or pathological evidence of bone disease. There is no single bone disease which occurs in renal failure; in most patients it is a combination of *osteomalacia* with a variable degree of *hyperparathyroidism*. Other features include:

• osteoporosis
• bone necrosis
• soft tissue calcification.

Table 25.1 Causes of hypercalcaemia	
Cause	Pathophysiology
Primary hyperparathyroidism	Abnormal PTH secretion from adenoma, hyperplasia or carcinoma of parathyroid glands
Malignant disease	Secondary deposits producing some destruction and calcium release or (rarely) inappropriate PTH secretion, usually squamous carcinoma of bronchus
Sarcoidosis	Probable secretion of vitamin D metabolites from granulomas
Miscellaneous causes: Drugs, e.g. thiazide diuretics Renal failure Thyrotoxicosis Immobility	

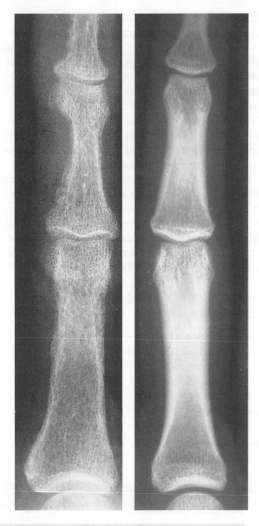

Fig. 25.5   X-ray of finger in primary hyperparathyroidism (left) and a normal patient (right)

The irregular outlines of the phalanges are the result of reabsorption of bone.

Table 25.2 Mechanisms of renal bone disease (renal osteodystrophy)	
Feature of renal failure	Pathological effect in bone
Inadequate renal tissue	Impaired conversion of 25(OH) D_3 to 1,25(OH)$_2$ D_3 → *Osteomalacia*
High serum phosphate	1. ?Inhibition of renal enzymes catalysing formation of 1,25(OH)$_2$ D_3 2. Decrease in ionised Ca^{++} in serum → *Hyperparathyroidism*
Prolonged haemodialysis	Inhibition of calcification of osteoid → *Osteomalacia*
Steroid therapy (e.g. for chronic glomerulonephritis)	Osteoporosis Avascular necrosis of bone

ated with aluminium deposition in organs such as brain and bone. In bone, aluminium inhibits the calcification of osteoid and contributes to osteomalacia in renal failure (Ch. 7).

Patients with chronic renal failure may have a low serum calcium. This is partly the result of impaired vitamin D metabolism, as vitamin D metabolites are essential for the proper absorption of calcium from the small intestine. The high serum phosphate also reduces the ionised fraction of plasma calcium. This acts as a stimulus to PTH production, and a degree of hyperparathyroidism is inevitable in severe renal failure. Patients with some forms of glomerulonephritis are treated with steroids and this may induce osteoporosis or, occasionally, areas of bone necrosis. Calcification of the soft tissues, or of blood vessel walls, is a further feature of chronic renal failure, particularly after prolonged haemodialysis.

The most important pathophysiological changes in renal bone disease are summarised in Table 25.2. Several mechanisms have been suggested to account for the osteomalacia. In all forms of renal failure there is a decrease in the amount of functional renal tissue, and this may be directly responsible for the inadequate production of active vitamin D metabolites. An increased blood phosphate level (hyperphosphataemia) is frequent in renal failure, and this may directly inhibit enzymes responsible for vitamin D metabolism in the kidneys. In the past, haemodialysis fluids rich in aluminium were associ-

OSTEOMYELITIS

- ► Inflammatory lesion due to bacterial infection of bone
- ► Bacteria enter bone either from blood (septicaemia) or directly through skin wound over a compound fracture
- ► Necrotic bone forms inner sequestrum; reactive new bone forms outer involucrum
- ► Most common in children, where *Staphylococcus aureus* is the usual cause
- ► A complication of advanced tuberculosis

Aetiology

Osteomyelitis is the result of a bacterial infection of bone. The typical patient is a young child who presents with pain in a long bone, sometimes with a misleading history of recent trauma. In the majority of cases the lesion develops in the metaphysis, the part of the shaft immediately adjacent to the epiphyseal plate. The rich capillary network and large venous channels in this area may favour the deposition of circulating micro-organisms and their subsequent growth. In children and adolescents, osteomyelitis is usually the result of *Staphylococcus aureus* bacteraemia, often secondary to a boil or other skin infections. Sometimes, the underlying cause of bacteraemia is not apparent. Osteomyelitis is also increasingly seen in elderly patients.

Before the introduction of antibiotics, tuberculous and even syphilitic osteomyelitis were common but these are now rare. Children with haemoglobinopathies, especially sickle cell disease, have an increased risk of osteomyelitis; unusual organisms, such as salmonella, are sometimes responsible.

Osteomyelitis is a well-recognised complication of compound fractures, particularly if the wound in the overlying skin is extensive and there are necrotic bone splinters at the fracture ends. Osteomyelitis is not a complication of closed fractures and, despite what some patients claim, direct trauma does not appear to predispose to infection of the underlying bone.

Pathogenesis

The sequence of changes in osteomyelitis is as follows:

1. Transient bacteraemia, e.g. *Staphylococcus aureus*.
2. Focus of acute inflammation in metaphysis of long bone.
3. Necrosis of bone fragments, forming the *sequestrum*.
4. Reactive new bone forms, the *involucrum*.
5. If untreated, sinuses form, draining pus to the skin surface via *cloacae*.

The initial focus of acute inflammation develops around small capillaries and veins in the metaphysis. The inflammatory process extends through the fine Haversian canals, compressing the adjacent veins and arteries. When the blood supply of bone trabeculae is compromised, bone death (*osteonecrosis*) results. Before antibiotic therapy was available, osteomyelitis was frequently a progressive condition. Large masses of dead bone developed and, because of their tendency to fragment and separate away from healthy bone,

were known as *sequestrum*. When the process is extensive, there is often a secondary thrombophlebitis of the larger veins draining towards the diaphysis and this contributes to ischaemia and bone necrosis.

When infection extends through the cortical bone to the periosteal layer, soft tissue swelling and periosteal elevation can be detected radiologically. In acute osteomyelitis there is marked oedema, fibrin deposition and acute inflammatory cell infiltration in the subperiosteal zones. If the lesion becomes chronic an enveloping layer of new bone is formed beneath the periosteum, and is known as *involucrum* (Fig. 25.6). As with any inflammatory process, there is a tendency for the pus and necrotic debris to drain towards the skin surface. In chronic osteomyelitis, these sinuses can persist for months or years. Their skin drainage sites are known as *cloacae*.

Brodie's abscess is a distinctive clinical form of subacute pyogenic osteomyelitis. The lesion is solitary and, as in typical acute osteomyelitis, localised to the metaphysis.

Clinical features, laboratory investigations and treatment

Most patients with acute osteomyelitis present with localised bone pain and some tissue swelling. A dull continuous back pain, which increases on straining, is typical of vertebral osteomyelitis. The radiological changes are usually characteristic. Blood cultures are positive in some patients, but open biopsy of the lesion may be needed to ensure accurate bacteriological diagnosis. The commonest organisms are *Staphylococcus aureus*, *Mycobacterium tuberculosis*, *Escherichia coli*, pneumococcus or group A streptococcus. Wherever possible a precise bacteriological diagnosis must be made and treatment continued for several weeks.

PAGET'S DISEASE

> ► Common disorder of unknown aetiology in which there is a localised increase in bone turnover
> ► May affect part of one bone, an entire bone, or many bones
> ► Most patients have few symptoms
> ► Complicated by pain, deformities, fractures, nerve compression, deafness, osteosarcoma and (rarely) heart failure

Incidence and epidemiology

Paget's disease is a common disorder in which there

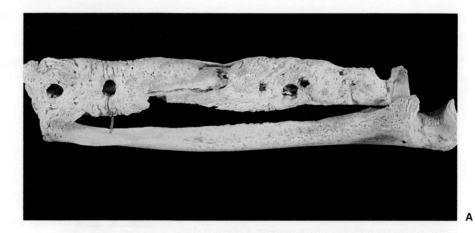

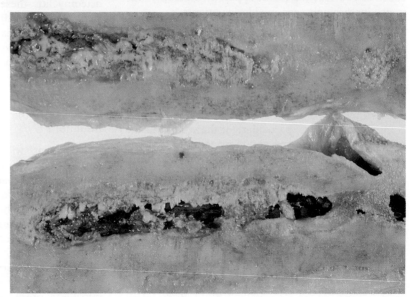

Fig. 25.6 Chronic osteomyelitis

A. The radius and ulna of an 18th-century sailor. The 'granular bone' is the involucrum and the circular defects are 'cloacae' through which pus drained. **B.** The cut surface of the femur of a 78-year-old male who received a shrapnel wound to his thigh in World War I. The pus drained through a sinus for the next 50 years! A thick bony involucrum surrounds a chronic inflammatory abscess in the marrow cavity.

is disorderly bony proliferation. If detected radiologically, it is present in at least 3%, and in some communities as many as 7–8%, of middle-aged and elderly patients. There is considerable variation in its incidence both within and between different countries and racial groups. Despite intensive study, little is known of the cause of Paget's disease and it is not regularly associated with any other common disorder. Electron microscopic studies have demonstrated probable viral inclusions in the nuclei of osteoclasts, possibly derived from measles, but no definite proof has been obtained.

Clinicopathological features

The usual presenting complaints of patients with Paget's disease are bone pain, deformities or frac-

tures. Although the pelvis and spine are most frequently affected, deformities are most obvious in the long bones such as the tibia, which is characteristically bowed, and in the skull.

Serum calcium concentration is usually normal, but the alkaline phosphatase is markedly elevated reflecting the osteoblastic activity. A variety of histological changes occur in Paget's disease and it is likely that these follow a sequence of bone breakdown (lysis), new bone formation and, later, bony sclerosis. Fractures may occur in the lytic phase. Large multinucleated osteoclasts are characteristic. In the later phases there is florid bony proliferation. Osteoblasts are present around thick and vascular trabeculae of new bone, and there may be wide seams of uncalcified osteoid. Eventually, this leads to dense bony sclerosis with wide and irregular trabeculae abutting upon each other forming a 'mosaic pattern'. It is this process which is responsible for the grossly thickened and deformed bone characteristic of Paget's disease (Fig. 25.7).

Complications

The complications of Paget's disease are:

- deformities
- bone pain
- fractures
- nerve or spinal cord compression
- deafness
- osteosarcoma, occasionally other bone tumours
- heart failure.

In many patients, Paget's disease is completely asymptomatic and is unlikely to be diagnosed unless discovered as an incidental finding on X-ray. The commonest complications are deformities (Fig. 25.8) and bone pain. In some cases, the pain is the result of

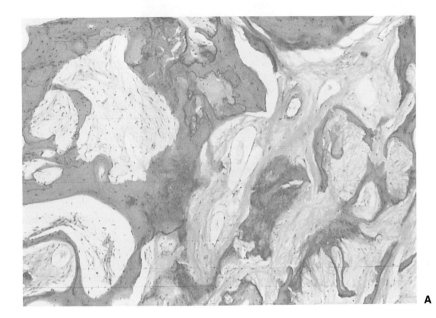

A

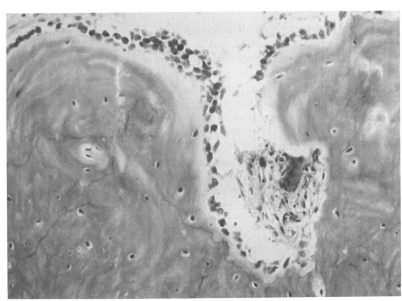

B

Fig. 25.7 Paget's disease

A. The typical disordered arrangement of bone trabeculae with intervening vascular fibrous tissue. **B.** A rim of osteoblasts surrounds dense pagetoid bone.

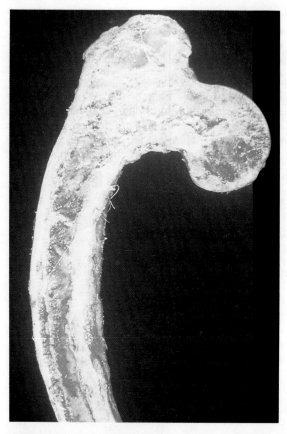

Fig. 25.8   Paget's disease

This affected femur shows characteristic thickening and deformity.

osteoarthritic degeneration of a related joint. The cause of the pain is uncertain, but in many bones with Paget's disease the subperiosteal zone is oedematous and highly vascular and there may be periosteal elevation. As the periosteum has a rich sensory innervation, these changes may be the cause of the pain. Pagetoid bone is particularly susceptible to fracturing in the initial lytic phase. Enlargement in the sclerotic stage can lead to nerve or spinal cord compression. Deafness is the result of both VIIIth cranial nerve compression and distortion of the middle ear cavity. Occasional patients develop other cranial nerve palsies and, in advanced cases, paraplegia can result.

The most sinister complication of Paget's disease is osteosarcoma; the majority of elderly patients with osteosarcoma do have Paget's disease. As in younger patients, osteosarcoma develops in the long bones, particularly the humerus. The prognosis of osteosar-

coma in Paget's disease is especially poor. There is also an increased incidence of fibrosarcomas, chondrosarcomas and giant cell tumours.

Patients with Paget's disease may also have heart failure. This is usually a simple coincidence of two common diseases of the elderly. However, the bone in patients with Paget's disease is extremely vascular (Fig. 25.7), and blood flow in these areas is markedly increased. This may contribute to the heart failure (Ch. 13).

MISCELLANEOUS BONE DISORDERS

Achondroplasia

Achondroplasia is a single gene disorder transmitted as an autosomal dominant with almost complete penetrance and occurs in approximately 1 in 25 000 births. The physical appearances of the patients are characteristic. The limbs are short, particularly the proximal portions of the arms, but the trunk is of normal length. There is usually a pronounced lumbar lordosis, a prominent forehead and depression of the nasal bridge. There is a failure of proper ossification in bones that have developed from a cartilagenous template (endochondral ossification). In contrast, bones which develop from connective tissue (intramembranous ossification), such as the vault of the skull, are normal. Epiphyses are abnormally wide and there are usually structural changes in the cartilagenous plates. Affected patients have normal intelligence and life-spans.

Avascular necrosis of bone

This usually presents with pain and limitation of joint movement. For anatomical reasons, fractures of bones such as the neck of the femur (Fig. 25.9) or the scaphoid deprive some areas of adjacent bone of their blood supply. Necrosis is then an inevitable consequence. Surgical treatment is therefore sometimes necessary to replace the fractured head of femur. The cause of other cases of avascular necrosis is less certain. Lesions occur in patients treated with corticosteroids, in sickle cell disease and other haemoglobinopathies. Similar lesions develop in divers and are probably the result of air embolism, associated with decompression.

Fibrous dysplasia

In this benign disorder of children and young adults,

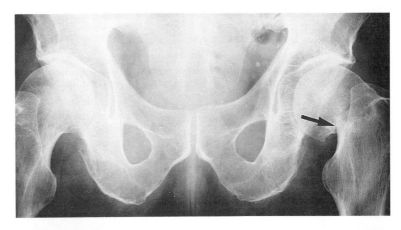

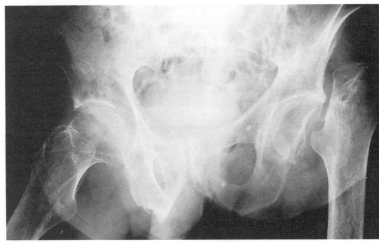

Fig. 25.9 Fractures of femoral head

A. Compare the normal contours of the femoral neck on the right with the fracture on the left (arrow). **B.** There is a displaced fracture of the left femoral head (detected 8 weeks after a fall!) resulting in necrosis of the bone deprived of its blood supply.

lesions composed of fibrous and bony tissue develop, usually in the ribs, femur, tibia or skull. Histologically, these lesions are composed of irregular masses of immature woven bone separated by a richly vascular fibrous stroma. Mature lamellar bone is not formed and this suggests that the lesion is a result of an arrest of bone maturation at the woven bone stage. Lesions do not usually enlarge after puberty, though some appear to be reactivated during pregnancy. Although the clinical and radiological findings are often diagnostic, lesions in long bones are often biopsied and the affected parts of ribs can be excised. In typical cases, the histological changes can be easily distinguished from true neoplastic disorders, such as osteosarcoma, fibrosarcoma or giant cell tumours.

Hypertrophic osteoarthropathy

This is an uncommon reactive condition in which there is clubbing, pain and swelling of the wrist and ankle joints, and subperiosteal new bone formation in the distal part of long bones. In the vast majority of affected patients there is an associated pulmonary carcinoma or a pleural mesothelioma. The underlying causes of both clubbing and hypertrophic osteoarthropathy are unknown, but in both cases there is a marked increase in blood flow in the distal portions of the limbs. Occasional cases regress after surgical treatment of the primary tumour.

Osteogenesis imperfecta

This is a genetically determined disorder of type 1 collagen. The responsible genes are at different sites, chiefly on chromosomes 7 and 17, and there is marked genetic heterogeneity. In some forms there is a high incidence of perinatal or intra-uterine death. In children who survive, bones are abnormally brittle and spontaneous fractures occur. The uveal pigment of the eye is visible through the thinned sclera which therefore appear blue.

BONE TUMOURS

> ▶ Commonest tumour in bone is metastatic carcinoma (commonly from breast, kidney, thyroid, lung or prostate)
> ▶ Important primary malignant bone tumours are osteosarcoma, chondrosarcoma and Ewing's sarcoma

Incidence and aetiology

Tumours of bone are uncommon and account for only 0.5% of all cancer deaths. Because of their rarity, these tumours are best managed in centres where there are orthopaedic surgeons, radiologists and histopathologists with sufficient experience of these lesions. Individual tumours tend to occur in particular age groups or in specific sites (Fig. 25.10).

In most cases, there are no obvious predisposing

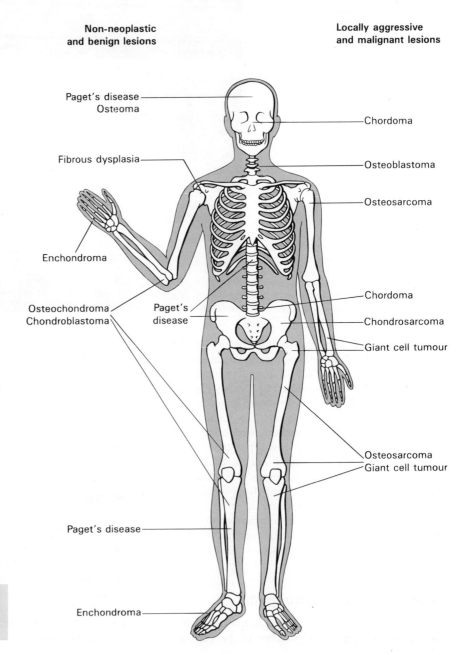

Non-neoplastic and benign lesions

Paget's disease
Osteoma

Fibrous dysplasia

Enchondroma

Osteochondroma
Chondroblastoma

Paget's disease

Paget's disease

Enchondroma

Locally aggressive and malignant lesions

Chordoma

Osteoblastoma

Osteosarcoma

Chordoma

Chondrosarcoma

Giant cell tumour

Osteosarcoma
Giant cell tumour

Fig. 25.10 The common sites of reactive, benign and malignant disorders of the skeleton

causes. Patients with Paget's disease and, to a lesser extent, fibrous dysplasia, have an increased incidence of malignant bone tumours, especially osteosarcoma. There is both clinical and experimental evidence that ionising radiation can induce bone tumours (Ch. 11).

Classification

Bone tumours are classified as follows:

1. *Benign tumours*:
   - osteochondroma (exostosis)
   - enchondroma
   - chondroblastoma
   - chondromyxoid fibroma
   - osteoma
   - osteoid osteoma
2. *Benign tumours* (locally aggressive or recurrent):
   - giant cell tumour ('osteoclastoma')
   - osteoblastoma
   - chordoma
   - adamantinoma
3. *Malignant tumours* (locally aggressive, frequently metastasise):
   - osteosarcoma
   - chondrosarcoma
   - fibrosarcoma
   - malignant fibrous histiocytoma
   - Ewing's sarcoma
4. *Metastases*, commonly from:
   - breast
   - lung
   - prostate
   - kidney
   - thyroid
5. *Myeloma* (plasmacytoma).

Benign tumours

The two commonest benign tumours of bone are the *osteochondroma* (*exostosis*) and the *chondroma* (*enchondroma*) which together make up over 50% of all benign bone tumours.

Osteochondroma

Patients with osteochondromas are usually less than 20 years of age and both sexes are affected. The lesions tend to develop near the epiphyses of limb bones although they can form in any bone that develops from cartilage. Solitary lesions are benign, though they may recur if incompletely excised. Histologically, a thick cartilagenous cap is present covering irregularly arranged bony trabeculae. There is an intermediate zone where the bone merges gradually into the overlying cartilage.

In *diaphyseal aclasis* there are multiple cartilage-capped exostoses and a substantial risk of associated chondrosarcoma. Malignancy should be suspected in any lesion which continues to grow after puberty. The incidence is approximately 1 per 2000 births and the lesion is transmitted as an autosomal dominant. Up to one-third of cases are the result of new mutations and the condition is probably a single gene disorder.

Chondroma (enchondroma)

Chondromas arise within the medullary cavity of the bones of the hands and feet and because of this are usually known as 'enchondromas'. They are thought to develop from small nests of cartilage that are sometimes found close to the metaphysis. They usually present in patients aged 20–50 years and are more common in men. There may be slight swelling of the affected bone but the lesions are sometimes discovered incidentally on X-ray. Simple curettage of the lesion is usually curative although some recur. *Enchondromatosis* (*Ollier's disease*) is the counterpart of multiple exostoses. Numerous enchondromas develop and there is a considerable risk of chondrosarcoma. This disorder has no obvious genetic basis.

Other benign tumours

Other benign bone tumours are uncommon. An *osteoma* is a mass of abnormally dense bone, usually in the paranasal sinuses or the skull.

An *osteoid osteoma* is a solitary and characteristically painful lesion which usually affects the femur or tibia. The pain may be severe, worse at night, and characteristically relieved by aspirin. Histologically there is a central 'nidus' of vascular fibrous tissue containing bone trabeculae formed by benign osteoblasts.

Chondroblastoma and *chondromyxoid fibroma* are rare tumours of long bones with distinctive histological appearances. They are most common in the femur, tibia or humerus in patients between 10 and 30 years of age.

Locally aggressive or recurrent benign tumours

Some benign tumours of bone, such as giant cell tumour ('osteoclastoma') and osteoblastoma are locally aggressive or may recur after surgery.

Giant cell tumours make up as much as 5% of all bone neoplasms and most often occur at the end of the long bones. They probably originate from undifferentiated mesenchymal cells in the connective tissue framework of bone. Their histological appearance is distinctive. Giant cells are conspicuous and for this reason the tumour has also been known as osteoclastoma, but these cells are not thought to be the neoplastic component. Giant cell tumours can also be confused histologically with the bone lesions of primary hyperparathyroidism ('von Recklinghausen's disease of bone'), in which osteoclasts are plentiful.

Osteoblastomas are uncommon solitary tumours which involve vertebrae and, to a lesser extent, the long bones of the extremities. The lesions are very vascular and show intense osteoblastic activity. Surgical treatment—usually by curettage—can be curative.

Chordomas arise from notochordal remnants, usually in the base of the skull or the sacral region. The constituent cells often have a characteristic 'bubbly' appearance due to cytoplasmic vacuolation. These tumours seldom metastasise but often recur locally.

Adamantinomas and *ameloblastomas* are histologically similar tumours. Ameloblastomas affect the jaw and have the capacity to produce tooth enamel but adamantinomas usually involve the tibia and do not produce enamel. The histological appearance is characteristic, with ribbons and cords of darkly staining cells arranged around a vascular fibrous stroma. Adequate surgical excision is often curative.

Malignant tumours

Although primary malignant tumours of bone are comparatively rare, they are always locally invasive and frequently metastasise. Patients are often young adults and, despite surgery and modern radio- and chemotherapy, the overall outlook remains poor (Table 25.3).

Osteosarcoma

This aggressive malignant tumour usually affects young adults and most often involves the distal femur, proximal tibia or humerus (Fig. 25.11). Occasional cases occur in the elderly, usually complicating Paget's disease or previous radiation. These tumours grow rapidly and often have a typical X-ray appearance. Osteosarcomas are characterised histologically by pleomorphic and mitotically active osteoblasts associated with osteoid (Fig. 11.13, p. 257); some variants are exceedingly vascular. Approximately 50% of patients can now be cured by a combination of surgery and intensive chemotherapy. Although amputation was previously necessary, local resection and the insertion of prosthetic joints is now sometimes possible.

Other malignant tumours

Chondrosarcomas, in contrast to osteosarcomas, grow slowly and arise not only in long bones but also in the pelvis, ribs and spine (Fig. 25.12). These tumours may be well differentiated and can resemble

Table 25.3 Malignant tumours of bone				
Tumour (% all primary malignant bone tumours)	Usual age and male: female sex ratio	Sites affected	Behaviour	Treatment and prognosis
Osteosarcoma (c. 30%)	Young adults 2:1	Long bones, esp. distal femur and proximal tibia	Rapid growth, pain and swelling, lung metastases	Surgery and chemotherapy 40% plus cure rate
Chondrosarcoma (c. 15%)	35–60 2:1	Pelvis, ribs, spine, long bones	Slow enlargement, eventual vascular invasion	Surgery c. 75% cure rate
Fibrosarcoma and malignant fibrous histiocytoma (c. 20%)	Any age, peak 30–40 3:2	Femur, tibia, humerus, pelvis	Local growth, vascular invasion	Surgery 40% cure rate
Ewing's sarcoma (c. 7%)	Children and teenagers 2:1	Long bones, pelvis and ribs	Widespread metastases	Chemotherapy 10% cure rate

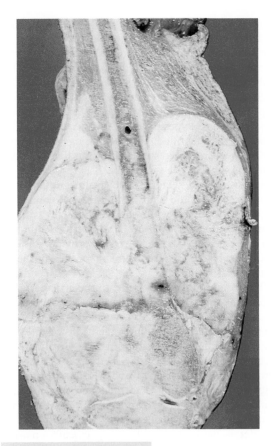

Fig. 25.11   Osteosarcoma

The cut surface of a rapidly growing tumour in the distal femur of a teenager.

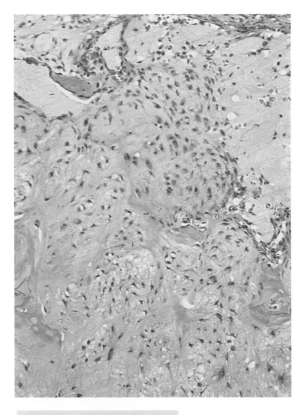

Fig. 25.12   Chondrosarcoma

The tumour has arisen in a pelvic bone of a 42-year-old female. Histologically the abnormal cartilage is much more cellular than normal.

normal cartilage. Surgical excision is the treatment of choice, as radiotherapy and chemotherapy are usually ineffective.

Fibrosarcomas and *malignant fibrous histiocytomas* are spindle cell malignant tumours with characteristic histological appearances. These lesions probably arise from fibroblasts and collectively they make up the majority of soft tissue sarcomas. They also occur as primary bone lesions, with the long bones and pelvis most often affected. With adequate surgical treatment up to 40% of patients can be cured. Death is usually the result of blood-borne metastases.

Ewing's sarcoma affects children and teenagers. The tumour is composed of small, darkly staining undifferentiated cells whose exact origin (histogenesis) has puzzled pathologists for many years. Males are affected more often than females, and the long bones, pelvis and ribs are the most frequent sites.

Widespread metastases are frequent and the bone marrow is often involved.

Metastases and multiple myeloma

The commonest malignant tumours of bone are secondary *metastatic deposits* from carcinomas in other sites. In Europe and North America, bronchus and breast are the commonest primary sites, but thyroid, prostate and kidney carcinomas also metastasise to bone. Widespread and extensive bony lesions are also a feature of *multiple myeloma*. Most secondary deposits in bone cause bone breakdown (osteolysis) but some, particularly from carcinoma of the prostate, stimulate bone formation (osteosclerosis; Fig. 25.13). Secondary deposits in bone are the commonest cause of hypercalcaemia in middle-aged and elderly patients and are a frequent cause of pathological fractures.

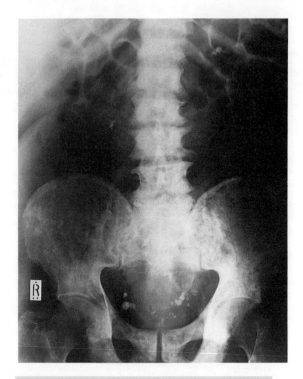

Fig. 25.13   Multiple bony metastases in a patient with widespread carcinoma of the prostate

Note the marked variation in density of the iliac bones. The vertebral bodies are uniformly dense. Deposits of prostatic carcinoma often induce this pattern of bony sclerosis. Other secondary metastases are usually osteolytic.

JOINTS

NORMAL STRUCTURE AND FUNCTION

Joints permit mobility, but not all junctions between bones are designed to allow movement. At one extreme, the cranial sutures in adults are rigidly fixed while, at the other, the shoulder joint has an almost unlimited range of movement. Joints such as the symphysis pubis and the lower tibiofibular joint have limited movement but are firmly bound by fibrous and cartilagenous tissue. In contrast, the articulating surfaces of *synovial joints* are in contact but not in continuity.

The articular surfaces of synovial joints are covered by a thin layer of hyaline or, occasionally, fibrous *cartilage*, up to 3 mm thick. In early life these surfaces are remarkably smooth, and slide and move against each other with very little friction. A viscous,

clear *synovial fluid* lubricates the joint surfaces and supplies essential nutrients to the chondrocytes of the articular cartilage. In a normal knee joint there is about 2 ml of synovial fluid, containing c.100 cells/mm^3, chiefly lymphocytes and macrophages.

Synovial joints are enclosed by a tough fibrous capsule, which in turn is lined by a thin *synovial membrane*. Two types of cells — type A and type B — have been identified in the lining membrane. Electron microscopic studies indicate that type A is primarily phagocytic while type B is responsible for synthesising and secreting the hyaluronic acid and other proteins of the synovial fluid. Loose connective tissue in the subsynovium merges gradually with the joint capsule. *Ligaments* are band-like thickenings of the joint capsule which not only provide stability, but, as with the cruciate ligaments of the knee joint, limit excessive mobility.

The bone immediately beneath the articular cartilage — the *subchondral bone plate* — provides the strength to withstand and cushion the repeated forces generated by joint movement. In weight-bearing joints, this plate is supported by an underlying 'scaffold' of bony trabeculae. If this supporting system is damaged, as in advanced osteoarthritis, the joint surfaces become deformed and movement is limited. The individual arteries and veins supplying joints and joint capsules have not been studied in detail and are seldom specifically named. Nevertheless, joints are richly vascular structures, particularly in acute inflammatory arthritis or during the active stages of rheumatoid disease. Joints such as the knee, the sternoclavicular and the temporomandibular have partial or complete discs of fibrocartilage called *menisci*, which either project into joint cavities or divide them into separate cavities. These may act as 'cushions' or 'shock absorbers'. When these discs are damaged or torn, there is acute limitation of joint movement and surgical removal or repair is often necessary.

Joints have a rich innervation, usually derived from nerves supplying the adjacent muscular tissue. This arrangement allows a local reflex arc to be established between movement in an individual joint and the actions of surrounding muscles. There are many sensory nerve endings in the fibrous capsule of joints and in the bone underlying the articular surfaces. In contrast, the synovial membrane has no specialised sensory receptors, apart from those associated with the adjacent blood vessels, and is therefore relatively insensitive to pain. However, any substantial pathological process involving a joint is likely to cause inflammatory cell infiltration and oedema of the adjacent joint capsule, if not of the articular surfaces themselves, and this leads to both pain and subsequent limitation of movement.

OSTEOARTHRITIS (OSTEOARTHROSIS)

▶ Common painful, disabling degenerative joint disease
▶ Primarily affects cartilage of weight-bearing joints (e.g. hips, knees)
▶ Erosion of cartilage leads to secondary changes in underlying bone
▶ Only limited inflammatory changes in synovial membrane
▶ Osteoarthritis of hip and knee can be treated surgically by joint replacement

Osteoarthritis is a remarkably common, disabling degenerative disease which usually affects large weight-bearing joints. The inevitable pain, and limitation of movement, associated with this disease is a major cause of morbidity in almost all societies. The development of surgical techniques for the treatment of osteoarthritis has been one of the most useful advances in medicine in the last 20 years.

Epidemiology

About 20% of elderly men and women have significant osteoarthritic joint disease. Pain and limitation of movement are the most important symptoms, particularly in the hip, the knee and the joints of the cervical spine (cervical spondylosis).

Pathological basis of clinical signs and symptoms of joint disease	
Sign or symptom	Pathological basis
Pain	Stimulation of nerve endings in joint capsule and synovium by inflammation (arthritis)
Deformity	Joint swelling due to: • synovial inflammation • effusion into joint space Erosion of articular surfaces
Restricted movement	Synovial swelling Fibrosis Limited by pain
Systemic features (e.g. subcutaneous nodules, lymphadenopathy)	Arthritis mediated by immune mechanisms

Certain occupations are associated with a high incidence of osteoarthritis in particular joints. Coal miners develop osteoarthritis in elbow joints, golfers in the first metatarsophalangeal joint of the foot, and footballers in the knees. Some patients with premature osteoarthritis of the hip have previous congenital dislocation in this joint. Similarly, any obvious deformity or previous fracture is an important predisposing cause. Patients with pre-existing bone disease, such as osteomalacia, gout or acromegaly, or other forms of arthritis such as rheumatoid disease, are at risk for secondary osteoarthritis. Nevertheless, in the majority of patients there are no obvious predisposing factors. This is particularly true of vertebral osteoarthritis which, although often asymptomatic, can produce severe pain and disability.

Pathogenesis

The earliest changes of osteoarthritis are in the articular cartilage, particularly in weight-bearing joints. These range from slight surface irregularity to full-thickness loss of cartilage. In the early stages, the articular cartilage becomes irregularly fragmented or fibrillated (Fig. 25.14). In some joints, such as the knee, changes are seen in the second or third decade of life and are part of normal wear and tear. They affect the edges of articular surfaces and do not necessarily progress to full-thickness loss of cartilage. This form of fibrillation is probably the result of repetitive everyday trauma, rather than the consequence of simple articular movement. In contrast, in osteoarthritic joints there are discrete areas of cartilagenous loss, well away from the articular margins. The underlying bone develops a shiny, ivory-like (eburnated) appearance.

Biochemical alterations have been detected in the articular cartilage in the early stages of osteoarthritis. The water content of the cartilgenous matrix is increased, and proteoglycans have a smaller molecular size and are synthesised at increased rates. These changes are associated with a decrease in both the elasticity and compliance of cartilage but why they should occur in the first instance is uncertain. Chondrocytes have an increased metabolic activity in early osteoarthritis and higher turnover. It has been suggested that the proteolytic enzymes that are released in this way produce the biochemical changes of early osteoarthritis. The stimulus to increased activity of chondrocytes is unknown. Cytokines secreted by synovial cells may stimulate chondrocytes, but how this could be related to repeated trauma and altered joint stresses is uncertain.

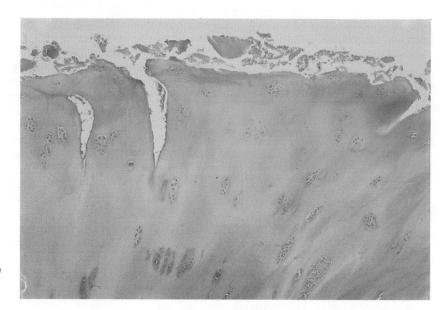

Fig. 25.14 Early osteoarthritis

Histology of a section through the articular surface showing 'fibrillation' and fissuring.

The second series of changes in the development of osteoarthritis involves the subchondral bone plate. This plate not only defines the contours of the articular surface but also contributes to the strength and resilience of the joint. Loss of articular cartilage is a stimulus to reactive proliferation of this plate. Although this increases the strength of the articular surface it reduces its ability to act as a 'shock absorber'. In turn, this leads to ever increasing damage to the residual articular cartilage.

Eventually, the articular surface becomes deformed and in many joints this is the major cause of limitation of movement. The normal pattern of bone trabeculae beneath the articular surface is lost and cystic lesions may develop. Bony outgrowths (osteophytes) develop at the margins of the articular surface (Fig. 25.15). These are a characteristic feature of osteoarthritis but serve no useful function. In joints such as the femur they limit the range of movement, and in the distal interphalangeal joints they produce characteristic nodular swellings called *Heberden's nodes*. In *cervical spondylosis*, a variant

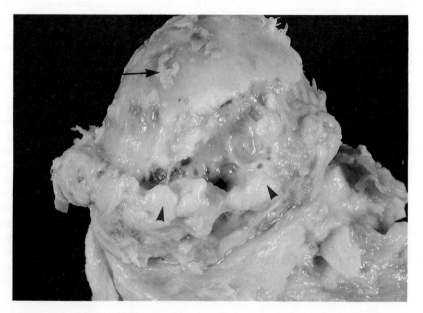

Fig. 25.15 Severe osteoarthritis

The articular surface of the femoral head is distorted and surrounded by a rim of osteophytes (arrowheads). Arrow indicates island of residual articular cartilage.

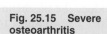

of osteoarthritis affecting the cervical spine, symptoms result from osteophytic outgrowths impinging on nerve roots as they leave the intervertebral foramina.

Clinicopathological features

The major symptoms of osteoarthritis are pain on joint movement, stiffness during inactivity and audible creaking of joints, often accompanied by a palpable crepitus. Although there is no primary synovial pathology in osteoarthritis, small joint effusions are common and histologically the synovium shows slight hyperplasia and focal areas of chronic inflammation, often as a reaction to calcified debris shed from the articular surfaces.

The diagnosis of osteoarthritis is made on the basis of clinical examination and characteristic radiological appearances. Almost all of the pathological features of osteoarthritis can be identified on a plain X-ray. One of the earliest changes is loss of joint space: the articular surfaces of the bone appear close together when articular cartilage has been lost. Reactive proliferation of the subchondral bone plate occurs and there are deformities of the articular surface.

In a typical patient, all routine laboratory investigations are normal. In particular, there is no evidence of anaemia, auto-antibody formation or any abnormality of calcium metabolism.

RHEUMATOID DISEASE

> ▶ Common systemic chronic inflammatory disorder invariably involving joints
> ▶ Associated with rheumatoid factor: an auto-antibody reactive with altered autologous immunoglobulin
> ▶ Chronic inflammation and proliferation of synovium gradually erodes articular cartilage
> ▶ Systemic features include subcutaneous rheumatoid nodules, anaemia, lymphadenopathy and splenomegaly, serositis (e.g. pericarditis), Sjögren's syndrome, uveitis, vasculitis, pulmonary changes, and amyloidosis

Rheumatoid arthritis is a common, systemic, progressive and often disabling chronic inflammatory disorder. Unlike osteoarthritis, the pathological changes are not restricted to joints. Inflammatory lesions can develop in many tissues, including the heart and pericardium, lungs, blood vessels, skin and subcutaneous tissues, eye, and salivary and lacrimal glands. For this reason, the disorder is more correctly termed rheumatoid *disease*, but the arthritis is the first and generally most disabling feature.

Aetiology

The main epidemiological and pathogenetic features of rheumatoid disease are:

- females affected more often than males
- occurs in all age groups; children can be affected (Still's disease)
- prevalence in most Caucasian populations at least 1%; less common and less aggressive in blacks and Asians
- slight familial tendency, especially in severe forms
- up to 75% of patients HLA-DR4 positive (normally only 25%)
- most adults have circulating auto-antibodies (rheumatoid factors) directed against autologous (native) immunoglobulins
- multisystem disease characterised by chronic inflammatory granulomatous lesions (rheumatoid nodules).

Immunological abnormalities

Rheumatoid disease is associated with a variety of immunological abnormalities. These involve both the cellular and the humoral arms of the immune system.

Humoral
Most patients have considerably raised levels of serum immunoglobulins and have a characteristic auto-antibody directed against autologous immunoglobulin, called *rheumatoid factor*. The exact role of this antibody in the pathogenesis of rheumatoid arthritis is uncertain but at the least it is associated with the progression of the disease. Generally, patients with severe arthritis and evidence of multisystem disease have high titres of this antibody. In contrast, seronegative patients often have a milder form of disease. With appropriate immunological techniques, rheumatoid factor can usually be demonstrated in plasma cells in the synovium of affected joints. There is less definite evidence that aggregates of these immunoglobulins can act as immune complexes and trigger acute and chronic inflammatory reactions in joints and other tissues. The nature of the underlying stimulus to rheumatoid factor production is completely unknown, but many patients with severe rheumatoid disease have generalised hyperplasia of lymphoid tissue with prominent lymphadenopathy and splenomegaly.

Cellular

Many of the inflammatory cells in rheumatoid synovium are T-cells, especially CD4, helper T-cells and macrophages. Polymorphs are present in the joint fluid and to a lesser extent in the synovium; there is also a population of mast cells. These all contribute to 'pannus' (Fig. 25.16) but there is argument as to which cells erode the articular cartilage. Careful studies using immunohistochemistry and in situ hybridisation have demonstrated a variety of cytokines in rheumatoid synovium. These include at least four of the interleukins, interferon γ and tumour necrosis factor alpha. As in many other disorders the exact ways in which these chemical signals 'network' to amplify each other and then induce the persistent and destructive inflammation are uncertain. When the underlying pathways are understood in more detail it may be possible to develop agents that specifically influence the nature and density of the synovial inflammation.

Infectious agents

Although the nature of the immunological abnormalities in rheumatoid disease is becoming clearer, very little progress is being made in identifying the factors which initiate these changes. Micro-organisms have been implicated for many years and it is now beyond doubt that Lyme arthritis (see below) is infectious and that parvovirus B19 can induce arthritis. Bacteria, viruses and mycoplasmas have been suggested as causes of rheumatoid disease. Although the synovial fluid of acutely inflamed rheumatoid joints contains both acute and chronic inflammatory cells, bacteriological cultures are usually sterile. There is indirect evidence that both Epstein–Barr and parvoviruses may infect rheumatoid synovium but whether this is a primary or secondary change is unresolved.

Pathogenesis

The wide variety of different hypotheses advanced to explain the progressive nature of rheumatoid arthritis is only one indication that the underlying pathology is poorly understood. The most reasonable overall view is that an as yet unidentified infectious agent initiates the disease process and that a complex series of immunological changes are responsible for its progression. In this way, rheumatoid arthritis has similarities to two other enigmatic chronic inflammatory disorders — sarcoidosis and Crohn's disease.

Clinicopathological features

The two major changes in rheumatoid arthritis are a chronic inflammatory synovitis and progressive erosion of the articular cartilage (Figs 25.16 and 25.17). In the early stages of the disease, there is pain and swelling, chiefly of the hands and the distal metatarsal joints of the foot. As the disease becomes established, the knees, ankles, hips, cervical spine and temporomandibular joints are affected. Joints are tender, and often swollen.

The synovial infiltrates include lymphocytes, plas-

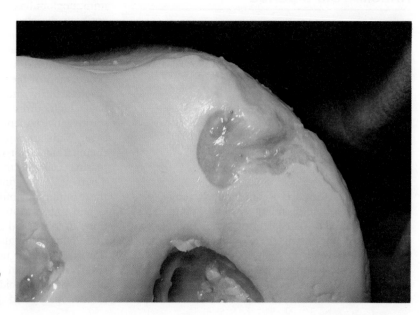

Fig. 25.16 Early rheumatoid disease

A layer of chronic inflammatory tissue ('pannus') has eroded the articular surface of the femoral condyle.

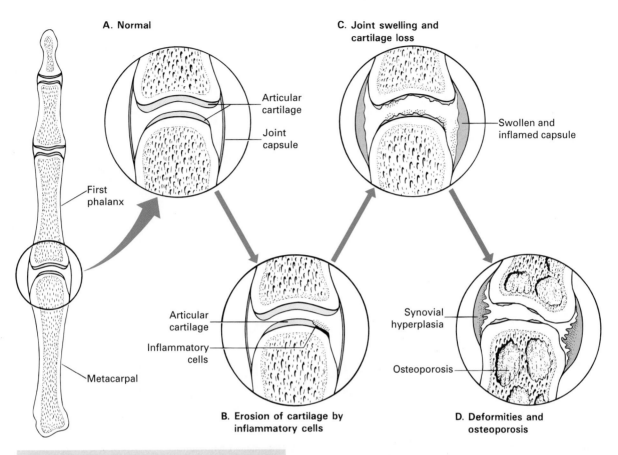

A. Normal

Articular cartilage

Joint capsule

First phalanx

Articular cartilage

Inflammatory cells

Metacarpal

B. Erosion of cartilage by inflammatory cells

C. Joint swelling and cartilage loss

Swollen and inflamed capsule

Synovial hyperplasia

Osteoporosis

D. Deformities and osteoporosis

Fig. 25.17   The progression of rheumatoid disease

ma cells, macrophages and occasional polymorphs (Fig. 25.18). In the earlier stages there is only a mild increase in inflammatory cells, but in the established disease large nodular masses of lymphocytes and macrophages are characteristic. True granulomas are not usually identified in the synovium but may occasionally be seen in the adjacent joint capsule. A layer of chronically inflamed fibrous tissue (pannus) slowly extends from the synovial margin, eroding the articular cartilage as it spreads (Fig. 25.16).

Osteoporosis often develops in the bones immediately adjacent to affected joints, particularly in the fingers. This is often the first radiological change of rheumatoid disease, but small pocket-like erosions of the periarticular surface are also seen (Fig. 25.19). In chronically diseased joints the articular cartilage is extensively eroded and fragmented and the resultant debris is a further source of synovial inflammation. The loss of articular cartilage causes deformities (Fig. 25.19) and secondary osteoarthritis can develop, particularly in the knee.

Extra-articular features

The extra-articular features of rheumatoid disease are:

- subcutaneous rheumatoid nodules
- anaemia
- lymphadenopathy and splenomegaly
- pericarditis
- dry eyes and mouth (Sjögren's syndrome)
- uveitis and scleritis
- vasculitis, especially fingers and nail beds
- pulmonary changes (nodules, interstitial fibrosis, obstructive airways disease)
- amyloidosis.

Subcutaneous *rheumatoid nodules* develop in up to one-third of patients with rheumatoid disease, but most of these are severe and progressive cases. Typically, they involve the extensor surfaces of the forearm, less commonly the dorsum of the foot. These locations suggest that everyday incidental

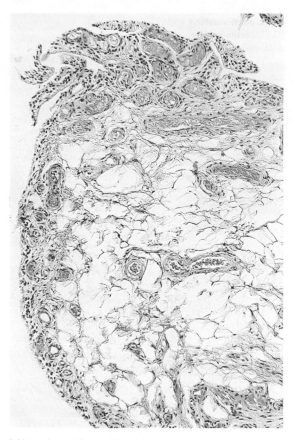

A Normal synovium

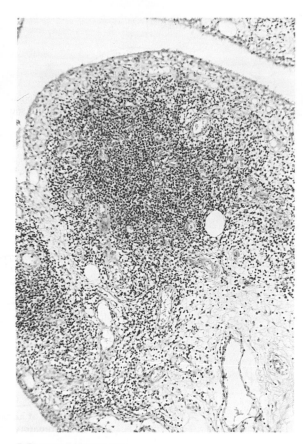

B Rheumatoid synovium

Fig. 25.18 Rheumatoid arthritis

Note the dense lymphocytic infiltrates in the synovial biopsy (**B**) from a patient with active rheumatoid arthritis.

trauma contributes to their development. The nodules vary in size but are usually 20–40 mm in maximum dimension. Their histological structure is characteristic: central areas of necrotic collagen are surrounded by palisades of fibroblasts and macrophages. It has been suggested that an immune complex vasculitis is the cause of rheumatoid nodule formation but there is very little evidence for this. Occasional patients with no evidence of rheumatoid disease have solitary subcutaneous lesions with the same microscopic features, and some uncommon skin disorders, such as granuloma annulare, have a somewhat similar histological appearance.

Many patients with rheumatoid disease have clinically obvious *lymphadenopathy*. In some, the spleen can be felt — rheumatoid disease is one of the commoner causes of *splenomegaly*. A chronic inflammatory fibrinous *pericarditis* is a frequent finding in

rheumatoid disease and occasionally chronic inflammatory granulomas can develop within the myocardium.

The wide range of *pulmonary pathology* includes rheumatoid nodule formation within the parenchyma of the lung and chronic interstitial fibrosis. Chronic inflammatory infiltrates can develop in both the lacrimal and salivary glands, impairing tear and saliva production. The resulting dryness in both the eyes and mouth (Sjögren's syndrome) is often persistent and irritating. Patients complain of a gritty feeling in the eyes and of photophobia. Both *uveitis* and *scleritis* are important ocular manifestations of rheumatoid disease (Fig. 25.20). The uveal tract, like the skin, the glomerulus of the kidney, and the joints, has a very high blood flow per unit mass of tissue and this may contribute to the deposition of immune complexes and the subsequent inflammatory reaction. Paradoxically, uveitis

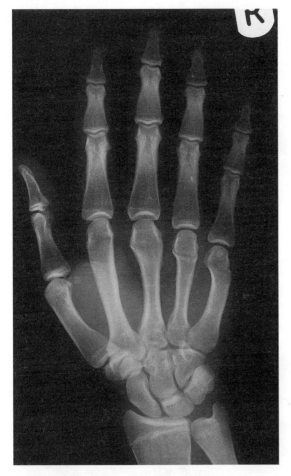

A Normal

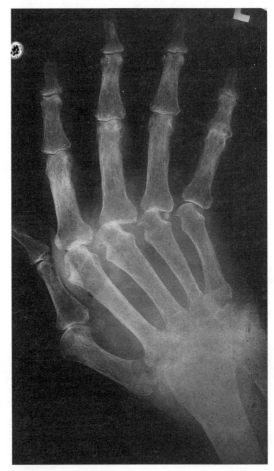

B Rheumatoid arthritis

Fig. 25.19 Radiological features of rheumatoid arthritis

There is prominent ulnar deviation in the patient (**B**) with longstanding rheumatoid disease. There are erosions of the distal metacarpal bones and of most of the carpal bones. Normal hand (**A**) for comparison.

can occur many years after the onset of rheumatoid arthritis, sometimes when the disease is in a quiescent phase. *Vasculitis* is a sinister feature and implies a poor prognosis. It is clinically most obvious in the fingers, particularly the nail beds (Fig. 25.21).

Iatrogenic ('doctor induced') disease is common in rheumatoid arthritis. Until recently, steroids were often used extensively in its treatment and Cushing's syndrome was commonplace. Rheumatologists are now reluctant to prescribe long-term corticosteroids, and use non-steroidal anti-inflammatory drugs in severe cases. Unfortunately, these and other second-line drugs also have significant side-effects, particularly gastric erosion and peptic ulceration.

Laboratory investigations

In contrast to the situation in osteoarthritis there are a wide range of haematological and immunological abnormalities in rheumatoid disease:

- normochromic, normocytic anaemia
- raised erythrocyte sedimentation rate (ESR) and acute phase proteins such as C reactive protein
- IgG and IgM rheumatoid factors are usually present in severe cases
- auto-antibodies, such as antinuclear factor (ANF), are identified in a higher proportion of patients than in the general population.

Patients with severe symptoms in the early stages of

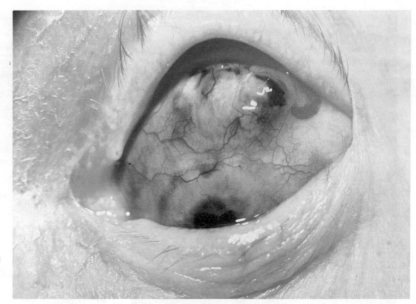

Fig. 25.20   Scleritis in rheumatoid arthritis

The inflammation has caused thinning of the scleral connective tissue revealing the underlying pigmentation of the choroid.

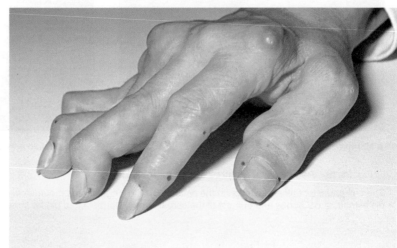

Fig. 25.21   Deformity and vasculitis in rheumatoid disease

There are deformities of the 3rd, 4th and 5th fingers, a rheumatoid nodule at the 2nd metacarpophalangeal joint and small dark red lesions of digital vasculitis.

the disease, or a poor response to anti-inflammatory drug therapy, tend to progress more rapidly. Careful evaluation of radiographs of the hand is also important, as the early development of bony erosions is another poor prognostic feature. Many severely affected patients require treatment with second-line drugs, such as gold, penicillamine, corticosteroids, or cytotoxic agents such as azathioprine or cyclophosphamide. If a remission of disease can be obtained with these agents it can sometimes be sustained for months or even years.

Prognosis and complications

At the onset of the disease it is very difficult to determine the prognosis for any individual patient. Approximately 10% of patients who develop rheumatoid arthritis will become severely disabled, dependent on others for some or all of their normal daily activities. In contrast, at least 20% of patients have only slight symptoms and relatively mild disability. They may have mild intermittent swelling of joints and difficulty in movements such as unscrewing lids or combing the hair at the back of the head. The remaining 70% of patients have varying degrees of disability and most will require some form of drug therapy, at least during exacerbations of disease.

Although rheumatoid disease can be relentless and progressive, it is seldom directly responsible for the death of an individual. Infections are more common in patients with rheumatoid disease than in the general population; these include septic arthritis, pneumonia, suppurative pericarditis and septicaemia. Blood culture is essential in a seriously ill patient with rheumatoid disease. Between 5 and 15% of patients with rheumatoid disease develop reactive systemic (AA) amyloidosis (Ch. 7).

Rheumatoid disease in children

At the turn of the century, chronic inflammatory arthritis with systemic manifestations was described by Sir George Still (1868–1941), a paediatrician at Great Ormond Street Hospital. He emphasised that the disease occurred 'between the first and second dentition' and that there were similarities to rheumatoid disease in adults. It is now appreciated that there are many different forms of juvenile chronic arthritis and that only some of these are strictly similar to rheumatoid disease in adults.

Clinicopathological features

In juvenile chronic arthritis there are prominent systemic manifestations, often early in the course of the disease. These include pyrexia, skin rashes, lymphadenopathy, splenomegaly, pericarditis and pleurisy, and some can occur even before the onset of the arthritis. As in the classical rheumatoid arthritis of adults, several joints are affected. The joint symptoms and synovial pathology are very similar to those of adult rheumatoid arthritis. A chronic inflammatory pannus may form and erode articular cartilage. Fortunately, articular cartilage is somewhat thicker in children and this tends to protect the underlying bone.

Laboratory investigations and prognosis

As in adults, the erythrocyte sedimentation rate (ESR) is raised and a normochromic normocytic anaemia may be present. Although there may be hyperglobulinaemia, specific tests for rheumatoid factor are usually negative; this is the most important laboratory investigation distinguishing juvenile

chronic arthritis from typical rheumatoid disease. A subgroup of adolescent children with chronic arthritis do have rheumatoid factor, and these children often have a progressive form of disease and require early treatment. In at least three-quarters of cases, the disease remits, either spontaneously or after drug treatment, and there is often no residual joint damage. In contrast, some patients may have a progressive arthritis and there can be substantial and permanent joint deformity.

Very little is known of the cause of juvenile chronic arthritis. The principles of treatment are much the same as in adult rheumatoid disease.

ANKYLOSING SPONDYLITIS, REITER'S DISEASE AND RELATED DISORDERS

This is a puzzling group of related disorders of unknown aetiology. In classical cases of ankylosing spondylitis and Reiter's disease, there are well-defined clinical signs and symptoms and, even if the pathogenesis is obscure, pathological changes have been identified in a number of different organs. In some systemic disorders, including psoriasis, ulcerative colitis, Crohn's disease, infectious dysentery and chlamydial urethritis, there may be a chronic and disabling arthropathy resembling true ankylosing spondylitis or Reiter's disease. Although most of these disorders have a familial tendency there is no clearly defined pattern of inheritance, and several different forms of arthropathy may occur in closely related individuals.

Ankylosing spondylitis

> ► Relatively uncommon inflammatory disorder of spinal joints
> ► 90% of cases have the HLA-B27 haplotype
> ► Systemic features include peripheral arthritis, uveitis, aortic valve incompetence and chronic inflammatory bowel disease

The term 'spondylitis' implies an inflammatory disorder of the spine, whereas 'spondylosis' is used to describe the commoner degenerative osteoarthritic change.

Epidemiology

Fully developed ankylosing spondylitis is rare and occurs in only 1 in 1000 middle-aged male adults, and rather fewer females. About 90% of patients with unequivocal ankylosing spondylitis have the HLA antigen B27—one of the strongest disease associations with a particular HLA haplotype. Once this association was established, surveys were undertaken to determine what proportion of the 5–10% of the Caucasian population who are B27-positive had signs of spondylitis. Depending on the stringency of the criteria used for diagnosis, up to 15% of these patients have some evidence of mild spondylitis but only 1–2% of severe spondylitis. The disease, particularly in its established form, is more common in males and the first symptoms usually occur before the age of 30 years.

Clinicopathological features

Information on the underlying pathological changes can be obtained only by sequential radiological studies or postmortem examination of the occasional patients who die in the early stages of the disease. The inflammatory process begins at the site where ligaments are attached to vertebral bone—the 'entheses'. As these lesions heal, there is reactive new bone formation in the adjacent ligaments and sclerosis of the underlying bone. The earliest changes are often present in the sacro-iliac joints and may be detected by careful radiological examination or computerised tomography. Pain may be produced if the lower portion of the sacrum is depressed forward with the patient lying face down. Fusion of the vertebral bodies inhibits both flexion and rotation, and this is particularly disabling when the cervical segment is affected. Some patients develop fixed spinal deformities.

The symptoms and lesions strongly associated with ankylosing spondylitis are:

- pelvic and back pain; chronic inflammatory changes in entheses, progressing to bony ankylosis
- peripheral arthritis (30%), often sparing the hands
- anterior uveitis
- aortic incompetence
- inflammatory bowel disease.

At least 30% of patients with typical ankylosing spondylitis have a peripheral arthropathy. There are no specific histological features that distinguish this from other low-grade forms of arthropathy, but the clinical distribution is distinctive. Lower limb joints and the shoulders are often involved, but the lower arm, and particularly the hands, are usually spared. The arthritis may begin before, together with, or some time after the first back symptoms.

Ankylosing spondylitis is one of the diseases that is associated with uveitis. In most cases, the anterior part of the eye, the iris and ciliary body, are affected, and choroidal changes are less common. The cause of the majority of cases of uveitis is unknown but between 10 and 20% will have some evidence of spondylitis. Uveitis is also associated with inflammatory bowel disease, and there is no doubt that both Crohn's disease and ulcerative colitis are more common in those with ankylosing spondylitis than in the general population. The best-recognised cardiovascular complication of spondylitis is aortic incompetence, but this is present in only 1–2% of longstanding cases. Pathologically, there is a chronic inflammatory aortitis, usually restricted to the valve ring and ascending aorta.

Reiter's disease

During World War I, a German physician, Hans Reiter, described the combination of arthritis, conjunctivitis and urethritis developing in a soldier shortly after an attack of dysentery. A century before, Benjamin Brodie had recognised the association of urinary tract infection with arthritis, and there are probably even earlier reports of this. Most of the patients are males and the onset of the illness is usually abrupt. The arthritis usually affects lower limb joints and classically there is swelling and inflammation at the insertion of the Achilles tendon. The urethritis is usually due to chlamydial infection, and the conjunctivitis only a minor feature of the illness.

The underlying pathological mechanisms in Reiter's disease are unknown. Chlamydial infections usually respond to tetracycline, but the arthritis can persist for months and occur at irregular intervals. Up to one-half of severely affected patients subsequently develop signs of spondylitis and, as most of these are HLA-B27 positive, it is very likely that the underlying disease process is the same as in true ankylosing spondylitis.

Psoriasis and arthritis

Psoriasis is a common and chronic skin disorder affecting up to 1% of Caucasians (Ch. 24). About 5% of patients with psoriasis have arthropathy, typically involving the distal interphalangeal joints. Again, if there is evidence of spondylitis, patients with arthropathy and psoriasis are usually HLA-B27 positive.

Arthritis and bowel disease

A low-grade peripheral arthropathy is well-recognised, though comparatively rare, complication of salmonella, shigella and yersinia gastroenteritis. HLA-B27-positive patients have a substantially increased risk of developing this complication. The underlying pathological mechanisms are unknown. Arthritis is seen at some stage in up to 20% of patients with ulcerative colitis and Crohn's disease. The knees and occasionally the ankles, elbows and the small digital joints are involved. A typical rash of erythema nodosum (Ch. 24) sometimes accompanies the joint lesions. Sacro-iliitis and, to a lesser extent, fully developed ankylosing spondylitis, occur much more frequently in patients with inflammatory bowel disease than in the general population. Spondylitis can occur before or after the onset of bowel symptoms and there may be a peripheral arthropathy and an anterior uveitis.

DEGENERATIVE DISEASE OF INTERVERTEBRAL DISCS

Degenerative softening of the fibrocartilagenous intervertebral discs is a very common cause of back pain. It usually affects adults and clinical symptoms are exacerbated by heavy straining when lifting or by poor posture. The degenerative change is characterised by the accumulation of connective tissue mucins within the central nucleus pulposus of the disc; discs in the lumbar spine are affected most commonly.

The softened nucleus pulposus can herniate vertically into an adjacent vertebral body, forming a *Schmorl's node* (Fig. 25.3) which may be radiologically evident. More seriously, the disc material may herniate posterolaterally through the surrounding annulus fibrosus forming a protrusion that impinges upon the nerve emanating from the intervertebral foramina. This is the *prolapsed intervertebral disc*, or so-called 'slipped disc', that causes severe pain radiating into the territory supplied by the compressed nerve (e.g. 'sciatica' when the pain radiates across the buttock and down the leg); motor nerve conduction may also be impaired. In many cases the symptoms resolve with analgesia, bed rest or wearing an orthopaedic corset, although gentle exercise is increasingly recommended. Recurrences are common. Surgical removal of the degenerate disc material may be necessary in some patients. With increasing age the naturally restricted movement of the spine reduces the probability of disc herniation.

INFECTIVE ARTHRITIS

Most cases of septic arthritis are the result of bacterial infection. In some viral diseases there is an associated arthritis, or at least arthralgia (joint pain) is a prominent symptom. In contrast, fungal infections of joints are extremely rare.

Organisms responsible include:

- *Staphylococcus aureus*
- *Staphylococcus albus* (prosthetic joints)
- *Streptococcus pyogenes*
- *Diplococcus pneumoniae*
- *Neisseria gonorrhoeae*
- *Haemophilus influenzae* (children)
- Gram-negative organisms (drug addicts)
- *Borrelia burgdorferi* (Lyme arthritis)
- *Mycobacterium tuberculosis*.

Septic arthritis is the result of blood-borne spread from a focus of infection elsewhere. The epiphyseal plate forms a very effective barrier and it is unusual for an area of osteomyelitis in the metaphysis to spread and involve adjacent joints. This occasionally occurs in the hip, where the metaphysis may lie within the joint capsule.

As with osteomyelitis, children are affected more commonly than adults but the reasons for this are uncertain. Most cases are the result of staphylococcal or streptococcal infection. Both pneumococci and gonococci have a tendency to involve joints, and a septic arthritis can follow a bacteraemia or septicaemia associated with these organisms. *Haemophilus influenzae* arthritis is restricted to young children. Gram-negative septicaemia may cause inflammatory arthritis, particularly in drug addicts.

Diabetes mellitus, rheumatoid arthritis and immunosuppressive treatment are all risk factors for septic arthritis. Similarly, intra-articular injections of corticosteroids can be followed by inflammatory arthritis, and rigorous asepsis is essential during these procedures, particularly in patients with rheumatoid disease.

Clinicopathological features

The symptoms of infective arthritis are pain, tenderness, swelling and erythema. Although the typical patient is a child aged 5–15 years, almost any age group can be affected, particularly if there is associated rheumatoid arthritis. Although most cases of bacterial arthritis involve a single joint (monoarthritis) a small proportion of staphylococcal infections, and the majority of cases of gonococcal arthritis involve two or more joints. As there is usually an associated septicaemia, patients are obviously ill, are usually pyrexial and may have rigors.

There are no diagnostic X-ray features, although radiographs are essential to exclude fractures or other bony injury. The diagnosis can be made only by aspirating and culturing the joint fluid. Special culture techniques are required for gonococci and mycobacteria, and full clinical details must therefore be given to the laboratory. Gram-stained preparations of synovial fluid may give a pointer to the causative organism and suggest appropriate antibiotic treatment before culture results are available. Initially, parenteral antibiotics should be given and oral antibiotics continued for 4–6 weeks. With adequate and prompt treatment, surgical drainage is not usually necessary, but should be considered if symptoms persist. The heavy polymorph infiltrates inevitably cause some superficial destruction of articular cartilage, and joint-space narrowing may become visible in radiographs. There may also be evidence of osteoporosis in the bones immediately adjacent to the joint.

Uncommon forms of infective arthritis

Gonococcal arthritis

This is usually a disorder of females or homosexual males, in which the primary genital infection has been overlooked. Characteristically, it is a polyarthritis, frequently involving the hands, wrists and knees. Gonococcal arthritis is probably the commonest cause of infective arthritis in teenagers and young adults. Only in a minority of cases can gonococci be isolated from the synovial fluid.

Tuberculous arthritis

Approximately 1% of patients with tuberculosis have bony involvement as a result of spread from an established focus in the lungs or elsewhere. Involvement of the synovial membrane and peri-articular tissues produces a persistent arthritis with typical caseating granulomatous lesions. An inflammatory pannus may form and erode the articular cartilage. Tuberculous arthritis affects the hip and knee in children, but the vertebral column is most commonly involved in adults. In the vertebral column the associated osteomyelitis causes extensive bony destruction, and wedging or complete collapse of vertebrae may result (Pott's disease of the spine). The lower thoracic and lumbar spine are most commonly affected. Infection may spread along fascial planes,

particularly around the psoas muscle, producing a full-blown psoas abscess. Synovial fluid culture may produce a diagnosis.

Arthritis due to spirochaetes

Lyme disease was first described in the eastern United States in 1977. Epidemics of the disease have now been reported in many different areas. The presenting symptom is a migratory erythematous rash — erythema chronicum migrans. An arthritis follows weeks, or months, after the initial infection. Epidemiological studies have now shown that ticks of the genus *Ixodes* are responsible for transmitting the causative agent, a spirochaete named *Borrelia burgdorferi*. Immune complexes containing antibody directed against this organism have been detected in joint fluid and may play a role in the development of the arthritis. Antibiotic therapy given early in the course of the disease can prevent the joint disease.

Virus-associated arthritis

Many different virus infections are associated with a transient arthritis, or at least distinct pain within joints. In rubella infections, arthritis of the hands and wrists is common and the virus has been isolated from affected joints. A mild arthralgia may persist for several weeks. Occasionally, transient arthritis follows rubella vaccination. An arthritis may be a feature early in the course of viral hepatitis and is more severe with hepatitis B infection. Arthralgia can also be a feature of infectious mononucleosis.

RHEUMATIC FEVER

> ► Characterised by joint pain, skin rashes and fever
> ► Due to a disordered immune reaction to a Lancefield group A β-haemolytic streptococcal pharyngeal infection
> ► Associated with pancarditis
> ► Commonest in children 5–15 years, boys more than girls

Rheumatic fever is a disease of disordered immunity characterised by inflammatory changes in the heart (Ch. 13) and joints and in some cases associated with neurological symptoms (chorea). The disease is common in India, the Middle East and Central Africa. Although it is now rare in Europe and North America occasional clusters of cases do occur and several recent outbreaks in the United States have emphasised that the disease must be considered in any child or adolescent with joint pain, skin rashes or unexplained fever. Polyarthritis is the presenting feature in over 75% of cases and usually involves the large joints of the wrists, elbows, knees and ankles. The arthritis characteristically 'flits' from joint to joint, involving each for 2–4 days, and may cause severe pain. In the acute phase the inflammation involves the endocardium, the myocardium and the pericardium ('pancarditis'). Heart murmurs are common and children can die from cardiac failure.

Most patients have had a recent sore throat, typically a group A β-haemolytic streptococcal infection. Disappointingly there have been no recent advances in the understanding of the underlying immunopathology. For many years it has been known that there is a strong antibody reaction to the streptococcus and it is thought that this may cross-react with as yet unknown antigens in connective tissues, especially in the heart and joints.

GOUT

> ▶ Painful acute inflammatory response to tissue deposition of urate crystals
> ▶ Most commonly affects metatarsophalangeal joint of first toe
> ▶ Much more common in males than in females
> ▶ Serum uric acid levels are raised
> ▶ May be associated with chronic renal damage

Gout is one of the most clearly documented conditions in medical history. Evidence of gouty arthritis has been detected in Egyptian mummies, and the condition is clearly described in the writings of Hippocrates and other Greek and Roman physicians. It appears to have been common in the 17th and 18th centuries and in the popular imagination is associated with corpulence and alcoholism.

Pathogenesis

The underlying biochemical mechanisms in gout are well understood (Ch. 7) although the exact reasons why the majority of patients develop a raised uric acid level are uncertain. The mechanisms and causes are:

- idiopathic decrease in uric acid excretion (c. 75% of cases of clinical gout)
- impaired uric acid excretion secondary to thiazide diuretics, chronic renal failure, etc.

- increased uric acid production due to increased cell turnover (e.g. tumours), increased purine synthesis (specific enzyme defects)
- high dietary purine intake.

At least 5% of middle-aged males have a serum uric acid greater than 0.5 mmol/l, but less than 5% of these will ever develop clinical signs of gout. In over 75% of patients who present with gout, there is a decrease in uric acid clearance by the kidney but the underlying cause of this is not known. In a few patients, there appears to be an idiopathic increase in the rate of purine synthesis leading in turn to increased uric acid production. The increased cellular turnover associated with a wide variety of different malignant disorders and other diseases is a common cause of secondary gout. Most patients receiving chemotherapy are now treated prophylactically with xanthine oxidase inhibitors in order to minimise the hyperuricaemia associated with the cellular necrosis induced by cytotoxic drugs.

The stimulus to the acute inflammatory reaction in acute gout is the deposition of monosodium urate crystals in the synovium and adjacent connective tissues of the joints. The exact mechanisms leading to this are poorly understood. Gout is most common in the metatarsophalangeal joint of the great toe, and gravitational factors could play a part in promoting crystal deposition. Acute gout also occurs in the ankle but is comparatively uncommon in the knee and hips. In acute gout, the joint fluid contains numerous polymorphs and in some of these crystals can be detected by polarised light microscopy. Microcrystals of monosodium urate can absorb a variety of immunoglobulins, complement components, fibrinogen and fibronectin, and these may encourage their phagocytosis by polymorphs. Regulatory cytokines, such as interleukin-1, almost certainly have some role in promoting inflammation. There is a rapid turnover of neutrophils within acutely inflamed gouty joints, largely because phagocytosed microcrystals have a toxic effect on cellular membranes. This is in itself a potent acute inflammatory stimulus, and in acute gout there is often an associated cellulitis.

Clinicopathological features

The clinicopathological features of gout are as follows:

- males usually affected (90%)
- onset 40–60 years, familial tendency
- acute inflammatory monoarthritis—more than one joint involved in 10%

- raised plasma uric acid (>0.5 mmol/l)
- deposition of monosodium urate crystals in joints
- variable incidence of uric acid renal calculi
- mild intermittent proteinuria with focal interstitial nephritis
- untreated patients may progress to chronic gouty arthritis and renal failure.

Gout presents as an acute inflammatory mono-arthritis. In over two-thirds of patients the metatarsophalangeal joint is affected. The onset can be surprisingly abrupt. Affected joints are warm and tender and exquisitely painful (Fig. 25.22). There may be associated pyrexia, and the white cell count and ESR are generally raised. The clinical diagnosis is usually obvious, and prompt treatment with non-steroidal anti-inflammatory drugs or colchicine relieves symptoms within hours. Occasionally, several joints can be involved simultaneously and this can be diagnostically misleading.

There may be long intervals between acute attacks in individual patients. Most patients are treated with allopurinol, which suppresses uric acid synthesis by inhibiting xanthine oxidase.

Renal disease is the most serious complication of gout. For poorly understood reasons, the incidence of renal calculi in gout varies from country to country. In Western Europe it is of the order of 10% and gout should be considered in any patient who presents with renal colic. Mild proteinuria is found in a proportion of patients but very few progress to chronic urate nephropathy and renal failure. Those that do so have usually received inadequate treatment or have a strong familial history of severe gout. Urate crystal deposition in renal tubular epithelium induces cellular necrosis, chronic interstitial nephritis and fibrosis.

In chronic *tophaceous gout*, large deposits of uric acid occur within joints or in the soft tissues, particularly around the pinna of the ear. In these patients, there are substantial X-ray changes, with soft tissue swelling, calcification of urate deposits and even erosions of phalangeal bone.

Gout is associated with obesity, alcoholism, hypertension, ischaemic heart disease, various forms of hyperlipoproteinaemia and impaired glucose tolerance. However, the majority of patients who have a raised blood uric acid level will never develop gout, or any of its complications.

PYROPHOSPHATE ARTHROPATHY

Pyrophosphate arthropathy, also known as 'pseudo-gout' or 'chondrocalcinosis', results from the deposition of calcium pyrophosphate crystals in joint cartilage. Occasionally, an acute arthritis results and this can mimic true gout.

The cause of the pyrophosphate deposition is unknown. It is very much an age-related phenomenon and is more common in the elderly. Pyrophosphate may be laid down in areas of previous cartilagenous damage but this accounts for only a minority of cases. There is an association with

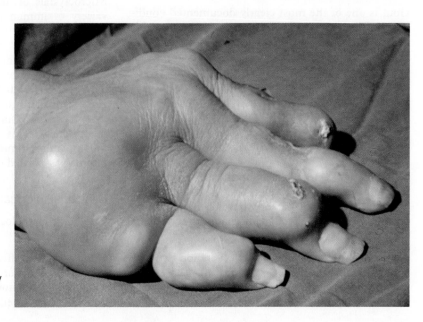

Fig. 25.22 Acute gout

Note the marked oedema and inflammation. There are areas of early ulceration at the tips of the index and ring fingers.

hyperparathyroidism and haemochromatosis and occasional familial cases are described.

Clinicopathological features

In most cases, pyrophosphate deposition produces no clinical symptoms. Minor degrees of cartilagenous calcification, particularly in the knee, are a common finding in X-rays taken in the elderly. In advanced cases, there is a characteristic linear area of calcification — evidence that the mid-zone of the articular fibrocartilage is particularly susceptible to pyrophosphate deposition. If crystals are shed into the joint cavity in sufficient numbers, an acute inflammatory arthritis results. This can usually be distinguished from true gout: the knee, rather than the foot, is usually involved; cartilagenous calcification should be obvious on X-ray; and if joint fluid is examined, the crystals do not have microscopic characteristics of urate.

There is a strong association between chondrocalcinosis and osteoarthritic joint disease. One explanation of this is that crystal deposition predisposes the articular cartilage to degenerative change and subsequent florid osteoarthritis. Alternatively, pyrophosphate crystals may be preferentially deposited in cartilage previously injured by early osteoarthritis. Most rheumatologists accept that there is a distinct form of osteoarthritis associated with crystal deposition, usually affecting the knees and shoulders of elderly women.

As most cases of chondrocalcinosis are asymptomatic, no particular treatment is indicated. Acute pseudogout is best treated by intra-articular corticosteroids. Anti-inflammatory drugs and colchicine are less effective than in true gout. No prophylactic measures are available to prevent recurrent attacks but these are uncommon.

JOINT INVOLVEMENT IN SYSTEMIC DISEASE

An arthritis, or at least some degree of joint involvement, is a common feature of many systemic disorders (Table 25.4). In some of these, the arthritis is the direct result of the primary pathological process involving the synovium.

Table 25.4 Systemic diseases and joint changes		
Underlying disease	Clinical features	Pathology
Acromegaly	Episodic painful swelling of small joints, e.g. in hands	Periosteal new bone formation
Amyloidosis	Arthropathy of shoulders, knees and wrists, usually secondary to myeloma	Amyloid deposition in synovium
Behçet's disease	Inflammatory arthropathy of knee (minor criterion)	Inflammatory synovitis
	Major features — oro-genital ulceration, uveitis and skin rashes	Underlying pathogenesis not understood
Clubbing	Characteristic swelling of nail beds	Increased blood flow to fingers and toes Associated with intra-thoracic pathology but mechanism unknown
Hypertrophic pulmonary osteoarthropathy (HPOA)	Arthropathy of wrists, ankles, feet	Periosteal new bone formation Same associations as clubbing, but less common
Haematological disorders		
Haemophilia	Recurrent joint haemorrhages Can progress to chronic painful deformative arthritis	Haemorrhage secondary to inherited deficiencies of factors VIII and IX
Haemoglobinopathies (esp. sickle cell disease)	Arthralgia, joint haemorrhages, aseptic necrosis of bone	Inherited defects in globin chain structure or synthesis
Acute leukaemia	Asymmetrical polyarthritis	Leukaemic infiltration of joints
Sarcoidosis	Small joint polyarthropathy, especially fingers	Sarcoidal granulomas in synovium

CONNECTIVE TISSUE DISEASES

There is no agreed definition of a 'connective tissue disease'. It is a convenient general term which covers a wide variety of disorders:

- rheumatoid arthritis
- systemic lupus erythematosus (SLE)
- polyarteritis nodosa
- ankylosing spondylitis, Reiter's disease and related disorders (p. 811)
- polymyositis and dermatomyositis
- polymyalgia rheumatica
- cranial (giant cell) arteritis
- systemic sclerosis (scleroderma)
- mixed connective tissue disease (MCTD).

These disorders have the following common features:

- multisystem disorders, often affecting joints, skin and subcutaneous tissues
- females preferentially affected (except in polyarteritis nodosa and ankylosing spondylitis), weak genetic tendency
- chronic clinical course, may respond to anti-inflammatory drugs
- first presentation may be during adolescent or early adult life
- immunological abnormalities often present, either circulating auto-antibodies or evidence of immune complex deposition.

These disorders were originally termed 'collagen diseases', and this emphasises that cutaneous and subcutaneous changes are often prominent clinical features. The clinical and pathological features of some of the more important connective tissue diseases are summarised in Table 25.5.

Pathological basis of clinical signs and symptoms of connective tissue diseases	
Sign or symptom	Pathological basis
Swelling	Tumour Oedema Inflammation
Joint pain	Synovial oedema and inflammation with stimulation of nerves in joint capsule
Ischaemic lesions	Vasculitis
Restricted mobility of tissues	Fibrosis or increased tissue tension due to inflammation

SYSTEMIC LUPUS ERYTHEMATOSUS

- ▶ Systemic disorder associated with auto-antibodies to DNA and other nuclear components
- ▶ Features include arthralgia, erythematous (butterfly) skin rash, anaemia, serositis (e.g. pericarditis), glomerular injury and neurological changes
- ▶ Can be provoked by drugs, especially hydralazine and procainamide

Systemic lupus erythematosus (SLE) is, more than any other connective tissue disease, a multisystem disorder. Females are affected more often than males, in some age groups by a ratio of up to 10:1. The incidence is higher in blacks and Asians than in Caucasians. The peak age of onset is usually between 20 and 30 years.

Aetiology and immunopathology

The cause of SLE is unknown. The first immunological abnormality was detected in the 1940s. It was found that leukocytes from patients with SLE phagocytosed nuclear debris produced by agitating a sample of freshly drawn blood. The characteristic 'LE cell' is a monocyte or polymorph which has phagocytosed a large mass of nuclear material. It was subsequently shown that most patients with SLE have circulating auto-antibodies directed against nuclear antigens. When serum containing these antibodies is added to tissue sections, such as liver or kidney, they bind to nuclear components and this can be visualised by immunofluorescence. Many other auto-antibodies have now been detected, reacting with both nuclear and cytoplasmic antigens. As these antibodies are characterised, it is becoming clear that they are directed against a relatively small range of epitopes, components of both nucleic acids and cytoplasmic phospholipids:

- anti-DNA (double or single stranded) — only 5% patients persistently negative
- antibodies to other nuclear components:
  — antihistones
  — anti-Ro, La and Sm★
- antiphospholipid antibodies (thrombotic tendency, recurrent abortions, false-positive tests for syphilis)
- red cell antibodies (autoimmune haemolytic anaemia)

★Ro, La, Sm refer to the names of patients in whom the auto-antibodies were first detected.

Table 25.5   Clinical and pathological features of the major connective tissue diseases

Disease	Sex ratio	Age at onset	Main clinical features	Immunological abnormalities	Pathology
Rheumatoid arthritis	3F:1M	Young or middle-aged adults Occasionally children	Chronic polyarthritis Subcutaneous nodules Splenomegaly	Auto-antibodies against native Ig (rheumatoid factors)	Chronic inflammatory synovitis Granulomatous lesions in subcutaneous tissues Fibrinous pericarditis
Systemic lupus erythematosus (SLE)	8F:1M	Young or middle-aged adults	Skin rashes Light sensitivity Arthritis Anaemia Leukopenia Renal disease	Auto-antibodies against nuclear and cytoplasmic proteins and many other cellular components	Inflammatory synovitis Glomerulonephritis Erythematous skin rashes, etc.
Polyarteritis nodosa (PAN)	3M:1F	Any age, chiefly middle-aged adults	Arthralgia Abdominal pain Hypertension Fever Leukocytosis and eosinophilia	Some patients: antinuclear antibodies and rheumatoid factors	Necrotising vasculitis affecting medium-sized arteries
Ankylosing spondylitis	2M:1F	Young adults	Back pain Arthritis Uveitis	No consistent changes Most patients HLA-B27 positive	Inflammatory changes progressing to partial bony fusion of spine and sacro-iliac joints
Polymyositis and dermato-myositis	3F:1M	Adults	Muscle weakness, pain and tenderness Skin rashes in dermatomyositis	Only if features of other connective tissue diseases present	Inflammatory myositis underlying malignancy in some cases
Polymyalgia rheumatica	2F:1M	Elderly	Malaise and weakness Muscular aching, esp. shoulders, pelvis and hips	No consistent changes Raised ESR	Limited and non-specific muscle biopsy changes Some cases overlap with temporal arteritis
Cranial (temporal or giant cell) arteritis	2F:1M	Elderly	Headache Visual loss Tender scalp	No consistent changes Raised ESR	Chronic granulomatous arteritis chiefly in head and neck arteries
Systemic sclerosis (scleroderma)	3F:1M	30–50 years	Raynaud's phenomenon Skin thickening Polyarthritis Dysphagia and dyspnoea Hypertension	Rheumatoid factor (25%) Antinuclear antibodies (50%)	Fibrosis of subcutaneous tissues Intimal and medial fibrosis of muscular arteries

- rheumatoid factors
- cell or organelle-specific antibodies (mitochondrial, smooth muscle, gastric parietal cell, etc.)

Why these auto-antibodies form in the first instance is unknown, and their role in the development of pathological lesions is equally uncertain. None is specific for SLE and most have been detected in other connective tissue disorders or in diseases with an immunological basis, such as pernicious anaemia or Hashimoto's thyroiditis. One of the antibodies directed against a phospholipid, the so-called 'cardiolipin antibody', is associated with arterial and venous thrombosis. These patients may develop cerebral infarcts and often have a history of recurrent spontaneous abortions (see below).

Many drugs have been suggested as causes of SLE, but in some instances the association is almost certainly fortuitous. The evidence is strongest for hydralazine, a potent vasodilator sometimes used in the treatment of hypertension. Oral contraceptives can exacerbate pre-existing SLE and must be used with caution in any patient with a suspected connective tissue disorder.

No other environmental or occupational factors have been implicated in SLE. It is not obviously associated with any particular HLA antigen but there is a strong familial tendency. Relatives of SLE patients have a substantially increased incidence of the disorder and there is a greater than 50% concordance in monozygotic twins.

Clinicopathological features

Spontaneous remissions and exacerbations are common in SLE and some patients can be managed for long periods without specific treatment. Signs and symptoms can occur in almost every system:

- mild arthralgia, especially hands, knees and ankles; low-grade inflammatory synovitis but few erosions
- erythematous ('butterfly') facial rash and alopecia; photosensitivity
- lymphadenopathy and splenomegaly
- myalgia
- anaemia and leukopenia
- pyrexia
- pleurisy and pericarditis
- glomerulonephritis with proteinuria and occasionally nephrotic syndrome
- psychological symptoms, headaches, fits and occasionally cerebral infarction with hemiplegia.

Arthralgia is often the presenting symptom and in the early stages may resemble rheumatoid arthritis. The hands, knees and ankles are most affected, and a series of joints may be involved in succession (flitting arthralgia). Synovial biopsy shows a low-grade inflammatory synovitis but, unlike the situation in rheumatoid disease, pannus does not form and cartilagenous erosions are rare.

The most characteristic *cutaneous change* in SLE is a symmetrical erythematous facial ('butterfly') rash (Fig. 25.23) which may be precipitated by exposure to sunlight (photosensitivity). Raynaud's phenomenon, urticaria, hyperpigmentation and cutaneous ulcers are other less common features.

Non-specific early signs in SLE include mild pyrexia, normochromic normocytic anaemia, leukopenia, muscle pain, lymphadenopathy and splenomegaly. Although pleurisy and pericarditis are common postmortem findings they rarely produce overt clinical symptoms. Non-bacterial thrombotic vegetations (Libman–Sacks endocarditis) may form on mitral or aortic valves and can be detected by echocardiography. Murmurs may result, but the vegetations seldom erode the valve leaflets or cause significant embolic disease.

Renal involvement is one of the most important fea-

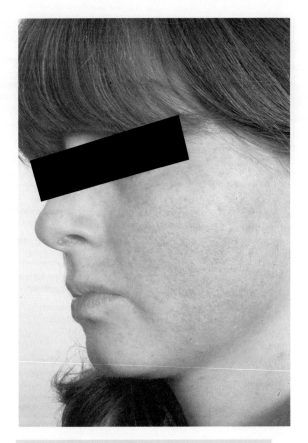

Fig. 25.23   The typical 'malar' flush of systemic lupus erythematosus

tures and patients should be regularly screened for proteinuria. The underlying lesion is glomerulonephritis which may be of minimal change, focal, membranous or diffuse proliferative type (Ch. 21). Although some patients do progress to renal failure, not all forms are necessarily associated with a poor prognosis.

Neurological changes are more common in SLE than in any other connective tissue disease. Psychiatric symptoms are the commonest abnormality but some of these may be the result of treatment with steroids. Severe headaches and convulsions occur in some patients. The small sub-group who present with recurrent transient ischaemic attacks or definite episodes of cerebral infarction generally have circulating antibodies to cardiolipin—the so-called 'antiphospholipid antibody syndrome'. The neuropathological changes in SLE are rather non-specific but occasional cases have evidence of cerebral arteritis or thrombosis.

Laboratory investigations

Abnormal findings in SLE include:

- raised ESR and C reactive protein
- mild normochromic normocytic anaemia
- leukopenia or thrombocytopenia
- circulating antinuclear antibodies
- reduced serum albumin, raised gamma globulins, low complement levels.

POLYARTERITIS NODOSA

> ▶ Inflammatory disorder of unknown aetiology affecting medium-sized arteries
> ▶ Causes muscle and joint pain, fever, ischaemic lesions in many organs, neuropathy and renal damage

Polyarteritis nodosa (PAN) is one of the most florid of the inflammatory disorders of arteries, collectively known as arteritis (Ch. 13). The main features are:

- medium-sized muscular arteries affected
- myalgia, polymyositis and arthralgia; fever and malaise
- abdominal pain, vomiting and diarrhoea
- mucosal ulcers, occasionally intestinal or splenic infarcts
- tender subcutaneous nodules (arteritic lesions), skin rashes and digital gangrene
- hypertension and pericarditis
- peripheral neuropathy — motor, sensory or mixed; usually single nerves involved (mononeuritis multiplex)
- haematuria and proteinuria; glomerulonephritis and hypertensive renal disease
- asthmatic symptoms, often with eosinophilia; haemoptysis; pulmonary infarcts due to pulmonary arteritis.

Almost any artery can be affected but because arthralgia and abdominal pain are frequent early symptoms, these patients are often referred to rheumatologists or gastroenterologists.

Aetiology and immunopathology

Very little is known about the cause of PAN or indeed any of the forms of systemic vasculitis. The incidence seems to be increasing but this may be because milder forms of vasculitis are now recognised. The florid acute inflammatory changes with associated fibrinoid necrosis resemble experimental models of immune complex vasculitis. Circulating immune complexes may be elevated in patients with vasculitis. Complement levels can be reduced and abnormal deposits of immunoglobulins are sometimes present in affected vessels in biopsy specimens. The nature of the associated antigen is quite uncertain. A small proportion of patients with PAN, and more rarely other forms of vasculitis, are hepatitis B virus surface antigen (HBsAg) positive. In some forms of vasculitis the lungs, and other parts of the respiratory tract, are affected early in the course of the disease and this might suggest that the responsible antigen was inhaled. Many patients with systemic vasculitis have circulating antibodies directed against different constituents of endothelial cells (antineutrophil cytoplasmic antibodies, ANCA). They are not specific for any particular disorder and may not be present in patients in clinical remission. It is not known whether these antibodies are involved directly in the disease process or are a secondary result of the associated vascular damage.

Clinicopathological features

Most patients present with non-specific signs of a generalised illness, such as pyrexia of unknown origin (PUO), malaise and myalgia. Arthralgia, abdominal pain, vomiting and diarrhoea are common in the early stages of the disease, and other non-specific signs include hypertension and pericarditis.

The underlying vasculitic process (Ch. 13) can involve almost any medium-sized artery. The disease was originally named because of the tender nodules produced by involvement of subcutaneous arteries, but these are quite different from rheumatoid nodules and occur in only a small proportion of cases. Peripheral gangrene can result from arteritis of digital vessels. Polyarteritis nodosa is a cause of mononeuritis multiplex — a pattern of peripheral neuropathy where individual nerves are affected because of disease of the nutrient arteries (Ch. 26). Symptoms can be motor, sensory or mixed.

Renal disease is one of the leading causes of death in PAN (see Ch. 21). There is a well-established association between PAN, pulmonary disease and eosinophilia. Classically, there are prominent asthmatic symptoms, with cough and dyspnoea. In severe cases, pulmonary arteritis leads to areas of infarction and there may be haemoptysis.

In contrast to the case in systemic lupus erythematosus, nervous system involvement is comparatively rare in PAN. Only occasional patients develop cerebral arteritis.

Laboratory investigations

Typical haematological findings in PAN include a mild normochromic normocytic anaemia, a moderate leukocytosis and an absolute eosinophilia. ESR and other acute phase reactants are raised. Although gamma globulin levels may be increased, auto-antibodies such as rheumatoid factor and antinuclear antibody are usually negative.

A firm diagnosis can be made histologically or by arteriography. Biopsy of a skin lesion or a nerve associated with an area of cutaneous anaesthesia or a muscle biopsy may show the histological appearances of necrotising arteritis (p. 326, Fig. 13.18). Selective angiography of the major abdominal branches, such as the coeliac axis or mesenteric artery, may reveal typical aneurysms.

The outlook in PAN is worst in patients with definite evidence of multisystem involvement. Patients with limited forms of the disease often do well and may need little or no treatment. It is quite possible that several disease processes are presently included under the label of 'polyarteritis nodosa'.

POLYMYALGIA RHEUMATICA

Polymyalgia rheumatica (PMR) is an important disorder of the elderly. It is more common in females than males, and patients usually present with persistent muscular pain in the shoulders and hips, lethargy and tiredness. These rather non-specific symptoms occur in most rheumatic disorders, and PMR may therefore be confused with rheumatoid arthritis, cranial arteritis (see below), polyarteritis nodosa or various forms of polymyositis. In most patients these disorders can be excluded, and PMR is considered to be a disease in its own right.

The underlying pathological changes are poorly understood. There are no specific histological changes in the muscles and, in particular, the inflammatory infiltrates characteristic of polymyositis (see below) are absent. In typical cases, the ESR is greater than 100 mm/h, but there are no other consistent laboratory abnormalities. There may be a mild normochromic or hypochromic anaemia and non-specific elevations of gamma globulins. Circulating auto-antibodies, such as rheumatoid factor and antinuclear antibody, are usually absent and creatine phosphokinase levels are normal.

Although PMR is a somewhat non-specific clinical and pathological entity, it is a common and important condition which can affect up to 1% of elderly patients. Clinical benefit can be obtained with steroid treatment, but there are inevitable side-effects if this is continued for long periods. At least 15% of patients with polymyalgia rheumatica have cranial arteritis and in these patients a positive temporal artery biopsy is of great value in justifying long-term treatment. In other patients steroids are usually given for at least a year and then discontinued gradually.

CRANIAL ARTERITIS

Cranial arteritis (also known as temporal or 'giant cell' arteritis) is an important, and not uncommon, disease of the elderly. It affects arteries of the head and neck region and, unlike almost all other arterial diseases, responds rapidly and predictably to treatment with anti-inflammatory drugs such as corticosteroids.

Aetiology and pathogenesis

Epidemiological surveys in different communities have demonstrated that the incidence of the disease varies between 50 and 150 cases per 100 000 population. The disease is commonest in Caucasians but occurs in all races. There is no satisfactory explanation for the preferential involvement of the arteries of the head and neck. Involvement of the superficial temporal artery is responsible for scalp tenderness, but it is disease of the ciliary and ophthalmic arteries which may produce blindness. The carotid arteries and, occasionally, the aorta may be affected but this is very much the exception. The disease appears to be a distinct entity, and the histological appearances and clinical course of the disorder are very different from those of other inflammatory conditions of arteries, such as polyarteritis nodosa. There is no obvious genetic basis, nor any strong familial incidence. Auto-antibodies cannot usually be detected in the serum, and immunological studies of affected arteries do not suggest that the disease has an immune complex origin.

Clinicopathological features

Because the superficial temporal artery is accessible for biopsy, the histological features are well described (Ch. 13).

Most patients with headache or scalp tenderness, and in any elderly patient these symptoms should suggest a diagnosis of cranial arteritis. There is a well recognised overlap between the symptoms of cranial arteritis and polymyalgia rheumatica. Careful palpation of the temporal arteries is essential in any patient with polymyalgia and, conversely, musculoskeletal symptoms are not uncommon in cases of cranial arteritis. The precise relationship between these disorders is uncertain, particularly as the pathological changes in the two disorders are rather dissimilar. Nevertheless, they are associated and many rheumatologists would suggest that temporal artery biopsy should be part of the normal management of patients with polymyalgia rheumatica. Fortunately, steroid therapy is the treatment of choice in each disorder.

Laboratory investigations

Temporal artery biopsy should be performed urgently in any patient with suspected cranial arteritis. Ideally, 20–30 mm of superficial temporal artery should be removed, preferably before steroid therapy has started. A high ESR is characteristic but in a few patients this may be only slightly elevated. There are no other characteristic laboratory findings, although a mild normochromic normocytic anaemia is sometimes present. Up to 40% of patients with good clinical evidence of cranial arteritis have a negative temporal artery biopsy. This merely indicates that the superficial temporal artery is only one of the many arteries that can be affected by disease and that the lesions are patchy.

POLYMYOSITIS AND DERMATOMYOSITIS

Polymyositis is a chronic inflammatory disorder of skeletal muscle of unknown cause. The typical patient is a female in late middle age with a history of progressive muscular weakness, often commencing in the shoulder or neck muscles. There is associated pain and tenderness but muscle wasting is not a feature in the early stages.

In active polymyositis there is a florid chronic inflammatory infiltrate in affected muscles (Fig. 25.24) with extensive associated degeneration of both type 1 and type 2 fibres (Ch. 26). Many of the clinical features suggest a viral infection but no particular virus has been consistently isolated. Autoantibodies to a variety of nuclear antigens have been detected in up to 25% of patients. Rheumatoid factor and antinuclear antibody are usually absent. The diagnosis is best made on a combination of clinical

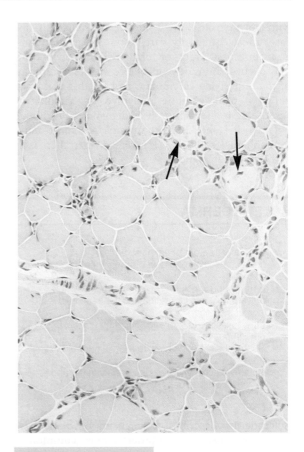

Fig. 25.24　Polymyositis

A low-power view of a muscle biopsy showing irregular infiltrates of inflammatory cells. Some muscle fibres are undergoing necrosis (arrows).

findings, raised levels of muscle enzymes such as creatine phosphokinase (CPK), electromyography and muscle biopsy. Serial estimation of CPK may give a clue to the prognosis in individual patients. The majority make an uneventful recovery, albeit over a period of months or years. Oesophageal disease produces a troublesome dysphagia, and cardiac involvement is not uncommon. The mortality rate is between 5 and 15% and is usually the result of respiratory failure, aspiration pneumonia or, occasionally, heart failure.

In *dermatomyositis* a variety of skin changes occur in association with an otherwise typical polymyositis. There is a diffuse erythema involving the upper part of the body, prominent swelling of the eyelids and a variable purple 'heliotrope' discolouration of the eyelids (Ch. 24). The muscular symptoms are more prominent in patients with dermatological changes.

At least 10% of middle-aged or elderly patients

with polymyositis have evidence of malignant disease, most commonly carcinoma of the bronchus, gastrointestinal tract or breast. The polymyositis may occur months or years before the first symptoms of the underlying carcinoma, and for this reason all patients with genuine polymyositis should be screened for the common malignancies. Although polymyositis and dermatomyositis are more common in females this ratio is reversed when there is an associated malignancy.

SCLERODERMA

> ▶ Systemic disorder of unknown aetiology characterised by sclerosis (hardening) of connective tissues
> ▶ Early features include Raynaud's phenomenon, polyarthritis, and induration and contraction of the skin of the fingers
> ▶ May be limited to skin and subcutaneous tissues ('morphoea')
> ▶ Submucosal fibrosis may develop in gastrointestinal tract
> ▶ Underlying changes include vascular injury and connective tissue deposition

Scleroderma describes a spectrum of diseases of uncertain cause. The disorder is most common in young and early middle-aged females who usually present with Raynaud's phenomenon, polyarthritis and thickening and tightness of the skin (Table 25.6). This affects the hands and fingertips first, and movements of the finger joints are impaired. Facial changes are also common; the mouth appears small and the peri-oral skin is taut and creased (Fig. 25.25). Careful observation of the progress of the disease gives a good indication of the prognosis. If the disease spreads to the upper arms, legs or the flank there is a strong chance that a generalised form of disease, *systemic sclerosis*, may develop. In contrast, in other patients the disease is entirely limited to the skin and is characterised by well-defined plaques or bands of subcutaneous fibrosis ('morphoea').

The underlying pathological changes include vascular injury, perivascular accumulation of mononuclear cells and deposition of connective tissue. In systemic sclerosis the process may extend to the gastrointestinal tract. A frequent symptom is dysphagia and there may be submucosal fibrosis and muscular atrophy in the lower oesophagus. Occasionally, the fibrosis can extend to the large or small intestine. Diarrhoea and malabsorption are possible clinical symptoms.

Little is known of the cause of scleroderma. Some circulating auto-antibodies have now been detected but they have not been as well characterised as in diseases such as systemic lupus erythematosus or

Table 25.6	Clinical and pathological features of scleroderma and systemic sclerosis	
Organ/system	Clinical features	Pathology
Skin	Tightness and tethering Pitting and induration, esp. finger tips Ulceration and calcification Telangiectasia, esp. face Fibrous plaques (morphoea)	Epidermal atrophy Loss of skin appendages Dense dermal fibrosis
Joints	Polyarthritis, esp. hands Lack of joint movement due to skin tethering	Low-grade inflammatory synovitis
Gastrointestinal tract	Dysphagia Occasionally malabsorption and diarrhoea	Submucosal fibrosis and muscular atrophy in lower oesophagus
Cardiovascular system	Raynaud's phenomenon Pericarditis	Intimal fibrosis of small and medium-sized arteries Pericarditis Patchy myocardial fibrosis Intimal thickening of arteries
Kidneys	Proteinuria Rapidly progessive renal failure (rare)	Ischaemic atrophy of tubules Fibrinoid necrosis of arterioles Widespread thickening of glomerular vessels
Lungs	Dyspnoea	Interstitial inflammation and fibrosis

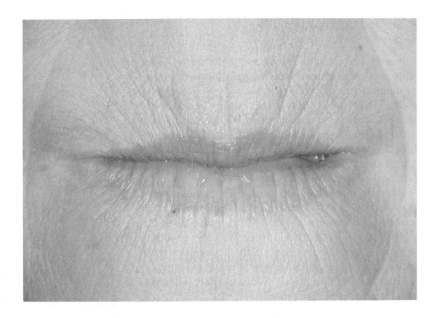

Fig. 25.25 Tightening of the peri-oral skin in scleroderma

rheumatoid disease. The pathological changes in small arteries and arterioles resemble those of systemic hypertension but only 20% of patients with scleroderma have raised blood pressure. Current research aims to identify the molecular signals which are responsible for the increased deposition of collagen.

MIXED CONNECTIVE TISSUE DISEASE (MCTD)

Connective tissue diseases share many common clinical and pathological features. In clinical practice, it is usually possible to attach a specific diagnostic label to the majority of patients. The term 'overlap syndrome' or mixed connective tissue disease (MCTD) is used when there are distinct overlapping features of systemic lupus erythematosus (SLE), systemic sclerosis, rheumatoid arthritis, polymyositis or even polyarteritis nodosa. The usual features are:

- occurrence in young adult females (75%)
- arthritis, suggestive of rheumatoid disease (>90%)
- Raynaud's phenomenon (>90%)
- swollen, puffy hands with skin changes suggestive of scleroderma (75%)
- anaemia and leukopenia (50%)
- disordered oesophageal motility (50%)
- lymphadenopathy, pleurisy and pericarditis (25%)
- antinuclear antibodies (100%)
- rheumatoid factor (>30%)
- *no* evidence of renal disease.

All patients with mixed connective tissue disease have a strongly positive fluorescent test for antinuclear antibodies. The exact nature of the nuclear antigen is unknown, but there is evidence that several different nuclear matrix proteins may be involved.

Because true MCTD is uncommon there is comparatively little information on clinical and pathological progression. In some patients a full clinical remission occurs, but others develop into typical scleroderma or SLE. In these patients the outlook is much the same as if a MCTD phase had not occurred.

CONNECTIVE TISSUE TUMOURS

Connective tissue tumours are, with few exceptions, relatively uncommon. However, those classified as malignant (i.e. sarcomas) are important because they are often deeply located, for example in the retroperitoneum, resulting in late clinical presentation and difficulties in ensuring complete surgical removal. As a general rule, the more deeply a connective tissue tumour is situated, the less likely it is to be benign.

Benign connective tissue tumours

Benign connective tissue tumours include:

- lipoma
- angioma
- leiomyoma

- fibrous histiocytoma
- granular cell tumour.

Lipomas are the commonest connective tissue tumours, usually subcutaneous and comprising morphologically mature adipocytes. They are usually solitary, but may be multiple, well circumscribed and located in subcutaneous fat. Uncommon variants include *angiolipoma* characterised by numerous blood vessels, *spindle cell lipoma* in which there is an admixture of fibroblasts, and *myelolipoma* containing haemopoietic cells.

Although *angiomas* are benign in the sense that they do not actively invade surrounding tissues, they can be troublesome clinically and prone to recurrences requiring further surgery. These problems arise because the margins of the lesion are often blurred, merging with the surrounding normal tissue, and foci of thrombosis within the neoplastic vessels result in endothelial proliferation.

Leiomyomas in connective tissues (they are commoner in the uterus and gut) arise from smooth muscle cells in the walls of blood vessels and, in the skin, from arrector pilae muscles.

Fibrous histiocytomas are neoplasms of cells, possibly of macrophage lineage, exhibiting fibroblastic and histiocytic morphology to varying degrees. Benign fibrous histiocytomas occur most commonly in the skin (dermatofibroma; Ch. 24).

Granular cell tumours are of uncertain histogenesis. Although benign, they are usually poorly circumscribed. They are usually located superficially and, curiously, when they occur beneath squamous epithelium (in skin, tongue, etc.) they often induce florid epithelial hyperplasia morphologically mimicking carcinoma.

Malignant connective tissue tumours (sarcomas)

Malignant connective tissue tumours include:

- liposarcoma
- malignant fibrous histiocytoma
- angiosarcoma
- leiomyosarcoma
- rhabdomyosarcoma
- synovial sarcoma
- epithelioid sarcoma
- peripheral neuroectodermal tumour
- fibrosarcoma.

Liposarcomas are the commonest. The incidence of tumours designated 'malignant fibrous histiocytoma' varies according to the belief of local histopatholo-

gists in this controversial entity; in places where its existence is accepted, the incidence is often as high as that of liposarcoma.

All sarcomas have the general properties of local invasion and a varying propensity for regional and distant metastasis, favouring the haematogenous route. Many of them grow as 'spindle cell tumours' or 'small blue round cell tumours', the latter particularly in children (the 'blue' refers to their appearance with haematoxylin and eosin staining), with few identifying characteristics to betray their true histogenesis; often they require immunocytochemistry or electron microscopy for precise classification.

Some of these tumours merit specific comments. *Synovial sarcomas* usually occur, as the name suggests, close to joints and have a biphasic growth pattern comprising spindle cells and clefts lined by cells with a more epithelial morphology. *Epithelioid sarcomas* are rare tumours occurring on the limbs and have an unusual tendency to arise from and grow along fascial sheaths. *Peripheral neuroectodermal tumours* occur most commonly in children and histologically resemble Ewing's tumour (p. 801). Indeed, the kinship is more than morphological for many of them show the same chromosomal translocation, designated as t(11;22)(q24;q12).

Tumour-like lesions of connective tissues

Some nodular connective tissue lesions are characterised by cellular proliferation but they do not fulfil all the criteria of neoplasia. These include:

- fibromatoses
- nodular fasciitis
- myositis ossificans.

Fibromatoses are tumour-like proliferations of myofibroblasts. These cells have contractile properties; this explains the puckering and tethering associated with some variants of fibromatoses. For example, *palmar fibromatosis* (Dupuytren's contracture) leads to permanent flexion of the fingers. Other variants of fibromatosis include *musculo-aponeurotic fibromatosis* and *desmoid tumours*.

Nodular fasciitis occurs superficially as a rapidly growing nodule with alarming histological appearances mimicking sarcoma. *Myositis ossificans* is characterised by, as its name suggests, inflammation in muscle and ossification. It is a benign lesion, but the newly-formed bone in these lesions can resemble that seen in osteosarcoma, a pitfall with which all histopathologists should be familiar.

FURTHER READING

Apley A G, Solomon L 1994 Concise system of orthopaedics and fractures, 3rd edn. Butterworth-Heinemann, London
Dieppe P, Cooper C, Kirwan J, McGill N 1991 Arthritis and rheumatism in practice. Gower Medical Publishing, London

Enzinger F M, Weiss S W 1994 Soft tissue tumours, 3rd edn. Mosby, St Louis
Revell P A 1985 Pathology of bone. Springer Verlag, Berlin

26

Central and peripheral nervous systems

NORMAL STRUCTURE AND FUNCTION

The central nervous system (CNS) is the most anatomically complex system in the body, able to function both as a self-contained unit and as the control unit which co-ordinates the activities of the peripheral nervous system (PNS), skeletal muscle and other main organ systems. Despite the structural and functional complexities of the CNS, the constituent cells can be divided into just five main groups:

- neurones
- glia
- microglial cells
- connective tissue
- blood vessels.

Neurones

Neurones, or nerve cells, vary considerably in size and appearance within the CNS. All possess a cell body and axons and dendrites.

The *cell body* or *perikaryon* is easily seen by light microscopy (Fig. 26.1). The perikaryon contains neurofilaments, microtubules, lysosomes, mitochondria, complex stacks of rough endoplasmic reticulum, free ribosomes and a single nucleus with a prominent nucleolus. Some groups of neurones contain the pigment neuromelanin and are readily identifiable with the naked eye as darkly coloured nuclei, e.g. in the substantia nigra.

Axons and dendrites are the neuronal processes which convey electrical impulses from and towards the perikaryon respectively. These processes vary enormously in size and complexity, and may be difficult to identify on routine microscopy.

Glia

Glia are specialised supporting cells of the CNS comprising four main groups:

- astrocytes
- oligodendrocytes
- ependymal cells
- choroid plexus cells.

Astrocytes are process-bearing cells which are poorly visualised by light microscopy (Fig. 26.1) unless special staining techniques are used. They perform several important roles:

- provision of a supportive framework for other cells in the CNS
- control of the neuronal environment by the intimate association of astrocyte processes with perikarya, influencing local neurotransmitter and electrolyte concentrations
- regulation of the blood–brain barrier by astrocyte foot processes which are closely applied around cerebral capillaries (see below).

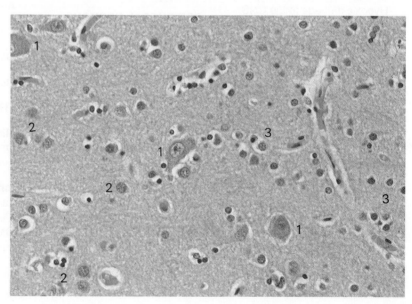

Fig. 26.1 Normal cerebral cortex

Figure shows the normal arrangement of neurones **(1)**, astrocytes **(2)**, oligodendrocytes **(3)** and capillaries in the cerebral cortex. Although the neuronal perikarya are visible, the cytoplasm of glial cells is best demonstrated by using special histological techniques.

Oligodendrocytes are the most numerous cells in the CNS. On light microscopy, they are visible as darkly staining nuclei located around neurones and nerve fibres (Fig. 26.1). The most important function of oligodendrocytes is the synthesis and maintenance of myelin in the CNS.

Ependymal cells form the single-cell lining of the ventricular system and the central canal of the spinal cord. They are short columnar cells which bear cilia on the luminal surface. Ependymal cells may participate in the absorption and secretion of cerebrospinal fluid (CSF).

Choroid plexus cells secrete CSF and contain large quantities of mitochondria, rough endoplasmic reticulum and Golgi apparatus within the cytoplasm. They form a cuboidal epithelial covering over the ventricular choroid plexus, and bear atypical microvilli.

Microglial cells

Microglial cells belong to the macrophage/monocyte system of phagocytic cells. They are normally quiescent, and inconspicuous on light microscopy, but are of major importance in reactive states, for example in inflammatory and demyelinating disorders.

Connective tissue

Connective tissue in the CNS is confined to two main structural groups: the meninges and perivascular fibroblasts.

The *meninges* comprise the pia, arachnoid and dura mater, and the arachnoidal granulations which are the main sites of CSF absorption. The meninges are composed of fibroblast-like cells which also extend around meningeal and cerebral blood vessels.

Pathological basis of neurological signs and symptoms

Sign or symptom	Pathological basis
Headache • intracranial cause	Raised or reduced intracranial pressure Stretching or pressure on intracranial vessels Distortion or inflammation of meninges
• extracranial cause	Referred from paranasal sinuses, cervical or temporomandibular joints, teeth, ears, etc.
Neck stiffness	Irritation or inflammation of meninges
Coma or impaired consciousness	Metabolic, e.g.: • hypoglycaemia • ketoacidosis • drug-induced • hepatic failure Brainstem lesions, e.g.: • infarction • haemorrhage Cerebral hemisphere lesions, e.g.: • intracerebral or extracerebral haemorrhage • infarction • infections • trauma
Dementia	Loss of functioning neurones due to ischaemia, toxic injury or primary disease

Sign or symptom	Pathological basis
Epileptic fits	Paroxysmal neuronal discharges, either idiopathic or emanating from focus of cortical disease or damage
Abnormal reflexes • exaggerated • impaired	Corticospinal tract lesion Peripheral neuropathy or cerebellar disease
Muscle deficit • wasting • weakness	Loss of trophic stimulus from lower motor neurones Myopathy Disease directly or indirectly affecting function of: • upper or lower motor neurones • neuromuscular conduction • muscle function
Sensory impairment and/or paraes-theslae	Disease directly or indirectly affecting function of: • cortical neurones • corticospinal tracts • peripheral nerves
Visual field defects or blindness	Disease involving either the eyes, optic nerves or visual cortex (e.g. cataracts, tumours intrinsic or extrinsic to optic neural pathways, ischaemia)
Tinnitus and/or deafness	Impaired transmission of sound through external meatus (e.g. wax) or through middle ear ossicles, or disease affecting the organ of Corti or the auditory nerve

Blood vessels

Blood vessels in the CNS are similar in structure and function to those elsewhere in the body, with the important exception of the capillaries. The capillaries within the CNS differ from most other capillaries in several respects:

- The vessels are non-fenestrated, and tight junctions are present between adjacent cells.
- The endothelial cells possess a thick layer of cytoplasm containing numerous organelles.
- Relatively few microvilli are present on the luminal surface of the endothelial cells, and only occasional pinocytotic vesicles are present in the cytoplasm.
- The endothelial cell basement membrane is intimately surrounded by a network of astrocyte processes.

These special structural features are important constituents of the *blood–brain barrier*: this is a functional unit which restricts the entry and exit of many substances — including proteins, ions, non-lipid-soluble compounds and drugs — to and from the CNS.

REACTIONS OF CNS CELLS TO INJURY

▶ Axonal damage results in central chromatolysis in neuronal perikarya, with anterograde degeneration of the damaged axon
▶ Axonal regeneration does not occur to a significant extent in the CNS
▶ Axonal degeneration results in breakdown of the myelin sheath around damaged fibres
▶ Hypertrophy and hyperplasia of astrocytes with fibrillary gliosis results in a glial scar around areas of tissue damage
▶ Microglia and recruited blood monocytes form a population of phagocytic cells

Neurones

Neurones can undergo various reactive changes to cell injury:

- central chromatolysis
- anterograde degeneration
- atrophy
- hypoxic cell damage
- neuronophagia.

Central chromatolysis is a distinctive reaction which usually occurs in response to axonal damage (Fig. 26.2). This reaction is maximal at around eight days following axonal damage, and is accompanied

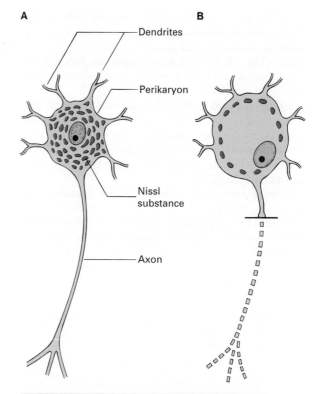

Fig. 26.2   Response to axonal injury: central chromatolysis and anterograde degeneration

A. In the normal neurone the nucleus is located centrally and surrounded by Nissl substance (RNA). **B.** Following axonal injury, the perikaryon swells and the nucleus migrates peripherally. The Nissl substance is dispersed to the periphery of the perikaryon, hence the term 'central chromatolysis'. Anterograde degeneration of the axon occurs distal to the site of injury.

by increased RNA and protein synthesis, suggestive of a regenerative response.

Anterograde degeneration occurs as a result of axonal transection, and is usually accompanied by central chromatolysis (see Fig. 26.2). Degeneration of the distal part of the axon will occur following its separation from the intact perikaryon, e.g. by transection. Within four days, the distal segment degenerates and becomes fragmented. The myelin sheath surrounding the axon also fragments, but this usually occurs only after axonal degeneration is established. Axonal and myelin debris is then phagocytosed by macrophages, which often remain around the site of injury for several months. Attempts at axonal regeneration do not occur to a significant extent in the CNS.

Atrophy of neurones occurs in many slowly progressive degenerative disorders, e.g. motor neurone disease. Such neurones appear shrunken, and often contain excess lipofuscin pigment. Trans-synaptic atrophy occurs in neurones following loss of the main afferent connections, e.g. in neurones of the lateral geniculate body following damage to the optic nerve or retina.

Hypoxic cell damage to neurones is described below.

Neuronophagia is a mononuclear phagocytic response to acute necrosis of neurones, for example in viral encephalitis. The phagocytic cells cluster around the dead neurones, thereby marking the sites of irreversible cell damage.

Astrocytes

Astrocytes undergo hyperplasia and hypertrophy following almost all forms of CNS damage, in a response known as 'reactive gliosis'. Gliotic tissue is translucent and firm, often forming a limiting barrier to sites of tissue damage, for example at the edge of a cerebral infarct.

Microglia

Microglia are also involved in the response to many forms of CNS damage, often acting as phagocytes (as in neuronophagia). When myelin is damaged, these cells ingest the breakdown products, resulting in an enlarged rounded cell body distended with droplets of neutral lipid.

Oligodendrocytes and ependymal cells

These cells show only a limited capacity to react to injury.

INTRACRANIAL SPACE-OCCUPYING LESIONS

▶ Brain swelling may be diffuse or focal
▶ Diffuse brain swelling is usually due to vasodilatation and vascular engorgement, or oedema (vasogenic, cytotoxic and interstitial types)
▶ Focal brain swelling may be due to inflammatory, traumatic, vascular or neoplastic lesions, and is often accompanied by vasogenic oedema in the adjacent tissue
▶ Result in intracranial shift and herniation (supracallosal, tentorial or tonsillar types) once a critical stage of mass expansion is reached
▶ Produce characteristic clinical signs and symptoms relating to raised intracranial pressure and intracranial shift or herniation

Intracranial space-occupying lesions may result from a variety of causes, but all share one common feature: an expansion in volume of the intracranial contents. Such brain swelling may be either diffuse or focal.

Diffuse brain swelling

Diffuse brain swelling denotes a generalised increase in the volume of the brain which results from either vasodilatation or oedema.

Vasodilatation
Vasodilatation in the brain occurs following changes in the calibre of intracerebral vessels, which cause an increase in cerebral blood volume resulting in brain swelling. This occurs particularly in response to hypercapnia and hypoxia, but may also result from failure of the normal vasomotor control mechanisms, for example in severe head injuries.

Oedema
Oedema in the brain is defined as an abnormal accumulation of fluid in the cerebral parenchyma which produces an increase in cerebral volume. Cerebral oedema can be classified into three main types:

- *vasogenic*: due to increased cerebral vascular permeability
- *cytotoxic*: due to cellular injury to neurones and glia
- *interstitial*: due to damage to the ventricular lining.

In many instances, cerebral oedema occurs due to a combination of mechanisms; for example, both vasogenic and cytotoxic mechanisms are involved in ischaemia. Cerebral oedema frequently accompanies focal lesions in the brain, thereby exaggerating the mass effect.

Focal brain swelling

Focal lesions of many types can produce an increase in cerebral volume, for example cerebral abscesses, intracranial haematomas and intrinsic neoplasms. Many extrinsic intracranial lesions, for example subdural haematomas and meningiomas, exert a mass effect within the cranial cavity and so act as space-occupying lesions.

Consequences of intracranial space-occupying lesions

The consequences of intracranial space-occupying lesions may be:

- raised intracranial pressure
- intracranial shift and herniation
- epilepsy
- hydrocephalus
- systemic effects.

Raised intracranial pressure

Raised intracranial pressure is an invariable consequence of enlarging intracranial lesions, since there is very little space within the rigid cranium to accommodate an expanding mass. Initially, however, there is a phase of spatial compensation, made possible in three ways:

- reduction in the CSF space within and around the brain
- pressure atrophy of the brain, which occurs most commonly with slow-growing extrinsic lesions, e.g. meningiomas
- reduction in blood volume, e.g. within the intracranial venous sinuses.

Once this phase is passed, there is a critical period in which a further increase in the volume of the intracranial contents will cause an abrupt increase in intracranial pressure. The characteristic clinical signs and symptoms of raised intracranial pressure and their likely causes are:

- papilloedema: due to accumulation of axoplasm in optic papilla when axonal flow is impeded
- nausea and vomiting: due to pressure on vomiting centres in the pons and medulla
- headache: due to compression and distortion of pain and stretch receptors around intracranial blood vessels and within the dura mater
- impairment of consciousness, ranging from drowsiness to deep coma, related to the level of increased intracranial pressure.

Intracranial shift and herniation

Intracranial shift and herniation are the most important consequences of raised intracranial pressure due to space-occupying lesions. They usually occur following a critical increase in intracranial pressure, which may inadvertently be precipitated by withdrawing CSF at lumbar puncture. Lumbar puncture is therefore contraindicated in any patient with raised intracranial pressure and a suspected intracranial space-occupying lesion to avoid the risk of precipitating a potentially fatal brainstem herniation.

Lateral shift of the midline structures is a common early complication of intracranial space-occupying lesions. However, patients with acute lateral displacement of the brain due to a hemispheric mass show a depressed level of consciousness even in the absence of an intracranial herniation. The clinical features are summarised in Table 26.1.

Herniations occur at several characteristic sites within the cranial cavity, depending on the site of the space-occupying lesion (Fig. 26.3). Transtentorial herniation is frequently fatal because of secondary haemorrhage into the brainstem (Fig. 26.4). This is a common mode of death in patients with large intrinsic neoplasms or intracranial haemorrhage.

Epilepsy

Seizures (fits) may be focal or generalised, and are particularly common in patients with cerebral abscesses and neoplasms. Focal sensory or motor

Table 26.1 Clinical consequences of intracranial herniation

Site of herniation	Effect	Clinical consequence
Transtentorial	Posterior cerebral artery compression	Cortical blindness
	Ipsilateral 3rd nerve compression	Ipsilateral fixed dilated pupil
	Ipsilateral cerebral peduncle compression	Ipsilateral upper motor neurone signs
	Ipsilateral 6th cranial nerve compression	Horizontal diplopia Convergent squint
	Brainstem compression and haemorrhage	Decerebrate posture Cardiorespiratory failure Death
Foramen magnum	Brainstem compression and haemorrhage	Decerebrate posture Cardiorespiratory failure Death
	Acute obstruction of CSF pathway	Decerebrate posture Cardiorespiratory failure Death

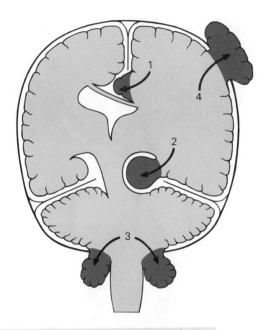

Fig. 26.3 Sites of intracranial herniation

Space-occupying lesions in the cerebral hemispheres may cause herniation of the cingulate gyrus under the falx cerebri (**1**) or of the hippocampal uncus and parahippocampal gyrus over the tentorium cerebelli (**2**). Cerebellar tonsillar herniation through the foramen magnum (**3**) can occur with lesions in the cerebrum or cerebellum. A swollen brain will herniate through any defect in the dura and skull (**4**).

seizures in adults are a common presenting feature of both primary and secondary CNS tumours.

Hydrocephalus

Hydrocephalus is a particularly common complication of space-occupying lesions in the posterior fossa which compress and distort the cerebral aqueduct and fourth ventricle.

Systemic effects

The systemic effects of raised intracranial pressure are of major clinical importance, since they may result in a life-threatening deterioration in an already ill patient. These are thought to result from autonomic imbalance and overactivity as a result of hypothalamic compression and include:

- hypertension and bradycardia
- pulmonary oedema
- gastrointestinal and urinary tract ulceration and haemorrhage
- acute pancreatitis.

CNS TRAUMA

> ▶ Classified as missile or non-missile injury: the latter is commoner
> ▶ CNS damage in non-missile injuries may occur as primary damage (immediate) or secondary damage (after the injury)
> ▶ Primary damage includes focal lesions (contusions and lacerations) and diffuse axonal injury
> ▶ Secondary damage includes intracranial haematomas, oedema, intracranial herniation, infarction and infection
> ▶ Important complications include epilepsy, persistent vegetative state and post-traumatic dementia

In the United Kingdom, 200–300 per 100 000 population present to hospital each year with head injuries, most of which are due to road traffic accidents and falls. Head injuries can be classified according to their aetiology: missile and non-missile (blunt) injuries. The latter are more common.

Missile injury to the brain

Missile injuries to the brain are typically caused by bullets or other small objects propelled through the air. Three main types of injury are recognised:

- *depressed injuries*, in which the missile causes a depressed skull fracture with contusions, but does not enter the brain
- *penetrating injuries*, which occur when the missile enters the cranial cavity but does not exit. Focal damage is common, and may be accompanied by infection
- *perforating injuries*, which are caused when a missile enters and exits from the cranial cavity, usually leaving a large exit wound. Brain damage around the missile tract is severe, with extensive haemorrhage. The risk of infection and epilepsy in survivors is high.

Non-missile injury to the brain

Non-missile injuries to the brain range from relatively minor injuries with spontaneous improvement (as in concussion injuries), to severe injuries which are rapidly fatal. These injuries occur most commonly in road traffic accidents (55%) and falls (35%), when rotational forces acting on the brain may be accompanied by impact-related forces. The latter often result in a skull fracture, but it is important to note that around 20% of fatal head injuries occur without a fracture. The types of brain damage occurring in

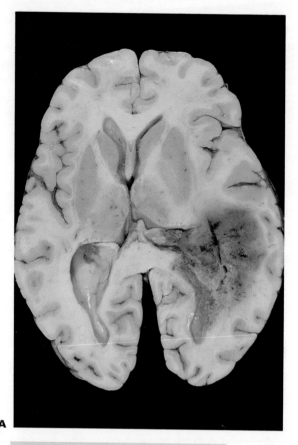

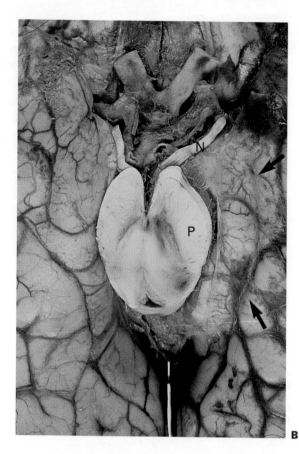

Fig. 26.4 Herniation effects in the brain

A. A large haemorrhagic neoplasm (glioblastoma) is present in the right cerebral hemisphere, causing shift of the midline structures to the left and compression of the right lateral ventricle. **B.** Transtentorial herniation at the base of the brain. A prominent groove surrounds the displaced parahippocampal gyrus (arrow). The adjacent 3rd nerve (N) is compressed and distorted and the ipsilateral cerebral peduncle (P) is distorted with small areas of haemorrhage.

non-missile injuries may be classified as either primary or secondary.

Primary brain damage

Primary brain damage occurs at the time of injury. There are two main forms: focal damage and diffuse axonal injury.

Focal damage

The commonest type of focal damage is contusions. These often occur at the site of impact, particularly if a skull fracture is present. Contusions are commonly asymmetrical and may be more severe on the side opposite the impact—the *'contrecoup' lesions* (Fig. 26.5). Movement of the brain within the skull brings these areas into contact with adjacent bone,

resulting in local injury. Large contusions may be associated with an intracerebral haemorrhage, or accompanied by cortical lacerations. Healed contusions are represented by wedge-shaped areas of gliosis and cortical rarefaction which are yellow–brown due to the presence of haemosiderin.

Other forms of focal damage, e.g. tears of cranial nerves, pituitary stalk or brainstem, occur less frequently.

Diffuse axonal injury

This type of damage occurs as a result of shearing and tensile strains on neuronal processes produced by rotational movements of the brain within the skull. It often occurs in the absence of a skull fracture and cerebral contusions. Two main components exist:

These complications often dominate the clinical picture, and are responsible for death in many cases:

- *Intracranial haemorrhage.* The mechanisms and clinical manifestations of traumatic intracranial haemorrhage are summarised in Table 26.2.
- *Traumatic damage to extracerebral arteries.* Although uncommon, this is of clinical importance since some cases can be treated surgically. The injuries encountered most frequently are dissection of the internal carotid artery and rupture of the vertebral artery.
- *Intracranial herniation.* The mechanisms and consequences of intracranial herniations are described above.
- *Hypoxic brain damage.* Hypoxic brain damage with cerebral infarction can often be related to a clinical episode of hypotension, for example cardiac arrest. Hypoxic damage may also occur as a consequence of raised intracranial pressure, fat emboli, traumatic damage to the main neck vessels or respiratory obstruction.
- *Meningitis.* This is well-recognised complication of head injury, particularly in patients with an open skull fracture.

Outcome of non-missile head injury

Most patients with minor head injuries make a satisfactory recovery. However, only 20% of survivors of severe head injuries make a good recovery, while 10% remain severely disabled. Important causes of persisting debility are:

- *post-traumatic epilepsy*, which is the commonest delayed complication of non-missile head injury
- *persistent vegetative state*, in which patients remain severely neurologically impaired; this occurs most often in patients with diffuse axonal damage and hypoxic brain damage
- *post-traumatic dementia*, due to neuronal loss and axonal damage following non-missile head injury.

Spinal cord injuries

Spinal cord injuries account for the majority of hospital admissions for paraplegia and tetraplegia. Over 80% occur as a result of road traffic accidents; most of the patients are males under 40 years of age. Two main groups of injury are recognised clinically: open injuries and closed injuries.

Open injuries

Open injuries cause direct trauma to the spinal cord

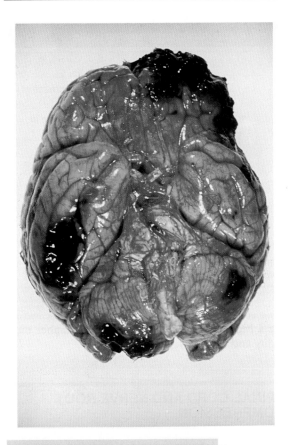

Fig. 26.5   Head injury: contusions and haematomas

A severe blow to the frontal bone has resulted in contusions and haematomas in the frontal lobes. 'Contrecoup' contusions are present in the parietal lobes, and in the cerebellum.

- *small haemorrhagic lesions* in the corpus callosum and dorsolateral quadrant of the brainstem; these heal by reactive gliosis (p. 833) and are represented by gliotic scars.
- *diffuse damage to axons*, which can only be detected microscopically in the form of axonal retraction balls; in long-term survivors, damaged axons undergo anterograde degeneration (p. 833), resulting in a loss of fibres in the white matter.

Modern neuropathological techniques reveal that diffuse axonal injury occurs in almost all fatal head injuries and may occur to a lesser degree in milder injuries (e.g. concussion).

Secondary brain damage

Secondary brain damage occurs as a result of complications developing after the moment of injury.

Table 26.2   Mechanisms and clinical manifestations of traumatic intracranial haemorrhage

Site	Mechanism	Clinical manifestations
Extradural space	Arterial rupture, e.g. middle meningeal artery	Lucid interval followed by a rapid increase in intracranial pressure
Subdural space	Rupture of venous sinuses or small bridging veins	Acute presentation with a rapid increase in intracranial pressure Chronic presentation with personality change, memory loss and confusion, particularly in the elderly
Subarachnoid space	Arterial rupture	Meningeal irritation with a rapid increase in intracranial pressure
Cerebral hemisphere	Cortical contusions	No special features
	Rupture of small intrinsic vessels with intracerebral haematoma	Increased intracranial pressure with focal deficits; usually fatal
	'Burst lobe' with intracerebral haematoma, contusions and subdural haematoma	Profound coma, usually rapidly fatal

and nerve roots. Perforating injuries can cause extensive disruption and haemorrhage, but penetrating injuries may result in incomplete cord transection which can be manifested clinically as the Brown-Séquard syndrome.

Closed injuries

Closed injuries account for most spinal injuries and are usually associated with a fracture/dislocation of the spinal column which is usually demonstrable radiologically. Damage to the cord depends on the extent of the bony injuries and can be considered in two main stages:

- primary damage: contusions, nerve fibre transection, haemorrhagic necrosis
- secondary damage: extradural haematoma, infarction, infection, oedema.

Complications and outcome

Late effects of cord damage include:

- ascending and descending anterograde degeneration of damaged nerve fibres
- post-traumatic syringomyelia
- systemic effects of paraplegia: urinary tract and chest infections, pressure sores and muscle wasting.

Outcome of cord injuries depends mainly on the site and severity of the cord damage. Patients with incomplete lesions in the cauda equina have an almost normal life expectancy, while patients surviv-

ing a high cervical lesion have a much higher morbidity and mortality.

SPINAL CORD AND NERVE ROOT COMPRESSION

The principal causes of spinal cord and nerve root compression are:

- intervertebral disc prolapse
- neoplasm (e.g. metastatic carcinoma, myeloma, schwannoma)
- skeletal disorder (e.g. spondylosis, rheumatoid arthritis, Paget's disease)
- infection (e.g. tuberculosis, abscess)
- vascular disease (e.g. arteriovenous malformation, haemorrhage)
- trauma.

The commonest causes of subacute or chronic nerve root and cord compression are intervertebral disc prolapse and spondylosis.

Intervertebral disc prolapse

Intervertebral disc prolapse (Ch. 25) occurs in two main ways:

- In young adults, disc rupture following strenuous exercise or sudden exertion is the main cause of disc herniation.
- In the middle-aged or elderly, disc herniation following minimal stress is due to degenerative disc

disease, usually accompanied by spondylosis (see below).

In both instances, a tear in the annulus fibrosus allows the soft nucleus pulposus to herniate posteriorly. This usually takes place in a lateral direction, causing nerve root compression. Central herniation is less common, but can cause direct cord damage and may also compress the anterior spinal artery, resulting in infarction. Disc prolapse occurs most commonly at the C5/C6 and L5/S1 levels; nerve root compression in the latter results in sciatica.

Spondylosis

Spondylosis due to osteoarthritis (Ch. 25) of the vertebral column occurs commonly with age. It affects around 70% of adults over 40 years of age, and is usually accompanied by degenerative disc disease. It is characterised by bony outgrowths, known as osteophytes, on the upper and lower margins of the vertebral bodies. These may encroach upon the spinal canal or intervertebral foramina to produce nerve root pain which is exacerbated by movement.

HYDROCEPHALUS

> ▶ A group of disorders resulting in excess CSF in the intracranial cavity
> ▶ Two main groups: primary hydrocephalus, usually accompanied by increased intracranial pressure; and secondary hydrocephalus, compensatory to loss of cerebral tissue
> ▶ Primary hydrocephalus usually due to obstruction of the CSF pathway; divided into communicating and non-communicating types
> ▶ Produces irreversible brain damage unless the raised intracranial pressure is relieved by surgical drainage

The cerebrospinal fluid (CSF) is secreted by the choroid plexus epithelium in an active process which carefully regulates its biochemical composition. In adults, the total volume of CSF is around 140 ml; this volume is renewed several times daily (Fig. 26.6).

CSF resorption occurs primarily at the arachnoid villi. Hydrocephalus is the term used to describe any condition in which an excess quantity of CSF is present in the cranial cavity. These conditions can be considered in two main groups:

- primary hydrocephalus
- secondary or compensatory hydrocephalus.

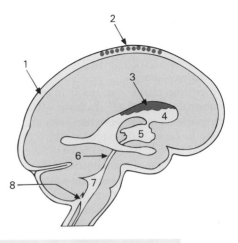

Fig. 26.6   Sites of obstruction in the cerebrospinal fluid (CSF) pathway

The circulation and absorption of CSF in the subarachnoid space (1) and arachnoid granulations (2) is readily impaired by inflammatory exudate and organising haemorrhage. CSF production in the choroid plexus (3) and flow through the lateral ventricles (4) and third ventricle (5) may be obstructed by intracranial or intraventricular neoplasms. The relatively narrow spaces of the cerebral aqueduct (6), and the fourth ventricle (7) and its exit foramina (8) are commonly obstructed by neoplasms, haemorrhage or inflammatory exudate.

Primary hydrocephalus

Primary hydrocephalus includes any disorder in which the accumulation of CSF is usually accompanied by an increase in intracranial pressure. It can be due to:

- obstruction to CSF flow (non-communicating hydrocephalus)
- impaired CSF absorption at the arachnoid villi (rare)
- excess CSF production by choroid plexus neoplasms (very rare).

Obstructive hydrocephalus

Obstructive hydrocephalus is by far the commonest form; it may be either congenital or acquired.

Congenital hydrocephalus
Congenital hydrocephalus occurs in around 1 per 1000 births and occasionally may be so marked as to considerably enlarge the fetal head and interfere with labour. The more severe forms may be diagnosed antenatally by ultrasound. Congenital malformations, for example *Arnold–Chiari malformation* (p. 859), are the principal causes of congenital hydrocephalus. A few cases in males are due to an X-linked disorder

which results in *aqueduct stenosis*. Aqueduct stenosis is more commonly due to acquired disorders, for example viral infections, which affect both sexes.

Acquired hydrocephalus
Acquired hydrocephalus can result from any lesion which obstructs the CSF pathway (Fig. 26.6). Expanding lesions in the posterior fossa are particularly prone to cause hydrocephalus, since the fourth ventricle and aqueduct are easily obstructed. Some lesions may cause intermittent obstruction, particularly colloid cysts of the third ventricle which may block the foramen of Monro. Obstructive hydrocephalus commonly results from the organisation of blood clot or inflammatory exudate in the CSF pathway following an episode of haemorrhage or meningitis. *Intermittent pressure hydrocephalus* is thought to result from defective CSF absorption at the arachnoid villi.

Secondary hydrocephalus

In secondary or compensatory hydrocephalus the increase in CSF volume occurs following a loss of brain tissue, for example cerebral infarction or atrophy, so that overall there is no increase in either intracranial volume or intracranial pressure (Fig. 26.22, p. 864).

Complications and treatment

The complications of hydrocephalus can be averted or relieved by the insertion of a ventricular shunt with a one-way valve system to drain CSF into the peritoneum. Untreated patients may suffer irreversible brain damage (Fig. 26.7). Ventricular

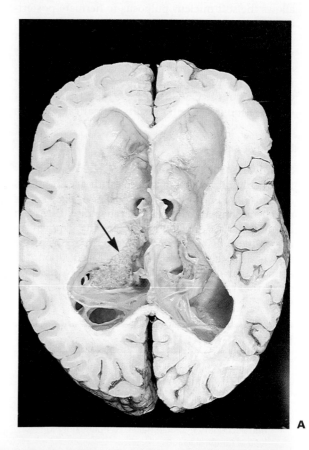

A

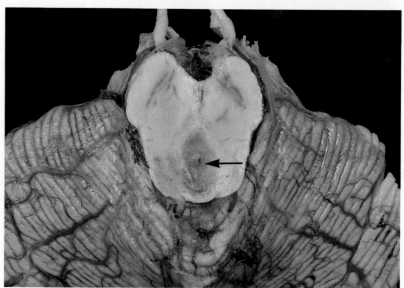

B

Fig. 26.7 Longstanding hydrocephalus

A. The lateral ventricles are very dilated and contain a prominent choroid plexus (arrow). The overlying white and grey matter are atrophic. Fibrous adhesions are present in the ventricles posteriorly, suggestive of previous infection. **B.** In the same case, the cerebral aqueduct in the midbrain is completely obliterated by glial tissue as a consequence of a previous viral infection (arrow). This has resulted in obstructive hydrocephalus.

shunts often need to be replaced in growing children and are prone to become infected with low-virulence bacteria, for example *Staphylococcus epidermidis*. Infection may result in shunt blockage and exacerbation of symptoms attributable to raised intracranial pressure.

SYRINGOMYELIA

Syringomyelia is an uncommon condition in which a cavity (syrinx) develops within the spinal cord, sometimes extending up into the brainstem (syringobulbia). The cavity is usually situated in the central region of the cord, posterior to the central canal. Syringomyelia occurs most frequently in the cervical region of the cord, and usually extends for several centimetres in a vertical direction. However, extensive cavities involving almost the entire length of the cord have been described. Modern radiological techniques are of great value in delineating the extent of the lesion (Fig. 26.20, p. 860).

Syringomyelia can arise in a variety of conditions which may be considered as follows:

- *maldevelopment of the cord*, with failure of fusion of the ventral and dorsal segments
- *disorders of CSF flow*, where CSF is propelled down the central canal; this mechanism is thought to operate in association with developmental abnormalities of the craniocervical junction, particularly the Arnold–Chiari malformation
- *tissue destruction* following a spinal cord injury, or as a consequence of an intrinsic neoplasm.

The cavities within the spinal cord in syringomyelia are lined by reactive astrocytes and their fibrillary processes. The CSF composition in syringomyelia is normal.

The clinical manifestations of syringomyelia are:

- muscle weakness and atrophy in upper limbs due to compression of anterior horn cells
- dissociated anaesthesia (loss of pain and temperature sensation) due to damage to nerve fibres crossing the cord in the lateral spinothalamic tracts.

These manifestations usually occur in adult life. Surgery can sometimes arrest or alleviate symptoms by decompression or draining the fluid in the cystic cavity.

CEREBROVASCULAR DISEASE

> - Third commonest cause of death in the United Kingdom and a major cause of morbidity in the elderly
> - CNS damage occurs in cerebrovascular disease as a result of hypoxia
> - Neurones are the cells most vulnerable to hypoxia; they become irreversibly damaged after 5–7 minutes
> - Important risk factors are atheroma, heart disease, hypertension and diabetes mellitus
> - Often presents clinically as a stroke or transient ischaemic attack
> - Most strokes (85%) are due to cerebral infarction; the remainder are due to intracerebral and subarachnoid haemorrhages

Cerebrovascular disease is the third commonest cause of death in the United Kingdom, after heart disease and cancer, and is a major cause of morbidity, particularly in the middle-aged and elderly. The ultimate effect of cerebrovascular disease is to reduce the supply of oxygen to the CNS, resulting in hypoxic damage to cells.

Hypoxic damage to the CNS

Hypoxic damage to the CNS occurs when the blood supply to the brain is reduced (oligaemia) or absent (ischaemia). It may also occur:

- when the blood supply is normal but oxygen is carried at a reduced tension (hypoxia)
- in anoxia
- in rare circumstances when cellular respiratory enzyme function is impaired, such as in cyanide poisoning.

The cells most vulnerable to hypoxia are the neurones, which depend almost exclusively on the oxidative metabolism of glucose for energy. Experimental evidence suggests that the early stage of hypoxic neuronal damage (microvacuolation) is reversible; in the final stages, however, the damaged neurones shrink and exhibit nuclear pyknosis and karyorrhexis.

The neurones most vulnerable to hypoxia are those in the 3rd, 5th and 6th layers of the cortex, in the CA1 sector of the hippocampus and in the Purkinje cells in the cerebellum. This pattern of selective vulnerability does not hold true at all ages; in infants, certain brainstem nuclei are also vulnerable. The basis of this selective vulnerability is unknown, but it may relate to differences in neuronal metabolism at these sites. Ischaemic neuronal death is characterised by activation of glutamate receptors, causing uncontrolled entry of calcium into the cell. This may be abolished or reduced in some cases by drugs which block glutamate receptors.

Complete cessation of the circulation, such as may occur following myocardial infarction, results in generalised cerebral ischaemia with focal accentuation of neuronal damage in the vulnerable zones. In less severe cases, a critical reduction of cerebral blood flow may result in boundary zone infarcts, which occur in zones between territories supplied by each of the main cerebral arteries.

Stroke

The term stroke denotes a sudden event in which a disturbance of CNS function occurs due to vascular disease. The annual incidence of stroke is 2 per 1000 of the general population in the United Kingdom, but is much commoner in the elderly. These events can be classified clinically into *completed strokes, evolving strokes,* or a *transient ischaemic attack* in which the CNS disturbance lasts for less than 24 hours. Transient ischaemic attack is a major risk factor for cerebral infarction; most attacks are due to circulatory changes in the CNS occurring as the result of disease in the heart or extracranial arteries.

The clinical features of stroke depend on the localisation and nature of the lesion (Table 26.3). Recurrent or multiple strokes often occur in patients with certain risk factors, particularly heart disease, hypertension and diabetes mellitus.

Cerebral infarction

The site and size of a cerebral infarct depend on the site and nature of the vascular lesion. Most infarcts occur within the cerebral hemispheres in the internal carotid territory, particularly in the distribution of the middle cerebral artery. Infarction of the corticospinal pathway in the region of the internal capsule is a common event, resulting in contralateral hemiparesis. Although many infarcts produce clinical symptoms, small infarcts may not result in any apparent neurological disturbance. These microinfarcts are often found in apparently normal elderly individuals, but are also numerous in the brains of hypertensive patients. Multiple infarcts involving the cerebral cortex may result in dementia (p. 863).

Pathogenesis
The following mechanisms may be responsible for cerebral infarction:

- *critical reduction of cerebral blood flow*, e.g. following cardiac arrest
- *critical reduction in arterial oxygenation*, e.g. in anoxia or profound hypoxia following respiratory arrest
- *arterial thrombosis* occurring as a complication of atheroma in the intracranial arterial tree or extracranial vessels supplying the CNS
- *embolic arterial occlusion* occurring as a complication of atheroma in the extracranial arterial supply (particularly around the carotid artery bifurcation) or mural thrombus in the heart following myocardial infarction. Fat and air emboli may also result in cerebral infarction following major trauma

Table 26.3 Comparison of the major causes of stroke					
Cause	No. of strokes (%)	Clinical presentation	30-day mortality (%)	Pathogenesis	Predisposing factors
Cerebral infarction	85	Slowly evolving signs and symptoms	15–45	Cerebral hypoperfusion Embolism Thrombosis	Heart disease (e.g. infective endocarditis, endocardial thrombus) Hypertension Atheroma Diabetes mellitus
Subarachnoid haemorrhage	5	Sudden headache with meningism	45	Rupture of saccular aneurysm	Hypertension Polycystic renal disease Coarctation of the aorta
Intracerebral haemorrhage	10	Sudden onset of stroke with raised intracranial pressure	80	Rupture of micro-aneurysm or arteriole	Hypertension Vascular malformation

- *head injury* may result in cerebral hypoxia, vascular occlusion or rupture, all of which may result in cerebral infarction
- *subarachnoid haemorrhage* following rupture of a saccular aneurysm may be accompanied by vascular spasm resulting in cerebral infarction
- *generalised arterial disease*, e.g. vasculitis, may affect both intra- and extracranial vessels and result in cerebral infarction
- *intraventricular haemorrhage in neonates* is often accompanied by infarction in the adjacent white matter (periventricular leukomalacia)
- *venous thrombosis* as a complication of local sepsis or drugs, e.g. oral contraceptives.

Pathological features

At a very early stage after cerebral infarction, no naked-eye abnormalities are apparent. However, 24 hours after infarction the affected tissue becomes softened and swollen, with a loss of definition between grey and white matter. There may be considerable oedema around the infarct, resulting in a local mass effect. Within four days, the infarcted tissue undergoes colliquative necrosis. Histology shows infiltration by macrophages which are filled with the lipid products of myelin breakdown. Reactive astrocytes and proliferating capillaries are often present at the edge of the infarct. Eventually, all the dead tissue is phagocytosed to leave a fluid-filled cystic cavity with a gliotic wall (Fig. 26.8). Some infarcts are haemorrhagic, possibly due to reflow of blood through anastomotic channels. Anterograde degen-eration of nerve fibres occurs distal to the site of infarction, for example in the ipsilateral cerebral peduncle in infarcts involving the internal capsule.

Venous infarction

Venous infarction is a consequence of venous thrombosis in the cranial cavity. This can occur at localised sites, most commonly in the lateral and sagittal sinuses, or as part of a generalised cortical venous thrombosis. Venous thrombosis results in a haemorrhagic infarction of the cerebral cortex and subcortical white matter. It usually occurs secondary to other disease processes, for example local sepsis, dehydration or drugs (e.g. oral contraceptives). Extensive infarcts are usually fatal.

Intracranial haemorrhage

Subarachnoid and intracerebral haemorrhage together account for around 15% of strokes. Extradural and subdural haemorrhages usually occur following trauma and are considered in Table 26.2 on page 838.

Subarachnoid haemorrhage

Subarachnoid haemorrhage usually occurs following rupture of a saccular 'berry' aneurysm on the circle of Willis. Other causes are uncommon, but include trauma, hypertensive haemorrhage, vasculitis, tumours and disorders of haemostasis.

Saccular aneurysms. Saccular aneurysms occur in 1–2% of the general population, but are commoner

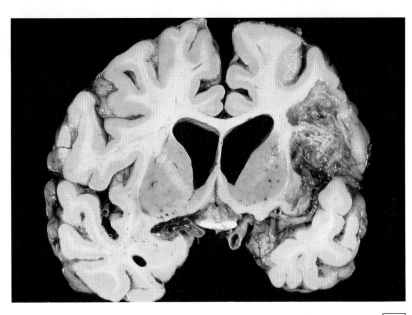

Fig. 26.8 Cerebral infarct: cystic change

In this old infarct in the territory of the right middle cerebral artery, the necrotic tissue has been phagocytosed to leave a cystic cavity lined by glial tissue.

in the elderly. Most cases of ruptured saccular aneurysms occur between 40 and 60 years of age; males in this age group are affected twice as often as females. Several predisposing factors for saccular aneurysms have been identified.

The role of hypertension in the pathogenesis of these lesions is uncertain, but it does appear that hypertensive patients are more likely to have multiple aneurysms than are normotensive patients. Local vascular abnormalities, such as atheroma, are important in the pathogenesis of saccular aneurysms by altering haemodynamics in affected vessels.

Saccular aneurysms are usually sited at proximal branching points on the anterior portion of the circle of Willis, particularly on the internal carotid, anterior communicating, and middle cerebral arteries. Most are less than 10 mm in diameter, but some may be partly filled by thrombus which can obscure their true size on radiological studies (Fig. 26.9). Their pathogenesis is thought to relate to congenital defects in the smooth muscle of the tunica media at the site of an arterial bifurcation, where local haemodynamic factors act to produce a slowly enlarging aneurysm.

Clinicopathological features and prognosis. Subarachnoid haemorrhage often presents with the characteristic clinical history of sudden onset of severe

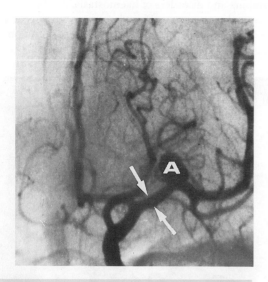

Fig. 26.9 Saccular aneurysm: demonstration in vivo

A saccular aneurysm (A) arises from the main trunk of the left middle cerebral artery (arrows). (Left internal carotid angiogram antero-posterior subtraction film: courtesy of Dr M Nelson, Leeds)

headache. Blood accumulates in the basal cisterns and around the brainstem following rupture of a saccular aneurysm. Subarachnoid haemorrhage may be instantly fatal in as many as 15% of cases, with some patients dying later due to rebleed at the site of rupture, or arterial spasm (see below). One-third of survivors are permanently disabled as a consequence of hypoxic brain damage following haemorrhage.

Arterial spasm in the distal cerebral vasculature following rupture causes cerebral ischaemia and infarction, which is often accompanied by brain swelling due to oedema.

Hydrocephalus can occur acutely following rupture as blood accumulates in the basal cisterns, or at a later stage in survivors, where fibrous obliteration of the subarachnoid space or arachnoid granulations may occur.

Intracerebral haemorrhage

The commonest cause of intracerebral haemorrhage is hypertensive vascular disease, in which haemorrhages occur most frequently in the basal ganglia (80% of cases), the brainstem, cerebellum and cerebral cortex. Most intracerebral haemorrhages occur in hypertensive adults over 50 years of age. The haematoma acts as a space-occupying lesion, causing a rapid increase in intracranial pressure and intracranial herniation (Fig. 26.10). In survivors, resorption of the haematoma eventually occurs, and a fluid-filled cyst with a gliotic wall is formed. The mortality from spontaneous intracerebral haemorrhage is greater than 80%, and many survivors suffer severe neurological deficit.

The pathogenesis of spontaneous intracerebral haemorrhage is not fully understood. For many years, it was thought that most intracerebral haemorrhages in hypertensive patients occurred following rupture of micro-aneurysms on small arterioles, particularly on the lenticulostriate branch of the middle cerebral artery. Recent studies, however, have found that in some cases of intracerebral haemorrhage in hypertensive patients, the site of vascular rupture is at, or close to, a bifurcation on a larger arteriole. These vessels often show replacement of smooth muscle by fibrous tissue at the site of bifurcation, which in hypertensive patients may predispose to rupture.

Systemic hypertension and the CNS

As well as being a major risk factor for stroke, systemic hypertension causes many other changes in the CNS which result in neurological dysfunction:

* alteration in autoregulation of cerebral blood flow

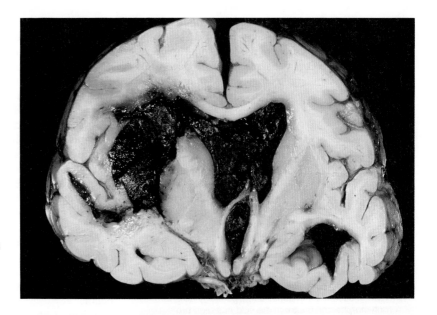

Fig. 26.10 Complications of intracerebral haemorrhage

An intracranial haemorrhage originating in the internal capsule on the left has ruptured into the ventricular system which is filled with blood. The mass effect of the haematoma has resulted in a shift of adjacent structures to the opposite site.

(e.g. a sudden drop in systemic blood pressure to normal levels may result in hypoperfusion)

- encephalopathy due to blood–brain barrier disruption and fibrinoid vascular necrosis
- vascular changes, especially atheroma
- aneurysms, including atheromatous aneurysms of the basilar artery, multiple saccular aneurysms on the circle of Willis, and micro-aneurysms on small arterioles in the basal ganglia
- dementia due to multiple infarcts in cerebral grey and white matter.

Spinal cord infarction

Spinal cord infarction is most often due to spinal cord trauma or compression, but may also result from ischaemia following myocardial infarction or aortic dissection. In such cases, the infarct occurs in the mid-thoracic region of the cord, in the distribution of the anterior spinal artery where the arterial blood supply is relatively poor. These infarcts result in paraplegia with a dissociated sensory loss, since the posterior columns are spared. Infarcts in the territory of the posterior spinal artery are very rare.

Intracranial haemorrhage in neonates

Intracranial haemorrhage in neonates has a markedly different pathology from intracranial haemorrhage in adults (Table 26.4). Haemorrhage from the subependymal germinal matrix is particularly important, and is the major cause of death in premature neonates.

Table 26.4 Intracranial haemorrhage in neonates

Site	Pathogenesis	Complication
Falx cerebri	Rupture of veins (birth trauma)	Acute subdural haematoma
Tentorium cerebelli		Cystic hygroma
Subdural space		
Subarachnoid space	Capillary or arterial rupture	Hydrocephalus
Subependymal germinal matrix	Prematurity, hypoxia (hyaline membrane disease)	Intraventricular haemorrhage
	Venous congestion	Venous infarction in white matter (periventricular leukomalacia)
	Arterial spasm	Hydrocephalus

Cerebrovascular malformations

Three main types of vascular malformation occur in the CNS:

- arteriovenous malformations
- cavernous angioma
- capillary telangiectasis.

Arteriovenous malformations are clinically the most important; these usually consist of an irregular plexus of dilated thick-walled vessels in the superficial grey matter of the cerebral hemispheres or spinal cord. Cerebral lesions may be associated with epilepsy, or may rupture to result in a subarachnoid or intracerebral haemorrhage. Cavernous angioma and capillary telangiectasis may also be associated with epilepsy, but are often clinically unapparent.

CNS INFECTIONS

Bacterial infections

> ▶ Follow direct spread of infection from the skull, or haematogenous spread
> ▶ Leptomeningitis is the commonest form of bacterial infection in the CNS; it occurs most frequently in children and the elderly
> ▶ CSF in bacterial meningitis contains many neutrophil polymorphs and bacteria; the fluid has high protein and low glucose concentrations
> ▶ Complications of bacterial meningitis include hydrocephalus, cerebral thrombophlebitis and cerebral abscess
> ▶ Cerebral abscesses are encapsulated foci of suppuration which act as space-occupying lesions
> ▶ Tuberculous infections occur as subacute meningitis or, rarely, as intracerebral tuberculomas

The CNS is normally sterile but, once bacteria gain access to it, spread of infection can occur rapidly, resulting in widespread meningitis. Bacteria gain access to the CNS by three main routes:

- *direct spread* from an adjacent focus of infection, such as the paranasal sinuses or middle ear; infections may also be established by direct spread from outside the body, for example in cases of head injury with open skull fractures
- *blood-borne spread*, which can occur as a consequence of septicaemia or as septic emboli from established infections elsewhere, for example bacterial endocarditis and bronchiectasis
- *iatrogenic infection*, following introduction of organisms into the CSF at lumbar puncture; a low-grade meningitis may occur in up to 20% of patients with a ventriculo-peritoneal shunt, usually due to *Staphylococcus epidermidis*, a skin commensal organism.

Bacterial meningitis

The clinical term 'meningitis' usually refers to inflammation in the subarachnoid space involving the arachnoid and pia mater, i.e. *leptomeningitis*.

However, inflammation of the meninges may involve predominantly the dura mater (*pachymeningitis*) under certain circumstances considered below.

Pachymeningitis
Pachymeningitis is usually a consequence of direct spread of infection from the bones of the skull following otitis media or mastoiditis, and is a well-recognised complication of skull fracture. Common bacterial pathogens include Gram-negative bacilli from the middle ear, α or β haemolytic streptococci from paranasal sinuses, or mixed organisms, often with *Staphylococcus aureus*, from skull fractures. An epidural or subdural abscess may then occur.

Epidural abscess. This is the result of suppuration between the dura mater and the skull or vertebral column. Epidural abscesses can act as space-occupying lesions, and usually require surgical drainage and antibiotic therapy before healing by fibrosis can occur.

Subdural abscess. In contrast to the above, a subdural abscess is seldom a localised lesion, since pus can readily spread in the subdural space over the cerebral hemispheres to form a subdural empyema. Involvement of subdural vessels may result in cerebral cortical thrombophlebitis and arteritis with infarction. Spontaneous resolution is rare, and surgical drainage and antibiotic therapy are usually required before healing can occur.

Leptomeningitis
Leptomeningitis is frequently a result of blood-borne spread of infection, particularly in children, but many cases arise from direct spread of infection from the skull bones. The most important organisms are:

- in neonates: *Escherichia coli*, *Streptococcus agalactiae*, *Listeria monocytogenes*, *Salmonella* spp.
- 2–5 years: *Haemophilus influenzae* type B
- 5–30 years: *Neisseria meningitidis*
- over 30 years: *Streptococcus pneumoniae* type 3.

Tuberculosis and syphilis are considered separately on pages 848–849.

Menigococcal meningitis is the commonest variety; it can occur in sporadic cases or as an epidemic outbreak in small communities. Subgroups A and C of *Neisseria meningitidis* are associated with epidemic disease, while subgroup B is usually responsible for solitary cases. The organism is spread in droplets from asymptomatic nasal carriers; the carriage rate in small communities may reach over 25%. The organism reaches the CNS by haematogenous spread, and the onset of the symptoms of meningitis may follow a short history of upper respiratory tract infection. A petechial rash may herald the onset of disseminated intravascular coagulation accompanied by adrenal haemorrhage (Waterhouse–Friderichsen syndrome) which is often fatal. Vigorous antibiotic therapy is essential: incomplete or inappropriate therapy can be fatal or may result in a chronic meningitis with marked meningeal thickening.

Diagnosis and complications of bacterial meningitis
Examination of the CSF by lumbar puncture is essential in each case; the main CSF changes in the CNS infections are listed in Table 26.5. The CSF in bacterial meningitis usually contains many organisms, although these are sometimes detected only on culture. In fatal cases, pus is present in the cerebral sulci and around the base of the brain extending down around the spinal cord (Fig. 26.11).

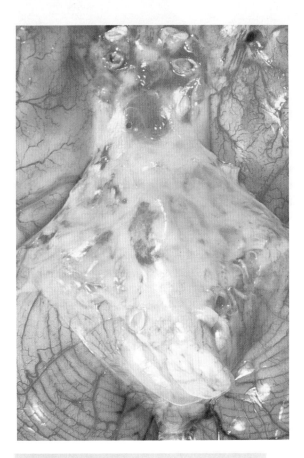

Fig. 26.11 Bacterial meningitis: basal exudate

In this example of pyogenic meningitis due to *Escherichia coli*, a dense acute inflammatory exudate is present around the brainstem, cerebellum and adjacent structures at the base of the brain. Obstruction of the fourth ventricle exit foramina resulted in acute hydrocephalus in this case.

The meningeal and superficial cortical blood vessels are congested, often with small foci of perivascular haemorrhage. The CSF is usually turbid, even in the ventricles which often show signs of acute inflammation with fibrin deposition. Common complications of bacterial meningitis are:

- cerebral infarction
- obstructive hydrocephalus
- cerebral abscess
- subdural empyema
- epilepsy.

Cerebral abscess

A cerebral abscess usually develops from an acute suppurative encephalitis following:

- *direct spread* of infection, usually Gram-negative bacilli, from the paranasal sinuses or middle ear
- *septic sinus thrombosis*, due to spread of infection from the mastoid cavities or middle ear via the sigmoid sinus
- *haematogenous spread*, for example in patients with infective endocarditis (particularly in association with congenital heart disease) or bronchiectasis. Haematogenous abscesses are most often found in the parietal lobes, but may occur in any region of the brain, and are often multiple.

Abscess formation in the brain, as in other tissues, occurs when pus formation is accompanied by local tissue destruction (Fig. 26.12). A pyogenic membrane is formed, and the abscess develops a capsule composed of granulation tissue, and reactive astrocytes and their fibrillary processes. The adjacent brain is markedly oedematous, containing a perivascular inflammatory infiltrate of lymphocytes and plasma cells. Cerebral abscesses frequently enlarge and become multiloculate.

The clinical presentation is similar to that of acute bacterial meningitis, but focal neurological signs, epilepsy and fever are common manifestations. Abscesses act as space-occupying lesions and it is important to remember that a lumbar puncture must never be performed as an initial investigation on a patient with a suspected cerebral abscess (or other space-occupying lesion) as this may precipitate a fatal intracranial herniation. Antibiotic therapy is useful in the treatment of abscesses at an early stage, but once a capsule has formed, surgical aspiration or excision is usually necessary. Complications of cerebral abscesses include:

- meningitis
- intracranial herniation

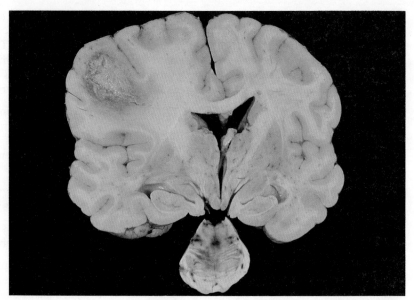

Fig. 26.12   Cerebral abscess: space-occupying lesion

A large abscess in the left parietal lobe is surrounded by oedematous white matter. This has acted as an expanding lesion and displaced the midline structures to the right. Death in this case resulted from a transtentorial brainstem herniation, with a characteristic haemorrhage in the central pons.

- focal neurological deficit
- epilepsy.

Tuberculosis

Tuberculous infection of the CNS is always secondary to infection elsewhere in the body; the lungs are the commonest site. CNS involvement takes two main forms: tuberculous meningitis and tuberculomas.

Tuberculous meningitis
Tuberculous meningitis is usually the result of haematogenous spread from a primary or secondary complex in the lungs. Rarely, it can result from direct spread of infection from a spinal vertebral body to the meninges. The resulting meningitis is characterised by a thick gelatinous exudate which is most marked around the basal cisterns and within cerebral sulci. The exudate often contains grey tubercles adjacent to

blood vessels. The findings in the CSF are listed in Table 26.5. On microscopy, the tubercles are seen to consist of granulomas with central caseation in which giant cells may be scanty or absent.

Patients usually present with signs and symptoms of a subacute meningitis, occasionally accompanied by isolated cranial nerve palsies. However, sometimes the clinical features are entirely non-specific and the diagnosis is made only following a lumbar puncture. This disorder is frequently fatal and requires intensive antituberculous chemotherapy.

Tuberculomas
Tuberculomas are uncommon in the United Kingdom, but are still encountered in patients originating from some other countries (particularly in Asia). These lesions consist of focal areas of granulomatous inflammation with caseation, and are surrounded by a dense, fibrous capsule. Tuberculomas occur most frequently in the cerebellum and present

Table 26.5 CSF parameters in health and infection				
	Cells	Protein (g/l)	Glucose (mmol/l)	Appearance
Normal	0–4 lymphocytes/mm^3	0.15–0.40	2.7–4.0	Clear and colourless
Bacterial meningitis	↑↑ polymorphs	↑	↓ or absent	Opaque and turbid
Tuberculous meningitis	↑ polymorphs initially, then lymphocytes	↑	↓ or absent	Clear or opalescent
Viral meningitis	↑ polymorphs initially, then ↑↑ lymphocytes	↑	Normal	Clear and colourless
Viral encephalitis	↑ polymorphs initially, then lymphocytes	↑	Normal	Clear and colourless

with signs and symptoms of raised intracranial pressure; features of meningitis are rarely present. As with pyogenic cerebral abscesses, surgical excision is often required.

Syphilis

Syphilis is now rare; it occurs most frequently in male homosexuals. After the initial infection, *Treponema pallidum* gains access to the CNS by haematogenous spread. CNS involvement includes:

- clinically silent *meningitis* during primary and secondary stages
- meningeal thickening in the tertiary stage, causing *cranial nerve palsies*
- *gummas*, causing cerebral or spinal compression
- *tabes dorsalis* due to degeneration of dorsal spinal columns
- *'general paralysis of the insane'* due to cerebral atrophy in chronic infections.

Viral infections

> ▶ Infections spread to the CNS by the haematogenous route or by retrograde neural transport
> ▶ Viral meningitis is a common, self-limiting illness with characteristic CSF changes
> ▶ Encephalitis is less frequent, but may result in death or severe disability
> ▶ Reactivation of a latent viral infection (e.g. herpes zoster) may damage the CNS
> ▶ CNS involvement in HIV infection is common and often accompanied by other viral, bacterial or parasitic infections
> ▶ 'Slow' virus infections are responsible for subacute spongiform encephalopathy, a rare cause of dementia
> ▶ Acute disseminated encephalomyelitis, a demyelinating disorder, may result from a virus-induced immune reaction

CNS infection by viruses can occur by the following mechanisms:

- *haematogenous spread* as part of a systemic infection with viraemia, usually causing meningitis or encephalitis
- *neural spread* along peripheral sensory nerves by retrograde axonal transport.

Certain viruses exhibit neurotropism—a tendency to spread specifically to the CNS from the initial site of infection, for example polio virus from the gut. Viruses can cause neurological dysfunction either as a result of viral multiplication within cells of the CNS, or as a result of an immunological response to a

viral infection (acute disseminated encephalomyelitis; see below). The former mechanism is much more common and is considered below under the main disease categories.

Viral meningitis

Although acute in onset, viral meningitis is usually clinically less severe than bacterial meningitis. In most instances, the viruses reach the CNS by haematogenous spread. Common organisms are:

- echovirus 7, 11, 24, 33
- coxsackie B 1–5
- coxsackie A9
- mumps virus
- other enteroviruses.

Characteristic changes are present in the CSF (Table 26.5) and serology is often used to confirm the diagnosis.

The histology of viral meningitis is poorly documented, since cases are rarely fatal. Infiltration of the leptomeninges by mononuclear cells (lymphocytes, plasma cells and macrophages) has been described, along with perivascular lymphocytic cuffing of blood vessels in the meninges and superficial cortex.

Viral encephalitis

Infection of the brain is a well-recognised complication of many common viral illnesses. Most cases are mild, self-limiting conditions but others, such as rabies and herpes simplex type I infections, result in extensive tissue destruction and are often fatal. Herpes simplex encephalitis is the commonest variety of acute viral encephalitis in the United Kingdom. Despite these differences in severity, all viral infections of the brain and spinal cord produce similar pathological changes in the CNS:

- *mononuclear cell infiltration* by lymphocytes, plasma cells and macrophages; this is often noticeable as perivascular cuffing which usually extends into the parenchyma (Fig. 26.13)
- *cell lysis* (cytolytic viral infection) and phagocytosis of cell debris by macrophages; when neurones are involved, for example as in polio virus infection, this process is known as neuronophagia
- *viral inclusions*, which can often be detected in infected neurones or glial cells; occasionally, these can be of diagnostic value, for example, 'owl-eye' inclusions in cytomegalovirus infection, or Negri bodies in rabies

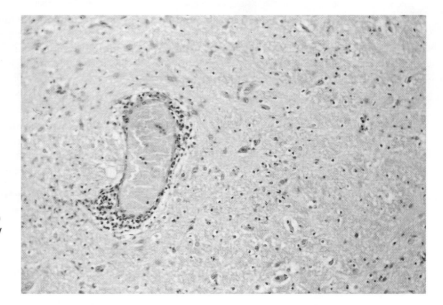

Fig. 26.13   Acute viral encephalitis due to herpes simplex virus

There is prominent lymphocytic cuffing around a blood vessel (left) with infiltration of the adjacent grey and white matter by lymphocytes and microglial cells. There is evidence of cerebral oedema with vacuolation in the perivascular tissue.

- *reactive hypertrophy* and hyperplasia of astrocytes and microglial cells, often forming cell clusters
- *oedema*, which is of vasogenic type.

Latent viral infections

Herpes zoster
Herpes zoster is an infection caused by the varicella zoster virus. It results from reactivation of latent virus within sensory ganglia in the CNS, the infection having been established following chickenpox in childhood. Reactivation usually occurs during periods of intercurrent illness or immunosuppression, particularly in the elderly. Acute inflammation of the sensory ganglion (usually a thoracic dorsal root ganglion or the trigeminal ganglion) is accompanied by pain and hyperalgesia along the nerve distribution, followed by erythema and vesicle formation.

Involvement of the ophthalmic division of the trigeminal nerve may result in blindness as a consequence of corneal ulceration and scarring.

Progressive multifocal leukoencephalopathy
Progressive multifocal leukoencephalopathy results from CNS infection by the JC papovavirus. Most cases occur in immunosuppressed patients, particularly those with Hodgkin's or non-Hodgkin's lymphomas. The virus produces a cytolytic infection of oligodendrocytes, and affected areas of the brain show multiple grey foci of demyelination in the white matter. The disease is uniformly fatal.

Antenatal viral infections

The commonest viruses to infect the CNS in utero are cytomegalovirus and rubella virus; the latter is becoming less common following the immunisation campaign in schoolgirls. Both viruses cause a necrotising encephalomyelitis resulting in developmental malformations and microcephaly, particularly when infection has occurred during the first trimester of pregnancy. Mild asymptomatic cases may occur when the organism has been acquired late in pregnancy.

Persistent viral infections

Persistent viral infections are uncommon diseases in which infection of the CNS occurs in early life, neurological disease occurring later and without an acute course.

Subacute sclerosing panencephalitis
An uncommon disease, subacute sclerosing panencephalitis usually affects children aged 7–10 years and is characterised by a progressive neurological deficit with dementia, myoclonus and focal signs leading to death. The disease is caused by the measles virus, which is usually acquired before the age of one year.

Large numbers of viral inclusion bodies are present within neurones, and high titres of measles antibody can be detected in the CSF. The pathogenesis of this prolonged disorder is not fully understood.

Progressive rubella panencephalitis

Progressive rubella panencephalitis is a very uncommon disease with clinical features similar to those of subacute sclerosing panencephalitis. It can occur as a sequel of congenital or postnatal rubella infection.

Human immunodeficiency virus (HIV) infection

The CNS is commonly involved in HIV infection both in the acquired immune deficiency syndrome (AIDS) and in pre-AIDS stages. The mechanisms by which HIV gains access to the CNS are uncertain; many research workers believe that the virus is carried across the blood–brain barrier in monocytes or macrophages (the 'Trojan horse' theory). Once in the CNS, the virus appears to reside predominantly in microglial cells and multinucleate cells of the macrophage/microglial type (Fig. 26.14). Evidence for direct infection of nerve cells and other glia is not fully established and awaits further research.

Patients with HIV infection frequently present with neurological abnormalities and at the time of death at least 80% of AIDS patients have CNS pathology resulting from:

- cerebral HIV infection (causing progressive dementia)
- multiple opportunistic infections (e.g. toxoplasma, fungi)
- other viral infections (e.g. cytomegalovirus, papovavirus)
- primary cerebral lymphoma (p. 870).

Other organisms important in infecting immunosuppressed patients are listed on page 853. Dementia may occur in the absence of overt immunodeficiency (i.e. AIDS); diagnosis can then be made by serology on the blood, examination of CSF and by viral isolation from a cerebral cortical biopsy.

'Slow' virus infections

'Slow' virus infections are responsible for the transmissible neurodegenerative disorders known as *subacute spongiform encephalopathies*. One of these disorders, kuru, was at one time restricted geographically to a small number of islands in the East Indies and appeared to result from ritual cannibalism; eating the brain of an infected individual resulted in the onset of the disease many years later. The disease is now extinct.

Creutzfeldt–Jakob disease

Creutzfeldt–Jakob disease usually presents in adult life as a rapidly progressive dementia often accompanied by pyramidal and extrapyramidal signs. It occurs as a sporadic disorder in 1 in 1 000 000 per year in the United Kingdom; familial and iatrogenic (see below) forms occur more rarely. No specific treatment is available and the disease is uniformly fatal.

In 1968, the disease was found to be transmissible to primates, and further studies have found the infectious agent to be of very small size and highly resistant to heat, ultraviolet light and most chemi-

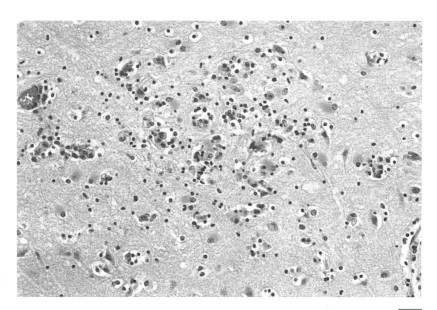

Fig. 26.14 Multinucleate giant cells in HIV encephalitis

These giant cells are derived from macrophages, contain HIV nucleic acids and express viral proteins on the cell surface.

cals. Its precise nature is as yet unknown; some investigators suggest a small encapsulated virus, others favour a 'novel proteinaceous particle' or prion. Cases of human–human transmission have been recorded, attributed to implantation of intracerebral electrodes, corneal grafts and, most recently, the administration of growth hormone extracted from human pituitary glands. These are, however, rare occurrences and the source of infection in most cases is unknown.

The brain from affected individuals often shows widespread cerebral cortical atrophy. Microscopy of the cortex shows a loss of neurones and a reactive proliferation of astrocytes. Numerous small vacuoles are present within neuronal and astrocytic processes, hence the term spongiform encephalopathy (Fig. 26.15). No inflammatory reaction occurs in this disorder.

Acute disseminated encephalomyelitis

Acute disseminated encephalomyelitis is an infrequent complication of measles, mumps and rubella infections, and may also occur following vaccination for smallpox and rabies. The onset of the disease is sudden, usually occurring 5–14 days after the initial infection or inoculation. Viruses are not detectable in the CNS, and the CSF shows minimal changes. Histologically, there is widespread perivascular lymphocytic cuffing and perivenous demyelination. This appears to be a T-cell-mediated delayed hypersensitivity response to a protein component of myelin, but the mechanism of sensitisation is unknown. The prognosis is good, with a complete recovery in 90% of cases.

Acute haemorrhagic leukoencephalitis is a related but more severe disorder which is accompanied by immune complex deposition in cerebral vessel walls and is usually rapidly fatal.

Fungal infections

Fungal infections of the nervous system are relatively uncommon; most occur as a consequence of haematogenous spread from the lungs, but direct spread of infection from the nose and paranasal sinuses also occurs. In the United Kingdom, most fungal infections of the CNS occur in immunosuppressed patients, but some organisms, for example *Cryptococcus neoformans*, are capable of producing disease in man in the absence of any predisposing illness. Cryptococcal infection usually presents as a subacute meningitis in which the inflammatory reaction is often remarkably mild. The organisms can be visualised, but serology is a more reliable method of diagnosis.

Opportunistic fungal infections with *Candida albicans* and *Aspergillus fumigatus* are usually accompanied by pulmonary infection. Both organisms may cause meningitis with haemorrhage due to vascular invasion, and characteristically produce multiple cerebral abscesses.

Mucormycosis is a rare fungal infection which particularly affects uncontrolled diabetics, producing a granulomatous mass in the paranasal sinuses which extends to involve directly the skull and

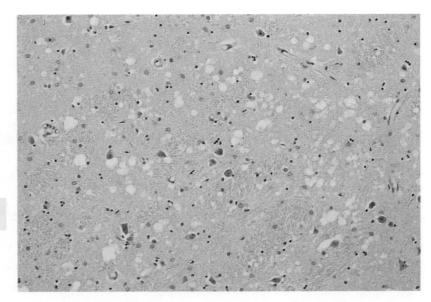

Fig. 26.15 Creutzfeldt–Jacob disease

The cerebral cortex shows a characteristic spongiform vacuolation, accompanied by neuronal loss and reactive astrocytosis.

frontal lobes. Vascular involvement is also common with this organism, resulting in cerebral infarction.

Parasitic infections

Parasitic infections of the CNS are uncommon except in countries in which human parasites are endemic. The most frequently encountered organisms are:

- *Toxoplasma gondii*, which may be congenital
- *Plasmodium falciparum*, causing one form of malaria
- *Trypanosoma rhodesiense*, causing chronic meningoencephalitis
- *Entamoeba histolytica*, causing solitary amoebic abscess
- *Taenia solium*, causing cerebral cysticercosis
- *Echinococcus granulosus*, causing solitary hydatid cyst
- *Toxocara canis*, causing eosinophilic meningitis, with granulomas around larvae.

Infections in immunosuppressed patients

CNS infections are common in immunosuppressed patients, whatever the nature of the underlying disease. The main varieties are:

- atypical mycobacteria
- cytomegalovirus
- papovaviruses
- *Candida albicans*
- *Aspergillus fumigatus*
- *Cryptococcus neoformans*
- *Toxoplasma gondii*
- *Entamoeba histolytica*.

Many of these infections prove fatal, and a diagnosis is often difficult to establish prior to death. Multiple infections are not uncommon, particularly in the acquired immune deficiency syndrome (AIDS).

DEMYELINATING CONDITIONS

> ▶ Can be due to viral, chemical or immunological mechanisms
> ▶ Axons are preserved while myelin disintegrates
> ▶ Myelin fragments are phagocytosed by macrophages and esterified into neutral lipids
> ▶ Commonest demyelinating condition is multiple sclerosis, in which the mechanism of demyelination is unknown
> ▶ Remyelination does not occur to any significant extent

In the CNS, most neuronal processes are ensheathed in myelin, which is formed from complex folds of oligodendrocyte cell membranes. CNS myelin differs slightly in structure and composition from peripheral myelin, but serves essentially the same functions:

- to protect and insulate neuronal processes
- to allow the rapid transmission of electrical impulses by saltatory conduction.

Most of the myelin in the CNS is located in the white matter, but neuronal processes in the grey matter are also surrounded by myelin.

Primary demyelination in the CNS occurs in several conditions where the myelin sheath is destroyed but the axons remain intact. Primary axonal damage results in the breakdown of myelin around damaged axons, a process referred to as *secondary demyelination*. Whenever myelin breakdown occurs, the debris is phagocytosed by macrophages. Intact myelin is rich in cholesterol and phospholipids, but following phagocytosis it is transformed into droplets of neutral lipids (mainly cholesterol esters).

Multiple sclerosis

Multiple sclerosis is the commonest demyelinating disorder affecting the CNS. It is most prevalent in populations living at latitudes remote from the equator; the prevalence is particularly high in northern Europe, but is low in the tropics (Table 26.6). Individuals who migrate from a high-prevalence to a low-prevalence area after the age of 15 remain at high risk; the disease risk is lower following migration at an earlier age. Studies of twins have shown a higher incidence of concordance in monozygous than in dizygous twins. An association between the disease and certain HLA antigens (A3, B7, DR2 and DQ1) has been found in European races, linking disease susceptibility to the HLA locus on chromosome 6.

Table 26.6 Geographical variance in the prevalence of multiple sclerosis	
Area	Crude prevalence per 100 000 population
North-east Scotland	144
Northumberland, England	50
North Italy	20
Israel	13
Mexico	1.5

The main theories as to the likely cause of multiple sclerosis are:

- abnormality in myelin lipid constituents
- autoimmune disorder (possibly virus-induced)
- circulating toxin in the CSF
- virus infection of the CNS (e.g. measles, canine distemper).

Multiple sclerosis may be an autoimmune disorder triggered by a virus infection (possibly measles) in a genetically susceptible host; this awaits proof. Clinical trials of cytokines, such as interferon, which modulate the immune response have reduced the frequency of disease relapse and progression in some patients.

Clinical features

Most cases present between 20 and 40 years of age. The disease is slightly commoner in females than in males, and the onset is usually characterised by the sudden development of a focal neurological deficit which spontaneously recovers. The relative incidences of initial manifestations are:

- limb weakness: 40%
- paraesthesiae: 20%
- optic neuritis: 20%
- diplopia: 10%
- bladder dysfunction: 5%
- vertigo: 5%.

The disease follows a characteristic relapsing and remitting course. Recovery from each episode of demyelination (relapse) is usually incomplete, and a progressive clinical deterioration ensues. The effects of demyelination may be detected electrophysiologically as delays in the latencies of visual and auditory evoked responses, since demyelinated axons conduct nerve impulses more slowly than normal. The progress of the disease is variable. Some patients (particularly children) follow a rapidly progressive course, while others may survive for over 20 years with only minor disability. Common complications of the disease include urinary tract infections, chest infections and pressure sores. Most patients die as a result of these problems rather than during an acute episode of demyelination.

Morphological features

The primary abnormalities in multiple sclerosis are confined to the CNS; the peripheral nervous system is not primarily involved. Patients dying with multiple sclerosis usually show numerous demyelinated

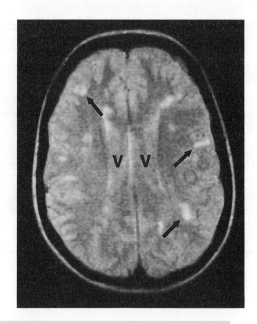

Fig. 26.16   Multiple sclerosis: demyelinated plaques

Multiple demyelinated plaques (arrows) are present in characteristic sites around the lateral ventricles (V) in the cerebral hemispheres of a patient with multiple sclerosis. (Magnetic resonance image: courtesy of Professor I Isherwood, Manchester)

plaques in the brain and spinal cord (Fig. 26.16), often closely related to veins and venules. In early lesions, the plaques are soft and pink with ill-defined boundaries. Histologically, there is myelin breakdown and phagocytosis by macrophages. Oedema is usually present, suggesting a local defect in the blood–brain barrier. Perivascular cuffing with inflammatory cells (plasma cells and T-lymphocytes) is widespread in the acute plaque. The plasma cells synthesise immunoglobulin, and oligoclonal bands of IgG are usually present in the CSF of patients with multiple sclerosis. T-lymphocytes have also been identified at the edges of acute plaques, whereas B-lymphocytes are usually found in areas of established demyelination.

As myelin breakdown eventually subsides, a reactive fibrillary gliosis is established, giving rise to the features of a chronic plaque. These lesions consist of sharply defined, grey, lucent areas of demyelination in which oligodendrocytes are scarce or absent. The inflammatory infiltrate also subsides, sometimes leaving small numbers of perivascular lymphocytes at the edge of chronic plaques (Fig. 26.17). Although it appears that oligodendrocytes have the capacity to proliferate, remyelination of established

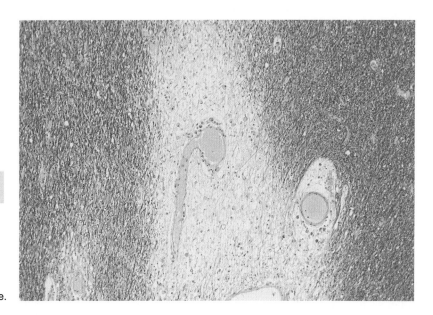

Fig. 26.17 Multiple sclerosis: chronic plaque

The chronic plaque consists of a sharply defined area of myelin loss (which appears pale in this preparation) containing fibrillary astrocytes. A few lymphocytes and macrophages are present around blood vessels in the plaque. Normal myelinated white matter appears blue.

plaques probably never occurs. Axons are usually preserved within chronic plaques.

Miscellaneous demyelinating conditions

Leukodystrophies
Although included as demyelinating conditions, it is known that most leukodystrophies result from a failure to synthesise normal myelin (sometimes called 'dysmyelination'). Two of these disorders — *metachromatic leukodystrophy* and *Krabbe's globoid cell leukodystrophy* — are due to inherited lysosomal enzyme deficiencies, and can be diagnosed antenatally. Others, such as *adrenoleukodystrophy*, are the result of an inherited abnormality in lipid metabolism, while in others the cause is unknown.

Metabolic disorders
Some metabolic disorders may result in demyelination. For example, in central pontine myelinolysis, which occurs most frequently in alcoholism and malnutrition, myelin breakdown occurs in the central brainstem and cerebrum. Its pathogenesis is unknown, but some cases appear to result from the rapid correction of hyponatraemia.

Toxins
Toxins may result in myelin breakdown in the CNS. One of the best-documented examples is hexachlorophene, an antiseptic agent which caused severe demyelination in infants by a direct effect on myelin.

Viruses
Viruses can cause demyelination, as in progressive multifocal leukoencephalopathy (p. 850), which produces a cytolytic infection of oligodendrocytes.

Immunological reactions
Immunological reactions may result in demyelination, as in acute disseminated encephalomyelitis (p. 852).

METABOLIC DISORDERS

▶ May be caused by toxins, deficiency states and metabolic disease
▶ Some toxins produce CNS damage directly; others produce liver damage causing secondary CNS changes
▶ Many of the early stages in toxic or deficiency states are reversible
▶ Many of the metabolic CNS diseases are inherited, and can be diagnosed antenatally

CNS toxins

The CNS can be affected by a large number of substances which act as toxins.

Methanol and ethanol

Both methanol and ethanol are toxic to the CNS. Acute poisoning with methanol can result in sudden death with multiple haemorrhageic lesions in the cerebral hemispheres, while chronic ingestion results in degeneration of neurones, e.g. in the retina, where loss of ganglion cells is accompanied by optic nerve atrophy. Ethanol can cause a wide range of CNS disorders (Table 26.7).

Drugs

Drugs affecting the CNS can be considered in two main groups:

- drugs affecting CNS development
- drugs affecting the mature CNS.

Drugs affecting CNS development include phenytoin and trimethadione which can cause microcephaly and other congenital abnormalities following maternal ingestion. Hexachlorophene caused vacuolation and degeneration of CNS myelin in premature infants when used in an antiseptic powder. Its use in such preparations is now discontinued. Drugs affecting the mature CNS include vincristine, which may cause axonal neuropathy.

Metal and industrial chemicals

Metals and industrial chemicals capable of affecting the CNS are listed in Table 26.8.

Deficiency states

In the developed countries of the world, the commonest deficiency states affecting the CNS are those involving vitamins, e.g. in chronic alcoholism. Elsewhere, the lack of an adequate food supply is responsible for a range of abnormalities which are still poorly understood in terms of their effects on the developing and mature CNS.

Malnutrition

Severe malnutrition may result in irreversible brain damage, particularly if it occurs in infancy during periods of CNS myelination since the lack of normal myelin development cannot be reversed at a later date. Malnutrition later in life, e.g. kwashiorkor (Ch. 7), may result in encephalopathy and ultimately lead to coma. The underlying mechanisms in these events are uncertain, but may result from severe electrolyte disturbances.

Vitamin deficiency

The major vitamin deficiency states (Ch. 7) affecting the nervous system are shown in Table 26.9. The most important of these are discussed below.

Vitamin B₁ (thiamine)

Vitamin B_1 (thiamine)
Vitamin B_1 deficiency is particularly common in chronic alcoholics and in patients with longstanding diseases of the upper gastrointestinal tract, for example, peptic ulcer and gastric carcinoma. Deficiency results in Wernicke's encephalopathy, which presents clinically with memory impairment, ataxia, visual disturbances and peripheral neuropathy. This disorder is often accompanied by Korsakoff's psychosis, in which case the term *Wernicke–Korsakoff syndrome* is used. Wernicke's encephalopathy is characterised by perivascular haemorrhages in the region

Table 26.7	Consequences of excessive ethanol intake on the CNS	
Disease	**Features**	**Mechanism**
Fetal alcohol syndrome	Cerebral malformations Facial and somatic malformations Growth retardation	Direct toxicity
Acute intoxication	Cerebral oedema Petechial haemorrhages	Direct toxicity
Cerebral and cerebellar atrophy	Neuronal loss	Direct toxicity
Nutritional disorders	Wernicke's encephalopathy	Deficiency of vitamin B_1
Hepatocerebral syndromes	Hepatic encephalopathy Chronic hepatocerebral degeneration	Hepatic toxicity with secondary effects on CNS
Demyelinating disorders	Central pontine myelinolysis	Electrolyte disturbances

Table 26.8 Metal and industrial chemical toxins affecting the CNS

Metal/Chemical	Source	Clinical manifestations of toxicity
Aluminium	Dialysis water from mains	Progressive encephalopathy in patients undergoing renal dialysis
Manganese	Mines	Degeneration of basal ganglia
Lead (inorganic)	Paint and petrol fumes	Encephalopathy in children
Mercury Inorganic Organic	 Industrial pollution Fungicides	 Progressive dementia Peripheral neuropathy, cerebellar and optic nerve degeneration (Minimata disease)
Acrylamide monomer	Construction industry	Encephalopathy and peripheral neuropathy with axonal degeneration
Hexacarbon compounds	Solvents	'Giant axonal neuropathy' affecting the CNS and peripheral nerves
Organophosphates	Insecticides	Anticholinesterase activity and distal axonopathy in CNS and peripheral nerves

Table 26.9 Major vitamin deficiency states affecting the nervous system

Vitamin	Deficiency state
A	Benign intracranial hypertension (rare)
B_1	Wernicke–Korsakoff syndrome
B_2	Peripheral neuropathy, ataxia, dementia
B_6	Convulsions in infants
B_{12}	Weakness and paraesthesiae in the lower limbs
C	Scurvy
E	Weakness, sensory loss, ataxia, nystagmus

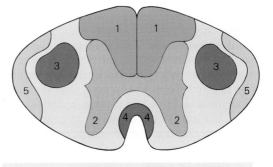

Fig. 26.18 Sites of degenerations in the spinal cord

1. Dorsal columns, involved in subacute combined degeneration, Friedreich's ataxia and tabes dorsalis. **2. Anterior horn cells**, involved in motor neurone disease and spinomuscular atrophy. **3. Lateral corticospinal tracts**, involved in motor neurone disease, subacute combined degeneration and Friedreich's ataxia. **4. Ventral corticospinal tracts**, involved in motor neurone disease. **5. Spinocerebellar tracts**, involved in Friedreich's ataxia.

of the fourth ventricle and aqueduct, particularly in the mammillary bodies. Fibrillary gliosis occurs in longstanding cases, when the affected structures appear shrunken. The pathogenesis of the lesions is uncertain.

Vitamin B_{12} (cyanocobalamin) deficiency
Vitamin B_{12} deficiency is an important condition which can result from a variety of disorders. The pathogenesis of the CNS damage is unknown; impairment of CNS amino acid and fatty acid metabolism has been implicated. In severe cases, there is extensive degeneration of the posterior columns and lateral corticospinal tracts in the spinal cord (Fig. 26.18); this process is referred to as *subacute combined degeneration of the spinal cord*. The cerebral hemispheres are involved to a lesser extent, and peripheral nerves may be affected. If replace-ment therapy is commenced at an early stage, the degenerative process is reversible. Longstanding cases show irreversible axonal damage accompanied by a reactive fibrillary gliosis.

Bilirubin toxicity

The term *kernicterus* is used to denote a yellow pigmentation of the brain in infants due to deposition of free bilirubin in its unconjugated form. This can occur in both premature and term neonates, when serum levels of unconjugated bilirubin are high, for example in materno-fetal rhesus or ABO blood group incompatibility. In fatal cases, bilirubin is deposited in the basal ganglia, thalamus and brainstem nuclei, which appear bright yellow. The CSF and meninges are also stained, to a lesser extent. A reduction in the incidence of rhesus haemolytic disease and the availability of exchange transfusions for jaundiced infants have greatly reduced the incidence of kernicterus.

Lysosomal storage diseases

Lysosomal storage diseases are uncommon inherited disorders characterised by a deficiency of various lysosomal enzymes which results in the accumulation of stored material in cells (Ch. 7). The CNS is involved in many lysosomal storage disorders (Table 26.10).

Hepatic encephalopathy

Hepatic encephalopathy may occur in patients with liver damage, due to a variety of agents. Encephalopathy in severe cases may progress to coma and result in permanent CNS damage in survivors. Increased levels of ammonia in the blood are associated with encephalopathy, possibly interfering with the function of certain neurotransmitters, such as gamma aminobutyric acid. Structural damage, including neuronal loss and reactive gliosis, occurs in longstanding cases. Two specific examples of hepatic encephalopathy are Wilson's disease and Reye's syndrome.

Wilson's disease

Wilson's disease, a disorder of copper metabolism, is inherited as an autosomal recessive condition. In some patients, liver disease is severe (Ch. 16) and may result in hepatic encephalopathy. In others, neurological signs predominate with tremor, rigidity and chorea; these abnormalities result from a marked loss of neurones in the basal ganglia, particularly the putamen, due to direct copper-induced damage. CNS damage in the early stages of the disease can be arrested by chelation therapy. Deposition of copper in the cornea results in the characteristic Kayser–Fleischer ring.

Reye's syndrome

Reye's syndrome usually affects children under 15 years of age who have a history of a preceding viral infection. It is characterised clinically by an acute onset of vomiting and seizures progressing to coma in severe cases. The liver may be enlarged, and there is usually biochemical evidence of hepatocellular damage and hypoglycaemia. Mortality rates of around 20% have been reported, even with intensive supportive therapy.

Epidemiological and biochemical studies have implicated salicylates (e.g. aspirin) in the pathogenesis of this disorder, although these compounds may not be the primary cause. Accordingly, salicylates for infants and children have been withdrawn from sale in the United Kingdom with a consequent decline in the incidence of this disorder.

CONGENITAL ABNORMALITIES

▶ Affect the CNS in 3–4 per 100 000 live births
▶ Neural tube defects and posterior fossa malformations are commonest
▶ Aetiology in most cases is unknown: genetic abnormalities and maternal infections account for many cases

Malformations of the CNS occur in 3–4 per 100 000 live births. The severe varieties cause considerable morbidity and mortality, but many of these abnormalities are of little clinical significance and may be detected only in later life as an incidental finding.

Table 26.10 Examples of lysosomal storage diseases affecting the CNS

Disease	Example	Enzyme deficiency
Sphingolipidosis	Tay–Sachs disease Niemann–Pick disease Metachromatic leukodystrophy	Hexosaminidase A Sphingomyelinase Arylsulphatase A
Mucopolysaccharidosis	Hurler's disease	α-L-iduronidase
Glycogenosis	Pompè's disease	Acid maltase
Ceroid lipofuscinosis	Batten's disease	Unknown

Some of the known causes of CNS malformations in humans are:

- genetic factors, such as in tuberous sclerosis (autosomal dominant), aqueduct stenosis (X-linked recessive), and Down's syndrome (trisomy 21)
- maternal infections, such as rubella and cytomegalovirus
- irradiation in utero
- toxic, as in fetal alcohol syndrome
- metabolic, such as phenylketonuria.

In many cases, the underlying causes are unknown. The most frequent malformations are the neural tube defects and posterior fossa malformations.

Neural tube defects

Neural tube defects are the commonest and most important congenital abnormalities of the CNS, occurring in 2–3 per 100 000 live births. Failure of the neural tube to close at 28 days' gestation, or damage to its structure after closure can be detected in utero by ultrasound. In 90% of cases, the level of alpha-fetoprotein in the maternal serum and amniotic fluid is increased; this investigation is often used as a screening procedure.

Both cranial and spinal involvement may occur; the term *spina bifida* is often used for the later, when the CNS malformation is usually accompanied by *rachischisis* — failure of the vertebral laminae to develop.

Spinal involvement

The major types of spinal involvement are illustrated in Figure 26.19.

Neural tube defects occur most frequently in the lumbosacral region. The more severe forms result in a considerable neurological deficit, with paraplegia and absence of sphincter control. The musculature of the lower limbs undergoes neurogenic atrophy, and meningitis and urinary tract infections are common. Hydrocephalus occurs in cases with an accompanying Arnold–Chiari malformation. These factors account for the generally poor prognosis in severe cases, even after early surgical repair of the spina bifida.

Cranial involvement

Encephalocele and *cranial meningocele* usually occur in the occipital region, with herniation of the posterior cerebral hemispheres and their coverings respectively through a defect in the skull.

Anencephaly is the commonest of the neural tube defects. It is thought to occur when the developing

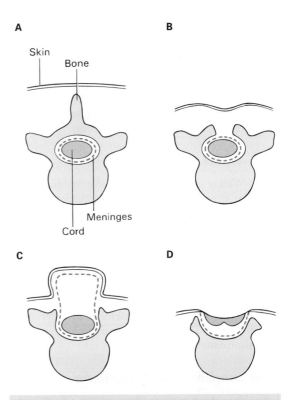

Fig. 26.19   Neural tube defects: spinal involvement

A. Normal arrangement. B. Spina bifida occulta: vertebral defect with a normal cord and meninges. The overlying skin is intact. **C. Myelocele:** the meningeal sac is usually covered by intact skin, but rupture of the sac may occur following birth. **D. Meningomyelocele:** the skin overlying the sac frequently ruptures, exposing the abnormal meninges and spinal cord.

brain is exposed to amniotic fluid as its coverings fail to develop. The calvaria is usually absent, but the base of the skull is thickened and partly covered by a mass of vascular granulation tissue. The anterior pituitary gland is present, but hypoplastic, and several associated visceral and limb abnormalities have been described. The condition is fatal and often results in spontaneous abortion.

A variety of factors, including environmental agents, social class, dietary conditions (particularly vitamin deficiencies) and genetic factors, have been implicated in the aetiology of neural tube defects, but their pathogenesis remains unknown.

Posterior fossa malformations

Arnold–Chiari malformation

Arnold–Chiari malformation is a complex disorder involving the cerebellum, brainstem and spinal cord, and is the commonest congenital malformation in the posterior fossa. It is often associated with a meningomyelocele. The main features are illustrated in Figure 26.20.

These abnormalities result in an obstructive hydrocephalus, usually of the communicating type (p. 839). There is no entirely satisfactory explanation for the Arnold–Chiari malformation.

Dandy–Walker malformation

Dandy–Walker malformation is the second most important congenital abnormality affecting the posterior fossa. The cerebellar hemispheres are of normal size, but the vermis is absent or hypoplastic. The fourth ventricle is markedly distended and forms a cyst-like structure between the cerebellar hemispheres. In most cases, the exit foramina of the fourth ventricle are imperforate. This results in obstructive hydrocephalus, usually of non-communicating type, which may be detectable antenatally by ultrasound. The aetiology and pathogenesis of this malformation are unknown.

Other congenital malformations

Many other congenital malformations affecting the

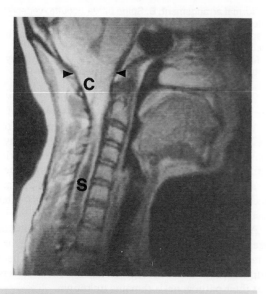

Fig. 26.20 Arnold–Chiari malformation: brain and cord abnormalities

The cerebellar tonsils (C) are displaced downwards from the shallow posterior fossa below the level of the foramen magnum (arrows). The brainstem is elongated and a syrinx (S) is present in the spinal cord commencing at the level of the third cervical vertebral body. (Magnetic resonance image: courtesy of Professor B S Worthington, Nottingham)

CNS have been described. Without being comprehensive, these can be considered in the following broad groups:

- agenesis and dysgenesis
- disorders of cell migration and corticogenesis
- destructive lesions
- phakomatoses
- chromosomal abnormalities.

Agenesis and dysgenesis

Agenesis and dysgenesis may involve almost any structure within the CNS, but the commonest sites affected are the corpus callosum and the olfactory bulbs and tracts (arhinencephaly). These lesions may occur in isolation or in association with other malformations, for example, agenesis of the corpus callosum with the Dandy–Walker malformation, and arhinencephaly with holoprosencephaly, a complex disorder of forebrain diverticulation.

Disorders of cell migration and corticogenesis

Failure of neuronal migration during CNS development results in a number of structural disorders, of which the most important are:

- *Agyria and pachygyria.* These result in defective formation of the cerebral cortex with complete failure (agyria) or partial failure of gyral development.
- *Polymicrogyria.* This is a complex disorder of neuronal distribution in the cerebral cortex. The cortical surface bears numerous small irregular gyri, imparting a wrinkled appearance to affected areas.
- *Heterotopias.* These occur when neuronal migration is arrested, and are seen most frequently in the white matter of the CNS. They can occur as an isolated finding, but occasionally occur as part of a more complex disorder, as in Down's syndrome.

Destructive lesions

Destructive lesions occur most frequently in the developing CNS as a consequence of maternal infections and hypoxia. Extensive destruction of tissue may result in microcephaly, but focal lesions may also occur, such as *ulegyria*, where a loss of neurones and axons in the cerebral cortex is accompanied by a reactive gliosis.

Phakomatoses

Phakomatoses are group of autosomal dominant

inherited neurocutaneous disorders which result in CNS malformations. Important members of this group include neurofibromatosis, tuberous sclerosis and von Hippel–Lindau syndrome.

Chromosomal abnormalities

Chromosomal abnormalities frequently result in mental retardation. CNS malformations are often present in such cases, and are sometimes of sufficient severity to cause permanent disability or death. The best characterised of these disorders include *Down's syndrome* ('mongolism'), the principal features of which are:

- trisomy 21
- abnormal facies and palmar creases
- mental retardation
- flattened cerebral contours
- abnormal myelination and neuronal heterotopias
- congenital heart defects
- development of Alzheimer-like changes from the fourth decade.

and can readily be detected in life by CT scanning. On average, the volume of the ventricular system increases from 35 ml in young adults to 60 ml in those over 60 years.

Other age-related changes in the CNS include:

- reduction in size, numbers and dendritic branches of neurones
- increase in number of astrocytes
- thickening of leptomeninges
- perivascular amyloid deposition
- arteriosclerosis.

Several other important age-related changes occur in relation to neurones, namely:

- senile plaques
- neurofibrillary tangles
- Lewy bodies
- alterations in the quantity and distribution of neurotransmitters (e.g. acetylcholine in the cerebral cortex and catecholamines in the basal ganglia).

AGE-RELATED CHANGES IN THE CNS

> ▶ Brain weight decreases slowly after the third decade and rapidly from the seventh decade
> ▶ Ageing is accompanied by cortical atrophy and loss of white matter with compensatory hydrocephalus
> ▶ The aged brain shows a variable loss of neurones with increased numbers of reactive astrocytes
> ▶ Surviving cortical neurones may exhibit a range of structural changes, e.g. neurofibrillary tangles
> ▶ Cerebrovascular disease is common, and may include amyloid deposition around small intracranial vessels

A wide variety of changes have been described in the CNS of normal elderly adults. The extent of these changes often relates to the age of the person, but there is considerable variation from one individual to another.

Brain weight progressively reduces from normal values of around 1450 g in males and 1300 g in females at about 40 years of age; these values decline more rapidly after the age of 60. The ratio of brain/skull volume is greater than 90% until the seventh decade, when it reduces to around 80%. This loss of brain substance appears to occur at an earlier age in females than in males, and is most evident in the white matter of the cerebral hemispheres. Ventricular enlargement (compensatory hydrocephalus; p. 840) is a variable finding in elderly brains

SYSTEM DEGENERATIONS

> ▶ Characterised by progressive loss of neurones in functionally related areas of the CNS
> ▶ Neuronal death is accompanied by neuronophagia and reactive fibrillary gliosis
> ▶ Considerable overlap of clinical and pathological features, but several well-defined entities exist, e.g. Parkinson's disease and motor neurone disease
> ▶ Several disorders show characteristic neurochemical abnormalities, for which replacement therapy may be clinically beneficial, e.g. Parkinson's disease
> ▶ Aetiology in most cases unknown, although some are inherited disorders, e.g. Friedreich's ataxia

Several degenerative conditions affecting the CNS are characterised by the progressive loss of certain groups of functionally related neurones and their associated pathways. These conditions can be considered as system degenerations; these disorders may occur in isolation or as part of a multiple systems degeneration. The pathogenesis of these disorders is unknown, but several occur as inherited conditions. It is therefore important to establish a diagnosis to allow genetic counselling of an affected family. Considerable overlap of both the clinical and pathological features occurs in this group of conditions, but several well-defined examples exist (Table 26.11).

Table 26.11   Examples of CNS system degenerations

Disease	Sites affected	Clinical features
Friedreich's ataxia	Spinal cord Sensory nuclei Cerebellum	Ataxia Sensory loss Deafness Autosomal recessive disorder
Cerebellar cortical atrophy	Purkinje cells Granular neurones Inferior olivary nuclei	Ataxia Nystagmus
Olivopontocerebellar atrophy	Purkinje cells Granular neurones Pontine nuclei Inferior olivary nuclei	Ataxia Rigidity Bulbar paresis
Multiple system atrophy (Shy–Drager syndrome)	Substantia nigra Purkinje cells Pontine nuclei Spinal autonomic nuclei	Ataxia Sensory loss Tremor Orthostatic hypotension

Motor neurone disease

This disorder affects 5/100 000 of the population, occurring most often in males over the age of 50 years. 5% of cases are familial, many of which have a mutation in the Cu/Mn superoxide dismutase gene on chromosome 21q. Three main disease patterns are recognised clinically:

1. *amyotrophic lateral sclerosis*, with distal and proximal muscle weakness and wasting, spasticity and exaggerated reflexes indicative of both upper and lower motor neurone involvement
2. *progressive muscular atrophy*, when predominantly lower motor neurone involvement results in weakness and wasting of distal muscles, fasciculation and absent reflexes
3. *progressive bulbar palsy*, when involvement of cranial nerve motor nuclei results in weakness of the tongue, palate and pharyngeal muscles.

Most patients die 3–5 years after diagnosis due to respiratory difficulties or the complications of immobility. Examination of the CNS shows loss of motor neurones (in patterns corresponding to the clinical groups listed above) and corticospinal pathway degeneration with reactive gliosis. Occasional surviving motor neurones contain filamentous cytoplasmic inclusions of unknown aetiology; in a minority of cases these inclusions may be widespread in the cerebral cortex and are associated with dementia.

Parkinson's disease

Parkinson's disease is characterised clinically by tremor, bradykinesia and rigidity, which usually become manifest between the ages of 45 and 60 years, affecting 1% of the population over 60. Similar clinical features may occur in unrelated conditions, such as cerebrovascular disease or phenothiazine drug therapy. This disorder affects pigmented neurones in the substantia nigra, the locus caeruleus and several other brainstem nuclei. At these sites there is progressive depigmentation and loss of neurones; surviving cells harbour round eosinophilic inclusions — Lewy bodies (Fig. 26.21) — containing cytoskeletal filaments, including neurofilaments. Lewy body inclusions may occasionally be widespread throughout the brain, particularly in the cerebral cortex, resulting in dementia due to 'diffuse Lewy body disease'.

The neurones of the substantia nigra synthesise dopamine, which acts as an inhibitory neurotransmitter at their axonal projection sites in the corpus striatum (putamen and globus pallidus). Loss of the pigmented neurones results in a relative deficiency of dopamine in the corpus striatum which can be overcome by replacement therapy, for example with L-dopa. This often relieves the clinical symptoms of the disease, but a permanent cure is not yet possible.

The cause of Parkinson's disease is unknown, but a similar disorder can be produced experimentally by the administration of MPTP (1–methyl-4-phenyl-1, 2, 3, 6-tetrahydropyridine). This compound

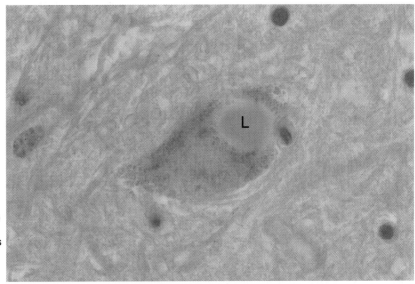

Fig. 26.21 Idiopathic Parkinson's disease

Surviving pigmented neurones in the substantia nigra contain intracytoplasmic inclusions known as Lewy bodies(L). These comprise a central pink hyaline core with a pale surrounding halo.

has also produced a severe disorder resembling Parkinson's disease in intravenous drug addicts when it is present as a contaminant in synthetic heroin preparations.

DEMENTIA

> ▶ Predominantly a disorder of the elderly; more than 15% of adults over 80 are demented
> ▶ Classified aetiologically into primary organic and secondary dementias
> ▶ Commonest cause of dementia in the United Kingdom is Alzheimer's disease, a progressive degenerative organic disorder
> ▶ Aetiology of most primary organic dementias is unknown; some are inherited as single gene defects, e.g. Huntington's disease

Dementia has been defined clinically as an acquired global impairment of intellect, reason and personality without impairment of consciousness. Emotional lability and memory dysfunction are prominent manifestations, implying a cerebral cortical disorder. Most patients with dementia exhibit both gross and histological abnormalities within the cerebral cortex, although some rarer causes of dementia appear to involve mainly subcortical structures. A variety of disorders affecting the CNS can result in dementia:

- primary organic dementia (e.g. Alzheimer's disease, Pick's disease, Huntington's disease, diffuse Lewy body disease)
- cerebrovascular disease (e.g. multi-infarct dementia, Binswanger's disease)
- infections (e.g. Creutzfeldt–Jakob disease, neurosyphilis, HIV infection)
- intracranial space-occupying lesions (e.g. neoplasms, chronic subdural haematoma)
- hydrocephalus
- drugs and toxins (e.g. barbiturates, digoxin, anticholinergic agents, alcohol, heavy metals)
- metabolic disorders (e.g. hypothyroidism, hypoparathyroidism, uraemia, hepatic failure)
- vitamin deficiencies (e.g. B_1 — Wernicke–Korsakoff syndrome, B_2, B_{12})
- paraneoplastic syndromes (e.g. limbic encephalitis).

These disorders may be considered in two main categories:

- primary degenerative disorders affecting the CNS (sometimes referred to as *organic dementias*)
- other disorders producing secondary changes in the CNS which result in dementia.

The commonest cause of dementia in Western countries is Alzheimer's disease (at least 50% of cases), followed by multi-infarct dementia (around 20% of cases). It is important to establish the cause of dementia in each patient, since in some cases an effective treatment is available. In other cases, dementia may be due to an inherited disorder, in which case genetic counselling is required for the affected family. The major causes of organic dementia are discussed below.

Alzheimer's disease

Alzheimer's disease is a degenerative condition which accounts for well over 50% of all cases of dementia in adults. In the United Kingdom, it is thought to affect 5% of people over the age of 65, rising to 15% of those over 80. As the number of elderly people in the population increases, so there is a concomitant increase in the number of patients suffering from Alzheimer's disease; this has been termed the 'silent epidemic'. Females are affected almost twice as frequently as males. Most cases occur sporadically, although a small proportion are inherited as an autosomal dominant disorder. Several gene loci are involved in familial cases, including the APP gene on chromosome 21 (see below) and chromosome 14. There is an increased incidence of sporadic Alzheimer's disease in individuals with the ApoE4 genotype on chromosome 19. The clinical presentation usually occurs after the age of 60 years, but a significant subgroup is affected between the ages of 50 and 60 years. The illness lasts from 2 to 8 years; most patients die from inanition and bronchopneumonia.

Morphological features

The changes in the CNS in Alzheimer's disease resemble those in the ageing, non-demented brain, but are much more severe. The brain is reduced in weight, often to 1000 g or less, and shows cortical atrophy which is often most marked in the frontal and temporal lobes. There is loss of both cortical grey and white matter, with compensatory dilatation of the ventricular system (secondary hydrocephalus; Fig. 26.22). The hindbrain structures and spinal cord appear normal.

The characteristic histological changes in Alzheimer's disease are most pronounced in the cerebral cortex, particularly in the hippocampus. The severity of these changes correlates with the clinical severity of the dementia. The histological hallmarks of Alzheimer's disease are *senile plaques* and *neurofibrillary tangles*. These are similar to those in the non-demented elderly brain (Fig. 26.23), but are far more numerous and extensive in their distribution.

Senile plaques

Senile plaques are best demonstrated in specially stained histological sections of the CNS (Fig. 26.23). They occur most frequently in the hippocampus, cerebral cortex and deep grey matter, for example the amygdaloid nucleus. Senile plaques can measure up to 200 μm in diameter, and in their earliest stages comprise a collection of dilated presynaptic neuronal processes which contain many organelles. As the plaques mature, they enlarge and develop a core of aluminosilicates and amyloid protein. The latter eventually forms the major component of the 'burnt-out' plaque. Reactive astrocytes and microglia are usually present at the periphery of the plaque.

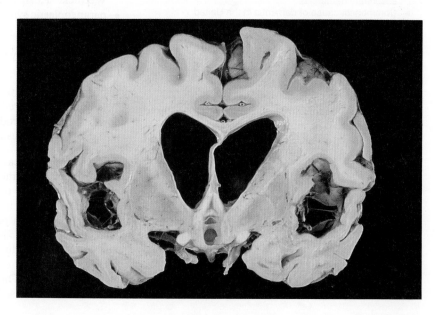

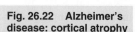

Fig. 26.22 Alzheimer's disease: cortical atrophy

The brain in Alzheimer's disease shows severe cortical atrophy with narrowing of the gyri and widening of the sulci. White matter loss is accompanied by dilatation of the ventricular system (compensatory hydrocephalus).

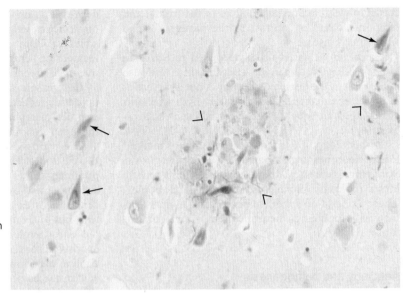

Fig. 26.23 Plaques and tangles: histology (immunocytochemistry)

Neurofibrillary tangles (arrows) are visible as dark brown linear structures in the perikaryon adjacent to the neuronal nucleus. Senile plaques (arrowheads) are extracellular lesions comprising brown-staining neuritic processes around a central amyloid core.

Neurofibrillary tangles

Neurofibrillary tangles are present within the neuronal perikarya and, like senile plaques, are most easily visualised in specially stained sections (Fig. 26.23). Affected neurones are most often found in the hippocampus, but may also occur in the cerebral cortex, subcortical grey matter and brainstem nuclei. This form of degeneration consists of a thickening of fibrils within the neuronal cytoplasm, to form a tortuous and elongated corkscrew-like structure. Electron microscopy has shown that each tangle consists of a mass of twisted tubules composed of paired helical filaments, each 10 nm in diameter, with a periodic narrowing at 80 nm. The nature of these filaments is unknown, but they bear antigenic resemblances to neurofilament and microtubule-associated proteins.

Neuronal loss

Neuronal loss is often widespread in the cerebral cortex, but is most severe in the hippocampus.

Perivascular amyloid

Amyloid is usually present around arterioles and capillaries within the brain. The precursor of this perivascular amyloid and of the amyloid core of senile plaques (p. 864) is a glycoprotein encoded by the APP gene on chromosome 21. This may explain why individuals with trisomy 21 (Down's syndrome) develop accelerated Alzheimer-like changes in the CNS as a consequence of their extra gene load.

Neurochemical abnormalities

The functional impairment in Alzheimer's disease is accompanied by a number of neurochemical abnormalities, the best known of which involve a reduction in cholinergic activity in the cerebral cortex. Replacement therapy, however, has not so far proved to be of major benefit.

Aetiology and pathogenesis

The aetiology and pathogenesis of this disorder are unknown. It has been suggested that an infectious agent might be responsible, but none has so far been identified. Other possibilities include toxins, for example aluminium which is present in the core of senile plaques, or an abnormality of regulation in the formation of the amyloid precursor protein.

Pick's disease

Pick's disease is an uncommon disorder which is sometimes inherited as an autosomal dominant condition. It usually presents as a relentlessly progressive dementia in late middle life, with a peak incidence around 60 years of age. Most patients die within 2–5 years of diagnosis.

Morphology

Naked-eye examination of the brain of an affected individual shows extreme atrophy of the cerebral cortex in well-circumscribed areas of the frontal and temporal lobes, in contrast to the pattern seen in Alzheimer's disease.

The brain weight is usually reduced to less than 1000 g. The basal ganglia and thalamus are also involved, but the degree of atrophy is not as severe as in the cerebral cortex. Compensatory hydrocephalus occurs as a consequence of the cortical and subcortical atrophy.

On histology, the affected areas show a marked loss of neurones, accompanied by a reactive gliosis. Surviving neurones may contain characteristic intracytoplasmic inclusions, known as Pick bodies. These consist of spherical masses of filamentous material including neurofilaments and microtubules.

Aetiology and pathogenesis

The aetiology and pathogenesis of Pick's disease are unknown and no specific treatment is available.

Huntington's disease

The degenerative condition known as Huntington's disease is inherited as an autosomal dominant disorder. It is uncommon, affecting 4–7 per 100 000 in the United Kingdom. The disease does not usually become clinically apparent until the fifth decade of life, when the onset of personality change and depression are later accompanied by choreiform movements, jerking and dementia. The gene responsible for Huntington's disease has recently been located on chromosome 4, allowing an effective means of preclinical and antenatal diagnosis.

The genetic abnormality is an excess number of tandemly repeated CAG nucleotide sequences. The number of repeats influences the age of onset: the more repeats, the earlier the onset.

The gross appearances are illustrated in Figure 26.24. Histology of the caudate nucleus and putamen shows a marked loss of small neurones, accompanied by a reactive fibrillary gliosis. The cerebral cortex in this disorder also shows neuronal loss, but to a variable extent.

Neurochemical abnormalities have been identified in this disorder, for example reduced levels of choline acetyltransferase and gamma aminobutyric acid in the basal ganglia. These changes are presumably secondary to the neuronal loss.

Dementia pugilistica

In the 'punch-drunk' syndrome seen in boxers, progressive dementia is accompanied by focal neurological signs. Characteristic findings in the brain are structural abnormalities of the septum pellucidum, thinning of the corpus callosum, degeneration of the substantia nigra and cerebral cortical neurofibrillary tangles. Unlike Alzheimer's disease, typical senile plaques are not present.

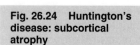

Fig. 26.24 Huntington's disease: subcortical atrophy

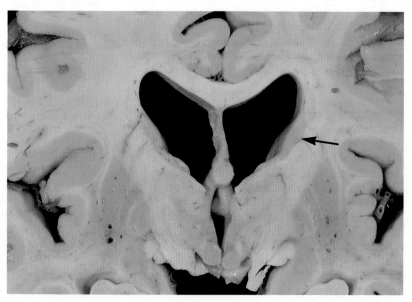

In Huntington's disease, cerebral atrophy is most marked in the caudate nucleus (arrow), which is markedly narrowed, and the adjacent putamen. These changes are accompanied by compensatory hydrocephalus involving the lateral ventricles.

CNS TUMOURS

► Second commonest tumours in children and the sixth commonest in adults
► Present clinically with localising signs due to tissue destruction, or with the non-specific effects of raised intracranial pressure
► Classified according to cell of origin and degree of differentiation
► In children, 70% are sited in the posterior fossa; most are intrinsic tumours
► In adults, 70% are sited supratentorially; intrinsic and extrinsic tumours both occur frequently
► Metatastic tumours occur more frequently with increasing age: most are carcinomas, which may form solid deposits in the CNS or spread by seeding in the CSF
► Survival depends on the age of the patient and the site, size and histology of the neoplasm

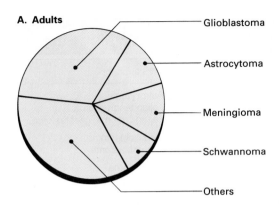

A. Adults
- Glioblastoma
- Astrocytoma
- Meningioma
- Schwannoma
- Others

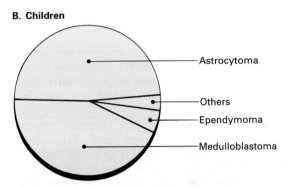

B. Children
- Astrocytoma
- Others
- Ependymoma
- Medulloblastoma

Fig. 26.25 Relative incidence of primary CNS neoplasms

The relative incidences of the commonest primary CNS neoplasms are illustrated for adults and children. Important differences in site also occur in relation to age. **A.** In adults, most neoplasms are supratentorial. **B.** In children, most arise in the posterior fossa.

Primary tumours of the CNS occur in approximately 8 per 100 000 of the general population. Two main peaks of incidence occur: in the first decade and in the fifth or sixth decades of life. In children, CNS tumours are the second commonest group of neoplasms (after leukaemias), but in adults they rate as the sixth commonest group. The relative incidences of the main groups of primary CNS tumours in adults and in children are shown in Figure 26.25.

Pathogenesis

The pathogenesis of most CNS neoplasms is unknown, but the following factors have been studied:

- *Genetic factors.* Primary CNS tumours are major components of several disorders inherited as autosomal dominant conditions including tuberous sclerosis, neurofibromatosis and von Hippel–Lindau syndrome.
- *Chemical and viral factors.* In animals, chemical and viral carcinogens resulting in the development of primary CNS neoplasms have been discovered but their relationship to tumours in humans is uncertain.
- *Radiation.* In man, irradiation of the CNS in childhood has very occasionally resulted in the development of a neoplasm in adult life.
- *Immunosuppression.* This is of major importance in the pathogenesis of primary CNS lymphomas.
- *Trauma.* The role of trauma in the pathogenesis of CNS neoplasms is unproven.

Classification

As in other organs, tumours of the CNS are classified according to their presumed cell of origin (Table 26.12).

Clinicopathological features

Brain tumours may present clinically in two main ways:

- *Local effects.* Epilepsy with a temporal lobe tumour or paraplegia with a spinal cord tumour are examples.
- *Mass effects.* Many tumours present with the non-specific signs and symptoms of space-occupying lesions, without any localising signs. Vasogenic oedema around CNS neoplasms is particularly common and may greatly potentiate the mass effect. Posterior fossa tumours present with the clinical features of hydrocephalus, particularly in children. Intracranial herniation is a common mode of death in patients with CNS neoplasms (Fig. 26.4).

Table 26.12 Classification of CNS tumours according to presumed cell of origin	
Cell of origin	CNS tumour
Glial cells	Astrocytoma, oligodendroglioma, ependymoma, glioblastoma
Primitive neuroectodermal cells	Medulloblastoma, neuroblastoma
Arachnoidal cell	Meningioma
Nerve sheath cells	Schwannoma, neurofibroma
Lymphoreticular cells	Lymphoma

Unlike neoplasms arising in other tissues, primary CNS neoplasms virtually never metastasise to other organs; the reasons for this are not clearly understood. However, infiltration of adjacent tissues both within the nervous system and its coverings (including the skull) is common, for example in meningioma, and seeding to remote parts of the nervous system by the CSF pathway is an important means of spread for certain intrinsic tumours, for example medulloblastomas. Spread by seeding can sometimes occur down a ventriculoperitoneal shunt, resulting in intra-abdominal tumour deposits.

Intrinsic tumours

The commonest group of primary CNS neoplasms are the intrinsic tumours of the brain, which account for all primary CNS neoplasms in children. In adults, intrinsic tumours account for around 65% of primary CNS neoplasms, the majority of which are of glial origin. Intrinsic tumours occur more frequently in male patients.

Astrocytomas

Astrocytomas account for 10% of all primary CNS tumours in adults, but are relatively more frequent in children (Fig. 26.25). They commonly arise in the cerebellum in children, and in the cerebral hemispheres in adults. Astrocytomas are usually classified according to the predominant cell type and degree of differentiation (Fig. 26.26). It is thought that many anaplastic astrocytomas arise as a consequence of dedifferentiation within a pre-existing astrocytic neoplasm. The prognosis for patients with astrocytomas (and gliomas generally) depends on the degree of tumour differentiation, the age of the patient at diagnosis, and the site and size of the neoplasm.

Glioblastoma

Glioblastoma accounts for 30% of all primary CNS tumours in adults, but is extremely rare in children. Most arise in the white matter of the cerebral hemispheres (Fig. 26.4). As its name implies, this neoplasm is characterised histologically by a

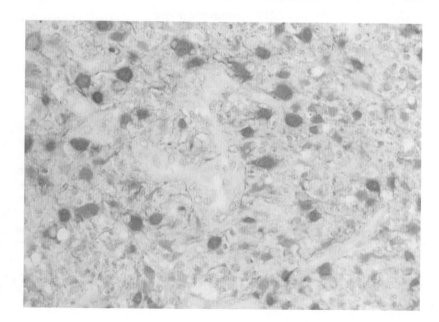

Fig. 26.26 Astrocytoma

In this well-differentiated cerebral astrocytoma, most of the cells bear numerous cytoplasmic processes which are arranged around blood vessels in a manner similar to astrocytic processes in normal grey matter.

pleomorphic cell population (Fig. 26.27). Although it is accepted that glioblastomas may arise de novo, it seems likely that many of these neoplasms arise as a consequence of dedifferentiation within a pre-existing astrocytic glioma. Dedifferentiation is accompanied by, or is the result of, a series of genetic events (Fig. 26.28). Mitotic activity in glioblastomas is abundant, and vascular endothelial proliferation is prominent. These features suggest a rapid growth rate; most patients die within one year of diagnosis.

Oligodendroglioma

Oligodendroglioma accounts for 3% of all primary CNS neoplasms in adults, but is rare in children. Oligodendrogliomas are usually ill-defined, infiltrating neoplasms, arising in the white matter of the cerebral hemispheres. Histologically, oligodendrogliomas present a spectrum of appearances which may be graded in a similar manner to astrocytomas. In a well-differentiated tumour, the neoplastic cells are small, rounded and uniform with a clear cytoplasm and prominent cell membrane. Small foci of calcification are common, and a characteristic interweaving vascular pattern is often present.

Ependymoma

An ependymoma arises from an ependymal surface, usually in the fourth ventricle, and projects into the CSF pathway (Fig. 26.29). Most ependymomas are well differentiated, and extensive invasion of adjacent CNS structures is uncommon. A special variant, the myxopapillary ependymoma, occurs in the cauda equina region in adults.

Choroid plexus papilloma

An uncommon intraventricular papillary growth, choroid plexus papilloma, is most often found in a lateral ventricle, and usually presents with obstructive hydrocephalus. Although showing little ten-

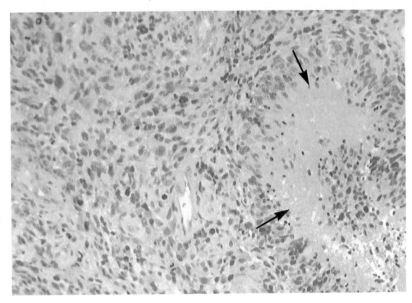

Fig. 26.27 Glioblastoma

Areas of necrosis (arrows) are a characteristic feature of this neoplasm, and are usually surrounded by the nuclei of small malignant cells. The neoplastic cell population is pleomorphic, and also includes multinucleate cells. Vascular endothelial proliferation is another characteristic histological feature.

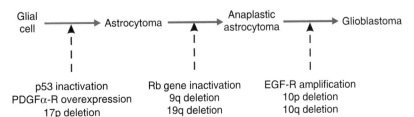

Fig. 26.28

Molecular genetic abnormalities in glioma progression.

Glial cell → Astrocytoma	Anaplastic astrocytoma	Glioblastoma
p53 inactivation PDGFα-R overexpression 17p deletion 22q deletion	Rb gene inactivation 9q deletion 19q deletion	EGF-R amplification 10p deletion 10q deletion

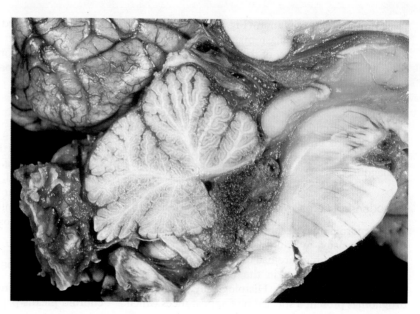

Fig. 26.29   Ependymoma: ventricular obstruction

The ependymoma arising from the lining of the fourth ventricle has almost totally obstructed the CSF pathway and produced obstructive hydrocephalus. This results in characteristic clinical features which are common presenting symptoms for this group of neoplasms.

dency to infiltrate locally, spread via the CSF may occur.

Primitive neuroectodermal tumours

The commonest variety of the primitive neuroectodermal group of tumours is the *medulloblastoma*, which arises in the cerebellum in children. The growth rate is rapid, and extensive local infiltration is common, often resulting in obstructive hydrocephalus. Meningeal infiltration frequently occurs and CSF seeding is common. As the name implies, these tumours are composed of poorly differentiated neuroepithelial cells which consist of small round nuclei surrounded by a scanty rim of cytoplasm. Mitotic figures are numerous, and evidence of differentiation into mature cell types, such as neurones or glia, is occasionally present. The prognosis for this group of tumours in children has improved in recent years, as a consequence of improved treatment with radiotherapy; the 5-year survival rate is around 60%.

Haemangioblastoma

Haemangioblastoma is an uncommon neoplasm arising most often in the cerebellum and forming a well-defined, frequently cystic mass. Histologically, the tumour is composed of blood vessels, separated by stromal cells with clear cytoplasm containing lipid. CNS haemangioblastomas are an important component of von Hippel–Lindau syndrome, an

autosomal dominant inherited disease with a genetic locus on chromosome 3p.

Lymphoma

Although an uncommon CNS tumour, there is much current interest in primary CNS lymphomas because of their greatly increased frequency of occurrence in immunosuppressed patients, for example in cardiac and renal transplant patients and in the acquired immune deficiency syndrome (AIDS). Recent studies have implicated the Epstein–Barr virus in the pathogenesis of these neoplasms. Most primary CNS lymphomas are ill-defined masses arising in the white matter or the cerebral hemispheres. Histologically, most are high-grade, non-Hodgkin's lymphomas of B-cell type. Accordingly, the prognosis is poor and most patients are dead within 2–3 years.

Tumours of neuronal cells

Tumours comprising neuronal elements are rare; they occur most commonly around the region of the third ventricle in children. In gangliocytomas, the neoplastic cells all resemble mature neurones, but gangliogliomas include neoplastic glial cells (usually astrocytic cells).

Miscellaneous cysts

A variety of cystic lesions occur in the CNS which,

although not all neoplastic, often present clinically with symptoms and signs similar to those of CNS tumours. Examples include:

- *craniopharyngioma* in the suprasellar region, causing pituitary dysfunction and visual disturbance
- *colloid cyst* in the third ventricle in children and young adults, causing intermittent hydrocephalus and sudden death
- *dermoid cyst* in the posterior fossa and lumbar spine in children and young adults, causing cerebellar signs and symptoms, and paraplegia
- *epidermoid cyst* in the cerebello-pontine angle and pituitary region in adults, causing cerebellar signs and symptoms of pituitary dysfunction respectively.

Extrinsic tumours

Tumours arising from the coverings of the brain and spinal cord, and from cranial and spinal nerve roots, are less common than intrinsic CNS tumours. Complete surgical removal of extrinsic neoplasms often results in a clinical cure.

Meningiomas

Meningiomas account for around 18% of intracranial neoplasms in adults; female patients outnumber males by 2:1. Meningiomas arise from cells of the arachnoid cap (a component of arachnoid villi). The most frequent sites are the parasagittal region, sphenoidal wing, olfactory groove and foramen magnum. Meningiomas are smooth lobulated masses, which are broadly adherent to the dura. Infiltration of the adjacent dura and overlying bone is not uncommon, but invasion of the brain is exceptionally rare. The brain, however, may be markedly compressed by a meningioma, resulting in considerable anatomical distortion (Fig. 26.30). Histologically, meningiomas display a variety of patterns, the most characteristic of which includes sheets of fusiform cells in a composite solid and whorled pattern. Small foci of calcification (psammoma bodies) are common.

Occasional meningiomas are frankly malignant and may metastasise outside the CNS, for example to the lung.

Schwannoma

As the name suggests, schwannomas derive from Schwann cells in the nerve sheath of the intracranial or intraspinal roots to sensory nerves. By far the commonest site is the vestibular branch of the 8th cranial nerve in the region of the cerebello-pontine angle; such neoplasms are often known as 'acoustic neuromas'. As with meningiomas, schwannomas occur most frequently in adults, and are commoner in females. Bilateral 8th nerve tumours commonly occur in patients suffering from central neurofibromatosis. Histologically, schwannomas exhibit two

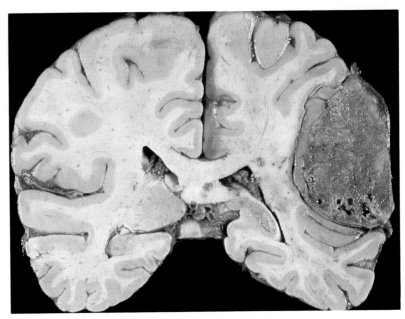

Fig. 26.30 Meningioma: cerebral compression

Meningiomas do not usually invade CNS structures, but may produce clinical manifestations by compression of the adjacent brain. This neoplasm has the lobulated surface characteristic of meningiomas, and is sharply demarcated from the cerebrum.

main patterns: densely packed spindle-shaped cells with frequent nuclear palisading (Antoni A tissue) and more loosely structured areas with a myxoid stroma which may contain cysts (Antoni B areas).

Neurofibromas

In the CNS, neurofibromas usually arise on the dorsal nerve roots of the spinal cord, and occur most frequently in patients suffering from neurofibromatosis. Unlike schwannomas, neurofibromas are not encapsulated but tend to involve an entire nerve root, producing a localised or diffuse expansion. Histologically, neurofibromas consist of a mixture of Schwann cells and fibroblasts, forming bundles of elongated cells with characteristically 'wavy' nuclei.

Secondary tumours

The CNS may be involved by other neoplasms in two main ways: compression and invasion, and metastasis.

Compression and invasion

Tumours arising in adjacent organs may compress and invade the CNS, producing localising clinical signs, or presenting as space-occupying lesions. The commonest examples involving the brain are pituitary adenomas, which frequently cause visual impairment due to pressure on the optic chiasm.

Metastasis

The CNS is a common site for metastases, which may occur by haematogenous or direct spread. The commonest neoplasms to metastasise to the CNS are carcinomas of the breast, bronchus, kidney and colon, and malignant melanomas. Metastases often occur at the boundary between grey and white matter (Fig. 26.31) and may present as space-occupying lesions with or without focal signs. Metastatic carcinoma sometimes infiltrates the subarachnoid space producing 'meningitis carcinomatosa'. Patients with this condition present with the symptoms of subacute meningitis, often with multiple cranial nerve palsies. Metastatic deposits within the spinal cord are uncommon, but extradural metastases occur frequently and may present with paraplegia. CNS involvement occurs commonly in acute leukaemias and non-Hodgkin's lymphomas (Ch. 22) with infiltration of the subarachnoid space and parenchyma. The prognosis for patients with a metastatic neoplasm within the CNS is extremely poor.

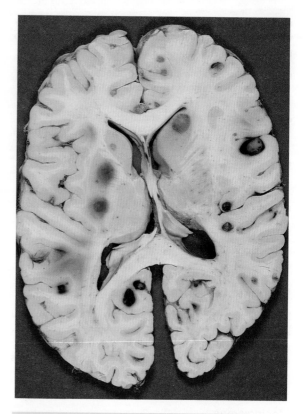

Fig. 26.31   Cerebral metastases: malignant melanoma

The darkly pigmented metastases from a malignant melanoma are present at several sites within the brain, mostly at junctions between grey and white matter. This is a characteristic pattern for metastases within the CNS.

PERIPHERAL NERVOUS SYSTEM

▶ Three main reactions to cell injury: Wallerian degeneration, segmental demyelination and distal axonal degeneration
▶ Peripheral neuropathies classified clinically according to distribution of lesions, and function of the nerve involved
▶ Commonest neoplasms arising in peripheral nerves are schwannomas and neurofibromas

NORMAL STRUCTURE AND FUNCTION

Peripheral nerves may be involved in many diseases, but because they can undergo only a limited number of pathological changes, it is important to consider their normal structure and general pathology before specific disorders are mentioned.

On histology, nerve fibres can be divided into two main groups: myelinated and non-myelinated.

Myelinated fibres

Myelinated fibres range in diameter from 2–17 μm, with myelin sheaths proportional in thickness to the diameter of the axon. Myelin is formed by the compaction of cell membranes from multiple Schwann cells along the length of the axon, to form a lamellar structure with a periodicity of 14 nm. The node of Ranvier is the site where adjacent Schwann cells meet and where their myelin sheaths terminate. This arragement allows the rapid transmission of electrical impulses by saltatory conduction, up to 10 m/s in the largest fibres.

Non-myelinated fibres

Non-myelinated fibres are much smaller in size (0.5–3 μm in diameter) and are surrounded by Schwann cell cytoplasm. The absence of myelin around these fibres results in slow conduction velocities (0.3–1.6 m/s).

REACTIONS TO INJURY

Although peripheral nerves may be involved by many disease processes, nerve fibres exhibit only three basic reactions to disease:

- axonal (Wallerian) degeneration
- segmental demyelination
- distal axonal degeneration.

These reactions may occur in combination in some peripheral neuropathies: this is usually referred to as combined or mixed degeneration.

Axonal (Wallerian) degeneration

Damage to the neuronal body, for example, anterior horn cells, spinal nerve roots or nerve trunks, results in degeneration of the axon distal to the site of the injury. In myelinated fibres, this is accompanied by breakdown of myelin around the degenerate axons (Fig. 26.32). This process is similar to anterograde degeneration in the CNS but occurs more rapidly.

Regeneration commences at 3–4 days following injury; the regenerating axonal sprouts grow at 2–3 mm/day. This is accompanied by central chromatolysis in the neuronal perikaryon, and remyelination by Schwann cells. If axonal regeneration and remyelination are successful, the re-innervation of the target organ, for example, motor end-plate of muscle, may occur. Re-innervation is hindered or prevented by factors which inhibit nerve growth, for example ischaemia or cytotoxic drugs, or disrupt the continuity of the perineurium, for example haematoma or scar tissue.

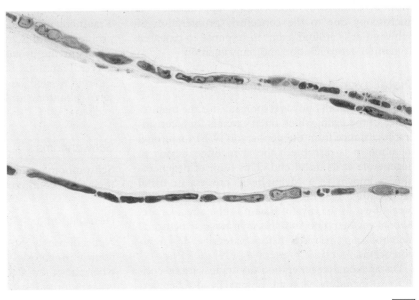

Fig. 26.32 Teased fibre preparations of peripheral nerves in Wallerian degeneration

These show a characteristic fragmentation of the myelin sheath (which appears dark) around the damaged axons.

Segmental demyelination

In segmental demyelination, the continuity of the axon is maintained, but the myelin sheath is broken down over various segments corresponding to the internodes. This results in a marked slowing of impulse conduction along the nerve fibres.

Primary segmental demyelination

Primary segmental demyelination occurs when damage to Schwann cells results in breakdown of the myelin sheath which they normally maintain. The myelin debris is eventually phagocytosed and digested by reactive macrophages. This can occur in many conditions, such as ischaemia, inherited metabolic disorders such as leukodystrophies, and the neuropathy of diphtheria.

Allergic segmental demyelination

Allergic segmental demyelination occurs when myelin sheaths are stripped and broken down by activated macrophages in the presence of lymphocytes. This mechanism is thought to operate in the Guillain–Barré syndrome. Remyelination of affected segments of nerve can occur in both allergic and primary segmental demyelination. Schwann cells in the affected internodes undergo mitosis within a few days following the injury, after which remyelination can commence.

Hypertrophic neuropathy

Certain chronic peripheral neuropathies, for example, leukodystrophies and hereditary sensorimotor neuropathy type III, are characterised by hypertrophic peripheral nerves. These are often thickened, with a distinctive 'onion-bulb' appearance on microscopy due to the concentric proliferation of Schwann cells around axons in response to repeated segmental demyelination and remyelination.

Distal axonal degeneration

The neuronal cell body is responsible for the maintenance of the axon, which often extends for a considerable distance from the perikaryon. When neuronal metabolism is disrupted, the axon often begins to degenerate at its distal end. This form of degeneration is known as a 'dying-back' process or distal axonopathy. It usually also results in secondary breakdown of the myelin sheath at the affected site. Axonal regeneration may occur if normal neuronal metabolism is restored before extensive degeneration occurs.

Distal axonal degeneration occurs in various conditions, including vitamin E and B_1 deficiencies, acute porphyria, isoniazid and hexacarbon neuropathies.

PERIPHERAL NEUROPATHY

Peripheral nerve disorders are often classified clinically according to the distribution of the lesions:

- *mononeuropathy*, e.g. carpal tunnel syndrome, diabetes: a single nerve is involved
- *mononeuritis multiplex*, e.g. polyarteritis nodosa, sarcoidosis: several isolated nerves are involved
- *polyneuropathy*, mainly motor, e.g. Guillain–Barré syndrome; mainly sensory, e.g. carcinomatous neuropathy; sensorimotor, e.g. alcoholism; autonomic, e.g. diabetes; or multiple nerve involvement.

Additional classifications include the predominant nerve fibre types involved, that is motor, sensory, autonomic or mixed. Many peripheral neuropathies are of a mixed type. Nerve biopsy will in some cases show diagnostic features, for example, in amyloid neuropathies or polyarteritis nodosa, but in many cases the aetiology of the neuropathy is not apparent on histology.

TUMOURS AND TUMOUR-LIKE CONDITIONS

Traumatic neuroma

Traumatic neuroma is not a neoplasm, but a reactive proliferation of Schwann cells and fibroblasts which occurs at the proximal severed end of a peripheral nerve. Traumatic neuromas contain disordered fascicles of twisted axons, and may produce severe pain (e.g. 'phantom limb' pain after amputation) until excised.

Schwannoma

Schwannomas are benign neoplasms that resemble their CNS counterparts histologically (p. 871).

Neurofibroma

Neurofibromas are a common manifestation of neurofibromatosis (see Phakomatoses, p. 860), when they may occur in large numbers and produce gross deformities.

Other tumours

Malignant peripheral nerve sheath tumours are rare; they occur most often in patients with neurofibromatosis, when they sometimes arise from a pre-existing neurofibroma. These neoplasms behave as sarcomas and are frequently fatal. Ganglion cell tumours occasionally arise from autonomic ganglia, particularly in the sympathetic chain. Phaeochromocytomas and neuroblastomas are discussed in Chapter 17.

- ▶ Diagnosis of skeletal muscle disorders requires clinicopathological liaison, and cannot be made on muscle biopsy histology alone
- ▶ Three groups of skeletal muscle disorders: neurogenic disorders, myopathies and disorders of neuromuscular transmission
- ▶ Neurogenic disorders and myopathies commonly occur in both children and adults; many of the latter are inherited, e.g. muscular dystrophies
- ▶ Neurogenic disorders may result from lesions affecting motor neurones, nerve roots or peripheral nerves
- ▶ Myopathic disorders include muscular dystrophies, polymyositis and other inflammatory conditions, and congenital, metabolic and toxic disorders
- ▶ Commonest disorder of neuromuscular transmission is myasthenia gravis, an autoimmune disease
- ▶ Commonest neoplasms arising in skeletal muscle are of connective tissue origin

The diagnosis of skeletal muscle diseases requires multidisciplinary investigation, often involving neurologists, neurophysiologists, neuropathologists, biochemists and geneticists. Muscle biopsy histology can contribute much important information, but it cannot alone be relied upon for a diagnosis. The innervation of muscle can be studied by electromyography and motor nerve conduction studies. Muscle fibres contain the enzyme creatine phosphokinase (CPK) which is released into the blood following muscle fibre damage; its measurement in serum is widely used in the investigation of muscle diseases.

Normal muscle consists of densely packed, uniformly-sized myofibres (40–80 μm diameter in adults) with peripheral nuclei (Fig. 26.33). The terminal axons supplying each fibre can also be studied using histochemical techniques, but the investigation of motor endplates and subcellular organelles requires electron microscopy. Muscle diseases can be classified clinically and pathologically into three main groups:

- neurogenic disorders
- myopathies
- disorders of neuromuscular transmission.

NEUROGENIC DISORDERS

Neurogenic muscle diseases all result from damage to the muscle innervation. This can occur as a consequence of lesions affecting the motor neurones in the spinal cord and brainstem, motor nerve roots or peripheral nerves. The denervated fibres undergo atrophy, and are eventually reduced to small clusters of nuclei with very little surrounding cytoplasm. Re-innervation may occur in some longstanding disorders, for example hereditary spinomuscular atrophy, producing the histological appearance of fibre type grouping (Fig. 26.34). In progressive disorders, for example motor neurone disease, the anterior horn cells responsible for re-innervation also eventually degenerate, resulting in atrophy of all the fibres in an affected muscle. Four main groups of disorders are responsible for neurogenic muscle disease:

- motor neurone disease
- spinal muscular atrophy
- peripheral neuropathies
- miscellaneous spinal disorders.

Motor neurone disease

Motor neurone disease is a progressive degenerative disorder affecting principally the anterior horn neurones in the spinal cord. (p. 860). This results in denervation atrophy (Fig. 26.34), fasciculation and weakness in affected muscles.

Spinal muscular atrophy

Spinal muscular atrophy is a group of inherited degenerative diseases affecting CNS motor neurones. The genetic locus for this group of diseases lies on the long arm of chromosome 5. It presents in four main forms which represent allelic variants:

- *Type 1 (Werdnig–Hoffmann disease)* has an onset before 3 months of age and is sometimes present at birth. This condition is rapidly progressive and usually results in death before the age of 18 months.

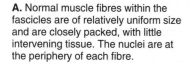

Fig. 26.33   Skeletal muscle histology

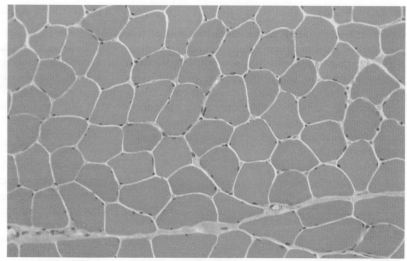

A. Normal muscle fibres within the fascicles are of relatively uniform size and are closely packed, with little intervening tissue. The nuclei are at the periphery of each fibre.

B. Histochemical preparation for myosin ATPase demonstrating the normal random mosaic pattern of fibre types within the fascicle (type 1 fibres are dark, type 2a pale and type 2b intermediate in colour).

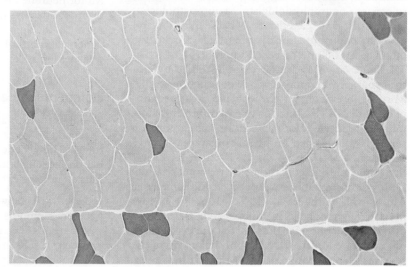

C. Histochemical preparation for myosin ATPase in a case of chronic spinal muscular atrophy showing a loss of the normal mosaic pattern, with fibre type 2b predominance and grouping.

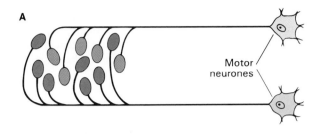

A

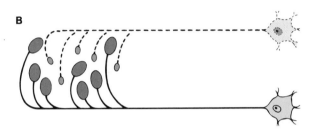

B

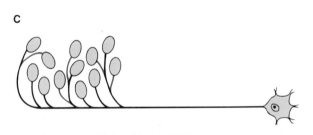

C

Fig. 26.34   Skeletal muscle: effects of denervation

A. In normal muscle, the two main fibre types are distributed in a mosaic pattern. The muscle fibre type is determined by its innervation from a motor neurone. A single motor neurone can supply many muscle fibres. **B.** Damage to a single motor neurone or its axon results in neurogenic atrophy of muscle fibres; each affected fibre is of the same fibre type. **C.** The atrophied denervated fibres can be re-innervated by axons from other motor neurones supplying adjacent fibres. This process can change the fibre type of the re-innervated muscle fibres, resulting in fibre type grouping with loss of the normal mosaic arrangement (see also Fig. 26.33C).

- *Type 2* also affects infants and children, with an onset between 6 and 12 months of age. It is more slowly progressive than Type 1, but causes severe disability with a variable life expectancy.
- *Type 3 (Kugelberg–Welander disease)* has an onset between 2 and 15 years of age. It is a slowly progressive disorder which usually allows survival into adult life with mild to moderate disability.
- *Type 4* affects adults, and pursues a very slow course, often causing mild disability. Its progress may become arrested after several decades.

Peripheral neuropathies

Peripheral neuropathies often present clinically with muscle wasting and weakness, accompanied by sensory loss in a 'glove and stocking' distribution. In chronic neuropathies, for example hereditary sensorimotor neuropathies, there is usually evidence of denervation and re-innervation on muscle biopsy.

Miscellaneous spinal cord disorders

There are a number of miscellaneous spinal cord disorders involving the anterior horn cells or ventral nerve roots, for example poliomyelitis, syringomyelia and spinal cord neoplasms.

MYOPATHIES

The main primary diseases of skeletal muscle may be classified as follows:

- muscular dystrophies
- inflammatory myopathies
- congenital myopathies
- metabolic myopathies
- toxic myopathies.

Muscular dystrophies

The muscular dystrophies form a group of inherited disorders which result in the progressive destruction of muscle fibres. The muscle innervation is normal in most cases. The most important examples are discussed below.

Duchenne dystrophy

Duchenne dystrophy is an X-linked disorder affecting 1 in 3000–5000 live male births. Approximately one-third of cases represent new mutations. The gene for this disorder has been located to the p21 region of the X chromosome. The gene product, *dystrophin*, is a protein normally present in the muscle cell membrane. Gene deletions in Duchenne dystrophy result in a deficiency of dystrophin in muscle fibre membranes, causing muscle fibre damage by the uncontrolled entry of calcium into the cell. Further understanding of the genetic defects in this disorder will allow for a fuller knowledge of its pathogenesis and hence potential for treatment.

The disease usually presents between 2 and 4 years of age, with proximal muscle weakness and pseudohypertrophy of the calves. The serum creatine phosphokinase (CPK) is elevated in the early stages of the disease, and is sometimes also elevated in female carriers. Most patients die before the age of 20, usually of the cardiomyopathy which occurs as part of this condition.

The characteristic biopsy findings are abnormal variation in the diameter of the muscle fibres, with many fibres showing hyaline degeneration or necrosis, with attempts at regeneration (Fig. 26.35). Partial or complete absence of dystrophin can be demonstrated by immunohistochemistry or Western blotting of muscle biopsies. Progressive endomysial fibrosis occurs, and eventually the muscle is almost totally replaced by fat and connective tissue.

Becker dystrophy

An X-linked disorder, Becker dystrophy, exhibits many similarities to Duchenne dystrophy, but the onset occurs at a later age and the progress of the disease is slower, many patients surviving into adult life. Genetic studies indicate that this disorder is an allelic variant of Duchenne dystrophy, involving deletions in the p21 region on the X chromosome.

Limb girdle dystrophy

The group of disorders known as limb girdle dystrophy are inherited as autosomal recessive conditions. The onset can occur in childhood or adult life, usually with weakness in the pelvic girdle and, later, the shoulder girdle. The progress of the disease is vari-able, many patients surviving with only mild to moderate disability. Muscle biopsy shows the typical dystrophic features of fibre destruction and regeneration, but to a lesser degree than occurs in Duchenne dystrophy.

Facioscapulohumeral dystrophy

Facioscapulohumeral dystrophy is an autosomal dominant disorder which usually presents in children and young adults with weakness of the face and shoulder girdle. The rate of progress is slow, and many patients survive with only mild disability. Muscle biopsy shows the features of a slowly progressive dystrophy, in which focal lymphocytic infiltration is occasionally present.

Myotonic dystrophy

Myotonic dystrophy is also an autosomal dominant condition, the gene for which has been localised to chromosome 19. The genetic abnormality is an unstable CTG repeat sequence in a cAMP-dependent protein kinase. It usually presents between 20 and 30 years of age with weakness and wasting of facial, limb girdle and proximal limb muscles. Myotonia (persistence of contraction after voluntary effort has ceased) is common in the involved muscles, and patients usually exhibit a number of systemic disorders, including cataract, balding, gonadal atrophy and diabetes mellitus. Characteristic changes are found on electromyography. Muscle

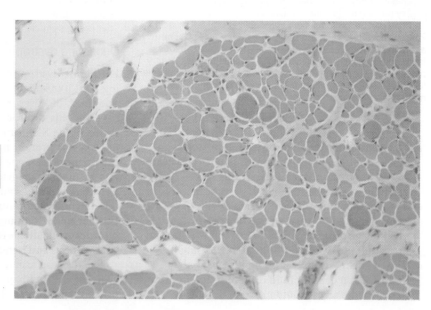

Fig. 26.35 Muscle biopsy in Duchenne muscular dystrophy

Several enlarged densely staining hyaline fibres with numerous small necrotic fibres are present throughout. There is an increased quantity of fibrous and adipose connective tissue (top left) which contributes to the muscular pseudohypertrophy noted clinically in this disease.

biopsy shows dystrophic changes, in which many fibres contain internal nuclei and exhibit a variety of cytoskeletal abnormalities.

Inflammatory myopathies

Muscle can be involved in a variety of infections, most of which are accompanied by a characteristic inflammatory reaction. The infecting organism may be:

- bacteria, such as streptococci (Group A), clostridia
- viruses, such as coxsackie B, influenza
- parasites, such as *Toxoplasma, Trichinella, Taenia solium.*

Several systemic inflammatory disorders frequently involve muscle, including sarcoidosis, systemic lupus erythematosus (SLE) and polyarteritis nodosa.

Polymyositis and dermatomyositis

Polymyositis is the commonest inflammatory muscle disorder, occurring most frequently in adults; females are affected more often than males. It may be associated with collagen vascular diseases (Ch. 25), for example systemic lupus erythematosus, or malignancies, for example bronchial carcinoma. Patients usually present with weakness, pain and swelling of proximal muscles. In dermatomyositis, the muscle inflammation is accompanied by skin involvement in the form of a characteristic violaceous facial rash, particularly in children. The serum CPK is usually elevated in the early stages of the disease, and characteristic changes are usually present on electromyography.

Histology shows muscle fibre necrosis with phagocytosis of degenerate fibres by macrophages. Lymphocytes are usually present within the endomysium and around blood vessels. Evidence of muscle fibre regeneration can usually be found, and fibre atrophy may be a striking feature in some cases, particularly in the perifascicular fibres in cases of childhood dermatomyositis.

The muscle fibre damage results from immunological injury by cytotoxic T-lymphocytes. The mechanism of sensitisation is unknown, but a coxsackievirus infection has been implicated in some cases. Treatment with immunosuppressive drugs, such as corticosteroids and azathioprine, is beneficial in many cases.

Inclusion body myositis

Inclusion body myositis is most frequent in elderly patients and clinically resembles polymyositis. Its aetiology is unknown, but affected muscles show inflammation and fibre necrosis associated with small filamentous intracellular inclusions and vacuoles. Unlike polymyositis, it responds poorly to corticosteroids and azathioprine.

Congenital myopathies

Congenital myopathies are uncommon; many of them occur as inherited disorders. Most cases present with hypotonia and floppiness in infancy; these features may prove fatal in severe cases. The diagnosis depends largely on the muscle biopsy appearances, which are thought to reflect delayed development and maturation of the muscle fibres, for example centro-nuclear myopathy, or congenital fibre type disproportion. Hypotonia in infancy is a common manifestation of muscle disease, but may be due to other disorders, including cerebral palsy, hypothyroidism and Down's syndrome.

Metabolic myopathies

Muscle involvement occurs in many inherited metabolic disorders, such as glycogenosis, carnitine deficiency and mitochondrial disorders. Most of these exhibit other systemic manifestations, for example retinitis pigmentosa in mitochondrial disorders. Other metabolic disorders involving muscle include:

- *Malignant hyperthermia.* This uncommon, dominantly inherited disorder results in an abnormal sensitivity to certain anaesthetic agents, such as halothane, which can result in a fatal hyperpyrexia on exposure.
- *Endocrine myopathies.* A large number of endocrine disorders may involve muscle, including hyper- and hypothyroidism and Cushing's syndrome. The changes are usually reversible with appropriate therapy.

Toxic myopathies

Many drugs, for example corticosteroids and penicillamine, can produce muscle damage which is usually reversible on withdrawal. One of the commonest toxins to affect skeletal muscle is ethanol. Two main patterns of damage are recognised:

- *Acute alcoholic myopathy* is induced by bouts of heavy drinking, which cause acute fibre necrosis. Release of myoglobin from the damaged fibres may result in acute renal failure.
- *Subacute alcoholic myopathy* occurs in chronic alcoholics, and presents with proximal muscle weakness and wasting. Biopsy shows selective atrophy of type 2b fibres, which is reversible in the early stages.

DISORDERS OF NEUROMUSCULAR TRANSMISSION

Two main conditions occur in this group: myasthenia gravis and Lambert–Eaton myasthenic syndrome.

Myasthenia gravis

Myasthenia gravis, an autoimmune disorder, usually presents in adults of 20–40 years of age, with fluctuating progressive weakness involving particularly the ocular, bulbar and proximal limb muscles. Females are affected more often than males. Over 90% of patients have antibodies against acetylcholine receptor proteins which bind to the post-synaptic receptor and block neurotransmission; anti-striated muscle antibodies are present in a smaller proportion of patients. Linkage with various HLA antigens has been demonstrated, for example A1, B7 and DRw3.

The thymus is hyperplastic in over 50% of patients, and a thymoma is present in a further 15%. The thymus appears to be the site of antigen presentation in this disorder, but the mechanism of sensitisation is unknown. Treatment with cholinergic drugs, immunosuppressive agents such as corticosteroids, plasmapheresis and thymectomy may be beneficial.

Lambert–Eaton myasthenic syndrome

Lambert–Eaton myasthenic syndrome is a rare, non-metastatic complication of malignancy (usually small cell carcinoma of the bronchus) which presents with limb girdle and proximal muscle weakness. Acetylcholine release from motor nerve terminals is impaired by the binding of an abnormal IgG class antibody to presynaptic calcium ion channels.

THE EYE

▶ Vascular disease of the retina in hypertension and diabetes mellitus is a common cause of visual impairment
▶ Inflammatory conditions include infectious disorders, sarcoidosis and autoimmune diseases
▶ Cataracts result from the formation of opaque proteins in the lens
▶ Glaucoma occurs when intra-ocular pressure is increased, usually due to obstruction to the outflow of aqueous fluid
▶ Commonest primary intraocular neoplasms are naevi, malignant melanomas and retinoblastomas

A brief summary of the anatomical features of the eye is given in Figure 26.36. The unique anatomy and function of the eye mean that the clinical and pathological manifestations of eye diseases often present features not encountered elsewhere.

TRAUMA

Damage to the eye can occur following direct or indirect injuries to the globe. The eye is also susceptible to damage by chemicals, for example ammonia, and physical agents, for example heat and irradiation. Direct injuries to the eye are the most important clinically, and may be classified according to the site and nature of the damage: in the perforating injuries, the sclera is only partially torn, but complete rupture occurs in penetrating injuries.

Penetrating and perforating injuries result in the most severe form of traumatic damage to the eye. The immediate complications of penetrating injuries include disruption of the globe, with haemorrhage and detachment of the lens and retina. Infection is a common complication, particularly if the missile is composed of organic material. *Sympathetic uveitis* and *ophthalmitis* are uncommon delayed complications of penetrating injuries (see below).

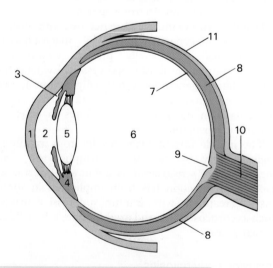

Fig. 26.36   Anatomy of the normal eye

Diagram shows cornea **(1)**, anterior chamber **(2)**, angle of the anterior chamber **(3)**, ciliary body **(4)**, lens **(5)**, posterior chamber **(6)**, retina **(7)**, choroid **(8)**, optic disc **(9)**, optic nerve **(10)**, and sclera **(11)**.

VASCULAR DISEASE

Vascular diseases are a major cause of visual impairment in the middle-aged and elderly. Two main categories are recognised: retinal ischaemia and retinal haemorrhages.

Retinal ischaemia

Retinal ischaemia usually occurs due to the occlusion of a blood vessel by atheroma, vasculitis, thrombosis or embolism. If the central retinal artery is involved, the inner two-thirds of the retina will undergo ischaemic degeneration; occlusion of the posterior ciliary artery damages the photoreceptor cells in the outer retinal layers.

Vascular occlusion in the retina causes exudation of plasma from capillaries. This is seen ophthalmoscopically as 'hard' exudates, which appear as discrete, well-defined, pale yellow retinal lesions. Ophthalmoscopy may also reveal 'soft' or 'cotton wool' exudates; these represent microinfarcts of the retina, involving both ganglion cells and nerve fibres. These lesions are most frequently seen in diabetic and hypertensive retinopathies, both of which are accompanied by changes in the retinal vessels which are readily detectable on ophthalmoscopy (Fig. 26.37).

Characteristic changes in *hypertensive retinopathy* include:

- decreased arteriolar tortuosity and calibre variation

- arteriovenous nipping
- flame-shaped haemorrhages
- soft exudates.

Characteristic changes in *diabetic retinopathy* include:

- increased tortuosity and dilatation of veins
- capillary dilatation and micro-aneurysms
- 'dot and blot' haemorrhages
- hard and soft exudates
- neovascularisation.

Retinal haemorrhages

Retinal haemorrhages may occur in a number of conditions, for example trauma or infection, but are most commonly found in diabetic and hypertensive retinopathy. Two main patterns of haemorrhage are seen on ophthalmoscopy:

- flame haemorrhages, originating from arterioles
- blot haemorrhages, focal accumulations of blood in the outer plexiform layer of the retina due to capillary rupture.

Neovascularisation

Neovascularisation is an important response to retinal ischaemia and haemorrhage, resulting in the proliferation of small vessels around the edge of the lesion. As well as proliferating in the retina, these small vessels may penetrate the vitreous fluid where the lack of supporting tissue renders them prone to

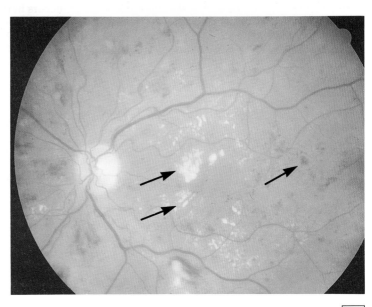

Fig. 26.37 Diabetic retinopathy

Using fundoscopy, multiple haemorrhages and exudates (arrows) are demonstrable throughout the retina in an adult with longstanding diabetes mellitus. (Courtesy of Mr B A Noble, Leeds)

rupture and haemorrhage. Neovascularisation can also occur in response to senile macular degeneration, causing a submacular fibrovascular mass which damages the overlying photoreceptor cells and results in loss of central vision.

INFLAMMATORY LESIONS

Micro-organisms, an important cause of ocular inflammation, can gain access to the eye by haematogenous spread from adjacent tissues, for example the paranasal sinuses, or from the external surface of the eye.

Bacterial infections

Bacterial infections can occur at any site within the eye, but are particularly liable to spread to the vitreous fluid and lens, where the local conditions favour growth of organisms. The cellular reactions to infection in the eye are similar to those elsewhere in the body and will not therefore be described in detail.

Inflammation of the uvea and ciliary body leads to exudation of protein and inflammatory cells into the posterior cornea which can be detected on ophthalmoscopy. Local inflammatory changes can result in adhesions within the anterior chamber, causing glaucoma (see below).

Viral infections

Important viral infections include:

- adenovirus 3,7, causing follicular conjunctivitis
- adenovirus 8,19, causing epidemic keratoconjunctivitis
- herpes simplex type 1 virus, causing superficial punctate keratitis and dendritic corneal ulcers
- varicella zoster virus, causing corneal vesicles with scarring.

Chlamydial infections

Two main forms of infection occur:

- *Chlamydia trachomatis A–C* cause *trachoma*, a tropical disease which is a common cause of blindness. The organism infects the conjunctival and corneal epithelium, and can be identified as intracytoplasmic inclusions on conjunctival smears.
- *Chlamydia trachomatis D–K* commonly infect the genital tract, but can cause a mild form of *keratoconjunctivitis*. The organism can be identified and cultured from conjunctival smears.

Parasitic infections

Acanthamoeba
Acanthamoeba is a free-living protozoan in mains water supplies. It can cause a corneal infection (keratitis) and may invade the eye, particularly in contact lens wearers. Antibiotic therapy is usually effective, although invasive infections are difficult to eradicate.

Toxoplasmosis
In congenital infections with the protozoan *Toxoplasma gondii*, the organism spreads to numerous sites in the body. Retinal involvement takes the form of chorioretinitis with extensive tissue destruction and microphthalmos in severe cases.

Toxocara canis
Toxocara canis infection is usually acquired in childhood from contact with ova from infected dogs. Ingestion of the ova is followed by liberation of larvae in the stomach and duodenum; the larvae migrate through the body but do not usually mature. A granuloma can develop in the retina around a dead larva, causing visual obstruction which clinically may mimic an intraocular neoplasm.

Sarcoidosis

Ocular involvement is often one of the main manifestations of sarcoidosis, along with erythema nodosum and hilar lymphadenopathy. The granulomatous inflammation characteristic of sarcoidosis occurs in three main forms:

- conjunctivitis
- iridocyclitis (the commonest form)
- retinitis, sometimes involving the optic nerve head.

Autoimmune disease

This group of uncommon disorders almost always arises as a consequence of ocular injury, particularly perforating wounds. Prompt clinical attention to such injuries has greatly reduced the incidence of these complications.

Lens-induced uveitis

Release of lens protein into the anterior chamber or vitreous (usually as a result of trauma) occasionally causes a giant cell granulomatous reaction involving the lens and uvea. This results from a delayed hypersensitivity reaction following sensitisation to lens antigens.

Sympathetic ophthalmitis

Trauma to one eye with damage to the iris or ciliary body may cause a delayed hypersensitivity reaction following sensitisation to uveal and retinal antigens. This results in a giant cell granulomatous inflammatory response in either the damaged eye or the second eye. Children are particularly susceptible to this uncommon complication.

CATARACT

The normal structure of the lens depends on the integrity of its elastic capsule, the viability of the lens fibre cells, which contain transparent proteins, and a supply of essential metabolites in the fluid.

Cataracts result from the formation of opaque proteins within the lens which usually also result in a loss of lens elasticity. This can occur in:

- rubella
- Down's syndrome
- senile degeneration
- tears in lens capsule
- irradiation
- uveitis
- diabetes mellitus
- corticosteroid therapy.

Mature cataracts can cause severe visual loss, but this can be treated surgically by removal of the affected lens and insertion of a synthetic plastic substitute. Cataracts occasionally cause glaucoma due to mechanical obstruction of the anterior chamber angle, or lens dislocation.

GLAUCOMA

The normal intra-ocular pressure is 15–20 mmHg. This pressure depends on:

- the rate of the production of aqueous fluid
- the resistance to fluid movement in the outflow system.

Glaucoma denotes a group of disorders in which the intra-ocular pressure is increased to a level which impedes blood supply to the retina, ultimately resulting in blindness. The increase in intra-ocular pressure is usually caused by obstruction to the outflow of aqueous fluid, for example at the trabecular meshwork, canal of Schlemm or the drainage angle of the anterior chamber (Fig. 26.36).

Closed-angle glaucoma

Closure of the irideocorneal angle, thus obstructing the drainage of aqueous humour from the anterior chamber, can occur when the iris is in mid-dilatation, particularly in middle-aged or elderly individuals. This results in acute glaucoma, with corneal oedema, congestion and pain. The next commonest cause of closed-angle glaucoma is neovascularisation around the irideocorneal angle (Fig. 26.38) following a variety of disorders, for example haemorrhage, ischaemia or infection.

Open-angle glaucoma

Open-angle glaucoma can occur as a primary degenerative condition in the elderly, when a progressive accumulation of collagen within the trabeculae and extracellular space of the outflow system increases resistance to the flow of aqueous fluid. This results in a slow increase in intra-ocular pressure which is often manifest clinically as a central visual field defect. The nerve fibres in the optic disc suffer compression and ischaemic damage, which can be visualised as cupping of the disc on ophthalmoscopy.

Open-angle glaucoma may also occur due to mechanical obstruction of the outflow system by inflammatory cells, haemorrhage or tumour infiltration. The effects of raised intra-ocular pressure are:

- central visual defect due to retinal ischaemia
- bullous keratopathy due to corneal oedema
- scleral bulges (staphylomas) due to scleral stretching
- in infants, expansion of the eye (buphthalmos).

OCULAR TUMOURS

A large variety of neoplasms may arise within the eye and its adnexa, tumours in the latter resembling those occurring in the skin, connective tissue and salivary glands. The most important intra-ocular tumours are naevi and malignant melanoma, and retinoblastoma.

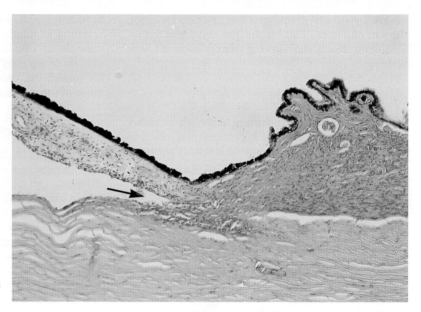

Fig. 26.38 Closed-angle glaucoma: neovascularisation

The aqueous outflow at the anterior chamber angle (arrow) is obstructed by a mass of fibrovascular tissue containing numerous capillaries. The resulting increase in intra-ocular pressure caused glaucoma, which eventually necessitated removal of the eye.

Naevi and malignant melanoma

Naevi and malignant melanoma occur most frequently in adults, and derive from the melanocytes of the uveal tract. *Naevi* are benign melanocytic lesions akin to those commonly occurring in skin. *Malignant melanomas* occur as a solitary mass in one eye, usually arising in the posterior choroid. The neoplasm often grows rapidly to form an intra-ocular mass which causes extensive retinal detachment and secondary glaucoma (Fig. 26.39). Histologically, two main patterns are recognised:

- *Spindle cell melanoma.* This has a relatively good prognosis, greater than 50% survival at five years.
- *Epithelioid melanoma.* This has a much worse prognosis. Blood spread to other organs (particularly the liver) can occur; these metastases sometimes present many years after enucleation of the affected eye.

Melanomas may also arise in the iris; these are associated with a better prognosis and seldom metastasise.

Retinoblastoma

There has been much recent interest in retinoblastoma. It is an uncommon neoplasm, with an incidence in the United Kingdom of around 1 per 20 000 live births. 5–10% of cases are familial, with affected individuals inheriting a deletion on the long arm of chromosome 13 which always involves a specific site (band q14). The same chromosomal abnormality occurs in tumour tissue (but not normal tissue) from patients with sporadic retinoblastomas (Ch. 11).

Children with retinoblastomas present with either visual loss, squint or enlargement of the eye, which is occupied by a tumour within the retina. On histology, the neoplasm has the features of a primitive neuroectodermal tumour, in which the cells tend to form rosettes. Local extension along the optic nerve or through the sclera is common, but distant metastases are rare. The results of early enucleation and radiotherapy are good, with a five-year survival of around 90%.

Optic nerve glioma

Optic nerve glioma is a rare neoplasm which occurs most frequently in children and young adults; it is a well-recognised complication of neurofibromatosis and tuberous sclerosis. Patients usually present with progressive visual failure, with proptosis and papilloedema. The histological features are those of a well-differentiated astrocytoma. The results of surgery and radiotherapy are good, with over 90% of patients surviving for five years or more.

Metastatic carcinoma

Metastatic carcinomas form the largest group of intra-ocular neoplasms. The commonest primary sources are breast carcinoma in females, and bronchial carcinoma in males.

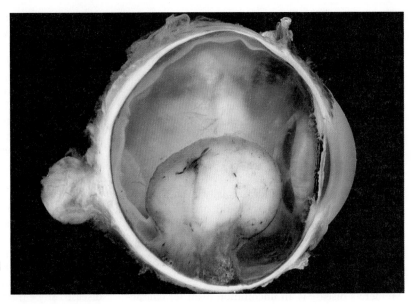

Fig. 26.39 Malignant melanoma: intra-ocular mass

In this eye, a large unpigmented malignant melanoma is arising from the choroid. The neoplasm has caused extensive retinal elevation and detachment.

THE EAR

MIDDLE EAR

The middle ear and mastoid air cells of the temporal bone are extensions of the upper respiratory tract, and are lined by ciliated epithelium. Infections in these sites are common, particularly in children, and may occur as part of a generalised upper respiratory tract infection.

Otitis media

Acute otitis media

Acute otitis media may result from primary or secondary bacterial infections; the latter occasionally complicate a viral illness. Acute bacterial otitis media is a suppurative inflammatory process most often caused by *Haemophilus influenzae* or *Streptococcus pneumoniae*. The inflammatory exudate can cause the tympanic membrane to bulge and rupture, and may spread to the mastoid air cells, causing acute mastoiditis. This condition usually responds rapidly to antibiotics.

Serous otitis media

Serous otitis media is a non-suppurative process in which fluid accumulates in the middle ear as a con-

sequence of Eustachian tube obstruction. It is an important cause of hearing difficulties in children ('glue ear') and can be relieved by removing the Eustachian obstruction, for example in patients with tonsillar hyperplasia.

Chronic otitis media

Chronic otitis media usually results from persistent or repeated acute bacterial infections. Common complications include:

- tympanic perforation and discharge
- aural polyps: granulation tissue in the middle ear
- disarticulation and resorption of ossicles, with conductive hearing loss
- cholesteatoma: accumulation of keratin derived from squamous epithelium spreading in from the external auditory canal following tympanic perforation.

Tumours

Middle-ear neoplasms are uncommon. The most frequently encountered are:

- adenomas: derived from the lining epithelium
- squamous cell carcinomas
- jugular paragangliomas: arising from paraganglia (chemoreceptor cells) in the glomus jugulare. These slow-growing neoplasms usually occur in women aged 40–60 years, and are characterised by relentless local invasion. Metastases are uncommon.

INNER EAR

The most important clinical manifestations of inner-ear disorders are deafness and dizziness. These occur in varying degrees, due to impaired cochlear and vestibular function. Amongst the commonest disorders affecting the inner ear are labyrinthitis, Menière's disease and otosclerosis.

Labyrinthitis

Infections of the labyrinth are usually viral; mumps, cytomegalovirus and rubella are the organisms most frequently involved. The inflammatory process usually subsides spontaneously.

Menière's disease

Menière's disease is an uncommon disorder charac-terised clinically by attacks of nausea, vertigo, nystagmus, tinnitus and hearing loss. The pathogenesis is unknown, but the disease results in distension of the endolymphatic system in the cochlear duct and saccule. The vestibular membrane of Reissner may rupture, and the distended saccule compresses adjacent structures. The aetiology of Menière's disease is uncertain, but similar symptoms may occur in post-infectious labyrinthitis following upper respiratory tract viral infections.

Otosclerosis

Otosclerosis is one of the commonest causes of hearing loss in young adults. It affects females more often than males, and is inherited as an autosomal dominant trait with variable penetrance. The conductive hearing loss results from bone deposition around the stapes footplate, which eventually results in ankylosis. The disease can be treated surgically by stapedectomy.

FURTHER READING

Adams J H, Graham D I 1994 An introduction to neuropathology, 2nd edn. Churchill Livingstone, Edinburgh
Anderson J R 1985 Atlas of skeletal muscle pathology (Current histopathology, vol 9). MTP Press, Lancaster
Burger P C, Scheithauer B W 1994 Atlas of tumor pathology, third series, fascicle 10: Tumors of the central nervous system. Armed Forces Institute of Pathology, Washington DC

Esiri M M, Oppenheimer D R 1989 Diagnostic neuropathology. Edward Arnold, London
Weller R O (ed) 1990 Systemic pathology, vol 4: Nervous system, muscle and eyes, 3rd edn. Churchill Livingstone, Edinburgh
Yanoff M, Fine B S 1992 Ocular pathology: A color atlas, 2nd edn. Gower Medical Publishing, New York

Glossary

Abscess Localised collection of pus resulting from an inflammatory reaction, often provoked by bacteria.

Acantholysis Separation of individual cells of the epidermis, often resulting in a bulla (blister).

Acanthosis Increased thickness of the stratum spinosum of the epidermis.

Achalasia Failure of a gut sphincter (usually) to relax causing dilatation proximally.

Achlorhydria Lack of gastric acid secretion.

Acidosis Disturbance of acid–base balance characterised by acidity (decreased pH) of body fluids (contrast with alkalosis).

Acquired Due to an event after birth (contrast with congenital).

Acute Appearing rapidly (e.g. acute inflammation), but not necessarily severe as in common usage (contrast with chronic).

Adenocarcinoma Malignant neoplasm of glandular or secretory epithelium.

Adenoma Benign glandular neoplasm.

Adenosis Glandular proliferation.

Adhesion Abnormal band or layer of connective tissue fixing two or more normally separate structures (e.g. between loops of bowel after peritonitis).

-aemia Suffix — of the blood.

Aetiology Cause of a disease.

Agenesis Failure of a tissue or organ to form during embryogenesis.

Agonal Terminal event, immediately prior to death.

Alkalosis Disturbance of acid–base balance characterised by alkalinity (increased pH) of body fluids (contrast with acidosis).

Allele One copy of a paired gene.

Allergy Excessive and/or inappropriate immunological reaction to an environmental antigen (allergen) as in hay fever, allergic asthma and some adverse drug reactions.

Allograft Tissue transplanted between two individuals of the same species.

Amyloid Insoluble extracellular material of variable composition (e.g. immunoglobulin light chains, amyloid protein A) causing hardening, enlargement and malfunction of the organs in which it is deposited.

Ana- Prefix — absent.

Anaemia Abnormally low blood haemoglobin concentration.

Anamnestic (response) Immunological reaction enhanced by previous exposure to the same agent.

Anaphylaxis Excessive and/or inappropriate type I immunological reaction; often used synonymously with hypersensitivity.

Anaplasia	Lack of differentiated features, usually in a tumour (i.e. anaplastic tumour).
Aneuploid	Abnormal chromosome numbers other than in exact multiples of the haploid state (i.e. not diploid, tetraploid, etc.); DNA aneuploidy is abnormal quantities of DNA per nucleus other than in exact multiples of the haploid quantity.
Aneurysm	Abnormal permanent dilatation of a blood vessel or part of a heart chamber.
Angiitis	Inflammation of a blood vessel.
Anisocytosis	Abnormal variation in size of red blood cells.
Ankylosis	Fusion of a joint, resulting in its impaired mobility.
Annular	Encircling the circumference of a hollow tube (e.g. annular carcinoma of the colon).
Anoxia	Lack of oxygen.
Antibody	Immunoglobulin with antigen specificity.
Antidote	Agent countering the harmful effects of a poison.
Antigen	A substance binding specifically to an antibody or T-cell antigen receptor.
Antiserum	Serum containing specific antibody.
Antitoxin	Antibody capable of neutralising a bacterial toxin.
Aplasia	Failure of growth of a tissue (e.g. aplastic anaemia).
Apoptosis	A form of normal or pathological individual cell death characterised by activation of endogenous endonucleases.
APUDoma	Neoplasm of APUD cells (APUD = amine content and/or precursor uptake and decarboxylation) (e.g. carcinoid tumour, insulinoma).
Arteriosclerosis	Hardening of the arteries caused by any condition.
Arteritis	Inflammation primarily within the wall of arteries (e.g. polyarteritis nodosa).
Ascites	Abnormal accumulation of fluid in the peritoneal cavity.
Aseptic	1. Performed in such a way as to avoid infection (e.g. by using sterile instruments); 2. inflammatory illness not due to any identifiable bacterium (e.g. 'aseptic' meningitis).
Asphyxia	Consequence of suffocation or mechanically impaired respiration.
Atelectasis	Failure to expand, usually of the lung.
Atheroma	Condition characterised by the focal accumulation of lipid in the intima of arteries causing their lumen to be narrowed, their wall to be weakened and predisposing to thrombosis.
Atherosclerosis	Atheroma causing hardening of arteries.
Atopy	Condition characterised by predisposition to allergies.
Atresia	Embryological failure of formation of the lumen of a normally hollow viscus or duct (e.g. biliary atresia).
Atrophy	Pathological or physiological cellular or organ shrinkage.

Atypia	Departure from the typical normal appearance, usually histological, either reactive or sometimes denoting pre-neoplastic change (i.e. dysplasia).
Auto-antibody	Antibody reactive with the body's own tissues or constituents.
Autocrine	Characteristic of a cell responding to growth factors, cytokines, etc. produced by it (contrast with endocrine and paracrine); when unregulated, a feature of neoplasia.
Autograft	Tissue transplanted in the same individual from which it is taken.
Autoimmunity	abnormal state in which the body's immune system reacts against its own tissues or constituents.
Autologous	Transplantation or transfusion in which the donor and recipient are the same individual.
Autolysis	Digestion of tissue by the enzymes contained within it.
Autopsy	Synonymous with necropsy or postmortem examination (autopsy = 'to see for oneself' rather than relying on signs and symptoms).
Autosomal (gene)	Residing on any autosome (autosomes are chromosomes other than sex chromosomes).
Bacteraemia	Presence of bacteria in the blood.
Bacteriuria	Presence of bacteria in the urine.
Benign	Relatively harmless though usually not without risk of serious consequences if untreated; as in benign hypertension (mild blood pressure elevation associated with insidious tissue injury), and benign neoplasm (tumour that does not invade or metastasise); (contrast with malignant).
Biopsy	The process of removing tissue for diagnosis, or a piece of tissue removed during life for diagnostic purposes.
'Blast' cell	Any primitive cell but especially a primitive haemopoietic cell such as a myeloblast, the presence of which in the blood is suspicious of acute leukaemia.
-blastoma	Suffix — tumour histologically resembling the embryonic state of the organ in which it arises and more commonly seen in young children (e.g. retinoblastoma).
Bronchiectasis	Permanent abnormal dilatation of bronchi.
Bulla	An abnormal thin-walled cavity filled with liquid (e.g. bulla of skin) or gas (e.g. emphysematous bulla of lung).
Cachexia	Extreme wasting of the body often associated with a malignant neoplasm.
Cadherin	Calcium-dependent cell surface adhesion molecule.
Calcification	Process occurring naturally in bone and teeth, but abnormally in some diseased tissues (dystrophic calcification) or as a result of hypercalcaemia ('metastatic' calcification).
Calculus	Stone (e.g. gallstone).
Callus	1. New immature bone formed within and around a bone fracture; 2. patch of hard skin formed at the site of repeated rubbing (also referred to as a "callosity")
Cancer	A general term, in the public domain, usually implying any malignant tumour.

Carbuncle

Large pus-filled swelling, usually on the skin, often discharging through several openings and invariably due to a staphylococcal infection.

Carcinogenesis

Mechanisms of the causation of malignant neoplasms (usually not just carcinomas).

Carcinoid

Tumour of usually low-grade malignancy arising from APUD cells but not characterised by the production of a peptide hormone from which an alternative name might be derived (e.g. insulinoma); often secretes 5-hydroxytryptamine (serotonin).

Carcinoma

A malignant epithelial neoplasm.

Carcinoma in situ

A malignant epithelial neoplasm that has not yet invaded through the original basement membrane; synonymous with intra-epithelial neoplasia (see CIN).

CD

Cluster of differentiation (or designation); a standard numerical coding scheme for antigens borne by different types and sub-types of leukocytes and some other cells; used for indentification of these cells by immunological methods.

Caruncle

Small fleshy nodule; whether normal or pathological depends on location.

Caseation

Type of necrosis, characteristically associated with tuberculosis, in which the dead tissue has a cheesey structureless consistency.

Cellulitis

Diffuse acute inflammation of the skin caused by streptococcal infection.

Centimorgan

Length of DNA estimated from exchange of homologous genetic material, between chromosomes during meiosis, averaging 1 cross-over per 100 gametes.

Centromere

Chromosomal constriction at which the chromatids are joined.

Cerebrovascular accident

Cerebral infarction, or haemorrhage within or around the brain.

CVA

Synonymous with 'stroke'.

Cestode

A tapeworm.

Chemotaxis

Migration of cells induced by some chemical influence such as complement components, and causing accumulation of leukocytes in inflamed tissues.

Cholestasis

Reduced or absent bile flow, thus leading to jaundice (cholestatic jaundice).

Chromatolysis (of nucleus)

Dissolution of the nucleus evident from the loss of its staining characteristics.

Chronic

Persisting for a long time (e.g. chronic inflammation) (contrast with acute).

CIN

Cervical intra-epithelial neoplasia, a precursor of invasive squamous cell carcinoma of the cervix uteri; graded I to III depending on the degree of severity.

Cirrhosis (liver)

Irreversible architectural disturbance characterised by nodules of hepatocytes with intervening fibrosis; a consequence of many forms of chronic liver injury.

Clot (blood)

Blood coagulated outside the cardiovascular system or after death (contrast with thrombus).

Coagulation

Solidification of material (e.g., blood coagulation, coagulative necrosis).

Coarctation

Congenital narrowing of the aorta.

Comedo(ne)	Plug of material (e.g. in some intraduct breast carcinomas, and in the lesions of acne vulgaris).
Comminuted (fracture)	Bone broken into fragments at fracture site.
Complement	Collective noun for a set of blood proteins which when activated in cascade by, for example, antigen–antibody reactions has various effects including leukocyte chemotaxis and cell lysis.
Complications	Events secondary to the primary disorder (e.g. complicated fracture involves adjacent nerves and/or vessels; cerebral haemorrhage is a complication of hypertension).
Compound	Involving more than one structure (e.g. compound naevus involves dermis and epidermis; compound bone fracture is associated with traumatic defect in the overlying skin).
Condyloma	Warty lesion often on genitalia.
Congenital	Condition attributable to events prior to birth, not necessarily genetic or inherited.
Congestion	Engorgement with blood.
Consolidation	Solidification of lung tissue, usually by an inflammatory exudate; a feature of pneumonia.
Cyst	Cavity with an epithelial lining and containing fluid or other material (contrast with pseudocyst).
Cytokines	Substances (e.g. interleukins) produced by one cell which influence the behaviour of another, thus effecting intercellular communication.
Cytopathic (virus effect)	Causing cell injury, not necessarily lethal.
Cytotoxic	Causing cell injury, not necessarily lethal.
Degeneration	Disorder, not otherwise classified, characterised by loss of structural and functional integrity of an organ or tissue.
Demyelination	Loss of myelin from around nerve fibres.
Desmoid (tumour)	A tumour-like connective tissue proliferation related to fibromatosis.
Desmoplasia	Proliferation of connective tissue, typically a stromal response to tumours.
Diapedesis	Passage of blood cells between endothelial cells into the perivascular tissue; characteristic of inflammation.
Diploid	Twice the haploid chromosome number or DNA content.
Differentiation	1. Embryological—process by which a tissue develops special characteristics; 2. pathological—degree of morphological resemblance of a neoplasm to its parent tissue.
Diffuse	Affecting the tissue in a continuous or widespread distribution.
Disease	Abnormal state causing or capable of causing ill health.
Diverticulum	Abnormal hollow pouch communicating with the lumen of the structure from which it has arisen.
Dominant	Characteristic of a gene of which only one copy is necessary for it it be expressed.

Dyskeratosis Disordered or premature keratinization; a feature of dysplasia in squamous epithelium.

Dysplasia Abnormal growth and differentiation of a tissue; in epithelia, often a feature of the early stages of neoplasia.

Dystrophy Abnormal development or degeneration of a tissue (e.g. muscular dystrophy, dystrophic calcification).

Ecchymoses Any bruise or haemorrhagic spot, larger than petechiae, on the skin (may be spontaneous in the elderly, usually due more to vascular fragility than to coagulation defects).

Ectasia Abnormal dilatation (e.g. lymphangiectasia — dilatation of lymphatics).

Ectopic Tissue or substance in or from an inappropriate site (but not by metastasis).

Effusion Abnormal collection of fluid in a body cavity (e.g. pleura, peritoneum, synovial joint).

Elastosis 1. Increase in elastin in a tissue; 2. altered collagen with staining properties normally characteristic of elastin.

Embolus Fluid (e.g. gas, fat) or solid (e.g. thrombus) mass mobile within a blood vessel and capable of blocking its lumen.

Emphysema Characterised by the formation of abnormal thin-walled gas-filled cavities; pulmonary emphysema — in lungs, 'surgical' emphysema — in connective tissues.

Empyema Cavity filled with pus (e.g. empyema of the gallbladder).

Endocrine Characteristic of cells producing hormones with distant effects (contrast with autocrine and paracrine).

Endophytic Tumour growing inwards from a surface, usually by invasion and thus malignant (contrast with exophytic).

Endotoxin Toxin derived from disruption of the outer membrane of gram-negative bacteria (contrast with exotoxin).

Epithelioid Histologically resembling epithelium; specifically as in epithelioid cells which are derived from macrophages and a distinctive feature of granulomas.

Eponym Name of a disease, etc. derived from its association with a place or person (e.g. Cushing's disease).

Erosion Loss of superficial layer (not full-thickness) of a surface (e.g. gastric erosion).

Erythema Abnormal redness of skin due to increased blood flow.

Essential (disease type) Without evident antecedent cause; synonymous with primary and idiopathic.

Exon Portion of a gene encoding the RNA and protein product (contrast with intron).

Exophytic Tumour growing outwards from a surface, usually because it lacks invasive properties (contrast with endophytic).

Exotoxin Toxin secreted by living bacteria (contrast with endotoxin).

Extrinsic 1. Outside the structure and, for example, compressing it (e.g. tumour outside the intestine, but compressing it and causing intestinal obstruction); 2. cause external to the body (e.g. extrinsic allergic alveolitis); (contrast with intrinsic).

Exudate	Extravascular accumulation of protein-rich fluid due to increased vascular permeability (contrast with transudate).
Fibrinoid	Resembling fibrin (e.g. fibrinoid necrosis).
Fibrinous	Rich in fibrin (e.g. fibrinous exudate).
Fibroid	Benign smooth-muscle tumour (leiomyoma) commonly arising from uterine myometrium.
Fibromatosis	A tumour-like infiltrative proliferation of fibroblasts and myofibroblasts.
Fibrosis	Process of depositing excessive collagen in a tissue.
Fibrous (tissue)	Connective tissue comprising predominantly fibroblasts and collagen.
Fistula	Abnormal connection between one hollow viscus and another or with the skin surface.
Fluke	A trematode (flatworm) of the order Digenea.
Focal	Localised abnormality (contrast with diffuse).
Follicular	Forming a circumscribed structure resembling a follicle (but not necessarily secretory, as would be the strict definition of follicular).
Forme fruste	Early stage of a disease, either at diagnosis or interrupted by treatment, before it has developed a complete set of characteristics.
Free radicals	Chemical radicals characterised by unpaired electrons in the outer shell and therefore highly reactive.
Fungating	Forming an elevated growth, usually neoplastic (and usually malignant).
Furuncle	A boil.
Ganglion (pathological)	Cystic lesion containing mucin-rich fluid associated with a joint or tendon sheath.
Gangrene	Bulk necrosis of tissues; 'dry' gangrene — sterile; 'wet' gangrene — with bacterial putrefaction.
Genotype	1. Genetic constitution of an individual; 2. Classification of organisms according to their genetic characteristics (contrast with serotype).
Giant cell	Abnormally large cell, often multinucleated.
Gliosis	Increase in glial fibres, within the central nervous system; analogous to fibrosis elsewhere in the body.
Goitre	Enlarged thyroid gland.
Grade	Degree of malignancy of a neoplasm usually judged from its histological features (e.g. nuclear size and regularity, mitotic frequency); (compare with stage).
Granulation tissue	Newly formed connective tissue often found at the edge or base of ulcers and wounds, comprising capillaries, fibroblasts, myofibroblasts and inflammatory cells embedded in mucin-rich ground substance.
Granuloma	An aggregate of epithelioid macrophages, often including giant multinucleate cells also derived from macrophages (histiocytes).

Gumma	Focal necrotic lesion in tertiary stage of syphilis.
Haematocrit	Volume fraction of blood consisting of cells.
Haematoma	Localised collection of blood or blood clot, usually within a solid tissue.
Haemostasis	Natural ability to arrest bleeding (e.g. by vascular spasm and blood coagulation) or its arrest by artificial means (e.g. by ligating a blood vessel).
Hamartoma	Congenital tumour-like malformation comprising two or more mature tissue elements normally present in the organ in which it arises.
Haploid	Single allocation of unpaired chromosomes, as found in ova and spermatozoa.
Hernia	Abnormal protrusion of an organ, or part of it, outside its usual compartment.
Heterologous	1. Transplantation or transfusion in which the donor and recipient are of different species (synonymous with xenogeneic); 2. Tissue not normally present at that site (contrast with homologous).
Heterotopia	Presence of normal tissue in an abnormal location, usually due to an error in embryogenesis.
Histiocyte	Macrophage within tissue.
Histogenesis	In the context of neoplasms, a term meaning the putative cell of origin.
Homeobox	Highly conserved DNA sequences usually present in genes controlling development.
Homograft	Transplantation from one individual to another of the same species.
Homologous	1. Transplantation or transfusion in which the donor and recipient are of the same species (synonymous with allogeneic); 2. Tissue normally present at that site (contrast with heterologous).
Hyaline	Amorphous texture, sometimes due to the deposition or accumulation of intra- or extracellular material (e.g. amyloid, Mallory's hyalin).
Hydrocele	Fluid-filled cavity, especially surrounding a testis.
Hyperaemia	Increased blood flow, usually through a capillary bed as in acute inflammation.
Hyperchromatic	Increased histological staining, usually of nucleus.
Hyperkeratosis	Formation of excess keratin on the surface of stratified squamous epithelium (e.g. epidermis).
Hyperplasia	Enlargement of an organ, or a tissue within it, due to an increase in the *number* of cells.
Hypersensitivity	Excessive or inappropriate reaction to an environmental agent, often mediated immunologically (see allergy).
Hypertrophy	Enlargement of an organ, or part of it, due to an increase in the *size* of cells.
Hypoxia	Reduction in available oxygen.
Iatrogenic	Caused by medical intervention (e.g. adverse effect of a prescribed drug).
Idiopathic	Unknown cause; synonymous with primary, essential and cryptogenic.
Immunity	A body defence mechanism characterised by specificity and memory.

Incompetence (valvular)	Allowing regurgitation when valve is closed.
Infarction	Death of tissue (an infarct) due to insufficient blood supply.
Infiltrate	Abnormal accumulation of cells (e.g. leukocytes, neoplastic cells) or acellular material (e.g. amyloid) in a tissue.
Integrins	Heterodimeric molecules responsible for cell—cell and cell—matrix adhesion.
Interleukins	Cytokines produced by leukocytes.
Intrinsic	1. Within a structure rather than compressing it from without; 2. defect without obvious external cause (e.g. intrinsic asthma); (contrast with extrinsic).
Intron	Portion of a gene not encoding the protein product (contrast with exon).
Intussusception	Invagination or telescoping of a tubular structure, especially bowel.
Invasion	Property of malignant neoplastic cells enabling them to infiltrate normal tissues and enter blood vessels and lymphatics.
Involution	Reduction in size of an organ or part of it; may be physiological (e.g. shrinkage of thymus gland before adulthood).
Ischaemia	An inadequate blood supply to an organ or part of it.
-itis	Suffix — inflammatory.
Junctional	At the interface between two structures (e.g. junctional naevus is characterised by naevus cells at the dermo-epidermal junction).
Karyolysis	Disintegration of the nucleus.
Karyorrhexis	Nuclear fragmentation seen in necrotic cells.
Karyotype	Description of the number and shape of chromosomes within a cell, normally characteristic of a species.
Keratinisation	Production of keratin by normal or neoplastic stratified squamous epithelium.
Keratosis	Excess keratin.
Koilocytosis	Vacuolation of the cells of stratified squamous epithelium (e.g. skin, cervix) often characteristic of human papillomavirus infection.
Latent (interval)	Period between exposure to the cause of a disease and the appearance of the disease itself (e.g. incubation period).
Leiomyo-	Prefix — of smooth muscle (e.g. leiomyosarcoma — malignant neoplasm of smooth muscle).
Lesion	Any abnormality associated with injury or disease.
Leukaemia	Neoplastic proliferation of white blood cells; classified into acute and chronic types, according to onset and likely behaviour, and from the cell type (e.g. lymphocytic, granulocytic).
Leukocytosis	Excessive number of white blood cells (leukocytes).
Leukopenia	Lack of white blood cells.
Lipo-	Prefix — of adipose tissue (e.g. lipoma — benign adipose tumour).
-lithiasis	Formation of calculi (stones) (e.g. cholelithiasis — gallstones).

Lobar	Affecting a lobe, especially of lung as in lobar pneumonia.
Lobular	Affecting or arising from a lobule (e.g. lobular carcinoma of the breast).
Loss of heterozygosity	Loss of constitutional maternal or paternal alleles of a gene which, if lost from all abnormal cells in a lesion, indicates a monoclonal proliferation; a molecular marker of neoplasia especially if at a tumour-suppressor gene locus.
Lymphokine	Cytokine produced by lymphocytes.
Lymphoma	Primary malignant neoplasm of lymphoid tissue classified according to cell type.
Lysis	Dissolution or disintegration of a cell, usually as a result of chemical effects.
Malformation	Congenital structural abnormality of the body.
Malignant	Condition characterised by relatively high risk of morbidity and mortality (e.g. malignant hypertension — high blood pressure leading to severe tissue damage; malignant neoplasm — invasive neoplasm with risk of metastasis); (contrast with benign).
Marantic (thrombus)	Occurring in association with severe wasting (marasmus), usually in infants.
Margination	Gathering of leukocytes on endothelial surface of capillaries and venules in acute inflammation.
Medullary (tumour)	Of a relatively soft consistency.
Melanoma	Malignant neoplasm of melanocytes (except 'juvenile' melanoma which is benign).
Metaplasia	Reversible change in the character of a tissue from one mature cell type to another.
Metastasis	Process by which a primary malignant neoplasm gives rise to secondary tumours (metastases) at other sites most commonly by lymphatic, vascular or transcoelomic spread.
Mole	1. Common benign skin lesion composed of melanocytes and/or melanocytic naevus cells; 2. hydatidiform mole—rare benign disorder of pregnancy characterised by swollen chorionic villi and hyperplastic trophoblast.
Monoclonal	Attributable to a single clone of cells and thus more characteristic of a neoplasm than of a reactive process (contrast with polyclonal).
Mononuclear cells	Vague histological term for leukocytes other than polymorphonuclear leukocytes and not otherwise identifiable precisely.
Mucocele	Mucus-filled cyst or hollow organ (e.g. mucocele of the gallbladder).
Mural	On the wall of a hollow structure (e.g. mural thrombus on the inner wall of the left ventricle after myocardial infarction).
Mutation	Alteration in the base sequence of DNA, possibly resulting in the synthesis of an abnormal protein product; often an early stage in carcinogenesis.
Mycosis	1. Mycosis — fungal infection; 2. mycosis fungoides — cutaneous T-cell lymphoma entirely unrelated to any fungal infection.
Myxoid	Having a mucin-rich consistency.
Naevus	Coloured lesion on skin, often congenital, most commonly consisting of melanin-containing cells, but may be vascular, etc.

Necrosis   Pathological cellular or tissue death in a living organism, irrespective of cause (compare with apoptosis, gangrene and infarction).

Nematode   A roundworm.

Neoplasm   Abnormal and uncoordinated tissue growth persisting after withdrawal of the initiating cause (synonymous in modern usage with 'tumour').

Neurogenic   Disorder attributable to interruption of nerve supply (e.g. neurogenic atrophy of muscle).

Normal   1. Statistical — distribution of a numerical variable in which the mode, median and mean are equal, 2. biological — natural state free of disease.

Nosocomial   Infection acquired in hospital or some other medical environment.

Occult   Abnormality present, but not observable.

Oedema   Abnormal collection of fluid within or, more usually, between cells.

-oma   Suffix — tumour (except 'granul*oma*', 'ather*oma*', 'st*oma*', etc.).

Oncocyte   Cell with swollen cytoplasm, commonly due to numerous mitochondria.

Oncofetal   Fetal characteristics expressed by tumours (e.g. carcinoembryonic antigen).

Oncogenesis   Mechanisms of the causation of tumours (almost synonymous with carcinogenesis).

Oncogene   A gene inappropriately, abnormally, or excessively expressed in tumours and responsible for their autonomous growth.

Opportunist (micro-organism)   Usually harmless, but causing disease in an individual with impaired immunity or some other susceptibility.

Opsonisation   Enhancement of phagocytosis by factors (opsonins) in plasma.

Organisation   Natural process of tissue repair.

-osis   Suffix — state or condition, usually pathological (e.g. osteoarthrosis, acidosis).

-penia   Suffix — deficiency (e.g. leukopenia — abnormally low white blood cell count).

p arm (of a chromosome)   Short arm (p=petit; contrast with q arm).

Papillary   Surface of a lesion characterised by numerous folds, fronds or villous projections.

Papilloma   Benign neoplasm of non-glandular epithelium (e.g. squamous cell papilloma).

Paracrine   Characteristic of neighbouring cells of different types influencing each other by secretion of cytokines, growth factors or hormones (contrast with autocrine and endocrine).

Parakeratosis   Excessive keratin in which nuclear remnants persist (a histological sign of increased epidermal growth).

Paraprotein   Abnormal plasma protein, usually a monoclonal immunoglobulin in multiple myeloma.

Parasite   Organism living on or in the body (the host) and dependent on it for nutrition.

Pathogenesis — Mechanism through which the cause (aetiology) of a disease produces the clinicopathological manifestations.

Pathogenicity — Ability (high, low, etc.) of a micro-organism to cause disease.

Pathognomonic — Pathological feature characteristic of a particular disease.

Pedunculated — On a stalk (contrast with sessile).

Peptic (ulcer) — Due to the digestive action of gastric secretions.

Petechiae — Minute haemorrhagic lesions.

Phagocytosis — Ingestion of micro-organisms or other particles by a cell, especially neutrophil polymorphonuclear leukocytes and macrophages.

Phlebitis — Inflammation of a vein.

Phlebothrombosis — Venous thrombosis.

Pleomorphism — Variation in size and shape, usually of nuclei and characteristic of malignant neoplasms.

Pleurisy — Painful inflammation of the pleura.

Pneumoconiosis — Lung disease due to dust inhalation.

Pneumonia — Inflammation of the lung.

Poikilocytosis — Abnormal erythrocyte shape.

Polyclonal — Indicative of more than one cell clone; feature of reactive rather than neoplastic proliferations (contrast with monoclonal).

Polycythaemia — Excessive number of red blood cells.

Polymorphic — Consisting of more than one cell type.

Polyp — Sessile or pedunculated protrusion from a body surface.

Polyposis — Numerous polyps.

Primary — 1. Initial event without apparent antecedent cause, synonymous with essential or idiopathic (e.g. primary hypertension); 2. a neoplasm arising in the organ in which it is situated; (contrast with secondary).

Primer — Short specific DNA or RNA sequence used to initiate the polymerase chain reaction.

Probe — 1. Specific RNA, DNA or antibody used to locate or detect a substance or organism in a tissue; 2. Mechanical device (e.g. rod) used to determine the route or patency of a track or orifice.

Prodromal — Any feature heralding the appearance of a disease.

Prognosis — Probable length of survival or disease-free state, especially after diagnosis and treatment of malignant neoplasms (e.g. 60% 5-year survival).

Prolapse — Protrusion or descent of an organ or part of it from its normal location (e.g. prolapsed intervertebral disc, rectal prolapse).

Psammoma (body) — Laminated calcified microspherule commonly found in meningiomas and papillary carcinomas of the thyroid and ovaries.

Pseudocyst — Cavity with a distinct wall but lacking an epithelial lining (contrast with cyst).

Pseudomembrane   'False' membrane consisting of inflammatory exudate rather than epithelium.

Punctum   Small orifice, especially where an epidermal cyst communicates with the skin surface.

Purpura   Small haemorrhages into the skin.

Pus   Creamy material consisting of neutrophil polymorphs, in various stages of disintegration, and tissue debris.

Pustule   Small abscess on skin.

Putrefaction   Decomposition or rotting of dead tissue due to bacterial action, often accompanied by unpleasant odours.

Pyaemia   Pus-inducing organisms in the blood.

Pyknosis   Shrinkage of nucleus in a necrotic cell.

Pyogenic   Inducing or forming pus (e.g. pyogenic bacteria).

q arm (of a chromosome)   Long arm (contrast with p arm).

Reactive (process)   Reversible response to an external stimulus.

Recessive   Characteristic of a gene of which both copies are necessary for it to be expressed.

Recurrence   Neoplasm growing at, or close to, site of previously treated primary neoplasm of identical type.

Regeneration   Formation of new cells identical to those lost.

Rejection   Damage to or failure of a tissue or organ transplant due to an immunological host-versus-graft reaction.

Relapse   Reappearance of the clinicopathological manifestations of a disease after a period of good health.

Remission   Period of good health prior to possible relapse.

Repair   Healing with replacement of lost tissue, but not necessarily by similar tissue.

Resolution   Restoration of normality.

Rhabdomyo-   Prefix — of striated muscle (e.g. rhabdomyosarcoma — malignant neoplasm of striated muscle).

Saprophyte   Organism deriving its nutrition from dead cells or tissue.

Sarcoma   Malignant connective tissue neoplasm.

Scirrhous   Of a scar-like consistency (i.e. firm, puckered) (e.g. scirrhous carcinoma of the breast).

Sclerosis   Hardening of a tissue often due to deposition of excess collagen.

Secondary   1. Attributable to some known cause (e.g. secondary hypertension);
2. neoplasm formed by metastasis from a primary neoplasm; (contrast with primary).

Septic   Infected.

Septum   Membrane or boundary dividing a normal or abnormal structure into separate parts.

Serotype	Classification of organisms according to their antigenic characteristics.
Serous	1. Serous exudate or effusion — containing serum or a fluid resembling serum; 2. serous cyst — containing fluid only resembling serum.
Sessile (polyp)	With a broad base rather than a discrete stalk (contrast with pedunculated).
Shock	State of cardiovascular collapse characterised by low blood pressure (e.g. due to severe haemorrhage).
Signet-ring cell	Neoplastic cell (usually adenocarcinoma) in which the nucleus shows crescentic deformation by a large globule of mucin within its cytoplasm.
Signs	Observable manifestations of disease (e.g. swelling, fever, abnormal heart sounds).
Sinus (pathological)	Abnormal track (tract) leading from an abscess to the skin surface and often discharging pus.
Spongiosis	Epidermal oedema causing partial separation of cells.
Stage	A recognised phase in the development or progression of a disease (usually a neoplasm); (compare with grade).
Stasis	Stagnation of fluid often due to obstruction (e.g. urinary stasis).
Steatorrhoea	Excess fat in the faeces, a manifestation of intestinal malabsorption.
Steatosis	Fatty change, especially in liver.
Stenosis	Narrowing of a lumen.
Stoma	Any normal, pathological or surgically constructed opening between one hollow structure and another or the skin.
Strangulation	Obstruction of blood flow by external compression (e.g. strangulated hernia).
Stroma	Non-neoplastic reactive connective tissue within a neoplasm.
Suppuration	Formation of pus; a feature of acute inflammation.
Symbiont	Close association of two living organisms which may be mutually or singly beneficial or detrimental.
Symptoms	The patient's complaints attributable to the presence of a disease (e.g. pain, malaise, nausea).
Syndrome	Combination of signs and symptoms characteristic of a particular disease, no one feature alone being diagnostic.
Systematic	Concerning each body system separately.
Systemic	Concerning all body systems as a whole.
Tamponade (cardiac)	Compression of heart, and therefore restriction of its movement, by excess pericardial fluid (e.g. haemorrhage, effusion) or by pericardial fibrosis (e.g. post-inflammatory scarring).
Telangiectasia	Dilated small blood vessels.
Telomere	End of a chromosome (contrast with centromere).
Teratoma	Germ-cell neoplasm in which there are representatives of endoderm, ectoderm and mesoderm; usually benign in the ovary, and malignant in the testis.

Thrombophlebitis   Venous inflammation associated with a thrombus.

Thrombus   Solid mass of coagulated blood formed *within* the circulation (contrast with clot).

Toxaemia   Presence of a toxin in the blood.

Toxin   Substance having harmful effects, usually of bacterial origin by common usage.

Trabeculation   Abnormal appearance of a surface characterised by ridges.

Transformation   Process in which cells are converted from normal to neoplastic.

Translocation   Exchange of chromosomal segments between one chromosome and another.

Transudate   Abnormal collection of fluid of low protein content due to either hypoproteinaemia or increased intravascular pressure in capillary beds (contrast with exudate).

Trauma   Injury.

Trematode   A flatworm.

Trisomy   Presence of three copies of a particular chromosome in otherwise diploid cells (e.g. trisomy 21, in which there are three copies of chromosome 21, is a feature of Down's syndrome).

Tumour   Abnormal swelling, now synonymous with neoplasm

Type (neoplasm)   Identity of a neoplasm determined from its differentiated features or assumed origin (histogenesis).

Ulcer   Full-thickness defect in a surface epithelium or mucosa.

Varicose   Distended and tortuous, especially referring to a blood vessel (e.g. varicose vein).

Venereal   Transmitted by sexual intercourse or intimate foreplay.

Vesicle (skin)   Small fluid-filled blister.

Villous   Characterised by numerous finger-like surface projections (villi) (e.g. villous adenoma of rectum).

Viraemia   Presence of a virus in the blood.

Virulence (micro-organism)   Relative ability to produce disease.

Volvulus   Loop of twisted intestine.

Xenograft   Transplantation from one species to another.

Index

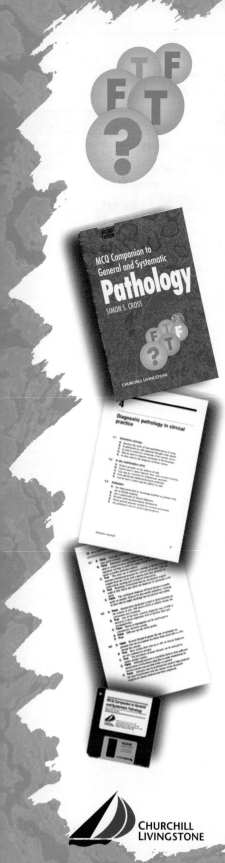

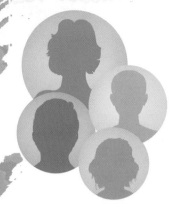
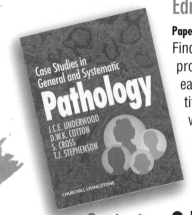